NEUROLOGY AND GENERAL MEDICINE

The Neurological Aspects of Medical Disorders

SECOND EDITION

NEUROLOGY AND GENERAL MEDICINE

The Neurological Aspects of Medical Disorders

SECOND EDITION

Edited By

MICHAEL J. AMINOFF, M.D., F.R.C.P.

Professor, Department of Neurology
University of California, San Francisco
School of Medicine
San Francisco, California

Churchill Livingstone
New York, Edinburgh, London, Madrid, Melbourne, Milan, Tokyo

Library of Congress Cataloging-in-Publication Data

Neurology and general medicine : the neurological aspects of medical
    disorders / edited by Michael J. Aminoff. — 2nd ed.
        p.   cm.
    Includes bibliographical references and index.
    ISBN 0–443–08933–7
    1.   Neurologic manifestations of general diseases.   I. Aminoff,
Michael J. (Michael Jeffrey)
    [DNLM: 1. Neurologic Manifestations.   2. Nervous System Diseases–
–complications.   WL 340 N4932 1995]
RC347.N479 1995
616.047—dc20
DNLM/DLC
for Library of Congress   94–13196

Distributed in the United Kingdom by Churchill Livingstone, Robert Stevenson House, 1–3 Baxter's Place, Leith
Walk, Edinburgh EH1 3AF, and by associated companies, branches, and representatives throughout the world.

Accurate indications, adverse reactions, and dosage schedules for drugs are provided in this book, but it is possible that they may change. The reader is urged to review the package information data of the manufacturers of
the medications mentioned.

The Publishers have made every effort to trace the copyright holders for borrowed material. If they have inadvertently overlooked any, they will be pleased to make the necessary arrangements at the first opportunity.

Acquisitions Editor: *Kerry Willis*
Copy Editor: *Donna C. Balopole*
Production Supervisor: *Christina Hippeli*
Cover Design: *Paul Moran*

Printed in the United States of America

First published in 1995   7 6 5 4 3 2 1

This book is dedicated to A. S. Aminoff, my father and friend.

Contributors

William K. Abend, M.D., Ph.D.
Assistant Clinical Professor, Department of Neurology, Harvard Medical School, Boston, Massachusetts

Gary M. Abrams, M.D.
Associate Professor of Clinical Neurology, Department of Neurology, Columbia University College of Physicians and Surgeons; Attending Neurologist, Neurology Service, Helen Hayes Hospital, West Haverstraw, New York

Michael J. Aminoff, M.D., F.R.C.P.
Professor, Department of Neurology, University of California, San Francisco, School of Medicine; Attending Physician, University of California Medical Center, San Francisco, California

Bruce O. Berg, M.D.
Professor, Departments of Neurology and Pediatrics, University of California, San Francisco, School of Medicine; Attending Physician, University of California Medical Center, San Francisco, California

Joseph R. Berger, M.D.
Thomas E. Whigham Professor, Departments of Neurology and Internal Medicine, University of Miami School of Medicine; Consultant, Department of Neurology, Jackson Memorial Hospital, Miami, Florida

Charles F. Bolton, M.D., F.R.C.P.(C)
Professor, Department of Clinical Neurological Sciences, University of Western Ontario Faculty of Medicine; Consultant Neurologist, Victoria Hospital, London, Ontario, Canada

David L. Brown, M.D.
Associate Professor, Department of Anesthesiology, Mayo Medical School; Consultant, Department of Anesthesiology, Mayo Clinic, Rochester, Minnesota

Michael Camilleri, M.D.
Professor, Department of Internal Medicine, Mayo Medical School; Consultant in Gastroenterology and Physiology and Biophysics, Mayo Clinic, Rochester, Minnesota

Gary M. Cox, M.D.
Fellow, Department of Medicine, Division of Infectious Diseases, Duke University School of Medicine, Durham, North Carolina

G. A. B. Davies-Jones, M.D.
Honorary Lecturer in Clinical Neurology, University of Sheffield; Consultant Neurologist, Department of Neurology, Royal Hallamshire Hospital, Sheffield, England

Larry E. Davis, M.D.
Professor, Departments of Neurology and Microbiology, University of New Mexico School of Medicine; Chief, Neurology Service, Veterans Affairs Medical Center, Albuquerque, New Mexico

Jean-Yves Delattre, M.D.
Professor, Department of Neurology, Hôpital de la Salpêtrière, Paris, France

Roger M. Des Prez, M.D.
Professor, Department of Medicine, Vanderbilt University School of Medicine; Chief, Medical Service, Veterans Affairs Medical Center, Nashville, Tennessee

William P. Dillon, M.D.
Professor of Radiology, Neurology, and Neurosurgery, Department of Radiology, University of California, San Francisco, School of Medicine; Chief, Diagnostic Neuroradiology Section, University of California Medical Center, San Francisco, California

Christopher F. Dowd, M.D.
Assistant Professor of Radiology and Neurosurgery, Department of Radiology, University of California, San Francisco, School of Medicine, San Francisco, California

David T. Durack, M.D., D. Phil.
Professor, Department of Medicine, Division of Infectious Diseases, Duke University School of Medicine, Durham, North Carolina

John W. Engstrom, M.D.
Assistant Professor, Department of Neurology, University of California, San Francisco, School of Medicine; Director, Neurology Outpatient Services, University of California Medical Center, San Francisco, California

Gerald M. Fenichel, M.D.
Professor and Chairman, Department of Neurology, and Professor, Department of Pediatrics, Vanderbilt University School of Medicine; Neurologist-in-Chief, Vanderbilt University Hospital and Children's Hospital, Nashville, Tennessee

Bruce J. Fisch, M.D.
Associate Professor and Director, Epilepsy and Sleep Disorders Programs, Department of Neurology, Louisiana State University School of Medicine in New Orleans, New Orleans, Louisiana

Clare J. Fowler, M.Sc., F.R.C.P.
Consultant Uro-neurologist, National Hospital for Neurology and Neurosurgery, Queen Square, London, England

P. C. Gautier-Smith, M.D., F.R.C.P.
Honorary Consultant Neurologist, National Hospital for Neurology and Neurosurgery, Queen Square, London, England

Douglas Gelb, M.D., Ph.D.
Clinical Assistant Professor, Department of Neurology, University of Michigan Medical School, Ann Arbor, Michigan

Christopher G. Goetz, M.D.
Professor, Department of Neurological Sciences, Rush Medical College of Rush University; Attending Physician, Rush-Presbyterian-St. Luke's Medical Center, Chicago, Illinois

Gerald S. Golden, M.D.
Vice President for Medical School Liaison, National Board of Medical Examiners; Adjunct Professor, Department of Neurology, University of Pennsylvania School of Medicine, Philadelphia, Pennsylvania

Douglas S. Goodin, M.D.
Associate Professor, Department of Neurology, University of California, San Francisco, School of Medicine; Attending Physician, University of California Medical Center, San Francisco, California

David A. Greenberg, M.D., Ph.D.
Professor and Vice-Chairman, Department of Neurology, University of Pittsburgh School of Medicine, Pittsburgh, Pennsylvania

Michael J. G. Harrison, D.M., F.R.C.P.
Professor in Clinical Neurology, Institute of Neurological Studies, University College London Medical School; Honorary Consultant Physician, National Hospital for Neurology and Neurosurgery, Queen Square, London, England

John R. Hotson, M.D.
Professor, Department of Neurology and Neurological Sciences, Stanford University School of Medicine, Stanford, California; Chief, Department of Neurology, Santa Clara Valley Medical Center, San Jose, California

Charles H. King, M.D.
Associate Clinical Professor, Department of Medicine, Division of Geographic Medicine, Case Western Reserve University School of Medicine; Attending Physician, University Hospitals of Cleveland, Cleveland, Ohio

Colin D. Lambert, B.M., F.R.C.P.(C)
Assistant Professor, Department of Medicine, Division of Neurology, University of Toronto Faculty of Medicine; Consultant Neurologist, Wellesley Hospital, Toronto, Ontario, Canada

J. William Langston, M.D.
Director, Parkinson's Institute, Sunnyvale, California

John M. Leonard, M.D.
Associate Professor, Department of Medicine, Vanderbilt University School of Medicine; Consultant, Department of Infectious Disease, Vanderbilt Hospital, Nashville, Tennessee

Phillip I. Lerner, M.D.
Professor, Department of Medicine, Case Western Reserve University School of Medicine; Chief, Infectious Disease Division, The Mount Sinai Medical Center, Cleveland, Ohio

Alan H. Lockwood, M.D.
Professor, Departments of Neurology and Nuclear Medicine, State University of New York at Buffalo School of Medicine and Biomedical Sciences; Director of PET Operations, Veterans Affairs Medical Center, Buffalo, New York

W. T. Longstreth, Jr., M.D., M.P.H.
Professor, Division of Neurology, Department of Medicine, University of Washington School of Medicine; Professor, Department of Epidemiology, University of Washington School of Public Health and Community Medicine; Head of Neurology Section, Harborview Medical Center, Seattle, Washington

Adel A. F. Mahmoud, M.D.
Professor, Departments of Medicine and Molecular Biology and Microbiology, and Chairman, Department of Medicine, Case Western Reserve University School of Medicine; Attending Physician, University Hospitals of Cleveland, Cleveland, Ohio

Elliott L. Mancall, M.D.
Professor and Chairman, Department of Neurology, Hahnemann University School of Medicine, Philadelphia, Pennsylvania

Frank L. Mastaglia, M.D., F.R.C.P., F.R.A.C.P.
Professor of Neurology, Department of Medicine, University of Western Australia; Deputy Director, Australian Neuromuscular Research Institute, Perth, Western Australia, Australia

Susan Mathers, M.B., Ch.B., M.R.C.P., F.R.A.C.P.
Neurologist, Monash Medical Centre and Bethlehem Hospital, Melbourne, Australia

Kathleen M. McEvoy, M.D., Ph.D.
Assistant Professor, Department of Neurology, Mayo Medical School; Consultant, Department of Neurology, Mayo Clinic, Rochester, Minnesota

Robert O. Messing, M.D.
Assistant Professor, Department of Neurology, University of California, San Francisco, School of Medicine; Investigator, Ernest Gallo Clinic and Research Center, San Francisco General Hospital, San Francisco, California

John W. Norris, M.D., F.R.C.P.(C)
Professor of Neurology, Department of Medicine, University of Toronto Faculty of Medicine; Director, Stroke Research Unit, Sunnybrook Health Science Centre, Toronto, Ontario, Canada

Richard K. Olney, M.D.
Associate Professor, Department of Neurology, University of California, San Francisco, School of Medicine; Attending Physician, University of California Medical Center, San Francisco, California

Stephen Oppenheimer, M.D., F.R.C.P., F.R.C.P.(C)
Director, Cerebrovascular Program and Neurocardiology Laboratory, Departments of Neurology and Cardiology, The Johns Hopkins University School of Medicine; Physician, The Johns Hopkins Hospital, Baltimore, Maryland

Andrew R. Pachner, M.D.
Professor, Department of Neurology, Georgetown University School of Medicine, Washington, D.C.

Gareth J. G. Parry, M.D., F.R.A.C.P.
Professor, Department of Neurology, University of Minnesota Medical School, Minneapolis, Minnesota

John R. Perfect, M.D.
Associate Professor, Department of Medicine, Division of Infectious Diseases, Duke University School of Medicine, Durham, North Carolina

Vincent G. Pons, M.D.
Clinical Professor of Medicine and Neurosurgery, Department of Medicine, University of California, San Francisco, School of Medicine; Attending Physician, University of California Medical Center, San Francisco, California

Jerome B. Posner, M.D.
Professor of Neurology and Neuroscience, Cornell University Medical College; Chairman, Department of Neurology, Memorial Sloan-Kettering Cancer Center, New York, New York

Neil H. Raskin, M.D.
Professor, Department of Neurology, University of California, San Francisco, School of Medicine; Attending Physician, University of California Medical Center, San Francisco, California

George A. Ricaurte, M.D., Ph.D.
Assistant Professor, Department of Neurology, The Johns Hopkins University School of Medicine, Baltimore, Maryland

Jack E. Riggs, M.D.
Professor, Departments of Neurology, Medicine, and Community Medicine, West Virginia University School of Medicine, Morgantown, West Virginia

Howard A. Rowley, M.D.
Assistant Professor of Radiology and Neurology, Department of Radiology, University of California, San Francisco, School of Medicine; Director, Biomagnetic Imaging Laboratory, University of California Medical Center, San Francisco, California

Thomas D. Sabin, M.D.
Professor, Departments of Neurology and Psychiatry, Boston University School of Medicine; Lecturer in Neurology, Harvard Medical School and Tufts University School of Medicine; Director, Neurological Unit, Boston City Hospital, Boston Massachusetts

Robert A. Salata, M.D.
Associate Professor, Department of Medicine, Division of Infectious Diseases, Case Western Reserve University School of Medicine; Attending Physician and Director, Traveler's Healthcare Center, University Hospital, Cleveland, Ohio

Hyman M. Schipper, M.D., Ph.D., F.R.C.P.(C)
Assistant Professor, Department of Neurology and Neurosurgery and Division of Geriatric Medicine and Aging, Department of Medicine, McGill University Faculty of Medicine; Attending Staff, Department of Neuroscience, Sir Mortimer B. Davis-Jewish General Hospital, Montreal, Quebec, Canada

Kathleen M. Shannon, M.D.
Assistant Professor, Department of Neurological Sciences, Rush Medical College of Rush University; Assistant Attending Physician, Rush-Presbyterian-St. Luke's Medical Center, Chicago, Illinois

Donald H. Silberberg, M.D.
Professor and Chairman, Department of Neurology, University of Pennsylvania School of Medicine, Philadelphia, Pennsylvania

Roger P. Simon, M.D.
Professor and Chairman, Department of Neurology, University of Pittsburgh School of Medicine, Pittsburgh, Pennsylvania

Michael Swash, M.D., F.R.C.P., F.R.C.Path.
Consultant Neurologist, The Royal London Hospital, St. Mark's Hospital, and The London Independent Hospital; Senior Lecturer in Neuropathology, The London Hospital Medical College, London, England

Thomas R. Swift, M.D.
Professor and Chairman, Department of Neurology, Medical College of Georgia School of Medicine, Augusta, Georgia

Michael R. Trimble, M.D., F.R.C.P., F.R.C.Psych.
Raymond Way Professor in Behavioural Neurology, Institute of Neurology, Queen Square; Consultant Physician in Psychological Medicine, National Hospital for Neurology and Neurosurgery, Queen Square, London, England

H. Richard Tyler, M.D.
Professor, Department of Neurology, Harvard Medical School; Senior Physician, Section of Neurology, Department of Medicine, Brigham and Women's Hospital, Boston, Massachusetts

Anthony J. Windebank, M.A., B.M., B.Ch., M.R.C.P.(UK)
Professor, Department of Neurology, Mayo Medical School; Dean, Mayo Graduate School; Consultant, Department of Neurology, Mayo Clinic, Rochester, Minnesota

Marc D. Winkelman, M.D.
Associate Professor, Department of Neurology, Case Western Reserve University School of Medicine; Attending Neurologist, MetroHealth Medical Center, Cleveland, Ohio

G. Bryan Young, M.D., F.R.C.P.(C)
Associate Professor, Department of Clinical Neurological Sciences, University of Western Ontario Faculty of Medicine; Director, EEG Laboratory, Victoria Hospital, London, Ontario, Canada

Preface to the Second Edition

Several years have passed since the first edition of *Neurology and General Medicine* was published by Churchill Livingstone. Over this time, major advances have been made in the fields of neurology and general medicine, especially in molecular biology, immunology, pharmacology, and imaging procedures. Changes have also occurred in the context in which clinical medicine is practiced in many of the developed countries, including the United States. It has therefore become more important than ever for clinical neurologists to have a clear appreciation of the neurological aspects of general medical disorders and to understand the medical complications that may punctuate the course of neurological diseases. At the same time, it remains essential for internists, family practitioners, and other non-neurologists to understand the many neurological disorders that may complicate general medical conditions. These circumstances, and the generous acceptance accorded the first edition, have prompted the preparation of this expanded and updated text.

The present volume includes several new chapters, broadening the scope of the book. At the same time, all of the other chapters have been revised and updated, and in some cases extensively rewritten, to provide a comprehensive account of relevance to the practicing clinician. The purpose of this book remains unchanged, however, namely to serve as a "bridge" between neurology and the other medical specialties.

I am indebted both to the new contributors and to those authors from the first edition who have revised their material to encompass advances in the field. I am also grateful to Dr. Kerry Willis and Ms. Donna Balopole of Churchill Livingstone for their advice and assistance during the preparation of this book. While the manuscript was in press, my father died unexpectedly in England, and I have chosen to dedicate the book to his memory. My wife, Jan, never failed to provide me with support, encouragement, and assistance and took on many extra domestic chores to allow me to work uninterrupted on this text. I am indebted to her and our three children—Alexandra, Jonathan, and Anthony— to a greater extent than they may ever appreciate, but which I nevertheless cannot let go unrecorded.

Michael J. Aminoff, M.D., F.R.C.P.

Preface to the First Edition

The increasing sophistication and complexity of modern medicine has led to greater specialization among practitioners and to more restricted communication between physicians in different disciplines. Perhaps inevitably, this trend has created certain major problems. These difficulties are particularly well exemplified by the relationship between neurology and general medicine.

For non-neurologists, evaluation of patients with neurological symptoms and signs has always been difficult because of the complexity of the anatomy and physiology of the nervous system and frustrating because the therapeutic options have seemed somewhat limited. Nevertheless, a number of neurological diseases are exacerbated by, or occur as specific complications of, general medical disorders. Appropriate management of these neurological disturbances requires their early recognition and an appreciation of their prognosis. It is equally important to recognize the manner in which such neurological disorders may influence the management of the primary or coexisting medical condition, as well as the manner in which systemic complications of neurological disorders may require somewhat different management than when these complications occur in other settings.

For neurologists, who are being asked increasingly to evaluate neurological disturbances presenting in the context of other medical disorders, the difficulty is equally apparent. The general background of cases is frequently confusing, the relationship of the neurological to the other medical problems is commonly not appreciated, and the manner in which treatment needs to be "tailored" to the specific clinical context is often not clear. Furthermore, neurological disturbances may themselves be the presenting feature of general medical disorders, or lead to general medical complications requiring speedy recognition and effective management.

I hope that the present volume will appeal to both neurologists and physicians in other specialties by providing a guide to the neurological aspects of general medical disorders, and to some of the medical complications of certain neurological diseases. It is not intended to be a textbook of neurology, but rather a "bridge" between neurology and the other medical specialties.

It is a pleasure to acknowledge the help that I received from various people in developing this book. I am grateful to the various contributors, who devoted a great deal of time and energy to reviewing developments in their own fields of interest, and showed considerable tolerance of the many demands that I made upon them. I am grateful also to Mr. Robert Hurley and Ms. Margot Otway at Churchill Livingstone for their help and advice during the preparation of this book. Finally, the support and encouragement of my wife, Jan, and of our children, Alexandra, Jonathan, and Anthony, did much to ease the burden involved in seeing this volume to its conclusion.

Michael J. Aminoff, M.D., F.R.C.P.

Contents

1
Breathing and the Nervous System

Roger P. Simon

The relation between breathing and the nervous system can be considered from two perspectives, both of which are important to neurologists as well as to general physicians. First, neurological dysfunction may lead to respiratory effects that are sometimes more disturbing than the underlying neurological disease. Second, primary respiratory dysfunction may affect the nervous system and lead to a request for neurological consultation. These interactions are considered in the present chapter.

RESPIRATORY EFFECTS OF NERVOUS SYSTEM DYSFUNCTION

Alteration of Pulmonary Gas Exchange

One of the most dramatic and life-threatening effects of nervous system dysfunction on respiration is the impairment of alveolar gas exchange by a neurologically induced increase in pulmonary interstitial and alveolar fluid: the phenomenon of *acute pulmonary edema*. The lung fluid producing pulmonary edema originates in the pulmonary capillaries. Fluid movement from the pulmonary capillary bed is governed by the variables in the classic Starling equation, which in its simplest form expresses transcapillary fluid flux as a balance between intravascular pressures (tending to push fluid out of the vascular lumen) and plasma osmotic forces (which tend to retain fluid within the vascular lumen) (Fig. 1-1).[1] The mechanisms by which neurogenically induced pulmonary edema occurs remain uncertain,[2] but the major factors are discussed below.

PULMONARY HYDROSTATIC PRESSURE

The main variable affecting pulmonary capillary fluid flux that is under the control of the nervous system is pulmonary vascular pressure. A marked increase in this pressure can force fluid from the vascular compartment, flood the interstitial space (Fig. 1-1), produce pulmonary edema, and impair oxygenation.

An *elevation in intracranial pressure* has often been suggested as a unifying factor that unbalances the Starling equation and results in neurogenic pulmonary edema.[3] Studies in patients with head injuries have failed to support this association. In the patients of Popp and associates, an elevation in pulmonary vascular resistance was highly associated with mortality, but neither pulmonary vascular resistance nor outcome correlated with intracranial pressure.[4] Careful experimental studies have demonstrated that the

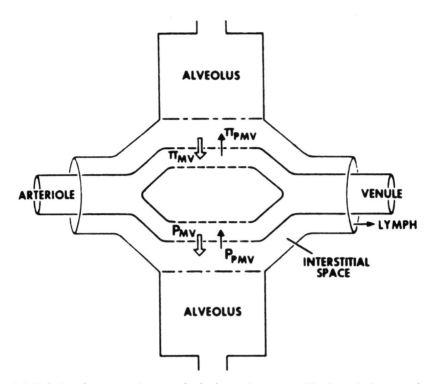

Fig. 1-1 Relations between microvascular hydrostatic pressure (Pmv), perimicrovascular hydrostatic pressure, i.e., within the interstitial space ($Ppmv$), plasma colloid osmotic pressure (πmv), and perimicrovascular pericolloid osmotic pressure (πpmv). Under the normal conditions the sum of forces is slightly positive, producing a small vascular fluid flux into the pericapillary interstitium of the lung, which is drained as lymph. (From Fein A, Grossman RF, Jones JG, et al: The value of edema fluid protein measurement in patients with pulmonary edema. Am J Med 67:32, 1979, with permission.)

effect of increased intracranial pressure on pulmonary vascular pressure and transcapillary fluid flux occurs only as intracranial pressure approaches systemic pressure. An increase in systemic pressure (the Cushing response) then occurs to protect cerebral perfusion. In most studies an increase in intracranial pressure has no effect on transcapillary fluid flux in the absence of the Cushing reflex. Pulmonary vascular pressure rises in concert with systemic pressure, and there is a resultant increase in pulmonary transcapillary fluid flux.[5] Therefore intracranial pressure elevation may result in an increase in fluid flux from the pulmonary capillaries, but only when the Cushing response has been induced. Only one experimental study has shown an increase in pulmonary transcapillary fluid flux in the absence of elevated pulmonary vascular pressure.[6]

Focal central nervous system (CNS) lesions can cause both an elevation of systemic vascular pressure and pulmonary edema. Although hemodynamic data in humans are lacking, there are many reports that the brainstem is the site of focal CNS injuries that result in pulmonary edema.[7-11] In unanesthetized small animals, brainstem lesions in the region of the nucleus tractus solitarius produce marked systemic hypertension and fulminant pulmonary edema; pulmonary vascular pressure cannot be measured in these small animals.[12] Following bilateral lesion placement in the ventral lateral nucleus tractus solitarius in sheep, however, pulmonary arterial pressures and transcapillary fluid flux in the lung may increase significantly without a change in systemic or left atrial pressures.[13] This pattern of response to a CNS injury is similar to that reported for neurogenic pulmonary edema in humans.[4,9] Furthermore, a patient has been reported in whom a unilateral injury occurred to the tractus solitarius during a neurosurgical procedure and in whom the contralateral tractus solitarius was absent because of a congenital brainstem syrinx. The patient died of pulmonary edema and hypoxemia 34 hours postoperatively.[7] The localization by magnetic resonance imaging (MRI) of a lesion at the obex (Fig. 1-2) in a patient with recently diagnosed multiple sclerosis supports this anatomical site as that inducing neurogenic pulmonary hypertension.[14]

Generalized seizures produce an abrupt, marked increase in sympathetic outflow from the brain,[15] and both systemic and pulmonary vascular pressures increase.[16] The degree of systemic pressure elevation correlates with the number of seizures and is maximal during status epilepticus. The magnitude of the pressure elevation in the pulmonary vasculature is independent of the number of seizures, however, although the duration of the elevation is maximal with status epilepticus (Fig. 1-3). The marked increase in systemic catecholamine concentrations induced by generalized seizures persists for hours, but the hemodynamic responses are transient, with pressure elevations returning to baseline in the systemic circulation within 30 minutes and in the pulmonary circulation within 15 minutes.[15] Nevertheless, the increase in transcapillary fluid flux resulting from this transient pulmonary vascular hypertension persists for hours after the pressure transient[17] and probably explains the phenomenon of pulmonary edema following seizures in man.[18,19]

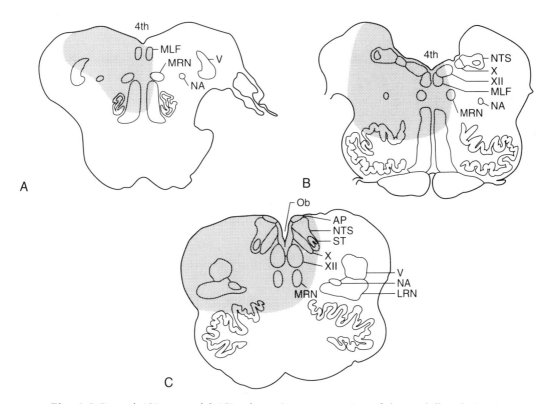

Fig. 1-2 Rostral **(A)** to caudal **(C)** schematic reconstruction of the medullary lesion in a patient with multiple sclerosis and pulmonary edema, based on the MRI, illustrating the major nuclear groups and tracts involved, *AP*, area postrema; *ST*, solitary tract; *NTS*, nucleus of the solitary tract; *V*, spinal trigeminal nucleus; *4th*, fourth ventricle; *X*, dorsal motor nucleus of the vagus; *XII*, hypoglossal nucleus; *LRN*, lateral reticular nucleus; *NA*, nucleus ambiguus; *MRN*, medial reticular nucleus; *MLF*, medial longitudinal fasciculus; *Ob*, obex. (From Simon RP: Respiratory manifestations of neurologic diseases. p. 496. In Goetz CG, Tanner CM, Aminoff MJ (eds): Handbook of Clinical Neurology. Vol 63. Elsevier, Amsterdam, 1993, with permission.)

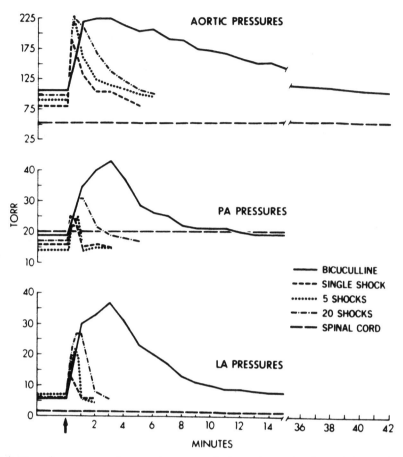

Fig. 1-3 Vascular pressure changes that occur during seizures in sheep. Mean values have been plotted at 10-second intervals. *Spinal cord* refers to animals with cervical spinal cord transection prior to seizures. *Single, 5,* and *20* shocks refer to the number of electroconvulsive seizures induced; *bicuculline* refers to bicuculline-induced status epilepticus. *PA,* pulmonary arterial; *LA,* left atrial. (From Bayne LL, Simon RP: Systemic and pulmonary vascular pressures during generalized seizures in sheep. Ann Neurol 10:566, 1981, with permission.)

CAPILLARY PERMEABILITY

Fulminant neurogenic pulmonary edema occurs in the setting of an alteration in pulmonary capillary permeability, either independent of[20] or in association with[21] an imbalance of the forces in the Starling equation. The classic explanation for the pathogenesis of the altered permeability is that the rapid elevation of pulmonary vascular pressures and blood flow mechanically disrupts the pulmonary capillary bed, resulting in a pulmonary capillary leak phenomenon and noncardiogenic pulmonary edema.[22] However, the exact mechanism of this alteration in permeability remains unknown and recent studies indicate the possibility of its occurrence in the absence of altered intravascular

pressure.[6] Other studies in animals have demonstrated an inverse correlation between maximum pulmonary vascular pressures and altered capillary permeability, suggesting that a combination of "cardiogenic" and "noncardiogenic" factors may be the most common cause of neurogenic pulmonary edema.[21]

Central Effects on Ventilatory Mechanisms

AUTONOMIC DYSFUNCTION

Neural pathways subserving volitional ventilation descend from cortex through the brainstem and spinal cord in the region of the corticospinal tract. The neuronal pools subserving rhythmic involuntary ventilation originate in the caudal medulla and give rise to descending pathways in the ventrolateral brainstem and spinal cord. Accordingly, appropriately placed focal lesions may interfere with voluntary or involuntary ventilation independently.

Impairment of autonomic but not volitional ventilation produces the phenomenon of sleep apnea, or "Ondine's curse."[23] This term was taken from a 1956 play by Jean Giraudoux, who recreated a German mythical legend. The sea nymph Ondine cursed the unfaithful knight Hans with the necessity of voluntary control over all of his autonomic functions: "He died, they will say, because it was a nuisance to breathe." In the brainstem, bilateral medullary infarctions (Fig. 1-4A) have resulted in sleep apnea, as has unilateral medullary infarction, reported in a single case (Fig. 1-4B). In the latter case the lesion depicted in Figure 1-4B will have destroyed primary ventilatory nuclei in and about the nucleus retroambigualis and the nucleus tractus solitarius as well as fibers from these nuclear groups, which descend contralaterally.

Primary involvement of autonomic ventilatory nuclei was a common consequence of bulbar poliomyelitis (Fig. 1-5) and has been reported as a consequence of near drowning.[24] As with lesions of the descending pathways from these nuclear groups, these lesions led to temporary or permanent sleep apnea. There are rare reports of hypoventilation in patients with systems degenerations,[25–27] and pathological material from such cases suggests that the causal abnormalities are located in the region of the solitary tracts in the caudal medulla. Iatrogenic sleep apnea occurs in some patients following bilateral cervical tractotomy per-

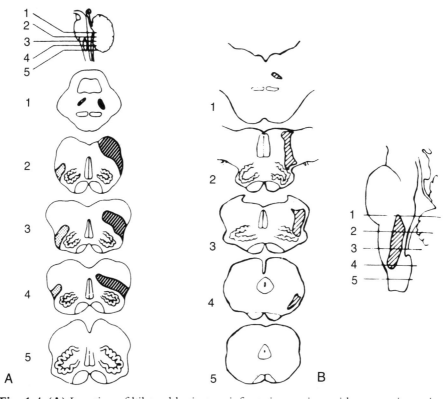

Fig. 1-4 **(A)** Location of bilateral brainstem infarcts in a patient with automatic respiratory failure. **(B)** Brainstem section showing a unilateral lesion that resulted in failure of autonomic respiration. (**A** from Devereaux MW, Keane JR, Davis RL: Automatic respiratory failure associated with infarction of the medulla. Arch Neurol 29:46, 1973, with permission. **B** from Levin BE, Margolis G: Acute failure of automatic respirations secondary to a unilateral brain stem infarct. Ann Neurol 1:583, 1977, with permission.)

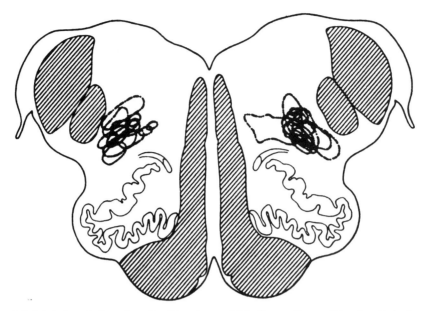

Fig. 1-5 Medullary lesions found in 17 patients with bulbar poliomyelitis who died of respiratory failure. (From Baker AB, Matzke HA, Brown JR: Poliomyelitis. III: Bulbar poliomyelitis; a study of medullary function. Arch Neurol Psychiatry 63:257, 1950, with permission.)

formed for intractable pain (6 of 112 patients reported by Tranmer and associates[28]). Figure 1-6 shows the most common site of the cordotomy lesion and the descending autonomic pathways in the reticulospinal tract. Descending pathways for voluntary ventilation are located in the corticospinal tract and thus are distant from the lesion site (Fig. 1-6).

Sleep apnea also occurs on an obstructive or mixed basis.[29] Such patients are usually obese, hypertensive men over the age of 40 years. Excessive daytime sleepiness and sleep attacks are associated symptoms. Nocturnal breath cessation is associated with prominent snoring, snorting, and gasping sounds. Obstructive sleep apnea has been associated with neurodegenerative diseases such as syringobulbia[30] and olivopontocerebellar degeneration,[31] which may produce oropharyngeal weakness. Treatment with continuous positive airway pressure (CPAP) during sleep is effective.[32] Further discussion of this syndrome can be found in Chapter 25.

Impairment of voluntary ventilatory efforts with preservation of autonomic ventilation may also occur. Cases have been reported from a demyelinating lesion in the high cervical cord[33] and a bilateral pyramidal tract lesion in the medulla resulting from syphilitic arteritis.[34] In another case an infarct of the basal pons produced quadriplegia; autonomic ventilation was modulated normally by laughing, crying, and anxiety, supporting a nonpyramidal location of descending pathways from limbic structures to medullary ventilatory nuclei.[27] The most common cause, however, is a midpontine lesion that produces the "locked in" syndrome. Patients may have a regular ventilatory pattern and a preserved response to CO_2 stimulation,[35] or a Cheyne-Stokes pattern that is volitionally unalterable.[26]

EXTRAPYRAMIDAL DISORDERS

Symptomatic or asymptomatic ventilatory dysfunction is an infrequently recognized but relatively common manifestation of extrapyramidal syndromes of multiple causes. Respiratory dysrhythmias are common in postencephalitic parkinsonism.[36] Tachypnea, the most common abnormality, may be episodic or continuous during sleep or wakefulness; rates as high as 100 per minute are reported. Ventilatory dysrhythmias are less common and manifest as breath-holding spells, sighing, forced or noisy expiration, inversion of the inspiration:expiration ratio, or the Cheyne-Stokes pattern. Respiratory tics occur as well, mani-

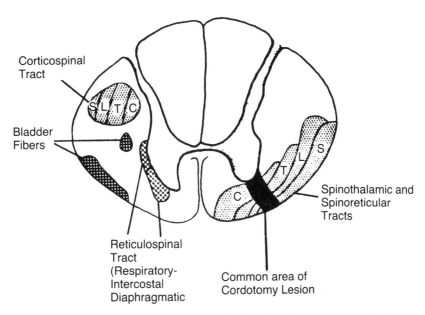

Fig. 1-6 Cervical spinal cord at the C1-C2 level, showing the area commonly damaged in cervical cordotomies and the site of the descending autonomic pathway subserving ventilation. (From Tranmer BI, Tucker WS, Bilbao JM: Sleep apnea following percutaneous cervical cordotomy. Can J Neurol Sci 14:262, 1987, with permission.)

festing as yawning, hiccuping, spasmodic coughing, and sniffing.

In a study by Kim, all of nine patients with postencephalitic parkinsonism had an increase in respiratory rate, and the normal variation in respiratory amplitude did not occur.[37] The most striking abnormality in these patients was their inability to alter the respiratory rhythm voluntarily so that, for instance, they were unable to hold their breath.

In an attempt to identify the site and cause of limitation of ventilatory airflow in patients with extrapyramidal disease, Vincken and colleagues used pulmonary function studies and direct fiberoptic visualization of the upper airway. They studied 27 patients with essential tremor, parkinsonian tremor, rigid parkinsonism, or dyskinesia.[38] Symptomatic stridor and ventilatory failure that could be reversed by endotracheal intubation were described in a number of these patients and suggested upper airway obstruction. Abnormal flow volume curves were commonly found, and at bronchoscopy rhythmic or irregular glottic and supraglottic involuntary movements were seen. Such upper airway dysfunction may be a factor in the retention of secretions and respiratory infections that occur in many patients. Respira-

tory distress and dyspnea have also been described in patients with extrapyramidal dysfunction in whom no cardiopulmonary source was found but in whom respiratory rates were irregular owing to involuntary respiratory dyskinesias that were either levodopa-induced or related to a tardive dyskinesia.[39] Respiratory dyskinesias, then, may be an accompaniment of choreiform movement disorders and may account for subjective complaints of dyspnea.[40]

FOREBRAIN INFLUENCES ON VENTILATION

That the forebrain influences both ventilatory rate and rhythm is documented by the volitional acts of overbreathing and breath-holding as well as by the coordinated semivoluntary or involuntary rhythmic alterations in ventilatory pattern that occur as part of speaking, singing, laughing, and crying. Furthermore, during sleep normal ventilatory patterns become more irregular, total ventilatory volume decreases, PCO_2 is elevated, and the CO_2 response curve shifts to the right.[41]

Focal destructive hemispheric lesions result in contralateral dysfunction of ventilatory muscles. In hemiplegia, chest wall movements are decreased on the side of the paralysis.[42] Furthermore, diaphragmatic excursion is depressed contralateral to the site of cortical injury.[43] Afferents from respiratory muscles have cortical connections.[44] The sensation of voluntary chest movements results from activation of receptors in the chest wall or respiratory muscles; airway and pulmonary receptors are not involved in the appreciation of these sensations.[45]

Cortical "readiness potentials" originating from supplementary motor and primary motor cortex can be recorded from humans prior to volitional inspiration or expiration.[44] Direct stimulation of the cortex in animals and humans provides additional evidence of the cortical influence on ventilation. The major effect of cortical stimulation on ventilation is inhibitory, although stimulation in the motor and premotor areas of the cortex may modestly increase ventilation.[46] In animals, mapping studies indicate that ventilation may be inhibited by stimulation of the uncus, fornix, amygdala, anterior cingulate gyrus, anterior insular cortex, inferior medial temporal cortex, and posterior lateral frontal cortex (Fig. 1-7).[47] In the main, these structures comprise the limbic system. Such limbic stimulation in primates (e.g., amygdala stimulation in squirrel monkeys) results in apnea and hypoxia sufficient to cause cardiac slowing and hypotension. The animals, however, make no attempt to increase ventilation and manifest no signs of dyspnea or distress despite asphyxial changes in arterial blood gases.[48]

Ventilatory arrest has been produced during cortical stimulation in humans; an apneic period of 56 seconds has been reported in one patient.[49] The cortical areas effective in inducing apnea in humans are similar to those in primates (Fig. 1-7) and include the anterior portion of the hippocampal gyrus, the ventral and medial surface of the temporal lobe, the anterior portion of the insula, and the anterior portion of the limbic gyrus. Phenomena associated with apnea include a feeling of tiredness, sleepiness, closure of the eyes, cessation of spontaneous movement, and depression of consciousness. The ventilatory arrest in humans usually occurs during expiration but rarely may be seen during inspiration.[50] Some patients can overcome the experimentally produced apnea when asked to speak, but the speech is markedly abnormal owing to poor breath control.[49]

Spontaneous seizures from limbic structures in hu-

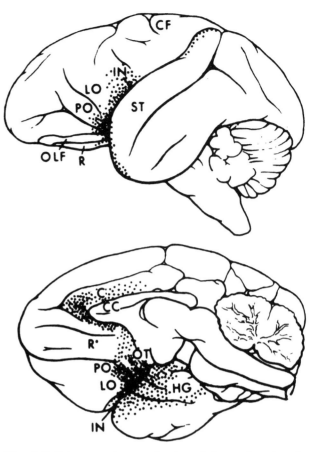

Fig. 1-7 Points on the anterior lateral (*upper figure*) and ventromedial (*lower figure*) cerebral cortex of *Macaca mulatta* where electrical stimulation elicited inhibition of respiration. *C*, cingulate gyrus; *HG*, hippocampal gyrus; *IN*, insula; *LO*, lateral orbital gyrus; *PO*, posterior orbital gyrus; *R*, gyrus rectus; *ST*, superior temporal gyrus. (From Kaada BR: Somato-motor, autonomic, and electrocorticographic responses to electrical stimulation of "rhinencephalic" and other structures in primates, cat and dog. Acta Physiol Scand 24:1, 1951, with permission.)

mans have produced apnea as an ictal event.[46] In one such patient nine episodes of apnea occurred, one of which required mechanical ventilation for 30 hours. The patient was studied with depth electrodes, and inspiratory or expiratory arrest could be reproduced by stimulation in the left amygdaloid nucleus.[50] Respiratory changes have also been associated with paroxysmal abnormalities in the electroencephalogram (EEG).[51]

Recent experiments involving transcranial magnetic stimulation in humans have shown that contralateral diaphragmatic contraction can be elicited by stimulation of a cortical area that is 3 cm off the midline and 3 cm anterior to the auricular plane.[52] Studies with positron emission tomography (PET) of cerebral blood flow during normal ventilation in human volunteers provide support for this localization in the motor strip and also indicate that blood flow is increased in the right premotor cortex, the supplementary motor cortex, and the cerebellum.[53] There were no differences between active and passive ventilation with regard to the pattern of cerebral blood flow.

APRAXIA OF VENTILATORY MOVEMENTS

The inability to take or hold a deep breath despite normal motor and sensory function is termed *respiratory apraxia*. This phenomenon is noted most often in elderly patients with evidence of mild or moderate cerebrovascular disease. Of the 15 patients reported by Plum, all were able to understand clearly the task and none had evidence of corticobulbar tract dysfunction, abnormalities of ventilation, or Cheyne-Stokes breathing.[46] Frontal release phenomena and paratonia were common, but corticospinal abnormalities and pseudobulbar palsy were not present. Other associated bulbar apraxias were frequently found, for example, an inability to swallow on command despite preservation of normal reflex swallowing of a bolus of food or water. Many of these patients would now fit the category of senile dementia of the Alzheimer's type; such patients commonly have apraxias. As no pyramidal abnormalities were found, an extrapyramidal motor dysfunction was postulated. Lesions of the nondominant hemisphere may also result in an inability to hold a breath.[54]

POSTHYPERVENTILATION APNEA

In 1867 Hering observed that brief periods of apnea followed hyperventilation in anesthetized animals.[55] Passive hyperventilation[56] produces a somewhat higher incidence of apnea than active (i.e., voluntary) hyperventilation.[57] Posthyperventilation apnea in awake normal human subjects is quite brief; a normal response to voluntary hyperventilation consists of regular ventilatory excursions at a reduced amplitude.[57] Apnea persisting for more than 12 seconds following five deep breaths (adequate to reduce the

arterial PCO_2 by 8 to 14 mmHg) was found in only 2 percent of normal subjects but occurred in 78 percent of patients with bilateral CNS disease of structural or metabolic cause.[58] It was therefore concluded that posthyperventilation apnea for more than 12 seconds suggests bilateral cerebral disease.

When these experiments were repeated in 1974 by Jennett and co-workers, apnea occurred for more than 10 seconds with equal frequency in patients with unilateral (67 percent) and bilateral (70 percent) damage.[59] No correlation was found between the decrease in end-tidal CO_2 and the occurrence of apnea. These authors suggested that level of consciousness rather than hypocapnia causes posthyperventilation apnea. Thus, 95 percent of the drowsy patients but only 48 percent of the alert patients became apneic following the period of hyperventilation. A depressed level of consciousness in normal subjects, as during drowsiness, sleep, or anesthesia, also leads to posthyperventilation apnea.[60] Accordingly this ventilatory response is best regarded as an indicator of depressed CNS function; its cause may be multifactorial, and its anatomical basis is uncertain.

HINDBRAIN CONTROL OF VENTILATION

The concept that the hindbrain controls ventilatory function, rate, and rhythm has grown from the experiments of Lumsden (Fig. 1-8).[61] These studies in anesthetized cats localized the brainstem ventilatory centers to regions below the inferior colliculus, because transection at this level did not alter the ventilatory pattern when the vagi were intact. Transection at the medullary-cervical junction produced the cessation of all ventilatory functions. Accordingly, the neuronal centers responsible for ventilation are located between these levels. Transection at the pontomedullary junction resulted in rhythmic breathing with a gasping quality unchanged by vagal transection, demonstrating that the most primitive respiratory oscillator is located within the medulla. The higher brainstem "centers" play a modulatory role. A more recent example of such experiments in anesthetized cats is found in Figure 1-9.

Cerebellum

The organization of the cerebellum is such that the ventilatory musculature is represented in the anterior lobe. The predominant effect of stimulation of this

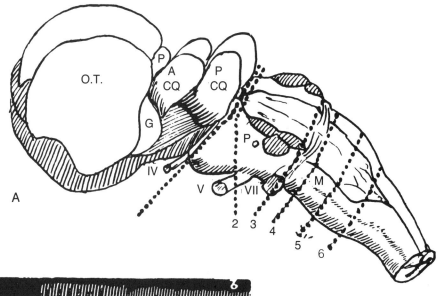

A

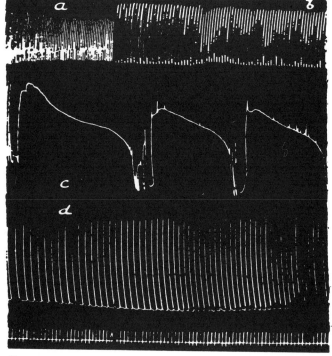

B

Fig. 1-8 (A) The original illustration from Lumsden (1923) showing the level of "crucial sections" producing ventilatory alteration in cats. Ventilatory effects produced with lesions: *1*, no alteration; *2*, apneusis; *4*, gasping; between *5* and *6*, cessation of all respiratory movements. **(B)** Respiratory tracings from Lumsden (1923). *a*, normal animal; *b*, after vagotomy; *c*, apneusis (transection 2); *d*, gasping (transection 4). (From Lumsden T: Observation on the respiratory centres in the cat. J Physiol (Lond) 57:153, 1923, with permission.)

region appears to be an inhibition of ventilation.[62] The effect of the cerebellum on ventilation is exerted via inspiratory and expiratory intercostal α and γ motor neurons and phrenic motor neurons. Motor neurons of intercostal muscles are inhibited with ipsilateral cerebellar stimulation and facilitated with contralateral stimulation.[63]

Pneumotaxic Center

Lumsden named the pneumotaxic center (*pneumotaxy:* normal rhythmic ventilation) and localized it to the rostral pons.[61] Transection at this level results in regular breathing; and the rate of this breathing but not the rhythm is slowed by vagotomy. Destruction of this region or transection below it produces the

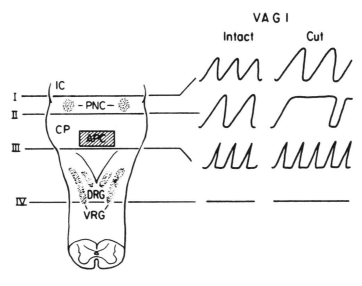

Fig. 1-9 Effects of brainstem and vagal transection on the ventilatory pattern in an unanesthe-tized cat. *APC*, apneustic center; *CP*, cerebellar peduncle; *DRG*, dorsal ventilatory group; *IC*, inferior colliculus; *PNC*, pneumotaxic center; *VRG*, ventral ventilatory groups. Tracings on right represent the tidal volume with inspiration upward. (From Berger AJ, Mitchell RA, Severinghaus JW: Regulation of respiration. N Engl J Med 297:139, 1977, with permission.)

phenomenon of apneusis (Fig. 1-8B), which is discussed below. Modern recording techniques have localized respiratory-related neuronal activity to circumscribed regions of the rostral pons bilaterally.[64] Electrical stimulation within this region produces premature switching of respiratory phases. This off-switching is modified at least in part by the classic Hering-Breuer (and possibly other) afferents carried within the vagus.[65,66] Neuroanatomical and neurophysiological studies in animals support the belief that the pneumotaxic center functions as a relay station, finely tuning the ventilatory pattern generator. The neurons in the pneumotaxic center appear to be driven from the dorsal ventilatory neuronal group in the medulla.[64]

Apneustic Center

The phenomenon of apneusis consists of prominent, prolonged end-inspiratory pauses, which can be produced by pontine transection in vagotomized animals (Fig. 1-8).[61,67] Although the phenomenon of apneusis is well recognized, anatomical definition of a neuronal aggregate that can reasonably be called the apneustic center is still lacking. Apneusis is defined operationally as a failure of activation of normal inspi-

ratory off-switching. The phenomenon of apneusis may result from one of a number of lesions or pharmacological manipulations.[67] Systemic but not local administration of antagonists of the *N*-methyl-D-aspartate (NMDA) subset of the glutamate receptor complex induces apneusis, thus defining the neurotransmitter system involved and the lack of a specific inducing site.[68,69]

Apneustic respiration is rare in humans. None of the 23 patients with brainstem infarction studied by Lee and associates, and who were specifically observed for respiratory rate and pattern, showed the apneustic phenomenon.[70] However, human cases have been reported.[71] Two patients of Plum and Alvord demonstrated apneustic breathing following basilar artery thrombosis.[71] The lesions at postmortem (Fig. 1-10) were similar to brainstem transections that result in apneusis in experimental animals and included regions associated with the pneumotaxic center in the cat.

Medullary Center

Rhythmic ventilatory excursions persist with brainstem transection at the pontomedullary level and all ventilatory movements are abolished by transection

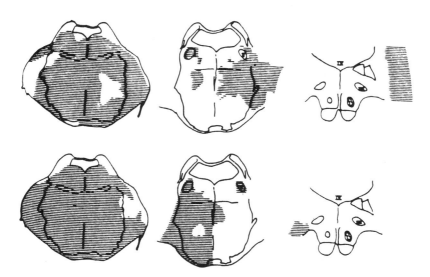

Fig. 1-10 Areas of brainstem infarction in two patients with apneustic breathing. (From Plum F, Alvord EC: Apneustic breathing in man. Arch Neurol 10:101, 1964, with permission.)

at the medullary-cervical junction. Accordingly, attention has been focused on the medulla as the generator of rhythmic ventilatory movements. Medullary centers responsible for inspiration and expiration were identified and were held to explain both ventilatory function and ventilatory rhythmicity. Experiments have provided a more complex picture of medullary ventilatory function.[64] Two major neuronal pools are responsible for ventilation. Primary inspiratory cells located in the ventrolateral nucleus tractus solitarius constitute the dorsal respiratory group (DRG), which receives all primary pulmonary afferents from the vagus nerves. Inspiratory and expiratory neurons are found in a separate grouping within the nucleus ambiguus and the nucleus retroambigualis, which together constitute the ventral respiratory group (VRG) (Fig. 1-11). Excitatory amino acid neurotransmitter function is necessary to modulate VRG function. NMDA receptors are the major mediators of VRG ventilatory drive, with modulation by non-NMDA glutamate systems.[72]

Thus ventilatory rhythmicity is mediated by the dorsal respiratory group, and projection to spinal respiratory motor neurons and vagally mediated auxiliary muscles of respiration occurs via the ventral respiratory group.[64]

Although rhythmic ventilatory responses occur from the medulla following pontomedullary transection, this respiratory pattern has a rather gasping quality and is not normal rhythmic ventilation. A gasping center has been found just rostral and ventral to the DRG.[73] Accordingly, the site of the primary ventilatory rhythm generator remains uncertain.[74]

Ventilatory Patterns of Uncertain Anatomical Basis

CHEYNE-STOKES BREATHING

Periodic, or Cheyne-Stokes, breathing commonly suggests nervous system dysfunction, but its original description by Cheyne was in a patient who died of heart failure.[75] In fact, both CNS and cardiac dysfunction (or a combination of the two) may produce this ventilatory pattern.

The Cheyne-Stokes pattern is that of escalating hyperventilation followed by decremental hypoventilation and finally apnea, which recurs in cycles. Cycle lengths of 40 to 100 seconds have been reported in humans.[76] Arterial blood gas assays during Cheyne-Stokes breathing indicate a rising pH and a falling PCO_2, which becomes maximal at the apnea point and never returns to normal values (Fig. 1-12). Cheyne-Stokes patterns have been seen in normal, premature infants,[77] during normal sleep,[78] and in subjects at high altitude.[79] Associated changes in arousal, pupillary size, cardiac rhythm, muscle tone, and consciousness may occur cyclically in patients

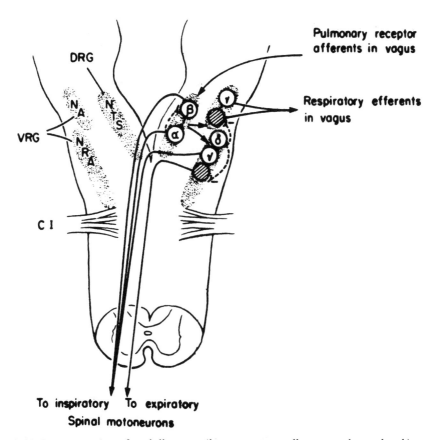

Fig. 1-11 Representation of medullary ventilatory groups, cell types, and postulated interconnections. The DRG is located in the ventrolateral NTS. The VRG consists of the NA and NRA. Inspiratory cells are open circles; expiratory cells are hatched circles. Solid lines are established, and dotted lines proposed connections. *DRG,* dorsal ventilatory group; *VRG,* ventral ventilatory group; *NA,* nucleus ambiguus; *NRA,* nucleus retroambigualis; *NTS,* nucleus tractus solitarius; *C1,* first cervical dorsal root; α, β, γ, δ represent inspiratory cell subtypes. (From Berger AJ, Mitchell RA, Severinghaus JW: Regulation of respiration. N Engl J Med 297:139, 1977, with permission.)

with Cheyne-Stokes breathing.[80] The alterations in PCO_2 also affect the cerebral vasculature, producing changes in the intracerebral volume of the vascular compartment. Alterations in cerebral blood flow and intracranial pressure are therefore seen.[81]

In one study of 28 patients with Cheyne-Stokes breathing due to CNS disease, each patient had a fixed respiratory alkalosis with an elevated PCO_2 and an O_2 saturation nadir at the peak of the Cheyne-Stokes ventilatory frequency (Fig. 1-12).[82] The study patients and elderly normal control subjects had equal circulation times, which were less than in patients with congestive heart failure, but no Cheyne-Stokes breathing pattern. It was suggested that the Cheyne-

Stokes pattern was the result of an increased respiratory drive in response to CO_2, resulting from bilateral CNS disease.

The possibility that a prolonged circulation time may itself produce ventilatory oscillations was evaluated by Guyton and colleagues, who noted in dogs that marked prolongation of transit time from carotid artery chemoreceptors to CNS receptors produced a pattern of ventilatory oscillation.[83] It was therefore suggested that a feedback loop delay to central receptors was the factor responsible for the Cheyne-Stokes ventilatory pattern. Lange and Hecht argued that a persistent respiratory alkalosis, which is characteristic of Cheyne-Stokes breathing, can be explained by the

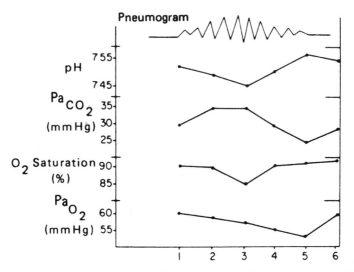

Fig. 1-12 Relation of blood gases to ventilatory cycle in Cheyne-Stokes breathing. (From Brown HW, Plum F: The neurological basis of Cheyne-Stokes respiration. Am J Med 30: 849, 1961, with permission.)

ventilatory oscillations alone,[76] without the requirement of central hypersensitivity to PCO_2 that had previously been suggested.[82] A third experimental study supported the induction of respiratory oscillations by the CNS regardless of afferent responses of baro- and chemoreceptors.[84] Further, Hoffman and associates, studying patients with cardiogenic pulmonary edema, found no differences in left ventricular ejection fractions in patients with or without Cheyne-Stokes breathing.[85]

The issue of an abnormal feedback to the CNS in the genesis of respiratory oscillations was studied in animals by Cherniack and associates, who used the normal phrenic nerve stimulus to trigger a mechanical ventilator that had been modified so that the gain could be varied to amplify or retard the induced tidal volume triggered by the phrenic stimulus.[86] This model produced periodic ventilations when the gain was increased. Supporting the concept of abnormal feedback loops generating Cheyne-Stokes breathing, ventilatory periodicity was eliminated by destruction of peripheral chemoreceptors but was unchanged by vagotomy. Furthermore, all animals had a persistent respiratory alkalosis. Duplicating observed clinical phenomena, the oscillations were enhanced by hypoxia and eliminated by increasing the oxygen or CO_2 content of inspired air. Hypoxemia (during sleep) also induces Cheyne-Stokes breathing in humans.[87]

Originally described as a variant of Cheyne-Stokes breathing, *Biot breathing* is characterized by clusters of breaths having equal and regular inspiratory and expiratory phases, rather than the spindle characteristics of Cheyne-Stokes breathing. The similarity to Cheyne-Stokes breathing is in the separation of the ventilatory periods by apnea, which in Biot breathing occurs in end-expiration. The location of the lesion in such cases is pontomedullary, in the region of the pneumotaxic center; superimposed vagal transection results in apneusis.[88] Hypoxia shortens and hyperoxia lengthens the period of apnea, as also occurs in sleep apnea. Accordingly, a similar autonomic substrate for these syndromes has been suggested.[88,89]

CENTRAL HYPERVENTILATION

In 1959 Plum and Swanson reported a patient with a mesencephalic reticular formation lesion and sustained tachypnea.[90] They suggested that lesions of the medial pontine and mesencephalic reticular formation permitted uninhibited stimulation of the medullary respiratory centers. Subsequently, McNealy and Plum included this respiratory pattern as a characteristic of midbrain dysfunction during transtentorial herniation.[91] In 1974 North and Jennett studied 227 neurosurgical patients for the presence of periodic (Cheyne-Stokes), irregular (ataxic), and tachypneic

Table 1-1 Incidence of Various Abnormal Ventilatory Patterns Associated with Lesions at Various CNS Sites

Lesion Site	Ventilatory Pattern		
	Periodic	Irregular	Tachypnea
Bilateral hemisphere	17	21	20
Single hemisphere	30	21	27
Suprasellar region	4	3	1
Midbrain	5	5	4
Pons	3	9[a]	5
Medulla	1	8[b]	4
Cerebellum	6	8	6

[a] Significant; $p = 0.01$ to 0.05.
[b] Highly significant; $p < 0.01$.
(From North JB, Jennett S: Abnormal breathing patterns associated with acute brain damage. Arch Neurol 31:338, 1974, with permission.)

(central hyperventilation) responses and sought a correlation between these ventilatory patterns and the site of CNS lesions (Table 1-1).[92] In their study, sustained tachypnea was much more common with unilateral or bilateral hemispheric lesions than with midbrain abnormalities. The major value of finding tachypnea in patients with neurological injury may be the poor prognosis that it signifies.[93] The exhaustion caused by such ventilatory efforts may be fatal; morphine or methadone will suppress this ventilatory drive.[94]

Cases of isolated brainstem tumors and sustained tachypnea offered the possibility of an unambiguous anatomical localization of the source of this ventilatory pattern. In two patients the tumors involved the lower pons and the medulla.[95,96] In a third patient the medulla was completely spared, and the tumor affected the midbrain and pons.[97] Extra-axial medullary compression may also cause central hyperventilation.[98] Accordingly, a specific midbrain localization for lesions producing this ventilatory pattern is unsupportable.

The cause of central hyperventilation remains uncertain. Plum reported the inability to induce this respiratory pattern by mesencephalic or pontine lesions in animals.[46] He suggested that pulmonary congestion of neurogenic cause (neurogenic pulmonary edema) might induce this respiratory pattern via stimulation of pulmonary receptors in the pulmonary interstitial space.[99] At the San Francisco General Hospi-

tal we have seen three patients with sustained tachypnea following stroke. Their in vivo lung water content was measured with a double indicator dilution technique (by Dr. Frank Lewis), and no elevation was found.

The possibility of central stimulation of medullary chemoreceptors[100] due to local lactate production from tumors[99] or stroke has been suggested to explain the lack of correlation between anatomical lesion site and ventilatory pattern. However PET studies have found an alkaline pH of CNS tumors.[101] Central hyperventilation has been associated particularly with CNS lymphoma, the infiltrating nature of which has been suggested as the common feature in such cases.[102]

Alveolar Hypoventilation

Hypoventilation, hypoxia, and apnea are major risks in diseases of the anterior horn cells, peripheral nerves, myoneural junctions, and muscles. Motor neuron disease, polyneuropathy, myasthenia gravis, and the muscular dystrophies are, respectively, the most common examples of such diseases that cause ventilatory disturbances. In part because of the decreased exercise demands induced by the disease processes, dyspnea is often absent and arterial blood gases may show little alteration immediately prior to fatal ventilatory compromise. Furthermore, the amount of muscle weakness in extremity and girdle muscles is often a poor predictor of ventilatory muscle function. Vincken and associates examined this point and documented that maximal inspiratory (diaphragmatic, intercostal, and accessory neck muscles) and expiratory (abdominal and intercostal muscles) pressure measurements were required to assess the risk of respiratory compromise in patients with chronic neuromuscular disease.[103] Unsuspected ventilatory dysfunction was found in one-half of the 30 patients studied, and in one-third of patients it was severe. In no case was the ventilatory dysfunction clinically suspected. A previous study reached similar conclusions but found the maximum expiratory pressure most sensitive; this measure correlated poorly with spirometry, which often underestimated ventilatory volumes in weak patients.[104] Accordingly, a maximal pulmonary expiratory pressure of less than 40 cm H_2O or pulmonary inspiratory pressure of less than 20 cm H_2O should replace spirometry (reduction in vital capacity to twice predicted tidal volume or less) as the means of determining the need for intubation and ventilatory support.[105]

Traumatic *myelopathies* or myelopathies resulting from infiltrative tumors produce ventilatory insufficiency with lesions above the cervical roots innervating the phrenic nerve (C3, C4). Such patients' ventilatory dysfunction has been successfully managed without mechanical ventilation by electrical pacing of the diaphragm. In patients with lesions between C3 and C5, this treatment is feasible if the C5 root is preserved below the level of the lesion. Each of eight patients with traumatic tetraplegia reported by Vanderlinden and co-workers were successfully weaned from ventilator support using this technique.[106] Glenn and colleagues reported bilateral pacing to be superior to unilateral diaphragmatic pacing because myopathic changes in the diaphragmatic muscle did not develop in the former group.[107]

Although ventilatory compromise is often the terminal event in advanced *motor neuron disease,* isolated respiratory insufficiency may be the presenting feature of the disease. In patients with primary bulbar disease, sleep apnea or nocturnal hypoventilation occurs, manifesting itself by both obstructive and central apnea. Orthopnea may be the presenting symptom of motor neuron disease. Such patients have predominantly diaphragmatic weakness, and this may be unilateral or bilateral. Paradoxical chest wall and abdominal movements are seen during inspiration, and vital capacity is reduced, especially when the patient is tested in the supine position. Of the patients studied by Howard and colleagues, predominant loss of anterior horn cells in the C3 to C5 region of the cord (corresponding to the area of the phrenic nerve nucleus) were found at autopsy.[108] In this patient group (clinical diaphragmatic weakness in the absence of bulbar impairment), symptomatic relief was obtained with ventilatory support (continuous positive airway pressure [CPAP] or nocturnal intermittent positive pressure ventilation) without unwarranted prolongation of life. The institution of ventilatory assistance most often requires continuation for the remaining life span. However, Braun and associates reported three patients with amyotrophic lateral sclerosis in whom intermittent negative pressure ventilation for 5 to 11 weeks stabilized or temporarily improved ventilatory status.[109] Therapy with a rock-ing bed at home may improve effective ventilatory assistance for as long as 1 to 2 years.[110]

Ventilatory failure requiring mechanical assistance has been reported in 10 to 80 percent of patients with *Guillain-Barré syndrome.* Intubation and ventilation were needed in 43 percent of the 111 patients from the French plasmapheresis study[111] and in 47 percent of the 123 patients in the American study.[112] The mean duration of the assisted ventilation was 31 days in the French study, and it was reduced to 18 days by plasmapheresis. Intubation is usually required when vital capacity falls below 18 ml/kg.[113] Sunderrajan and Davenport analyzed the presenting and early stages of their patients' illness and were unable to identify any characteristics or neurological features that would predict the need for assisted ventilation.[114] While the mean hospital day during which intubation was required was 4.4, the range was broad (0 to 21 days). The hospital day on which the patient was extubated had an equally wide range: hospital day 5 to 90. Two unusual cases required ventilatory support for more than a year. This experience suggests that extubation will be successful when vital capacities exceed 1 L. A detailed study of diaphragmatic performance in patients with Guillain-Barré syndrome suggested that improvement in the maximum transdiaphragmatic pressure was the best predictor of recovery, and this measure was correlated with maximal inspiratory force but not forced vital capacity.[115] The duration of mechanical ventilatory support required in patients with the Guillain-Barré syndrome was nearly halved by treatment with plasma exchange. How efficient infusion of gamma globulin will be in regard to this aspect remains to be determined,[113] although initial reports are promising.[116]

An acute, primary axonal, degeneration of motor and sensory fibers occurs in the setting of prolonged sepsis (approximately 2 weeks) with multiple organ failure.[117] This syndrome has been termed *critical illness neuropathy,* and is described in detail in Chapter 44. The neuropathy is characterized clinically by distal weakness with reduced or absent tendon reflexes; when it is severe, there is paralysis with areflexia. The syndrome is frequently recognized only because of unexpected difficulty in weaning patients from assisted ventilation. Phrenic nerve conduction velocities have been abnormal and autopsy studies have shown axonal degeneration of the phrenic nerve, with denervation atrophy in the intercostal muscles and diaphragm.[118] Complete recovery over a period of 6 months is the rule in mild and moderate cases, but patients with severe polyneuropathy may fail to improve and have a fatal outcome.

Temporary ventilatory support may be required in *myasthenia gravis.* Indications include the post-thymectomy period and failure of outpatient pharmacological therapy. Of 22 such patients seen at the Mayo Clinic, the duration of ventilatory support required was 1 to 32 days,[119] with 1 to 41 days reported by O'Donohue and colleagues.[105]

In patients with *myopathy,* ventilatory dysfunction may occur and may be disproportionate to the severity of the muscle weakness. Although the poor prognosis in the *muscular dystrophies* usually commits patients to ventilatory support for the remainder of their lives, two patients with Duchenne's muscular dystrophy were weaned from continual positive pressure ventilation with intermittent negative pressure techniques.[109] Recurrent episodes of ventilatory failure independent of muscle weakness have been reported in patients with mitochondrial myopathies.[120] Patients have depressed respiratory responses to hypoxia, and often to hypercapnea as well. Life-threatening hypoventilation often occurs in the setting of surgery, sedation, or infection. Reported cases include typical Kearns-Sayre syndrome, MERRF (myoclonic epilepsy and ragged red fibers) syndrome, and familial mitochondrial myopathy. No specific biochemical defect has been found, although a defect in cytochrome *c* oxidase has recently been suggested.[120] The cause of the hypoventilation may be central rather than muscular.

NERVOUS SYSTEM EFFECTS OF RESPIRATORY DYSFUNCTION

Hypoxia

ACUTE HYPOXIA

The terms *hypoxic* and *anoxic encephalopathy* are frequently used to describe neurological syndromes that occur following cardiac arrest. The encephalopathy, however, is due primarily to cerebral ischemia. Acute hypoxia results in transient alterations of cognitive function similar to those due to intoxication with al-

cohol. Hallucinations and alterations in judgment and behavior are well known in mountain climbers at high altitudes. Climbers to the Mt. Everest summit, at 8,854 m (29,000 feet) have been studied to determine the potential acute and long-term neurological deficits from hypoxia at these altitudes. The results of simple tests of short-term memory (number recall) and simple motor tasks (finger tapping) are shown in Figure 1-13. Significant reductions in performance in both tests were found immediately after the expedition, and significant impairments persisted 12 months later.[121] Ascent to high altitudes will eventually prove fatal: Two of three balloonists who ascended to 7,000 m (23,000 feet) died.[122]

The mechanisms of death and CNS injury in hypoxia have been studied physiologically and neuropathologically. In dogs, heart failure and systemic hypotension were produced with arterial PO$_2$ below 45 mmHg. They were not prevented by perfusing the coronary arteries with normally oxygenated blood but were averted by perfusion of the carotid arteries with oxygenated blood. A PO$_2$ below 15 mmHg was then required for heart failure to occur. Accordingly, a CNS-induced reflex depression of cardiac function

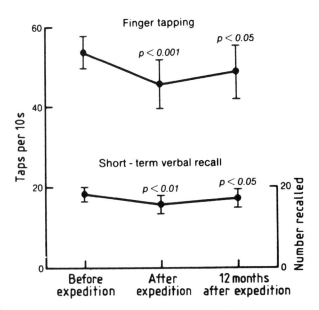

Fig. 1-13 Results of finger-tapping and short-term memory tests performed before, immediately after, and 1 year following an expedition to Mt. Everest. (From West JB: Do climbs to extreme altitude cause brain damage? Lancet 2:387, 1986, with permission.)

explains circulatory compromise in acute hypoxia.[123] Neuropathological studies of the CNS in primates subjected to hypoxia have generated similar conclusions. Neuropathological change is found only in the watershed distribution between major arterial territories. Thus the effects of acute hypoxia on the brain are those of cerebral hypoperfusion.[124]

HIGH ALTITUDE SICKNESS

Several days after ascending rapidly to altitudes of 2,400 to 3,600 m (8,000 to 12,000 feet), a syndrome of headache, insomnia, anorexia, nausea, vomiting, and impaired cognitive function may develop. Concomitant hypoventilation, such as may occur with sleep, sedatives, or alcohol, worsens these symptoms. A more marked syndrome of severe headache with delirium, hallucinations, ataxia, and, occasionally, seizures occurs at elevations of more than 3,000 m (10,000 feet). Cerebral edema is responsible, and papilledema and retinal hemorrhages may be seen.[125] The cause of the cerebral edema remains uncertain, but the delay of hours to days between rapid ascent to high altitude and the development of symptoms rules out simple hypoxia as a cause. Acute mountain sickness may be prevented by prophylaxis with acetazolamide[126] or dexamethasone.[127] The fully developed syndrome is also rapidly attenuated by dexamethasone.[128] The reason for the effectiveness of these agents is uncertain, but a decrease in interstitial pulmonary edema, with resultant improvement in oxygenation, may be responsible.[128,129]

Hypercapnia

CHRONIC HYPERCAPNIA

A reversible syndrome of headache, papilledema, and impaired consciousness with "tremor of the extremities" has been described in patients with chronic pulmonary insufficiency.[130,131] Tremulousness is most prominent with the fingers outstretched and has the characteristics of an action tremor or the features of asterixis; in some patients it resembles myoclonus. The headaches are attributed to the increased intracranial pressure. Arterial oxygen saturations in one study[131] ranged from 81 to 94 percent (but may be as low as 40 percent), and the PCO_2 levels ranged from 39 to 68 mmHg (but can be higher). The EEG

shows slowing in the theta or delta range. The etiology of such CO_2 narcosis is probably multifactorial, including hypercapnia, hypoxia, and elevated intracranial pressure. The increased intracranial pressure may produce papilledema that can progress to blindness.[132] Ventilatory support and discontinuation of sedative drugs constitute effective treatment. Vigorous hyperventilation is to be avoided as renewed obtundation, seizures, and even death may result, presumably from hyperventilation-induced cerebral vasoconstriction.[133]

ACUTE HYPERCAPNIA

Nervous system abnormalities from hypercapnia are related in significant measure to the rate of increase of PCO_2. With slow elevations of PCO_2 and maintenance of oxygenation, CNS symptoms may be absent. Neff and Petty reported ten such patients with a mean PCO_2 of 90 mmHg (range 75 to 110 mmHg).[134] Carbon dioxide inhalation in normal patients produces alteration of consciousness, and CO_2 has been used as an anesthetic.[130] In animals a biphasic effect is seen before this anesthetic phase. Initially, there is an increase in the threshold for electrical and chemically induced seizures that is maximal at CO_2 concentrations of about 10 to 15 percent.[135] Subsequently, seizure threshold decreases. Seizures have been noted in patients with CO_2 intoxication.[130]

The role of cerebrospinal fluid (CSF) acidosis in brain dysfunction was raised by Posner and associates.[136] The rapid diffusibility of carbon dioxide across the blood-brain barrier produces a prompt fall in CSF pH in respiratory acidosis, a decrease that does not occur in metabolic acidosis.[137] The mechanism of the depressive effect of this acidosis remains uncertain. Cerebral metabolic rate is altered minimally, but glucose utilization is depressed.[138] The mechanism of the depressive effect of this acidosis has previously been unexplained. However, a potent inhibitory effect of H^+ upon the postsynaptic receptor for glutamate, the brain's major excitatory neurotransmitter, has recently been described and is probably responsible for the acute encephalopathy of hypercapnia.[139] Ultrastructurally, hypercapnia produces an increase in water content of white matter structures.[140] The role of vasodilatation in the production of this edema is uncertain.

Hypocapnia

ACUTE HYPOCAPNIA

Acute hypocapnia occurs during hyperventilation. The symptom complex of dizziness, light-headedness, faintness, paresthesias, and impaired consciousness can be reproduced in normal subjects during hyperventilation, supporting a cause-and-effect relation between acute hypocarbia and the symptoms of the hyperventilation syndrome (Table 1-2).[141] This syndrome is somewhat more common in women than men and has its maximal incidence during the third decade. Distal paresthesias are notable and may be asymmetrical, prompting evaluation for a more sinister cause. Alteration or loss of consciousness is common (31 percent in the series of Perkin and Joseph[141]), leading to an inappropriate diagnosis of epilepsy. Symptoms can often be reproduced by voluntary hyperventilation, and the EEG findings while the patient is symptomatic can help to exclude a diagnosis of seizure disorder.

The effects of hypocapnia include cerebral vasoconstriction, alteration in the ionic balance of calcium, and a shift in the oxyhemoglobin dissociation curve

Table 1-2 Symptoms in 78 Patients During the Hyperventilation Syndrome[a]

Symptoms	No.	Percent
Neurological		
Giddiness	46	59
Paraesthesiae	28	36
Loss of consciousness	24	31
Visual disturbance	22	28
Headache	17	22
Ataxia	14	18
Tremor	8	10
Tinnitus	2	3
Cardiorespiratory		
Dyspnea	41	53
Palpitations	33	42
Chest discomfort	6	8
Gastrointestinal		
Nausea	15	19
Abdominal pain	1	1
Vomiting	1	1

[a] Most patients had more than one symptom.
(From Perkin GD, Joseph R: Neurological manifestations of the hyperventilation syndrome. J R Soc Med 79:448, 1986, with permission.)

with reduced delivery of oxygen to peripheral tissues. A combination of these events is responsible for the clinical symptoms. Perhaps the most distinctive neurological symptom of hyperventilation is tetany. The pathogenesis of this phenomenon has been investigated in dogs by Edmondson and colleagues.[142] Respiratory alkalosis or hypocalcemia alone were poor inducers of tetany, but hypocalcemia combined with alkalosis invariably produced it. No relation was found between CSF calcium ion content and tetany, nor was the rate of calcium decrease a critical factor.

CHRONIC HYPOCAPNIA

Fixed respiratory alkalosis is a common or even diagnostic finding in a number of metabolic disorders, the most prominent being hepatic encephalopathy; sepsis and salicylate poisoning are additional examples. However, the role of the alkalosis itself in causing CNS dysfunction is uncertain. Potential mechanisms by which alkalosis may affect the brain include a shift of the oxyhemoglobin dissociation curve (which decreases oxygen availability to tissues), a decrease in cerebral blood flow resulting from cerebral vasoconstriction, and alkalosis-induced hypophosphatemia.[143] Such marked decreases in serum phosphate may produce a neuromuscular syndrome similar to the Guillain-Barré syndrome.[144] Nevertheless, Mazzara and colleagues, reporting 114 patients with extreme respiratory alkalosis, found that although hypocapnia had clear prognostic implications, controlled ventilation to alter the fall in arterial blood pH did not influence the survival statistics.[145] Again, control of the alkalosis by mechanical ventilation did not alter the encephalopathic manifestations in patients with hepatic failure.[146] Accordingly, alkalosis per se appears to have a minimal effect on the CNS.

HICCUP

Persistent or intractable hiccup is an abnormality resulting from many CNS causes, including brainstem neoplasm,[147] multiple sclerosis,[148] and thoracic herpes zoster.[149] It may also occur with cortical pathology.[150,151] Idiopathic cases of intractable hiccup are much more common in men than women; for example, 118 of 220 such patients seen at the Mayo Clinic were men.[152] Hiccup results from CNS-induced synchronous contraction of the diaphragm and the external (inspiratory) intercostal muscles, followed rapidly by inhibition of expiratory intercostal muscles and glottal closure.[153] The glottal closure minimizes air exchange. However, with tracheostomy the induced ventilatory movements of hiccup cause air exchange, and a respiratory alkalosis is produced.[153]

The frequency, but not amplitude of hiccuping is modulated by arterial PCO_2. Hiccup frequency is reduced with elevated PCO_2 levels and increased with a fall in arterial PCO_2.[153] This observation is in keeping with the traditional cure for hiccups—breath-holding. Another common lay remedy for hiccups is swallowing or pharyngeal stimulation, maneuvers that may increase vagal tone. Vagal mucosal and laryngotracheal afferents are known to inhibit hiccups.[154] Accordingly, hiccups are most common at maximal inspiration because these vagal afferents are inhibited by maximal lung inflation. High-frequency diaphragmatic flutter, responsive to carbamazepine, is responsible for hiccups in some patients.[151] Chlorpromazine remains the most popular pharmacological treatment, although a host of other approaches has been suggested.[155]

SNEEZING

The coordinated act of sneezing arises from a caudal brainstem center near the nucleus ambiguus.[156] Cortical input has long been recognized.

The central mediation of sneezing was noted by Penfield and Jasper in a patient during temporal lobe stimulation when both sneezing and chewing movements were induced.[157] Rare additional cases of CNS dysfunction with sneezing have also been reported.[158] A common reflex that induces sneezing is that which occurs on sudden exposure to bright light. In a report by Everett, the incidence of this reflex was 30 percent in male medical students and 50 percent in women.[159] Furthermore, it was found in 80 percent of the families of medical students in whom the phenomenon of light-induced sneezing was reported. It has been suggested that this reflex is inherited in an autosomal dominant manner.[160]

YAWNING

Yawning is coordinated from uncertain brainstem sites via extrapyramidal pathways. This reflex may occur in patients "locked in" from pontine transection who have nonvolitional mouth opening with spontaneous yawns.[161] Yawning in the setting of a pyramidal lesion (capsular infarction) may be associated with arm stretching in the paretic limb, supporting the involvement of extrapyramidal circuitry.[162] Cortical input also occurs, as reflected by the yawning related to boredom and somnolence. Yawning has been seen to initiate a temporal lobe seizure.[157]

REFERENCES

1. Taylor AE: Capillary fluid filtration: Starling forces and lymph flow. Circ Res 49:557, 1981
2. Simon RP: Neurogenic pulmonary edema. Neurol Clin 11:309, 1993
3. Ducker TB, Simmons RL: Increased intracranial pressure and pulmonary edema. II: The hemodynamic response of dogs and monkeys to increased intracranial pressure. J Neurosurg 29:118, 1968
4. Popp JA, Gottlieb ME, Paloski WH, et al: Cardiopulmonary hemodynamics in patients with serious head injury. J Surg Res 32:416, 1982
5. Simon RP, Bayne LL: Pulmonary lymphatic flow alterations during intracranial hypertension in sheep. Ann Neurol 15:188, 1984
6. McClellan MD, Dauber IM, Weil J: Elevated intracranial pressure increases pulmonary vascular permeability to protein. J Appl Physiol 67:1185, 1989
7. Brown RH, Beyeri BD, Iseke R, Lavyne MH: Medulla oblongata edema associated with neurogenic pulmonary edema. J Neurosurg 64:494, 1986
8. Yamour BJ, Sridharan MR, Rice JF: Electrocardiographic changes in cerebrovascular hemorrhage. Am Heart J 99:294, 1980
9. Harari A, Rapin M, Regnier B, et al: Normal pulmonary-capillary pressures in the late phase of neurogenic pulmonary oedema. Lancet 1:494, 1976
10. Schlesinger B: Neurogenic pulmonary edema due to puncture wound of the medulla oblongata. J Nerv Ment Dis 102:247, 1945
11. Baker AB: Poliomyelitis: a study of pulmonary edema. Neurology 7:743, 1957
12. Doba N, Reis DJ: Acute fulminating neurogenic hypertension produced by brainstem lesions in the rat. Circ Res 32:584, 1973

13. Darragh TM, Simon RP: Nucleus tractus solitarius lesions elevate pulmonary arterial pressure and lymph flow. Ann Neurol 17:565, 1985
14. Simon RP, Gean MA, Sander JE: Medullary lesion inducing pulmonary edema: a magnetic resonance imaging study. Ann Neurol 30:727, 1991
15. Benowitz NL, Simon RP, Copeland JR: Status epilepticus: divergence of sympathetic activity and cardiovascular response. Ann Neurol 19:197, 1986
16. Bayne LL, Simon RP: Systemic and pulmonary vascular pressures during generalized seizures in sheep. Ann Neurol 10:566, 1981
17. Simon RP, Bayne LL, Tranbaugh RF, Lewis FR: Elevated pulmonary lymph flow and protein content during status epilepticus in sheep. J Appl Physiol 52:91, 1982
18. Darnell JC, Jay SJ: Recurrent postictal pulmonary edema: a case report and review of the literature. Epilepsia 23:71, 1982
19. Terrence CF, Rao GR, Perper JA: Neurogenic pulmonary edema in unexpected, unexplained death of epileptic patients. Ann Neurol 9:458, 1981
20. Cameron GR, De SN: Experimental pulmonary oedema of nervous origin. J Pathol Bacteriol 61:375, 1949
21. Maron MB: Analysis of airway protein concentration in neurogenic pulmonary edema. J Appl Physiol 62:470, 1987
22. Theodore J, Robin ED: Speculations on neurogenic pulmonary edema (NPE). Am Rev Respir Dis 113:405, 1976
23. Severinghaus JW, Mitchell RA: Ondine's curse—failure of respiratory center automaticity while awake. Clin Res 10:122, 1962
24. Beal MF, Richardson EP, Brandstetter R, et al: Localized brainstem ischemic damage and Ondine's curse after near-drowning. Neurology 33:717, 1983
25. Lockwood AH: Shy-Drager syndrome with abnormal respirations and antidiuretic hormone release. Arch Neurol 33:292, 1976
26. Plum F, Leigh RJ: Abnormalities of central mechanisms. p. 989. In Hornbein TF (ed): Regulation of Breathing, Part II. Marcel Dekker, New York, 1981
27. Munschauer FE, Loh L, Bannister R, Newsom-Davis J: Abnormal respiration and sudden death during sleep in multiple system atrophy with autonomic failure. Neurology 40:677, 1990
28. Tranmer BI, Tucker WS, Bilbao JM: Sleep apnea following percutaneous cervical cordotomy. Can J Neurol Sci 14:262, 1987
29. Kales A, Vela-Bueno A, Kales JD: Sleep disorders: sleep apnea and narcolepsy. Ann Intern Med 106:434, 1987
30. Haponik EF, Givens D, Angelo J: Syringobulbia-myelia with obstructive sleep apnea. Neurology 33:1046, 1983
31. Adelman S, Dinner DS, Goren H, et al: Obstructive sleep apnea in association with posterior fossa neurologic disease. Arch Neurol 41:509, 1984
32. Bradley TD, Shapiro CM: ABC of sleep disorders: unexpected presentations of sleep apnoea: use of CPAP in treatment. Br Med J 306:1260, 1993
33. Newsom-Davis J: Autonomous breathing. Arch Neurol 30:480, 1974
34. Meyer J, Herndon RM: Bilateral infarction of the pyramidal tracts in man. Neurology 12:637, 1962
35. Feldman MH: Physiological observations in a chronic case of locked-in syndrome. Neurology 18:1166, 1968
36. Turner WA, Critchley M: Respiratory disorders in epidemic encephalitis. Brain 48:72, 1925
37. Kim R: The chronic residual respiratory disorder in post-encephalitic parkinsonism. J Neurol Neurosurg Psychiatry 31:393, 1968
38. Vincken W, Gauthier SG, Dolfuss RE, et al: Involvement of upper-airway muscles in extrapyramidal disorders: a cause of airflow limitation. N Engl J Med 311:428, 1984
39. Zupnick HM, Brown LK, Miller A, Moros DA: Respiratory dysfunction due to L-dopa therapy for parkinsonism: diagnosis using serial pulmonary function tests and respiratory inductive plethysmography. Am J Med 89:109, 1990
40. Weiner WJ, Goetz CG, Nausieda PA, et al: Respiratory dyskinesias: extrapyramidal dysfunction and dyspnea. Ann Intern Med 88:327, 1978
41. Robin ED, Whaley RD, Crump CH, Travis DM: Alveolar gas tensions, pulmonary ventilation and blood pH during physiologic sleep in normal subjects. J Clin Invest 37:981, 1958
42. Fluck DC: Chest movements in hemiplegia. Clin Sci 31:383, 1966
43. Keltz H, Kaplan S, Stone DJ: Effect of quadriplegia and hemidiaphragmatic paralysis on thoracoabdominal pressure during respiration. Am J Phys Med 48:109, 1969
44. Gandevia SC, Macefield G: Projection of low-threshold afferents from human intercostal muscles to the cerebral cortex. Resp Physiol 77:203, 1989
45. Sears TA: Breathing: a sensorimotor act. p. 129. In Gilliland I, Francis J (eds): The Scientific Basis of Medicine: Annual Reviews. Athlone Press, London, 1971
46. Plum F: Neurological integration of behavioral and metabolic control of breathing. p. 168. In Porter R (ed): Breathing: Hering-Breuer Centenary Symposium. Churchill Livingstone, London, 1970
47. Kaada BR: Somato-motor, autonomic and electrocor-

ticographic responses to electrical stimulation of "rhinencephalic" and other structures in primates, cat and dog. Acta Physiol Scand 24:1, 1951

48. Reis DJ, McHugh PR: Hypoxia as a cause of bradycardia during amygdala stimulation in monkey. J Appl Physiol 214:601, 1968

49. Kaada BR, Jasper H: Respiratory responses to stimulation of temporal pole, insula and hippocampal and limbic gyri in man. Arch Neurol Psychiatry 68:609, 1952

50. Nelson DA, Ray CD: Respiratory arrest from seizure discharges in limbic system. Arch Neurol 19:199, 1968

51. Johnson LC, Davidoff RA: Autonomic changes during paroxysmal EEG activity. Electroencephalogr Clin Neurophysiol 17:25, 1964

52. Maskill D, Murphy K, Mier A, et al: Motor cortical representation of the diaphragm in man. J Physiol (Lond) 443:105, 1991

53. Colebatch JG, Adams L, Murphy K, et al: Regional cerebral blood flow during volitional breathing in man. J Physiol (Lond) 443:91, 1991

54. Atack EA, Suranyi L: Respiratory inhibitory apraxia. Can J Neurol Sci 2:37, 1975

55. Hering P. Cited in Plum F, Brown HW, Snoep E: Neurologic significance of post-hyperventilation apnea. JAMA 181:1050, 1962

56. Bainton CR, Mitchell RA: Posthyperventilation apnea in awake man. J Appl Physiol 21:411, 1966

57. Fink BR: Influence of cerebral activity in wakefulness on regulation of breathing. J Appl Physiol 16:15, 1961

58. Plum F, Brown HW, Snoep E: Neurologic significance of post-hyperventilation apnea. JAMA 181:1050, 1962

59. Jennett S, Ashbridge K, North JB: Post-hyperventilation apnoea in patients with brain damage. J Neurol Neurosurg Psychiatry 37:288, 1974

60. Fink BR, Hanks EC, Ngai SH, Papper EM: Central regulation of respiration during anesthesia and wakefulness. Ann NY Acad Sci 109:892, 1963

61. Lumsden T: Observation on the respiratory centres in the cat. J Physiol (Lond) 57:153, 1923

62. Moruzzi G: Paleocerebellar inhibition of vasomotor and respiratory carotid sinus reflexes. J Neurophysiol 3:20, 1940

63. Corda M, Eklund G, von Euler C: External intercostal and phrenic motor responses to changes in respiratory load. Acta Physiol Scand 63:391, 1965

64. Mitchell RA, Berger AJ: Neural regulation of respiration. p. 541. In Hornbein TF (ed): Regulation of Breathing, Part I. Marcel Dekker, New York, 1981

65. Gautier H, Bertrand F: Respiratory effects of pneumotaxic center lesions and subsequent vagotomy in chronic cats. Respir Physiol 23:71, 1975

66. St. John WM, Zhou D: Rostral pontile mechanisms regulate durations of expiratory phases. J Appl Physiol 71:2133, 1991

67. Sears TA: The respiratory motoneuron and apneusis. Fed Proc 36:2412, 1977

68. Foutz AS, Champagnat J, Denavit-Saubie M: Involvement of N-methyl-D-aspartate (NMDA) receptors in respiratory rhythmogenesis. Brain Res 500:199, 1989

69. Monteau R, Gauthier P, Rega P, Hilaire G: Effects of N-methyl-D-aspartate (NMDA) antagonist MK-801 on breathing pattern in rats. Neurosci Lett 109:134, 1990

70. Lee MC, Klassen AC, Heaney LM, et al. Respiratory rate and pattern disturbances in acute brain stem infarction. Stroke 7:382, 1976

71. Plum F, Alvord EC: Apneustic breathing in man. Arch Neurol 10:101, 1964

72. Abrahams TP, Hornby PJ, Walton DP, et al: An excitatory amino acid(s) in the ventrolateral medulla is (are) required for breathing to occur in the anesthetized cat. J Pharmacol Exp Ther 259:1388, 1991

73. St John WM: Neurogenesis, control, and functional significance of gasping. J Appl Physiol 68:1305, 1990

74. Von Euler C: Brain stem mechanisms for generation and control of breathing pattern. p. 1. In Cherniack NS, Widdicombe JG (eds): Handbook of Physiology, Vol 2: The Respiratory System. American Physiological Society, Bethesda, MD, 1986

75. Cheyne J: A case of apoplexy in which the fleshy part of the heart was converted to fat. Dublin Hosp Rep 2:216, 1818

76. Lange RI, Hecht HH: The mechanism of Cheyne-Stokes respiration. J Clin Invest 41:42, 1962

77. Chernick V, Avery ME: Response of premature infant with periodic breathing to ventilatory stimuli. J Appl Physiol 21:434, 1966

78. Webb P: Periodic breathing during sleep. J Appl Physiol 37:899, 1974

79. Luft UC: Aviation physiology: the effects of altitude. p. 1345. In Magoun HW (ed): Handbook of Physiology. Section III, Vol 2. American Physiological Society, Washington, DC, 1960

80. Dowell AR, Buckley CE, Cohen R, et al: Cheyne-Stokes respiration. Arch Intern Med 127:712, 1971

81. Karp HR, Sieker HO, Heyman A: Cerebral circulation and function in Cheyne-Stokes respiration. Am J Med 30:861, 1961

82. Brown HW, Plum F: The neurologic basis of Cheyne-Stokes respiration. Am J Med 30:849, 1961

83. Guyton AC, Crowell JW, Moore JW: Basic oscillating mechanism of Cheyne-Stokes breathing. Am J Physiol 187:395, 1956

84. Preiss G, Iscoe S, Polosa C: Analysis of a periodic breathing pattern associated with Mayer waves. Am J Physiol 228:768, 1975

85. Hoffman R, Agatston A, Krieger B: Cheyne-Stokes respiration in patients recovering from acute cardiogenic pulmonary edema. Chest 97:410, 1990

86. Cherniack NS, von Euler C, Homma I, Kao FF: Experimentally induced Cheyne-Stokes breathing. Respir Physiol 37:185, 1979

87. Hanly PJ, Millar TW, Steljes DG, et al: Respiration and abnormal sleep in patients with congestive heart failure. Chest 96:480, 1989

88. Webber CL, Speck DF: Experimental Biot periodic breathing in cats: effects of changes in P_ICO_2 and P_ICO_2. Resp Physiol 46:327, 1981

89. Motta J, Guilleminault C: Effects of oxygen administration in sleep-induced apneas. p. 137. In Guilleminault C, Dement W (eds): Sleep Apnea Syndromes. Alan R. Liss, New York, 1978

90. Plum F, Swanson AG: Central neurogenic hyperventilation in man. Arch Neurol Psychiatry 81:535, 1959

91. McNealy DE, Plum F: Brainstem dysfunction with supratentorial mass lesions. Arch Neurol 7:10, 1962

92. North JB, Jennett S: Abnormal breathing patterns associated with acute brain damage. Arch Neurol 31:338, 1974

93. Leigh RJ, Shaw DA: Rapid regular respiration in unconscious patients. Arch Neurol 33:356, 1976

94. Jaeckle KA, Digre KB, Jones CR, et al: Central neurogenic hyperventilation: pharmacologic intervention with morphine sulfate and correlative analysis of respiratory, sleep, and ocular motor dysfunction. Neurology 40:1715, 1990

95. Goulon M, Escourolle R, Augustin P, et al: Hyperventilation primitive par gliome bulbo-protuberantiel. Rev Neurol (Paris) 121:636, 1969

96. Rodriguez M, Baele PL, Marsh HM, et al: Central neurogenic hyperventilation in an awake patient with brainstem astrocytoma. Ann Neurol 11:625, 1982

97. Lange LS, Laszlo G: Cerebral tumour presenting with hyperventilation. J Neurol Neurosurg Psychiatry 28:317, 1965

98. Dubayo BA, Afridi I, Hussain M: Central neurogenic hyperventilation in invasive laryngeal carcinoma. Chest 99:767, 1991

99. Plum F: Mechanisms of "central" hyperventilation. Ann Neurol 11:636, 1982

100. Mitchell RA, Loeschcke HH, Massion WH, et al: Respiratory responses mediated through superficial chemosensitive areas on the medulla. J Appl Physiol 18:523, 1963

101. Rottenberg DA, Ginos JZ, Kearfott KJ, et al: In vivo measurement of brain tumor pH using dimethyloxa-

zolidinedione and positron emission tomography. Ann Neurol 16:132, 1984

102. Shibata Y, Meguro K, Narushima K, et al: Malignant lymphoma of the central nervous system presenting with central neurogenic hyperventilation. J Neurosurg 76:696, 1992

103. Vincken W, Elleker MG, Cosio MG: Determinants of respiratory muscle weakness in stable chronic neuromuscular disorders. Am J Med 82:53, 1987

104. Griggs RC, Donohoe KM, Utell MJ, et al: Evaluation of pulmonary function in neuromuscular disease. Arch Neurol 38:9, 1981

105. O'Donohue WJ Jr, Baker JP, Bell GM, et al: Respiratory failure in neuromuscular disease. JAMA 235:733, 1976

106. Vanderlinden RG, Epstein SW, Hyland RH, et al: Management of chronic ventilatory insufficiency with electrical diaphragm pacing. Can J Neurol Sci 15:63, 1988

107. Glenn WWL, Hogan JF, Loke JSO, et al: Ventilatory support by pacing of the conditioned diaphragm in quadriplegia. N Engl J Med 310:1150, 1984

108. Howard RS, Wiles CM, Loh L: Respiratory complications and their management in motor neuron disease. Brain 112:1155, 1989

109. Braun SR, Sufit RL, Giovannoni R, et al: Intermittent negative pressure ventilation in the treatment of respiratory failure in progressive neuromuscular disease. Neurology 37:1874, 1987

110. Parhad IM, Clark AW, Barron KD, Staunton SB: Diaphragmatic paralysis in motor neuron disease. Neurology 28:18, 1978

111. French Cooperative Group on Plasma Exchange in Guillain-Barré Syndrome: Efficiency of plasma exchange in Guillain-Barré syndrome: role of replacement fluids. Ann Neurol 22:753, 1987

112. The Guillain-Barré Syndrome Study Group: Plasmapheresis and acute Guillain-Barré syndrome. Neurology 35:1096, 1985

113. Ropper AH: The Guillain-Barré syndrome. N Engl J Med 326:1130, 1992

114. Sunderrajan EV, Davenport J: The Guillain-Barré syndrome: pulmonary-neurologic correlations. Medicine (Baltimore) 64:333, 1985

115. Borel CO, Tilford C, Nichols DG, et al: Diaphragmatic performance during recovery from acute ventilatory failure in Guillain-Barré syndrome and myasthenia gravis. Chest 99:444, 1991

116. van der Meche FG, Schmitz PI: A randomized trial comparing intravenous immune globulin and plasma exchange in Guillain-Barré syndrome: Dutch Guillain-Barré Study Group. N Engl J Med 326:1123, 1992

117. Zochodne DW, Bolton CF, Wells GA, et al: Critical

illness polyneuropathy: a complication of sepsis and multiple organ failure. Brain 110:819, 1987

118. Witt NJ, Zochodne DW, Bolton CF, et al: Peripheral nerve function in sepsis and multiple organ failure. Chest 99:176, 1991

119. Gracey DR, Divertie MB, Howard FM: Mechanical ventilation for respiratory failure in myasthenia gravis. Mayo Clin Proc 58:597, 1983

120. Barohn RJ, Clanton T, Sahenk Z, Mendell JR: Recurrent respiratory insufficiency and depressed ventilatory drive complicating mitochondrial myopathies. Neurology 40:103, 1990

121. Townes BD, Horbein TF, Schoene RB, et al: Human cerebral function at extreme altitude. p. 32. In West JB, Lahiri S (eds): High Altitude and Man. American Physiological Society, Bethesda, MD, 1984

122. Tissandier G. Cited in Tavel FV: Die Auswirkungen des Sauerstoffmangels auf den menschlichen Organismus bei kurzfristigem Aufenthalt in grosser Hohe. Helv Physiol Acta, suppl 1:1, 1943

123. Cross CE, Rieben PA, Barron CI, Salisbury PF: Effects of arterial hypoxia on the heart and circulation: an integrative study. Am J Physiol 205:963, 1963

124. Brierley JB, Graham DI: Hypoxia and vascular disorders of the central nervous system. In Adams JH, Corsellis JAN, Duchen LW (eds): Greenfield's Neuropathology. 4th Ed. John Wiley & Sons, New York, 1984

125. Sutton JR: Classification and terminology of altitude illness. Semin Respir Med 5:129, 1983

126. Forwand SA, Landowne M, Follansbee JN, Mansen JE: Effect of acetazolamide on acute mountain sickness. N Engl J Med 279:839, 1968

127. Johnson TS, Rock RB, Fulco CS, et al; Prevention of acute mountain sickness by dexamethasone. N Engl J Med 310:683, 1984

128. Ferrazzini G, Maggiorini M, Kriemler S, et al: Successful treatment of acute mountain sickness with dexamethasone. Br Med J 294:1380, 1987

129. Sutton JR, Lassen N: Pathophysiology of acute mountain sickness and high altitude pulmonary oedema. Bull Eur Physiopathol Respir 15:1045, 1979

130. Sieker HO, Hickam JB: Carbon dioxide intoxication. Medicine (Baltimore) 35:389, 1956

131. Austen FK, Carmichael MW, Adams RD: Neurologic manifestations of chronic pulmonary insufficiency. N Engl J Med 257:579, 1957

132. Reeve P, Harvey G, Seaton D: Papilloedema and respiratory failure. Br Med J 291:331, 1985

133. Faden A: Encephalopathy following treatment of chronic pulmonary failure. Neurology 26:337, 1976

134. Neff TA, Petty TL: Tolerance and survival in severe chronic hypercapnia. Arch Intern Med 129:591, 1972

135. Woodbury DM, Karler R: The role of carbon dioxide in the nervous system. Anesthesiology 21:687, 1960

136. Posner JB, Swanson AG, Plum F: Acid-base balance in cerebrospinal fluid. Arch Neurol 12:479, 1965

137. Mitchell RA, Singer MM: Respiration and cerebrospinal fluid pH in metabolic acidosis and alkalosis. J Appl Physiol 20:905, 1965

138. Miller AL, Hawkins RA, Veech RL: Decreased rate of glucose ultilization of rat brain in vivo after exposure to atmospheres containing high concentrations of CO_2. J Neurochem 25:553, 1975

139. Tang CM, Dichter M, Morad M: Modulation of the N-methyl-D-aspartate channel by extracellular H+. Proc Natl Acad Sci USA 87:6445, 1990

140. Bakay L, Lee JC: The effect of acute hypoxia and hypercapnia on the ultrastructure of the central nervous system. Brain 91:697, 1968

141. Perkin GD, Joseph R: Neurological manifestations of the hyperventilation syndrome. J R Soc Med 79:448, 1986

142. Edmondson JW, Brashear RE, Ting-Kai L: Tetany: quantitative interrelationships between calcium and alkalosis. Am J Physiol 228:1082, 1975

143. Saltzman HA, Heyman A, Sieker HO: Correlation of clinical and physiologic manifestations of sustained hyperventilation. N Engl J Med 268:1431, 1963

144. Weintraub MI: Hypophosphatemia mimicking acute Guillain-Barré-Strohl syndrome. JAMA 235:1040, 1976

145. Mazzara JT, Ayres SM, Crate WJ: Extreme hypocapnia in the critically ill patient. Am J Med 56:450, 1974

146. Posner JB, Plum F: Toxic effects of carbon dioxide and acetazolamide in hepatic encephalopathy. J Clin Invest 39:1246, 1980

147. Stotka UL, Barcay SJ, Bell HS, et al: Intractable hiccoughs as the primary manifestation of brain stem tumor. Am J Med 32:313, 1962

148. McFarling DA, Susac JO: Hoquet diabolique: intractable hiccups as a manifestation of multiple sclerosis. Neurology 29:797, 1979

149. Efrati P: Obstinate hiccup as a prodromal symptom in thoracic herpes zoster. Neurology 6:601, 1956

150. Jansen PHP, Joosten EMG, Vingerhoets HM: Persistent periodic hiccups following brain abscess: a case report. J Neurol Sci 103:144, 1991

151. Vantrappen G, Decramer M, Harlet R: High-frequency diaphragmatic flutter: symptoms and treatment by carbamazepine. Lancet 339:265, 1992

152. Souadjian JV, Cain JC: Intractable hiccups. Postgrad Med 43:72, 1968

153. Newsom-Davis J: An expermental study of hiccup. Brain 93:851, 1970

154. Salem MR, Baraka A, Rattenborg CC, et al: Treat-

ment of hiccups by pharyngeal stimulation in anesthetized and conscious subjects. JAMA 202:32, 1967

155. Kolodzik PW, Eilers MA: Hiccups (singultus): review and approach to management. Ann Emerg Med 20: 565, 1991

156. Nonaka S, Unno T, Ohta Y, Mori S: Sneeze-evoking region within the brainstem. Brain Res 511:265, 1990

157. Penfield W, Jasper H: Epilepsy and the Functional Anatomy of the Human Brain. Little, Brown, Boston, 1954

158. Co S: Intractble sneezing: case report and literature review. Arch Neurol 36:111, 1979

159. Everett HC: Sneezing in response to light. Neurology 14:483, 1964

160. Peroutka SJ, Peroutka LA: Autosomal dominant transmission of the "photic sneeze reflex." N Engl J Med 310:599, 1984

161. Gschwend J: Gahnen als einziges Verhaltensmuster der Gesichts- und Kiefermuskulatur bei einem Patienten mit Ponsgliom. Fortschr Neurol Psychiatr 45:652, 1977

162. Wimalaratna HSK, Capildeo R: Is yawning a brainstem phenomenon? Lancet 1:300, 1988

2

Neurological Complications of Aortic Disease and Surgery

Douglas S. Goodin

The aorta is the main conduit through which the heart supplies blood to the body, including the brain, brainstem, and spinal cord. In addition, this vessel is situated close to important neural structures. In consequence, both disease of the aorta and operations on it may have profound but variable effects on nervous system function. Often the neurological syndrome produced by aortic disease or surgery depends more on the part of the aorta involved than on the nature of the pathological process itself. For example, either syphilis or atherosclerosis may produce symptoms of cerebral ischemia if the pathology affects the aortic arch, or of spinal cord ischemia if the pathology is in the descending thoracic aorta. Even when the nature of the pathological process is important in determining the resultant neurological syndrome, several diseases may result in the same pathology. Thus atherosclerosis, infection, inflammation, and trauma may each result in the formation of aortic aneurysms; similarly, coarctation of the aorta may be congenital, a result of Takayasu's arteritis, or a sequela of radiation exposure during childhood.

The present chapter initially focuses on the three major areas of neurological dysfunction resulting from aortic disease and surgery: spinal cord ischemia,

cerebral ischemia, and peripheral neuropathy. Specific conditions that merit special consideration are then discussed individually. The normal anatomical relations are also considered in order to provide insight into the pathogenesis of the resulting neurological syndromes.

CLINICAL NEUROLOGICAL SYNDROMES DUE TO AORTIC PATHOLOGY

Aortic disease may produce a variety of neurological syndromes. The specific syndrome depends to a large extent on the site of involvement along the aorta.

Spinal Cord Ischemia

ANATOMY

Embryological Development
During embryological development, primitive blood vessels arise along the spinal nerve roots bilaterally and at each segmental level.[1] Each of these segmental vessels then divides into anterior and posterior

branches, which ramify extensively on the surfaces of the developing spinal cord. As development proceeds, most of these vessels regress and a few enlarge, so that by birth the blood supply to the spinal cord depends on a small but highly variable number of persisting segmental vessels (Fig. 2-1).[1–12] In the thoracic region, where the aorta is situated to the left of the midline, the persisting vessels entering the spinal canal are those from the left in 70 to 80 percent of cases.[1,6–8]

Anterior Spinal Artery

The anterior spinal artery is formed rostrally from paired branches of the intracranial vertebral arteries that descend from the level of the medulla (Fig. 2-1).

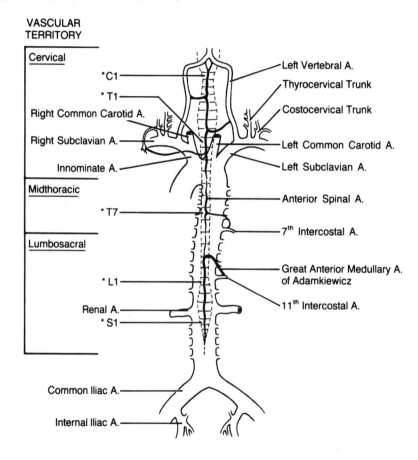

VASCULAR
TERRITORY

Cervical
- *C1 — Left Vertebral A.
- * T1 — Thyrocervical Trunk
- Right Common Carotid A. — Costocervical Trunk
- Right Subclavian A. — Left Common Carotid A.
- Innominate A. — Left Subclavian A.

Midthoracic
- * T7 — Anterior Spinal A.
- 7th Intercostal A.

Lumbosacral
- * L1 — Great Anterior Medullary A. of Adamkiewicz
- Renal A. — 11th Intercostal A.
- * S1

- Common Iliac A.
- Internal Iliac A.

* *Segmental Levels*

Fig. 2-1 Extraspinal contributions to the anterior spinal arteries showing the three arterial territories. In the cervical region an average of three arteries (derived from the vertebral arteries and the costocervical trunk) supply the anterior spinal artery. The anterior spinal artery is narrowest in the midthoracic region, often being difficult to distinguish from other small arteries on the anterior surface of the cord; occasionally it is discontinuous with the anterior spinal artery above and below. In addition, this region is often supplied by only a single small radiculomedullary vessel. The lumbosacral territory is supplied by a single large artery, the great anterior medullary artery of Adamkiewicz, which turns abruptly caudad after joining the anterior spinal artery. If it gives off an ascending branch, that branch is generally a much smaller vessel. This artery is generally the most caudal of the anterior radiculomedullary arteries, but when it follows a relatively high thoracic root there is often a small lumbar radiculomedullary artery below. In this and subsequent illustrations, *A.* indicates artery, *N.* indicates nerve, and *M.* indicates muscle.

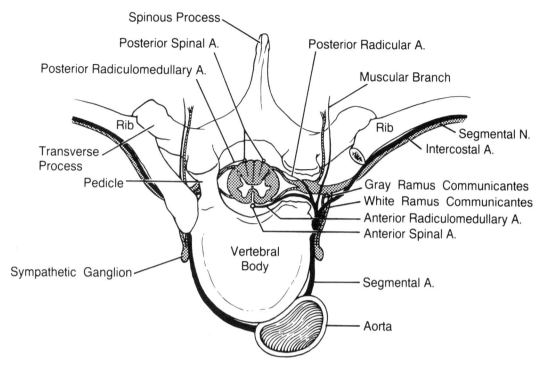

Fig. 2-2 Anatomy of the spinal cord circulation, showing the relation of the segmental arteries and their branches to the spinal canal and cord. The left rib and the left pedicle of the vertebra have been cut away to show the underlying vascular and neural structures.

These two arteries fuse to form a single anterior spinal artery, which overlies the anterior longitudinal fissure of the spinal cord.[1] This artery is joined at different levels by anterior radiculomedullary arteries, which are branches of certain segmental vessels (Fig. 2-2). The number of these vessels is variable among individuals, ranging from 2 to 17, although 85 percent of individuals have between 4 and 7.[1,8,11]

The anterior spinal artery in the region that includes the cervical enlargement (C1 to T3) is particularly well supplied, receiving contributions from an average of three segmental vessels.[8] One constant artery arises from the costocervical trunk and supplies the lower segments; the others arise from the extracranial vertebral arteries and supply the middle cervical segments.[11] In addition, branches of the vertebral arteries have rich anastomotic connections with other neck vessels, including the occipital artery, deep cervical artery, and ascending cervical artery.[11]

The anterior spinal artery in the midthoracic portion of the cord (T4 to T8) often receives only a single contribution from a small artery located at about T7,

most often on the left.[8,11] The anterior spinal artery has its smallest diameter in this region, and it is sometimes discontinuous with the vessel in more rostral or caudal regions.[1,7,11]

The anterior spinal artery in the region of the lumbar enlargement (T9 to the conus medullaris) is, as at the cervical enlargement, richly supplied, deriving its blood supply predominantly from a single large (1.0 to 1.3 mm in diameter) artery, the great anterior medullary artery of Adamkiewicz. This artery almost always accompanies a nerve root between T9 and L2, generally on the left, although rarely it may accompany a root above or below these levels.[1,7,8,11] Caudally, at the conus medullaris, the anterior spinal artery anastomoses with both posterior spinal arteries.[11]

Posterior Spinal Arteries

The paired posterior spinal arteries are formed rostrally from the intracranial portion of the vertebral arteries. They are distinct paired vessels only at their

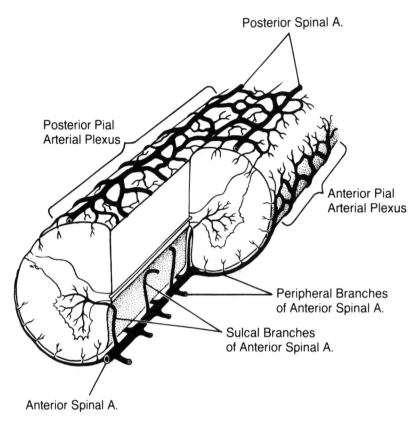

Fig. 2-3 Vascular anatomy of the spinal cord. The anterior spinal artery gives off both peripheral and sulcal branches. The sulcal branches pass posteriorly, penetrating the anterior longitudinal fissure. On reaching the anterior white commissure, they turn alternately to the right and to the left to supply the gray matter and deep white matter on each side.[12] Occasionally two adjacent vessels pass to the same side, and on other occasions a common stem vessel bifurcates to supply both sides. Terminal branches of these vessels overlap those from vessels above and below on the same side of the cord. The peripheral branches of the anterior spinal artery pass radially and form an anastomotic network of vessels, the anterior pial arterial plexus, which supplies the anterior and lateral white matter tracts via penetrating branches. The posterior pial arterial plexus is formed as a rich anastomotic network from the paired posterior spinal arteries. Penetrating branches from this plexus supply the posterior horns and posterior funiculi.

origin, however, and thereafter become intermixed with an anastomotic posterior pial arterial plexus (Fig. 2-3).[1,7,11] This plexus is joined at different levels by a variable number (10 to 23) of posterior radiculomedullary vessels that accompany the posterior nerve roots.[1]

Intrinsic Blood Supply of the Spinal Cord

In contrast to the extreme interindividual variability in the extraspinal arteries that supply the spinal cord, the intrinsic blood supply of the cord itself is more consistent. The anterior spinal artery gives off central (sulcal) arteries that pass posteriorly, penetrating the anterior longitudinal fissure and supplying most of the central gray matter and the deep portion of the anterior white matter (Fig. 2-4). The number of these sulcal vessels is variable, with 5 to 8 vessels per centimeter in the cervical region, 2 to 6 vessels per centimeter in the thoracic region, and 5 to 12 vessels per centimeter in the lumbosacral region.[1,9,11]

The anterior spinal artery also gives off peripheral arteries that pass radially on the anterior surface of the spinal cord to supply the white matter tracts ante-

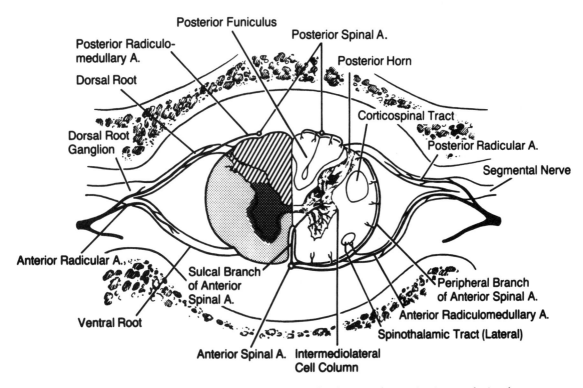

Fig. 2-4 Intrinsic blood supply of the spinal cord. The vascular territories are depicted on the right half of the cord. The hatched lines indicate the territory supplied by the posterior spinal arterial system. The stippled area is that supplied by the anterior circulation, with the darker stippling indicating the area supplied exclusively by the sulcal branches of the anterior spinal artery.

riorly and laterally. These arteries form the anterior pial arterial plexus, which is often poorly anastomotic with its posterior counterpart.[1] The posterior horns and posterior funiculi are supplied by penetrating vessels from the posterior pial arterial plexus.

ISCHEMIC CORD SYNDROMES

Ischemia of the spinal cord may be produced either by the interruption of blood flow through critical feeding vessels or by aortic hypotension. The resulting neurological syndrome depends on the location of ischemic lesions along and within the spinal cord, which depends, in turn, on the vascular anatomy discussed above. A wide variety of pathological disturbances of the aorta result in spinal cord ischemia. They include both iatrogenic causes, such as surgery or aortography,[13–16] and intrinsic aortic diseases, such as dissecting and nondissecting aneurysms,[17,18] inflammatory aortitis,[19] occlusive atherosclerotic dis-

ease,[20] infective and noninfective emboli,[21,22] and congenital coarctation.[23] Spinal cord ischemia is a rare complication of pregnancy,[10,24] possibly due to aortic compression, which can occur toward the end of gestation.[25]

Some authors have suggested that the midthoracic region (T4 to T8) is particularly vulnerable to ischemia because of the sparseness of vessels feeding the anterior spinal artery in this region and its poor anastomotic connections.[11] Others have stressed the vulnerability of the watershed areas between the three anterior spinal arterial territories.[10] Although the concept is theoretically appealing, documentation of the selective vulnerability of these regions is not completely convincing. For example, a review of 61 case reports[17,26–29] with respect to the distribution of ischemic myelopathies resulting from surgery on the aorta does not especially suggest that either of these areas is more vulnerable than other cord segments (Table 2-1). Even when the operation was performed

Table 2-1 Influence of Location of Aortic Surgery on the Vascular Territory of Resulting Spinal Cord Ischemia

	Location of Surgery	
Vascular Territory of Ischemia	Abdominal Aorta	Thoracic Aorta
Cervical region (C1–T3)	0	0
Midthoracic region (T4–T8)	1	14
Lumbosacral region (T9–conus)	25	21

(Based on 61 reported cases.[17,26–29])

on the thoracic aorta (and thus the proximal clamp was placed above the midthoracic cord feeder), the lumbosacral cord segments were the site of the ischemic damage more often than the supposedly more vulnerable midthoracic segments (Table 2-1). Similarly, the watershed area between these two arterial territories (T8–T9) does not seem particularly vulnerable. In fact, the most frequently affected cord segment within each vascular territory in these 61 cases

was centrally placed—T6 in the midthoracic territory and T12 in the lumbosacral territory—rather than at the borders, as would be anticipated with watershed vulnerability (Fig. 2-5).

Moreover, in an unselected autopsy series of 300 cases, Mannen found 25 cases of spinal cord infarction, two-thirds of which were in cervical cord segments[8]; the most commonly affected segment was C6. Such a distribution would be unexpected if either the midthoracic or the watershed area was particularly vulnerable. The poorly vascularized thoracic cord has much less gray matter than the cervical and lumbar enlargements, and it may be that the sparse blood supply to this cord region matches its reduced metabolic requirements.[7,30]

The site of aortic pathology also plays an important role in the location of the lesion along the spinal cord. For example, distal aortic occlusion often presents with lumbosacral involvement,[20,31] whereas dissecting aneurysm of the thoracic aorta commonly presents with infarction in the midthoracic re-

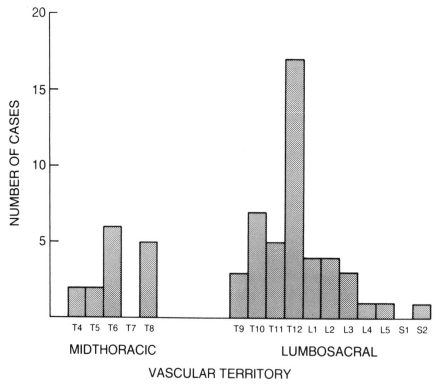

Fig. 2-5 Upper segmental level of spinal cord involvement in 61 cases of spinal cord ischemia following surgery on the aorta (based on previously published reports[17,26–29]).

gion.[18,32] Similarly, cord ischemia following surgery on the abdominal aorta is essentially confined to the lumbosacral territory, whereas surgery on the thoracic aorta not infrequently involves the midthoracic segments (Table 2-1). Regardless of the pathological process affecting the aorta, however, it generally involves the suprarenal portion if there is cord ischemia,[10,33] because the important radiculomedullary arteries usually originate above the origin of the renal arteries.

Anterior Spinal Artery Syndrome

Ischemic injury of the spinal cord at a particular segmental level may present with a complete transverse myelopathy.[11] Within the spinal cord, however, there are certain vascular territories that can be affected selectively. In particular, the territory of the anterior spinal artery, especially its sulcal branch, is prone to ischemic injury.[7,11] This increased vulnerability probably relates to two factors. First, the anterior circulation receives a much smaller number of feeding vessels than the posterior circulation.[1,7,8,11] Second, the posterior circulation is a network of anastomotic channels[1,7,11] and therefore probably provides better collateral flow than the single anterior artery, which in some patients is discontinuous along its length. The relative constancy of the resulting syndrome[11,34,35] presumably reflects the relative constancy of the intrinsic vascular anatomy of the cord.

As mentioned earlier, the anterior spinal artery supplies blood to much of the spinal gray matter and to the tracts in the anterior and lateral white matter. Ischemia in this arterial territory therefore gives rise to a syndrome of diminished pain and temperature sensibility with preservation of vibratory and joint position sense. Weakness (either paraparesis or quadriparesis, depending on the segments involved) occurs below the level of the lesion and may be associated with other evidence of upper motor neuron involvement, such as Babinski signs, spasticity, and hyperreflexia. Bowel and bladder functions are affected, owing to interruption of suprasegmental pathways. Segmental gray matter involvement may also lead to lower motor neuron deficits and depressed tendon reflexes at the level of the lesion. Thus a lesion in the cervical cord may produce flaccid areflexic paralysis with amyotrophy in the upper extremities, spastic paralysis in the lower extremities, and disso-

ciated sensory loss in all limbs. In contrast, a lesion in the thoracic cord typically presents with only spastic paraplegia and dissociated sensory loss in the legs. The syndrome generally comes on abruptly, although occasionally it is more insidious and progressive.[36]

Motor Neuron Disease

On occasion, diseases of the aorta (e.g., dissecting aneurysms or atherosclerosis) that interfere with the blood supply to the anterior spinal artery result in more restricted cord ischemia, perhaps because of better anastomotic connections between the anterior and posterior pial arterial plexuses in some individuals or because of greater vulnerability of the anterior horn cells with their greater metabolic activity.[11,15,36–43] The ischemic injury is limited to the gray matter supplied by the sulcal branches (Fig. 2-6). Clinical impairment is then confined to the motor system and is associated with amyotrophy. When the onset is abrupt,[37–39] the ischemic nature of the lesion is generally apparent, but when the onset is more gradual,[36,40–43] and especially when pyramidal signs are also present, it may mimic other diseases, such as amyotrophic lateral sclerosis or spinal cord tumors.

Posterior Spinal Artery Syndrome

In contrast to the anterior spinal artery syndrome, selective ischemia of the posterior circulation, characterized by prominent loss of posterior column func-

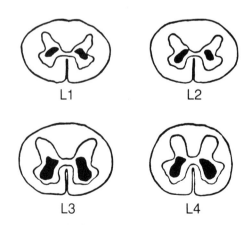

Fig. 2-6 Area of infarction within the spinal cord over four adjacent spinal segments in a patient reported by Herrick and Mills.[38] The infarction was extensive but limited to the gray matter, particularly the anterior horns.

tion with relative sparing of other functions, is rarely if ever recognized clinically[11,15] and only occasionally reported pathologically.[20,44] This presumably relates to the more abundant feeding vessels and better anastomotic connections in this arterial system.

Intermittent Claudication

Intermittent claudication (limping) refers to a condition in which a patient experiences difficulty in walking that is brought about by use of the lower extremities. Charcot initially described this syndrome in 1858 and related it to occlusive peripheral vascular disease in the lower extremities.[45] In 1906, Dejerine distinguished claudication caused by ischemia of the leg muscles from that caused by ischemia of the spinal cord.[46] In the latter condition the arterial pulses in the legs tend to be preserved; pain tends to be dysesthetic or paresthetic in quality and may not occur; and neurological signs are frequently present, especially after exercise. In 1961, Blau and Logue identified another form of neurogenic claudication caused by ischemia or compression of the cauda equina and resulting from a narrowed lumbosacral canal (either congenital or due to degenerative disease).[47] This condition is similar to that produced by ischemia of the spinal cord; however, the sensory complaints tend to have a more radicular distribution, and signs of cord involvement (e.g., Babinski signs) are not present.

The clinical distinction between various types of claudication, particularly between the two neurogenic varieties, is sometimes difficult. The cauda equina variety, however, is far more common than the spinal form.[48] Intermittent spinal ischemia, when it occurs, is often associated with intrinsic diseases of the aorta, such as coarctation or atherosclerotic occlusive disease.[49–52]

Bony erosion through vertebral bodies from an abdominal aortic aneurysm with direct compression of the spinal nerve roots has also been reported to produce intermittent neurological symptoms.[53] The clinical details of the single reported case, however, are not sufficient to determine if the symptoms resemble those of intermittent claudication.

Cerebral Ischemia

ANATOMY

The aortic arch gives rise to all of the major vessels that provide blood to the brain, brainstem, and cervical spinal cord (Fig. 2-7). The first major branch is the innominate (brachiocephalic) artery, which subsequently divides into the right common carotid and right subclavian arteries. The latter artery subsequently gives rise to the right vertebral artery, which ascends through the foramina of the transverse processes of the upper six cervical vertebrae to join with its counterpart on the left and form the basilar artery. The basilar artery provides blood to the posterior fossa and posterior regions of the cerebral hemispheres. The second major branch of the aortic arch is the left common carotid artery, and the third is the left subclavian artery, which, in turn, gives rise to the left vertebral artery.

STROKES AND TRANSIENT ISCHEMIC ATTACKS

Diseases of the aortic arch—such as atherosclerosis, aneurysms, or aortitis—as well as surgery on this segment of the aorta may give rise to symptoms of cerebrovascular insufficiency, such as strokes or transient ischemic attacks (TIAs).[14,19,32,54–58] A young woman has even been reported with a stroke secondary to an occlusion of the aorta that was associated with the use of birth control pills and recurrent venous thromboses.[59] Cerebral ischemia is produced either by occlusion of a major vessel or by embolization of atheromatous or other material to more distal arteries. The resulting neurological syndromes are not specific for any disease process but depend on the location and duration of the vascular occlusion.

Atherosclerosis

Atherosclerosis of the aortic arch and its branches, compared to atherosclerosis at the origin of the internal carotid artery, is an infrequent cause of stroke or TIAs, probably for two reasons. First, atherosclerosis is much less common in this location than at the carotid bifurcation[60] (Table 2-2). Second, the anastomotic connections between the major vessels in the neck are extensive,[11,61] and an occlusion at their origin from the aortic arch is therefore less likely to be associated with symptoms of ischemia than a more peripheral obstruction.

Transient Emboligenic Aortoarteritis

Transient emboligenic aortoarteritis has been reported by Wickremasinghe and colleagues to be a cause of stroke in young patients.[62] They described

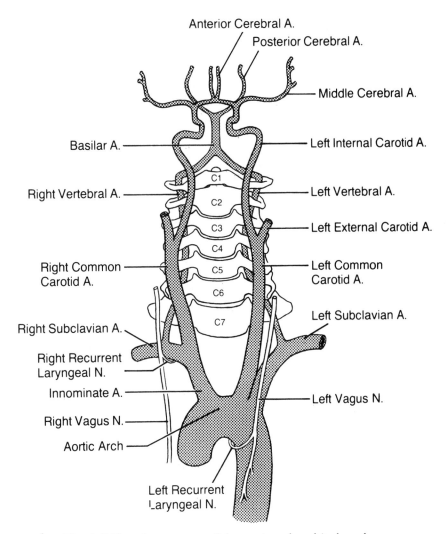

Fig. 2-7 Vascular anatomy of the aortic arch and its branches.

Table 2-2 Distribution of Atherosclerosis in the Aorta and Its Branches

Location	No. of Lesions
External carotid artery	9
Internal carotid artery	256
Common carotid artery	16
Innominate artery	16
Subclavian artery	29
Vertebral artery	55
Aortoiliac region	952
Femoropopliteal region	772

(Based on a study by Crawford and associates.[60])

ten patients (aged 16 to 36 years), all of whom had presented with pathologically verified thromboembolic strokes, and three of whom had a history of TIAs preceding the event by as many as 4 years. All of these patients had both active and healed inflammatory lesions of the central elastic arteries, such as the aorta, innominate, common carotid, and proximal subclavian arteries. Active lesions were small (200 to 300 μm in diameter) and associated with a mural thrombus on the intimal surface. Healed lesions were generally associated with fibrous plaques but not with a mural thrombus. More peripheral arteries supplying the brain were normal. This condition seems to be distinct from segmental aortitis of the Takayasu type.

Clinically it is an acute, intermittent disorder with an approximately equal sex incidence, whereas Takayasu's disease is more chronic and has a strong female predominance. The systemic symptoms of Takayasu's disease are absent, and occlusion of the central arteries does not occur in this condition.[63]

Subclavian (Cerebral) Steal

Disease of the aortic arch may result in occlusion of either the innominate artery or the left subclavian artery proximal to the origin of the vertebral artery. This, in turn, may result in the reversal of the usual cephalad direction of blood flow in the ipsilateral vertebral artery (Fig. 2-8), depending on individual variations in the collateral circulation, and may result in ischemia in the posterior cerebral circula-

tion.[61,63–67] In some patients this is particularly evident when the metabolic demand (and therefore the blood flow) of the affected arm is increased during exercise.[64] If the innominate artery is blocked proximally, it may also cause a reversal of blood flow in the right common carotid artery, resulting in anterior circulation ischemia (Fig. 2-8).[65]

Killen and colleages reviewed the clinical features of a series of patients with demonstrated reversals of arterial blood flow in a vertebral artery (i.e., with flow from the vertebral artery into the ipsilateral subclavian artery).[64] The left subclavian artery was affected more than twice as often as the right subclavian and innominate arteries combined, probably as a result of the more frequent involvement of this artery by atherosclerosis (Table 2-2). Men were affected

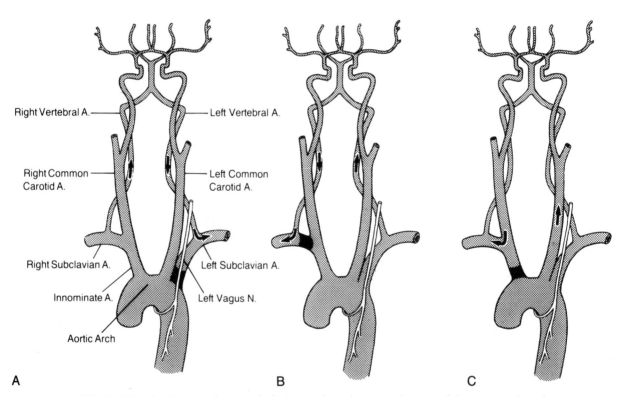

Fig. 2-8 Mechanisms producing subclavian steal syndrome in diseases of the aortic arch and its branches. **(A)** Obstruction of left subclavian artery at its origin, resulting in reversal of blood flow in the left vertebral artery. **(B)** Obstruction of the right subclavian artery distal to the takeoff of the right common carotid artery, resulting in reversal of blood flow in the right vertebral artery. **(C)** Obstruction of the innominate artery at its origin, producing reversal of blood flow in the right common carotid artery.

three times as often as women, probably reflecting the greater prevalence of atherosclerosis in men. Of the 87 patients in this series with symptoms that were adequately described, 75 (86 percent) had symptoms referable to the central nervous system (CNS). These symptoms were generally transient, lasting seconds to a few minutes, although the deficits were sometimes permanent. The neurological manifestations of steal were varied but most frequently included motor difficulties, vertigo, visual deficits, or syncope. Ischemic symptoms in the arms occurred in only a few patients, and precipitation of CNS symptoms by exercise of the arm ipsilateral to the occlusion was uncommon. The pulse in the affected arm was diminished or absent in all patients, and the systolic blood pressure in this arm was reduced by 20 mmHg or more in all but one patient. The clinical signs were otherwise generally unhelpful for establishing the diagnosis. Reconstructive surgery eliminated symptoms in most patients in this series, and this has also been the experience of others.[61,65]

More recently, noninvasive techniques such as Doppler ultrasonography have been used to define the direction of blood flow in the great vessels in a large spectrum of patients with vascular disease who previously would not have been imaged. These studies have generally shown a high prevalence (50 to 75 percent) of patients with asymptomatic subclavian steal.[66,67] When symptoms did occur, they were suggestive of transient vertebrobasilar insufficiency in only 7 to 37 percent of patients with steal; the occurrence of infarcts in this vascular territory was distinctly rare.[66,67] Such factors must be weighed carefully when considering surgical treatment of patients with subclavian steal.

Peripheral Neuropathy

The peripheral nervous system is sometimes affected by aortic disease or surgery. The syndromes produced may be the presenting manifestations of aortic disease and may mimic less life-threatening conditions.

MONONEUROPATHIES

Left Recurrent Laryngeal Nerve
The left recurrent laryngeal nerve descends in the neck as part of the vagus nerve and wraps around the aortic arch just distal to the ligamentum arteriosum (Fig. 2-7) before reascending in the neck to innervate all of the laryngeal muscles on the left side except the cricothyroideus. It may be compressed by disease of the aortic arch, such as dissecting and nondissecting aneurysms or aneurysmal dilatation proximal to a coarctation of the aorta.[56,68] The resulting hoarse, low-pitched voice may be one of the earliest presenting symptoms of these conditions, although it is often overshadowed by other symptoms or signs, such as chest pain, shortness of breath, congestive heart failure, or hypertension.[68]

Femoral Nerve
The femoral nerve arises from the nerve roots of L2, L3, and L4. It forms within the belly of the psoas muscle and then exits on its lateral aspect to innervate the quadriceps femoris, iliacus, pectineus, and sartorius muscles and the skin of the anterior thigh and medial aspect of the leg. The nerve is located considerably lateral to the aorta (Fig. 2-9) and thus is rarely involved by direct compression. It may, however, be compressed by a hematoma from a ruptured aortic aneurysm into the psoas muscle and thereby signal a life-threatening condition that requires an urgent operation.[69–71]

The femoral nerve may also be injured as a consequence of aortic surgery. Boontje and Haaxma reported this complication in 3.4 percent of 1,006 abdominal aortic operations for atherosclerotic or aneurysmal disease, the left femoral nerve being involved unilaterally in two-thirds of the cases and jointly with the right femoral nerve in another 6 percent.[72] The mechanism of injury in these cases was presumed to be ischemic and related to poor collateral blood supply to the intrapelvic portions of the femoral nerves, especially on the left.

Obturator Nerve
The obturator nerve also forms within the belly of the psoas muscle by the union of fibers from the L2, L3, and L4 segments but, in contrast to the femoral nerve, exits medially from this muscle (Fig. 2-9). It innervates the adductors of the leg and the skin on the medial aspect of the thigh. It too is lateral to the aorta and not usually involved by direct compression. Like the femoral nerve (and often together with it),

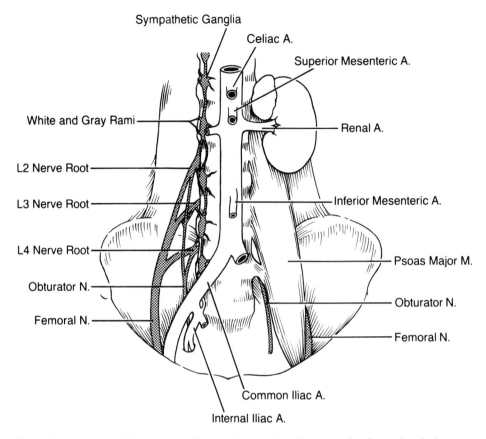

Fig. 2-9 Anatomy of the abdominal aorta showing its relation to the femoral and obturator nerves, which form within the psoas muscle from branches of the L2, L3, and L4 segmental nerves.

the obturator nerve may be compressed by a hematoma in the psoas muscle.[69,70]

RADICULOPATHIES

Nerve roots, particularly L4, L5, S1, and S2, which lie almost directly underneath the terminal aorta and iliac arteries (Fig. 2-10), may be directly compressed by an aortic aneurysm in this region. The syndromes produced are typical of radicular disease, with unilateral radiating pain and a radicular pattern to the sensory and motor findings.[69,73]

Radiculopathies may also be produced by erosion of one or more vertebral bodies by an aortic aneurysm, with consequent compression of the nerve roots in the cauda equina or at the root exit zones. The syndrome produced is not necessarily associated with back pain; it may result in multisegmental involvement on one side or even in paraplegia.[74,75]

POLYNEUROPATHIES

Ischemic Monomelic Neuropathy

Ischemic monomelic neuropathy was described in detail by Wilbourn and co-workers, who reported 3 patients (and alluded to another 11) who had a distal "polyneuropathy" in one limb following sudden occlusion of a major vessel.[76] One of their patients had a saddle embolus to the distal aorta that occluded the right common iliac artery; another had a superficial femoral artery occlusion following placement of an intra-aortic balloon pump; and the third had upper extremity involvement. The syndrome consists of a predominantly sensory neuropathy with a distal gradient. It affects all sensory modalities and is associated

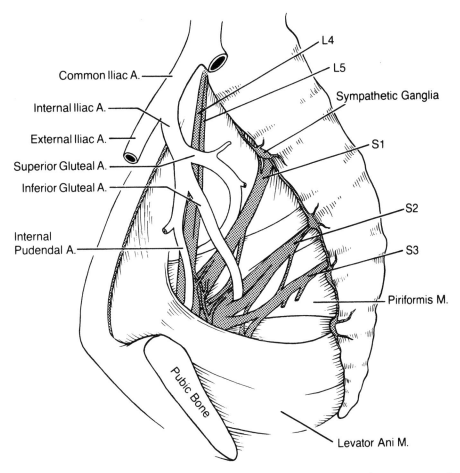

Fig. 2-10 Anatomy of the terminal branches of the aorta in relation to the nerve roots that subsequently join to form the sciatic nerve. Aneurysmal dilatation of the abdominal aorta often includes dilatation of these branch vessels, which can compress the nerve roots, particularly the L4, L5, S1, and S2 nerve roots, which lie directly underneath.

with a constant, deep, causalgia-like pain. The symptoms persist for months, even after revascularization or without evidence of ongoing ischemia. The results of nerve conduction studies and needle electromyography suggest an axonal neuropathy. There is no evidence of ischemic muscle injury, such as induration, muscle tenderness, or elevated serum creatine kinase levels. This condition is rare, but occasional case reports are reminiscent of the syndrome[77] and it may be that it is more prevalent than currently appreciated.

AUTONOMIC NEUROPATHIES

Anatomy

The autonomic nerves, particularly the lower thoracic and lumbar sympathetic fibers that lie close to the aorta and its branches, may be injured by disease of or surgery on the aorta. The preganglionic efferent sympathetic nerve fibers originate in the intermediolateral cell column in the spinal cord (Fig. 2-4) and exit segmentally between T1 and L2 with the ventral roots.[78] The sympathetic fibers part company with the segmental nerves via the white rami communicantes (Fig. 2-2), which enter the paravertebral sympathetic ganglia and trunks to form bilateral sympathetic chains; these chains are situated lateral to and parallel with the vertebral column (Fig. 2-11). Some of these fibers synapse on postganglionic neurons in the ganglia of their segmental origin, whereas others ascend or descend in the trunk to different segmental levels before making such synapses. In the lumbosa-

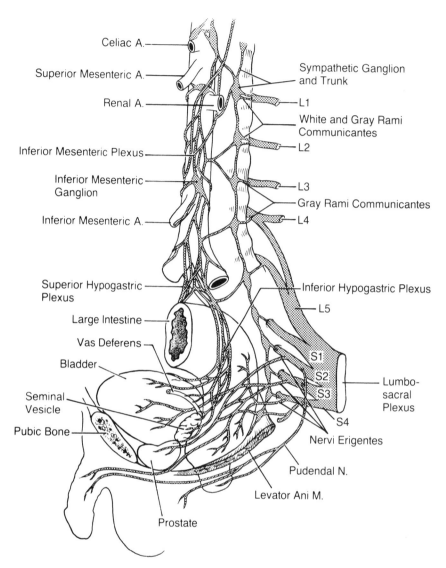

Celiac A.
Superior Mesenteric A.
Renal A.
Inferior Mesenteric Plexus
Inferior Mesenteric Ganglion
Inferior Mesenteric A.
Superior Hypogastric Plexus
Large Intestine
Vas Deferens
Bladder
Seminal Vesicle
Pubic Bone
Prostate

Sympathetic Ganglion and Trunk
L1
White and Gray Rami Communicantes
L2
L3
Gray Rami Communicantes
L4
Inferior Hypogastric Plexus
L5
S1
S2
S3
Lumbo-sacral Plexus
S4
Nervi Erigentes
Pudendal N.
Levator Ani M.

Fig. 2-11 Anatomy of the terminal aorta and pelvis in the male in relation to the sympathetic and parasympathetic nerves in the region.

cral and cervical segments, where there are no white rami (i.e., below L2 or above T1), the segmental ganglia receive preganglionic contributions only from cord segments either above them (lumbosacral ganglia) or below them (cervical ganglia).[78] The postganglionic fibers rejoin the segmental nerves via the gray rami communicantes (Fig. 2-2) to provide vasomotor, sudomotor, and pilomotor innervation throughout the body.

Some of the preganglionic fibers, in contrast, do not synapse in the paravertebral ganglia but pass through them to form splanchnic nerves, which then unite in a series of prevertebral ganglia and plexuses (many of which overlie the thoracic and abdominal aorta). These structures, in turn, provide sympathetic innervation to the viscera. The plexus that overlies the aorta in the region of its bifurcation, the superior hypogastric plexus (Fig. 2-11), is responsible (via the inferior hypogastric and other pelvic plexuses) for sympathetic innervation of the pelvic organs, includ-

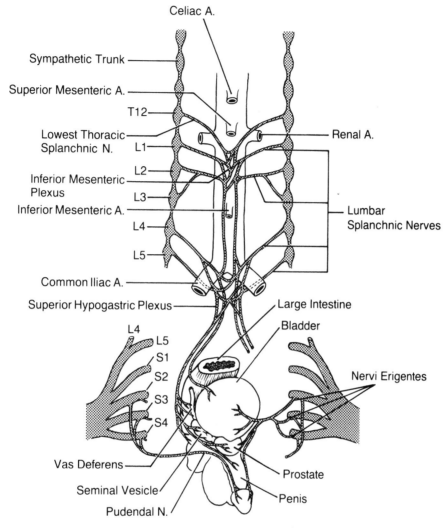

Fig. 2-12 Distribution of sympathetic *(left)* and parasympathetic *(right)* nerves to the pelvic viscera and sexual organs in the male.

ing the prostate, prostatic urethra, bladder, epididymis, vas deferens, seminal vesicles, and penis in men (Fig. 2-12) and the uterus, bladder, fallopian tubes, vagina, and clitoris in women. This plexus is formed by the union of the third and fourth lumbar splanchnic nerves with fibers from the more rostral inferior mesenteric plexus. Its segmental contribution generally derives from T11 to L2.[78]

The visceral afferent fibers accompany the efferent autonomic fibers and pass uninterrupted back through the trunk, ganglia, and white rami to reach their nerve cells of origin in the dorsal root.

Postsympathectomy Neuralgia

Operations on the distal aorta to treat symptomatic aortic disease from atherosclerosis or other causes frequently include intentional sympathectomy as part of the effort to improve blood flow to the legs. It is generally done by dividing the sympathetic chain below the last white ramus at L2, thereby depriving the lower lumbar and sacral ganglia of their preganglionic innervation. Such an operation is often followed by a distinctive pain syndrome,[79,80] which Raskin and associates termed postsympathectomy neuralgia.[79] In their experience with 96 such operations, this syndrome occurred in 35 percent of the patients. In each case the sympathetic chain was interrupted at L3 by removal of the segmental ganglion. The pain was characterized as deep, boring, nonrhythmic, and nonradiating; it had an abrupt but delayed onset. The mean delay from sympathectomy to onset of pain was 12 days. The pain was located predominantly in the thigh, either medially or laterally, and was associated with tenderness in the area of pain. The course was always self-limited, with an average duration of 3 weeks.

Disorders of Sexual Function

Normal male sexual function has two distinct components. The first, erection, is a response mediated predominantly through the parasympathetic nervous system via the pelvic splanchnic nerves (nervi erigentes) arising from segments S2, S3, and S4 (Fig. 2-12). Activation of these nerves causes vasodilatation and engorgement of the penile musculature and sinuses.[81,82] The blood supply to the penis is provided by the internal pudendal artery via the internal iliac artery (Fig. 2-10). The sympathetic nervous system, however, must have at least a modifying influence on erection, since sympathectomy may disturb it.[81,82] The second component, ejaculation, can be divided into two phases. The first phase, expulsion of seminal fluid into the prostatic urethra, is a response predominantly mediated by the sympathetic nervous system through the superior hypogastric plexus.[81,82] The second phase, emission, is produced by the clonic contraction of penile musculature (bulbocavernosus and ischiocavernosus) innervated by somatic (pudendal) nerves (Fig. 2-12).

Male sexual function may be disturbed by aortic disease or surgery.[83–90] Female sexual function in these circumstances has not been well studied, mainly because of the lack of objective signs of dysfunction in women. Because the superior hypogastric plexus lies in close proximity to the aortic bifurcation (Fig. 2-11), most pre- and postoperative sexual disturbances occur with disease of this portion of the aorta, and most involve ejaculation (Table 2-3). The pelvic splanchnic nerves are not situated near the aorta (Fig. 2-11) and are not generally affected by aortic disease or surgery. Disturbances in erection, however, do occur, possibly due to either sympathetic dysfunction or a reduction in blood flow to the internal pudendal artery and penis.[83–90] To determine whether blood flow or sympathetic function was more important in this regard, Ohshiro and Kosaki examined the outcome of (1) terminal aortic operations either done traditionally or designed to spare the superior hypogastric plexus and (2) operations that did or did not preserve internal iliac blood flow.[89] Their results indicated that preservation of the hypogastric plexus appeared to be more important for maintenance of normal erection and ejaculation than was preservation of internal iliac artery blood flow (Table 2-4). Other authors have also found that modification of operative technique to spare the superior hypogastric plexus considerably improves postoperative sexual function.[85,86,88]

Despite the importance of operative technique in preserving sexual function, preservation of blood flow is probably also important. Thus, Nevelsteen and colleagues reported a clear relationship between the occurrence of preoperative impotence and the ad-

Table 2-3 Male Sexual Dysfunction in Disease of and Surgery on the Aorta

Patient Status	No. of Patients	Sexual Function	
		Normal (%)	Abnormal (%)
Preoperative status (all patients)			
Iliac occlusion	22	82	18
Terminal aortic occlusion	10	40	60
Abdominal aortic aneurysm	12	83	17
Postoperative status (patients with normal preoperative sexual function)		Impaired ejaculation (%)	Impaired erection (%)
Iliac occlusion	18	28	17
Terminal aortic occlusion	4	75	25
Abdominal aortic aneurysm	10	70	30

(Based on a study by Ohshiro and colleagues.[87])

Table 2-4 Influence of Blood Flow and Sympathetic Function on Male Sexual Function Following Abdominal Aortic Operations

Parameter	No. of Patients	Postoperative Sexual Disturbance	
		Ejaculation (%)	Erection (%)
Internal iliac blood flow			
Bilaterally good	29	31	21
Unilaterally good	12	42	8
Bilaterally poor	4	50	25
Type of surgery			
Classic	32	47	25
Nerve sparing	13	8	8

(Based on a study by Ohshiro and Kosaki.[89])

equacy of blood flow through the internal iliac arteries.[90] In this study, however, no special attempt was made to improve blood flow in the internal iliac artery during surgery, so that it is unclear whether a different operative approach might have been beneficial in restoring postoperative sexual function.

AORTIC DISEASES AND SURGERY

Certain conditions affecting the aorta merit special consideration because of the variety of nervous system syndromes that each can produce.

Aortitis

Injury to the aorta by a variety of infectious, toxic, allergic, or idiopathic causes may produce similar inflammatory pathological changes within the elastic media[19] (Table 2-5). Such aortic damage may lead to neurological syndromes either primarily through direct involvement of important branch arteries by the pathological process or secondarily through the development of aneurysms, aortic stenosis, or atherosclerosis. The neurological syndromes produced either primarily or secondarily by aortitis depend on both the nature and the location of the resulting aortic lesion.

Table 2-5 Causes of Aortitis

Stenosing aortitis
  Takayasu's arteritis
  Postirradiation during infancy
Nonstenosing aortitis
  Syphilis
  Mycotic aneurysms
  Rheumatic fever
  Rheumatoid arthritis
  Giant cell arteritis
  Collagen vascular and other diseases[a]
  Ankylosing spondylitis
  Reiter's syndrome
  Relapsing polychondritis

[a] Systemic lupus erythematosus, scleroderma, psoriasis, and ulcerative colitis.

SYPHILITIC AORTITIS

During the prepenicillin era, syphilis was a common cause of aortitis,[19,91] although by the 1950s its occurrence had markedly declined.[91] A report in 1958 on the relative occurrence of atherosclerotic and syphilitic thoracic aortic aneurysms showed cases of syphilis outnumbering atherosclerosis by a ratio of 1.3:1.0.[92] A similar report published in 1982 gave this ratio as 0.13:1.0.[93] The pathology in syphilitic aortitis is almost always in the thoracic aorta,[19,91] in contrast to the distribution of atherosclerosis, which is more prevalent in the abdominal aorta (Table 2–2). The aortitis is accompanied by aneurysmal dilatation of the aorta in approximately 40 percent of cases.[91] Rarely it presents with multiple arterial occlusions and mimics Takayasu's arteritis,[56] although patients are generally older than those with Takayasu's arteritis and are usually men.

TAKAYASU'S ARTERITIS

Takayasu's arteritis, an idiopathic condition, occurs in young patients, with its onset generally before 30 years of age.[56,94–97] More than 85 percent of affected individuals are women. In the early (prepulseless) phase the disease may be characterized by systemic symptoms such as fever, night sweats, weight loss, myalgia, arthralgia, arthritis, and chest pain. In some patients, however, the systemic symptoms are either inconspicuous or absent. The later (pulseless) phase of the disease is characterized by occlusion of the major

44 NEUROLOGY AND GENERAL MEDICINE

vessels of the aortic arch, producing symptoms such as Takayasu's retinopathy, secondary hypertension, aortic regurgitation, and aortic aneurysms. Symptoms of cerebral ischemia can occur but are present in only a few patients.[56,95,96] Other patients may present with symptoms related to a coarctation of the aorta secondary to more restricted aortic involvement.[19] The disorder is discussed further in Chapter 23.

Aortic Aneurysms

NONDISSECTING ANEURYSMS

Nondissecting aortic aneurysms can be caused by any pathological process that weakens the arterial wall, such as inflammation, infection, or atherosclerosis.[16,19,53,60,91–93,98–101] In the past, syphilis was an important cause,[102] but at the present time almost all of these aneurysms are caused by atherosclerosis. As a result, the distribution of aortic aneurysms essentially parallels the distribution of atherosclerosis within the aorta, with most occurring in the abdominal aorta (Tables 2-2 and 2-6). The prognosis of untreated aneurysms is grave, with 80 percent of patients dying of rupture within 12 months of the onset of symptoms.[98] Disturbances of neurological function in aortic aneurysms are uncommon, but when they occur they are variable in nature and depend in part on the location and extent of the lesion. Abdominal aneurysms may result in sexual dysfunction or compressive neuropathies[69–75,83–90]; descending thoracic aneurysms may produce spinal cord ischemia[17]; and aortic arch aneurysms may result in cerebral ischemia or recurrent laryngeal nerve dysfunction.[56,68] Most commonly, neurological symptoms are produced by either rupture or direct compression. Even when an-

Table 2-6 Distribution and Nature of Aortic Aneurysms

Site	No. of Cases
Nondissecting aneurysms	
Aortic arch	56
Descending thoracic aorta	116
Thoracoabdominal aorta	25
Abdominal aorta	829
Dissecting aneurysms	
Thoracic aorta	62

(Based on a review by Crawford and colleagues.[60])

eurysms result in paraplegia, the neurological deficit is often caused by bony erosion through the vertebral bodies and direct compression of the spinal cord or cauda equina, rather than by ischemia.[75,103]

DISSECTING AORTIC ANEURYSMS

Dissecting aortic aneurysms, in contrast to nondissecting aortic aneurysms, predominantly involve the thoracic aorta, either at the beginning of the ascending segment or immediately distal to the left subclavian artery.[18,32,55,68,77,104,105] Their etiology has not been established. Atherosclerosis is probably not a major factor, as atherosclerosis is seldom found in the region of the intimal tear, and the distribution of these aneurysms along the aorta is unlike that of atherosclerosis.[105] Dissecting aortic aneurysms have been associated with cystic medial necrosis (a degenerative condition focally affecting the arterial media, which may itself be related to hypertension). This condition is increased in patients with Marfan's syndrome, as are dissecting aneurysms. Most aneurysms, however, do not occur in patients with Marfan's syndrome or other identifiable collagen disorders, and the pathophysiology remains unknown.[105] Neurological involvement from dissecting aneurysms (due to the cutoff of important arteries by the dissection or by embolization) is well described but uncommon, and usually involves either spinal or cerebral ischemia. In one large series of 527 patients,[68] stroke occurred preoperatively in 4 percent, and paraparesis occurred in another 2 percent. Aortic dissection usually presents with acute chest pain, which generally leads to the proper diagnosis.[68] On occasion, however, pain is absent, and the neurological syndrome is the presenting feature.[77,104] Moreover, the neurological deficit produced by the dissecting aneurysm is sometimes only transient, lasting for several hours, and thereby mimicking other transient disturbances of neurological function.[104]

TRAUMATIC AORTIC ANEURYSM

Brutal deceleration injuries to the chest, especially from motor vehicle accidents, may result in traumatic rupture of the thoracic aorta, often just distal to the left subclavian artery. Many of these patients die immediately, but some present with an acute paraplegia.[106–111] Still others develop a chronic aortic aneurysm that may present years later with acute spinal cord ischemia[107] or other neurological symptoms.[108]

Coarctation of the Aorta

Coarctation of the aorta is a relatively common congenital condition,[112] that typically results in constriction of the thoracic aorta just distal to the origin of the left subclavian artery. Less commonly it occurs as part of Takayasu's arteritis, and this condition should be suspected if the location of the coarctation is atypical.[19] It may also follow radiation exposure during infancy[113,114]; in these cases the pathology is focal and limited to the segment of aorta that was in the field of irradiation. Coarctation can result in a variety of neurological symptoms[15,112,115–119] (Table 2-7). Cerebral infarcts probably result from embolization of thrombotic material in the dilated aorta proximal to the obstruction.[112]

Subarachnoid hemorrhage from ruptured saccular aneurysms can occur with coarctation. In the general population, aneurysmal hemorrhage has an annual incidence of approximately 8 per 100,000[120] and rarely occurs before the age of 20 years.[121] Accordingly, the reported occurrence of ruptured aneurysms in 2.5 percent of patients with coarctation of the aorta[112] suggests an association of these two disorders, although the coincidental occurrence of the two conditions cannot be completely excluded.[121]

Headache is a common accompaniment of coarctation, perhaps as a result of secondary hypertension; but again the incidental occurrence of two unrelated conditions cannot be excluded.

Table 2-7 Neurological Sequelae of Coarctation of the Aorta

Sequela	Incidence (%)
Ruptured intracerebral aneurysms	2.5
Ischemic stroke during childhood	1.0
Neurogenic intermittent claudication[a]	7.5
Headache	25.0
Episodic loss of consciousness	3.0
Intracerebral hemorrhage[b]	<1.0
Spinal cord compression[b]	<1.0

[a] Patients with exercise-induced motor or sensory disturbances in the lower extremities.
[b] These complications were not found in the series reported by Tyler and Clark[112] but have been reported by others.[115–119]
(Based on a review of 200 patients with coarctation of the aorta by Tyler and Clark.[112])

Episodic loss of consciousness may also occur in patients with coarctation of the aorta. It may result either from syncope due to associated cardiac abnormalities[112] or from seizures.[112,115] It is unclear, however, if seizures unrelated to cerebrovascular disease are more prevalent in these patients than in the general population.[112]

Neurogenic intermittent claudication can result from aortic coarctation. In patients with coarctation of the aorta, blood flow to the legs is often provided by collateral connections between the spinal arteries and the distal aorta. In these situations the blood flow through the radiculomedullary and intercostal arteries distal to the obstruction is reversed,[52,121] and the exercise-related spinal ischemia may be related to "steal" by the increased metabolic demands (and thus increased blood flow) of the legs,[52] rather than from aortic hypotension distal to the coarctation (Fig. 2-13). These collaterals are sometimes so extensive that they cause spinal cord compression and mimic (clinically and radiologically) vascular malformations of the spinal cord.[15,116–119]

Surgery and Other Procedures on the Aorta

SURGERY

As with diseases of the aorta, the risks of aortic surgery depend in part on the site of operation. Thus operations on the aortic arch may produce cerebral ischemia either by intraoperative occlusion of major vessels or embolization of material such as calcified plaque loosened during surgery.[14,56–58] Operations on the suprarenal aorta may result in spinal ischemia,[14] whereas operations on the distal aorta may result in sexual dysfunction or ischemia of the femoral nerve.[74,83–90]

The major complication of all aortic operations, however, is intraoperative spinal cord ischemia with resultant paraplegia or paraparesis. The occurrence of this complication varies with the location of the surgery and the nature of the pathological process affecting the aorta (Table 2-8). Thus, surgery on dissecting or nondissecting aortic aneurysms that are entirely abdominal is associated with a lower incidence of this complication than operations on aneurysms confined to the thoracic aorta.[26,92,122–126] Surgery on

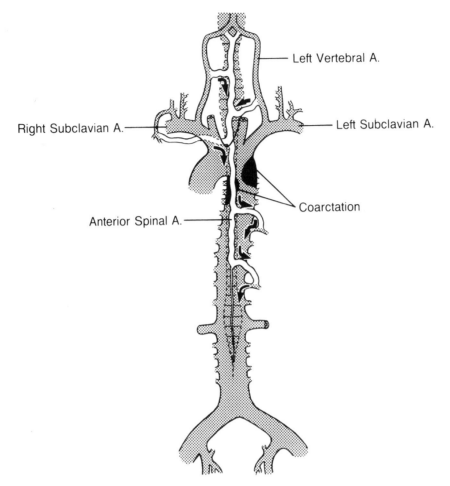

Fig. 2-13 Mechanism of steal in coarctation of the aorta. Obstruction of the aorta at the isthmus causes dilatation of the anterior spinal artery and reversal of blood flow in anterior radiculomedullary arteries distal to the obstruction. In this circumstance the blood flow to the lower extremities is provided by these (and other) collaterals, and use of the lower extremities may cause shunting of blood from the spinal circulation to the legs, which, in turn, sometimes results in spinal cord ischemia.

aneurysms involving the entire abdominal and thoracic aorta carries the highest risk of producing cord ischemia.[122] Operations on the distal aorta for occlusive disease only rarely result in spinal ischemia, especially when confined to the infrarenal portion.[26,33] This variability presumably occurs because important feeding arteries to the spinal circulation are more likely to be ligated during surgery, included within the segment of the aorta that is cross-clamped, or subjected to distal hypotension when the aortic pathology is above the level of origin of the renal arteries.

Operations on the thoracic aorta for coarctation are much less frequently complicated by spinal ischemia than thoracic operations done for other reasons.[23] There are probably at least two reasons for this difference. First, the former patients are younger, and the extent of overall arterial pathology is therefore less. Second, as mentioned above, the flow in the radiculomedullary vessels below the coarctation is frequently reversed,[52,127] so obstruction of blood flow in them (either by ligation or cross-clamping the aorta above and below their origin) may actually result in an increased blood supply to the spinal cord.

Table 2-8 Spinal Cord Ischemia During Surgery and Procedures on the Aorta

Problem	No. of Patients	Percent with Spinal Cord Damage
Nondissecting aortic aneurysm		
Abdominal[a]	1,724	0.46
Thoracic[b]	585	6.3
Thoracoabdominal[c]	102	21.6
Dissecting aortic aneurysm[d]	102	30.4
Abdominal aortic occlusion[e]	1,089	0
Coarctation of aorta[e]	12,532	0.41
Aortography[a]	17,949	0.01

[a] Based on a report by Szilagyi and associates.[26]

[b] Based on reports by DeBakey and associates,[92] Kahn and Sloan,[126] Livesay and associates,[123] Crawford and associates (Group I),[122] Bloodwell and associates,[125] and Neville and associates.[124]

[c] Based on a report by Crawford and associates (Group II).[122]

[d] Based on a report by Crawford and associates.[122] The relative risk of operation in these patients depended on the location along the aorta and essentially paralleled the experience in nondissecting aneurysms, although the numbers in each subcategory were too small to be included separately.

[e] Based on a report by Brewer and associates.[23]

AORTOGRAPHY AND OTHER PROCEDURES ON THE AORTA

Aortography may be associated with either spinal[128–130] or cerebral[131] ischemia, depending on the portion of the aorta visualized. This complication, however, is distinctly rare (Table 2-8). Paraplegia may also occur during intra–aortic balloon assistance following myocardial revascularization.[132]

INTRAOPERATIVE ADJUNCTS TO AVOID SPINAL CORD ISCHEMIA

Several adjuncts are commonly employed intraoperatively in an attempt to avoid spinal cord injury. They include the use of hypothermia, thiopental anesthesia, and intraoperative corticosteroids, which are thought to reduce the metabolic requirements of the cord or otherwise enhance the tolerance to ischemia.[133–136] In addition, many authors have reported that minimization of cross-clamp time results in a lower incidence of spinal ischemia.[122,123]

Other adjunctive methods, such as the reattachment of intercostal arteries or the use of shunts to maintain distal aortic perfusion pressure, have not proved consistently effective at preventing cord ischemia.[53,133–135,137] Failure of these procedures may relate to the extreme variability of the blood supply to the spinal cord. For example, if a crucial spinal artery leaves the aorta within the cross-clamped section, the preservation of distal blood flow is irrelevant. Furthermore, since the important intercostal arteries are few in number and unpredictably situated, the random reattachment of a few intercostal arteries may be fruitless.

There has been considerable interest in the use of somatosensory evoked potentials (SEPs) and motor evoked potentials (MEPs) for assessing spinal cord function during operations on the aorta.[133,138–145] In general, the reported studies have been of limited clinical relevance because they have not correlated specific intraoperative SEP changes with the likelihood of postoperative paraplegia, but a study by Kaplan and co-workers[140] does suggest that SEPs will ultimately prove to be of use in this regard. The combined use of SEPs and MEPs may prove better than either technique alone.[145] Another approach that may be helpful is the use of MEP amplitude to identify intraoperatively those feeding vessels that perfuse the spinal cord and therefore need reattachment.[144]

REFERENCES

1. Turnbull IM: Blood supply of the spinal cord. p. 478. In Vinken PJ, Bruyn GW (eds): Handbook of Clinical Neurology. Vol 12. North Holland, Amsterdam, 1972

2. Adamkiewicz A: I. Die Gefasse der Ruckenmarkersubstanz. Sitzungsb Akad Wissensch Wien Math-Naturw 84:469, 1881

3. Adamkiewicz A: Die Blutgefasse des menschlichen Ruckenmarkes: II. Die Gefasse der Ruckenmarksoberflache. Sitzungsb Akad Wissensch Wien Math-Naturw 85:101, 1882

4. Kadyi H: Uber die Blutgefasse des menschlichen Ruckenmarker. Anat Anz 1:304, 1886

5. Kadyi H: Uber die Blutfegasse des menschlichen Ruckenmarkes: Nach einer im XV Bande der Denkschriften d Math-Naturw C1 d Akad d Wissensch in Krakau erschienenen Monographie aus dem Polnischen Ulsersatzt vom Verfasser. Grubrynowicz & Schmidt, Lemberg, 1889

6. Suh TH, Alexander L: Vascular system of the human spinal cord. Arch Neurol Psychiatry 41:659, 1939
7. Gillilan LA: The arterial blood supply of the human spinal cord. J Comp Neurol 110:75, 1958
8. Mannen T: Vascular lesions in the spinal cord in the aged. Geriatrics 21:151, 1966
9. Hassler O: Blood supply to human spinal cord—a microangiographic study. Arch Neurol 15:302, 1966
10. Henson RA, Parsons M: Ischaemic lesions of the spinal cord: an illustrated review. Q J Med 36:205, 1967
11. Lazorthes G: Pathology, classification and clinical aspects of vascular diseases of the spinal cord. p. 492. In Vinken PJ, Bruyn GW (eds): Handbook of Clinical Neurology. Vol 12. North Holland, Amsterdam, 1972
12. Herren RY, Alexander L: Sulcal and intrinsic blood vessels of human spinal cord. Arch Neurol Psychiatry 41:678, 1939
13. Skillman JJ: Neurological complications of cardiovascular surgery: I. Procedures involving the carotid arteries and abdominal aorta. Int Anesthesiol Clin 24:135, 1986
14. Shaw PJ: Neurological complications of cardiovascular surgery: II. Procedures involving the heart and thoracic aorta. Int Anesthesiol Clin 24:159, 1986
15. Aminoff MJ: Vascular disorders of the spinal cord. p. 259. In Davidoff RA (ed): Handbook of the Spinal Cord. Marcel Dekker, New York, 1987
16. Ross RT: Spinal cord infarction in disease and surgery of the aorta. Can J Neurol Sci 12:289, 1985
17. Kewalramani LS, Orth MS, Katta RSR: Atraumatic ischaemic myelopathy. Paraplegia 19:352, 1981
18. Leramo OB, Char G, Coard K, Morgan OS: Spinal stroke as a presentation of dissecting aneurysm of the aorta. West Indian Med J 35:203, 1986
19. Lande A, Berkmen YM: Aortitis: pathologic, clinical and arteriographic review. Radiol Clin North Am 14:219, 1976
20. Rudar M, Urbanke A, Radonic M: Occlusion of the abdominal aorta with dysfunction of the spinal cord. Ann Intern Med 56:490, 1962
21. Dickson AP, Lum SK, Whyte AS: Paraplegia following saddle embolism. Br J Surg 71:321, 1984
22. Syrjanen J, Iivanainen M, Kallio M, et al: Three different pathogenic mechanisms for paraparesis in association with bacterial infections. Ann Clin Res 18:191, 1986
23. Brewer LA, Fosburg RG, Mulder GA, Verska JJ: Spinal cord complications following surgery for coarctation of the aorta. J Thorac Cardiovasc Surg 64:368, 1972
24. Barré JA, D'Andrade C: Paraplegie par ramollissement aigu unisegmentaire de la moelle survenne au cours de la grossesse: étude anatomo-clinique. Rev Neurol (Paris) 69:133, 1938
25. Bieniarz J, Maqueda E, Caldeyro-Barcia R: Compression of aorta by the uterus in late human pregnancy. Am J Obstet Gynecol 95:795, 1966
26. Szilagyi DE, Hageman JH, Smith RF, Elliott JP: Spinal cord damage in surgery of the abdominal aorta. Surgery 83:38, 1978
27. Lynch C, Weingarden SI: Paraplegia following aortic surgery. Paraplegia 20:196, 1982
28. Costello TG, Fisher A: Neurological complications following aortic surgery. Anaesthesia 38:230, 1983
29. Picone AL, Green RM, Ricotta JR, et al: Spinal cord ischemia following operations on the abdominal aorta. J Vasc Surg 3:94, 1986
30. Gelfan S, Tarlov IM: Differential vulnerability of spinal cord structures to anoxia. J Neurophysiol 18:170, 1955
31. Cook AW: Occlusion of the abdominal aorta and dysfunction of the spinal cord: a clinical syndrome. Bull NY Acad Med 35:479, 1959
32. Moersch FP, Sayre GP: Neurologic manifestations associated with dissecting aneurysm of the aorta. JAMA 144:1141, 1950
33. Adams HD, Geertruyden HH: Neurologic complications of aortic surgery. Ann Surg 144:574, 1956
34. Steegmann AT: Syndrome of the anterior spinal artery. Neurology 2:15, 1952
35. Peterman AF, Yoss RE, Corbin KB: The syndrome of occlusion of the anterior spinal artery. Proc Mayo Clin 33:31, 1958
36. Skinhoj E: Arteriosclerosis of the spinal cord. Acta Psychiatr Neurol Scand 29:139, 1954
37. Kepes JJ: Selective necrosis of spinal cord gray matter: a complication of dissecting aneurysm of the aorta. Neuropathologica 4:293, 1965
38. Herrick MK, Mills PE Jr: Infarction of the spinal cord. Arch Neurol 24:228, 1971
39. Beattie EJ Jr, Nolan J, Howe JS: Paralysis following surgical correction of coarctation of the aorta. Surgery 33:754, 1950
40. Jellinger K: Spinal cord arteriosclerosis and progressive vascular myelopathy. J Neurol Neurosurg Psychiatry 30:195, 1967
41. Gruner J, Lapresle J: Etude anatomo-pathologique des médullopathies d'origine vasculaire. Rev Neurol (Paris) 106:592, 1962
42. Jellinger K, Neumayer E: Myélopathies progressives d'origine vasculaire. Rev Neurol (Paris) 106:666, 1962
43. Jellinger K, Neumayer E: Myélopathie progressive d'origine vasculaire: contribution anatomoclinique aux syndromes d'une hypovascularisation chronique de la moelle. Acta Neurol Belg 62:944, 1962

44. Garland H, Greenberg J, Harriman DGF: Infarction of the spinal cord. Brain 89:645, 1966

45. Charcot JM: Sur la claudication intermittente observée dans un cas d'oblitèration complète de l'une des artères iliaques primitives. C R Mem Soc Biol 5:225, 1858

46. Dejerine J: Sur la claudication intermittente de la moelle épinière. Rev Neurol (Paris) 14:341, 1906

47. Blau JN, Logue V: Intermittent claudication of the cauda equina. Lancet 1:1081, 1961

48. Wilson CB: Significance of the small lumbar spinal canal: cauda equina compression syndromes due to spondylosis. J Neurosurg 31:499, 1969

49. Bergmark G: Intermittent spinal claudication. Acta Med Scand 138, suppl. 246:30, 1950

50. Gilfillan RS, Jones OW Jr, Roland SI: Arterial occlusions simulating neurological disorders of the lower limbs. JAMA 154:1149, 1954

51. Ratinov G, Jimenez-Pabon E: Intermittent spinal ischemia. Neurology 11:546, 1961

52. Kendall BE, Andrew J: Neurogenic intermittent claudication associated with aortic steal from the anterior spinal artery complicating coarctation of the aorta. J Neurosurg 37:89, 1972

53. Crawford ES, Snyder DM, Cho GC, Roehm JOF: Progress in treatment of thoracoabdominal and abdominal aortic aneurysms involving celiac, superior mesenteric, and renal arteries. Ann Surg 188:404, 1978

54. Jex RK, Schaff HV, Piehler JM, et al: Early and late results following repair of dissections of the descending thoracic aorta. J Vasc Surg 3:226, 1986

55. Frist WH, Baldwin JC, Starnes VA, et al: A reconsideration of cerebral perfusion in aortic arch replacement. Ann Thorac Surg 42:273, 1986

56. Currier RD, DeJong RN, Bole GC: Pulseless disease: central nervous system manifestations. Neurology 4:818, 1954

57. Culliford AT, Colvin SB, Rohrer K, et al: The atherosclerotic ascending aorta and transverse arch: a new technique to prevent cerebral injury during bypass: experience with 13 patients. Ann Thorac Surg 41:27, 1986

58. Landymore RW, Kinley CE, Murphy DA, et al: Prevention of neurological injury during myocardial revascularization in patients with calcific degenerative aortic disease. Ann Thorac Surg 41:293, 1986

59. Bogousslavsky J, Regli F: Ischemic stroke in adults younger than 30 years of age. Arch Neurol 44:479, 1987

60. Crawford ES, DeBakey ME, Cooley DA, et al: Surgical considerations of aneurysms and atherosclerotic occlusive lesions of the aorta and major arteries. Postgrad Med 29:151, 1961

61. Wylie EJ, Effeney DJ: Surgery of the aortic arch branches and vertebral arteries. Surg Clin North Am 59:669, 1979

62. Wickremasinghe HR, Peiris JB, Thenabadu PN, et al: Transient emboligenic aortoarteritis. Arch Neurol 35:416, 1978

63. Reivich M, Holling HE, Roberts B, et al: Reversal of blood flow through the vertebral artery and its effect on cerebral circulation. N Engl J Med 265:878, 1961

64. Killen DA, Foster JH, Walter GG Jr, et al: The subclavian steal syndrome. J Thorac Cardiovasc Surg 51:539, 1966

65. Williams SJ: Chronic upper extremity ischemia: current concepts in management. Surg Clin North Am 66:355, 1986

66. Ackermann H, Diener HC, Dichgans J: Stenosis and occlusion of the subclavian artery: ultrasonographic and clinical findings. J Neurol 234:396, 1987

67. Hennerici M, Klemm C, Rautenberg W: The subclavian steal phenomenon: a common vascular disorder with rare neurologic deficits. Neurology 38:669, 1988

68. DeBakey ME, McCollum CH, Crawford ES, et al: Dissection and dissecting aneurysms of the aorta: twenty-year follow-up of five hundred twenty-seven patients treated surgically. Surgery 92:1118, 1982

69. Kubacz GJ: Femoral and sciatic compression neuropathy. Br J Surg 58:580, 1971

70. Fletcher HS, Frankel J: Ruptured abdominal aneurysms presenting with unilateral peripheral neuropathy. Surgery 79:120, 1976

71. Owens ML: Psoas weakness and femoral neuropathy: neglected signs of retroperitoneal hemorrhage from ruptured aneurysm. Surgery 91:363, 1982

72. Boontje AH, Haaxma R: Femoral neuropathy as a complication of aortic surgery. J Cardiovasc Surg 28:286, 1987

73. Wilberger JE: Lumbosacral radiculopathy secondary to abdominal aortic aneurysms. J Neurosurg 58:965, 1983

74. Rothschild BM, Cohn L, Aviza A, Yoon B-H: Aortic aneurysm producing back pain, bone destruction, and paraplegia. Clin Orthop 164:123, 1982

75. Higgins R, Peitzman AB, Reidy M, et al: Chronic contained rupture of an abdominal aortic aneurysm presenting as a lower extremity neuropathy. Ann Emerg Med 17:284, 1988

76. Wilbourn AJ, Furlan AJ, Hulley W, Ruschhaupt W: Ischemic monomelic neuropathy. Neurology 33:447, 1983

77. Gerber O, Heyer EJ, Vieux U: Painless dissections of the aorta presenting as acute neurologic syndromes. Stroke 17:644, 1986

78. Williams PC, Warwick R: Functional Neuroanatomy of Man. WB Saunders, Philadelphia, 1975

79. Raskin NH, Levinson SA, Hoffman PM, et al: Post-sympathectomy neuralgia: amelioration with diphenylhydantoin and carbamazepine. Am J Surg 128:75, 1974

80. Smead WL, Vaccaro PS: Infrarenal aortic aneurysmectomy. Surg Clin North Am 63:1269, 1983

81. Whitelaw GP, Smithwick R: Some secondary effects of sympathectomy with particular reference to disturbance of sexual function. N Engl J Med 245:121, 1951

82. Quayle JB: Sexual function after bilateral lumbar sympathectomy and aortoiliac by-pass surgery. J Cardiovasc Surg 21:215, 1980

83. O'Conor VJ Jr: Impotence and the Leriche syndrome: an early diagnostic sign; consideration of the mechanism; relief by endarterectomy. J Urol 80:195, 1958

84. Harris JD, Jepson RP: Aorto-iliac stenosis: a comparison of two procedures. Aust NZ J Surg 34:211, 1965

85. DePalma RG, Levine SB, Feldman S: Preservation of erectile function after aortoiliac reconstruction. Arch Surg 113:958, 1978

86. DePalma RG: Impotence in vascular disease: relationship to vascular surgery. Br J Surg 69, suppl:S14, 1982

87. Ohshiro T, Takahashi A, Kosaki G: Sexual function in patients with aortoiliac vascular disorders. Int Surg 67:49, 1982

88. Flanigan DP, Schuler JJ, Keifer T, et al: Elimination of iatrogenic impotence and improvement of sexual function after aortoiliac revascularization. Arch Surg 117:544, 1982

89. Ohshiro T, Kosaki G: Sexual function after aortoiliac vascular reconstruction. J Cardiovasc Surg 25:47, 1984

90. Nevelsteen A, Beyens G, Duchateau J, Suy R: Aorto-femoral reconstruction and sexual function: a prospective study. Eur J Vasc Surg 4:247, 1990

91. Heggtveit HA: Syphilitic aortitis: a clinicopathologic autopsy study of 100 cases, 1950 to 1960. Circulation 29:346, 1964

92. DeBakey ME, Cooley DA, Crawford ES, et al: Aneurysms of the thoracic aorta: analysis of 179 patients treated by resection. J Thorac Surg 36:393, 1958

93. Bickerstaff LK, Pairolero PC, Hollier LH, et al: Thoracic aortic aneurysms: a population-based study. Surgery 92:1103, 1982

94. Strachan W, Wigzell FW, Anderson JR: Locomotor manifestations and serum studies in Takayasu's arteriopathy. Am J Med 40:560, 1966

95. Nakao K, Ikeda M, Kimata S, et al: Takayasu's arteritis: clinical report of eighty-four cases and immunological studies of seven cases. Circulation 35:1141, 1967

96. Ishikawa K: Natural history and classification of occlusive thromboaortopathy (Takayasu's disease). Circulation 57:27, 1978

97. Morooka S, Saito Y, Nonaka Y, et al: Clinical features and course of aortitis syndrome in Japanese women older than 40 years. Am J Cardiol 53:859, 1984

98. Haimovici H: Abdominal aortic aneurysm. p. 685. In Haimovici H (ed): Vascular Surgery. Appleton-Century-Crofts, East Norwalk, CT, 1984

99. Johansen K, Devin J: Mycotic aortic aneurysms: a reappraisal. Arch Surg 118:583, 1983

100. Bennett DE: Primary mycotic aneurysms of the aorta. Arch Surg 94:758, 1967

101. Schneider JA, Rheuban KS, Crosby IK: Rupture of postcoarctation mycotic aneurysms of the aorta. Ann Thorac Surg 27:185, 1979

102. Brindley P, Schwab EH: Aneurysms of the aorta, with a summary of pathological findings in 100 cases at autopsy. Tex State J Med 25:757, 1930

103. Lucke B, Rey MH: Studies on aneurysms: II. Aneurysm of the aorta. JAMA 81:1167, 1923

104. Rosen SA: Painless aortic dissection presenting as spinal cord ischemia. Ann Emerg Med 17:840, 1988

105. Dalen JE, Pape LA, Cohn LH, et al: Dissection of the aorta: pathogenesis, diagnosis, and treatment. Prog Cardiovasc Dis 23:237, 1980

106. Gschaedler R, Dollfus P, Loeb JP, et al: Traumatic rupture of the aorta and paraplegia. Paraplegia 16:123, 1978

107. Conti VR, Calverley J, Safley WL, et al: Anterior spinal artery syndrome with chronic traumatic thoracic aortic aneurysm. Ann Thorac Surg 33:81, 1982

108. Mitchell RL, Enright LP: The surgical management of acute and chronic injuries of the thoracic aorta. Surg Gynecol Obstet 157:1, 1983

109. Schmidt CA, Jacobson JG: Thoracic aortic injury: a ten-year experience. Arch Surg 119:1244, 1984

110. Woolsey RM: Aortic laceration after anterior spinal fusion. Surg Neurol 25:267, 1986

111. Mattox KL, Holzman M, Pickard LR, et al: Clamp/repair: a safe technique for treatment of blunt injury to the descending thoracic aorta. Ann Thorac Surg 40:456, 1985

112. Tyler HR, Clark DB: Neurologic complications in patients with coarctation of aorta. Neurology 8:712, 1958

113. Rotman M, Seidenberg B, Rubin I, et al: Aortic arch syndrome secondary to radiation in childhood. Arch Intern Med 124:87, 1969

114. Cologuhoun J: Hypoplasia of the abdominal aorta following therapeutic irradiation in infancy. Radiology 86:454, 1966

115. Woltman HW, Shelden WD: Neurological complications associated with congenital stenosis of the isthmus of the aorta. Arch Neurol Psychiatry 17:303, 1927

116. Wyburn-Mason R: The Vascular Abnormalities and Tumours of the Spinal Cord and Its Membranes. Henry Kimpton, London, 1943
117. Herron PW, Foltz EL, Plum F, et al: Partial Brown-Sequard syndrome associated with coarctation of the aorta: review of literature and report of a surgically treated case. Am Heart J 55:129, 1958
118. Lerberg DB, Hardesty RL, Siewers RD, et al: Coarctation of the aorta in infants and children: 25 years of experience. Ann Thorac Surg 33:159, 1982
119. Weenink HR, Smilde J: Spinal cord lesions due to coarctatio aortae. Psychiatr Neurol Neurochir 67:259, 1964
120. Bailey WL, Loeser JD: Intracranial aneurysms. JAMA 216:1993, 1971
121. McCormick WF: The natural history of intracranial saccular aneurysms. Weekly Update Neurol Neurosurg 1:2, 1978
122. Crawford ES, Crawford JL, Safi HJ, et al: Thoracoabdominal aortic aneurysms: preoperative and intraoperative factors determining immediate and long-term results of operations in 605 patients. J Vasc Surg 3:389, 1986
123. Livesay JJ, Cooley DA, Ventemiglia RA, et al: Surgical experience in descending thoracic aneurysmectomy with and without adjuncts to avoid ischemia. Ann Thorac Surg 39:37, 1985
124. Neville WE, Cox WD, Leininger B, et al: Resection of the descending thoracic aorta with femoral vein to femoral artery oxygenation perfusion. J Thorac Cardiovasc Surg 56:39, 1968
125. Bloodwell RD, Hallman GL, Cooley DA: Partial cardiopulmonary bypass for pericardiectomy and resection of descending thoracic aortic aneurysms. Ann Thorac Surg 6:46, 1968
126. Kahn DR, Sloan H: Resection of descending thoracic aneurysms without left heart bypass. Arch Surg 97:336, 1968
127. Krieger KH, Spencer FC: Is paraplegia after repair of coarctation of the aorta due principally to distal hypotension during aortic cross-clamping? Surgery 97:2, 1985
128. Boyarsky S: Paraplegia following translumbar aortography. JAMA 156:599, 1954
129. Grossman LA, Kirtley JA: Paraplegia after translumbar aortography. JAMA 166:1035, 1958
130. Killen DA, Foster JH: Spinal cord injury as a complication of aortography. Ann Surg 152:211, 1960
131. Galbreath C, Salgado ED, Furlan AJ, et al: Central nervous system complications of percutaneous transluminal coronary angioplasty. Stroke 17:616, 1986
132. Tyras DH, Willman VL: Paraplegia following intraaortic balloon assistance. Ann Thorac Surg 25:164, 1978
133. Laschinger JC, Cunningham JN, Cooper MM, et al: Prevention of ischemic spinal cord injury following aortic cross-clamping: use of corticosteroids. Ann Thorac Surg 38:500, 1984
134. Robertson CS, Foltz R, Grossman RG, et al: Protection against experimental ischemic spinal cord injury. J Neurosurg 64:633, 1986
135. Casthely PA, Fyman PN, Abrams LM, et al: Anaesthesia for aortic arch aneurysm repair: experience with 17 patients. Can Anaesth Soc J 32:73, 1985
136. Oldfield EH, Plunkett RJ, Nylander WA Jr, et al: Barbiturate protection in acute experimental spinal cord ischemia. J Neurosurg 56:511, 1982
137. Crawford ES, Rubio PA: Reappraisal of adjuncts to avoid ischemia in the treatment of aneurysms of descending thoracic aorta. J Thorac Cardiovasc Surg 66:693, 1973
138. Laschinger JC, Cunningham JN Jr, Nathan IM, et al: Experimental and clinical assessment of the adequacy of partial bypass in maintenance of spinal cord blood flow during operations on the thoracic aorta. Ann Thorac Surg 36:417, 1983
139. Cunningham JN Jr, Laschinger JC, Merkin HA, et al: Measurement of spinal cord ischemia during operations upon the thoracic aorta. Ann Surg 196:285, 1982
140. Kaplan BJ, Friedman WA, Alexander JA, et al: Somatosensory evoked potential monitoring of spinal cord ischemia during aortic operations. Neurosurgery 19:82, 1986
141. Mizrahi EM, Crawford ES: Somatosensory evoked potentials during reversible spinal cord ischemia in man. Electroencephalogr Clin Neurophysiol 58:120, 1984
142. Cheng MK, Robertson C, Grossman RG, et al: Neurological outcome correlated with spinal evoked potentials in a spinal cord ischemia model. J Neurosurg 60:786, 1984
143. Coles JG, Wilson GJ, Sima AF, et al: Intraoperative detection of spinal cord ischemia using somatosensory cortical evoked potentials during thoracic aortic occlusion. Ann Thorac Surg 34:299, 1982
144. Svensson LG, Patel V, Robinson MF, et al: Influence of preservation or perfusion of intraoperatively identified spinal cord blood supply on spinal motor evoked potentials and paraplegia after aortic surgery. J Vasc Surg 13:355, 1991
145. Reuter DG, Tacker WA, Badylak SF, et al: Correlation of motor-evoked potential response to ischemic spinal cord damage. J Thorac Cardiovasc Surg 104:262, 1992

3

Neurological Complications of Cardiac Surgery

John R. Hotson

Neurological complications can nullify or limit the potential benefits of open heart surgery. Early retrospective studies of open heart surgery found that severe stroke and anoxic encephalopathy were the common postoperative neurological complications that occurred in more than 20 percent of patients.[1-4] Improvements in surgery and extracorporeal circulation may have initially reduced the frequency of permanent, disabling neurological sequelae.[5-7] However, subsequent prospective, sensitive studies have shown that neurological sequelae remain a common consequence of cardiac surgery.[8-27] At the same time the use of coronary artery bypass graft surgery for treatment of ischemic heart disease has increased and heart transplantation programs have expanded. It is estimated that in the United States over 70,000 patients per year have minor or major neurological sequelae from cardiopulmonary bypass and cardiac surgery.[28] Therefore, prevention of perioperative neurological complications is an important clinical problem.

EXTRACORPOREAL CIRCULATION

Cardiopulmonary bypass was first used successfully in cardiac surgery in 1953 and was the pivotal development that led to modern cardiac surgery.[29,30]

Its early use in humans resulted in frequent complications, which restricted its use to seriously ill patients with progressive heart failure. The safety of extracorporeal circulation, however, increased over the subsequent two decades. Independent of the heart surgery itself, extracorporeal circulation remains a potential though low-risk cause of neurological complications.

Technique

During open heart surgery, cardiopulmonary bypass begins with exposure of the heart, usually by a median sternotomy, followed by cannulation of the ascending aorta and vena cava or right atrium.[30] Insertion of the aortic cannula can dislodge atheromatous material in a severely diseased aorta, thereby leading to cerebral embolization. In addition, this combined procedure can produce rotational torsion or compression of the brachial plexus, with subsequent injury.[31-34]

Extracorporeal circulation is used in association with systemic heparinization, hypothermia, and hemodilution.[30] Anticoagulation is used to prevent clot formation when blood is exposed to the nonendothelial surfaces of the bypass pump oxygenator and microaggregation filtration system. Core hypothermia of 26° to 30°C is often used in combination with selective cooling of the heart, or cold cardioplegia, in order to protect the heart, brain, and other vital organs from ischemic damage.[16,30] Neuropsychological performance after normothermic cardiopulmonary bypass, however, may not differ from that after hypothermic procedures.[35] Infusion of ice slush solutions into the pericardium is one technique for inducing cold cardioplegia, but it occasionally produces focal phrenic nerve injuries.[36–40] Normovolemic hemodilution is used in part to conserve blood loss. It also compensates for the progressive hemoconcentration, decrease in plasma volume, and reduced blood flow that is associated with hypothermia.[30]

During cardiac surgery with extracorporeal circulation, the ascending aorta is routinely cross-clamped; during valvular replacement surgery, congenital heart disease repair, or left ventricular aneurysm resection, the cardiac chambers are entered.[30] These procedures may disrupt diseased tissue and produce emboli.

Arterial systolic, diastolic, and mean pressure; pump pressure and flow rate; and central venous pressure are monitored during cardiopulmonary bypass. Mean arterial pressure is usually maintained between 50 and 100 mmHg by vasodilators, pressors, or volume expanders.[8,21,30]

Consequences During "Normal" Convalescence

Extracorporeal circulation has predictable effects that result in a postperfusion syndrome during "normal" convalescence.[30,41] This syndrome includes the following conditions.

1. *Reduced clotting factors.* Exposure of blood to an abnormal environment during cardiopulmonary bypass leads to consumption of platelets and coagulation factors. Platelets adhere to the unphysiological surface of the oxygenators and filtration system of the bypass pump.[42] This clumping of platelets not only predisposes to platelet emboli but can reduce the number of circulating platelets. The exposure to foreign surfaces also causes release and depletion of granule-stored aggregating proteins in surviving platelets.[43] Therefore, remaining platelets have decreased adhesiveness.

    Coagulation factors are also consumed during cardiopulmonary bypass. A variety of carrier pro-

teins and lipoproteins are denatured when blood passes through the bypass pump oxygenator.[30,44] Even with adequate heparin levels, these damaged proteins can initiate a cascade in several coagulation and inflammatory systems.[45] The clinical significance of these hematological changes is usually minor. They may contribute, however, to the intracranial hemorrhages that are occasionally observed after open heart surgery.[1]

2. *Cardiovascular response.* During the early postoperative period, the degree of peripheral vasoconstriction provides a clinical estimate of cardiac output.[30] If the pedal pulses are absent and the feet are cold, cardiac output may be reduced, a condition that may be associated with organ dysfunction during convalescence. Transient atrial fibrillation, which carries a risk for cardiac emboli, is common during the convalescent period. A metabolic acidosis is also common during the 2 hours immediately after operation and reflects a washout of lactic acid from regions of poor perfusion during extracorporeal circulation. Persistence of a metabolic acidosis may indicate inadequate tissue perfusion secondary to low cardiac output.[30]

3. *Red blood cell fragmentation.* Exposure of blood to nonendothelial surfaces during bypass surgery causes a breakdown of red blood cells, with subsequent anemia, hemoglobinemia, and hemoglobinuria.[30]

4. *Mild mental confusion.* Transient mild disturbances of orientation, memory, and level of alertness that resolve within the first few days after open heart surgery with cardiopulmonary bypass are frequent.[21,30] Whether the changes in mentation are totally reversible events that accompany most major operations or indicate long-term sequelae is an area of evolving interest.[10,11,14,16,18,22]

These expected consequences of cardiopulmonary bypass are functionally reversible and compensated for during convalescence. However, they also create numerous potential hazards that may be augmented by procedural error, so that they then lead to permanent injury of the central nervous system. Cardiac operations using extracorporeal circulation carry the risks of cerebral hypoperfusion, embolus formation (from platelets, fibrin, tissue or surgical debris, air, or fat), and even hemorrhage.

NEUROLOGICAL SEQUELAE OF CARDIAC SURGERY

Diffuse or multifocal anoxic-ischemic damage, focal cerebral infarction, and lower brachial plexus injuries remain the major cause of permanent, disabling neurological complications after cardiac surgery (Table 3-1).[8,11,46-48] Therefore the common, obvious postoperative symptoms include diffuse impairment of cognition and level of consciousness, focal deficits from stroke, and isolated peripheral weakness and sensory loss in one arm and hand.

Brain Disorders

Stroke, encephalopathy, coma, and seizures are the major brain disorders complicating cardiac surgery.[46] Stroke occurs more frequently with valvular heart surgery than with coronary artery bypass graft operations (Table 3-1). A permanent neurological disability after valve replacement occurs in 5 to 10 percent of patients.[5,15] In contrast, the risk of a severe disability complicating coronary artery bypass graft surgery is less than 2 to 5 percent,[47,48] and ischemic complications after percutaneous transluminal coronary angioplasty, which does not involve cardiopulmonary bypass, occur with a frequency of less than 0.2 percent.[49] This difference is due to the greater risk of cardiac macroemboli with operations that require opening a heart chamber. Removal or repair of diseased, calcified mitral or aortic valves is associated with the disbursement of tissue and surgical debris in the cardiac chambers. There is a high risk that some of this debris may form multiple cerebral emboli. Imaging studies, including cerebral arteriograms, suggest that the main cause of cerebral infarction with both valvular and coronary artery bypass surgery is embolization and not hypoperfusion.[50]

Intracranial hemorrhage is an infrequent cause of stroke, but its rapid identification is important so that surgical evacuation can be undertaken if necessary.[51-53] Hematomas may be located in the brain parenchyma or in subdural or epidural spaces. Intracranial hemorrhage may be related to reduced platelet adhesion and coagulation factors during cardiopulmonary bypass.

The global encephalopathy that can follow heart surgery varies from coma to confusion or a psychotic delirium with impaired cognition. Stupor or coma after uncomplicated surgery is infrequent, occurring in less than 1 percent of patients.[22,46] It may be due to global anoxia-ischemia, massive stroke, or multiple brain infarctions. Additional, rarely reported causes of encephalopathy or coma include hypoglycemia,[54] a hypernatremic hyperosmolar state,[55] and acute obstructive hydrocephalus.[56]

When anoxia-ischemia is the cause of coma, myoclonus, at times accompanied by seizures, may be prominent. Postanoxic myoclonus and seizures are often poorly responsive to anticonvulsant therapy. The outcome in these comatose patients is usually extremely poor, with only a rare patient making a meaningful recovery.[22]

A confusional state that persists for days after uncomplicated surgery is much more common than coma, occurring in 3 to over 10 percent of patients. These encephalopathic patients may be slow to emerge from anesthesia, are often agitated, have

Table 3-1 Major Neurological Sequelae of Cardiac Surgery

Sequela[a]	Valvular Replacement		Coronary Artery Bypass Graft	
	Early Complication (%)	1-Year Deficit (%)	Early Complication (%)	6-Month Deficit (%)
Prolonged encephalopathy	6	4	9	1
Stroke	32	3	9	4
Peripheral nerve disorder	12	2	12	4
Severe disability or death from any neurological cause	—	7	—	2

[a] Prolonged encephalopathy varied from obtundation to impaired mental status. Stroke included mild to severe hemiparesis, aphasia, and homonymous hemianopia. Peripheral nerve disorder included brachial plexus injuries and other focal neuropathies.
(Data compiled from Breuer and colleagues,[8] Shaw and associates,[11] and Sotaniemi.[17])

moderate to severe impairment of cognitive function, and occasionally have bilateral Babinski signs. Improvement often occurs during the first postoperative week.[23] In comparison, patients who are matched for age and clinical condition but who have major surgery for peripheral vascular disease without cardiopulmonary bypass rarely develop such an impairment of intellectual function.[12] Therefore, exposure to cardiopulmonary bypass appears to be a major contributing factor to the encephalopathic state in otherwise uncomplicated cardiac surgery. Disseminated microemboli during extracorporeal circulation may be a cause of this encephalopathy.

A psychotic delirium after open heart surgery has been attributed to a situational psychiatric reaction if the level of alertness and memory remain intact.[57] When the latter processes are also impaired, the psychotic behavior has been called an organic delirium. In patients undergoing cardiac surgery, this differentiation may be incorrect. When the psychotic response has cleared and neuropsychological testing is performed, both groups have similar, multiple cognitive impairments compared to patients without neurobehavioral complications.[58] The diagnosis of an intensive care unit psychosis is usually restricted to reactions that begin 2 to 5 days after surgery, are associated with preserved memory and alertness, and rapidly resolve after treatment with neuroleptic agents or discharge from the intensive care unit. A reduced availability of tryptophan, the precursor to the cerebral neurotransmitter serotonin, may be associated with postoperative delirium.[59] Psychotic reactions that occur during the first 48 postoperative hours in a previously stable patient probably represent a behavioral response to an anoxic-ischemic insult associated with cardiac surgery and cardiopulmonary bypass.[57,60,61]

Seizures may accompany coma, encephalopathy, or delirium, or they may occur independently after cardiac surgery.[46] They occur in less than 1 percent of patients, usually early in the postoperative period and often within the first 24 hours. Tonic-clonic or partial motor seizures are clinically apparent, but partial complex seizures in an encephalopathic patient may be difficult to recognize clinically. Choreoathetosis after heart surgery, a complication that occurs mainly in children, sometimes raises the question of a seizure disorder.[62] Nonconvulsive status epilepticus may occur with stroke complicating cardiac surgery

and will then contribute to a prolonged confusional state that is treatable with anticonvulsant drugs.[63] Therefore the electroencephalographic (EEG) evaluation of patients with a persistent encephalopathy may be valuable.

Peripheral Nerve Disorders

The brachial plexus and phrenic nerves are the most frequent peripheral nerves injured during cardiac surgery. A polyneuropathy may also occur under certain circumstances.

A persistent brachial plexopathy after median sternotomy has been reported to occur in more than 5 percent of patients.[5,11,31–34] Transient and minor brachial plexus injuries may be even more common. Most frequently the lower trunk of the brachial plexus is injured. Therefore, the intrinsic hand muscles are often most severely impaired, and the triceps reflex may be decreased in the affected arm. Sensory loss is sometimes present in the affected hand. Pain is prominent in some patients, and a minority have Horner's syndrome. Injuries of the upper brachial plexus can also occur but are less frequent. The plexus injuries may be due to torsional traction or compression during the open heart surgery.[31–35] Although not life-threatening and usually reversible in 1 to 3 months, a brachial plexus injury may produce permanent disability, particularly if it affects the dominant hand or produces intractable causalgia. Such injuries may be prevented by minimizing the opening of the sternal retractor, placing the retractor in the most caudal location, and avoiding asymmetrical traction.[33,34] Specific attempts to reduce the occurrence of these injuries with intraoperative electrophysiological monitoring techniques are rarely mentioned in published accounts.

Unilateral phrenic nerve injuries with hemidiaphragmatic paralysis occur in at least 10 percent of patients during open heart surgery.[37–40] The location of the phrenic nerve adjacent to the pericardium makes it particularly vulnerable to injury from manipulation, ischemia, or hypothermia associated with topical cold cardioplegia. Unilateral phrenic nerve injury causes atelectasis and inspiratory muscle weakness, predisposing to postoperative respiratory complications. In most patients, however, there is low morbidity. Some recovery is usually evident by about 6 months after injury, but there may be a more protracted course consistent with axonal injury and regeneration.[39,40]

Severe, bilateral phrenic nerve injury is a rare complication of heart surgery and leads to prolonged mechanical respiration. Phrenic nerve electrodiagnostic studies may help to assess the severity of injury and the rate of recovery of unilateral or bilateral phrenic nerve disorders.[36,38]

Mononeuropathies resulting from compression or trauma during surgery may involve the accessory, facial, lateral femoral cutaneous, peroneal, radial, recurrent laryngeal, saphenous, and ulnar nerves.[31,64–66] A recurrent laryngeal nerve injury with vocal cord paralysis[31,67] and a persistent peroneal neuropathy[31] are the most disabling. Ischemia to the cochlea-auditory nerve can result in severe hearing loss.[68] Most compressive mononeuropathies are transient. This reversibility, usually with 4 to 8 weeks, may reflect the focal selective injury to myelin, with relative sparing of nerve axons, which occurs with compression neuropathies.[69] Awareness of possible intraoperative compression sites helps to prevent these complications.

Diffuse paralysis as a result of the Guillain-Barré syndrome may follow otherwise uncomplicated cardiac surgery as well as other surgical procedures.[70] Persistent paralysis also occurs after cardiac surgery in critically ill patients who have renal failure and require days of vecuronium to facilitate mechanical respiration.[71] If heart surgery is complicated by sepsis and multiorgan failure lasting for over a week, a "critical illness" polyneuropathy may develop, with difficulty in weaning from a respirator, distal weakness, and reduced tendon reflexes.[72] This syndrome is discussed further in Chapter 44.

Neuro-Ophthalmological Disorders

Visual disorders from cardiac surgery are frequent but usually asymptomatic and reversible. Retinal disorders include multifocal areas of retinal nonperfusion in almost all patients, cotton wool spots consistent with retinal infarctions in 10 to 25 percent of patients, and visualization of retinal emboli in fewer individuals. These retinal disorders are infrequently associated with reduced visual acuity.[73–75]

An anterior ischemic optic neuropathy is an uncommon, disabling complication of heart surgery. It produces infarction of the optic nerve head, with a painless and usually permanent decrease in visual acuity. An ischemic optic neuropathy may produce a monocular altitudinal, arcuate, or central scotoma.[75] Homonymous visual field defects occur with focal ischemic injury of the visual cortex or retrochiasmal visual pathways.

An occasional patient is found to be cortically blind after heart surgery, usually from bilateral ischemia of the occipital cortex. These patients may sometimes deny any visual impairment. At least partial recovery from cortical blindness is possible.[73,75,76]

Horner's syndrome occurs predominantly in association with injuries to the lower brachial plexus and results from concomitant injury to the preganglionic sympathetic fibers that travel through the eighth cervical and first thoracic ventral roots.[73]

Gaze deviations, gaze paralysis, and dysconjugate gaze may occur in postoperative patients who have a brainstem or large hemispheric stroke involving eye movement systems. Intermittent gaze deviation with nystagmoid movements raises concerns about postoperative focal seizures.[77]

Pituitary apoplexy resulting from acute hemorrhage or infarction of a pituitary tumor is a rare complication of cardiopulmonary bypass.[78,79] Most reported patients have had pituitary tumors that were not recognized prior to surgery. After heart surgery, they awakened with headache, ptosis, ophthalmoplegia, and visual impairment from compression of the adjacent cranial nerves and the anterior visual pathways. Transsphenoidal surgical decompression has been used safely in some patients. Pituitary tumors may be particularly susceptible to the ischemic and hemorrhagic risks associated with cardiopulmonary bypass.

Visual hallucinations solely on eye closure have been reported following cardiovascular surgery.[80] Patients are otherwise fully alert and lucid and can stop the hallucinations simply by opening their eyes. Atropine or lidocaine toxicity and partial complex seizures have been associated with such hallucinations.

INJURED NEURONAL RESERVE AND MICROEMBOLI

Sensitive prospective studies have shown that subtle neurological changes are common during the early postoperative period. Between 40 and 60 percent of patients may develop new, usually minor neurological signs after coronary artery bypass graft surgery.[10,11,14,16,18,21,24] These signs most commonly include the appearance of primitive reflexes and ischemic changes in the retina. Magnetic resonance imaging (MRI) of the brain, however, often reveals no ischemic changes,[81] and more than 90 percent of these minor neurological signs resolve within 6 months without obvious disabling sequelae.

There is concern and evidence, nevertheless, that these new minor neurological signs represent an anoxic-ischemic insult to a neuronal reserve that is needed to adapt to future processes such as brain aging.[82] The initial effect of this insult may consist only of subtle changes in personality or memory. There are reports that patients with reversible postoperative neurological signs have a persistently poor performance on neuropsychological testing even a year after surgery.[11–14,16,18,22,24] Even though most minor neurological signs resolve within 6 months, cognitive limitation may persist.

Patients who develop abnormal psychometric test scores postoperatively also have an associated elevation in adenylate kinase in the cerebrospinal fluid (CSF).[19,21] Adenylate kinase, an intracellular enzyme that provides a CSF marker of cell membrane integrity, is increased by brain ischemia.[19] Its concentration in the CSF is elevated in more than 50 percent of patients after cardiac surgery, providing evidence of brain cell injury.

Cerebral blood flow studies using single photon emission computed tomography (SPECT) also provide evidence of diffuse brain ischemia during cardiac operations.[10] Most patients have a persistent reduction in cerebral blood flow during the first postoperative week. This decrease in brain perfusion correlates positively with increasing age, duration of mean arterial pressure below 40 to 50 mmHg, and duration of cardiopulmonary bypass.[10] The reduced cerebral blood flow improves over the subsequent year but does not return to preoperative levels.

Retinal fluorescein angiograms during cardiopulmonary bypass demonstrate multifocal areas of retinal ischemia in almost all patients.[74] Areas of capillary nonperfusion occur in isolation or in association with arteriolar occlusion. Retinal histology from an animal model suggests that intravascular platelet-fibrin microemboli contribute to these areas of retinal ischemia. In most patients, areas of nonperfusion are re-

perfused in postoperative retinal angiograms without clinical sequelae. These observations suggest that, during cardiopulmonary bypass, there is a continuous process of microvascular occlusions followed by reperfusion.[74]

Transcranial Doppler ultrasonography can detect microemboli of 50 to several hundred micrometers in size.[23,83] Air emboli produce more intense signals than particulate emboli. Transcranial Doppler has shown that showers of air microemboli occur routinely during aortic cannulation, at the inception of cardiopulmonary bypass, and during the redistribution of blood from the heart-lung machine to the empty beating heart when it is beginning to eject blood actively. There is a higher frequency of microembolic events associated with bubble oxygenators than with the membrane oxygenators used in cardiopulmonary bypass.[83]

There is also pathological evidence of disseminated brain microemboli during cardiac surgery.[28] The brain's microvasculature, unlike the larger cerebral vessels, stains strongly for alkaline phosphatase. An alkaline phosphatase map of the afferent cerebral microvasculature reveals thousands to millions of focal, small capillary and arteriolar dilatations in patients and dogs who have recently undergone cardiopulmonary bypass. Subjects who die without exposure to cardiopulmonary bypass do not have these microaneurysms. These capillary and arteriolar dilatations are usually empty, suggesting that gas bubbles or fat emboli are a prime cause. Whether these microaneurysms persist or resolve in the postoperative weeks is unclear.

The permanent functional significance of the frequent minor neurological signs, impairments in neuropsychological scores, biochemical evidence of ischemia, reduced cerebral blood flow, and markers of microemboli that follow cardiac surgery is unclear. Fewer than half of the patients with early neurological sequelae of cardiac surgery return to employment,[11] for a variety of reasons that are usually not related to intellectual impairment.[14] A direct comparison of preoperative and postoperative work performance has not been made. It is not uncommon, however, for patients' families to note changes in memory and personality after cardiac surgery that are not detected by surgical observers. The above observations raise an important concern that cardiopulmonary bypass surgery has a higher than recognized risk of limiting maximum cognitive performance.

RISK FACTORS

Attempts to prevent neurological sequelae after cardiac surgery have focused on improved surgical and cardiopulmonary bypass techniques.[5–7] There have been additional attempts at identifying patient characteristics that indicate a high risk for a complication. As noted previously, it is known that individuals who require surgical opening of a heart chamber, as for aortic or mitral valve repair, have a relatively high rate of stroke from cardiac emboli.[15] Other preoperative clinical factors, however, are less well defined (Table 3-2).

Age, severe carotid artery stenosis, preoperative stroke, severe aortic atheroma, and profound, sustained intraoperative hypotension are probable risk factors for neurological sequelae, but the supporting evidence is often inconsistent. One prospective study found that patients over the age of 60 years had 4.5 times the frequency of neurological sequelae than did younger patients.[15] Another study demonstrated a progressive increase in the risk of stroke during coronary artery surgery with each decade above 50 years of age. The occurrence of obvious stroke was 1.3, 3.0, and 6.3 percent in patients in their fifties, sixties, and seventies, respectively.[26] Most other studies also concluded that increasing age was a risk factor for neurological sequelae.[3,8,14,47,84,85] In the past decade, an expanding number of patients above 75 years of age have received coronary artery bypass grafts. These very old patients have a fourfold increase in stroke and neurological complications when compared to younger patients.[86–88]

It seems reasonable to assume that hemodynamically significant carotid artery disease is a risk factor

Table 3-2 Risk Factors for Neurological Sequelae of Cardiac Surgery

Probable	Possible
Opening cardiac chambers	Prolonged cardiopulmonary bypass
Sustained mean arterial pressure <30–40 mmHg	Severe carotid or cerebrovascular disease
Older age	Postoperative atrial fibrillation
Recent stroke	Congestive heart failure
Severe atheroma of the aorta	Diabetes mellitus
	Protein C deficiency

for cerebral ischemia during coronary artery bypass graft surgery. This assumption provides the basis for advocating carotid endarterectomy when it is believed that there is possible hemodynamic compromise from a carotid stenosis, even if the patient is asymptomatic. In this situation it is common surgical practice to recommend combined carotid and coronary artery surgery in a staged or simultaneous procedure.[89–91]

There is a lack of unanimity, however, concerning carotid disease as a risk factor for perioperative stroke.[9,25–27] Some studies suggest that the presence of carotid disease increases the risk of stroke during heart surgery,[25,92–94] whereas other studies fail to confirm this observation.[9,27] Intraoperative transcranial Doppler studies have not demonstrated reduced middle cerebral artery blood flow ipsilateral to severe carotid stenosis or occlusion during coronary artery bypass surgery.[95] Furthermore, perioperative stroke in association with severe carotid stenosis commonly occurs 2 or more days after cardiac surgery.[94] Perioperative strokes in association with general surgery also usually occur with a similar delay.[95] These observations suggest that the collateral circulation that is effective for cortical perfusion prior to surgery usually remains effective during cardiopulmonary bypass. Factors other than hypoperfusion, such as postoperative coagulation changes or atrial fibrillation, may be related to these delayed postoperative strokes. Even if hemodynamically significant carotid disease is a risk factor for perioperative stroke, there is only meager evidence that a carotid endarteretomy decreases this risk.[25,94] The conclusion that prior occlusive carotid artery disease increases the risk of cerebral hypoperfusion and intraoperative stroke is intuitively persuasive. However, the conflicting reports outlined above indicate that this conclusion may be deceptive.

A prior history of stroke of transient ischemic attack is often associated with arteriosclerotic cerebrovascular disease. Most investigators have reported an increased frequency of perioperative stroke in individuals who have a history of cerebral ischemia.[26,27,48,85,96–98] Others, however, have not confirmed this conclusion.[8,25,92] Current evidence suggests that cardiac surgery within 3 months of a stroke carries a particular risk for worsening preoperative neurological deficits.[97]

Dislodgement of atheroma during instrumentation of the aorta has been identified as a risk factor for stroke.[99-103] Approximately 20 percent of patients receiving a coronary artery bypass graft have moderate to severe atherosclerotic plaques in their ascending aorta identified intraoperatively. The frequency of such aortic disease increases with age.[101] Atheromatous disease can be identified with intraoperative ultrasonographic scanning of the ascending aorta or by transesophageal echocardiography of the aortic arch. These observations have led to a recent recommendation that intraoperative ultrasonographic imaging be considered in all patients who are 70 years of age or older and in selected young patients with risk factors for atheroma formation.[99] Identification of a moderately to severely atheromatous aorta may alter surgical management.[103]

Other possible risk factors may be minor or inconsistent contributors to postoperative neurological sequelae. These possible risk factors include long-duration operations that require more than 2 hours of extracorporeal circulation,[3,47] a history of congestive heart failure,[47,48] postoperative atrial fibrillation,[47,85,98] diabetes mellitus,[47,48,85] and perhaps protein C deficiency.[104,105] The risk of a mean arterial pressure below 40 to 50 mmHg during cardiopulmonary bypass remains unclear.

PREVENTION OF NEUROLOGICAL COMPLICATIONS

Identification of surgical and technical factors that carry particular risks of neurological complications after cardiac surgery has led to the adoption of preventive measures.[5,6,30] An arterial line microfilter system has been incorporated into extracorporeal circulation with the aim of reducing cerebral embolization. Improved surgical techniques reduce the time and opportunity for a complication. Systemic heparinization, hemodilution, and use of an acellular priming solution for the oxygenator prevents clot formation and microcoagulation. Maintenance of the mean arterial blood pressure above 50 mmHg provides a safety margin against periods of relative hypoperfusion. The use of a membrane oxygenator decreases the magnitude of air emboli. Identification of a severely atheromatous aorta allows surgical attempts to avoid dislodging emboli. Delaying heart surgery for 3 months

after a recent stroke has been recommended if the cardiac condition allows such a delay.

Almost all physicians would concur that preoperative carotid endarterectomy is indicated when a patient has had recent transient ischemic symptoms ipsilateral to a high-grade (≥ 70 percent) stenosis. Many would also agree that bilateral, severe carotid disease, even if asymptomatic, is also an indication for carotid endarterectomy before cardiac surgery.[9] Others would recommend maintaining a higher intraoperative mean arterial pressure and, perhaps, monitoring hemispheric perfusion in patients with high-grade, unilateral carotid stenosis if it is asymptomatic. The results of recent and pending studies of the benefit of carotid endarterectomy in individuals with asymptomatic carotid stenosis in the general population may influence such decisions.[106,107] The evidence that carotid endarterectomy is of any value in reducing the neurological morbidity of cardiac surgery is incomplete.

The magnitude of cerebral microemboli and the frequent neuropsychological and anoxic-ischemic findings associated with cardiac surgery suggest a need and opportunity to study brain protective agents. These agents are effective in animal models when given before or immediately after anoxic-ischemic brain injury.[108] Barbiturates, in doses sufficient to produce an isoelectric EEG, may reduce neuropsychological dysfunction associated with cerebral embolism and valvular heart disease.[92] Barbiturates at such doses have not gained wide acceptance during coronary artery bypass surgery, in part due to side effects of cardiovascular instability and slow emergence from anesthesia.[108] Nimodipine is a calcium channel blocker that may increase cerebral blood flow; in a preliminary study, its use as a cerebral protective agent was inconclusive.[109] Neuronal death due to overstimulation of glutamate receptors forms the basis of the excitotoxic hypothesis of anoxic-ischemic brain injury. If this applies in the clinical setting, then glutamate receptor antagonists should reduce neuronal death. Proposals to test this protective strategy in patients undergoing cardiac surgery await fulfillment.[110]

Monitoring the peripheral and central nervous systems during cardiac surgery is technically possible but expensive and of unproved value.[111-113] Somatosensory evoked potentials that depend on the integrity of the brachial plexus can be monitored. It would be valuable to know whether such monitoring will permit detection of plexus compression during sternal retraction and thereby lead to corrective maneuvers that prevent subsequent injury. Routine EEG monitoring during cardiac surgery has not proved useful except for detecting unexpected events leading to profound decreases in cerebral perfusion.[22,108] EEG recordings may be used to monitor hemispheric perfusion in patients with hemodynamically significant but asymptomatic carotid stenosis. Transcranial Doppler ultrasonography can monitor blood flow in the middle cerebral artery.[23] It remains unclear whether neural or cerebrovascular monitoring can alter outcome on a routine basis.

CARDIAC TRANSPLANTATION

Cardiac transplantation is an established treatment for selected patients with progressive, preterminal heart failure. Survival has improved with advances such as endomyocardial biopsy to assess organ rejection, use of antithymocyte antiglobulin to treat rejection, and administration of cyclosporine as a relatively selective immunosuppressive agent. Cardiac transplant centers now report survival rates at 1 year of greater than 80 to 85 percent and at 5 years of 60 to 80 percent.[114–116] Neurological sequelae occurring in either the perioperative period or as a late complication may negate an otherwise successful heart transplant. The early identification of treatable complications offers the best opportunity to prevent severe disability.

The perioperative neurological sequelae from cardiac transplantation are similar to the complications associated with valvular or bypass graft surgery, discussed above.[117–120] Anoxic-ischemic encephalopathy, stroke, headaches, psychosis, seizures, and peripheral nerve disorders are the most common problems. Neuropathological examination in patients with impaired mentation usually reveals changes consistent with multiple embolic cerebral infarcts; anoxic changes occur less frequently.

Vascular headaches accompanied by nausea and vomiting may occur in the first week after transplantation.[22] The headaches are associated with a rapid shift from low preoperative to high postoperative mean arterial pressures. Similar headaches may rarely precede an intraparenchymal hemorrhage. These vascular headaches respond to β-adrenergic receptor blocking agents.

Seizures have been reported in up to 15 percent of patients with cardiac transplants.[120] They commonly occur in the perioperative period. They also occur as a side effect of cyclosporine or as a late complication from a brain infection or tumor. Seizures in the perioperative period are usually due to stroke and may not require chronic anticonvulsant therapy. When anticonvulsant drugs are indicated, selection of the best agent may be difficult.[121] Phenytoin, phenobarbital, and carbamazepine decrease the blood levels and immunosuppressive effect of cyclosporine. When these agents are used, cyclosporine and corticosteroid doses may have to be increased. Valproic acid does not induce the metabolism of cyclosporine or corticosteroids and may be preferred after cardiac transplantation.

Psychotic behavior with hallucinations, delusional thought processes, and disorganized behavior can occur during the first 2 weeks after transplantation or as a late complication. When it occurs during the postoperative period, multiple causal factors may be present; but with time the psychotic behavior usually resolves. When psychotic behavior occurs as a late complication, it is often a manifestation of an intracranial infection, most commonly viral. A thorough neurological evaluation is therefore indicated when a cardiac transplant recipient develops an acute, late psychosis.[118,119]

Immunosuppression remains the major cause of late neurological complications after cardiac transplantation. Opportunistic infections can occur as early as 2 weeks after surgery and immunosuppression, but usually there is an interval of at least a month. Focal meningoencephalitis or brain abscess, meningitis, and diffuse encephalitis are three common presentations of infections in cardiac transplant recipients.[119,122,123]

Aspergillosis is the most frequent fungal infection, producing a necrotizing meningoencephalitis and single or multiple brain abscesses.[123,124] Cerebral aspergillosis is almost always disseminated from a preceding pulmonary infection. The abscesses appear as low-density lesions with no or irregular contrast enhancement on computed tomographic (CT) scans. Aspergillosis also causes an invasive necrosis of intracranial vessels that may lead to hemorrhagic infarction. Therefore focal hemorrhage on brain imaging is suggestive of *Aspergillus* infection. The diagnosis can be confirmed only by direct needle aspiration or biopsy; serological and CSF studies and cultures usually are not helpful. If the diagnosis is made late, the disease is fatal; early diagnosis and treatment in an immunosuppressed patient, however, can lead to recovery.[124]

Toxoplasma gondii is the second most common cause of focal or multifocal meningoencephalitis and abscess formation following cardiac transplantation.[123,125] It can produce multiple ring-enhancing lesions, seen with contrast CT scans. MRI may demonstrate additional lesions not apparent on CT scans and may also show a rapid response to antibiotic therapy. Serological evidence of *T. gondii* is supportive evidence, particularly if there is seroconversion after transplantation or a rise in titer compared to the preoperative baseline serology.[125] Examination of immunoperoxidase-stained material aspirated from an abscess is diagnostic.[126] Consideration of the diagnosis is mandatory because of the excellent therapeutic response to pyrimethamine in combination with sulfonamides or other antitoxoplasmic antibiotics.[127]

Other, less frequent opportunistic infections that produce focal meningoencephalitis or brain abscess include the rhinocerebral phycomycotic organisms, *Candida albicans, Nocardia asteroides,* and *Klebsiella* (abscess).[118,123,128,129]

Meningitis after cardiac transplantation is most commonly due to *Cryptococcus neoformans* when the white blood count in the CSF is mildly to moderately elevated with predominantly mononuclear cells. *Listeria monocytogenes* is the most common organism when there is a prominent CSF pleocytosis consisting of polymorphonuclear and mononuclear cells. *Coccidioides immitis* and *Pseudoallescheria boydii* as well as previously mentioned fungi are less frequent causes of meningitis.[119,120,130]

Cytomegalovirus, herpes simplex, and herpes zoster encephalitis also occurs, in association with a disseminated viremia, in patients who have undergone cardiac transplantation.[119,122,131] Immunosuppression, however, transforms the acute necrotizing focal herpes simplex encephalitis into a more diffuse and slowly progressive process. Immunosuppression for cardiac transplantation also predisposes to the development of a primary or secondary lymphoma of the brain.[132,133] Brain imaging that reveals bilaterally symmetrical lesions in the periventricular or basal ganglia regions or involvement of the corpus callosum suggests lymphoma.[119] Lymphoma of the brain may regress with radiotherapy and reduction of immunosuppressive therapy.[134]

Immunosuppressive agents can also cause neurological side effects more directly. Prior to the use of cyclosporine, high-dose prednisone in combination with azathioprine was commonly used. The main side effect of the prednisone was weakness of the proximal lower extremities, osteoporosis with lower thoracic and lumbosacral compression fractures, or alterations of mood.[118] With the use of cyclosporine, the dose of prednisone has been lowered, reducing its side effects. Cyclosporine itself, however, may cause tremor, a lowered seizure threshold, and paresthesias. Mental confusion, muscle weakness, ataxia, paresthesias, visual hallucinations, and a leukoencephalopathy with cortical blindness have also been observed. These neurotoxic side effects rapidly remit with reduction of the cyclosporine dose.[135]

The monoclonal anti-CD3 antibody (OKT3) is used to prevent and treat graft rejection following cardiac transplantation. Aseptic meningitis with fever, headache, seizures, and a variable encephalopathy occurs in 5 percent of patients as a reaction to it. This aseptic meningitis may occur during the course of OKT3 therapy or in the weeks immediately subsequent to it.[135,136]

As noted above, most of the neurological complications of cardiac transplantation with immunosuppression may present with a confusional state in which headache and focal neurological findings may be present or absent. It is not uncommon, however, for more than one complication of immunosuppression to cause symptoms in an individual cardiac transplant recipient.[118,119,123]

REFERENCES

1. Brierley JB: Neuropathological findings in patients dying after open-heart surgery. Thorax 18:291, 1963
2. Gilman S: Cerebral disorders after open-heart operations. N Engl J Med 272:489, 1965
3. Tufo HM, Ostfeld AM, Shekelle R: Central nervous system dysfunction following open-heart surgery. JAMA 212:1333, 1970
4. Stockard JJ, Bickford RG, Schauble JF: Pressure-dependent cerebral ischemia during cardiopulmonary bypass. Neurology 23:521, 1973

5. Branthwaite MA: Prevention of neurological damage during open-heart surgery. Thorax 30:258, 1975

6. Kritikou PE, Branthwaite MA: Significance of changes in cerebral electrical activity at onset of cardiopulmonary bypass. Thorax 32:534, 1977

7. Aberg T, Kihlgren M: Cerebral protection during open-heart surgery. Thorax 32:525, 1977

8. Breuer AC, Furlan AJ, Hanson MR, et al: Central nervous system complications of coronary artery bypass graft surgery: prospective analysis of 421 patients. Stroke 14:682, 1983

9. Furlan AJ, Crachiun AR: Risk of stroke during coronary artery bypass graft surgery in patients with internal carotid artery disease documented by angiography. Stroke 16:797, 1985

10. Henriksen L: Evidence suggestive of diffuse brain damage following cardiac operations. Lancet 1:816, 1984

11. Shaw PJ, Bates D, Cartlidge NEF, et al: Neurological complications of coronary artery bypass graft surgery: six month follow-up study. Br Med J 293:165, 1986

12. Shaw PJ, Bates D, Cartlidge NEF, et al: Neurologic and neuropsychological morbidity following major surgery: comparison of coronary artery bypass and peripheral vascular surgery. Stroke 18:700, 1987

13. Shaw PJ, Bates D, Cartlidge NEF, et al: Early intellectual dysfunction following coronary bypass surgery. Q J Med 58:59, 1986

14. Shaw PJ, Bates D, Cartlidge NEF, et al: Long-term intellectual dysfunction following coronary artery bypass graft surgery: a six month follow-up study. Q J Med 62:259, 1987

15. Slogoff S, Girgis KZ, Keats AS: Etiologic factors in neuropsychiatric complications associated with cardiopulmonary bypass. Anesth Analg 61:903, 1982

16. Smith PLC, Treasure T, Newman SP, et al: Cerebral consequences of cardiopulmonary bypass. Lancet 1:823, 1986

17. Sotaniemi KA: Brain damage and neurological outcome after open-heart surgery. J Neurol Neurosurg Psychiatry 43:127, 1980

18. Sotaniemi KA, Mononen H, Hokkanen TE: Long-term cerebral outcome after open-heart surgery: a five-year neuropsychological follow-up study. Stroke 17:410, 1986

19. Aberg T, Ronquist G, Tyden H, et al: Release of adenylate kinase into cerebrospinal fluid during open-heart surgery and its relation to postoperative intellectual function. Lancet 1:1139, 1982

20. Aberg T, Ahlund P, Kihlgren M: Intellectual function late after open-heart operation. Ann Thorac Surg 36:690, 1983

21. Aberg T, Ronquist G, Tyden H, et al: Adverse effects on the brain in cardiac operations as assessed by biochemical, psychometric, and radiologic methods. J Thorac Cardiovasc Surg 87:99, 1984

22. Furlan AJ, Sila CA, Chimowitz MI, Jones SC: Neurologic complications related to cardiac surgery. Neurol Clin 10:145, 1992

23. Brillman J: Central nervous system complications in coronary artery bypass graft surgery. Neurol Clin 11:475, 1993

24. Townes BD, Bashein G, Hornbein TF, et al: Neurobehavioral outcomes in cardiac operations. J Thorac Cardiovasc Surg 98:774, 1989

25. Kartchner MM, McRae LP: Carotid occlusive disease as a risk factor in major cardiovascular surgery. Arch Surg 117:1086, 1982

26. Gardner TJ, Horneffer PJ, Manolio TA, et al: Major stroke after coronary artery bypass surgery: changing magnitude of the problem. J Vasc Surg 3:684, 1986

27. Brener BJ, Brief DK, Alpert J, et al: The risk of stroke in patients with asymptomatic carotid stenosis undergoing cardiac surgery: a follow-up study. J Vasc Surg 5:269, 1987

28. Moody DM, Bell MA, Challa VR, et al: Brain microemboli during cardiac surgery or aortography. Ann Neurol 28:477, 1990

29. Gibbon JH Jr: Application of a mechanical heart and lung apparatus to cardiac surgery. Minn Med 37:171, 1959

30. Kirklin JW, Barratt-Boyes BG: Cardiac Surgery: Morphology, Diagnostic Criteria, Natural History, Techniques, Results, and Indications. 2nd Ed. Churchill Livingstone, New York, 1993

31. Lederman RJ, Breuer AC, Hanson MR, et al: Peripheral nervous system complications of coronary artery bypass graft surgery. Ann Neurol 12:297, 1982

32. Tomlinson DL, Hirsch IA, Kodali SV, et al: Protecting the brachial plexus during median sternotomy. J Thorac Cardiovasc Surg 94:297, 1987

33. Vahl CF, Carl I, Muller-Vahl H, Struck E: Brachial plexus injury after cardiac surgery. J Thorac Cardiovasc Surg 102:724, 1991

34. Vander Salm TJ, Cutler BS, Okike ON: Brachial plexus injury following median sternotomy. Part II. J Thorac Cardiovasc Surg 83:914, 1982

35. Wong BI, McLean RF, Naylor CD, et al: Central-nervous-system dysfunction after warm or hypothermic cardiopulmonary bypass. Lancet 339:1383, 1992

36. Chandler KW, Rozas CJ, Kory RC, Goldman AL: Bilateral diaphragmatic paralysis complicating local cardiac hypothermia during open heart surgery. Am J Med 77:243, 1984

37. Markland ON, Moorthy SS, Mahomed Y, et al: Postoperative phrenic nerve palsy in patients with open-heart surgery. Ann Thorac Surg 39:68, 1985

38. Werner RA, Geiringer SR: Bilateral phrenic nerve palsy associated with open-heart surgery. Arch Phys Med Rehabil 71:1000, 1990

39. Wilcox PG, Pare PD, Pardy RL: Recovery after unilateral phrenic injury associated with coronary artery revascularization. Chest 98:661, 1990

40. De Vita MA, Robinson LR, Rehder J, et al: Incidence and natural history of phrenic neuropathy occurring during open heart surgery. Chest 103:850, 1993

41. Chenoweth DE, Cooper SW, Hugli TE, et al: Complement activation during cardiopulmonary bypass. N Engl J Med 304:497, 1981

42. Wsmonsa LH Jr, Soxena NC, Hellyer P, et al: Relationship between platelet count and cardiotomy suction return. Ann Thorac Surg 25:306, 1978

43. Addonizio VP Jr, Smith JB, Strous JF III, et al: Thromboxane synthesis and platelet secretion during cardiopulmonary bypass with bubble oxygenator. J Thorac Cardiovasc Surg 79:91, 1980

44. Lee WH, Krumbhoar D, Fonkalsrud EW, et al: Denaturation of plasma proteins as a cause of morbidity and death for intracardiac operations. Surgery 50:29, 1961

45. Butler J, Rocker GM, Westaby S: Inflammatory response to cardiopulmonary bypass. Ann Thorac Surg 55:552, 1993

46. Coffey CE, Massey EW, Roberts KB, et al: Natural history of cerebral complications of coronary artery bypass graft surgery. Neurology 33:1416, 1983

47. Reed GL, Singer DE, Picard EH, DeSanctis RW: Stroke following coronary-artery bypass surgery. A case-control estimate of the risk from carotid bruits. N Engl J Med 319:1246, 1988

48. Shaw PJ, Bates D, Cartlidge NEF, et al: An analysis of factors predisposing to neurological injury in patients undergoing coronary bypass operations. Q J Med 72:633, 1989

49. Galbreath C, Salgado ED, Furlan AJ, et al: Central nervous system complications of percutaneous transluminal coronary angioplasty. Stroke 17:616, 1986

50. Hise JH, Nipper ML, Schnitker JC: Stroke associated with coronary artery bypass surgery. AJNR 12:811, 1991

51. Yokote H, Itakura T, Funahashi K, et al: Chronic subdural hematoma after open heart surgery. Surg Neurol 24:520, 1985

52. Song XL, Wang C, Yang XD, Zhang C: Diabetes insipidus caused by epidural hematoma as a complication of extracorporeal circulation. Int J Cardiol 5:219, 1984

53. Humphreys RP, Hoffman HJ, Mustard WT, et al: Cerebral hemorrhage following heart surgery. J Neurosurg 43:671, 1975

54. Criado A, Dominguez E, Carmona J, et al: Hypoglycemic coma after cardiac surgery. Crit Care Med 12:409, 1984

55. Hiramatsu Y, Sakakibara Y, Mitsui T, et al: Clinical features of hypernatremic hyperosmolar delirium following open heart surgery. Nippon Kyobu Geka Gakkai Zasshi 39:1945, 1991

56. Gonzalez-Santos JM, Gonzalez-Santos ML, Vallejo JL: Acute obstructive hydrocephalus: an unusual complication after cardiopulmonary bypass. Thorac Cardiovasc Surg 34:201, 1986

57. Dubin WR, Field HL, Gastfriend DR: Postcardiotomy delirium: a critical review. J Thorac Cardiovasc Surg 77:586, 1979

58. Juolasmaa A, Outakoski J, Hirvenoja R, et al: Effect of open heart surgery on intellectual performance. J Clin Neuropsychol 3:181, 1981

59. van der Mast RC, Fekkes D, Moleman P, Pepplinkhuizen L: Is postoperative delirium related to reduced plasma tryptophan? Lancet 338:851, 1991

60. Heller SS, Frank KA, Malm JR, et al: Psychiatric complications of open-heart surgery. N Engl J Med 283:1015, 1970

61. Smith LW, Dimsdale JE: Postcardiotomy delirium: conclusions after 25 years? Am J Psychiatry 146:452, 1989

62. DeLeon S, Ilbawi M, Arcilla R, et al: Choreoathetosis after deep hypothermia without circulatory arrest. Ann Thorac Surg 50:714, 1990

63. Fagan KJ, Lee SI: Prolonged confusion following convulsions due to generalized nonconvulsive status epilepticus. Neurology 40:1689, 1990

64. Marini SG, Rook JL, Green RF, Nagler W: Spinal accessory nerve palsy: an unusual complication of coronary artery bypass. Arch Phys Med Rehabil 72:247, 1991

65. Parsonnet V, Karasakalides A, Gielchinsky I, et al: Meralgia paresthetica after coronary bypass surgery. J Thorac Cardiovasc Surg 101:219, 1991

66. Lavee J, Schneiderman J, Yorav S, et al: Complications of saphenous vein harvesting following coronary artery bypass surgery. J Cardiovasc Surg 30:989, 1989

67. Horn KL, Abouav J: Right vocal-cord paralysis after open-heart operation. Ann Thorac Surg 27:344, 1979

68. Plasse HM, Mittleman M, Frost JO: Unilateral sudden hearing loss after open heart surgery: a detailed study of seven cases. Laryngoscope 91:101, 1981

69. Aguayo AJ: Neuropathy due to compression and entrapment. p. 688. In Dyck PJ, Thomas PK, Lambert EH (eds): Peripheral Neuropathy. 1st Ed. Vol 1. WB Saunders, Philadelphia, 1975

70. Hogan JC, Briggs TP, Oldershaw PJ: Guillain-Barré

syndrome following cardiopulmonary bypass. Int J Cardiol 35:427, 1992

71. Segredo V, Caldwell JE, Matthay MA, et al: Persistent paralysis in critically ill patients after long-term administration of vecuronium. N Engl J Med 327:524, 1992

72. Witt NJ, Zochodne DW, Bolton CF, et al: Peripheral nerve function in sepsis and multiple organ failure. Chest 99:176, 1991

73. Shaw PJ, Bates D, Cartlidge NEF, et al: Neuro-ophthalmological complications of coronary artery bypass graft surgery. Acta Neurol Scand 76:1, 1987

74. Blauth CI, Arnold JV, Schulenberg WE, et al: Cerebral microembolism during cardiopulmonary bypass. J Thorac Cardiovasc Surg 95:668, 1988

75. Shahian DM, Speert PK: Symptomatic visual deficits after open heart operations. Ann Thorac Surg 48:275, 1989

76. Hoyt WF, Walsh FB: Cortical blindness with partial recovery following acute cerebral anoxia from cardiac arrest. Arch Ophthalmol 60:1061, 1958

77. Tusa RJ, Kaplan PW, Hain TC, Naidu S: Ipsiversive eye deviation and epileptic nystagmus. Neurology 40:662, 1990

78. Slavin ML, Budabin M: Pituitary apoplexy associated with cardiac surgery. Am J Ophthalmol 98:291, 1984

79. Cooper DM, Bazaral MG, Furlan AJ, et al: Pituitary apoplexy: a complication of cardiac surgery. Ann Thorac Surg 41:547, 1986

80. Laloux P, Osseman M: Visual hallucinations on eye closure after cardiovascular surgery. J Clin Neuro Ophthalmol 12:242, 1992

81. Schmidt R, Fazekas F, Offenbacher H, et al: Brain magnetic resonance imaging in coronary artery bypass grafts: a pre- and postoperative assessment. Neurology 43:775, 1993

82. Gilston A: Brain damage after cardiac surgery. Lancet 1:1323, 1986

83. van der Linden J, Casimir-Ahn H: When do cerebral emboli appear during open heart operations? A transcranial Doppler study. Ann Thorac Surg 51:237, 1991

84. Stephenson LW, MacVaugh H, Edmunds LH: Surgery using cardiopulmonary bypass in the elderly. Circulation 58:250, 1978

85. Lynn GM, Stefanko K, Reed JF, et al: Risk factors for stroke after coronary artery bypass. J Thorac Cardiovasc Surg 104:1518, 1992

86. Weinstraub WS, Jones EL, Craver J, et al: Determinants of prolonged length of hospital stay after coronary bypass surgery. Circulation 80:276, 1989

87. Glower DD, Christopher TD, Milano CA, et al: Performance status and outcome after coronary artery bypass grafting in persons aged 80 to 93 years. Am J Cardiol 70:567, 1992

88. Salomon NW, Page US, Bigelow JC, et al: Coronary artery bypass grafting in elderly patients: comparative results in a consecutive series of 469 patients older than 75 years. J Thorac Cardiovasc Surg 101:209, 1991

89. Jones EL, Craver JM, Michalik RA, et al: Combined carotid and coronary operations: when are they necessary? J Thorac Cardiovasc Surg 87:7, 1984

90. Matar AF: Concomitant coronary and cerebral revascularization under cardiopulmonary bypass. Ann Thorac Surg 41:431, 1986

91. Babu SC, Pravin MS, Sing BM, et al: Coexisting carotid stenosis in patients undergoing cardiac surgery: indications and guidelines for simultaneous operations. Am J Surg 150:207, 1985

92. Nussmeier NA, Arlund C, Slogoff S: Neuropsychiatric complications after cardiopulmonary bypass: cerebral protection by a barbiturate. Anesthesiology 64:165, 1986

93. Hertzer NR, Loop FD, Beven EG, et al: Surgical staging for simultaneous coronary and carotid disease: a study including prospective randomization. J Vasc Surg 9:455, 1989

94. Faggioli GL, Curl GR, Ricotta JJ: The role of carotid screening before coronary artery bypass. J Vasc Surg 12:724, 1990

95. von Reutern G-M, Hetzel A, Birnbaum D, Schlosser V: Transcranial Doppler ultrasonography during cardiopulmonary bypass in patients with severe carotid stenosis or occlusion. Stroke 19:674, 1988

96. Landercasper J, Merz BJ, Cogbill TH, et al: Perioperative stroke risk in 173 consecutive patients with a past history of stroke. Arch Surg 125:986, 1990

97. Rorick MB, Furlan AJ: Risk of cardiac surgery in patients with prior stroke. Neurology 40:835, 1990

98. Taylor GJ, Malik SA, Colliver JA, et al: Usefulness of atrial fibrillation as a predictor of stroke after isolated coronary artery bypass grafting. Am J Cardiol 60:905, 1987

99. Wareing TH, Davila-Roman VG, Barzilai B, et al: Management of the severely atherosclerotic ascending aorta during cardiac operations: a strategy for detection and treatment. J Thorac Cardiovasc Surg 103:453, 1992

100. Bar-El Y, Goor DA: Clamping of the atherosclerotic ascending aorta during coronary artery bypass operations: its cost in strokes. J Thorac Cardiovasc Surg 104:469, 1992

101. Blauth CI, Cosgrove DM, Webb BW, et al: Atheroembolism from the ascending aorta: an emerging problem in cardiac surgery. J Thorac Cardiovasc Surg 103:1104, 1992

102. Ribakove GH, Katz ES, Galloway AC, et al: Surgical implications of transesophageal echocardiography to

grade the atheromatous aortic arch. Ann Thorac Surg 53:758, 1992

103. Wareing TH, Davila-Roman VG, Daily BB, et al: Strategy for the reduction of stroke incidence in cardiac surgical patients. Ann Thorac Surg 55:1400, 1993

104. Ridley PD, Ledingham SJ, Lennox SC, et al: Protein C deficiency associated with massive cerebral thrombosis following open heart surgery. J Cardiovasc Surg 31:249, 1990

105. Camerlingo M, Finazzi G, Casto L, et al: Inherited protein C deficiency and nonhemorrhagic arterial stroke in young adults. Neurology 41:1371, 1991

106. Hobson RW, Weiss DG, Fields WS, et al: Efficacy of carotid endarterectomy for asymptomatic carotid stenosis. N Engl J Med 328:221, 1993

107. Moore WS: Carotid endarterectomy for prevention of stroke. West J Med 159:37, 1993

108. Wong DHW: Perioperative stroke. Part II: Cardiac surgery and cardiogenic embolic stroke. Can J Anaesth 38:471, 1991

109. Forsman M, Olsnes BT, Semb G, Steen PA: Effects of nimodipine on cerebral blood flow and neuropsychological outcome after cardiac surgery. Br J Anaesth 65:514, 1990

110. Albers GW, Goldberg MP, Choi DW: N-methyl-D-aspartate antagonists: ready for clinical trial in brain ischemia? Ann Neurol 25:398, 1989

111. Malone M, Prior P, Scholtz CL: Brain damage after cardiopulmonary by-pass: correlations between neurophysiological and neuropathological findings. J Neurol Neurosurg Psychiatry 44:924, 1981

112. Bolsin SNC: Detection of neurological damage during cardiopulmonary bypass. Anaesthesia 41:61, 1986

113. Jones SJ: Investigation of brachial plexus traction lesions by peripheral and spinal somatosensory evoked potentials. J Neurol Neurosurg Psychiatry 42:107, 1979

114. Grattan MT, Moreno-Cabral CE, Starnes VA, et al: Eight-year results of cyclosporine-treated patients with cardiac transplants. J Thorac Cardiovasc Surg 99:500, 1990

115. Hunt S, Billingham M: Long-term results of cardiac transplantation. Annu Rev Med 42:437, 1991

116. Keogh AM, Kaan A: The Australian and New Zealand Cardiothoracic Organ Transplant Registry: first report 1984–1992. Aust NZ J Med 22:712, 1992

117. Schober R, Hermann MM: Neuropathology of cardiac transplantation: survey of 31 cases. Lancet 1:962, 1973

118. Hotson JR, Pedley TA: The neurological complications of cardiac transplantation. Brain 99:673, 1976

119. Hotson JR, Enzmann DR: Neurologic complications of cardiac transplantation. Neurol Clin 6:349, 1988

120. Sila CA: Spectrum of neurologic events following cardiac transplantation. Stroke 20:1586, 1989

121. Gilmore RL: Seizures and antiepileptic drug use in transplant patients. Neurol Clin 6:279, 1988

122. Conti DJ, Rubin RH: Infection of the central nervous system in organ transplant recipients. Neurol Clin 6:241, 1988

123. Britt RH, Enzmann DR, Remington JS: Intracranial infection in cardiac transplant recipients. Ann Neurol 9:107, 1981

124. Burton JR, Zachary JB, Bessin R, et al: Aspergillosis in four renal transplant patients: diagnosis and effective treatment with amphotericin B. Ann Intern Med 77:383, 1972

125. Luft BJ, Naot Y, Araujo FG, et al: Primary and reactivated toxoplasma infection in patients with cardiac transplants. Ann Intern Med 99:27, 1983

126. Navia BA, Petito CK, Gold JWM, et al: Cerebral toxoplasmosis complicating the acquired immune deficiency syndrome: clinical and neuropathological findings in 27 patients. Ann Neurol 19:224, 1986

127. Renold C, Sugar A, Chave J-P, et al: Toxoplasma encephalitis in patients with the aquired immunodeficiency syndrome. Medicine (Baltimore) 71:224, 1992

128. Montero CG, Martinez AJ: Neuropathology of heart transplantation: 23 cases. Neurology 36:1149, 1986

129. Hjall WA, Martinez AJ, Dummer JS, et al: Nocardial brain abscess: diagnostic and therapeutic use of stereotactic aspiration. Surg Neurol 28:114, 1987

130. Alsep SG, Cobbs CG: Pseudo-Allescheria boydii infection of the central nervous system in a cardiac transplant recipient. South Med J 79:383, 1986

131. Pollard RB, Arvin AM, Gamberg P, et al: Specific cell-mediated immunity and infections with herpes viruses in cardiac transplant recipients. Am J Med 73:679, 1982

132. Helle TL, Britt RH, Colby T: Primary lymphoma of the central nervous system. J Neurosurg 60:94, 1984

133. Patchell RA: Primary central nervous system lymphoma in the transplant patient. Neurol Clin 6:297, 1988

134. Starzl TE, Nalesnik MA, Porter KA, et al: Reversibility of lymphomas and lymphoproliferative lesions developing under cyclosporin-steroid therapy. Lancet 1:583, 1984

135. Walker RW, Brochstein JA: Neurologic complications of immunosuppresive agents. Neurol Clin 6:261, 1988

136. Adair JC, Woodley SL, O'Connell JB, et al: Aseptic meningitis following cardiac transplantation: clinical characteristics and relationship to immunosuppressive regimen. Neurology 41:249, 1991

4

Neurological Manifestations of Congenital Heart Disease

Gerald S. Golden

Congenital heart defects are among the most common serious congenital anomalies, occurring with an incidence of between 7 and 10 per 1,000 live births.[1] The relative frequency of specific malformations is indicated in Table 4-1.

During the prenatal period the oxygen needs of the fetus are supplied through the placenta. The fetal circulation utilizes shunts through the ductus venosus, ductus arteriosus, and foramen ovale; congenital malformations of the heart are not associated at this time with the pathophysiological problems that they present during postnatal life. Any developmental abnormality of the heart that is severe enough to compromise the fetal circulation is likely to lead to fetal death.

Many of these lesions require corrective surgery; and although surgical morbidity and mortality have been remarkably reduced, operations often must be performed with hypothermia and cardiac arrest or with cardiovascular bypass. Thus, the risk of complications involving the central nervous system remains high.

Even without surgery, there is a great risk of impairment of brain function because of the abnormal hemodynamics produced by the cardiac defect, chronic hypoxia in some conditions, and embolic and thrombotic complications. This chapter concentrates on these issues. Specific syndromes in which there are developmental malformations involving both the brain and the heart are not discussed.[2]

NEUROPATHOLOGY

The study of neuropathological changes in the brains of patients with congenital heart disease is complicated by the variety of cardiac lesions and the fact that many of the patients studied at autopsy have had surgery at some time in the past. Damage to the white matter is most common in children under 3 months of age.[3] The major abnormality in these infants is a leukoencephalopathy with the accumulation of astrocytes, most severe in the subependymal and subpial regions and the deep white matter. Focal areas of white matter necrosis are present as well, and are most obvious in the subependymal region. These lesions do not appear to be embolic in origin but are due to a reduction of capillary blood flow and the formation of fibrin thrombi. Lipid-containing glial cells and macrophages are seen also.

Gliotic changes in the white matter appear to increase with age.[4] Thirty-nine percent of those infants who die before 4 months of age show these changes, and the changes are present in 72 percent of those who are older than 1 year at the time of death. Older children also have a higher incidence of gliosis in the anterior temporal lobes.

Older patients are more likely to show either focal neuronal damage or bilateral symmetrical cortical necrosis. Hypoxia, acidosis, and hypotension seem to

Table 4-1 Relative Frequency of Congenital Heart Lesions

Lesion	Percent
Cyanotic lesions	
Tetralogy of Fallot	10
Transposition of the great vessels	6
Other cyanotic lesions	6
Acyanotic lesions	
Isolated ventricular septal defect	25
Atrial septal defect	10
Patent ductus arteriosus	10
Coarctation of aorta	6
Pulmonary stenosis	5
Aortic stenosis	5
Atrioventricular canal	4
Other acyanotic lesions	5
Rare or complex lesions	8

(Modified from Moller J: Acyanotic congenital heart disease. Ch. 25, p. 2. In Kelley VC (ed): Practice of Pediatrics. Harper & Row, Philadelphia, 1987, with permission.)

be involved in the etiology of these lesions.[3] A watershed distribution of necrosis is seen in those patients with long-standing hypotension, and cardiac arrest is associated with necrosis in the pyramidal layer of the hippocampus. Evidence of embolization is rare, even following cardiac catheterization.

Embolic strokes can occur in patients with either cyanotic or acyanotic congenital heart disease and in those with abnormalities of the valves, especially the mitral and aortic valves. Ischemia develops acutely and is usually severe; progressive narrowing of the artery, as is seen with thrombotic lesions, does not occur, and collateral circulation does not develop. Normal thrombolytic processes then degrade the embolus, allowing reentry of blood into the damaged area. The integrity of the blood vessels and blood-brain barrier is compromised from the anoxia, and the area then becomes hemorrhagic.

Primary venous thromboses, common in infants with cyanotic congenital heart disease, are associated with dramatic pathological changes. There is severe cerebral edema and multiple areas of hemorrhagic infarction. Ischemic damage to neurons is also present. Patients may also have evidence of both subarachnoid and subdural bleeding.

In patients with hypoplastic left heart syndrome, the major lesions correlate with specific physiological abnormalities.[5] Intracranial hemorrhage is associated with low diastolic blood pressure, thrombocytopenia, and cardiac surgery. Hypoxic-ischemic lesions follow hypoxia, hypercapnia, and cardiac surgery. Fifty-five percent of these infants have a normal brain or only minimal findings at the time of autopsy.

Cerebral abscesses also complicate cyanotic congenital heart disease, especially in older children and young adults. The abscesses, usually solitary, may be present in any area of the brain, but most typically involve the cerebral hemispheres. Initially, cerebritis is present. The brain is edematous and hyperemic, and an inflammatory infiltrate is seen microscopically. The center of the infected area then liquefies, and fibrosis and gliosis begin and then encapsulate the abscess. Abscesses tend to track through white matter and may rupture into the ventricular system or, less commonly, the subarachnoid space before encapsulation occurs. This complication is usually lethal.

CYANOTIC CONGENITAL HEART DISEASE

The neurological complications of cyanotic congenital heart disease are related directly to the pathophysiology of the cardiac lesions. The cyanosis is an indicator of arterial oxygen desaturation resulting either from a right-to-left shunt or, in the case of transposition of the great arteries, from two largely independent circulatory loops with desaturated blood recirculating through the systemic circulation. The chronic arterial desaturation stimulates the release of erythropoietin from the kidney, which, in turn, causes increased production of red blood cells with resultant polycythemia. When the hematocrit rises to levels of 65 to 70 percent, hyperviscosity develops and leads to an increase in vascular resistance and decreased tissue perfusion, which then decreases the delivery of oxygen to the tissues. As infants have limited iron stores and limited ability to absorb dietary iron, there is also relative anemia with microcytosis and hypochromia, a situation that also compromises tissue oxygenation.

Hyperviscosity is also a factor in the etiology of thrombosis of cerebral veins and dural sinuses. These complications are most common in children under 1 year of age. Paradoxically, these patients also may have associated abnormalities in coagulation mechanisms, so subarachnoid and subdural bleeding often accompany these venous thromboses. The coagulopathy is a result of thrombocytopenia, hypofibrinogenemia, and increased fibrinolysis.

Children with severe hyperviscosity, especially those with hematocrits above 65 percent, also tend to have more symptoms related to their cardiac disease. They have decreased exercise tolerance and an increase in cyanotic spells. Cardiac failure may also be more common. If treatment of the problem appears to be necessary, the recommended procedure is an exchange transfusion, using albumin or fresh frozen plasma as the replacement fluid. Phlebotomy without replacement of the circulating blood volume is not tolerated well.

A second pathophysiological feature placing the patient at high risk for neurological complications is the loss of the filtering action of the pulmonary vasculature that results from the right-to-left shunt. This situation has the potential of allowing thrombi and bacteria in the venous circulation to gain access to the arterial circulation and the blood supply of the brain. Both cerebral infarction and brain abscess can result. The only specific treatment is surgical closure of the shunt. Most cases of bacterial endocarditis can be prevented by the institution of antimicrobial prophylaxis prior to any procedure (e.g., dental surgery) that is associated with a high risk of bacteremia.

Based on these considerations, it can be seen that the neurological problems found in patients with cyanotic congenital heart disease can be caused by chronic hypoxia, circulatory abnormalities resulting from the polycythemia, and loss of the pulmonary filter because of the right-to-left shunt. In addition, these children usually have frequent intercurrent illnesses and decreased exercise tolerance, and they may not be able to share the life experiences of their peers, a situation that may adversely affect developmental progress as well.

Cyanotic Spells

Sudden spells of increased cyanosis and dyspnea occur frequently in children with tetralogy of Fallot and may be seen as well in those with tricuspid atresia or any condition in which there is a right-to-left shunt and severe pulmonary tract outflow obstruction. The spells occur most frequently during the first and second years of life and may be precipitated by feeding or crying. They are usually brief but may be prolonged for an hour or more. Severe spells are associated with syncope; seizure-like motor activity may be associated if the anoxic episode is severe or sufficiently prolonged. Cerebrovascular accidents also may follow a spell but are uncommon. The pathophysiological mechanism is not clear, but spasm of the right ventricular outflow tract has been postulated. Hyperpnea also may trigger spells.

Treatment of a cyanotic spell consists of putting the child in the knee-chest position and administering oxygen. It has been noted that many children with tetralogy of Fallot spontaneously assume a squatting position, which accomplishes the same ends. If the episode continues, administration of morphine is useful. A prolonged spell also produces a severe acidosis, and intravenous administration of sodium bicarbonate is indicated at that time. Propranolol has been used prophylactically, but its use may be limited by the development of bradycardia.

Venous Thrombosis

Children with cyanotic congenital heart disease are susceptible to primary venous or venous sinus thrombosis, especially during the first year of life.[6,7] The child typically is polycythemic, but red blood cell indices show hypochromia and microcytosis. The onset, often precipitated by dehydration, is calamitous, with seizures, hemiparesis or bilateral hemipareses, and increased intracranial pressure. The level of consciousness is impaired, and the child may become comatose.[7] Examination of the cerebrospinal fluid shows elevated pressure and signs of subarachnoid hemorrhage. If the venous infarction is extensive, the mortality rate is high.

Treatment is difficult, and if the thrombosis is extensive, the mortality rate is high. General supportive treatment includes correcting dehydration and treating any systemic infection that might be present. Overhydration should be avoided, as severe cerebral edema is usually present. The latter is treated, if necessary, with endotracheal intubation and hyperventilation, the judicious use of osmotic agents such as mannitol, and the administration of corticosteroids. Surgical removal of the thrombus has been suggested but has never been proved to be a useful technique. Experience with newly developed thrombolytic agents is limited, and no conclusions concerning their usefulness are possible at this time. Anticoagulants should be avoided because of the underlying coagulopathy in many of these patients.

Arterial occlusions are less common but also are most likely to occur in the child with severe polycythemia.[7] Like venous thrombosis, they are a rare complication in older children.

Brain Abscess

Brain abscess is the most common acute neurological complication of cyanotic congenital heart disease. A number of etiological hypotheses have been put forward, most of which point to predisposing hemodynamic risk factors, including passage of bacteria through the right-to-left shunt, paradoxical septic emboli, and cerebral embolization or thrombosis with subsequent infection of the infarcted area by blood-borne bacteria. Microorganisms enter the circulation several times daily, following such everyday activities as tooth-brushing. In the presence of a right-to-left intracardiac shunt, the bacteria are not removed in the pulmonary capillary bed.[8]

Abscesses are extremely rare in children under 2 years of age[8]; they have a bimodal peak incidence between 4 and 7 years of age and between 20 and 30 years of age.[9] Among adults, men are affected more frequently than women, but this discrepancy is not seen in children. The most common underlying lesion is tetralogy of Fallot, which accounts for 60 percent of cases; transposition of the great vessels accounts for an additional 10 percent.[9] It is most unusual to find brain abscesses in children with acyanotic congenital heart disease.[9]

Cerebral abscess can present with the acute onset of focal neurological signs, seizures, increased intracranial pressure, or any combination of these findings. Frequently the clinical characteristics are more suggestive of a stroke or space-occupying lesion than of an infection.

Examination of the cerebrospinal fluid reveals elevated pressure and increased protein concentration. Pleocytosis is variable. Neuroimaging helps to differentiate infarction from abscess. Multiple abscesses are present in approximately 20 percent of patients.[9]

Initial treatment of brain abscess depends heavily on antibiotics, which must cover a wide spectrum of organisms, as abscesses often have a mixed bacterial flora. Anaerobic organisms commonly are present,

either as the sole infectious agent or as part of a mixed infection. If bacterial endocarditis is present, unusual organisms may be found. The drugs must be given in high doses to ensure that adequate concentrations penetrate to the abscess and surrounding brain. The duration of treatment should be sufficient to sterilize the abscess and cure the underlying bacterial endocarditis, if this is present.

Brain abscesses produce severe cerebral edema, and management of this problem is of utmost importance. Seizures commonly occur and should be treated vigorously. Seizures are the most common long-term complication and may require continuous anticonvulsant prophylaxis.

The role of surgery in treatment has been a source of controversy. It now appears that many abscesses can be cured with the use of antibiotics alone or with antibiotics and aspiration of the lesion.[10] This regimen reduces the risk of surgical removal of brain tissue that is edematous but would be functional following resolution of the infection. If the abscess produces a significant mass effect that cannot be controlled with physiological and pharmacological treatment methods, surgery may be life-saving, although the mortality rate is high. Another controversial area is the need for delayed surgery following sterilization of the abscess, with removal of the abscess wall if the initial treatment consisted of antibiotics alone or antibiotics and aspiration. Despite optimal treatment, the mortality rate is high, ranging between 25 and 50 percent in early series; it was 37 percent in a more recent report.[9]

Because of the evidence that abscesses may form in a previously infarcted brain, it has been recommended that antibiotic therapy be begun in any patient with congenital heart disease who develops focal neurological signs or seizures.[11] If repeated neuroimaging studies do not show evidence of abscess formation over the course of the following week, the antibiotics can be discontinued.

Developmental Outcome

Children with cyanotic congenital heart disease have a lower intelligence level, a higher incidence of mental retardation, delayed motor development, and deficits in perceptual function and motor coordination when compared to those with acyanotic lesions.[12–15] Risk factors include prolonged hypoxia, congestive heart failure, the failure of surgery to correct the hypoxia, growth failure, and intercurrent neurological complications such as stroke or infection of the central nervous system.[14] The differences in intelligence quotient (IQ) are not related to the child's age or to the degree of general illness and disability, but seem to relate specifically to the presence of cyanosis.[15] Group differences in mean IQ are approximately 10 points. The incidence of mental retardation is approximately 6.5 percent in the cyanotic group of children and 2.2 percent in the acyanotic group.

Psychosocial variables also relate to developmental outcome and adaptation. The most significant are the socioeconomic status of the family and the life stresses at the time of evaluation.[14] The overall outcome seems to be reasonably good for the child with a single risk event, either medical or psychosocial, but is less good if two or more risk factors are present.

Cyanotic children have delayed motor development compared to acyanotic children; this is especially noted by the age at which they become capable of independent walking. The two groups also differ in that a higher proportion of cyanotic children have abnormalities on neurological examination and abnormal electroencephalograms than acyanotic patients.

Surgery that improves the cardiovascular status of the child and reduces or eliminates the hypoxia may improve cognitive function. Patients with tetralogy of Fallot who undergo a Blalock procedure have IQ scores 10 points higher than those of the unoperated group: an average increase of 4.5 points in IQ is seen following surgery.[16] Children with transposition of the great vessels and an intact ventricular septum demonstrate IQ scores that are inversely related to the age at surgical correction. In addition to the effect on the overall IQ, similar significant findings are present for tests of visual and auditory association.[17] These data have been interpreted as demonstrating progressive impairment in cognitive function in children with uncorrected transposition of the great vessels. There is not a similar correlation between age of repair and cognitive status in children with acyanotic congenital heart disease.

ACYANOTIC CONGENITAL HEART DISEASE

A number of entities are subsumed by the term *acyanotic congenital heart disease,* and each is associated with complications that arise from specific patho-

physiological features. The presence of a left-to-right shunt can be associated with cerebral embolization, which results from thrombi in the region of the defect of the ventricular septum or on malformed mitral or aortic valves. These valvular abnormalities commonly accompany septal defects. Although brain abscess is much less common than in patients with cyanotic lesions, it can occur if the emboli are infected.

Congenital lesions of the mitral or aortic valves without associated septal defects also can lead to the development of thrombi and subsequent embolization. Infection of these thrombi with the development of subacute bacterial endocarditis is a long-term risk in these patients. Antibiotic prophylaxis prior to dental surgery is mandatory.

Aortic or muscular subaortic stenosis may be so severe that cardiac output is insufficient to provide adequate cerebrovascular perfusion during exertion. This may produce attacks of syncope (Adams-Stokes attacks), sometimes associated with seizure-like motor activity. If these incidents occur, cardiac surgery with correction of the aortic outlet obstruction or placement of a prosthetic valve must be carried out.

Artificial valves in children do not entirely eliminate the risk of cerebrovascular accidents.[18] In children less than 15 years of age, the use of a xenograft is associated with a risk of stroke of 4 percent per patient-year; mechanical valves have a risk of 2 percent per patient-year.

Intracavitary cardiac tumors (e.g., atrial myxomas) are extremely rare during childhood. If they occur in the left atrium, signs similar to those of mitral valve dysfunction are seen. Embolization to the brain with one or more episodes of stroke is the most common neurological complication. The diagnosis can be suspected on auscultation of the heart and is easily proved with echocardiography.

Disturbances of Cardiac Rhythm

Congenital atrioventricular block may occur as an isolated lesion or in association with other forms of congenital heart disease. It also occurs frequently as a complication of cardiac surgery, especially following repair of a ventricular septal defect or atrioventricular canal. The patient may have Adams-Stokes attacks consisting of episodes of dizziness followed by syncope. In less severe cases, spells of dizziness may be the sole manifestation. Similar episodes occur in the sick-sinus syndrome in which bradycardia and supraventricular tachycardia alternate in unpredictable fashion.

Two hereditary syndromes are associated with a prolonged Q-T interval on the electrocardiogram. The patient often presents with episodes of syncope with or without some convulsive activity, although sudden death may occur and often is found in the family history. The syncope or sudden death probably is caused by ventricular fibrillation. The Jervell-Lange-Nielsen syndrome is the association of a prolonged Q-T interval and congenital deafness. In the Romano-Ward syndrome there is no hearing loss.[19,20]

Developmental Outcome

Children with acyanotic lesions do not seem to suffer the same progressive loss of cognitive function that has been documented for those with transposition of the great vessels.[17] Some authors have reported that acyanotic children with a history of congestive heart failure demonstrate lower IQ scores and more difficulties in tasks of perceptual motor and fine motor coordination than those without such a history.[13] These children are not as compromised as those with cyanotic congenital heart disease, however. Other investigators have documented the difference in cognitive function between the cyanotic and acyanotic groups but have not demonstrated an adverse effect of cardiac failure in either group.[15]

COMPLICATIONS OF CARDIAC SURGERY

Data concerning improvement in intelligence following surgery for acyanotic congenital heart disease are not as clear as those for cyanotic lesions. Preoperative testing shows generalized impairment of functioning similar to that following anoxia.[21] Improvement following surgery may be due to practice effects.

Acute neurological impairment following surgery is most common in children in whom cardiopulmonary bypass is used and is mainly the result of either embolism or hypoxia and ischemia.[22] Seizures occur in 9 percent of children following surgery that involves profound hypothermia and circulatory arrest.[23] In two-thirds of these patients there is no obvious etiology for the seizures, which occur 24 to 48 hours following surgery. There is no relation to the type of cardiac lesion or to the duration of the hypothermia and circulatory arrest. These seizures respond rapidly to anticonvulsant therapy, and the children have neither seizures nor neurological abnormalities on long-term follow-up. There have been some reports, however, that suggest a correlation between the duration of cardiopulmonary bypass and the occurrence of seizures. It has also been reported that focal seizures may be difficult to stop, despite the use of large doses of antiepileptic medication.[22]

Surgery for coarctation of the aorta, especially if clamping of collateral vessels or prolonged cross-clamping of the aorta is required, may be followed by an acute myelopathy. Recovery is poor in most patients, with residual paraparesis and bladder dysfunction.

Anticoagulation is required during and following surgery and can be associated with hemorrhage into the brain, subarachnoid space, or subdural space. Patients with cyanosis and polycythemia have abnormalities of their coagulation mechanisms and are particularly prone to develop this complication.

Although, as noted, there can be an increase in the patient's measured IQ following the correction of a cardiac lesion associated with cyanosis, the operation itself may be associated with damage to the central nervous system and impairment of cognitive function. The frequency of these problems is difficult to ascertain because of differences in the cardiac lesions represented in many series, differences in the surgical techniques and duration of cardiac bypass, and lack of adequate neuropsychological studies pre- and postoperatively.

Deep hypothermia was used during surgery for complex cardiac defects in a group of 49 children; in one-half of the cases cardiac arrest was used also.[24] Study of the survivors (81 percent) showed that there was a negative correlation between the early postoperative cerebral blood flow and the duration of surgery but no abnormality in cerebral uptake of either glucose or oxygen. Follow-up (limited to interviews) for 3 years gave no evidence of neurological symptoms or psychological disorders. Three children may have had problems with fine motor skills.

A more extensive study compared children whose operations were performed under conditions of profound hypothermia and cardiac arrest with those whose operations were performed with moderate hypothermia and continuous cardiopulmonary bypass.[25] Sibling controls were used for each group. Those treated with total cardiac arrest showed significantly lower IQ scores than their siblings as a result of deficits in verbal, quantitative, and general cognitive abilities. The authors estimated a loss of 0.53 IQ points per minute of arrest time.

Surgical correction of congenital heart lesions using cardiopulmonary bypass and deep hypothermic circulatory arrest may be followed by choreoathetosis.[26] This tends to be transient and less severe in younger patients. Older children have more severe and persistent choreoathetosis and a high mortality rate. Factors associated with development of severe symptoms include cyanotic heart disease with systemic-to-pulmonary collaterals and excessive duration of the cooling period. A syndrome of choreoathetosis associated with oral-facial dyskinesias, hypotonia, pseudobulbar signs, and affective changes also may occur following surgery with profound hypothermia and circulatory arrest.[27]

Phrenic nerve paralysis following surgery may reduce breathing capacity to the extent that assisted ventilation is required. The risk of this complication is highest in patients undergoing cardiopulmonary bypass.[28]

Major catastrophic events occur during surgery, although they are uncommon. Hypoxic-ischemic encephalopathy can be avoided, especially if the child is observed closely postoperatively for problems with insufficient cardiac output or arrhythmias. Air embolism is always a hazard when cardiopulmonary bypass is instituted or discontinued or when the heart is opened at surgery, and it may be an important cause of postoperative stroke.

REFERENCES

1. Moller J: Acyanotic congenital heart disease. Ch. 25, p. 2. In Kelley VC (ed): Practice of Pediatrics. Harper & Row, Philadelphia, 1987
2. Moller JH, Anderson RC: 1,000 consecutive children with a cardiac malformation with 26- to 37-year follow-up. Am J Cardiol 70:661, 1992
3. Bozoky B, Bara D, Kertesz E: Autopsy study of cerebral complications of congenital heart disease and cardiac surgery. J Neurol 231:153, 1984
4. Gilles FH, Leviton A, Jammes J: Age-dependent changes in white matter in congenital heart disease. J Neuropathol Exp Neurol 32:179, 1973
5. Clancy RR, Glauser TA, Rorke LB, Weinberg P: Acquired neuropathological lesions associated with the hypoplastic left heart syndrome. Ann Neurol 18:388, 1985
6. Parsons CG, Astley R, Burrows FGO, Singh SP: Transposition of great arteries: a study of 65 infants followed for 1 to 4 years after balloon septostomy. Br Heart J 33:725, 1971
7. Cottrill CM, Kaplan S: Cerebral vascular accidents in cyanotic congenital heart disease. Am J Dis Child 125:484, 1973
8. Takeshita M, Kagawa M, Yonetani H, et al: Risk factors for brain abscess in patients with congenital cyanotic heart disease. Neurol Med Chir (Tokyo) 32:667, 1992
9. Kagawa M, Takeshita M, Yato S, Kitamura K: Brain abscess in congenital cyanotic heart disease. J Neurosurg 58:913, 1983
10. Aebi C, Kaufmann F, Schaad UB: Brain abscess in childhood—long-term experiences. Eur J Pediatr 150:282, 1991
11. Kurlan R, Griggs RC: Cyanotic congenital heart disease with suspected stroke: should all patients receive antibiotics? Arch Neurol 40:209, 1983
12. Feldt RH, Ewert JC, Stickler GB, Weidman WH: Children with congenital heart disease: motor development and intelligence. Am J Dis Child 117:281, 1969
13. Silbert A, Wolff PH, Mayer B, et al: Cyanotic heart disease and psychological development. Pediatrics 43:192, 1969
14. O'Dougherty M, Wright FS, Garmezy N, et al: Later competence and adaptation in infants who survive severe heart defects. Child Dev 54:1129, 1983
15. Aram DM, Ekelman BL, Ben-Shachar G, Levinsohn MW: Intelligence and hypoxemia in children with congenital heart disease: fact or artifact? J Am Coll Cardiol 6:889, 1985
16. Finley KH, Buse ST, Popper RW, et al: Intellectual functioning of children with tetralogy of Fallot: influence of open-heart surgery and earlier palliative operations. J Pediatr 85:318, 1974
17. Newburger JW, Silbert AR, Buckley LP, Fyler DC: Cognitive function and age at repair of transposition of the great arteries in children. N Engl J Med 310:1495, 1984
18. Wada J, Yokoyama M, Hashimoto A, et al: Long-term follow-up of artificial valves in patients under 15 years old. Ann Thorac Surg 29:519, 1980

19. Bricker TJ, Garson AS, Gillette PC: A family history of seizures associated with sudden cardiac deaths. Am J Dis Child 138:866, 1984

20. Horn CA, Beekman RH, Dick M, Lacina SJ: The congenital long QT syndrome: an unusual cause of childhood seizures. Am J Dis Child 140:659, 1986

21. Zuo C, Yang L: Neuropsychological status of patients with congenital and rheumatic heart diseases: preoperative and postoperative comparison. Int J Neurosci 26:59, 1985

22. Ferry PC: Neurologic sequelae of cardiac surgery in children. Am J Dis Child 141:309, 1984

23. Ehyai A, Fenichel GM, Bender HW: Incidence and prognosis of seizures in infants after cardiac surgery with profound hypothermia and circulatory arrest. JAMA 252:3165, 1984

24. Settergren G, Ohqvist G, Lundberg S, et al: Cerebral blood flow and cerebral metabolism in children following cardiac surgery with deep hypothermia and circulatory arrest: clinical course and follow-up of psychomotor development. Scand J Cardiovasc Surg 16:209, 1982

25. Wells FC, Coghill S, Caplan HL, Lincoln C: Duration of circulatory arrest does influence the psychological development of children after cardiac operation in early life. J Thorac Cardiovasc Surg 86:823, 1983

26. Wong PC, Barlow CF, Hickey PR, et al: Factors associated with choreoathetosis after cardiopulmonary bypass in children with congenital heart disease. Circulation 86, suppl:II118, 1992

27. Wical BS, Tomasi LG: A distinctive neurologic syndrome after induced profound hypothermia. Pediatr Neurol 6:202, 1990

28. Mok Q, Ross-Russell R, Mulvey D, et al: Phrenic nerve injury in infants and children undergoing cardiac surgery. Br Heart J 65:287, 1991

5

Neurological Manifestations of Acquired Cardiac Disease and Dysrhythmias and of Interventional Cardiology

Colin D. Lambert

The neurological manifestations of acquired cardiac disease fall into several categories:

1. The sudden onset of a focal neurological deficit due to occlusion of a cerebral artery by an embolus that has arisen within the heart (cardiogenic embolism)
2. Transient, self-limiting episodes of generalized cerebral ischemia that occur as a consequence of brief failures of cardiac output, due to either rhythm disturbances or outflow obstruction, resulting in syncopal events
3. Generalized cerebral ischemia consequent upon a more prolonged period of circulatory arrest
4. The complications of invasive techniques for the investigation or management of cardiac disease

The major exceptions to these generalizations occur with atrial fibrillation, which is associated with embolus formation rather than syncopal disturbances, and with chronic sinoatrial disorder, which predisposes to both syncopal and embolic disturbances. Increasing interest has recently come to be focused upon cardiac dysrhythmias that are secondary to a cerebral event, either vascular or epileptic.

Topics that are the specific focus of other chapters within this book are not considered here. In this chapter the term *stroke* is used to mean the sudden onset of a focal neurological deficit of ischemic origin. *Cerebral embolus* is used where the deficit is thought to be of embolic origin. The term *cardiogenic embolism* is reserved for events in which the embolic occlusion is considered to be the result of a cardiac disorder. This chapter will address three major situations: (1) cardiogenic embolism, (2) dysrhythmias and their manifestations (syncope), and (3) interventional processes.

CARDIOGENIC EMBOLISM

In 1992, it could still be stated that "the lack of valid criteria for the clinical diagnosis of cardiogenic embolism is a major problem in both patient care and research."[1] In the absence of a "gold standard" for clinical diagnosis, features suggesting cardioembolism are usually derived from analysis of the clinical presentation and computed tomography (CT) scan features of acute ischemic strokes that occur in patients with cardiac abnormalities known to predispose to thrombus formation. These have been divided into high- and medium-risk groups,[2] which are shown in Table 5-1.

It has been suggested that stroke can be classified into five major groups—large artery atherosclerosis, cardioembolism, small artery occlusion (lacune), stroke of other determined etiology, and stroke of undetermined etiology.[2] The level of confidence with which a stroke can be attributed to a specific process has shown wide variations in recent large studies. In a prospective analysis of 1,273 ischemic infarcts in the United States, a surprising 508 cases (40 percent) were

Table 5-1 Cardiac Abnormalities Predisposing to Thrombus Formation and Embolism

High-risk sources
　　Mechanical prosthetic valve
　　Mitral stenosis with atrial fibrillation
　　Atrial fibrillation (other than lone atrial fibrillation)
　　Left atrial/atrial appendage thrombus
　　Sick sinus syndrome
　　Recent myocardial infarction (less than 4 weeks)
　　Left ventricular thrombus
　　Dilated cardiomyopathy
　　Akinetic left ventricular segment
　　Atrial myxoma
　　Infective endocarditis

Medium-risk sources
　　Mitral valve prolapse
　　Mitral annulus calcification
　　Mitral stenosis without atrial fibrillation
　　Left atrial turbulence
　　Atrial septal aneurysm
　　Patent foramen ovale
　　Atrial flutter
　　Lone atrial fibrillation
　　Bioprosthetic cardiac valves
　　Nonbacterial thrombotic endocarditis
　　Congestive heart failure
　　Hypokinetic left ventricular segment
　　Myocardial infarction (after 4 weeks but within 6 months)

(From Adams HP, Bendixen BH, Kappelle LJ, et al: Classification of subtype of acute ischemic stroke: definitions for use in a multicenter clinical trial. Stroke 24:35, 1993, with permission.)

labeled as infarcts of undetermined cause. By contrast, among the first 1,000 patients from the Lausanne Stroke Registry, no cause of infarction was found in only 8 percent; in another 18 percent, the sole determined etiology was "a minor arterial lesion."[3,4] In the US study, 9 percent were considered of atherosclerotic origin, compared with 43 percent of cases so classified in the Lausanne study. Both studies, however, concluded that approximately 20 percent of strokes were of cardioembolic origin. Coexistent pathology (i.e., arterial and heart disease in the same patient) compounds the problem, and this can be seen in as many as one-quarter of those patients with a potential cardiac source of embolism. In the Lausanne series, a similar proportion of those with a potential cardiac source of embolism showed a lacunar syndrome.[5]

Differences may exist in nonwhite populations. In Asians, hemorrhage and lacunar infarction appear more prominent.[6,7] Atrial fibrillation remains an equally significant contributor to fatal stroke in elderly Japanese.[8]

In the young stroke population (generally regarded as patients who have their first stroke before the age of 45 years), the annual incidence of stroke also varies throughout the world from a low of 9 to a high of 40 per 100,000 population. The lowest values have been found in Italy and England and the highest in Japan and Libya.[9] A similar proportion of strokes in this age group were considered cardioembolic: 17 percent in a study from Spain,[9] and 23 percent in a Swiss population.[10] In this latter series of 202 patients, the 23 percent figure was the same in the group between ages 16 and 30 years and in the group ranging from ages 31 to 45 years. Atrial fibrillation was not seen in any of the younger group, and was reported in only 2 of the older group, which comprised 146 patients.[10] In the largest study reported, 333 young patients were prospectively evaluated after a transient ischemic attack (TIA) or stroke. There was a low prevalence of atrial fibrillation, conventional sources of cardiac emboli were found in 7.5 percent of cases, and an additional 24 percent of cases were attributed to "potential" cardiac causes (with mitral valve prolapse and chronic ischemic heart disease accounting for the majority of these cases).[11] A French study attributed 12 percent of infarcts to cardiac embolism.[12]

Comparison of etiological factors for TIAs in younger as opposed to older patients disclosed that only two cardiac sources were encountered more frequently in the younger age group: valvular heart disease and mitral valve prolapse. The study was a prospective one over a 10-year period, with 75 of the 798 patients in the younger age group.[13]

Clinical Features

Analysis of neurological clinical criteria, taken from the older literature, for the diagnosis of embolic stroke produced 10 features regarded as suggestive. Application of these criteria to strokes thought to be of cardioembolic origin demonstrated that "only rapidity and loss of consciousness at onset were associated with the presence of a cardiac source of embolus to a significant degree. Although these symptoms were highly specific for a cardiac source of embolus, they were not sensitive. A distinct clinical neurological profile from the symptoms and mode of onset was not identified."[14]

A subsequent study confirmed these observations and also found that evidence of systemic embolism occurred significantly more often with a high-risk cardiac source, but only in 5 percent of cases. Earlier work had suggested that previous TIA in the ipsilateral territory was a negative predictor for cardiogenic embolism, but this was not confirmed[15]; similarly TIAs in another territory have not been found suggestive of a potential cardiac source of embolism.[5]

Features on the neurological examination that are statistically significant with regard to a high-risk cardiac source are diminished level of consciousness at onset, aphasia, neglect, or a visual field deficit.[5,16]

Emboli may lodge in either the anterior (carotid) or posterior (vertebrobasilar) circulation. The anterior circulation is affected four times more commonly than the posterior. Least likely to be affected are the entire internal carotid artery, deep branches of the middle cerebral artery, and brainstem.[4] Although the posterior circulation is less commonly affected, studies of the mechanism of infarction in specific territories (e.g., those of the posterior inferior cerebellar artery and superior cerebellar artery) implicate cardiogenic embolism in 50 percent of cases.[17] A cardioembolic mechanism occurred in 67 percent of cases with isolated cerebellar infarcts (i.e., without concomitant brainstem or occipital infarcts).[18] Embolism is also a common mechanism of infarction within the territory of the posterior cerebral artery.[19]

Investigation

The first neurological investigation in stroke is usually a CT scan of the head. This was found to be normal in 38 percent of cases in one series of 1,254 cases.[3] Analysis of those in the "high-risk" group for cardioembolism (244 cases) disclosed that these infarcts were more likely to involve one-half of a lobe or more, or the infarcts involved both superficial and deep structures. Deep small infarcts were underrepresented and were considered to have a predictive value of 90 percent for the absence of a major cardiac source.[1] Similar conclusions were drawn in an earlier study—namely, that the mechanism underlying lacunes is rarely if ever embolic and that infarctions in the pial (superficial) artery territory are usually indicative of an embolic mechanism.[20]

The potential for embolic infarcts to show hemorrhagic transformation remains a source of concern when anticoagulant therapy has to be considered. A hemorrhagic infarct was seen on the initial CT scan of 6 percent of patients in a series of 244 cases, none of whom were on anticoagulants.[1] In a series of scans performed within 48 hours of onset, the figure rose to 24 percent.[21] With prospective follow-up scanning, a total of 40 percent was found at 1 month.[22] With the more sophisticated technology of magnetic resonance imaging (MRI), the figure rose to nearly 70 percent at 3 weeks. Both the latter studies showed that larger infarcts were more liable to demonstrate hemorrhagic transformation, with a figure of 90 percent for infarcts with a volume greater than 10 cm^3.[23] Thus the key factors that determine whether hemorrhagic transformation is seen appear to be the time of the study, the size of the infarct, and the technology applied. The age of the patient may also be a factor, in that elderly patients (those over 70 years of age) may be more liable to hemorrhagic transformation.[22]

At this time, angiography remains the definitive method for assessing structural abnormalities of the carotid circulation. Use of this invasive procedure requires recognition of the associated risks. A review of 15 studies (8 prospective) concluded that the mortality rate was very low (less than 0.1 percent), but that the risk of a neurological complication (TIA or stroke) was approximately 4 percent and that of a permanent neurological deficit was 1 percent.[24] These figures, therefore, require consideration before such studies are obtained, especially in an era where noninvasive studies have gained increasing importance. The characteristic angiographic appearance of an embolic occlusion is that of a proximal, meniscus-like filling defect in an artery that is otherwise normal and lacks evidence of atherosclerotic change. Emboli tend to fragment. In a study of 142 patients who underwent angiography, the initial procedure, performed at a median of 1.5 days after the precipitating event, revealed an occlusion in 82 percent. Follow-up angiography, at a median of 20 days, showed reopening of the vessels in 95 percent of the repeat studies.[22] Distal branch occlusions are often also considered to be embolic manifestations.

In young patients with stroke, although embolic features may be identified angiographically in up to 40 percent of cases, an underlying cardiac cause was found in only 13 and 16 percent in two recent studies comprising 251 patients.[25,26]

The role of MRI is still being defined. It is more sensitive than CT scanning in the early detection of infarction. Initial changes have been noted within the first 3 hours of a stroke and consist of increased signal intensity in the gray matter on proton density–weighted images.[27] Magnetic resonance angiography will probably play an increasing role in noninvasive diagnosis.[18] CT scanning remains the method of choice to rule out intracerebral bleeding.[28]

Echocardiography has come to occupy a preeminent place in the structural evaluation of the heart. Transthoracic echocardiography (TTE) is noninvasive but has limitations that can be overcome by using the transesophageal route (TEE). For the latter procedure, the patient is usually mildly sedated and topical anesthetic is applied to the posterior pharynx. The use of anticoagulants is considered a relatively minor contraindication. Antibiotics are used as for the prophylaxis of endocarditis, but their efficacy remains unproved. A history of dysphagia or esophageal disease is a contraindication to TEE. The technique employed (TEE or TTE) depends on the area to be visualized (Table 5-2). In some respects the two procedures can be considered complementary.[29]

The yield from conventional (TTE) echocardiography is generally very low for patients who do not have clinical evidence of heart disease. Criteria vary in different studies. An overview suggests a range of abnormality at about 1.5 percent (range, 0 to 6 percent).[30] In contrast, the yield from TEE is high—e.g., 39 percent potential cardiac sources of

Table 5-2 Echocardiographic Evaluation of the Heart

Type of Echocardiography	Preferred Clinical Applications
Transthoracic (TTE)	Left ventricular thrombus Myxomatous mitral valvopathy with prolapse Mitral annular calcification Mitral stenosis Aortic stenosis Aortic valve vegetations
Transesophageal (TEE)	Atrial myxoma Atrial septal aneurysm Atrial septal defect Atrial thrombus Atrial appendage thrombus Patent foramen ovale Mitral valve vegetations Pathology in the aortic arch

embolism in patients with no clinical heart disease.[31] Comparisons of the two methods show that TEE identified atrial septal aneurysm, with or without a patent foramen ovale, significantly more frequently. Another study found widespread thoracic aortic atherosclerotic plaques by TEE but not TTE in 32 of the 72 patients.[32]

An algorithm has been suggested for the use of echocardiography in stroke. If the patient is a candidate for anticoagulation or surgery and is under the age of 45 years, TEE should be performed. In the older patient with no clinical cardiac signs, TEE is also recommended. In the presence of clinical cardiac signs with atrial fibrillation, echo is not required unless it is needed to clarify cardiac pathology. In the absence of atrial fibrillation, TTE is performed; if it is negative, TEE should be considered.[29]

The role of other, noninvasive technologies, such as transcranial Doppler for the detection of solid cerebral emboli, remains to be established.[33] In patients with patent foramen ovale, an unexpectedly high percentage have been shown to have emboli both in the basilar and in the middle cerebral territories (75 percent).[34]

It remains necessary for the clinician to balance extensive investigation against its impact on patient management, usually the justification for lifelong anticoagulant therapy and its consequent risks. In sev-

Table 5-3 Major Cardiac Sources of Embolic Stroke

Source	Percent of Embolic Strokes
Nonvalvular atrial fibrillation	45
Ischemic heart disease	
Acute myocardial infarct	15
Ventricular aneurysm	10
Rheumatic heart disease	10
Prosthetic cardiac valves	10
Other sources	10
Total	100

(From Cerebral Embolism Task Force: Cardiogenic brain embolism. Arch Neurol 43:71, 1986, with permission.)

eral situations there are no established guidelines for management. The onus remains on the clinician to determine the significance of "potential" sources of emboli and their implications for management.

Aggregate clinical data suggest that, in the developed western world, the major cardiac sources of embolic stroke are as shown in Table 5-3.[35]

ATRIAL FIBRILLATION

Chronic atrial fibrillation without valvular disease is an age-related disorder. In The Framingham Study, after 30 years of follow-up, age-specific incidence rates increased from 0.2 per 1,000 for ages 30 to 39 years to 39 per 1,000 for ages 80 to 89. There was a corresponding increase in the proportion of strokes associated with this dysrhythmia, from 7 percent in the age group 50 to 59 to 36 percent in the age group 80 to 89 years.[36]

It is well established that the risk of stroke in atrial fibrillation is related to the presence or absence of associated structural cardiac disease. In the absence of rheumatic heart disease (nonvalvular atrial fibrillation) there is a 5-fold increase in stroke incidence, whereas—in association with rheumatic heart disease—this increase is 17-fold.[37] Only in "lone" atrial fibrillation (i.e., fibrillation in the absence of overt cardiovascular disease or precipitating illness) developing in middle age is the prognosis relatively benign. Follow-up, at 15 years, disclosed a rate of thromboembolic events of 0.55 per 100 person-years.[38] This was equivalent to 1.3 percent of the patients experiencing a stroke on a cumulative actuarial basis. There was no difference among the groups of patients with isolated, recurrent, or chronic atrial fibrillation.[38]

It is now well established, from four studies, that anticoagulation significantly reduces the risk of stroke in atrial fibrillation. A fifth, Canadian, study was terminated prior to completion because the other studies had shown clear evidence of benefit (Table 5-4).

Each study was randomized and had a control group, but two studies also incorporated an aspirin arm. In the Veterans Administration study, all patients were men. The target level of anticoagulation varied and ranged from a target international normalized ratio (INR) of between 1.4 and 4.2. There were differences in outcome measures, although all included stroke. These studies also differed in the percentage of patients with intermittent atrial fibrillation, which ranged between 0 and 34 percent. No differences in thromboembolic risk were found between the groups with intermittent and constant atrial fibrillation. In the Danish study, the age of patients, at 75 years, was significantly higher than in the other studies, in which the mean age was between 66 and 68 years. There was no statistically significant increase in major bleeding events in either the warfarin- or aspirin-treated patients.

Aspirin, in a dosage of 325 mg daily, provided a 42 percent reduction of relative risk compared to placebo[40]; but at a dosage of 75 mg per day, no benefit was found.[39] In the Boston study, the aspirin group, derived from nonrandomized "treatment received" analyses, did worse than the placebo group.[44]

There remains skepticism among physicians concerning the cost-benefit ratio of anticoagulant therapy, especially in the elderly, in whom the response to warfarin appears to be exaggerated.[45,46] This skep-

Table 5-4 Effect of Anticoagulation on Risk of Stroke in Patients With Atrial Fibrillation

Site/Origin of Study	Percent Risk Reduction	Reference Number
Denmark	66	39
San Antonio	69	40
Boston area	85	41
United States, Veterans Administration	71	42
Canada	53	43

Table 5-5 Cumulative Risk of Hemorrhage in Anticoagulated Patients Over an 8-Year Period[a]

Year	Life-Threatening Bleed (%)	Serious Bleed (%)
1	1	12
2	2	20
4	5	28
8	9	40

[a] There was a recurrence of bleeding in 32 percent of patients with life-threatening or serious bleeds.
(Based on data from Fihn and co-workers.[47])

ticism is supported by what tends to be forgotten after large controlled trials: the number of patients excluded. The figure for two recent studies was a remarkable 93 percent.[40,42] Of 26,358 patients screened, only 1,901 were entered into the trials. One major reason for noninclusion was a contraindication to anticoagulation. The Canadian[43] and Danish studies[39] excluded 74 and 61 percent of those screened. The clinician must therefore be equally thoughtful in deciding which patients should be anticoagulated on a long-term basis.

Analysis of a cohort of patients attending five anticoagulation clinics documented the cumulative risk of bleeding over an 8-year period (Table 5-5).[47] Points that emerged were that the incidence of bleeding and thromboembolic complications remained approximately constant, with a prothrombin time ratio (PTR) of 1.3 to 2.0, but it increased sharply above or below those limits (i.e., thromboembolism was much more likely with a PTR of less than 1.3). No increase in bleeding complication was found related to any specific indication for therapy, including cerebrovascular disease. Older patients did not have a greater risk of bleeding. The highest risk of bleeding was seen during the first 3 months of therapy; then it tended to plateau somewhat. Of particular note was the high risk of recurrence (32 percent) in those patients who experienced one serious bleed. It was also noted that patients who had more than four dosage adjustments per year bled 25 percent more often than those who had fewer adjustments.

It remains necessary to individualize management strategies for specific patients, taking into account compliance and other medical conditions. Stratification of risk may help the decision process. This was attempted in four of the studies referred to above, but predictors varied. The Danish study found that only

a history of previous myocardial infarction increased stroke risk.[48] The Veterans Administration study found angina to be a risk factor.[42] The Boston group found that age, clinical heart disease, and mitral annular calcification increased stroke risk.[41] The Stroke Prevention in Atrial Fibrillation Investigators identified the clinical features of congestive heart failure, hypertension, and previous thromboembolism as independent risk factors. In the absence of these features, rates of thromboembolism were 2.5 percent per year; in the presence of 2 or 3 risk factors, this increased to 17.6 percent. Echocardiography, to assess left ventricular dysfunction and size of the left atrium, altered risk stratification in 38 percent of those without clinical risk factors.[49,50]

A scheme of stratification of risk of thromboembolism in patients with atrial fibrillation has been proposed, pooling these and other data, as shown in Table 5-6.[51]

Table 5-6 Risk of Thromboembolism in Patients with Atrial Fibrillation

High risk (5 percent or more per year)
Valvular heart disease (e.g., mitral stenosis, prosthetic mechanical valves)
Recent onset of congestive heart failure (within 3 months)
Prior thromboembolism
Thyrotoxicosis
Systolic hypertension
Severe left ventricular dysfunction by echocardiography
Demonstration of cardiac thrombus

Moderate risk (3 to 5 percent per year)
Age of 60 years or more
Mitral annulus calcification
Diuretic therapy
Silent cerebral infarction by CT brain scan

Low risk (less than 3 percent per year)
Lone atrial fibrillation (chronic or paroxysmal)
Age of 60 years or less

Uncertain risk
Diabetes mellitus
Left atrial enlargement
Coexistent carotid artery disease
Recent onset (rather than chronic) atrial fibrillation
Reduced cerebral blood flow

(From Kelley RE: Rationale for antithrombotic therapy in atrial fibrillation. Neurol Clin 10:233, 1992, with permission.)

The conclusions reached by the Third Consensus Conference on antithrombotic therapy[52] were as follows:

1. It is strongly recommended that long-term oral warfarin therapy (INR 2.0 to 3.0) be used in patients with atrial fibrillation who are eligible for anticoagulation except in those less than 60 years of age with no associated cardiovascular disease ("lone atrial fibrillation").

2. Patients with atrial fibrillation who are poor candidates for anticoagulation therapy should be treated with aspirin at a daily dosage of 325 mg.

CARDIOVERSION IN ATRIAL FIBRILLATION

Review of 22 series published over a 30-year period shows an overall risk of embolism of 1.5 percent (55 of 3,798 patients).[53] Figures have changed little in recent years, with an incidence rate of 1.3 percent.[54] An earlier prospective study noted a difference in patients who were not anticoagulated; they showed 5.3 percent embolic events compared to 0.8 percent among those on anticoagulants.[55] It does not appear, at this time, that TEE prior to cardioversion is adequate to determine which cases require anticoagulants. No left atrial thrombus had been seen on precardioversion TEE in 40 patients; among these, 4 had emboli 1 to 7 days after cardioversion. It was suggested that cardioversion itself may promote thrombus formation.[56] It appears that up to 3 weeks may be required for atrial mechanical activity to recover.[57] It is therefore "strongly recommended that warfarin therapy (INR of 2.0 to 3.0) should be given for 3 weeks before elective cardioversion of patients who have been in atrial fibrillation for more than 2 days and be continued until normal sinus rhythm has been maintained for 4 weeks."[52]

PAROXYSMAL ATRIAL FIBRILLATION

An early (1930) report of 200 patients with paroxysmal auricular fibrillation documented a benign prognosis with regard to cerebral events. Only one stroke was reported; another patient experienced a femoral embolus. Complete loss of consciousness in association with a paroxysm occurred in eight patients; faintness or giddiness was common. Duration of follow-up was not specifically stated; it was for 10 years or more in some cases, and as many as 200 paroxysms were thought to have occurred in one patient. The majority of patients had underlying heart disease. Conversion to chronic atrial fibrillation occurred in 28 percent.[58]

Recent studies show a much less favourable prognosis. Arterial emboli (nearly 60 percent of which were cerebral) occurred in 79 of 426 patients (18.5 percent). Chronic atrial fibrillation developed in 33 percent of the patients.[59] A later review concluded that the risk of embolism was less in paroxysmal as opposed to chronic atrial fibrillation and found that the number of paroxysms was of no significance with regard to risk of embolization.[60] Other studies have failed to show a difference between paroxysmal and chronic cases of atrial fibrillation.[40,41,61–63] At this time it is therefore recommended that patients with intermittent atrial fibrillation "should be considered" for antithrombotic therapy.[52]

CHRONIC SINOATRIAL DISORDER

In a study comparing age- and sex-matched controls suffering from atrioventricular heart block and those with chronic sinoatrial disorder, a prevalence of systemic embolism was found in 16 percent of those with sick-sinus syndrome compared to 1.3 percent of those with atrioventricular block.[64] Other studies have disclosed similar figures; patients with the "bradytachy" form of the disorder appear to be particularly at risk.[65,66] Insertion of a pacemaker does not protect against embolic phenomena. In one series, 6 out of 10 strokes developed after pacemaker insertion. Only one of these patients was anticoagulated at the time.[67] Concern has been raised that, although ventricular pacing provides symptomatic relief, this modality may worsen the underlying disease process by increasing the rate at which atrial fibrillation, congestive heart failure, and thromboembolism occur.[68] A literature review showed that, during a $2\frac{1}{2}$ year observation period, atrial fibrillation occurred in 22.3 percent of cases after ventricular pacing, compared with 4 percent in those with an atrial demand pacemaker. There was a corresponding difference in systemic embolism in the two groups, at 13 percent and 1.6 percent, respectively.[69] A retrospective, nonrandomized study did show that single-chamber ventricular pacing carried a more than 40 percent increased risk for both total and cardiovascular death, but this difference was of borderline statistical significance.[70] It was concluded that a large randomized study was necessary to confirm whether physiological pacing provided a substantial reduction in mortality as compared with ventricular pacing.[70] Recommendations have recently been published concerning the most appropriate choice of pacemaker.[71] Inappropriate choices may lead to the so-called pacemaker syndrome, which includes the "neurological" symptoms of dizziness, near-fainting, and confusion. A spectrum of cardiac symptoms may also be observed.[72] No specific recommendations with regard to anticoagulation have been made, but it is evident that, since atrial fibrillation may develop, patients with this disorder should be considered for such therapy.

THYROTOXICOSIS

Atrial fibrillation is said to complicate thyrotoxicosis in between 10 and 30 percent of patients.[73] Occult thyrotoxicosis should also be considered as a cause of "idiopathic atrial fibrillation."[74] Embolic complications occur in between approximately 10 and 20 percent of those patients who develop fibrillation in association with thyrotoxicosis. These events occur under three sets of conditions: (1) during the phase of acute thyrotoxicosis, (2) at the time of reversion of atrial fibrillation to sinus rhythm, and (3) in a euthyroid patient who remains in atrial fibrillation.[75,76] If reversion from atrial fibrillation to sinus rhythm occurs, it will probably do so within 4 months of the euthyroid state being reached, but it is unlikely to occur if the fibrillation was present for 13 months or more prior to reaching a euthyroid status.[77] Warfarin therapy is therefore recommended in patients with thyrotoxicosis who are in atrial fibrillation and should be continued for 4 weeks after conversion to normal sinus rhythm has occurred.[52]

CARDIOMYOPATHY

This heterogeneous group of disorders has in common dysfunction, primarily affecting heart muscle, that is not attributable to hypertension, ischemia, or valvular disease. There is considerable variation throughout the world in the prevalence and etiology of the cardiomyopathies—disorders that are more commonly encountered in underdeveloped and tropical countries than in the developed world.

In South India, cardiomyopathy was noted to account for 12 percent of cardiac admissions.[78] In South Africa, among Zulus, the disorder was found in 14 percent of 1,000 consecutive cases of heart disease.[79] In Uganda, endomyocardial fibrosis, producing a restrictive cardiomyopathy, accounted for 15 percent of deaths due to congestive cardiac failure.[80] At autopsy, intracardiac thrombosis was common and was, in fact, found three times more frequently than in subjects with rheumatic heart disease. Embolic problems were found in 15 percent of 117 cases, the descending order of frequency being to the lungs, spleen, kidneys, and brain.[81] In western countries, the corresponding disorder is that of Loffler's endocarditis, also known as the hypereosinophilic syndrome.[82,83] A male predominance is evident in western but not tropical cases. Although mural thrombosis, either atrial or ventricular, is common at autopsy, clinically evident events are seen in only 6 percent of cases. In South America, Chagas' disease (American trypanosomiasis) has been estimated to affect, in its chronic form, up to 18 million people. Population movements will result in increasing recognition of that disorder in the United States.[84] The characteristic cardiac feature is aneurysmal dilatation at the apex of the left ventricle, with thrombus formation.[85] This is often associated with endocardial thrombosis. Stroke has been documented in association with this process and may affect individuals in early adult life, one series showing a mean patient age of 33 years.[86] In spite of the common occurrence of this process, stroke has not been documented in this disorder in any extensive or systematic manner.[87]

In the United States, the most common form of cardiomyopathy is of the dilated (or congestive) type.[88] A clinicopathological correlation showed evidence of embolic events (systemic or pulmonary) in 60 percent of instances. Curiously, patients with atrial fibrillation had a lower frequency both of embolic events and of intracardiac thrombi,[89] confirming an earlier report that severity of the cardiomyopathy was the major risk factor of embolism.[90] Current recommendations "argue strongly" for the use of warfarin in these patients.[52] Hypertrophic cardiomyopathy is of relatively recent recognition, but since 1957 some 46 different terms have been used to describe variations of this process.[91] Cerebral complications are much less common than in the dilated form, so that a recent overview makes no reference to neurological events.[92] Atrial fibrillation may develop in this disorder, in which case the risk of embolism is increased and cerebral events may be the presenting feature.[93,94] An early paper, which reported eight cases, showed a possible "neurological" presentation in three: a boy of 14 who had a blackout, a 19-year-old man who had a stroke during reversion of atrial fibrillation to normal sinus rhythm, and a 25-year-old man who had a series of convulsions, from which he died.[95]

MYOCARDIAL INFARCTION

Three large studies in the immediate prethrombolytic era from different countries (Australia,[96] the United States,[97] and Israel[98]) reached similar conclusions concerning the incidence of stroke related to myocardial infarction:

1. The overall risk of stroke is low (1.7, 2.4, and 0.9 percent respectively).
2. Morbidity and mortality are substantially higher in the stroke group.
3. Stroke is more liable to occur in the presence of apical or anterolateral infarcts, rather than the inferior group.
4. The size of the myocardial infarction is a significant factor. In the Australian study, this was reflected by peak elevations of serum creatine kinase to more than 8 times the upper limit of normal. This relationship was not confirmed in the US study, which did, however, note that cardiac pump failure, defined as low cardiac output up to the fifth day, increased the risk of stroke from 4 to 20 percent. In the Israeli study, congestive heart failure and paroxysmal atrial fibrillation were more often present in the stroke (or TIA) group. This study also implicated age as a significant factor.

Most strokes (51 out of the total of 85 in the three series) occurred on or before the fourth day. Echocardiographic studies show that left ventricular thrombi appear mainly between the second and seventh days after an acute myocardial infarct, and this can occur in spite of prophylactic anticoagulation.[99] Thrombi may persist despite anticoagulation, but the risk of embolism is only increased in the first 2 months after a myocardial infarct.[100]

In a prospective study of 94 consecutive patients who had a stroke more than 3 months after a myocardial infarction, it was noted that all had an akinetic left ventricular segment, but thrombus was seen in only 12 percent. In 14 percent of cases, this was the only stroke risk factor identified. Other mechanisms encountered were atrial fibrillation (15 percent), hypertension with lacunar infarction (12 percent), and significant carotid stenosis (21 percent).[101]

The present recommendation, in the absence of thrombolytic therapy, is that, after an acute myocardial infarct, heparin therapy should be initiated and followed by warfarin for 3 months in patients considered to be at increased risk of embolism, either pulmonary or systemic. The high-risk patients are those with severe left ventricular dysfunction, congestive heart failure, a history of previous pulmonary or systemic embolism, echocardiographic evidence of mural thrombosis, or the presence of atrial fibrillation. Because of the recognized increased frequency of mural thrombosis in anterior as opposed to inferior myocardial infarcts, it is also recommended that patients with an anterior Q-wave infarction receive heparin followed by warfarin.[102]

THROMBOLYTIC THERAPY

Concern that the introduction of aggressive thrombolytic therapy for myocardial infarction would result in an increase in stroke was not substantiated by the results of the initial large Italian trial into which nearly 12,000 patients were enrolled. Stroke rate was 0.77 percent in the streptokinase group, compared with 0.92 percent in the control group. An excess of stroke was evident only during the first day after randomization to streptokinase. After this time, patients in the control group had more stroke or TIA events. The study did not include CT scan results.[103] Extended experience from this group, specifically stressing stroke risk rate, found that stroke occurred in 1.14 percent (236 cases) of 20,768 patients. Autopsy or CT scanning enabled the cause of stroke to be identified in 74 percent. Ischemia was the most common mechanism (42 percent), followed by intracerebral hemorrhage (31 percent). Cause remained unknown in 26 percent. Patients receiving recombinant tissue plasminogen activator (t-PA) showed a small but significant excess of stroke.[104] Comparison of four thrombolytic strategies confirmed a slight excess of hemorrhagic stroke in those receiving t-PA and in those receiving combined thrombolytic agents. This excess risk was in the order of 2 to 3 per 1,000 treated.[105] In the four groups, stroke risk rate ranged from a low of 1.22 percent in those treated with streptokinase and subcutaneous heparin to 1.64 percent in those treated with intravenous heparin and both tPA and streptokinase. Overall, it will be noted that these percentages are equal to or less than those documented in recent large prethrombolytic studies of acute myocardial infarction.

RHEUMATIC HEART DISEASE

Extensive experience has accumulated over several decades concerning the association of systemic embolism with rheumatic heart disease. This material was published mostly before the era of CT scans and controlled clinical trials. A 1973 review concisely summarized relevant features.[106] A minimum of 20 percent of patients with rheumatic heart disease experience a thromboembolic complication at some time, and 40 percent of these arterial emboli involve the brain. Embolic events are the cause of death in 16 to 35 percent of adults dying of rheumatic heart disease, and subgroups of patients having a much greater frequency of embolic complication can be identified.

The risk of embolism is substantially increased when atrial thrombosis is present (risk increases from 16 to 41 percent) or atrial fibrillation develops (risk increases from 7 to 30 percent). The proportion of patients developing left atrial thrombosis increases from 9 to 41 percent when atrial fibrillation is present; conversely, 80 percent of patients with atrial thrombosis are in atrial fibrillation. Embolism is most likely to occur when the dominant valvular lesion is that of mitral stenosis, either alone or in combination with aortic valve disease or mitral insufficiency. Isolated aortic valve disease is rarely associated with embolic events. Older patients more frequently have atrial fibrillation, atrial thrombosis, and embolic events.

Studies of atrial thrombosis were initially done by the transthoracic route. This is an insensitive method. Of 293 patients in one study who were to undergo open heart surgery, TTE studies disclosed thrombi in the left atrium in 33. At surgery, this was confirmed in 30 of those cases, but the study had missed 21 additional patients, including all 11 in whom thrombus was located in the left atrial appendage.[107]

Once embolization has occurred, recurrence rate is high, approaching 60 percent.[108] Current recommendations are therefore strongly in favor of the use of long-term warfarin (to prolong the INR to 2.0 to 3.0) in patients with rheumatic mitral valve disease who have a history of systemic embolism or who develop atrial fibrillation, either chronic or paroxysmal. It is also recommended that the same treatment be given to patients in normal sinus rhythm if the left atrial diameter is in excess of 5.5 cm. It is further recommended that if recurrent systemic embolism occurs despite adequate warfarin therapy, the addition of aspirin be considered.[109] The beneficial effect of the addition of aspirin, 100 mg daily, to warfarin has been demonstrated in the context of prosthetic heart valves.[110]

ATRIAL MYXOMA

Atrial myxomas have long been recognized as a cause of cerebral embolism. They are uncommon, one large institution reporting 24 cases over a 50-year period.[111] Classically the presentation is either of cardiac, obstructive, or constitutional symptoms; a primary neurological event is infrequently the presenting problem. Myxomas may occur at any age but are most common between the ages of 30 and 60 years, and some studies show a female preponderance. Echocardiography is the method of choice for diagnostic screening, and the treatment of choice is early surgical resection.[112] A neurological event may be the presenting feature.[113]

MEDIUM-RISK SOURCES OF CARDIAC EMBOLISM

Mitral Valve Prolapse

Mitral valve prolapse is a common abnormality. Using echocardiographic data, The Framingham Study found it in 5 percent of 4,967 unselected subjects. Prevalence was determined by both age and sex. In women, a prevalence as high as 17 percent was found in subjects in their 20s, but this figure declined steadily, to 1 percent, in 80-year-old women. In contrast, prevalence in men remained between 2 and 4 percent throughout adult life.[114]

A causal relationship between mitral valve prolapse

and cerebral ischemic events (stroke or TIA) was first suggested in 1974; a 1987 review of six series, in adults, confirmed the association.[115] Of the 114 patients, 68 were women and 46 men, with an average age range between 37 and 51 years in the different series. Two-thirds of the patients had a stroke; the remaining one-third presented with a TIA. Events recurred in about 20 percent of patients at intervals ranging from months to years.

The prognosis of isolated mitral valve prolapse in children was considered excellent in 119 patients in whom the disorder was identified by auscultation; in most (91 percent) of these, it was confirmed by echocardiography. The mean age at time of diagnosis was 10 years, with a mean follow-up of 7 years. Only one child experienced a stroke, at the age of 10.[116] An early study in adults comprised 760 patients followed up by cardiologists for an average of 2 years. During that time only one patient, an 82-year-old woman, developed a pure motor hemiparesis. In contrast, it was noted that of 43 patients with stroke admitted to the neurology service, 9 showed mitral valve prolapse on echocardiography. In these patients, no evidence of carotid or other cardiac disease was found.[117] During long-term follow-up of 237 adults with echocardiographically documented mitral valve prolapse, 10 (mean age 50 years) sustained a stroke; of these cases, 6 were in atrial fibrillation and showed left atrial enlargement, 2 had other factors predisposing to stroke, and only 2 had no other predisposing factors. Both were women, aged 24 and 34 years respectively.[118] Follow-up was for a mean of 6.2 years. A Dutch study followed 300 patients for a similar period of time. Stroke occurred in 11 patients with an average age of 40 years. Little in the way of clinical details was provided, but they were "not in paroxysmal atrial fibrillation."[119]

Overall it has been calculated that the stroke rate in young adults with mitral valve prolapse is 1 in 6,000 per year.[120] Recommendations are that long-term warfarin be used only in patients with prolapse who have had a documented systemic embolism or are in atrial fibrillation, either chronic or paroxysmal. In the absence of embolic events or atrial fibrillation, prophylaxis is thought to be unjustified; if a TIA or stroke does occur, initial treatment is with aspirin, 325 to 975 mg daily. Ticlopidine would be an alternative.[109]

The association of infective endocarditis with mitral valve prolapse has been documented in several studies. This process represents an alternative mechanism for cerebral events. The absolute risk is low; it has been estimated at 1 person per 1,920 per annum if a systolic murmur is present, declining to 1 in 21,950 in the absence of such a murmur.[121]

Atrial Septal Aneurysm

Atrial septal aneurysm occurs in between 1 and 6 percent of the population. Transesophageal echocardiography has facilitated identification of this abnormality. It is frequently associated with interatrial defects (patent foramen ovale or atrial septal defect) and also occurs in association with mitral valve prolapse.[122] Atrial septal aneurysm has been found more commonly in patients with stroke (20 of 133 cases) than in those without (12 of 277).[123] Stroke or TIA has been noted in up to 25 percent of cases.[124,125] Mechanisms postulated are paradoxical embolization or local thrombus formation related to the defect itself, but the appropriate management for these cases has yet to be established. Surgical repair of the defect or anticoagulation requires consideration.[122]

Patent Foramen Ovale

Patent foramen ovale is a common finding in patients with stroke, with an overall prevalence of 18 percent. In the subgroup of cryptogenic stroke, however, the figure is 31 percent in all age groups even with correction for other recognized risk factors for stroke. Thus this abnormality is considered an independent risk factor for stroke.[126] Both transcranial Doppler and contrast TEE may identify the disorder, but the latter technique is more sensitive.[127] It has been suggested that paradoxical embolism is the mechanism responsible.[128] Other studies have refuted this conclusion.[129]

Left Atrial Spontaneous Echo Contrast

Left atrial spontaneous echo contrast (smoke) may be detected in transesophageal echocardiography and is thought to represent stasis of blood within the left atrium. The finding may thus indicate a predisposition to thrombus formation. It is most commonly encountered in patients with either atrial fibrillation or mitral stenosis and has been found to be highly associated with previous stroke or peripheral embolism in this context.[130]

Mitral Annulus Calcification

Mitral annulus calcification has been shown in an elderly population to be associated with a doubled risk of stroke, but it is unclear whether this relationship is causal or a marker for other risk factors.[131]

Anticoagulation After Cardiogenic Embolism

The purpose of anticoagulant therapy, initially with heparin and then by long-term warfarin, is to prevent recurrence of an embolic event of cardiac origin. The frequently quoted figure of an approximate 12 percent recurrence in the first 2 or 3 weeks seems likely to be an overestimate.[35] The Stroke Data Bank experience was of a 4.3 percent recurrence of cardio-embolic infarction at 30 days; with prospective follow-up for 2 years, the cumulative recurrence rate became 13 percent. Atrial fibrillation was not associated with a higher risk.[132] Another study showed an even lower recurrence rate of 2 percent at 30 days.[133] The risk of death in patients with a cardiac source of embolus was 14 times that of a recurrent stroke—it was therefore concluded that treatment in this group should be directed toward the underlying cardiac process, especially congestive heart failure or myocardial infarction. Independent predictors of recurrent stroke were found to be cardiac valve disease and congestive heart failure.[134]

Because embolic infarcts are often hemorrhagic, there has been concern that conversion into a frank hemorrhage may occur and lead to clinical deterioration. Factors found to increase this possibility in one study were large infarct size and initiation of anticoagulation after CT scanning performed less than 12 hours from presentation.[135] The present recommendation is that in nonhypertensive patients without evidence of hemorrhage on CT scan performed 24 to 48 hours after stroke, immediate anticoagulation should be undertaken; anticoagulation should be delayed for 7 days in those with large infarcts. Continued anticoagulant therapy was shown not to result in clinical deterioration in a small number of patients in whom this therapy was maintained despite CT scan findings of a hemorrhagic infarct.[136]

SYNCOPE

Transient, self-limiting interruptions of cardiac output result in generalized cerebral ischemia, a condition that is termed *syncope* when it results in a loss of consciousness. Syncope is discussed in Chapter 8 but is considered further here with particular regard to its occurrence in patients with acquired cardiac disease and dysrhythmias.

In normal volunteers the effects of acute arrest of the cerebral circulation have been studied by the sudden inflation of a cervical pressure cuff.[137] A consistent sequence of events followed. Subjects noted blurring of vision, with narrowing of the visual fields that progressed to complete loss of vision. They often experienced paresthesias, and consciousness was then lost. On recovery, the subjects felt dazed and somewhat confused; some were unaware that they had lost consciousness. The first objective finding noted by observers was fixation of eye movement, followed by upward turning of the eyes and then loss of consciousness, sometimes followed by generalized motor activity that was reportedly mild and lasted for 6 to 8 seconds. Changes first appeared within 5 to 10 seconds of cuff inflation. Electrocardiograms showed only minimal changes, whereas the electroencephalogram (EEG) showed large slow waves.

A modern study noted that consciousness was lost after 9 or more seconds from induction of a ventricular dysrhythmia (fibrillation or tachycardia).[138] Patients felt distant, dazed, or as if they were "fading out" before loss of consciousness. Motor activity was noted in 10 of 15 episodes, with generalized tonic contraction of axial muscles followed or accompanied by irregular jerking of the extremities, generalized rigidity without clonic activity, or irregular facial movement or eyelid flutter without tonic activity. None of the patients bit their tongues or were incontinent.

During the recovery phase, tonic flexion of the trunk was seen in three patients. Patients remained dazed or confused for up to 30 seconds or more after restoration of the circulation. This study confirmed that motor phenomena occur in association with syncope without corresponding EEG evidence of epileptic discharges. The EEG findings were those of slowing and relative loss of electrocerebral activity. The authors noted variability in EEG findings and poor correlation of these changes with the clinical ones.[138]

The clinical spectrum of abnormalities that occur with generalized ischemia is thus an extended one, ranging from nonspecific "dizziness" through a variety of sensory disturbances including paresthesias and alterations of vision, to loss of consciousness, perhaps with some convulsive features. This has long been recognized in the context of blood donation, where 12 percent of syncopal reactions were shown to have some convulsive features.[139] Confusion may occur on recovery. Focal symptoms are rare with cardiac dysrhythmia. Evaluation of 290 patients who required pacemaker insertion disclosed that only 4 had focal neurological symptoms or signs; among these, only 2 had focal symptoms that could be related to a specific episode of cardiac dysfunction.[140] Rarely, features suggestive of complex partial seizures may be seen.[141]

Syncope is common. In The Framingham Study, at least one syncopal episode had occurred in over 3 percent of patients. The disorder is more common in the elderly, who show a high recurrence rate.[142,143] A recent considered overview of the subject reviews several large series. A cardiac cause was assigned in between 8 and 39 percent of patients, but in some series almost 50 percent of events remain unexplained.[144] The role of psychiatric disorder in syncope may perhaps have been underestimated. Depression and panic disorder should be considered prior to expensive invasive electrodiagnostic test procedures. Suggestive features are younger age group, multiple prodromal symptoms, and frequent episodes of syncope.[145,146] The history and examination remain the cornerstone for diagnosis and will identify the potential cause in 49 to 89 percent of cases.

A cardiac basis for syncope may occur either because of acquired heart disease with aortic tract outflow stenosis or because of intermittent obstruction to outflow, e.g., by a mobile thrombus or tumor in the left atrium.[147,148] The associated cardiac symptoms and signs usually draw attention to the presence of a structural lesion that is readily confirmed by further investigation. A second group of cardiac disturbances resulting in syncope consists of disorders of cardiac rhythm; these are not necessarily associated with structural disease of the heart and are often intermittent. The disorders represent dysfunction of the conduction tissues: the sinoatrial or atrioventricular pathways, or ventricular dysrhythmias.

The association of a slow pulse with syncopal attacks has long been recognized; the term *Adams-Stokes attack* is used for such events, which subsequently came to be associated with atrioventricular block.[149] The slow pulse of the disorder is usually well tolerated, and the syncopal episodes are rarely due to extreme bradycardia as such; rather, they are secondary to episodic ventricular standstill, ventricular tachycardia or fibrillation, or a combination of these events.[150] Disturbance of sinoatrial function with normal atrioventricular conduction may also result in syncope; a variety of terms have been used to describe this situation, including *chronic sinoatrial disorder, sick-sinus syndrome,* and *bradycardia-tachycardia*.[151] Both chronic sinoatrial and chronic atrioventricular disease affect mainly the elderly, although in chronic sinoatrial disorder a smaller peak in incidence is also seen in young adults.[152,153]

A third group of disorders associated with syncope is that of the paroxysmal tachycardias. Those of supraventricular origin infrequently cause syncope and it appears that, in this context, syncope is related to vasomotor factors and not to length of the tachycardia cycle.[154] Ventricular tachycardia or fibrillation usually occurs in the context of serious heart disease but may occur in the absence of or at an early stage of such a process. This situation infrequently occurs in young adults.[155,156] A syndrome of sudden nocturnal death due to ventricular fibrillation has also been reported in young men from southeast Asia. These individuals are free from overt coronary disease and may have nocturnal episodes suggestive of seizures; they die from a presumed ventricular dysrhythmia.[157]

The long Q-T interval syndrome is a rare disorder, usually of congenital origin and familial in nature. It may be asssociated with deafness. The ventricular dysrhythmias that occur may be provoked by emotion or physical distress and may result in sudden death or in seizure-like events. Prospective follow-up of 196 patients disclosed a mean patient age of 24 years, a slight female preponderance, and evidence of Q-T prolongation in family members.[158] Measurement of the Q-T interval may be insufficient for identifying family members; in some cases DNA markers enable the diagnosis to be made.[159] Treatment options include therapy with β-blocking drugs and left stellate ganglionectomy.

If the history and physical examination fail to disclose an etiology for syncope, investigations are usually instigated. Indiscriminate use of "neurological" studies is to be discouraged. EEG and CT scanning of the head have a low diagnostic yield but should be considered if focal features are present or if an epileptic process is suspected.[144]

An electrocardiogram (ECG) may be abnormal in 50 percent of cases but will only establish a cause for syncope in between 2 and 11 percent of cases. Prolonged ECG (Holter) monitoring has a similarly low yield, estimated at 4 percent of a composite series of 2,612 cases. No arrhythmia was seen in 69 percent, an arrhythmia without syncope occurred in 13 percent, and there was arrhythmia during symptoms in 17 percent.[144] Holter monitoring may therefore be useful in excluding a dysrhythmia as a relevant factor. It was concluded that little benefit was gained from extending monitoring beyond 24 hours. Frequent or repetitive ventricular ectopy or sinus pauses of greater than 2 seconds were considered potentially significant, because these abnormalities are rarely found in asymptomatic individuals. Loop ECG recorders may come to be a more useful diagnostic device. Clinically useful information was found in one series in 68 percent of cases,[160] but the procedure is not without its disadvantages. Human error or machine malfunction resulted in a failure to diagnose 18 of 32 events in one series of 57 cases; diagnosis was made in 14 patients, in 7 of whom a dysrhythmia was identified.[161] Invasive electrophysiological testing may be required in selected cases. Features associated with a negative study have been the absence of structural heart disease, normal ECG and normal ambulatory ECG monitoring, and an ejection fraction greater than 0.40.[162] The noninvasive signal-averaged ECG may be useful in identifying patients with ventricular tachycardia. Absence of a late potential identifies patients with a very low incidence of that dysrhythmia.[163]

Recently there has been increasing interest in cardiac arrhythmias resulting from vascular or epileptic cerebral events. Sinoauricular heart block was reported as an epileptic manifestation in 1954.[164] Tachycardia is the most commonly observed rhythm disturbance, and two studies suggested that it is a common occurrence during temporal lobe seizures. The relation of the tachycardia to the epileptic discharge was different in these series. In one the seizure discharge occurred several seconds after the onset of tachycardia,[165] whereas in the other the reverse sequence was seen.[166] In some cases it is therefore necessary to obtain simultaneous ECG and EEG recordings in order to determine whether cardiac or cerebral features are primary in the genesis of attacks of loss of consciousness.[167] Sinus bradycardia, complete atrioventricular block, and cardiac arrest have all been documented as epileptic effects.[168–170] Atrial fibrillation itself may be the product of stroke, especially of infarcts in the parietoinsular and brainstem regions.[171] Finally, it should be noted that anticonvulsant drugs themselves result in disorders of cardiac rhythm.[172] The topic of cardiac arrhythmias of cerebral origin has been the subject of a recent detailed review.[173]

INTERVENTIONAL PROCESSES

Coronary angiography carries a small (0.2 percent) risk of central nervous system (CNS) complications. An unexplained observation is the preponderance of embolic events within the posterior circulation, regardless of the route of catheterization.[174] The corresponding clinical features are those of visual disturbances, which may be migrainous, transient, or persistent; confusion may also occur.[175–177] *Percutaneous transluminal coronary angioplasty* carries a similar neurological complication rate (0.2 percent) but events were not noted to be visual.[178] If *intra-aortic balloon pump* support is required after surgery, the rare complication of a spinal cord lesion may occur either as a consequence of aortic dissection or from localized occlusion of a feeding artery.[179]

Coronary artery bypass graft is a very frequently performed operation; more than 300,000 procedures are undertaken annually in the United States.[180] Stroke is a recognized complication and was documented in about 5 percent of cases in two prospective studies.[181] Imaging, by CT scanning, confirmed the impression that most infarcts were of embolic origin. Of the 22 patients studied, 15 had single lesions, 5 multiple lesions, and only 2 had scans suggestive of watershed infarction related to hypoperfusion.[182] Attempts to identify risk factors for this complication were notable for the failure of multiple parameters to predict stroke. The only feature to emerge as a clear risk factor was prior stroke. It was therefore recommended that coronary artery bypass surgery be delayed for 3 months in patients who had experienced a recent stroke. The finding of a carotid bruit prior to surgery may give rise to concern. A recent review of the subject concludes that there is no evidence that asymptomatic patients with less than 90 percent stenosis of one carotid artery are at increased risk of stroke, that there is no evidence that either staged or combined endarterectomy lowers stroke risk in asymptomatic stenosis, and that the great majority of patients with asymptomatic unilateral stenosis do not sustain a stroke.[181] The means to identify the patients who do develop a stroke in this context remains elusive.[181]

Encephalopathy may occur in up to 12 percent of cases. It is characterized by delay in emerging from anesthesia, agitation and restlessness, poor visual fixation, small reactive pupils, and occasional Babinski signs. Duration is on the order of 4 days. The mechanism remains uncertain; the encephalopathy is not clearly related to intraoperative hypoperfusion but appears multifactorial.[180,181]

The global cerebral consequences of coronary artery bypass surgery may in part reflect the occurrence of generalized microembolism to the brain, a complication that persists in spite of advances in technique over several years. Fluorescein angiograms performed 5 minutes before discontinuation of cardiopulmonary bypass have shown evidence of retinal microvascular occlusions in all patients studied.[183] Prospective clinical analysis has identified a 20 percent rate of ophthalmological abnormality.[184] In a study comparing patients undergoing coronary artery bypass surgery with those undergoing peripheral vascular surgery in whom parameters were otherwise similar with regard to age, duration of operation, and so on, it was concluded that the bypass procedure itself was the relevant factor in explaining the common occurrence of neuropsychological complications, which were seen in 38 percent of patients at the time of hospital discharge.[185] Follow-up at 6 months showed that although neurological signs were common, these were minor and of little functional importance; neurological problems contributed minimally to failure to resume work at that time.[186]

The neuropathological correlate of microembolism may be the occurrence of small capillary and arteriolar dilations or of microaneurysms, which have been observed both in the context of cardiac surgery and aortography.[187] Studies on dogs disclosed that the lesions were intravascular platelet-fibrin microaggregates.[183] Microemboli may also consist of air particles. Transcranial Doppler demonstrates waves of these at various stages of the procedure: aortic cannulation and inception of bypass.[188] Microemboli may be a contributory factor to the brain swelling that can be shown by MRI scanning at the end of surgery.[189] Further details of the relationship between neurological problems and cardiac surgery are provided in Chapter 3.

REFERENCES

1. Kittner SJ, Sharkness CM, Sloan MA, et al: Features on initial computed tomography scan of infarcts with a cardiac source of embolism in the NINDS stroke data bank. Stroke 23:1748, 1992
2. Adams HP, Bendixen BH, Kappelle LJ, et al: Classification of subtype of acute ischemic stroke: definitions for use in a multicenter clinical trial. Stroke 24:35, 1993
3. Sacco RK, Ellenberg JH, Mohr JP, et al: Infarcts of undetermined cause: the NINCDS stroke data bank. Ann Neurol 25:382, 1989
4. Bogousslavsky J, Van Melle G, Regli F: The Lausanne Stroke Registry: analysis of 1,000 consecutive patients with first stroke. Stroke 19:1083, 1988
5. Bogousslavsky J, Cachin C, Regli F, et al: Cardiac sources of embolism and cerebral infarction–clinical consequences and vascular concomitants: The Lausanne Stroke Registry. Neurology 41:855, 1991
6. Huang CY, Chan FL, Yu YL, et al: Cerebrovascular disease in Hong Kong Chinese. Stroke 21:230, 1990
7. Suzuki K, Kutsuzawa T, Takita J, et al: Clinico-epidemiologic study of stroke in Akita, Japan. Stroke 18:402, 1987
8. Yamanouchi H, Tomonaga M, Shimada H, et al: Nonvalvular atrial fibrillation as a cause of fatal massive cerebral infarction in the elderly. Stroke 20:1653, 1989
9. Leno C, Berciano J, Combarros O, et al: A prospective study of stroke in young adults in Cantabria, Spain. Stroke 24:792, 1993
10. Bogousslavsky J, Pierre P: Ischemic stroke in patients under age 45. Neurol Clin 10:113, 1992
11. Carolei A, Marini C, Ferranti E, et al: A prospective study of cerebral ischemia in the young. Analysis of pathogenic determinants. Stroke 24:362, 1993
12. Gautier JC, Pradat-Diehl P, Lascault G, et al: Accidents vasculaires cerebraux des sujets jeunes. Rev Neurol (Paris) 145:437, 1989
13. Giovannoni G, Fritz VU: Transient ischemic attacks in younger and older patients: a comparative study of 798 patients in South Africa. Stroke 24:947, 1993

14. Ramirez-Lassepas M, Cipolle RJ, Bjork RJ, et al: Can embolic stroke be diagnosed on the basis of neurologic clinical criteria? Arch Neurol 44:87, 1987

15. Kittner SJ, Sharkness CM, Price TR, et al: Infarcts with a cardiac source of embolism in the NINCDS stroke data bank: historical features. Neurology 40: 281, 1990

16. Kittner SJ, Sharkness CM, Sloan MA, et al: Infarcts with a cardiac source of embolism in the NINDS stroke data bank: neurological examination. Neurology 42:299, 1992

17. Kase CS, Norrving B, Levine SR, et al: Cerebellar infarction: clinical and anatomic observations in 66 cases. Stroke 24:76, 1993

18. Bogousslavsky J, Regli F, Maeder P, et al: The etiology of posterior circulation infarcts: a prospective study using magnetic resonance imaging and magnetic resonance angiography. Neurology 43:1528, 1993

19. Pessin MS, Lathi ES, Cohen MB, et al: Clinical features and mechanism of occipital infarction. Ann Neurol 21:290, 1987

20. Ringelstein EB, Koschorke S, Holling A, et al: Computed tomographic patterns of proven embolic brain infarctions. Ann Neurol 26:759, 1989

21. Weisberg LA: Computerized tomographic findings in cardiogenic cerebral embolism. Comput Radiol 9:189, 1985

22. Okada Y, Yamaguchi T, Minematsu K, et al: Hemorrhagic transformation in cerebral embolism. Stroke 20:598, 1989

23. Hornig CR, Bauer T, Simon C, et al: Hemorrhagic transformation in cardioembolic cerebral infarction. Stroke 24:465, 1993

24. Hankey GJ, Warlow CP, Sellar RJ: Cerebral angiographic risk in mild cerebrovascular disease. Stroke 21:209, 1990

25. Smoker WRK, Biller J, Hingtgen WL, et al: Angiography of nonhemorrhagic cerebral infarction in young adults. Stroke 18:708, 1987

26. Lisovoski F, Rousseaux P: Cerebral infarction in young people: a study of 148 patients with early cerebral angiography. J Neurol Neurosurg Psychiatry 54: 576, 1991

27. Shimosegawa E, Inugami A, Okudera T, et al: Embolic cerebral infarction: MR findings in the first 3 hours after onset. AJR 160:1077, 1993

28. Kertesz A, Black SE, Nicholson L, Carr T: The sensitivity and specificity of MRI in stroke. Neurology 37: 1580, 1987

29. DeRook FA, Comess KA, Albers GW, Popp RL: Transesophageal echocardiography in the evaluation of stroke. Ann Intern Med 117:922, 1992

30. Cerebral Embolism Task Force: Cardiogenic brain embolism. Arch Neurol 46:727, 1989

31. Pearson AC, Labovitz AJ, Tatineni S, Gomez CR: Superiority of transesophageal echocardiography in detecting cardiac source of embolism in patients with cerebral ischemia of uncertain etiology. J Am Coll Cardiol 17:66, 1991

32. Pop G, Sutherland GR, Koudstaal PJ, et al: Transesophageal echocardiography in the detection of intracardiac embolism sources in patients with transient ischemic attacks. Stroke 21:560, 1990

33. Markus H: Transcranial doppler detection of circulating cerebral emboli: a review. Stroke 24:1246, 1993

34. Venketasubramanian N, Sacco RL, Di Tullio M, et al: Vascular distribution of paradoxical emboli by transcranial Doppler. Neurology 43:1533, 1993

35. Cerebral Embolism Task Force: Cardiogenic brain embolism. Arch Neurol 43:71, 1986

36. Wolf PA, Abbott RD, Kannel WB: Atrial fibrillation: a major contributor to stroke in the elderly: The Framingham Study. Arch Intern Med 147:1561, 1987

37. Wolf PA, Dawber TR, Thomas HE, Kannel WB: Epidemiologic assessment of chronic atrial fibrillation and risk of stroke: The Framingham Study. Neurology 28:973, 1978

38. Kopecky SL, Gersh BJ, McGoon MD, et al: The natural history of lone atrial fibrillation: a population-based study over three decades. N Engl J Med 317: 669, 1987

39. Petersen P, Boysen G, Godtfredsen J, et al: Placebo-controlled, randomised trial of warfarin and aspirin for prevention of thromboembolic complications in chronic atrial fibrillation. Lancet 1:175, 1989

40. Stroke Prevention in Atrial Fibrillation Investigators: Stroke prevention in atrial fibrillation study: final results. Circulation 84:527, 1991

41. The Boston Area Anticoagulation Trial for Atrial Fibrillation Investigators: The effect of low-dose warfarin on the risk of stroke in patients with nonrheumatic atrial fibrillation. N Engl J Med 323:1505, 1990

42. Ezekowitz MD, Bridgers SL, James KE, et al: Warfarin in the prevention of stroke associated with nonrheumatic atrial fibrillation. N Engl J Med 327:1406, 1992

43. Connolly SJ, Laupacis A, Gent M, et al: Canadian atrial fibrillation anticoagulation (CAFA) study. J Am Coll Cardiol 18:349, 1991

44. Singer DE, Hughes RA, Gress DR, et al: The effect of aspirin on the risk of stroke in patients with nonrheumatic atrial fibrillation: the BAATAF study. Am Heart J 124:1567, 1992

45. Kutner M, Nixon G, Silverstone F: Physicians' attitudes towards oral anticoagulants and antiplatelet

agents for stroke prevention in elderly patients with atrial fibrillation. Arch Intern Med 51:1950, 1991

46. Gurwitz JH, Avorn J, Ross-Degnan D, et al: Aging and the anticoagulant response to warfarin therapy. Ann Intern Med 116:901, 1992

47. Fihn SD, McDonell M, Martin D, et al: Risk factors for complications of chronic anticoagulation: a multicenter study. Ann Intern Med 118:511, 1993

48. Petersen P, Kastrup J, Helweg-Larsen S, et al: Risk factors for thromboembolic complications in chronic atrial fibrillation: the Copenhagen AFASAK study. Arch Intern Med 150:819, 1990

49. The Stroke Prevention in Atrial Fibrillation Investigators: Predictors of thromboembolism in atrial fibrillation: I. Clinical features of patients at risk. Ann Intern Med 116:1, 1992

50. The Stroke Prevention in Atrial Fibrillation Investigators: Predictors of thromboembolism in atrial fibrillation: II. Echocardiographic features of patients at risk. Ann Intern Med 116:6, 1992

51. Kelley RE: Rationale for antithrombotic therapy in atrial fibrillation. Neurol Clin 10:233, 1992

52. Laupacis A, Albers G, Dunn M, Feinberg W: Antithrombotic therapy in atrial fibrillation. Chest 102, suppl:426S, 1992

53. Stein B, Halperin JL, Fuster V: Should patients with atrial fibrillation be anticoagulated prior to and chronically following cardioversion? Cardiovasc Clin 21:231, 1990

54. Arnold AZ, Mick MJ, Mazurek RP, et al: Role of prophylactic anticoagulation for direct current cardioversion in patients with atrial fibrillation or atrial flutter. J Am Coll Cardiol 19:851, 1992

55. Bjerkelund CJ, Orning OM: The efficacy of anticoagulant therapy in preventing embolism related to DC electrical conversion of atrial fibrillation. Am J Cardiol 23:208, 1969

56. Fatkin D, Kuchar D, Thorburn C, et al: Transesophageal echocardiography before and during direct current cardioversion of atrial fibrillation: evidence for "atrial stunning" as a mechanism of thromboembolic complications. J Am Coll Cardiol 21:28A, 1993

57. Manning WJ, Leeman DE, Gotch PJ, Come PC: Pulsed Doppler evaluation of atrial mechanical function after electrical cardioversion of atrial fibrillation. J Am Coll Cardiol 13:617, 1989

58. Parkinson J, Campbell M: Paroxysmal auricular fibrillation: a record of two hundred patients. Q J Med 24:67, 1930

59. Petersen P, Godtfredsen J: Embolic complications in paroxysmal atrial fibrillation. Stroke 17:622, 1986

60. Petersen P: Thromboembolic complications in atrial fibrillation. Stroke 21:4, 1990

61. Roy D, Marchand E, Gagne P, et al: Usefulness of anticoagulant therapy in the prevention of embolic complications of atrial fibrillation. Am Heart J 112:1039, 1986

62. Cabin HS, Clubb KS, Hall C, et al: Risk for systemic embolization of atrial fibrillation without mitral stenosis. Am J Cardiol 65:1112, 1990

63. Moulton AW, Singer DE, Haas JS: Risk factors for stroke in patients with nonrheumatic atrial fibrillation: a case-control study. Am J Med 91:156, 1991

64. Fairfax AJ, Lambert CD, Leatham A: Systemic embolism in chronic sinoatrial disorder. N Engl J Med 295:190, 1976

65. Bathen J, Sparr S, Rokseth R: Embolism in sinoatrial disease. Acta Med Scand 203:7, 1978

66. Simonsen E, Nielsen JS, Nielsen BL: Sinus node dysfunction in 128 patients. Acta Med Scand 208:343, 1980

67. Fisher M, Kase CS, Stelle B, Mills RM: Ischemic stroke after cardiac pacemaker implantation in sick sinus syndrome. Stroke 19:712, 1988

68. Camm AJ, Katritsis D: Ventricular pacing for sick sinus syndrome—a risky business? PACE 13:695, 1990

69. Sutton R, Kenny RA: The natural history of sick sinus syndrome. PACE 9:1110, 1986

70. Sgarbossa EB, Pinski SL, Maloney JD: The role of pacing modality in determining long-term survival in the sick sinus syndrome. Ann Intern Med 119:359, 1993

71. Clarke M, Sutton R, Ward D, et al: Recommendations for pacemaker prescription for symptomatic bradycardia. Br Heart J 66:185, 1991

72. Ausubel K, Furman S: The pacemaker syndrome. Ann Intern Med 103:420, 1985

73. Presti CF, Hart RG: Thyrotoxicosis, atrial fibrillation, and embolism, revisited. Am Heart J 117:976, 1989

74. Forfar JC, Miller HC, Toft AD: Occult thyrotoxicosis: a correctable cause of "idiopathic" atrial fibrillation. Am J Cardiol 44:9, 1979

75. Yuen RWM, Gutteridge DH, Thompson PL, Robinson JS: Embolism in thyrotoxic atrial fibrillation. Med J Aust 1:630, 1979

76. Staffurth JS, Gibberd MC, Ng Tang Fui S: Arterial embolism in thyrotoxicosis with atrial fibrillation. Br Med J 2:688, 1977

77. Nakazawa HK, Sakurai K, Hamada N, et al: Management of atrial fibrillation in the post-thyrotoxic state. Am J Med 72:903, 1982

78. Reddy CRR, Parvathi G, Rao NR: Pathology of cardiomyopathy from South India. Br Heart J 32:226, 1970

79. Cosnett JE: Heart disease in the Zulu: especially car-

diomyopathy and cardiac infarction. Br Heart J 24: 76, 1962

80. Shaper AG, Wright DH: Intracardiac thrombosis and embolism in endomyocardial fibrosis in Uganda. Br Heart J 25:502, 1963

81. Shaper AG, Hutt MSR, Coles RM: Necropsy study of endomyocardial fibrosis and rheumatic heart disease in Uganda 1950–1965. Br Heart J 30:391, 1968

82. Davies J, Spry CJF, Vijayaraghavan G, De Souza JA: A comparison of the clinical and cardiological features of endomyocardial disease in temperate and tropical regions. Postgrad Med J 59:179, 1983

83. Parrillo JE, Borer JS, Henry WL, et al: The cardiovascular manifestations of the hypereosinophilic syndrome: prospective study of 26 patients, with review of the literature. Am J Med 67:572, 1979

84. Kirchhoff LV: American trypanosomiasis (Chagas' disease)—a tropical disease now in the United States. N Engl Med 329:639, 1993

85. Oliveira JSM, Correa De Araujo RR, Navarro MA, Muccillo G: Cardiac thrombosis and thromboembolism in chronic Chagas' heart disease. Am J Cardiol 52:147, 1983

86. Nussenzveig I, Wajchemberg BL, Macruz R, et al: Acidentes vasculares cerebrais embolicos na cardiopatia chagasica cronica. Arq Neuro-Psiquiat (Sao Paulo) 11:386, 1953

87. Lambert CD: Neurological complications of cardiomyopathies. p. 131. In Goetz CG, Tanner CM, Aminoff MJ (eds): Handbook of Clinical Neurology. Vol 63. Elsevier, Amsterdam, 1993

88. Gillum RF: Idiopathic cardiomyopathy in the United States, 1970–1982. Am Heart J 111:752, 1985

89. Roberts WC, Siegel RJ, McManus BM: Idiopathic dilated cardiomyopathy: analysis of 152 necropsy patients. Am J Cardiol 60:1340, 1987

90. Kyrle PA, Korninger C, Gossinger H, et al: Prevention of arterial and pulmonary embolism by oral anticoagulants in patients with dilated cardiomyopathy. Thromb Haemost 54:521, 1985

91. McKenna WJ, Goodwin JF: The natural history of hypertrophic cardiomyopathy. Curr Probl Cardiol 6: 1, 1981

92. Spirito P, Chiarella F, Carratino L, et al: Clinical course and prognosis of hypertrophic cardiomyopathy in an outpatient population. N Engl J Med 320: 749, 1989

93. Glancy DL, O'Brien KP, Gold HK, Epstein SE: Atrial fibrillation in patients with idiopathic hypertrophic subaortic stenosis. Br Heart J 32:652, 1970

94. Russell JW, Biller J, Hajduczok ZD, et al: Ischemic cerebrovascular complications and risk factors in idiopathic hypertrophic subaortic stenosis. Stroke 22: 1143, 1991

95. Teare D: Asymmetrical hypertrophy of the heart in young adults. Br Heart J 20:1, 1958

96. Thompson PL, Robinson JS: Stroke after acute myocardial infarction: relation to infarct size. Br Med J 2: 457, 1978

97. Komrad MS, Coffey CE, Coffey KS, et al: Myocardial infarction and stroke. Neurology 34:1403, 1984

98. Behar S, Tanne D, Abinader E, et al: Cerebrovascular accident complicating acute myocardial infarction: incidence, clinical significance, and short- and long-term mortality rates. Am J Med 91:45, 1991

99. Visser CA, Kan G, Lie KI, Durrer D: Left ventricular thrombus following acute myocardial infarction: a prospective serial echocardiographic study of 96 patients. Eur Heart J 4:333, 1983

100. Dexter DD, Whisnant JP, Connolly DC, O'Fallon WM: The association of stroke and coronary heart disease: a population study. Mayo Clin Proc 62:1077, 1987

101. Martin R, Bogousslavsky J: Mechanisms of late stroke after myocardial infarct: the Lausanne Stroke Registry. J Neurol Neurosurg Psychiatry 56:760, 1993

102. Cairns JA, Hirsh J, Lewis HD, et al: Antithrombotic agents in coronary artery disease. Chest 102, suppl: 456S, 1992

103. Maggioni AP, Franzosi MG, Farina ML, et al: Cerebrovascular events after myocardial infarction: analysis of the GISSI trial. Br Med J 302:1428, 1991

104. Maggioni AP, Franzosi MG, Santoro E, et al: The risk of stroke in patients with acute myocardial infarction after thrombolytic and antithrombotic treatment. N Engl J Med 327:1, 1992

105. The GUSTO Investigators: An international randomized trial comparing four thrombolytic strategies for acute myocardial infarction. N Engl J Med 329:673, 1993

106. Abernathy WS, Willis PW: Thromboembolic complications of rheumatic heart disease. Cardiovasc Clin 5: 131, 1973

107. Shrestha NK, Moreno FL, Narciso FV, et al: Two-dimensional echocardiographic diagnosis of left-atrial thrombus in rheumatic heart disease: a clinicopathologic study. Circulation 67:341, 1983

108. Carter AB: Prognosis of cerebral embolism. Lancet 2:514, 1965

109. Levine HJ, Pauker SG, Salzman EW, Eckman MH: Antithrombotic therapy in valvular heart disease. Chest 102, suppl:434S, 1992

110. Turpie AGG, Gent M, Laupacis A, et al: A comparison of aspirin with placebo in patients treated with warfarin after heart-valve replacement. N Engl J Med 329:524, 1993

111. Bulkley BH, Hutchins GM: Atrial myxomas: a fifty year review. Am Heart J 97:639, 1979

112. Markel ML, Waller BF, Armstrong WF: Cardiac myxoma: a review. Medicine (Baltimore) 66:114, 1987

113. Knepper LE, Biller J, Adams HP, Bruno A: Neurologic manifestations of atrial myxoma: a 12-year experience and review. Stroke 19:1435, 1988

114. Savage DD, Garrison RJ, Devereux RB, et al: Mitral valve prolapse in the general population: I. Epidemiologic features: The Framingham Study. Am Heart J 106:571, 1983

115. Wolf PA, Sila CA: Cerebral ischemia with mitral valve prolapse. Am Heart J 113:1308, 1987

116. Bisset GS, Schwartz DC, Meyer RA, et al: Clinical spectrum and long-term follow-up of isolated mitral valve prolapse in 119 children. Circulation 62:423, 1980

117. Jones HR, Naggar CZ, Seljan MP, Downing LL: Mitral valve prolapse and cerebral ischemic events: a comparison between a neurology population with stroke and a cardiology population with mitral valve prolapse observed for five years. Stroke 13:451, 1982

118. Nishimura RA, McGoon MD, Shub C, et al: Echocardiographically documented mitral-valve prolapse: long-term follow-up of 237 patients. N Engl J Med 313:1305, 1985

119. Duren DR, Becker AE, Dunning AJ: Long-term follow-up of idiopathic mitral valve prolapse in 300 patients: a prospective study. J Am Coll Cardiol 11:42, 1988

120. Hart RG, Easton JD: Mitral valve prolapse and cerebral infarction. Stroke 13:429, 1982

121. MacMahon SW, Roberts JK, Kramer-Fox R, et al: Mitral valve prolapse and infective endocarditis. Am Heart J 113:1291, 1987

122. Belkin RN, Kisslo J: Atrial septal aneurysm: recognition and clinical relevance. Am Heart J 120:948, 1990

123. Pearson AC, Nagelhout D, Castello R, et al: Atrial septal aneurysm and stroke: a transesophageal echocardiographic study. J Am Coll Cardiol 18:1223, 1991

124. Belkin RN, Hurwitz BJ, Kisslo J: Atrial septal aneurysm: association with cerebrovascular and peripheral embolic events. Stroke 18:856, 1987

125. Zabalgoitia-Reyes M, Herrera C, Gandhi DK, et al: A possible mechanism for neurologic ischemic events in patients with atrial septal aneurysm. Am J Cardiol 66:761, 1990

126. Di Tullio M, Sacco RL, Gopal A, et al: Patent foramen ovale as a risk factor for cryptogenic stroke. Ann Intern Med 117:461, 1992

127. Di Tullio M, Sacco RL, Venketasubramanian N, et al: Comparison of diagnostic techniques for the detection of a patent foramen ovale in stroke patients. Stroke 24:1020, 1993

128. Lechat P, Mas JL, Lascault G, et al: Prevalence of patent foramen ovale in patients with stroke. N Engl J Med 318:1148, 1988

129. Ranoux D, Cohen A, Cabanes L, et al: Patent foramen ovale: is stroke due to paradoxical embolism? Stroke 24:31, 1993

130. Chimowitz MI, DeGeorgia MA, Poole RM, et al: Left atrial spontaneous echo contrast is highly associated with previous stroke in patients with atrial fibrillation or mitral stenosis. Stroke 24:1015, 1993

131. Benjamin EJ, Plehn JF, D'Agostino RB, et al: Mitral annular calcification and the risk of stroke in an elderly cohort. N Engl J Med 327:374, 1992

132. Sacco RL, Foulkes MA, Mohr JP, et al: Determinants of early recurrence of cerebral infarction: The Stroke Data Bank. Stroke 20:983, 1989

133. Hier DB, Foulkes MA, Swiontoniowski M, et al: Stroke recurrence within 2 years after ischemic infarction. Stroke 22:155, 1991

134. Broderick JP, Phillips SJ, O'Fallon WM, et al: Relationship of cardiac disease to stroke occurrence, recurrence, and mortality. Stroke 23:1250, 1992

135. Cerebral Embolism Study Group: Cardioembolic stroke, early anticoagulation, and brain hemorrhage. Arch Intern Med 147:636, 1987

136. Pessin MS, Estol CJ, Lafranchise F, Caplan LR: Safety of anticoagulation after hemorrhagic infarction. Neurology 43:1298, 1993

137. Rosen R, Kabat H, Anderson JP: Acute arrest of cerebral circulation in man. Arch Neurol Psychiatry 50:510, 1943

138. Aminoff MJ, Scheinman MM, Griffin JC, Herre JM: Electrocerebral accompaniments of syncope associated with malignant ventricular arrhythmias. Ann Intern Med 108:791, 1988

139. Lin JTY, Ziegler DK, Lai CW, Bayer W: Convulsive syncope in blood donors. Ann Neurol 11:525, 1982

140. Reed RL, Siekert RG, Merideth J: Rarity of transient focal cerebral ischemia in cardiac dysrhythmia. JAMA 223:893, 1973

141. Pearson RSB: Sinus bradycardia with cardiac asystole. Br Heart J 7:85, 1945

142. Savage DD, Corwin L, McGee DL, et al: Epidemiologic features of isolated syncope: The Framingham Study. Stroke 16:626, 1985

143. Lipsitz LA, Wei JY, Rowe JW: Syncope in an elderly, institutionalised population: prevalence, incidence, and associated risk. Q J Med 55:45, 1985

144. Kapoor WN: Diagnostic evaluation of syncope. Am J Med 90:91, 1991

145. Katon W: Panic disorder and somatization: review of 55 cases. Am J Med 77:101, 1984

146. Linzer M, Felder A, Hackel A, et al: Psychiatric syn-

cope: a new look at an old disease. Psychosomatics 31:181, 1990

147. Schwartz LS, Goldfischer J, Sprague GJ, Schwartz SP: Syncope and sudden death in aortic stenosis. Am J Cardiol 23:647, 1969

148. Myerson RM, Vivacqua RJ, Pastor BH: Obstructing intracardiac thrombi. Arch Intern Med 118:478, 1966

149. MacMurray FG: Stokes-Adams disease: a historical review. N Engl J Med 256:643, 1957

150. Parkinson J, Papp C, Evans W: The electrocardiogram of the Stokes-Adams attack. Br Heart J 3:171, 1941

151. Lambert CD, Fairfax AJ: Cerebral effects of cardiac dysrhythmias. p. 259. In Vinken PJ, Bruyn GW (eds): Handbook of Clinical Neurology. Vol 39. North Holland, Amsterdam, 1980

152. Fairfax AJ, Lambert CD: Neurological aspects of sinoatrial heart block. J Neurol Neurosurg Psychiatry 39:576, 1976

153. Siddons H: Deaths in long-term paced patients. Br Heart J 36:1201, 1974

154. Leitch JW, Klein GJ, Yee R, et al: Syncope associated with supraventricular tachycardia. An expression of tachycardia rate or vasomotor response? Circulation 85:1064, 1992

155. Lemery R, Brugada P, Della Bella P, et al: Nonischemic ventricular tachycardia: clinical course and long-term follow-up in patients without clinically overt heart disease. Circulation 79:990, 1989

156. Deal BJ, Miller SM, Scagliotti D, et al: Ventricular tachycardia in a young population without overt heart disease. Circulation 73:1111, 1986

157. Otto CM, Tauxe RV, Cobb LA, et al: Ventricular fibrillation causes sudden death in Southeast Asian immigrants. Ann Intern Med 101:45, 1984

158. Moss AJ, Schwartz PJ, Crampton RS, et al: The long QT syndrome: a prospective international study. Circulation 71:17, 1985

159. Vincent GM, Timothy KW, Leppert M, Keating M: The spectrum of symptoms and QT intervals in carriers of the gene for the long-QT syndrome. N Engl J Med 327:846, 1992

160. Brown AP, Dawkins KD, Davies JG: Detection of arrhythmias: use of a patient-activated ambulatory electrocardiogram device with a solid-state memory loop. Br Heart J 58:251, 1987

161. Linzer M, Pritchett ELC, Pontinen M, et al: Incremental diagnostic yield of loop electrocardiographic recorders in unexplained syncope. Am J Cardiol 66:214, 1990

162. Krol RB, Morady F, Flaker GC, et al: Electrophysiologic testing in patients with unexplained syncope: clinical and noninvasive predictors of outcome. J Am Coll Cardiol 10:358, 1987

163. Kuchar DL, Thorburn CW, Sammel NL: Signal-averaged electrocardiogram for evaluation of recurrent syncope. Am J Cardiol 58:949, 1986

164. Phizackerley PJR, Poole EW, Whitty CWM: Sinoauricular heart block as an epileptic manifestation. Epilepsia 3:89, 1954

165. Marshall DW, Westmoreland BF, Sharbrough FW: Ictal tachycardia during temporal lobe seizures. Mayo Clin Proc 58:443, 1983

166. Blumhardt LD, Smith PEM, Owen L: Electrocardiographic accompaniments of temporal lobe epileptic seizures. Lancet 1:1051, 1986

167. Gilchrist JM: Arrhythmogenic seizures: diagnosis by simultaneous EEG/ECG recording. Neurology 35:1503, 1985

168. Constantin L, Martins JB, Fincham RW, Dagli RD: Bradycardia and syncope as manifestations of partial epilepsy. J Am Coll Cardiol 15:900, 1990

169. Wilder-Smith E: Complete atrio-ventricular conduction block during complex partial seizure. J Neurol Neurosurg Psychiatry 55:734, 1992

170. Liedholm LJ, Gudjonsson O: Cardiac arrest due to partial epileptic seizures. Neurology 42:824, 1992

171. Vingerhoets F, Bogousslavsky J, Regli F, Van Melle G: Atrial fibrillation after acute stroke. Stroke 24:26, 1993

172. Boesen F, Andersen EB, Jensen EK, Ladefoged SD: Cardiac conduction disturbances during carbamazepine therapy. Acta Neurol Scand 68:49, 1983

173. Valeriano J, Elson J: Electrocardiographic changes in central nervous system disease. Neurol Clin 11:257, 1993

174. Keilson GR, Schwartz WJ, Recht LD: The preponderance of posterior circulatory events is independent of the route of cardiac catheterization. Stroke 23:1358, 1992

175. Vik-Mo H, Todnem K, Folling M, Rosland GA: Transient visual disturbance during cardiac catheterization with angiography. Cathet Cardiovasc Diagn 12:1, 1986

176. Oliva A, Scherokman B: Two cases of occipital infarction following cardiac catheterization. Stroke 19:773, 1988

177. Kosmorsky G, Hanson MR, Tomsak RL: Neuro-ophthalmologic complications of cardiac catheterization. Neurology 38:483, 1988

178. Galbreath C, Salgado ED, Furlan AJ, Hollman J: Central nervous system complications of percutaneous transluminal coronary angioplasty. Stroke 17:616, 1986

179. Riggle KP, Oddi MA: Spinal cord necrosis and paraplegia as complications of the intra-aortic balloon. Crit Care Med 17:475, 1989

180. Brillman J: Central nervous system complications in coronary artery bypass graft surgery. Neurol Clin 11: 475, 1993

181. Furlan AJ, Sila CA, Chimowitz MI, Jones SC: Neurologic complications related to cardiac surgery. Neurol Clin 10:145, 1992

182. Hise JH, Nipper ML, Schnitker JC: Stroke associated with coronary artery bypass surgery. AJNR 12:811, 1991

183. Blauth CI, Arnold JV, Schulenberg WE, et al: Cerebral microembolism during cardiopulmonary bypass. J Thorac Cardiovasc Surg 95:668, 1988

184. Shaw PJ, Bates D, Cartlidge NEF, et al: Early neurological complications of coronary artery bypass surgery. Br Med J 291:1384, 1985

185. Shaw PJ, Bates D, Cartlidge NEF, et al: Neurologic and neuropsychological morbidity following major surgery: comparison of coronary artery bypass and peripheral vascular surgery. Stroke 18:700, 1987

186. Shaw PJ, Bates D, Cartlidge NEF, et al: Neurological complications of coronary artery bypass graft surgery: six months follow-up study. Br Med J 293:165, 1986

187. Moody DM, Bell MA, Challa VR, et al: Brain microemboli during cardiac surgery or aortography. Ann Neurol 28:477, 1990

188. Pugsley W, Klinger L, Paschalis C, et al: Microemboli and cerebral impairment during cardiac surgery. Vasc Surg (Lond) 24:34, 1990

189. Harris DNF, Bailey SM, Smith PLC, et al: Brain swelling in first hour after coronary artery bypass surgery. Lancet 342:586, 1993

6

Neurological Manifestations of Infective Endocarditis

Phillip I. Lerner

Reviews of the neurological manifestations of infective endocarditis often refer to Osler's historic Gulstonian Lectures on Malignant Endocarditis, delivered to the Royal College of Physicians over a century ago.[1] However, earlier nineteenth-century investigators first called attention to emboli,[2] neurological involvement,[3] and aneurysms[4] in infective endocarditis. Virchow in 1847 recognized embolism in cases of infective endocarditis and noted destruction of vascular walls at embolic sites.[2] Tufnell recognized the importance of embolism in the production of aneurysms.[4] However, it was Osler's celebrated triad—fever, heart murmur, and stroke—and his observation that a "considerable number of cases. . .come under observation. . . .for the first time with symptoms of cerebral or even cerebrospinal trouble"[1] that established an enduring fascination with the neurological manifestations of endocarditis, a topic addressed repeatedly over the past 65 years.[5-17]

Neurological complications in infective endocarditis relate to embolic occlusion of cerebral (occasionally peripheral) arteries; expansion, leakage, or rupture of infected arteries (arteritis) or mycotic aneurysms; or metastatic infection in the form of meningitis or brain abscess. Occasionally infection (abscess) is present in the wall of an aneurysm or surrounds an aneurysm, or both may be present separately but adjacent to each other.[18-20] Each of these conditions derives ultimately from emboli, large or small, infected or bland, that separate from endocardial vegetations. Major cerebral emboli, the most common neurological complications seen in infective endocarditis, account for 50 percent of all neurological complications. The mortality rate of patients with central nervous system (CNS) complications has been recorded to be as high as 50 to 83 percent,[10,11,13,14] which is generally, and sometimes considerably, higher than the mortality in cases without CNS complications.

The incidence and spectrum of nervous system complications in infective endocarditis today is remarkably similar to the picture described before antibiotics became available and in the early years of the antibiotic era. So common is hemiplegia that Jochmann, in 1924, put forth in his textbook the still valid clinical maxim: "*Bei Hemiplegien in jugendlichen Alter denke Man immer an eine Endocarditis lenta.*" (In hemiplegia in young adults, one always thinks of subacute bacterial endocarditis.)[21]

The clinical profile and expression of infective endocarditis has undergone profound changes in the past half-century due to a natural evolution of the disease, although some changes relate to newer therapies and different populations at risk.[22-24] The average age of patients with infected heart valves has increased strikingly and, outside the developing and Third World countries, rheumatic heart disease has virtually disappeared as an underlying cardiac abnormality. Infective endocarditis today includes many nosocomial infections, an epidemic of cases associated with illicit intravenous drug use,[23,24] and the emergence of an entirely new category, prosthetic valve endocarditis.[25,26] The nervous system manifestations of infective endocarditis remain the only expression of this fascinating infection, which maintains the "traditional" picture first emphasized by Osler[1] and described and catalogued by many others in the first half of this century.[5-9] Since the first edition of this textbook, important clinical experiences and observations have been reported from a number of centers,[27-35] further supplementing and updating a number of recent important reviews[10-17] and augmenting the earlier classic reports.[5-9]

The evolving sophistication of echocardiography[24,36,37] enhances our ability to diagnose and, to a certain extent, prognosticate in infective endocarditis. Vegetation size and location, valve function, and serial changes in these features all play a role, albeit somewhat controversial, in the management of this disorder. Similarly, the rapidly evolving scanning technologies of computed tomography (CT) and magnetic resonance imaging (MRI) help to clarify some previously mystifying "toxic" and "neuropsychiatric" syndromes and to select those patients most likely to benefit from four-vessel cerebral angiography. Many of the current data and recommendations, drawn from reports cited in this review, will soon yield to still further clarification as larger numbers of successfully treated patients become the beneficiaries of these dramatic new technologies.

General reviews[22,23,38-40] often consider only the major neurological categories of CNS complications; minor or atypical abnormalities are addressed more often in reports where neuropsychiatric features are highlighted.[5-15,41] The incidence of nervous system compromise recognized during the course of infective endocarditis ranges between 20 and 40 percent (average 30 percent).[16,33] For example, at St. Thomas Hospital in London (1968–1987), neurological presentations (meningitis, toxic confusion, thromboemboli, headache) occurred in 54 percent of all cases of staphylococcal endocarditis, but in only 19 percent of episodes of *viridans* streptococcal and enterococcal endocarditis among 178 episodes of native valve

endocarditis, yielding an overall 33 percent incidence of neurological complications.[29] A higher incidence of cerebral involvement often emanates from major referral centers whose series include autopsy material, since death in endocarditis not infrequently results from brain damage[12] and autopsies disclose clinically "silent" emboli in many organs including the CNS.[22] Minor neurological complications are easily overlooked.[42] A comprehensive review from the Massachusetts General Hospital (MGH) in Boston analyzed the records of 218 patients with infective endocarditis (1964–1973).[13] Among this group, 84 patients (39 percent) experienced clinically evident neurological complications, a very high incidence influenced by that institution's referral pattern.[13] Patients exhibiting neurological complications ranged in age from 3 months to 89 years and were equally distributed between the sexes; 58 percent died, compared to a 20 percent mortality among the 134 patients without neurological involvement ($p < 0.001$). Mortality was similarly increased among the patients with CNS involvement in the St. Thomas Hospital experience.[29]

LeCam and colleagues also recorded a high incidence (56 percent) of neurological events in 48 of 86 cases of bacterial endocarditis.[14] Mortality increased from 26 percent in patients without neurological problems to 83 percent in patients with them ($p < 0.01$). Two factors significantly affected the incidence of neurological complications: (1) the location of vegetations, with 76 percent of neurological complications seen in mitral valve endocarditis compared with 37 percent in other cases ($p < 0.005$), and (2) the infecting organism—71 percent in *Staphylococcus aureus* endocarditis compared to 45 percent with other bacteria ($p < 0.02$). When the mitral valve was infected by *S. aureus,* the frequency of neurological complications was 87.5 percent, significantly higher than in other forms of endocarditis (43.5 percent; $p < 0.001$). (Remarkably similar figures emerged also from a more recent survey of 166 cases in San Antonio, Texas.[33]) Intracerebral hemorrhages were significantly more likely to occur in staphylococcal endocarditis (10 of 35) than in endocarditis of other bacterial etiology (5 of 51) ($p < 0.05$).[14] Fatal acute suppurative meningitis (6 patients) was mainly associated with staphylococcal mitral endocarditis.[14,33] Cerebral emboli and intracranial hemorrhages were the most common complications. Staphylococcal mitral valve endocarditis carried the highest risk of neurological complication and death, confirming the MGH experience.[13,14]

Neurological complications were also analyzed recently in 175 patients with infective endocarditis seen at the Cleveland Clinic from 1974 to 1986.[43] They occurred with the same frequency (35.3 percent and 38.7 percent, respectively) and distribution among 113 patients with native valve endocarditis and 62 patients with prosthetic valve endocarditis. *S. aureus* endocarditis correlated statistically with the development of neurological complications ($p < 0.01$) and death ($p < 0.01$). Mortality among patients in this series with (20.6 percent) and without (13.6 percent) neurological complications was not significantly different ($p = 0.23$).

Approximately 25 years ago, Ziment labeled symptom complexes in endocarditis as follows: toxic, psychiatric, stroke, meningoencephalitis, cranial neuropathy, myelopathy, dyskinesia, and peripheral neuropathy.[12] He acknowledged difficulty in determining the proportion of patients with "toxemic" symptoms (I would add psychiatric) that might actually have had organic brain lesions secondary to infective endocarditis. Imaging by CT scanning and MRI now permits more precision in assigning anatomical diagnoses to patients with these more obscure presentations.[33,44] This review concentrates on complications relating to or deriving from embolization (ischemic and hemorrhagic "strokes"), hemorrhage from arteritis or mycotic aneurysm, and metastatic infection (meningitis, brain abscess). Included also is a brief discussion of nonbacterial thrombotic endocarditis.

EMBOLIC EVENTS

Embolic occlusion of major cerebral arteries leads to cerebral infarction in 10 to 30 percent of all patients with infective endocarditis and accounts for one-half the total number of neurological complications; at the MGH, the most recent figure was 17 percent.[13]

A recent survey of six hospitals from San Antonio, Texas (212 episodes, 1978 to 1986) revealed 21 percent of cases complicated by stroke.[32] In native valve endocarditis, most (74 percent) ischemic strokes had occurred by the time of presentation, and an additional 13 percent occurred within 48 hours after diagnosis. Control of infection dramatically reduces the risk of subsequent embolism in patients with infective endocarditis.[32,34,43] Subsequent or recurrent stroke (0.5 percent/day) often heralds relapse or uncontrolled infection.[32]

More than 90 percent of large emboli lodge in the middle cerebral artery, leading to contralateral hemiparesis or hemiplegia and a hemisensory deficit; occlusion of the middle cerebral artery or its branches may also produce parietal lobe signs of sensory loss, neglect, dyspraxia, hemianopia, and—when the dominant hemisphere is involved—aphasia.[41] Embolization to branches of the anterior or posterior cerebral artery occurs less often. Patients with lesions of the basal ganglia may develop signs of parkinsonism or chorea.[45] Lesions of the median longitudinal fasciculus may produce unilateral internuclear ophthalmoplegia.[46] Brainstem lesions can cause dysphagia, intractable hiccups, or vomiting. Less often, one encounters myelitis, acute mononeuropathy,[42,47,48] mononeuropathy multiplex, optic neuritis, or unilateral blindness due to retinal artery embolus. Pseudobulbar palsy may dominate the clinical picture.[49] Generalized multifocal peripheral neuropathy can sometimes be seen with multifocal septic emboli.[50]

In the recent MGH series, 11 percent of the patients had multiple microemboli resulting in punctate cerebral infarctions,[13] expressed most commonly as an "altered level of consciousness"; more specific findings were seizures or fluctuating focal neurological signs, often mimicking the picture of a transient ischemic attack (TIA), presumably from emboli that disintegrate after initial lodgement.[13,51] Particularly in the elderly, aphasia, hemiplegia, confusion, delirium, psychoses, or TIAs are likely to be attributed to arteriosclerotic cerebrovascular disease.[51] Autopsy-proven microemboli may be clinically silent or may provoke only an altered level of consciousness not otherwise explained by metabolic, cardiac, or other neurological abnormalities.[13]

Emboli occur more commonly in patients infected with virulent organisms, an event very likely to occur early (within 2 weeks) in the course of such infections, in contrast to the later embolic events (third or fourth week or after 1 to 3 months) seen in subacute bacterial endocarditis (SBE) caused by organisms such as *viridans* streptococci or when infections due to more virulent organisms have been modified by prior antibiotic therapy. Significant metastatic abscess formation may occur on occasion even in the infective endocarditis associated with *viridans* streptococci.[42,52] Patients infected with virulent organisms now survive more frequently, and long enough to experience cerebral emboli. Fortunately, late emboli—i.e., sterile fragments of valve material that detach many months (occasionally 1 to 2 years) after cure of infection—are no longer common; nine such examples were noted in an early series at the MGH (prior to 1959),[38] in contrast to the single case in their more recent experience.[13] Among 50 patients with native valve endocarditis not receiving anticoagulants or antiplatelet agents after discharge from the Cleveland Clinic, only one had a "stroke" during a mean follow-up period of 48 months.[43]

Emboli to the cerebrum, lungs, and peripheral vessels are more often clinically apparent, in contrast to those directed to the spleen, kidneys, and myocardium, which are more often discovered only at autopsy.[11,12,22] In the MGH experience, cerebral emboli occurred more commonly in patients with mitral valve infection than in those with aortic valve involvement, although systemic (noncerebral) emboli occurred with equal frequency.[13] Almost 50 percent of patients with cerebral emboli deposit emboli in other organs as well.[13] Since the foramen ovale may be patent in up to 18 percent of the normal population, paradoxical embolism should be considered in intravenous drug abusers with tricuspid valve endocarditis who develop neurological complications.[53–55] Septic pulmonary lesions, such as a septic pulmonary arteriovenous fistula, may also explain cerebrovascular events in intravenous drug abusers with only tricuspid valve endocarditis.[56]

Pathological examination of valve vegetations readily explains the increased incidence of embolization seen in more virulent infections. In subacute disease, valvular lesions progress slowly, with evidence of early healing; in acute endocarditis, by contrast, the process is rapidly destructive, with little or no evidence of healing and larger, more friable lesions. Streptokinase (fibrinolytic) therapy in experimental canine *Streptococcus sanguis* endocarditis significantly reduces the size of aortic valve vegetations at the expense of a considerable increase in the volume of infarcted brain due to embolism.[57] The most extreme examples of large vegetations are found in fungal (especially *Aspergillus* and *Candida*) endocarditis, in which patients characteristically suffer a high incidence of embolic phenomena. Infections with *Pseu-*domonas aeruginosa and other gram-negative "coliform" bacilli, the capnophilic gram-negative rods (*Haemophilus* species, *Cardiobacterium hominis, Actinobacillus actinomycetemcomitans*), the group B β-hemolytic streptococcus (*Streptococcus agalactiae*), and nutritionally deficient streptococci also produce notably large vegetations with enhanced embolic potential.[58–60] In patients surviving the first week of antibiotic treatment with control of their infection, subsequent embolic events occur at a rate of less than 0.5 percent/day.[32] Novel approaches to prevent or minimize the growth of vegetations and subsequent emboli (e.g., aspirin administration) are under consideration.[61] Anticoagulants are contraindicated in native valve endocarditis because they do not prevent growth of vegetations or recurrent embolization but do increase the risk of hemorrhagic complications.[32,33]

In the San Antonio experience of native valve endocarditis, most ischemic strokes (74 percent) had occurred by the time of presentation and an additional 13 percent occurred during the 48 hours after diagnosis; the incidence of brain ischemia was 13 percent on presentation, 3 percent during the first 48 hours, and 2 to 5 percent during the remainder of the acute course.[32] Stroke recurred at the rate of 0.5 percent/day, often heralding relapse or uncontrolled infection. Only 9 percent of ischemic infarcts were large (all in patients with *S. aureus* infection), whereas 8 percent were small and subcortical. The authors concluded that anticoagulants and surgery are not warranted to prevent recurrent stroke in these patients because control of infection virtually eliminated the risk of recurrent stroke.

Immunological Abnormalities and Vasculitis

Microbial antigens in infected heart valves stimulate a wide range of antibodies (antiglobulins) and provoke a number of immunological abnormalities, including hyperglobulinemia, generally relating to a polyclonal immunoglobulin G (IgG) or, in rare instances, a monoclonal immunoglobulin, rheumatoid factor in 30 to 50 percent of cases, reduced complement levels, the presence of cryoglobulins, and the formation of immune complexes.[62,63] High levels of circulating immune complexes (complement and immunoglobulins) in the active phase of infective endocarditis are associated with deposition of these complexes in capillary walls in the kidneys (proliferative glomerulonephritis) and skin (leukocytoclastic angiitis), at times with palpable purpura; they may also explain, in part, the pathogenesis of some of the traditional peripheral vascular manifestations of infective endocarditis, such as Osler nodes, Janeway lesions, Roth spots, and petechiae.[62,63]

The relation of these immunological phenomena and immune complex–mediated vasculitis to various neurological complications has received little attention.[64] Alajouanine and associates described patients with delayed late focal neurological abnormalities; affected vessels demonstrated a "proliferative endarteritis" resulting in thrombotic occlusion.[64] Bayer and colleagues described two young patients with thrombotic thrombocytopenic purpura and endocarditis who displayed prominent neuropsychiatric complaints that cleared entirely, as did all evidence of the hematological disorder and of hypocomplementemic immune complex–mediated renal failure, following successful treatment of the underlying endocarditis.[65] In both cases, high levels of circulating immune complexes declined as the thrombotic thrombocytopenic purpura abated. Immune complex–mediated vasculitis superimposed on a subclinical radiation vasculitis contributed to the neurological deterioration reported by others in a patient with streptococcal endocarditis; dexamethasone therapy produced prompt improvement in the face of continued deterioration despite antibiotic therapy.[66]

Nonbacterial Thrombotic Endocarditis

Nonbacterial thrombotic endocarditis (previously called marantic endocarditis), currently recognized in 1 percent of all autopsy cases, also serves as an important source of CNS emboli; when associated with fever, seizures, or disseminated intravascular coagulation (DIC), it may be confused with culture-negative infective endocarditis.[67] Initially described as a terminal event associated with disseminated mucus-secreting adenocarcinomas, this form of endocarditis (usually on the aortic or mitral valves) not only gives rise to systemic emboli but also occurs in the course of many disorders other than malignancy (e.g., rheumatic heart disease, pregnancy, drug overdose, vasculitis, and cirrhosis).[68] It may also complicate localized cancer and may even precede that diagnosis.

Adenocarcinomas comprise more than 50 percent of associated malignancies—mostly lung and pancreas—but hematopoietic malignances, including non-Hodgkin's lymphoma, Hodgkin's disease, acute leukemia, multiple myeloma, and bone marrow transplantation have also been implicated.[69,70]

The pathophysiology of nonbacterial thrombotic endocarditis involves three factors:

1. Coagulopathy (20 to 30 percent of patients evidence a chronic form of DIC) predisposes to deposition of platelets and fibrin on cardiac valves.
2. Abnormal cardiac valves present a fertile surface for fibrin deposition.
3. Mucin may promote either fibrin deposition on the valves or embolism.

Thromboembolism is usually the first sign, but systemic thromboembolism may be asymptomatic, with pulmonary and myocardial infarcts found only at autopsy. Stroke (often causing hemiplegia) or encephalopathy is often the first clinical manifestation. Cancer patients with seemingly reactive psychological symptoms may actually be suffering from organic emboli secondary to nonbacterial thrombotic endocarditis.[71] The small vegetations do not interfere with valve function sufficiently to produce murmurs in most patients; echocardiographic visualization is not helpful because the vegetations are usually less than 2 mm in size. It is not an easy diagnosis to establish clinically. Rarely, the disorder is complicated by colonization with organisms, so that infective endocarditis results.

CEREBRAL MYCOTIC ANEURYSMS

The term *mycotic aneurysm,* designating an arterial lesion of infectious origin, was coined by Osler in 1885 to describe mushroom-shaped aneurysms that developed in patients with SBE, when the term *mycotic* (now restricted to fungal infections) more broadly referred to infection with any microorganism.[1]

Intracranial hemorrhage, either intracerebral or subarachnoid, occurs in 2.7 to 7.0 percent of patients with infective endocarditis.[11,13,32,43] It is usually attributed to a ruptured mycotic aneurysm, even when no aneurysm can be demonstrated.[13,72,73] Mycotic aneurysms may, in fact, be obliterated by the hemorrhages that they produce, so that neither angiographic nor pathological examination reveals them.[28] Intracranial hemorrhage in infective endocarditis may also result from a septic arteritis that erodes and ruptures the arterial wall without a well-defined aneurysm ever having formed.[28,31,35,74] Additionally, hemorrhagic transformation of ischemic brain infarcts has been well documented.[28,35]

Hart and associates have analyzed the mechanisms of intracranial hemorrhage in infective endocarditis, both in their own series of 209 patients and in a detailed review of the literature.[28] They argue persuasively that mycotic aneurysms no longer account for the approximately 5 percent of recognized intracranial hemorrhages in infective endocarditis, as previously believed,[13,72,73] but are proven in only about 1.7 percent (range 0.8 to 2.8 percent) of cases. In only 2 of their 17 patients with infective endocarditis and intracranial hemorrhage was an aneurysm present; hemorrhagic infarct or septic necrosis of the arterial wall accounted for the remaining cases.[28]

Two mechanisms are currently proposed to explain the pathogenesis of cerebral mycotic aneurysms.[75–77] In the first, septic embolism initiates inflammatory destruction of the cerebral arterial wall from within the lumen, at the endothelial surface (embolic-mycotic process).[72] In the second, infected embolic material lodges in the adventitial layer of the artery, entering through the vasa vasorum and subsequently destroying the adventitia and muscularis, resulting in aneurysmal dilatation. Animal studies support the vasa vasorum pathway.[75,77]

The consequences of a cerebral embolus thus depend upon the anatomical location of the embolus, the presence or absence of accompanying bacteria, the virulence of the transported organism, and the effectiveness of antimicrobial therapy. Symptomatic intracranial hemorrhage associated with *S. aureus* endocarditis usually develops prior to hospitalization or within 48 hours of admission and prior to control of infection, as observed by many reviewers.[13,28] Organisms are not routinely found in the Gram stain of presumed mycotic aneurysms,[72] but abscess formation and bacterial colonies may be present when virulent organisms are involved.[78]

Although infection via the vasa vasorum pathway is currently accepted as the major cause of aneurysm formation, the embolic-mycotic process apparently operates in some instances where intraluminal occlu-sion can be documented prior to aneurysm formation[13,79] or even in the rare instance where a brain abscess surrounds an aneurysm.[20]

Atherosclerosis, especially when associated with an intraluminal thrombus, is an important cause of mycotic aneurysms in the aorta and other large systemic vessels, as it diminishes the normal resistance of the arterial intima to invasion by passing bacteria, such as *Salmonella* species. Atherosclerosis plays no role in CNS mycotic aneurysms associated with infective endocarditis, except perhaps in unusual instances where a proximal (circle of Willis) congenital aneurysm is involved or where carotid artery aneurysms (not usually associated with infective endocarditis, although there are rare exceptions[80,81]) are involved. The internal carotid artery, close to the pharynx, develops mycotic aneurysms secondary to tonsillitis, mastoiditis, pharyngitis, or periodontal disease, whereas mycotic aneurysms of the common carotid artery derive from hematogenous sources or adjacent lymph nodes.[82,83] Rarely, intracranial mycotic aneurysms of extravascular origin may develop secondary to trauma, otitis media, or meningitis.[76]

Frazee and associates estimated that approximately 3 to 4 percent of patients with infective endocarditis develop intracranial mycotic aneurysms, but many of their reviewed cases antedated CT scanning and refined angiographic techniques.[73] There were only 3 recognized cases among 150 patients with infective endocarditis at the Cleveland Clinic (since 1974), indicating a 2 percent incidence.[15] Nevertheless, this complication remains a significant cause of morbidity and mortality in developing and Third World countries, where acute rheumatic fever and rheumatic heart disease are still prevalent.[84]

Cerebral mycotic aneurysms, recognized clinically in approximately 2 percent of cases, have been found at autopsy in approximately 5 to 10 percent of cases.[13,15,73,85] Because many aneurysms remain totally asymptomatic and heal quietly during antibiotic therapy, whereas those that rupture may obliterate evidence of their presence during the massive hemorrhagic injury that follows,[72,76,86] the recorded incidence in many series must be inappropriately low. Even at autopsy, unless cerebral or subarachnoid bleeding has occurred, small lesions may be missed without careful dissection of the circle of Willis and examination of the entire vascular tree. Cerebral mycotic aneurysms usually occur earlier but less often in acute endocarditis, in comparison with SBE. As mentioned previously, however, effective therapy of acute infective endocarditis has improved the survival rate, so this pattern may no longer apply. Although it has been stated that mycotic aneurysms occur more often with low-virulence organisms,[87] other studies suggest a greater risk with more virulent organisms such as *S. aureus*.[13,75] Morbidity and mortality associated with experimental mycotic aneurysms also relate to organism virulence.[75]

The middle cerebral artery is involved four times more often than either the anterior or posterior cerebral artery. Mycotic aneurysms develop at the bifurcation of small, secondary branch, peripheral arteries, in contrast to congenital cerebral aneurysms, which are usually found near the circle of Willis.[72] The preponderance of mycotic aneurysms at peripheral sites, particularly at sites of vessel branching, is probably due to fragmentation of the friable emboli that ultimately impact in small-caliber peripheral vessels. Though usually small and single, multiple aneurysms may be present and, occasionally, a mycotic aneurysm develops in a more proximal location, thus mimicking a congenital (berry) aneurysm.[88] Infection of congenital aneurysms (usually located near the circle of Willis) also occurs; these are frequently fusiform and present major problems in management.[72,76,88,89]

Infectious intracranial aneurysms not associated with infective endocarditis may have unusual and atypical features, including uncharacteristic locations (e.g., on the posterior cerebral artery, the vertebral artery at the origin of the posterior inferior cerebellar artery, the mid- and distal basilar artery, or the intracavernous internal carotid artery) and predisposing medical conditions (e.g., bacterial meningitis, immunocompromised state, or the postoperative period). Unusual organisms (e.g., *Pseudomonas aeruginosa* and fungi) are often involved.[90]

Cerebral embolization frequently but not invariably precedes recognition of a cerebral mycotic aneurysm[15,76,86] and is a much more common cause of "stroke" in infective endocarditis than is intracranial hemorrhage.[13] Aneurysms often remain asymptomatic until or unless they rupture, although prior to rupture an enlarging aneurysm may compromise cranial nerve function by compression or produce a nonspecific premorbid phase with unilateral headache or nuchal rigidity. Some aneurysms leak slowly before rupture, provoking intense perivascular inflammation, which can produce a mild or moderate meningeal irritation; the cerebrospinal fluid (CSF) is sterile but shows several hundred erythrocytes and leukocytes, with modest elevation of protein concentration.[41,76]

Rupture of a cerebral mycotic aneurysm is a catastrophic event, producing either subarachnoid hemorrhage, intraventricular hemorrhage, or destruction of cerebral tissue.[91] This event may be the initial manifestation of infective endocarditis or may occur after the disease has been treated or even cured by antibiotic therapy. Some authors suggest that the more peripheral location results in less destructive effects than occur with berry lesions and may also make mycotic aneurysms more amenable to excision and safe clipping of the parent vessel without severe infarction. Rarely, a subdural hematoma forms.

Among 29 patients with cerebral mycotic aneurysms gathered from the literature (1955 to 1974), 13 presented with rupture.[76] In the remaining 16, where infective endocarditis preceded evidence of a ruptured aneurysm, 4 were suspected of having antecedent embolization and 3 had focal arteritis proximal to a thrombosed vessel.[76] In some patients the embolus is heralded by a TIA.[51] The staff of the Cleveland Clinic compared 150 patients with infective endocarditis seen there since 1974, including 3 cases with documented cerebral mycotic aneurysm, with 65 documented cases of cerebral mycotic aneurysms reported in the English literature since 1957.[15] A neurological prodrome, prior to rupture or angiographic discovery of the aneurysm, was present in 29 of the 68 cases (42.6 percent) with mycotic aneurysms. The most common prodome was a focal deficit indicating embolic infarction (16 cases); the time interval between the first neurological complaint and discovery or rupture of the mycotic aneurysm ranged from 2 days to 18 months. No specific profile distinguished patients with and without mycotic aneurysm. The authors recommended four-vessel angiography for all patients with infective endocarditis who develop a focal deficit during the acute phase of the illness, indicating that this procedure should be performed within 2 weeks of the event but not before 48 hours (the minimum time necessary for aneurysm formation, according to experimental studies).

The value of angiography lies in (1) demonstrating that aneurysms are probably mycotic because of their peripheral location; (2) confirming that acute episodes are either embolic or hemorrhagic; (3) documenting the multiplicity of aneurysms, if present; and (4) providing a baseline for serial studies if medical management is elected.[15,76] It is currently unclear whether angiography should be repeated, if initially negative, when long-term anticoagulation is planned.[30,31] Cerebral angiography is recommended in patients with headache and red blood cells in the CSF and should be considered in any patient with nonfocal neurological symptoms before initiating anticoagulation therapy.[15] Although more than 50 percent of patients with cerebral mycotic aneurysms have no recognizable prodrome, patients who successfully complete a course of parenteral antibiotic therapy without experiencing neurological symptoms have a low risk of subsequent subarachnoid hemorrhage. Such patients can probably be safely anticoagulated without angiography,[15] although some disagree and recommend angiography at the conclusion of antibiotic therapy in patients requiring long-term anticoagulation.[30] Thus, the presence or suspicion of cerebral emboli during an episode of infective endocarditis should be an indication to perform a CT scan or MRI of the head and to consider cerebral angiography.

The variable interval between septic embolization and arterial wall destruction reflects the virulence of the organism, the intensity of the host response, and the influence of antibiotic therapy. As an increasing number of patients with acute infective endocarditis are rescued by prosthetic valve surgery, the incidence of mycotic aneurysm may be expected to rise.[92] Untreated, dogs bleed from mycotic aneurysms within 2 days of septic cerebral embolization to the vasa vasorum.[75] In treated patients the average interval between symptoms suggesting cerebral embolization and intracranial hemorrhage is highly variable[15] but is in the order of 10 days.[12,73]

The natural history of cerebral mycotic aneurysms remains uncertain. Antibiotic therapy unquestionably delays rupture of some mycotic aneurysms without necessarily preventing their development.[72,73,93,94] In the largest single series of documented intracranial mycotic aneurysms reported to date—28 aneurysms in 17 patients—20 aneurysms were followed angiographically or with CT scans during medical treatment; 10 became smaller or disappeared and 10 remained unchanged or enlarged, 1 with a fatal rupture.[30] Unfortunately, the total number of patients treated for endocarditis at that medical center

during the 18-year study period was not indicated. The authors of the study concluded that all patients with infective endocarditis should undergo neurological evaluation, CT scan of the head, and (unless contraindicated) a lumbar puncture, and that all patients with neurological abnormalities not attributable to systemic toxicity or with CSF pleocytosis or apparent infarction on CT scan should undergo four-vessel cerebral angiography.[30] They further recommended that single, accessible mycotic aneurysms in medically stable patients should be promptly excised and that angiography should be repeated at the conclusion of antibiotic therapy in patients requiring long-term anticoagulation even if initial angiograms were normal, because aneurysms may form during treatment. This aggressive approach, suggested in the early literature by others[30,72,73,85] and based on anecdotal reports and selected case series that emphasize the often tragic consequences of rupture, conflicts with the recent Cleveland Clinic experience.[43] It was strongly challenged also by the group from San Antonio, Texas,[28,31] whose data led to the more conservative recommendation that it is unjustified to perform lumbar puncture and CT scan of the head in all patients with infective endocarditis because presymptomatic detection of aneurysms is of little therapeutic benefit—hemorrhagic presentations, either early or late, correlate better with the presence of pyogenic arteritis[28,31] or hemorrhagic transformation of ischemic cerebral infarcts.[32] They would restrict arteriography to those with subarachnoid hemorrhage or, perhaps, severe headache persisting in the face of adequate control of infection. Based on my own experience, I would favor this conservative approach.

All patients with sterile meningitis and focal neurological symptoms or unilateral headache should undergo sequential thin-slice CT scanning or MRI of the head, as well as angiography if indicated, particularly when there is infection with virulent organisms or if there has been previous clinical evidence of an embolus and a sudden, unexplained neurological deterioration occurs.[13] CT scans may demonstrate small focal areas of cortical enhancement that correspond to peripheral aneurysms seen on subsequent angiography[95] (Fig. 6-1A&B). CT scan or MRI demonstration of small, round peripheral areas of focal enhancement associated with an intracerebral hemorrhage suggests that a mycotic aneurysm is the cause.[44,96] Abnormal CSF formulas, in the absence of focal neurological abnormalities, may not always warrant routine angiography with its attendant risks,[13] but these patients should at least undergo CT scanning or MRI. Rarely, left atrial myxoma gives rise to peripherally situated "mycotic" aneurysms caused by tumor invasion of the vessel walls[97] (Fig. 6-1C&D). Another uncommon primary neoplasm, choriocarcinoma, produces this picture as well.[98]

Serial angiographic studies have demonstrated the resolution of mycotic aneurysms with successful antibiotic therapy,[76,86,92,93] although it may occur only in 50 percent of cases.[30,72] Sequential thin-slice CT scans or MRI can safely and accurately monitor the course of infectious intracranial aneurysms identified angiographically, sometimes reducing the need for serial angiography with its attendant risks.[99]

Late rupture of a cerebral mycotic aneurysm occurs uncommonly. The Cleveland Clinic group reported only 1 late intracranial hemorrhage in 122 survivors of infective endocarditis followed for a mean of 40 months: the single patient with hemorrhage was excessively anticoagulated at the time.[15] Bamford and associates successfully resected a peripheral aneurysm that ruptured 6 months after bacteriological cure of streptococcal mitral valve endocarditis.[100] Cases of unruptured mycotic aneurysms have been reported as long as 24 months after successful treatment of infective endocarditis.[38,60,73,101]

INFECTION (ABSCESS, MENINGITIS, MENINGOENCEPHALITIS)

Infected embolic material may be deposited in cerebral or meningeal vessels, causing arteritis, abscess, or meningitis. Toone considered the fundamental CNS complication in endocarditis to be a diffuse embolic meningoencephalitis and emphasized a meningeal syndrome with neck rigidity and spinal fluid pleo-

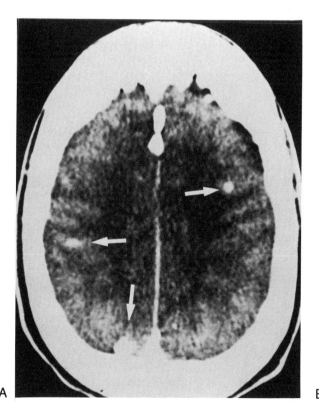 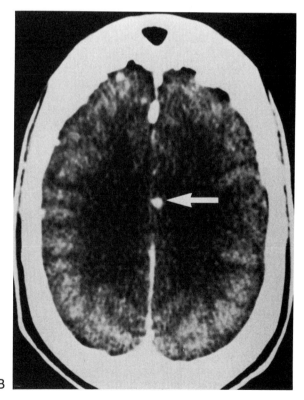

A B

Fig. 6-1 (A&B) CT scans with contrast, demonstrating multiple peripheral enhancing lesions *(arrows)* that correspond to multiple peripheral aneurysms demonstrated on a subsequent bilateral carotid angiogram. *(Figure continues.)*

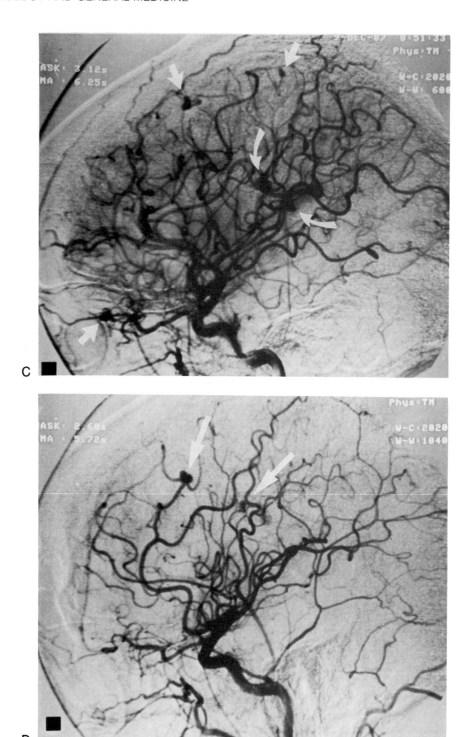

Fig. 6-1 *(Continued)* **(C)** Right carotid arteriogram; **(D)** left carotid arteriogram. Arrows indicate aneurysms. The patient had a left atrial myxoma; these tumor-derived aneurysms mimic the picture seen with true mycotic aneurysms. (Courtesy of Dr. T. J. Masaryk, Cleveland, OH.)

cytosis (polymorphonuclear or lymphocytic).[9] Persistent encephalopathy related to infective endocarditis probably results from multifocal brain ischemia due to multiple small septic emboli, usually occurring during uncontrolled infection with virulent organisms.[33] Macroscopic brain abscess is an uncommon complication and relates to the level and duration of bacteremia, the virulence of the infecting organism, and the occurrence of preceding septic emboli. There was a far greater incidence of cerebral abscess and purulent meningitis in acute infective endocarditis than in SBE when Pankey examined these two aspects among cases seen from 1939 to 1959; the incidence figures were 62 percent and 4 percent, respectively.[39,40] Some abscesses were small and found only at autopsy. Under appropriate circumstances, even a *viridans* streptococcus (e.g., *S. sanguis*) can provoke the suppurative picture usually associated with *S. aureus*.[52] At the MGH, most lesions were multiple and microscopic, associated with a fulminant course and with miliary microabscesses in other organs, and usually due to virulent organisms, particularly *S. aureus*.[13] In 9 of the 218 patients (4.1 percent) there was no suspicion of brain abscess until autopsy; in 8 of these cases the abscesses were less than 1 cm^3, mainly microscopic, and of insufficient size either to create a mass effect or to require surgery (Fig. 6-2). In one patient only, a large (cerebellar) staphylococcal abscess extended directly from adjacent otitis media and mastoiditis. Thus, the single cerebral abscess warranting surgical drainage among 218 patients derived from an otitic focus rather than a bacteremia.[13] Macroscopic brain abscess due to infective endocarditis was seen in only 4 of 830 patients (0.5 percent) in four combined series.[13,22,33,43] Multiple small abscesses or diffuse changes, often labeled *cerebritis* on CT studies, usually resolve uneventfully with antibiotic therapy[102] (Fig. 6-3). Little can or need be done for microscopic lesions except to treat the underlying endocarditis with appropriate antimicrobial therapy.

The clinical picture is highly variable. Headache, confusion, increased intracranial pressure, and focal signs, often developing slowly over a period of days, are noted with large abscesses. The CSF may contain a modest number of cells and a slightly elevated protein content, consistent with a "sterile" meningitis. Occasionally, suppurative meningitis is present and the organisms can be isolated.[13,33] Infective endocarditis is present in approximately one-third of patients with spontaneous staphylococcal meningitis (not related to trauma), who generally experience a more fulminant course.[33,103]

Meningoencephalitis—characterized by confusion, stiff neck, headache, and a "sterile" spinal fluid (with a minimal pleocytosis)—has at times been designated as "acute brain syndrome" or placed within a "toxic" category ("toxic encephalopathy"). These imprecise designations should be abandoned, since a meningoencephalitic picture can be caused by infection, embolization with bland infarction(s), or even a mycotic aneurysm under appropriate circumstances. Confusion or delirium may be due to systemic metabolic abnormalities, e.g., azotemia, or to arteriosclerotic vascular disease, especially in the elderly, in whom paranoia, hallucinations, or personality changes, sometimes associated with a TIA, misdirects the clinician who fails to consider the possibility of infective endocarditis in all febrile patients with cardiac disease and acute neuropsychiatric signs and symptoms. Even amnesia may herald the diagnosis of infective endocarditis.[104] MRI in confused patients with infective endocarditis and normal CT scans has shown multiple focal areas of abnormality consistent with ischemia.[44] In patients with persistent "encephalopathy," incompletely controlled infection is often the explanation, and the patient should be investigated fully (MRI, CSF examination, evaluation for DIC).

SEIZURES

Seizures may be focal or generalized; most focal seizures in this setting are due to cerebral emboli,[13] although metabolic abnormalities may trigger a preexisting focus. In contrast, causes of generalized seizures during the course of infective endocarditis include hypoxia, uremia, purulent meningitis, or even drug administration (e.g., lidocaine or large doses of penicillin).[13] Penicillin neurotoxicity was thought to have provoked the onset of seizures, both focal and generalized, in seven patients in the recent MGH experience, particularly in those exhibiting myoclonus.[13] Overall, 24 (11 percent) of the 218 patients in that series experienced seizures; in 5, they were part of the presenting symptom complex.

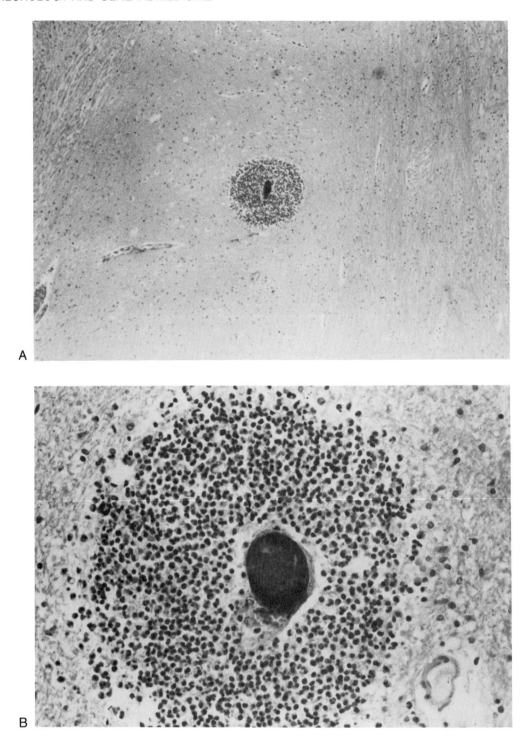

Fig. 6-2 (A&B) Micrographs of a microscopic embolomycotic cerebral abscess in a fatal case of fulminant staphylococcal endocarditis. There were multiple microembolic abscesses in the brain and throughout the body. (Original magnifications: **A** ×450; **B** ×1,000)

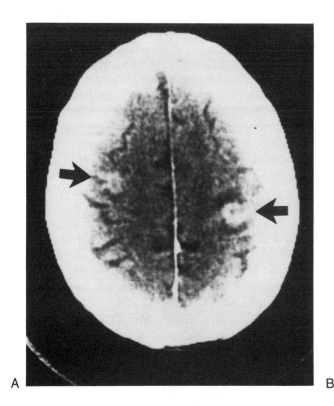

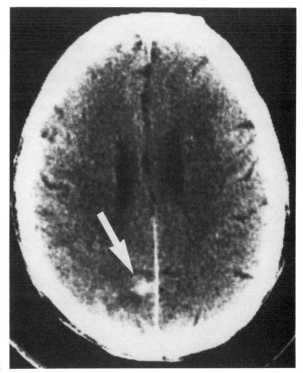

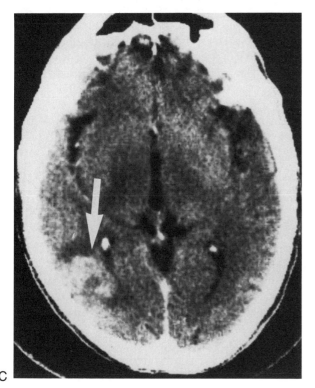

Fig. 6-3 Multiple CT contrast-enhancing lesions *(arrows)* in a young male intravenous drug addict with staphylococcal mitral valve endocarditis. All lesions resolved after a 6-week course of intravenous antibiotic. (Courtesy of Dr. A. Pearlstein, Cleveland, OH.)

INTRAVENOUS DRUG ABUSE

Neurological presentations in abusers of intravenous drugs who have developed infective endocarditis add further diagnostic confusion. Many chronic heroin addicts present with delirium or altered states of consciousness resulting from an acute reaction to the intravenous mixture. Both focal and generalized seizures can accompany this "overdose syndrome," and persistent organic mental changes, parkinsonian features, and hemiparesis in the absence of infection have been recorded. Autopsies reveal both septic and nonseptic cerebral emboli, purpura cerebri, and a variety of meningitides (fungal, bacterial, and tuberculous). Paradoxically, addicts with staphylococcal endocarditis are less prone to develop congestive heart failure and exhibit fewer neurological manifestations as compared with nonaddicts with staphylococcal infective endocarditis, probably because of predominant tricuspid valve involvement in the addicted group.[105]

PROSTHETIC VALVE ENDOCARDITIS

Neurological complications are a major source of morbidity and mortality among patients with prosthetic valve endocarditis (PVE), particularly of the late variety (more than 60 days after surgery),[25,26] but they occur no more frequently than in patients with native valve endocarditis (NVE).[35,43]

The management of anticoagulation in patients with PVE is a crucial and unresolved issue. Except for patients with porcine valves in normal sinus rhythm and, in some centers, patients with cloth-covered prostheses, most patients with prosthetic valves receive anticoagulants. Anticoagulation decreases the incidence of thromboembolic phenomena in noninfected patients, but there is uncertainty and disagreement about continuing anticoagulant therapy once PVE is diagnosed.[35] The incidence of CNS thromboembolic phenomena in patients with PVE ranges from 50 to 70 percent[23,26] when they are inadequately anticoagulated.[27] However, patients with PVE who receive anticoagulants have an increased incidence of CNS bleeding as compared with noninfected patients.[35]

At the MGH, 43 percent of the thromboembolic phenomena occurring in patients with PVE were hemorrhagic[13]; the figure at the Mayo Clinic was only 11 percent.[26] Among 43 patients at the MGH, 12 (28 percent) anticoagulated patients with PVE suffered major CNS complications.[25] In contrast, only 20 percent of 283 adequately anticoagulated noninfected patients with prosthetic valves experienced cerebral thromboembolic complications. Fatal CNS hemorrhage or hemorrhagic infarction occurred in 5 infected patients, highlighting the risks of anticoagulation during active PVE. At the Mayo Clinic a 71 percent incidence of clinical CNS symptoms was noted among 14 patients with PVE who were not receiving anticoagulants, compared with an 8 percent incidence of such symptoms among 38 patients who were adequately anticoagulated.[26] Autopsy data from the Mayo Clinic disclosed a higher frequency of CNS emboli or infarction in cases without anticoagulation (7 of 8; bland infarcts in 4 and multiple bland and hemorrhagic infarcts in 3) in comparison to the 14 patients with PVE who died after adequate anticoagulant treatment (6 had thromboemboli: multiple bland infarcts in 5 and multiple hemorrhagic infarcts in 1).[26] At the MGH, anticoagulation is continued in patients with late PVE unless CNS complications arise, at which point anticoagulation is temporarily reversed.[25] Care is taken, however, to maintain the prothrombin time at approximately 1.5 times the control value. Neurological complications may be more frequent in PVE when control of anticoagulation is inadequate.[27] Anticoagulation must be maintained in a narrow therapeutic range; some therefore advocate heparin sodium in this setting.[27,35] Thus, available data have yet to clarify the role of anticoagulants in PVE.[28]

CEREBROSPINAL FLUID

Spinal fluid pleocytosis is a frequent neurological abnormality in patients with infective endocarditis, who most commonly display an "aseptic" or "sterile" CSF formula with a modest lymphocytic (occasionally polymorphonuclear) pleocytosis, moderately elevated protein content, a normal glucose level, and negative Gram stain and culture. With virulent organisms, particularly *S. aureus,* purulent meningitis has been recorded more commonly.[13,33] Infective endocarditis was associated with one-third of the cases of spontaneous *S. aureus* meningitis—not related to neurosurgery, trauma, cerebrospinal defects, or indwelling shunts—seen in six Toronto hospitals over a 15-year period.[103] This group of patients experienced a more fulminant illness.[103] One-third of patients with native valve staphylococcal endocarditis may present with clinical features of meningitis (40 percent with no cardiac murmur).[29] Although the percentage of cases of infective endocarditis due to *Streptococcus pneumoniae* (pneumococcus) has declined from the 10 to 15 percent figures of the preantibiotic era to 1 to 2 percent today, the incidence of concomitant meningitis remains as high as 70 percent.[106]

CSF examination was performed in 69 of 84 patients with neurological complications at the MGH and was normal in 30 percent, purulent (polymorphonuclear leukocytic pleocytosis with reduced glucose and elevated protein levels) in 28 percent, "aseptic" (lymphocytic pleocytosis, with normal glucose and normal or slightly elevated protein levels) in 25 percent, and hemorrhagic in 13 percent.[13] In 35 patients with nuchal rigidity, disorientation, or both, the CSF was purulent in 16, "aseptic" in 8, normal in 9, and hemorrhagic in 2. Unsuspected lumbar epidural abscess was found in 1 patient. Among 25 patients with new focal neurological signs, the CSF was normal in 8, "aseptic" in 8, hemorrhagic in 6, purulent in 2, and both hemorrhagic and purulent in 1. Finally, 9 patients underwent lumbar punctures because of seizures; CSF was normal in 5 and purulent, "aseptic," and hemorrhagic in 1 each; in the ninth patient, the fluid was normal but under increased pressure. Therefore, except for finding a purulent CSF more frequently in patients with meningeal signs, no single clinical or neurological event or setting was associated with a characteristic CSF formula. By contrast, CSF findings did correlate with the nature of the infecting organism, since virulent organisms (*S. aureus,* enteric gram-negative bacilli, and *S. pneumoniae*) were frequently associated with a purulent CSF, whereas relatively avirulent organisms (e.g., *viridans* streptococci) were associated with a normal or "aseptic" picture. In only 11 specimens among the 69 CSF samples was the culture positive; in each case, the CSF was purulent, yielding *S. aureus* in 8; 1 each grew *S. pneumoniae, Proteus mirabilis,* and a *viridans* streptococcus.[13] Occasionally, however, even a CSF sample with an "aseptic" formula yields a pathogen, even a *viridans* streptococcus.[107] Therefore, CSF examination aids in the differential diagnosis of specific neurological complications only when hemorrhage or a purulent meningitis is present.

DIAGNOSIS AND THERAPY

Most patients with neurological involvement improve as appropriate antimicrobial therapy suppresses and ultimately eliminates the endocardial focus of infection. Any patient with infective endocarditis who has persistent or evolving neurological findings or an abnormal CSF should undergo a CT scan or, preferably, MRI of the head, which may disclose areas of inflammation or leakage around intact aneurysms or small hematomas, infarcts, or other changes suggesting (early) formation of an aneurysm.[95,99] Although many reports suggest that most patients with cerebral mycotic aneurysms are asymptomatic and rarely have a "warning leak" prior to a sudden, massive, often fatal subarachnoid or intracerebral hemorrhage,[11,72,85] some reports suggest otherwise.[15,60] At the Mayo Clinic, six of eight patients with cerebral mycotic aneurysms were diagnosed antemortem when complaints of severe, unremitting, localized headache were investigated with head CT scans and angiography.[60] Although a neurological prodrome prior to the rupture or angiographic discovery of a cerebral mycotic aneurysm was present in 42.6 percent of published reports reviewed by Cleveland Clinic investigators, a headache "alarm" syndrome was notably less frequent than an antecedent focal deficit syndrome (13.2 compared with 23.5 percent),[15] and there was no significant difference in the overall frequency of neurological symptoms between patients with and without mycotic aneurysms.

The natural history of cerebral mycotic aneurysms, as reviewed previously, is incompletely understood; some believe that most will rupture if not resected, whereas others claim that effective medical therapy leads to cure (resolution) in most cases.[30,72,79,86,93] Angiography should be performed as early as possible, when the suspicion of aneurysm first arises, and may even be indicated when only an embolic event has been documented, since, as previously noted, clinically apparent emboli often precede the appearance of a mycotic aneurysm.[73,76] Rarely, even a four-vessel angiogram fails to disclose a mycotic aneurysm that is discovered on a later study, at autopsy, or by subsequent hemorrhage.[94] Serial studies can now be performed at reasonable intervals (7 to 10 days) with reduced amounts of contrast dye by use of arterial digital subtraction angiography. Serial angiography demonstrates that mycotic aneurysms can increase or decrease in size rapidly, within days or weeks, with no corresponding change in clinical status.[30] Since an aneurysm may heal without leakage or rupture following appropriate antimicrobial therapy, surgery is not routinely recommended when one is discovered.[72,86,101] Aggressive resection is nevertheless pursued in some centers,[30] particularly in patients who need cardiac valve replacement.[73] The aneurysm is resected first, unless the cardiac hemodynamic status is deteriorating too rapidly, because the effect or likelihood of aneurysmal rupture may be augmented during the heparinization associated with cardiopulmonary bypass[102,108] or by increased systemic perfusion and greater patient mobility following valve replacement.[108] When cerebral mycotic aneurysms are present (or suspected) in a patient requiring urgent valve replacement, bioprosthetic (porcine) tissue valves are preferred to avoid the need for postoperative anticoagulation.[101]

Wilson and colleagues suggested an approach based on their experiences at the Mayo Clinic.[60] They recommended serial angiography to monitor a single aneurysm peripheral to the first bifurcation of a major vessel, with prompt excision if it enlarges or bleeds. When multiple aneurysms are present, close monitoring with CT scans and serial angiograms is recommended to detect enlargement of one or more of these lesions, with prompt surgical excision when indicated. Excision of the aneurysm is preferred to clipping. Aneurysms proximal to the first bifurcation are more difficult to excise and are approached more cautiously, because ligation may result in severe neurological deficits. These may stabilize or resolve by thrombosis with antibiotic therapy and therefore may have a favorable outcome even without surgery.[30,60,72,86,101]

Standard surgical technique for mycotic aneurysms includes ligation of the affected arterial segment (where there is no involvement by suppuration) followed by excision of the necrotic aneurysm and the adjacent vessel wall.[60,85] Surgical intervention may require aggressive and imaginative maneuvers to avoid or minimize neurological damage, such as extracranial-intracranial bypass grafting, in the case of aneurysms that are located in critical areas or on deep proximal vessels.[109,110]

Occasionally a large solitary brain abscess may require surgical drainage, but most patients have small microabscesses (often multiple) that require no surgical intervention (Fig. 6-3). Even relatively large presumptive brain abscesses (possibly focal cerebritis) that have been monitored by serial CT scans or MRI may resolve partially or completely with antimicrobial therapy.[102,111] Despite concerns about placing a prosthetic valve in patients with infective endocarditis and an undrained intracerebral abscess (and the risk of subsequently seeding that valve, with resultant PVE), a major problem does not generally result.[102] The duration of antimicrobial therapy should probably be extended to 6 or 8 weeks in such individuals. Corticosteroids may be necessary in the presence of acute cerebral edema. All other therapeutic interventions (except for anticoagulation) fall into the surgical realm, including evacuation of an intracerebral hematoma, shunting a developing hydrocephalus (secondary to either meningitis or hemorrhage), and, occasionally, providing emergency decompression in the event of acute cerebral edema.[60]

Since all neurological complications derive from emboli, is there a role for prophylactic valve replacement or debridement when echocardiography discloses large vegetations on either the mitral or aortic valve?[60] Patients experiencing a single clinically evident embolic event or those with no history of emboli but simply large vegetations demonstrated echocardiographically are considered candidates for valve replacement or debridement by some authorities.[24,36,37] Patients with large vegetations have an incidence of congestive heart failure and a requirement for surgery similar to that of patients with smaller vegetations, and they do not necessarily experience a greater incidence of stroke or death.[32] Aortic valve endocarditis has a high complication rate, particularly of congestive heart failure, and large aortic valve vegetations may be associated with an even greater complication rate of both heart failure and stroke.[54]

The presence of a valvular vegetation on echocardiogram places a patient with infective endocarditis at increased risk of systemic embolization and congestive heart failure, especially when large (i.e., exceeding 1 cm diameter) aortic and mitral valve lesions due to *S. aureus* are present.[24,36] Since echocardiography detects valvular vegetations in 75 to 80 percent of patients with infective endocarditis, it is obvious that all patients are not at increased risk to the same degree, even though we recognize that patients without demonstrable vegetations represent a lower risk group in terms of embolic complications. At present, there are insufficient data to define the subset with the highest risk, those patients who would benefit from preventive surgical valvular debridement or replacement,[111] although aortic valve endocarditis and large (greater than 1 cm) vegetations due to "virulent" pathogens represent such a subset to some investigators.[54,111] Others find more emboli associated with mitral valve lesions.[13,14,37] Despite isolated dramatic cases of delayed cerebral emboli occurring late in the course of successful antibiotic therapy,[112] each case requires separate consideration. Hemorrhagic transformation of an ischemic infarct should be sought whenever the infarct is large or previous signs worsen,[35] although 75 percent of cases lack clinical clues to transformation. Repeat CT scan is the optimal method, 2 to 4 days after the initial scan. It should also not be forgotten that a single clinically evident embolus is accompanied by clinically inapparent emboli in most patients, so the criterion of multiple emboli as an indication for valve surgery seems wholly inappropriate by itself.

The role of anticoagulants in patients with infective endocarditis remains controversial.[27,28,32] Anticoagulants used in the early stages of cerebral embolism deriving from noninfected cardiac sources exert a beneficial effect on both morbidity and mortality,[113] but they have traditionally been considered to be contraindicated in patients with infective endocarditis because of the danger of bleeding from an unrecognized mycotic aneurysm or following embolic infarction of the brain. Paschalis and colleagues found no difference in the incidence of cerebral embolism among 61 patients with infective endocarditis seen at the Middlesex Hospital (1981 to 1987) when comparing patients on long-term anticoagulants (30 percent) with those who were not anticoagulated (29 percent).[34] They concluded that once antibiotic treatment is begun and infection is brought under control, the embolic risk is reduced so profoundly that anticoagulation is unlikely to exert any beneficial effects. Although anticoagulants may not increase the risk of primary hemorrhage, they increase the risk of hemorrhagic transformation of an infarct.[28] If patients with infective endocarditis develop clear evidence of thromboembolic disease not related to vegetations (e.g., femoral vein phlebitis) or if an intracardiac prosthesis is present, anticoagulation may be required. Anticoagulation is of no benefit in the management of the valvular infection per se because it not only fails to prevent growth and separation of small fragments from the infected vegetation but also probably enhances fragmentation. During the prepenicillin era, heparinization in the face of inadequate antimicrobial therapy was associated with a catastrophic incidence of major hemorrhagic episodes. Heparin sodium, however, may have a role in "fine tuning" anticoagulation in late PVE.[27,35] In the recent experience at the MGH, despite relatively small numbers, 23 percent of the hemorrhagic events occurred in the 3 percent of patients who were receiving anticoagulants.[13] A very similar pattern was seen in Lyon, France, where 50 percent of brain hemorrhages (6 of 12) occurred among the 13 percent (35 of 269) of patients who were anticoagulated ($p < 0.001$).[35] The available data concerning anticoagulation and PVE have already been discussed.[13,25–27,35]

The timing of cardiac surgery following an acute embolic stroke raises concerns about the risk of secondary bleeding into an ischemic infarct when the patient is anticoagulated during cardiopulmonary bypass, and concerns that ischemic edema may be encouraged during hypotension/nonpulsatile blood flow.[33] In one report, among 5 patients with infective endocarditis undergoing surgery, 2 experienced hemorrhagic worsening when surgery was performed at 1 and 4 days after their strokes.[114] In contrast, no neurological deterioration occurred in 14 patients with infective endocarditis who underwent cardiac surgery at a mean of 12 days after an acute stroke.[115] Despite such meager data to guide management, it seems prudent, whenever possible, to prevent or minimize the risk of secondary hemorrhagic transformation or accentuation of brain edema by delaying cardiac surgery for 3 to 4 days or (especially with large infarcts) until there is evidence by CT of resolution of the edema.[33]

REFERENCES

1. Osler W: Gulstonian lectures on malignant endocarditis. Lancet 1:415, 459, 505 (three parts), 1885
2. Virchow R: Uber die akute Entzündung der Arterien. Virchows Arch (Pathol Anat) 1:272, 1847

3. Kirkes WS: Principal effects resulting from detachment of fibrinous deposits from the interior of the heart, and their mixture with the circulating blood. Med Chir Trans 35:281, 1852

4. Tufnell J: On the influence of vegetations on the valves of the heart in the production of secondary arterial diseases. Dublin Q J Med Sci 15:371, 1853

5. Winkelman NW, Eckel JL: The brain and bacterial endocarditis. Arch Neurol Psychiatry 23:1161, 1930

6. Neal JB, Jackson HW, Appelbaum E: Neurological complications of subacute bacterial endocarditis. NY State J Med 36:1818, 1936

7. Krinsky CM, Merritt HH: Neurologic manifestations of subacute bacterial endocarditis. N Engl J Med 218:563, 1938

8. Kernohan JW, Woltman HW, Barnes AR: Involvement of the nervous system associated with endocarditis. Arch Neurol Psychiatry 42:789, 1940

9. Toone EC: Cerebral manifestations of bacterial endocarditis. Ann Intern Med 14:1551, 1941

10. Harrison MJ, Hampton JR: Neurological presentation of bacterial endocarditis. Br Med J 2:148, 1967

11. Jones HR, Siekert RG, Geraci JE: Neurological manifestations of bacterial endocarditis. Ann Intern Med 71:21, 1969

12. Ziment I: Nervous system complications in bacterial endocarditis. Am J Med 47:593, 1969

13. Pruitt AA, Rubin RH, Karchmer AW, Duncan GW: Neurologic complications of bacterial endocarditis. Medicine (Baltimore) 57:329, 1978

14. LeCam B, Guivarch G, Boles JM, et al: Neurologic complications in a group of 86 bacterial endocarditis. Eur Heart J 5, suppl C:97, 1984

15. Salgado AV, Furlan AJ, Keys TF: Mycotic aneurysm, subarachnoid hemorrhage, and indications for cerebral angiography in infective endocarditis. Stroke 18:1057, 1987

16. Jones HR, Siekert RG: Neurological manifestations of infective endocarditis: review of clinical and therapeutic challenges. Brain 112:1295, 1989

17. Salgado AV: Central nervous system complications of infective endocarditis. Stroke 22:1461, 1991

18. Amine ARC: Neurosurgical complications of heroin addiction: brain abscess and mycotic aneurysm. Surg Neurol 7:385, 1977

19. Sato T, Sakuta Y, Suzuki J, et al: Successful surgical treatment of intracranial mycotic aneurysm with brain abscess: report of a case. Acta Neurochir (Wien) 47:53, 1979

20. Pozzati E, Tognetti F, Padovani R, et al: Association of cerebral mycotic aneurysm and brain abscess. Neurochirurgia 26:18, 1983

21. Nocht B, Paschen E, Hegler C: Jochmann's Lehrbuch der Infektions-krankenheiten. p. 144. Springer, Berlin, 1924

22. Lerner PI, Weinstein L: Infective endocarditis in the antibiotic era. N Engl J Med 274:199, 259, 323, 388 (four parts), 1966

23. Garvey GJ, Neu HC: Infective endocarditis—an evolving disease. A review of endocarditis at the Columbia-Presbyterian Medical Center, 1968–1973. Medicine (Baltimore) 57:105, 1978

24. Bayer AS: Infective endocarditis. Clin Infect Dis 17:313, 1993

25. Karchmer AW, Dismukes WE, Buckley MJ, et al: Late prosthetic valve endocarditis: clinical features influencing therapy. Am J Med 64:199, 1978

26. Wilson WR, Geraci JE, Danielson GK, et al: Anticoagulant therapy and central nervous system complications in patients with prosthetic valve endocarditis. Circulation 57:1004, 1978

27. Leport C, Vilde JL, Bricaire F, et al: Fifty cases of late prosthetic valve endocarditis: improvement in prognosis over a 15 year period. Br Heart J 58:66, 1987

28. Hart RG, Kagan-Hallet K, Joerns SE: Mechanisms of intracranial hemorrhage in infective endocarditis. Stroke 18:1048, 1987

29. Gransden WR, Eykyn SJ, Leach RM: Neurological presentations of native valve endocarditis. Q J Med 73:1135, 1989

30. Brust JCM, Dickinson PCT, Hughes JEO, Holtzman RNN: The diagnosis and treatment of cerebral mycotic aneurysms. Ann Neurol 27:238, 1990

31. Kanter MC, Hart RG: Cerebral mycotic aneurysms are rare in infective endocarditis. Ann Neurol 28:590, 1990

32. Hart RG, Foster JW, Luther MF, Kanter MC: Stroke in infective endocarditis. Stroke 21:695, 1990

33. Kanter MC, Hart RG: Neurologic complications of infective endocarditis. Neurology 41:1015, 1991

34. Paschalis C, Puglsey W, John R, Harrison MJG: Rate of cerebral embolic events in relation to antibiotic and anticoagulant therapy in patients with bacterial endocarditis. Eur Neurol 30:87, 1990

35. Delahaye JP, Poncet P, Malquarti V, et al: Cerebrovascular accidents in infective endocarditis: role of anticoagulation. Eur Heart J 11:1074, 1990

36. Jaffe WM, Morgan DE, Pearlman AS, Otto CM: Infective endocarditis, 1983–1988: echocardiographic findings and factors influencing morbidity and mortality. J Am Coll Cardiol 15:1227, 1990

37. Rohmann S, Erbel R, Gorge G, et al: Clinical relevance of vegetation localization by transoesophageal echocardiography in infective endocarditis. Eur Heart J 12:446, 1992

38. Morgan WL, Bland EF: Bacterial endocarditis in the antibiotic era. Circulation 19:753, 1959

39. Pankey GA: Subacute bacterial endocarditis at the University of Minnesota Hospitals 1939 through 1959. Ann Intern Med 55:550, 1961

40. Pankey GA: Acute bacterial endocarditis at the University of Minnesota Hospitals 1939 through 1959. Am Heart J 64:583, 1962

41. Greenlee JE, Mandell GL: Neurological manifestations of infective endocarditis: a review. Stroke 4:958, 1973

42. Barrett AP, Smith MW: Maxillary nerve involvement in bacterial endocarditis. J Oral Maxillofac Surg 43: 816, 1985

43. Salgado AV, Furlan AJ, Keys TF, et al: Neurologic complications of endocarditis: a 12-year experience. Neurology 39:173, 1989

44. Bertorini TE, Laster RE, Thompson BF, Gelfand M: Magnetic resonance imaging of the brain in bacterial endocarditis. Arch Intern Med 149:815, 1989

45. Medley DRK: Chorea and bacterial endocarditis. Br Med J 1:861, 1963

46. Ross AT, DeMyer WE: Isolated syndrome of the medial longitudinal fasciculus in man. Arch Neurol 15: 203, 1966

47. Jones HR, Siekert RG: Embolic mononeuropathy and bacterial endocarditis. Arch Neurol 19:535, 1968

48. Andreas S, Tebbe U, Holzgraef M, Kreuzer H: Embolic mononeuropathy in subacute bacterial endocarditis. Clin Cardiol 13:666, 1990

49. Shafar J: Bacterial endocarditis presenting as pseudobulbar palsy. Br Med J 4:338, 1967

50. Pamphlett R, Walsh J: Infective endocarditis with inflammatory lesions in the peripheral nervous system. Acta Neuropathol (Berl) 78:101, 1989

51. Seikert RG, Jones HR: Transient cerebral ischemic attacks associated with subacute bacterial endocarditis. Stroke 1:178, 1970

52. Young SG, Davee T, Fierer J, Morey MK: Streptococcus sanguis II (viridans) prosthetic valve endocarditis with myocardial, splenic and cerebral abscesses. West J Med 146:479, 1987

53. Hubbel G, Cheitlin MD, Rapaport E: Presentation, management and follow-up evaluation of infective endocarditis in drug addicts. Am Heart J 102:85, 1981

54. Wong D, Chandrarathna AN, Wishnow RM, et al: Clinical implications of large vegetations in infectious endocarditis. Arch Intern Med 143:1874, 1983

55. Shenoy MM, Greif E, Friedman SA, et al: Paradoxical embolism secondary to tricuspid valve endocarditis. Am J Cardiol 54:1374, 1984

56. Stagaman DJ, Presti C, Rees C, Miller DD: Septic pulmonary arteriovenous fistula. Chest 97:1484, 1990

57. Dewar HA, Jones MR, Barnes WS, et al: Fibrinolytic therapy in bacterial endocarditis: experimental studies in dogs. Eur Heart J 7:520, 1986

58. Lerner PI, Gopalakrishna KV, Wolinsky E, et al: Group B streptococcus (S. agalactiae) bacteremia in adults: analysis of 32 cases and review of the literature. Medicine (Baltimore) 56:457, 1977

59. Ellner JJ, Rosenthal MS, Lerner PI, et al: Infective endocarditis caused by slow-growing, fastidious, gram-negative bacteria. Medicine (Baltimore) 58:145, 1979

60. Wilson WR, Giuliani ER, Danielson GK, et al: Management of complications of infective endocarditis. Mayo Clin Proc 57:162, 1982

61. Taha TH, Durrant SS, Mazeika PK, et al: Aspirin to prevent growth of vegetations and cerebral emboli in infective endocarditis. J Intern Med 231:543, 1992

62. Rubenfield S, Min KW: Leukocytoclastic angiitis in subacute bacterial endocarditis. Arch Dermatol 113: 1073, 1977

63. Kauffmann RH, Thompson J, Valentijn M, et al: The clinical implications and the pathogenetic significance of circulating immune complexes in infective endocarditis. Am J Med 71:17, 1981

64. Alajouanine T, Castaigne P, Lhermitte F, et al: L'arterite cerebrale de la maladie d'Osler: ses complications tardives. Sem Hop Paris 35:1160, 1959

65. Bayer AS, Theofilopoulos AN, Eisenberg R, et al: Thrombotic thrombocytopenic purpura-like syndrome associated with infective endocarditis. JAMA 238:408, 1977

66. Groothuis DR, Mikhael MA: Focal cerebral vasculitis associated with circulating immune complexes and brain irradiation. Ann Neurol 19:590, 1986

67. Biller J, Challa VR, Toole JF, et al: Nonbacterial thrombotic endocarditis: a neurologic perspective of clinicopathologic correlations of 99 patients. Arch Neurol 39:95, 1982

68. Macdonell RAL, Kalnins RM, Donnan GA: Nonbacterial thrombotic endocarditis and stroke. Clin Exp Neurol 22:123, 1986

69. Ojeda VJ, Frost F, Mastaglia FL: Non-bacterial thrombotic endocarditis associated with malignant disease: a clinicopathological study of 16 cases. Med J Aust 142:629, 1985

70. Rogers LR, Cho E, Kempin S, et al: Cerebral infarction from non-bacterial thrombotic endocarditis. Am J Med 83:746, 1987

71. MacKenzie TB, Popkin MK: Psychological manifestations of nonbacterial thrombotic endocarditis. Am J Psychiatry 127:972, 1980

72. Bohmfalk GL, Story JL, Wissinger JP, et al: Bacterial intracranial aneurysm. J Neurosurg 48:369, 1978

73. Frazee JG, Cahan LD, Winter J: Bacterial intracranial aneurysms. J Neurosurg 53:633, 1980

74. Masuda J, Yutani C, Waki R, et al: Histopathological

analysis of the mechanisms of intracranial hemorrhage complicating infective endocarditis. Stroke 23:843, 1992

75. Molinari GF, Smith L, Goldstein MN, Satran R: Pathogenesis of cerebral mycotic aneurysms. Neurology 23:325, 1973

76. Moskowitz MA, Rosenbaum AE, Tyler HR: Angiographically monitored resolution of cerebral mycotic aneurysms. Neurology 24:1103, 1974

77. Nakata Y, Shionoya S, Kamiya K: Pathogenesis of mycotic aneurysm. Angiology 19:593, 1968

78. Bell WE, Butler C: Cerebral mycotic aneurysms in children: two case reports. Neurology 18:81, 1968

79. Katz RI, Goldberg HI, Selzer ME: Mycotic aneurysm: case report with novel sequential angiographic findings. Arch Intern Med 134:939, 1974

80. Hardin CA, Thompson R: Mycotic aneurysm of the innominate artery with supravalvular aortic stenosis. J Cardiovasc Surg 17:489, 1976

81. Jebara VA, Acar C, Dervanian P, et al: Mycotic aneurysms of the carotid arteries—case report and review of the literature. J Vasc Surg 14:215, 1991

82. Lansky LL, Maxwell JA: Mycotic aneurysm of the internal carotid artery in an unusual intra-cranial location. Dev Med Child Neurol 17:79, 1975

83. Plotkin GR, O'Rourke JN: Mycotic aneurysm due to Yersinia enterocolitica. Am J Med Sci 281:35, 1981

84. Bullock R, Van Dellen JR, Van Den Heever CM: Intracranial mycotic aneurysms: a review of 9 cases. S Afr Med J 60:970, 1981

85. Roach MR, Drake CG: Ruptured cerebral aneurysms caused by microorganisms. N Engl J Med 273:240, 1965

86. Cantu RC, LeMay M, Wilkinson HA: The importance of repeated angiography in the treatment of mycotic-embolic intracranial aneurysms. J Neurosurg 25:189, 1966

87. Weinstein LW, Schlesinger J: Pathoanatomic, pathophysiologic and clinical correlation in endocarditis. N Engl J Med 291:1122, 1974

88. Rah H, Wahal KM: Subarachnoid hemorrhage in subacute bacterial endocarditis. Neurology 7:265, 1957

89. Sypert GW, Young HF: Ruptured mycotic pericallosal aneurysm with meningitis due to Neisseria meningitidis infection. J Neurosurg 37:467, 1972

90. Barrow DL, Prats AR: Infectious intracranial aneurysms: comparison of groups with and without endocarditis. Neurosurgery 27:562, 1990

91. Vincent FM, Zimmerman JE, Auer TC: Subarachnoid hemorrhage—the initial manifestation of bacterial endocarditis. Neurosurgery 7:488, 1980

92. Nelson RJ, Harley DP, French WJ, et al: Favorable ten-year experience with valve procedures for active infective endocarditis. J Thorac Cardiovasc Surg 87:493, 1984

93. Bingham WF: Treatment of mycotic intracranial aneurysms. J Neurosurg 46:428, 1977

94. Schold C, Earnest MP: Cerebral hemorrhage from a mycotic aneurysm developing during appropriate antibiotic therapy. Stroke 9:267, 1978

95. Simmons KC, Sage MR, Reilly PL: CT of intracerebral hemorrhage due to mycotic aneurysms—case report. Neuroradiology 19:215, 1980

96. Bohmfalk G, Story JL, Wissinger JP, et al: Treatment of mycotic aneurysms. J Neurosurg 54:566, 1981

97. Desousa AL, Muller J, Campbell RL, et al: Atrial myxoma: a review of the neurological complications, metastases and recurrences. J Neurol Neurosurg Psychiatry 41:1119, 1978

98. Olmsted WW, McGee TP: The pathogenesis of peripheral aneurysms of the central nervous system: a subject review from the AFIP. Radiology 123:661, 1977

99. Ahmadi J, Tung H, Giannotta SL, Destian S: Monitoring of infectious intracranial aneurysms by sequential computed tomographic/magnetic resonance imaging studies. Neurosurgery 32:45, 1993

100. Bamford J, Hodges J, Warlow C: Late rupture of a mycotic aneurysm after "cure" of bacterial endocarditis. J Neurol 233:51, 1986

101. Morawetz RB, Karp RB: Evolution and resolution of intracranial bacterial (mycotic) aneurysms. Neurosurgery 15:43, 1984

102. Magilligan DJ Jr: Neurologic complications in endocarditis. p. 187. In Magilligan DJ, Quinn EL (eds): Endocarditis: Medical and Surgical Management. Marcel Dekker, New York, 1986

103. Fong IW, Ranalli P: Staphylococcus aureus meningitis. Q J Med 53:289, 1984

104. Grillo RA, Olson NH: Amnesia as a presenting symptom in subacute bacterial endocarditis. J Clin Psychiatry 47:383, 1986

105. Chambers HF, Korzeniowski DM, Sande MA: Staphylococcus aureus endocarditis: clinical manifestations in addicts and nonaddicts. Medicine (Baltimore) 62:170, 1983

106. Powderly WG, Stanley SL Jr, Medoff G: Pneumococcal endocarditis: report of a series and review of the literature. Rev Infect Dis 8:786, 1986

107. Lerner PI: Meningitis caused by streptococcus in adults. J Infect Dis 131, suppl:S9, 1975

108. Bullock R, Van Dellen JR: Rupture of bacterial intracranial aneurysms following replacement of cardiac valves. Surg Neurol 17:9, 1982

109. Day AL: Extracranial-intracranial bypass grafting in the surgical treatment of bacterial aneurysms: report of two cases. Neurosurgery 9:583, 1981

110. Steinberg GK, Guppy KH, Adler JR, Silverberg GD: Stereotactic, angiography-guided clipping of a distal, mycotic intracranial aneurysm using the Cosman-Roberts-Wells system: technical note. Neurosurgery 30:408, 1992

111. Fredericka DN: Endocarditis and brain abscess due to Bacteroides oralis. J Infect Dis 145:918, 1982

112. Lee WL, Dooling EC: Acute Kingella kingae endocarditis with recurrent cerebral emboli in a child with mitral prolapse. Ann Neurol 16:88, 1984

113. Levine HJ, Pauker SG, Salzman EW: Antithrombotic therapy in valvular heart disease. Chest 95, suppl:98S, 1989

114. Maruyama M, Kuriyama Y, Sawada T, et al: Brain damage after open heart surgery in patients with acute cardioembolic stroke. Stroke 20:1305, 1989

115. Zisbrod Z, Rose DM, Jacobowitz IJ, et al: Results of open heart surgery in patients with recent cardiogenic embolic stroke and central nervous system dysfunction. Circulation 76, suppl V:V-109, 1987

7

Neurological Complications of Hypertension

Michael J. G. Harrison

The heart was larger than ordinary, especially the walls of the left ventricle, which were as thick as the breadth of two fingers. When I opened his head I found in the cavity of the right ventricle of the brain, an extravasation of about two pints of black clotted blood which was the cause of his apoplexy and death.

Baglivi thus described the autopsy of Malpighi in 1694, in which the association between hypertensive cardiac disease and cerebral hemorrhage was clearly made.[1] It is now realized that arterial hypertension is the single most important etiological risk factor in the genesis of strokes of all types. This chapter reviews the role of hypertension in the epidemiology, pathology, and clinical phenomenology of stroke.

EPIDEMIOLOGY

Hypertension as a Risk Factor

All major population studies reveal hypertension to be quantitatively the second most important risk factor for stroke (after age) and therefore the most important potentially reversible etiological factor.[2] The presence of hypertension in the Rochester Study increased the risk of stroke about sixfold, and a similar figure was obtained by The Framingham Study.[3] All types of stroke (cerebral infarction, cerebral hemor-

rhage, and subarachnoid hemorrhage) appear to be involved, though no controlled prospective study using computed tomography (CT) has yet been reported. Both diastolic and systolic readings prove predictive of stroke during follow-up, and there is no evidence in the Framingham data of a "cutoff" level. The risk appears to be graded according to the absolute value of the pressure. This adverse effect of hypertension applies in both sexes and at all ages. There is no evidence for the widely held clinical belief that women and the elderly "tolerate" elevated pressure better than other groups. The traditional obsession with diastolic pressure readings is also misguided. Systolic pressures are probably an even better predictor of risk.[4] The importance of realizing that systolic pressures are predictive of stroke risk becomes clear when it is realized that 25 percent of subjects over 65 years of age have a systolic blood pressure of more than 160 mmHg. Such individuals have twice the stroke risk of those with lower systolic pressures.[3] The belief that labile hypertension does not matter and that the lowest level reached is the "real" value also proves unfounded. The Framingham data show that the average pressure in such situations represents the correct assessment of risk.

The size of the risk is highlighted by the calculation that stroke risk doubles for each increment of about 7.5 mmHg in mean diastolic blood pressure across the whole range of population pressures.[5] The interaction of hypertension and other risk factors in determining the incidence of stroke is obvious in the British regional heart study, which followed 7,735 men aged 40 to 59 years in 24 towns in England, Wales, and Scotland. The relative risk of stroke for men with a systolic pressure exceeding 160 mmHg who were also smokers was 12.1.[6] Death rates are further increased if the hypertensive patient is also a smoker and has a high cholesterol level. Thus a man aged between 46 and 57 years with a diastolic pressure greater than 90 mmHg has a relative risk (of mortality) of 1.3 compared to someone with a diastolic pressure less than 90 mmHg. If he also smokes and has a serum cholesterol concentration over 250 mg/dl, this risk rises to 1.5.[7]

Other proven risk factors for stroke, such as electrocardiographic abnormalities, heart disease, and hematocrit level, are partly active through their associations with hypertension. In practice, an elevated arterial pressure is recorded in some 35 percent of subjects with transient ischemic attacks (TIAs)[8] and in more than 50 percent of patients with cerebral infarction or cerebral hemorrhage.[9] Hypertension also proves to be a risk factor for second or multiple strokes and adversely affects prognosis after stroke.[10]

Stroke mortality appears to be declining, especially in North America.[11] This trend dates back approximately 50 years, and it has been suggested that the decline in the use of salt as a food preservative has been beneficial in reducing the prevalence of hypertension in the population. The reduction in stroke mortality accelerated around 1972 to 1973 and is now running at 4 percent per year. This change may be related to the introduction during the early 1970s of a program for the detection and treatment of hypertension in North America.

Primary Prevention Trials

The connection between hypertension and stroke is confirmed by the success of primary prevention trials, in which the treatment of hypertension reduces the incidence of stroke during follow-up. A meta-analysis[12] of these trials shows a reduction in stroke of 42 percent for a mean reduction in blood pressure of 5 to 6 mmHg, closely paralleling predictions from the epidemiological data of the theoretically reduction in stroke risk.[5]

Does the severity of the hypertension influence the results? The only trial that specifically considered *severe* hypertension was that run by the Veterans Administration (VA) in North America, which included only compliant male patients with a settled pretrial diastolic blood pressure of 115 to 129 mmHg.[13] Among these patients, 70 received a placebo and 73 a mixture of hydrochlorothiazide, reserpine, and hydralazine. Fatal and nonfatal morbid events were reduced from 27 to 2, necessitating stopping the trial. By this time there had been only five strokes, so a statistically significant conclusion cannot be drawn (though four occurred in the placebo group).

Large trials have been necessary for *mild* hypertension, since the event rate is lower and the power of such trials is critically dependent on the number of endpoints. The Australian Therapeutic Trial in Mild Hypertension screened 104,171 subjects to find 3,427 with mild hypertension.[14] After equal division of subjects into treated and untreated groups, 12 treated and 25 untreated subjects had strokes or TIAs. These primary prevention trials show that stroke is less likely in the treated groups at all pressure levels. One problem when translating these studies to present-day clinical practice is that they were carried out with what Mitchell has called "yesterday's drugs."[15] This is important, as it is possible though unproved that the regimen employed may have an important effect on outcome. Thus thiazide diuretics, although lowering blood pressure, may adversely affect other risk factors, such as the uric acid and blood glucose levels and the hematocrit. Despite these theoretical changes, however, the therapeutic success of the trials, which mostly employ thiazide as the first agent in stepped care, indicate that such influences must be minor. The success of β-blockers in the secondary prevention of myocardial infarction suggests that they might be the preferred method of lowering blood pressure. This issue is the subject of several trials. The Medical Research Council trial in the United Kingdom revealed that thiazides and propranolol both reduced stroke risk but that the β-blocker possibly also reduced coronary events, at least in nonsmokers.[16]

There has always been controversy over whether treatment of blood pressure is appropriate in the elderly. The European Working Party on Hypertension in the Elderly (EWPHE) recruited patients over the age of 60 with a diastolic pressure of between 90 and 119 mmHg and a systolic blood pressure of 160 to

239 mmHg.[17] Active treatment consisted of a combination of hydrochlorothiazide and triamterene. In all, 840 patients were randomized to treatment or placebo. Although deaths from cerebrovascular disease were not significantly reduced, nonfatal cerebrovascular events were halved (a reduction of 11 strokes per thousand patient-years in the treated group). This result compared favorably with the much smaller beneficial effect in the mild hypertension in younger subjects seen in the Medical Research Council trial (1.2 fewer strokes per 1,000 patient-years).[16] In 1991 the final results of the Systolic Hypertension in the Elderly Program (SHEP) were reported.[18] These showed that in persons over 60 years with systolic pressures of 160 to 219 mmHg (4,736 recruited from 447,921 screened), stepped care with chlorthalidone and atenolol reduced the incidence of stroke by 36 percent. This represented a prevention of 30 events per 1,000 subjects over a 5-year period. TIAs were also less frequent in the treated group (with a reduction of 25 percent).

There is thus good evidence that reduction in blood pressure over all ranges and at all ages reduces the risk of stroke. The absolute benefit is small when mild hypertension is treated; if 850 mildly hypertensive patients are treated with antihypertensive medication for 1 year, chronic side effects will occur in a substantial number of patients and only about one stroke will be prevented.[16] This raises questions about the cost-benefit of such an approach. The absolute benefit is greater in patients with more severe hypertension and in the elderly, in whom the risks are high. It remains to be seen whether calcium channel blockers and an-giotensin converting enzyme inhibitors have anything to offer over and above the proved success of thiazides and β-blockers.

Another strategy for reducing the incidence of stroke in the community would be to produce a general reduction in blood pressure by nonpharmacological means. Thus, lifestyle and dietary changes (including a reduced consumption of salt and alcohol, dietary supplementation with potassium and fish oils, and increased exercise) might be expected to bring about small reductions in pressure. Rose calculated that a 2- to 3-mmHg reduction in the blood pressure of the UK population would theoretically prevent as many vascular deaths as is achieved by all drug treatment of hypertension.[19]

PATHOLOGY AND PATHOPHYSIOLOGY

Cerebral blood flow (CBF) is normally regulated by a tight coupling between metabolic demand and oxygen delivery[20] and is independent of blood pressure over a wide range (Fig. 7-1). This phenomenon of autoregulation is believed to depend on local changes in vessel caliber as a direct "myogenic" response to intraluminal pressure, though sympathetic activity plays a role in "setting" the level. Hypertensive patients show a shift of the autoregulatory curve so that the mean arterial pressure at which CBF falls is higher than normal. They are thus more vulnerable to seemingly modest falls in pressure. This shift in curve presumably reflects a change in the myogenic

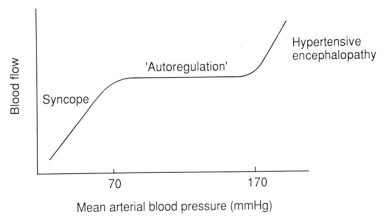

Fig. 7-1 Autoregulation of cerebral blood flow (CBF).

response due to vessel wall changes. Treatment of hypertension is believed to return the autoregulatory curve toward normal. In the presence of cerebral infarction (and hemorrhage), there is focal and sometimes widespread loss of autoregulation. This produces a potentially dangerous situation in the aftermath of acute stroke in which lowered blood pressure aggravates the fall in CBF and may extend the area of infarction. There is some evidence that autoregulation returns after 2 to 3 weeks, though experimentally it may persist for much longer. Patients who have sustained a brainstem infarct may have particularly persistent loss of autoregulation, leaving them vulnerable to episodes of hypotension.

If pressure rises above the upper limit of the autoregulatory curve, blood flow "breaks through" and increases steeply.[21] It produces congestion and, at sites where the vessel wall gives way, edema fluid leaks out. Patchy congestion and edema produce elevated intracranial pressure, papilledema, and the signs and symptoms of hypertensive encephalopathy. If pressure is reduced below the lower limit of autoregulation, infarction in a watershed territory may occur (Fig. 7-2).

The cause of cerebral hemorrhage was suggested by Charcot and Bouchard to be rupture of a small aneurysm (Fig. 7-3). They observed "while studying an apoplectic focus . . . two small spherical masses each attached to a vascular filament. They represented two small aneurysms one of which had ruptured." There was great controversy over these aneurysms, which many thought were spurious. In 1963, Ross Russell restored respectability to the Charcot-Bouchard aneurysms by showing that they were dilatations on small penetrating arteries.[22] Importantly, he also showed that they were found in the basal ganglia, pons, and cerebellum in sites commonly affected by hemorrhage, and that their presence or absence depended on the presence or absence of hypertension. Cole and Yates confirmed their presence in the brains of hypertensive patients and showed that hemorrhagic lesions were common at autopsy only in hypertensive individuals with these aneurysms.[23] The appearance of aneurysms also depended on age. It is now generally accepted that hypertension leads to vessel wall changes that allow the development of Charcot-Bouchard aneurysms and that rupture of these aneurysms underlies many cases of cerebral hemorrhage (Fig. 7-4). However, penetrating arteries

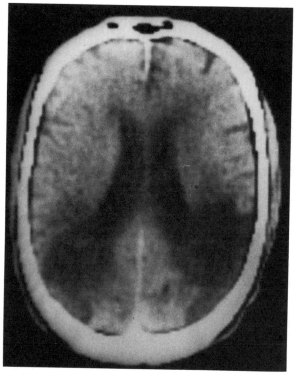

Fig. 7-2 CT scan showing infarction in the watershed area between the territories of the middle and posterior cerebral arteries, due to prolonged hypotension.

affected by lipohyalinosis or fibrinoid change may also rupture.

The influence of hypertension on cerebral infarction is more complicated. Most infarcts are secondary to occlusion of cerebral or cervical vessels resulting either from thrombosis on atheromatous plaques or from thromboembolism from the heart or stenosed neck vessels. The effect of hypertension on the incidence of myocardial infarction would be expected to increase the risk of cardioembolic stroke. Hypertension also causes accelerated development of experimental atheroma and can be shown to increase the rate of progression of angiographically followed carotid stenosis in patients.[24] At autopsy atheromatous changes are found more distally in intracerebral vessels in hypertensive individuals than in normotensive subjects. The tendency to thrombus formation may also be affected by hypertension, there being some evidence of enhanced platelet aggregation in hypertensive individuals.[25] Finally, hypertension affects small intracerebral vessels in a variety of ways in addi-

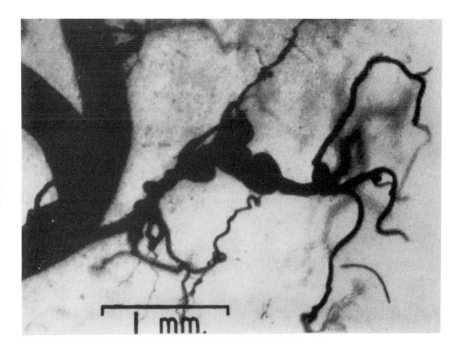

Fig. 7-3 Microaneurysms (Charcot-Bouchard type) on penetrating vessels in the brain of a hypertensive subject. (From Ross Russell RW: Observations on intracranial aneurysms. Brain 86:425, 1963, with permission.)

tion to the production of Charcot-Bouchard aneurysms. Mural hypertrophy occurs with thickening of the media and insudation of plasma proteins, leading to hyalinosis and fibrin deposition.[23] With malignant hypertension, fibrinoid change is seen in small cerebral vessels. Such mural changes are believed to predispose to thrombotic occlusion.

Lacunae are small infarcts that, in their chronic state, appear as simple slit-like cavities in basal ganglia, the deep white matter of the hemispheres, and

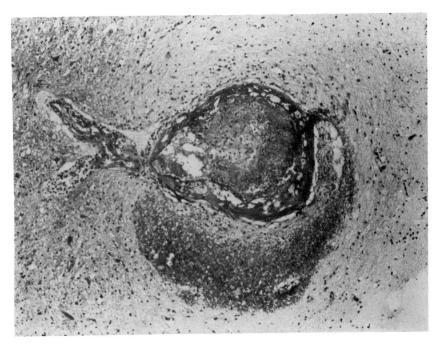

Fig. 7-4 Microaneurysm that has bled. (From Tavcar D: Hyalinosis as the cause of massive cerebral hemorrhage. Acta Med Iugosl 28:403, 1974, with permission.)

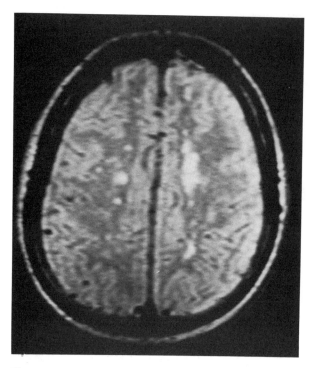

Fig. 7-5 MRI showing small, deep lacunar infarcts in a hypertensive patient.

the pons[23] (Fig. 7-5). Fisher's study revealed that they were strongly associated with the finding of atherosclerotic changes in intracerebral and pial vessels.[26] Elevated blood pressure was documented in 111 of his 114 cases. The distribution of lacunae closely paralleled the distribution of atherosclerosis and lipohyalinosis of small vessels. These changes could be demonstrated in association with individual lacunae in most cases, but in a few the local vessel was open, suggesting embolism. Plaque and embolism appeared to account for most lacunae over 10 mm in size, and lipohyalinosis accounted for most small ones. The area of ischemia at the time of vessel occlusion is probably two to three times larger than the eventual lacuna. Most lacunae in the lenticular nucleus, putamen, or caudate affect the internal capsule at their periphery; lacunae disrupting all the capsular fibers are rare. These two features probably account for the restricted and often reversible neurological deficit associated with them. The distribution of hyalinosis[27] and aneurysm[22] parallels that of lacunae[26] and cerebral hemorrhage[28] (Table 7-1).

Demyelination of hemispheric white matter may occur in hypertensive individuals (Binswanger's encephalopathy), especially in the occipital and temporal lobes.[29] Extensive hyaline change in cerebral vessels is usually found, but whether that is the responsible lesion or both changes are the sequelae of patchy ischemic edema is uncertain. Reversible changes are not infrequently seen in the white matter on CT scans and magnetic resonance imaging (MRI) in hypertensive individuals, favoring the second hypothesis.

CLINICAL PROBLEMS

Transient Ischemic Attacks

The brief episodes of focal neurological deficit due to transient regional ischemia (TIAs) are often the result of embolism from the heart or neck vessels,

Table 7-1 Distribution of Lacunae, Microaneurysms, Hyalinosis (Severe), and Intracerebral Hemorrhage

Site	Lacunae (%) (376 lacunae[26])	Microaneurysms (%) (53 cases[23])	Severe Hyalinosis (%) (100 cases[27])	Intracerebral Hemorrhage (%) (164 cases[28])
Lenticular	37	26	42	⎫
Caudate	9	8	9	⎬ 68
Thalamus	14	17	27	⎪
Internal capsule	11	15	⎫	⎭
Centrum semiovale	6	2	⎬ 6	10
Pons	16	7	5	7
Cerebellum	⎫ 7	⎫ 23	⎫ 11	13
Other (including subcortical)	⎭	⎭	⎭	2

though no cause is found in as many as one in four instances.[8] As noted before, some 35 percent of patients have hypertension. The Rochester community data reveal that the increase in stroke risk in TIA patients is further increased by elevated arterial pressure, an effect that is obliterated by successful treatment (though this conclusion is rather insecurely based on the use of historical controls rather than on a randomized study).[30] In practice, few patients' TIAs appear to be triggered by an increase in blood pressure.

A fall in blood pressure (e.g., as a result of treatment of hypertension) may rarely cause a TIA, but syncopal symptoms are more usual. Focal ischemia is likely only if blood pressure falls in the context of a hemodynamically significant stenosis (e.g., of a carotid artery). A hemodynamic cause for such a TIA is suggested by the description of accompanying features, such as the coincidence of palpitations or the adoption of the upright posture, and should always be considered in a treated hypertensive patient in case the problem is a reflection of iatrogenic hypotension.

Although symptoms of TIAs reverse within 24 hours and commonly in just a few minutes, investigation sometimes reveals evidence of cerebral infarction. CT or MRI not infrequently shows small lesions indicative of infarction, though these are more frequently encountered when the neurological episode lasts days or weeks.

Clinical management involves control of hypertension and other risk factors and a search for a source of emboli in the heart or neck vessels. Carotid stenosis is more likely in those with brief hemispheric attacks affecting face or arm, amaurosis fugax, visible retinal emboli, or a localized bruit.[31] Noninvasive screening of all patients with carotid-territory TIAs is advised, however, as long as they are candidates for surgery if an operable stenosis of 70 percent or more is found on the symptomatic side.[32] With or without surgery, such patients should receive antiplatelet agents in the form of aspirin or ticlopidine, as both have been shown to reduce stroke risk in TIA patients by about 25 percent. In the presence of a potential cardiac source of emboli, such as atrial fibrillation, anticoagulants may well be indicated. A series of primary prevention trials have conclusively shown a reduction in the incidence of stroke with anticoagulation.[33] The risk of stroke in such trials seems to be higher in the presence of hypertension.[34] Because hypertension is believed to increase the risk of hemorrhage, its con-

trol is particularly important if a patient is to be anticoagulated in an attempt to prevent stroke.

Lacunar Strokes

Lacunae probably account for about 20 percent of cerebral ischemic lesions and are often found at autopsy in the brains of hypertensive individuals. Their clinical counterparts were recognized early in the century, but detailed clinicopathological descriptions awaited the studies of Fisher.[26] As discussed earlier, many lacunar strokes are due to occlusion of penetrating arteries affected by lipohyalinosis or atheroma, though some are due to embolism. With the advent of CT and MRI, their recognition has become easier, and the occasional association of a lacuna with internal carotid or middle cerebral artery occlusion has been demonstrated[35] (Table 7-2). Though Fisher thought virtually all these patients were hypertensive, many lacunar infarcts are now seen (by CT or MRI) in normotensive individuals. The clinical syndromes often but not exclusively seen with lacunar infarction include the following.

1. *Pure Motor Hemiplegia*. Fisher described patients whose hemiparesis was perhaps complicated by dysarthria but who showed no sensory change, regardless of whether there were any sensory symptoms. There was no field defect, dysphasia, or other cortical disturbance. Almost one-third had had a prior TIA, and most recovered well, often within a few weeks. Capsular or basal ganglia lacunae were held responsible, though a lesion in the basis pontis can also produce the same picture. Nelson and colleagues have shown, from CT

Table 7-2 Radiological Findings in 37 Cases of Lacunar Stroke

Finding	No.
CT scans	
Small infarcts	18
Large infarcts	6
Normal	13
Angiography	
Carotid occlusion	4
Carotid stenosis	3
Middle cerebral abnormalities	2

(Data from Nelson and colleagues.[35])

data, that the same picture occasionally occurs with a cortical infarct[35] and rarely from a small hematoma.

2. *Pure Sensory Stroke.* Unilateral dysesthesias may develop suddenly or insidiously, often after TIAs. The lesion lies in the thalamus, and the prognosis is usually good.

3. *Homolateral Ataxia and Crural Paresis.* This well-recognized syndrome consists of cerebellar ataxia on the same side as a hemiparesis, which is more marked distally in the lower limb. The responsible lacuna may prove to be in the pons or in the thalamocapsular region.

4. *Dysarthria—Clumsy Hand Syndrome.* In this syndrome, dysarthria is associated with clumsiness of the hand that appears to be the result of a loss of fine movements from a pyramidal tract lesion, combined with a cerebellar deficit. Again, capsular or pontine lesions may be responsible. CT scans are more likely to reveal the capsular lesion than that in the pons. Identification of small infarcts in the brainstem is easier with MRI.

5. *Other Syndromes.* Isolated hemichorea, dysarthria, and facial weakness or combinations of ocular and limb signs implying a brainstem lesion may all be due to lacunar infarction.

MANAGEMENT

Although clinical recognition of these syndromes was thought to be sufficiently secure that their treatment could be devised without recourse to angiography, it is now clear that the clinical material is heterogeneous. Before deciding that regulation of arterial blood pressure alone will suffice to reduce the risk of recurrence, CT scan or MRI studies should be obtained. If a cortical lesion or a large infarct (more than 10 mm) is seen, the possibility of a thromboembolic event should be considered to determine whether vascular surgery is appropriate. The SHEP study shows that treatment of hypertension can reduce the incidence of lacunar strokes. As lacunar strokes are a marker of the presence of systemic vascular disease, it is probably also appropriate to prescribe antiplatelet agents to all patients shown not to have had a hemorrhage.

Lacunar strokes have a somewhat different natural history than other types of ischemic stroke. Thus the recurrence of lacunar strokes is evenly spread across the subsequent year, rather than showing a peak in the first month after the stroke, as is typical in cardioembolism. Although most lacunar strokes cause only a modest deficit, residual disability is common.[36]

"ETAT LACUNAIRE"

Multiple lacunae are unusual but represent a cause of pseudobulbar palsy with dysarthria, emotional lability, and a *marche à petit pas* gait. CT scans in some of these patients, as well as showing multiple lacunae, may reveal diffuse white matter change. This is even more striking on MRI, and there appears to be a lot of overlap between the multiple lacunar state and the more diffuse-looking damage attributed to demyelination (leukoariosis). The differential diagnosis includes multiple embolic infarcts with multi-infarct dementia and hydrocephalus. Treatment depends on blood pressure control and antiplatelet agents, although no focused trial has sought to discover whether aspirin or ticlopidine affects this condition. The role of lacunar infarcts in causing dementia is uncertain unless there is widespread white mater damage as well.

Binswanger Encephalopathy

A progressive dementia and pseudobolbular palsy (Binswanger encephalopathy) has been recognized in hypertensive patients with diffuse demyelination of hemispheric white matter, especially posteriorly.[29] As the small intracerebral vessels in such hypertensive patients show diffuse hyaline change, the process has been attributed to diffuse ischemic edema, though without the breakthrough of autoregulation or congestion seen with acute hypertensive encephalopathy. The demyelination may alternatively result from impaired nutritional blood supply to oligodendrocytes secondary to small vessel disease in the presence of poor collateral support of the white matter circulation. Binswanger encephalopathy was considered a rare condition, but the advent of CT scanning and MRI has suggested that the white matter changes (leukoariosis) are common in elderly arteriopathic individuals and especially in those who are hypertensive (Fig. 7-6). Dementia is particularly likely when the changes are severe. Such changes are not uncommonly found in combination with one or two lacunar infarcts when an elderly hypertensive person is inves-

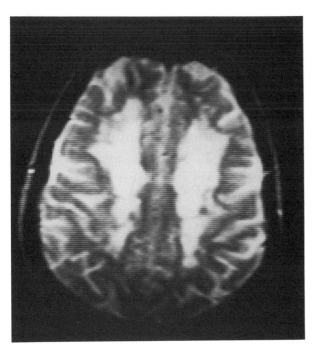

Fig. 7-6 T_2-weighted MRI showing high signal in the white matter, associated with systemic hypertension.

of the patient's previous state, since a secondary rise often accompanies the acute stroke event.[38] It may be partly a stress reaction; a compensatory rise, if intracranial pressure is increasing, may also play a role. The presence of hypertension on admission may even have a good effect on prognosis, perhaps because collateral flow is encouraged in the area of damaged autoregulation. Later, however, high arterial pressure probably aggravates vasogenic edema, which contributes to the brain swelling and herniation that account for most deaths during the first week after stroke (Fig. 7-7). A theoretical risk of hemorrhage into an infarct if pressure remains high does not seem to be realized in practice.

Treatment of hypertension in the acute aftermath of cerebral infarction is potentially hazardous. Anecdotal evidence confirms that deterioration in neurological deficit may follow precipitous falls in blood pressure. Such deterioration is also encountered if orthostatic hypotension or a hemodynamically significant cardiac arrhythmia develops during convalescence.

The reason for deterioration if blood pressure falls

tigated for minor complaints. Until there is better clinicopathological correlation, it is uncertain whether the current tendency to diagnose Binswanger's encephalopathy on imaging criteria is fully justified. The practical implication is clear, however. Such patients need close control of their blood pressure, and management of any other risk factors for arterial disease. A series of studies by Meyer and colleagues has shown better preservation of cognitive function (and cerebral blood flow) with control of blood pressure and with the prescription of aspirin in impaired elderly subjects followed for some months. Although blood flow and cognition were improved by control of the blood pressure, this was not the case if pressures fell too low (e.g., below a mean of 135 mmHg).[37]

Cerebral Infarction—Ischemic Stroke

As noted earlier, some 50 percent of patients with a completed stroke due to cerebral infarction prove to be hypertensive. Blood pressure levels during the first 24 hours may not, however, be representative

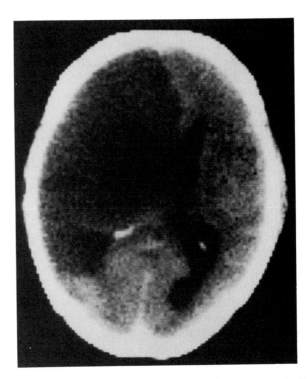

Fig. 7-7 CT scan of patient with an edematous cerebral infarction showing a mass effect.

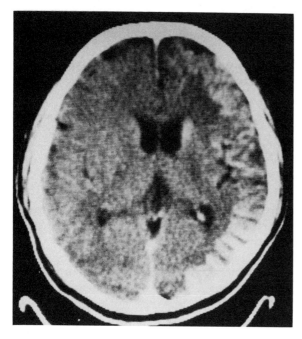

Fig. 7-8 Gyral pattern of enhancement in the territory of a middle cerebral artery infarct.

or is reduced is the reduction of CBF that occurs in dilated collateral channels and in the penumbra around an infarct where autoregulation is defective.[39] In such areas, metabolism and blood flow are mismatched, and ischemia may progress to infarction if flow is further lowered. Preservation of flow and reduction of tissue pressure by controlling edema are more logical aims, though to date the results of clinical trials of dexamethasone and hyperosmolar agents have been disappointing.[40] Increasing flow by isovolemic hemodilution has also proved ineffective.[41] If there are other pressing indications to lower the arterial pressure (e.g., the development of left ventricular failure), the risk of extending a cerebral infarct must be taken. If not, most authorities recommend delaying hypotensive treatment until 2 to 3 weeks after the ictus. If a CT scan shows enhancement of an infarct (Fig. 7-8), a disturbance of the blood-brain barrier is implied, and it may tentatively be concluded that autoregulation is still likely to be impaired. If blood pressure reduction is deemed necessary during this acute stage of stroke, agents that produce a smooth subacute effect are preferred (e.g., oral β-blockers). The precipitous fall in blood pressure that may occur

with intravenous agents makes their use unsatisfactory. Since hemodilution is safe in this context,[41] venisection may be the preferred method for rapidly lowering the pressure in a patient with an infarct who is developing left ventricular failure and pulmonary edema.

Secondary Prevention Trials

Does subsequent lowering of blood pressure prevent stroke recurrence? There have been two secondary prevention trials (Table 7-3). Carter randomized 99 patients with a diastolic pressure above 110 mmHg (phase 4) after stroke.[42] During follow-up 20.5 percent of treated and 42 percent of untreated patients became victims of a second stroke. In the other comparable study many patients had less severe hypertension (diastolic blood pressure 90 to 115 mmHg, phase 5); 37 of 233 treated patients had a second stroke, compared with 41 of 219 controls, a difference that was not significant.[43] There were, however, some peculiarities in this second trial: a large number of the total group had syphilis, and the mean diastolic blood pressure of the group was only 100 mmHg. Hutchinson and Acheson found no difference in the time to second stroke according to blood pressure, though their study was not a controlled trial.[10]

The benefit from treating mild hypertension after stroke has not, therefore, been well documented. There is evidence, however, that the quality of blood pressure control influences stroke recurrence. Thus, in the study reported by Beevers and co-workers, blood pressure control was considered good if the mean standing diastolic blood pressure was under 100

Table 7-3 Secondary Prevention Trials

Study Group	No. of Patients	Second Stroke	%
Carter[42]: Diastolic BP >110 mmHg (phase 4)			
Treated	49	10	20.5
Control	50	21	42.0
		$p < 0.05$	
Hypertension Stroke Cooperative Group[43]: Diastolic BP 90–115 mmHg (phase 5)			
Treated	233	37	15.9
Control	219	42	19.2
		N.S.	

mmHg, fair if the average level was 100 to 110 mmHg, and poor if it was above 110 mmHg.[44] Second strokes occurred in 52 percent with poor control, 32 percent with fair control, but only 16 percent of those with good control. A second Glasgow study suggested that recurrences were even fewer if the achieved diastolic pressure level was below 90 mmHg. The success of primary prevention trials also encourages most physicians to treat moderate or severe hypertension after stroke. There is some evidence that recurrent strokes are more likely to be hemorrhages if the blood pressure is high (e.g., a diastolic pressure over 120 mmHg).[45]

Cerebral Hemorrhage

Most textbooks imply that virtually all cerebral hemorrhages occur in hypertensive individuals, but modern series suggest a figure of about 60 percent. Anticoagulant medication accounts for another 10 to 20 percent, and angiomas, aneurysms, tumors, substance abuse, and other hematological disorders account for the remainder. Hemorrhage in a dementing patient suggests the possibility of amyloid angiopathy. The reason that some patients have a cerebral hemorrhage and others an infarct is not clear. There is a suggestion that depressed platelet function is common among patients with cerebral hemorrhage when compared with the victims of ischemic stoke.[46] It is tempting to speculate that the combination of hypertensive vessel damage and impaired platelet function permits hemorrhage.

Hemorrhages are responsible for about 15 percent of adult strokes. It is important that they be identified, because some require surgical management. Bedside diagnosis is often faulty, as proved by autopsy and CT scan studies, but use of a weighted clinical score is correct in more than 80 percent of cases. Detection of a hemorrhage depends basically on the presence of coma, vomiting, and neck stiffness on a background of hypertension; infarcts, by contrast, are suggested by the presence of TIAs and the absence of the factors that suggest hemorrhage (e.g., vomiting).[47] Problems remain with hemorrhagic infarction and in comatose patients with an incomplete history. Since the advent of CT scanning, it has also become clear that small hematomas may occur asymptomatically or with only a brief deficit (e.g., 5 days) (Fig. 7-9). Such

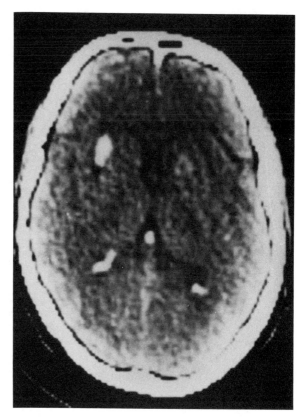

Fig. 7-9 CT scan of a small frontal hematoma.

hemorrhages were documented pathologically by Cole and Yates in the brains of hypertensive subjects.[23]

Common to large cerebral hemorrhages (Fig. 7-10) are the development of headache, vomiting, neck stiffness, and coma; the presence and nature of focal features depend on the site of the bleeding. The onset is usually during activity; recovery in the first few hours is extremely rare. Most hematomas arise in the basal ganglia, encroaching on the internal capsule and often rupturing into the ventricular system. Alternatively, they may track into the external capsular region or into a hemispheric lobe ("lobar" hematoma). In general, massive ganglionic hematomas are rapidly fatal, the patient being comatose and hemiplegic, with deviation of the eyes toward the side of the clot (Fig. 7-10). Signs of "coning" supervene, with a third-nerve palsy or fixed pupils, decerebrate posturing, and irregular respiration.[48] Smaller collections in the same site may not cause coma, but the patient has a hemianopia, hemiplegia, and hemisensory deficit

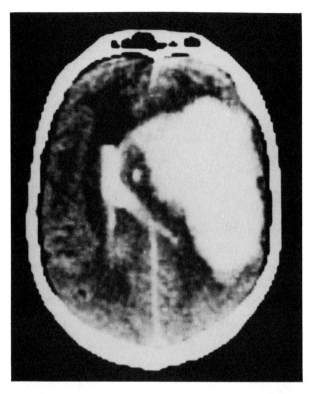

Fig. 7-10 CT scan of a massive, fatal hematoma showing a mass effect and rupture into the ventricular system.

affecting all modalities, with impaired contralateral conjugate gaze. The deficit usually develops smoothly and steadily.

When the hematoma is sited in the thalamus, a rapidly fatal outcome may also result, as with putaminal bleeds; but a smaller collection may produce hemisensory loss, hemiparesis, dysphasia if on the dominant side, and, because of involvement of the top of the brainstem, eye signs. The pupils are often unequal and may become unreactive. The eyes may be in forced down-gaze or show skew deviation (one up and one down), or there may be lateral gaze palsies. Later, hemichorea or the thalamic syndrome may develop.

Lobar hematomas cause drowsiness and confusion, and often a subacute evolution as the hematoma tracks through the white matter, separating rather than destroying fiber tracts.[49] Occipital hemorrhage causes pain around the ipsilateral eye and dense hemianopia. Left temporal hemorrhage produces fluctuating fluent aphasia and partial hemianopia. Parietal bleeds begin with headache and hemisensory loss.

Frontal clots cause headache and a hemiparesis that is maximal in the arm.

Hemorrhage into a cerebellar hemisphere (Fig. 7-11) accounts for perhaps 10 percent of hematomas and so is not common. However, cerebellar hematomas deserve close attention, since they are frequently fatal yet potentially reversible by surgical evacuation.[50] Some patients present with the rapid onset of headache, vomiting, and vertigo; they may demonstrate unilateral limb ataxia, making clinical localization relatively easy. Others present in coma, with small pupils and loss of eye movements due to rapid pontine compression, thereby mimicking pontine hemorrhage. Hyperpyrexia is said not to occur with cerebellar hemorrhage, but in practice the clinical distinction cannot be made. Finally, some patients present with depressed consciousness and deviation of eyes (due to pontine disturbance) without hemiplegia, though there may be facial weakness. This combination should cause suspicion of cerebellar hemorrhage (or infarct with edema). "Stroke somewhere, stroke nowhere, stroke in the cerebellum" is an adage that reflects the need to consider cerebellar hemorrhage when the acuteness of onset suggest a stroke but the signs fail to provide confirmatory evidence of hemisphere or brainstem localization.

Pontine hemorrhage also occurs in hypertensive individuals. Coma is present from the onset in one-half of cases, and hyperthermia often develops early (too soon to be due to complications such as bronchopneumonia). The pupils are classically pinpoint though reactive; horizontal eye movements, as tested by counterrolling of the head or cold-water caloric stimulation, are lost. Ocular bobbing may occur however, as may inequality of pupils and skew deviation. There is usually quadriparesis. The differential diagnosis includes thalamic hemorrhage and cerebellar hematoma; a definite diagnosis can be made safely only by CT scanning or MRI.

In general, surgery is necessary for hematomas of 3 cm or more in the cerebellum. Similarly, large lobar hematomas and external capsular bleeds may be considered for surgery, especially if the neurological deficit increases despite recovery of consciousness. The overall surgical policy is receiving increasing scrutiny, however, since conservative management may be preferable, especially for small hematomas.[51] The prognosis for patients in coma is poor, and little benefit seems to accrue from surgery in comatose subjects except in the case of cerebellar hematomas.

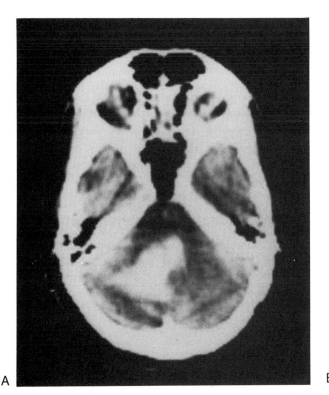
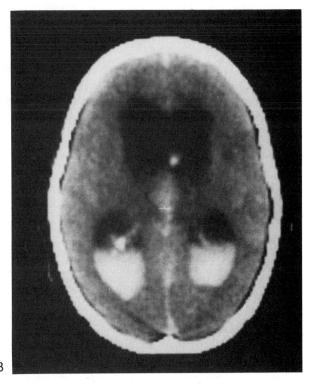

A   B

Fig. 7-11 CT scans showing **(A)** a posterior fossa hematoma and **(B)** a secondary hydrocephalus with blood entering the CSF.

Subarachnoid Hemorrhage

Although 80 percent of subarachnoid hemorrhages are due to rupture of aneurysms or to arteriovenous malformations, hypertension probably plays a role in both the development of aneurysms and their rupture. Approximately one-third of patients with aneurysmal rupture are hypertensive. Headache of sudden onset with vomiting, clouding of consciousness, and neck stiffness may be complicated by focal deficit due to a local hematoma at the site of the bleeding. The clinical onset presents few diagnostic difficulties when there is a clear history of a sudden explosive headache, especially if accompanied by neck stiffness and subhyaloid preretinal hemorrhage on fundoscopy.

CT scanning is the first investigation of choice. It shows the presence of blood in the subarachnoid space in more than 80 percent of cases (Fig. 7-12). It may also reveal the cause of any associated focal deficit to be a hematoma around the site of bleeding. If the CT scan fails to make the diagnosis, lumbar puncture should be performed. Blood staining of lumbar spinal fluid may not be detectable in the first 12 hours, so a judicious delay may be sensible if the patient is seen before this; if the differential diagnosis includes meningitis, however, no such delay is permissible. Xanthochromia excludes a traumatic tap as the cause for bloody cerebrospinal fluid and should be confirmed by spectroscopy. It may be detectable for 2 weeks after a bleed. Management depends on early four-vessel angiography followed by early aneurysm surgery in patients whose general state is good.[52] Patients with focal deficits may need evacuation of a hematoma. If focal deficit or clouding of consciousness is due to vasospasm, however, some authorities prefer to delay surgery for a few days. A focal deficit developing in the early days after an aneurysmal bleed usually results from vasospasm due to the effect of shed blood around the site of bleeding. Its incidence is reduced by nimodipine prescribed prophylactically from the moment that subarachnoid hemorrhage is confirmed and continued for the following 3 weeks.[53]

Loss of autoregulation combined with vasospasm makes these patients vulnerable to deterioration if the

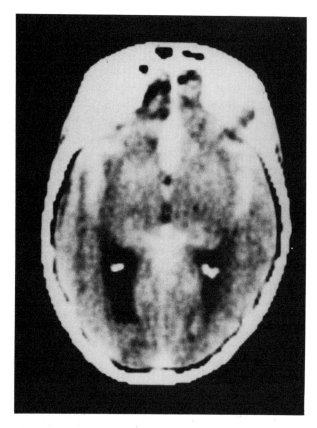

Fig. 7-12 CT scan showing blood in the CSF spaces in a patient with a subarachnoid hemorrhage.

surges of hypertension may be an indication for the use of β-blockers, in addition to the use of nimodipine to combat vasospastic ischemic deficits. Long-term management of any hypertension should continue, as with any other form of cerebrovascular disease. The initial mortality from subarachnoid hemorrhage is about 25 percent, and this occurs in the first 24 hours. Another 25 percent succumb to rebleeding or ischemic damage in the first month. The risk of hemorrhage from an unruptured aneurysm is between 1 and 3 percent per annum.

Hypertensive Encephalopathy

The term *hypertensive encephalopathy* should be restricted to the diffuse cerebral effects of severe hypertension that reverse with control of the blood pressure and are not due to focal infarction or hemorrhage.[54] Some use the term loosely and erroneously to include virtually any neurological mishap in a hypertensive individual. The condition is rare, and personal experience accords with the published findings that other conditions account for most episodes attributed to hypertensive encephalopathy. As discussed in the section on pathophysiology, this condition is characterized by cerebral edema and congestion due to a breakthrough at the upper limit of autoregulation of CBF. MRI and CT scans show diffuse edema of the hemispheres. Measurements of cerebral blood volume and of CBF have not been reported.

Patients—usually with a known history of hypertension—develop increasing headache, visual blurring, confusion, and drowsiness, with superadded seizures and recurrent focal deficits such as occipital blindness or dysphasia. When examined, they show a depressed level of consciousness and usually but not invariably have bilateral papilledema. The blood pressure is very high (e.g., 250/150 mmHg) and there are often focal deficits. Retinal edema and hemorrhages are common and help in the differentiation from raised intracranial pressure due to mass lesions. The blood urea concentration is usually elevated. If the cerebrospinal fluid is examined, it is commonly found to be under increased pressure, but lumbar puncture is not advised.

The differential diagnosis may include uremia, subarachnoid hemorrhage, cerebral infarction or hemorrhage, and subdural hematoma. Prompt diagnosis is vital, since the condition is reversible if arterial blood

mean arterial blood pressure falls. Fears that a high blood pressure will increase the risk of rebleeding must therefore be moderated by appreciation of the risk of hypotension. Once the aneurysm has been clipped, ischemic deficits due to vasospasm can be treated by inducing hypertension, making use of the loss of autoregulation.[51] Dopamine or metaramine are usually used in this context. If there is no aneurysm or angioma, or surgery is not possible because of technical factors or the poor state of the patient, conservative management is advised and usually consists of bed rest. There was, for a time, an enthusiasm for the use of antifibrinolytic agents such as epsilon-aminocaproic acid (EACA) to reduce the risk of rebleeding. However, this treatment carries the risk of an increased frequency of complications and thrombotic ischemia, and control trials were inconclusive with regard to the overall value of such agents; they are therefore advocated no longer. Prevention of pressure is controlled. Lowering of blood pressure is generally contraindicated in the acute aftermath of subarachnoid hemorrhage, cerebral infarction, or cerebral hemorrhage, so this differential diagnosis requires prompt attention and usually necessitates urgent CT scanning or MRI. Epilepsy and mental impairment may persist despite energetic treatment, and rarely blindness or some other deficit develops if pressure is reduced too enthusiastically.[55] The aim, therefore, is to lower pressure over 18 to 48 hours and avoid vasodilatation, which may aggravate cerebral congestion. Intravenous sodium nitroprusside or oral β-blockers may be used. Improvement should be appreciable within 36 hours. Patients with seizures should also be given anticonvulsants. It appears logical to prescribe corticosteroids in view of the damaged blood-brain barrier, but this has not been studied formally. There is clinical belief that the blood-brain barrier may be damaged at a relatively lower mean arterial pressure in acute renal failure, in which situation hypertensive encephalopathy may develop at modest levels of blood pressure. This would be in keeping with a lower upper limit of autoregulation in a previously normotensive subject.

Eclampsia

This may be considered a form of hypertensive encephalopathy.[56] If the early rise of pressure to levels of more than 145/90 mmHg after the 24th week of pregnancy (preeclampsia) is not detected and reversed, further rises may trigger encephalopathic symptoms, with irritability, headache, and seizures before, during, or within 24 hours of delivery.

Paroxysmal Hypertension

PHEOCHROMOCYTOMA

These tumors arise in the chromaffin cells. Ninety percent arise in the adrenal medulla, although rare examples arise in the neck, para-aortic region, and bladder. They are occasionally familial and associated with medullary carcinoma of the thyroid or other components of the multiple endocrine neoplasia (MEN) syndrome. Patients with neurofibromatosis or von Hippel-Lindau disease should also be screened for pheochromocytoma.

The tumors secrete catecholamines (predominantly norepinephrine but also epinephrine and dopamine), producing paroxysmal or sustained hypertension. Surges in the levels of circulating catecholamines cause attacks in which headache, sweating, palpitations, nausea, anxiety, and angina mimic panic attacks, ischemic heart disease, and hypoglycemia. Rare patients have attacks which simulate brain tumors (headache, vomiting) or transient ischemic attacks of cardioembolic origin (headache, focal weakness, palpitations). If the patient is seen during an attack or one is inadvertently triggered by palpation of the abdomen or during investigation, a rise in both systolic and diastolic blood pressure is recorded. Whether the pulse rate rises depends on the proportion of different catecholamines secreted.

The diagnosis is made by detecting high levels of catecholamines or their metabolites in the urine or plasma. The best yield for urine assays follows spontaneous attacks; otherwise there is a significant false-negative rate. A high index of suspicion (based on the clinical picture) and repeated assays is the best strategy. CT imaging or scintigraphy with ^{131}I-labeled metaiodobenzylguanidine (MIBG) will usually locate the tumors for surgical removal. If surgery is not possible, alpha and beta blockade may control attacks. Rarely, the tumor is malignant, though usually slow-growing.

CONCLUDING COMMENT

The occurrence of stroke or TIA should be regarded as a failure of prevention. The detection of risk factors can identify the 15 percent of the population in whom some 40 percent of strokes will occur. Among these risk factors, hypertension predominates. The risk is graded and affects both sexes and all ages and races. Systolic blood pressure may well be even more important than the diastolic pressure. Primary prevention trials have shown that a reduction in pressure of about 6 mmHg almost halves stroke risk. Secondary prevention also appears to be related to the quality of blood pressure control. Acute but not precipitous lowering of blood pressure is indicated in the increasingly rare condition of hypertensive encephalopathy, but it is contraindicated in the immediate aftermath of stroke. Hypertension contributes to the etiology of all types of stroke, including TIAs and lacunar strokes, but patients should also be investigated for an embolic source. Most cerebral hemorrhages occur in hypertensive patients, some of whom require neurosurgical management. Therefore, all stroke victims, particularly if hypertensive, deserve CT scanning or MRI to exclude hemorrhage and to characterize the cause of their neurological deficit. The overall incidence of stroke in the community should respond to a policy of detection of hypertension and its management by a combination of nonpharmacological means and appropriate drug therapy.

Further understanding of the various stroke syndromes associated with hypertension and of their pathophysiology promises to be obtained from positron emission tomography and new developments in MRI. Interest in these new technological advances must not, however, divert attention from the simple fact that the detection and treatment of hypertension prevents strokes.

REFERENCES

1. Baglivi G: The Practice of Physick. Bell, London, 1704
2. Kurtzke JF: Epidemiology and risk factors in thrombotic brain infarction. p. 27. In Harrison MJG, Dyken ML (eds): Cerebral Vascular Disease. Butterworths, London, 1983
3. Kannel WB, Wolf PA: Epidemiology of cerebrovascular disease. p. 1. In Ross Russell RW (ed): Vascular Disease of the Central Nervous System. 2nd Ed. Churchill Livingstone, Edinburgh, 1983
4. Rutan GH, McDonald RH, Kuller LH: A historical perspective of elevated systolic vs diastolic blood pressure from an epidemiological and clinical trial viewpoint. J Clin Epidemiol 42:663, 1989
5. McMahon S, Peto R, Cutler J, et al: Blood pressure, stroke and coronary heart disease. Lancet 335:765, 1990
6. Shaper AG, Phillips AN, Pocock SJ, et al: Risk factors for stroke in middle aged British men. Br Med J 302:1111, 1991
7. Browner WS, Hulley SB: Effect of risk status on treatment criteria: implications of hypertension trials. Hypertension 13, suppl I:I-51, 1989
8. de Bono DP, Warlow CP: Potential sources of emboli in patients with presumed transient cerebral and retinal ischaemia. Lancet 1:343, 1981
9. Harrison MJG: Clinical distinction of cerebral haemorrhage and cerebral infarction. Postgrad Med J 56:629, 1980
10. Hutchinson EC, Acheson EJ: Strokes: Natural History, Pathology and Surgical Treatment. WB Saunders, London, 1975
11. Hachinski V, Norris JW: The Acute Stroke. FA Davis, Philadelphia, 1985
12. Collins R, Peto R, MacMahon S, et al: Blood pressure, stroke, and coronary heart disease. Part 2. Short-term reductions in blood pressure: overview of randomised drug trials in their epidemiological context. Lancet 335:827, 1990
13. Veterans Administration Cooperative Study Group on Antihypertensive Agents: Effects of treatment on morbidity in hypertension: results in patients with diastolic pressure averaging 115 through 129 mmHg. JAMA 202:1028, 1967
14. Report by the Management Committee: The Australian therapeutic trial in mild hypertension. Lancet 1:1261, 1980
15. Mitchell JRA: Hypertension and stroke. p. 46. In Harrison MJG, Dyken ML (eds): Cerebral Vascular Disease. Butterworths, London, 1983
16. Medical Research Council Working Party: MRC trial of treatment of mild hypertension: principal results. Br Med J 291:97, 1985
17. European Working Party: Mortality and morbidity results from the European Working Party on high blood pressure in the elderly trial. Lancet 1:1349, 1985
18. SHEP Cooperative Research Group: Prevention of stroke by antihypertensive drug treatment in older persons with isolated systolic hypertension. JAMA 265:3255, 1991
19. Rose G: Strategy of prevention: lessons from cardiovascular disease. Br Med J 282:1847, 1981
20. Frackowiak RSJ: The pathophysiology of human cerebral ischaemia: a new perspective obtained with positron tomography. Q J Med 57:713, 1985
21. Strandgaard S, Olesen J, Skinhøj E, Lassen NA: Autoregulation of brain circulation in severe arterial hypertension. Br Med J 1:507, 1973
22. Ross Russell RW: Observations on intracranial aneurysms. Brain 86:425, 1963
23. Cole FM, Yates PO: The occurrence and significance of intracerebral micro-aneurysms. J Pathol Bacteriol 93:393, 1967
24. Schneidau A, Harrison MJG, Hurst C, et al: Arterial disease risk factors and angiographic evidence of atheroma of the carotid artery. Stroke 20:1466, 1989
25. Winther K, Gleerup G, Hender T: Enhanced risk of thromboembolic disease in hypertension from platelet hyperfunction and decreased fibrinolytic activity: has antihypertensive therapy any influence? J Cardiovasc Pharmacol 19, suppl 3:S1, 1992
26. Fisher CM: Lacunes: small deep cerebral infarcts. Neurology 15:774, 1965

27. Tavcar D: Hyalinosis as the cause of massive cerebral haemorrhage. Acta Med Iugosl 28:403, 1974

28. Adams RD, Van der Eecken HM: Vascular disease of brain. Annu Rev Med 4:213, 1953

29. Loizou LA, Kendall BE, Marshall J: Subcortical arteriosclerotic encephalopathy: a clinical and radiological investigation. J Neurol Neurosurg Psychiatry 44:294, 1981

30. Whisnant J: A population study of stroke and TIA: Rochester, Minnesota. p. 21. In Gillingham FJ, Mawdsley C, Williams AE (eds): Stroke. Churchill Livingstone, Edinburgh, 1976

31. Harrison MJG: Carotid endarterectomy. p. 57. In Rice Edwards JM (ed): Topical Reviews in Neurosurgery. PSG Wright, Bristol, 1982

32. NASCET Collaborators: Beneficial effect of carotid endarterectomy in symptomatic patients with high grade stenosis. N Engl J Med 325:445, 1991

33. The Boston Area Anticoagulant Trial for Atrial Fibrillation Investigators: The effect of low dose warfarin on the risk of stroke in patients with nonrheumatic atrial fibrillation. N Engl J Med 323:1505, 1990

34. SPAF Investigators: Predictors of thromboembolism in atrial fibrillation: 1. Clinical features of patients at risk. Ann Intern Med 116:1, 1992

35. Nelson RF, Pullicino P, Kendall BE, Marshall J: Computed tomography in patients presenting with lacunar syndromes. Stroke 11:256, 1980

36. Bamford J: Clinical examination in diagnosis and subclassification of stroke. Lancet 339:400, 1992

37. Meyer JS, Judd BW, Tawaklna T, et al: Improved cognition after control of risk factors for multi-infarct dementia. JAMA 256:2203, 1986

38. Wallace JD, Levy LL: Blood pressure after stroke. JAMA 246:2177, 1981

39. Hommel M, Guell A, Bess A: The extent of autoregulation impairment in acute ischaemic stroke—in man. p. 45. In Meyer JS, Lechner H, Reivich M, Ott EO (eds): Cerebrovascualr Disease 4. Excerpta Medica, Amsterdam, 1983

40. Norris JW, Hachinski VC: High dose steroid treatment in cerebral infarction. Br Med J 292:21, 1986

41. Italian Acute Stroke Study Group: Haemodilution in acute stroke: results of the Italian haemodilution trial. Lancet 1:318, 1988

42. Carter AB: Hypertensive therapy in stroke survivors. Lancet 1:485, 1970

43. Hypertension Stroke Cooperative Group: Effect of antihypertensive treatment on stroke recurrence. JAMA 229:409, 1974

44. Beevers DG, Fairman MJ, Hamilton M, Harpur JE: Antihypertensive treatment and the course of established cerebral vascular disease. Lancet 1:1407, 1973

45. Marquardsen J: The natural history of acute cerebrovascular disease. Acta Neurol Scand 45, suppl 38:90, 1969

46. Mulley GP, Heptinstall S, Taylor PM, Mitchell JRA: ADP-induced platelet release reaction in acute stroke. Thromb Haemost 50:524, 1983

47. Allen C: Clinical diagnosis of the acute stroke syndrome. Q J Med 52:515, 1983

48. Ojemann RG, Heros RC: Spontaneous brain hemorrhage. Stroke: 14:468, 1983

49. Ropper AM, Davis KR: Lobar cerebral hemorrhages: acute clinical syndromes in 26 cases. Ann Neurol 8: 141, 1980

50. Muller HR, Radue EW: Intracerebral haematoma. p. 320. In Harrison MJG, Dyken ML (eds): Cerebral Vascular Disease. Butterworths, London, 1983

51. Brown SD, Hanlon K, Mullins S: Treatment of aneurysmal hemiplegia with dopamine and mannitol. J Neurosurg 49:525, 1978

52. Haley EC, Kassell NF, Torner JC: The international cooperative study on the timing of aneurysm surgery: the North American experience. Stroke 23:205, 1992

53. Pickard JD, Murray GD, Illingworth R, et al: Effect of oral nimodipine on cerebral infarction and outcome after subarachnoid hemorrhage: British aneurysm nimodipine trial. Br Med J 298:636, 1989

54. Jellinek EH, Painter M, Prineas J, Ross Russell RW: Hypertensive encephalopathy with cortical disorders of vision. Q J Med 33:239, 1964

55. Ledingham JGG, Rajagopalan B: Cerebral complications in the treatment of accelerated hypertension. Q J Med 48:25, 1979

56. Dinsdale HB: Hypertensive encephalopathy. p. 787. In Barnett HJM, Mohr JP, Stein BM, Yatsu FM (eds): Stroke, 2nd Ed. Churchill Livingstone, New York, 1992

8

Postural Hypotension

Michael J. Aminoff

When a normal person stands up after being recumbent, about 500 ml of blood (or more) pools in the vessels of the legs and abdomen, causing a reduction in filling pressure of the right atrium and thus a decrease in cardiac output and systemic blood pressure. This leads to changes in baroreceptor activity and thus to changes in impulse traffic in the ninth and tenth cranial nerves. These changes affect the activity of the brainstem vasomotor center, which, in turn, influences the autonomic neurons in the intermediolateral cell columns of the thoracolumbar spinal cord, producing reflex peripheral vasoconstriction and an increase in force and rate of myocardial contraction (Figs. 8-1 and 8-2). Standing up also leads to release of norepinephrine. In addition, there is secretion of antidiuretic hormone (arginine vasopressin) and activation of the renin-angiotensin-aldosterone system, so that salt and water are conserved and blood volume increases. These, however, are typically long-term rather than immediate control mechanisms.

Postural hypotension is defined as a decrease of at least 20 mmHg in systolic pressure or 10 mmHg in diastolic pressure on standing. It occurs when there is a failure of the autoregulatory mechanisms that maintain the blood pressure on standing. It may therefore occur with any neurological disorder that impairs baroreceptor function, disturbs the afferent input from these receptors, directly involves the brainstem vasomotor center or its central connections, or interrupts the sympathetic outflow pathway either centrally or peripherally. It may also occur with

a number of nonneurological disorders, and it is important to consider these disorders if patients are to be managed correctly.

NONNEUROLOGICAL CAUSES OF POSTURAL HYPOTENSION

Cardiovascular Disorders

A variety of cardiac disorders may lead to postural hypotension or even syncope. Pathology such as mitral valve prolapse, aortic stenosis, or hypertrophic cardiomyopathy may limit cardiac output. Cardiac outflow may also be blocked in rare instances by a thrombus or myxoma when the patient is in the upright position. Certain paroxysmal cardiac dysrhythmias may occur with activity or on standing and produce episodic hypotension or syncope; however, disturbances of cardiac rhythm are common in asymptomatic elderly persons, and their presence must be interpreted with caution. In patients with congestive heart failure, the heart rate and level of sympathetic tone may be such that compensatory adjustments cannot be made when the patient stands, and postural hypotension therefore results.

Alterations of Effective Blood Volume

Postural hypotension can occur because of loss of effective blood volume. Normal adults can withstand the loss of 500 ml of blood or bodily fluids with few

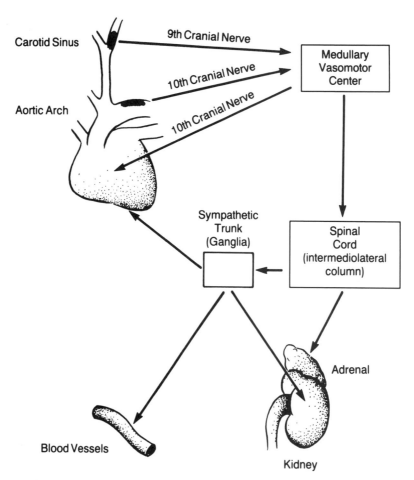

Fig. 8-1 Anatomy of the autonomic pathways involved in maintaining the blood pressure on standing.

if any symptoms, but greater volume depletion may occur acutely for a variety of reasons (e.g., hemorrhage or burns) and cause a postural drop in blood pressure. Hyponatremia and Addison's disease may also lead to an absolute reduction in blood volume. Postural hypotension may occur owing to venous pooling in patients with severe varicose veins or congenital absence of venous valves, or because of poor peripheral resistance and reduced muscle tone in patients with paralyzed limbs. Similarly, it may occur during the late stages of pregnancy owing to obstructed venous return by the gravid uterus. Marked vasodilatation, such as occurs in the heat or with the use of certain drugs or alcohol, sometimes causes postural hypotension.

Drugs

Numerous drugs may produce postural hypotension, including those given to treat neurological disorders (e.g., bromocriptine and levodopa) and psychiatric disturbances (e.g., tranquilizing, sedative, hypnotic, and antidepressant agents).[1] Antihypertensive drugs, diuretics, and vasodilators commonly lead to postural hypotension as a side effect. Insulin may cause nonhypoglycemic postural hypotension in diabetics with autonomic neuropathy, possibly due to vasodilatation and reduced venous return in the absence of functioning compensatory mechanisms or to impaired baroreceptor responses to changes in arterial

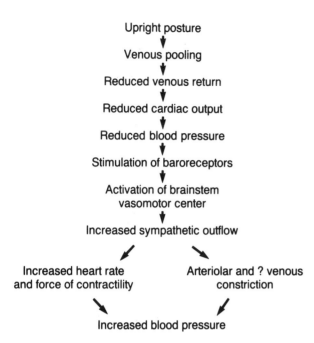

Upright posture
↓
Venous pooling
↓
Reduced venous return
↓
Reduced cardiac output
↓
Reduced blood pressure
↓
Stimulation of baroreceptors
↓
Activation of brainstem
vasomotor center
↓
Increased sympathetic outflow

Increased heart rate   Arteriolar and ? venous
and force of contractility   constriction

Increased blood pressure

Fig. 8-2 Sequence of events that ensure maintenance of the blood pressure following adoption of the upright posture. Only the immediate cardiovascular changes are shown. As indicated in the text, a variety of other humoral mechanisms are also activated.

pressure.[2] Iatrogenic and toxic autonomic neuropathy is considered below.

Endocrine and Metabolic Disorders

Autonomic neuropathy, with consequent postural hypotension, is a major and common complication of diabetes. Postural hypotension may be a feature of Addison's disease, hypopituitarism, myxedema, thyrotoxicosis, pheochromocytoma, carcinoid syndrome, and hypokalemia. It may also occur with anorexia nervosa. Anemia may exacerbate or cause postural hypotension. A patient who developed marked postural hypotension and extreme lability of the blood pressure in association with severe hypophosphatemia has been described.[3]

Inadequate Postural Adjustments

Prolonged bed rest may result in postural hypotension when patients first begin standing again, but this problem is self-limiting. Its cause is poorly under-

stood, but it may relate to the redistribution of body fluids.[4] In otherwise healthy subjects, vigorous exercise to the point of exhaustion may also cause a postural decline in blood pressure, possibly because of marked peripheral vasodilatation.[5]

Age

Johnson and associates found that 17 percent of patients over 70 years of age had a drop in systolic pressure of 20 mmHg or more on standing.[6] Baroreflex sensitivity reportedly declines with age. Phenylephrine-induced increases in blood pressure cause less reduction in heart rate in old people than young persons.[7] Again, old people are more sensitive than the young to the hypotensive effects of nitroprusside and show a blunting of the reflex tachycardia that occurs in response to the decline in blood pressure.[8] Elderly people therefore are more sensitive to vasodilators, and it is more difficult for them to compensate for sudden drops in blood pressure that occur for any reason. Age-related changes in the carotid artery and aortic arch may also influence baroreflex sensitivity. MacLennan and associates suggested that arterial and arteriolar rigidity directly affect both the ability of these vessels to constrict and baroreceptor sensitivity.[9]

However, Robinson and co-workers did not find any evidence of reduced tachycardia on standing in elderly patients with postural hypotension compared to age-matched patients without a significant orthostatic drop in blood pressure.[10] Moreover, the norepinephrine response on standing in the patients with postural hypotension was not consistent with reduced baroreceptor sensitivity or peripheral denervation.[10] Other factors, such as loss of blood vessel elasticity and adrenoreceptor sensitivity, occur in the elderly and may cause postural hypotension; mechanical factors (e.g., varicose veins) may also be contributory.

There is some evidence that, in the elderly, urinary sodium excretion takes longer to come into equilibrium with restricted intake than in young subjects,[11] and this may sometimes lead to volume depletion and postural hypotension. There is also some evidence that elderly patients with basal systolic hypertension are more likely to have poor postural blood pressure control.[9]

Syncope is a common problem in the elderly. Often no precise explanation for it can be found, but postural hypotension is probably responsible in many instances. However, it is best not to ascribe patients' symptoms to postural hypotension unless they can be reproduced by a demonstrable fall in blood pressure on standing. Many of the homeostatic mechanisms that maintain intravascular volume and blood pressure may be impaired with advancing age, as discussed above, so that syncope is more likely to occur. Indeed, in many elderly patients a number of factors can be found to account for syncope, and it is then difficult to determine which of these factors is responsible in any individual instance.

AUTONOMIC REGULATION OF THE HEART AND BLOOD VESSELS

The central nervous system (CNS) is important in regulating cardiovascular function. Various lower brainstem centers receive inputs from both the periphery and other central structures such as the cerebral cortex, temporal lobe, amygdala, hypothalamus, cerebellum, and pontine nuclei.[12,13] The nucleus tractus solitarius is the site of termination of baroreceptor and chemoreceptor afferent fibers; it connects with the dorsal nucleus of the vagus and with neurons in the lateral reticular formation that project to the cord in the bulbospinal pathway, thereby influencing the cardiovascular system.

The vagus nerve has a major role in regulating the heart rate responses to various maneuvers. The sympathetic nervous system is important in influencing vasomotor tone and peripheral vascular resistance, but the sympathetic outflow to different regions and structures is regulated separately. The sympathetic nervous system causes a vasoconstriction in response to the release of norepinephrine. The occurrence of vasodilatation in the limbs probably depends on reduced sympathetic activity, and, to a lesser extent, on axon reflexes and antidromic conduction, but some of the vessels in limb muscles are probably also supplied by sympathetic vasodilator cholinergic fibers.

Microneurographic studies in humans have shown that bursts of impulses occur rhythmically in sympathetic efferent vasomotor fibers to the skin and muscles and are time-locked to the pulse. This rhythmic activity is dependent on supraspinal mechanisms and is not seen below the level of a complete cord transec-

tion. Such sympathetic impulse traffic to vessels in the limb muscles is markedly affected by baroreceptor activity but not by brief mental stress,[14] whereas the traffic in human cutaneous nerves is markedly increased by mental stress. High-pressure arterial baroreceptors are located primarily in the carotid sinus and aortic arch, from which afferent fibers pass to the brainstem in the glossopharyngeal and vagus nerves respectively.

Sympathetic efferent activity is inhibited by an increase in the pressure in the carotid sinus and aortic arch, while a reduced pressure causes increased sympathetic activity and a peripheral vasoconstriction. The heart rate is also influenced by the baroreceptors, so that a bradycardia occurs when the pressure is increased and a tachycardia when the blood pressure declines.

Change from recumbency to an erect posture causes blood to pool in the legs and lower abdomen. There is a slight fall in systolic blood pressure; this leads to baroreceptor activation, a peripheral vasoconstriction, and an increase in heart rate and contractile force. Compensatory changes in the splanchnic vasculature, constriction of venous beds, and activation of the renin-angiotensin system also occur.

When physical activity is initiated spontaneously, there is an immediate increase in cardiac and respiratory rates as well as in blood pressure, due to a central command that arises above the level of the pons.[15]

NEUROLOGICAL CAUSES OF POSTURAL HYPOTENSION

Central Lesions and Spinal Injury

A few weeks after transection of the cervical cord, activity returns to the isolated spinal segment, but the brain is no longer able to control the sympathetic nervous system. Loss of regulation during postural change leads to orthostatic hypotension, whereas overactivity occurs if spinal sympathetic reflexes are activated and leads to the syndrome of autonomic hyperreflexia and hypertension. In general, spinal cord transection produces postural hypotension if the lesion is above about the T6 level. Intramedullary and extramedullary tumors, transverse myelitis, and syringomyelia[16] involving the cord above T6 may also produce autonomic failure.

A variety of brainstem lesions can impair autonomic function and affect control of the blood pressure, including syringobulbia[16] and posterior fossa tumors.[17] Impairment in Wernicke's encephalopathy may relate to central or peripheral involvement.[18,19] The extent to which autonomic function, and particularly cardiovascular regulation, is impaired in Parkinson's disease is disputed. The preponderance of evidence suggests that cardiovascular reflexes are preserved in patients with Parkinson's disease; reflex responses may be reduced slightly but are usually in the normal range.[20–22] In some patients, however, there seems to be an alteration in the "set" of baroreceptor reflexes without loss of their integrity.[23,24] The findings in certain other disorders with parkinsonian features (such as Shy-Drager syndrome, olivopontocerebellar atrophy, and striatonigral degeneration) are discussed on p. 142. Mild postural hypotension occurs occasionally in progressive supranuclear palsy, but cardiovascular reflexes are preserved or show only minor abnormalities of dubious significance.[21,25] A variety of dysautonomic symptoms may occur in Huntington's disease,[22] but any abnormalities of blood pressure regulation are usually mild and subclinical[26] except when related to neuroleptic medication taken for chorea or behavioral disturbances. Postural hypotension and other disturbances of cardiovascular autonomic function occur occasionally in patients with multiple sclerosis[27] or cerebrovascular disease.

Root and Peripheral Nerve Lesions

Postural hypotension may occur in patients with tabes dorsalis, due to interruption of circulatory reflexes. In patients with polyneuropathies, autonomic involvement is not uncommon. It is particularly conspicuous in diabetic neuropathy, and insulin may contribute to the severity of the postural hypotension,[1] as discussed earlier. Other polyneuropathies associated with postural hypotension include those of alcoholism, Guillain-Barré syndrome, bronchogenic carcinoma,[28,29] primary amyloidosis, and acute porphyria. In many patients with chronic alcoholism, however, there is no excessive decline in blood pressure on standing,[30] although the cardiovascular re-

sponses to various maneuvers are often abnormal and indicate chronic vagal damage.[31]

Autonomic dysfunction with abnormal cardiovascular responses may occur in patients with chronic renal failure on intermittent hemodialysis,[32] but the site of autonomic involvement is unclear.[33] Vitamin B_{12} deficiency may lead to autonomic neuropathy and postural hypotension that improves or resolves completely after vitamin supplementation.[34,35] Autonomic involvement, with impairment of sweating and cardiovascular responses, may occur in leprosy, sometimes without conspicuous features of peripheral nerve involvement.[36] Symptoms of autonomic impairment, including postural hypotension, may be a presenting feature of systemic autoimmune disorders.[37] In Fabry disease, disturbed sweating, reduced saliva and tear production, impaired pupillary responses, and gastrointestinal symptoms are common, but postural hypotension does not usually occur, and postural cardiovascular reflexes are normal.[38]

Autonomic involvement in Guillain-Barré syndrome may be fatal, due sometimes to cardiac arrhythmia or asystole.[39] The severity of autonomic involvement in the Guillain-Barré syndrome is not related to the degree of sensory or motor disturbance, and a wide variety of autonomic abnormalities is found if patients are studied in detail.[40]

Autonomic neuropathy of acute or subacute onset,[41,42] possibly on an autoimmune basis, sometimes occurs in isolation or with associated sensory[43] or motor involvement. It has occurred in the context of bronchial[28] or testicular malignancy,[44] Hodgkin's disease,[45] infectious mononucleosis,[46] rheumatoid arthritis,[47] and ulcerative colitis.[48] Recovery occurs to a variable degree and at different rates in different patients.

Autonomic involvement may occur in a variety of hereditary polyneuropathies. In familial dysautonomia, or Riley-Day syndrome, many parts of the nervous system are affected. Presentation during infancy may be with inability to suck, but episodic vomiting, recurrent pulmonary infections, hypertension, tachycardia, and diaphoresis occur, especially after 3 years of age. There may also be emotional outbursts, difficulty in swallowing, hypo- or hyperthermia, poor flow of tears, postural hypotension, and syncope. Sensory abnormalities include impaired pain and temperature appreciation, and the tendon reflexes are depressed. The tongue is smooth and lacks fungiform papillae. Cardiac arrest may occur on tracheal intubation. No firmly established data account for the etiology of the developmental changes in this recessively inherited disease.[49] Postural hypotension is generally not a feature of the other hereditary sensory and autonomic neuropathies, whereas sudomotor function is often markedly impaired.[50]

Autonomic symptoms or signs may occur in patients with Charcot-Marie-Tooth disease, and abnormal vascular reflex responses may be present.[51] Postural hypotension is generally not a conspicuous feature of the disorder.

A familial disorder characterized by progressive distal weakness and muscle atrophy, distal sensory loss, pyramidal and visual pathway lesions, and dysautonomia has been reported.[52] Patients had a sensorimotor polyneuropathy. The dysautonomia consisted of postural hypotension, lack of normal sinus arrhythmia, an abnormal sweat test, abnormal pupillary responses with denervation supersensitivity, and low serum norepinephrine levels in both the recumbent and upright positions.

Iatrogenic polyneuropathies are not uncommon, and in the neuropathy caused by perhexiline maleate there may be conspicuous autonomic involvement with marked postural hypotension.[53] Postural hypotension may also occur in patients receiving vincristine, and the response to the Valsalva maneuver may be abnormal.[54]

Toxic Exposure

Autonomic dysfunction may result from occupational or other exposure to certain neurotoxins but does not usually lead to postural hypotension. Disturbances of bladder and sexual function have resulted from exposure to dimethylaminoproprionitrile[55,56] and prolonged exposure to nitrous oxide.[57] One study suggested that long-term occupational exposure to a mixture of organic solvents causes subtle disturbances of peripheral parasympathetic nerves as well as sensorimotor peripheral neuropathies, as reflected by cardiovascular reflex studies,[58] but other reports of autonomic involvement in this context are lacking. Acrylamide neuropathy is usually accompanied by hyperhidrosis and cold cyanotic extremities; and in intoxicated rats, but not in humans, there is evidence that acrylamide alters common measures of cardiovascular function.[59] A variety of autonomic symptoms (including tachycardia, hypertension, disturbances of sweating) may occur with thallium, arsenic, or mercury poisoning, but postural hypotension is not usually a feature.

McFarlane and associates described a patient who developed severe postural hypotension and neurological signs that were attributed to styrene intoxication.[60] The rodenticide N-3-pyridylmethyl-N-p-nitrophenyl urea (Vacor) has caused severe dysautonomia with disabling postural hypotension[61,62] as well as sensorimotor peripheral neuropathy and encephalopathic states. Iatrogenic postural hypotension was considered earlier.

Primary Degeneration of the Autonomic Nervous System

Postural hypotension resulting from primary degeneration of the autonomic nervous system is well described.[63,64] Two distinct groups of patients are now recognized. In one, primary autonomic failure leads to idiopathic orthostatic hypotension and other evidence of dysautonomia without peripheral neuropathy or CNS involvement. In the other, autonomic failure is associated with more widespread neurological degeneration (i.e., with evidence of multisystem atrophy) such that there may be clinical features of parkinsonism (or striatonigral degeneration), and often of pyramidal, cerebellar, and lower motor neuron lesions as well (Shy-Drager syndrome). A disorder similar to olivopontocerebellar atrophy may also occur. The autonomic deficit may precede the somatic neurological one, or vice versa, but within a short period there is clinical evidence of both. Occasionally there is a family history of dysautonomia.[65]

In patients of both groups, plasma renin activity is generally subnormal. There are, however, a number of reported pharmacological differences between them. Patients with *idiopathic orthostatic hypotension* have low plasma norepinephrine levels when lying down, and these levels fail to increase appropriately on standing; they also have a lower threshold for the pressor response to infused norepinephrine.[66,67] The increase in plasma norepinephrine level in response to tyramine (see p. 150) is significantly less than in normal subjects or patients with multiple system atrophy.[68] Extensive cell loss has been reported in the intermediolateral cell columns of the thoracic cord,[69] and the autonomic dysfunction has been attributed primarily to loss of these preganglionic sympathetic neurons. However, the pharmacological studies described above indicate that loss of postganglionic noradrenergic neurons also occurs, and norepinephrine may be depleted from sympathetic nerve endings.

By contrast, in *multiple system atrophy,* in which lesions are situated at multiple sites in the CNS, circulating norepinephrine levels are normal, suggesting that peripheral sympathetic neurons are intact, but plasma norepinephrine fails to increase appropriately with standing, implying that these neurons have not been activated.[66-68] There is also an exaggerated pressor response to infused norepinephrine, but only patients with idiopathic orthostatic hypotension show a shift to the left in their dose-response curve, reflecting true adrenergic receptor supersensitivity.[68]

Some investigators have not found any clear pattern in the resting level of plasma norepinephrine that distinguishes between these two types of autonomic failure. They have emphasized that low levels probably indicate the severity of sympathetic dysfunction rather than the site of lesions.[70]

Endogenous arginine vasopressin is a powerful vasoconstrictor agent; it also acts on the kidney to control urinary concentrating mechanisms.[71] The cardiovascular responses generally associated with arginine vasopressin are reduced cardiac output, reduced heart rate and plasma renin activity, and increased vascular resistance and blood pressure.[72] Arginine vasopressin helps maintain arterial pressure in certain hypotensive situations such as hemorrhage or volume depletion, but increased levels of arginine vasopressin do not normally affect the blood pressure significantly because the acute vasoconstrictor effects are buffered by the baroreceptor reflex. The chronic effects of vasopressin on renal function do not produce sustained retention of sodium and water, and so produce only minimal changes in mean arterial pressure.

Vasopressin release is influenced by the plasma's osmotic pressure and by the activity of vascular stretch receptors. In normal subjects, plasma arginine vasopressin increases in response to standing, presumably because a decrease in venous return influences afferent activity from these stretch receptors. In patients with progressive autonomic failure and multiple system atrophy, plasma levels similar to control values are found in the horizontal position, but the postural rise is only 10 percent that in normals.[73] If hypertonic saline is infused intravenously

into such patients, plasma arginine vasopressin increases in a manner comparable to that in normal controls.[74] This suggests normal function of the efferent connections from the osmoreceptors within the hypothalamus and implies that in this clinical context the loss of vasopressin response with head-up tilt is due to lesions in ascending pathways from cardiovascular receptors.[74]

Miscellaneous Disorders

Patients with Holmes-Adie syndrome may present with or develop postural hypotension or abnormalities of thermoregulatory sweating. Studies in two patients with orthostatic hypotension have suggested an afferent or central block of impulses from baroreceptors, with normal function of efferent vasomotor pathways.[75]

Postural hypotension may occur in botulism, but blurred vision, dry mouth, and constipation are much more common autonomic manifestations.

Rare cases of postural hypotension due to excessive amounts of endogenous bradykinin (a vasodilator) have been reported,[76] as has a patient with a congenital defect of norepinephrine release.[77] In patients with dopamine beta-hydroxylase deficiency, norepinephrine and epinephrine cannot be synthesized, and dopamine is released from central and peripheral adrenergic nerve terminals.[78] Severe postural hypotension is accompanied by other autonomic disturbances.

SYMPTOMS OF DYSAUTONOMIA

Postural hypotension is usually the most disabling feature of autonomic failure. Symptoms induced by postural hypotension reflect cerebral hypoperfusion and include faintness, light-headedness, blurred vision, and syncope. They may be particularly troublesome after exercise or a heavy meal, or in the morning, when the blood pressure tends to be at its lowest. However, in some patients marked postural hypotension may be clinically asymptomatic or may be accompanied by symptoms not usually regarded as suggestive of postural hypotension—for example, nausea, breathlessness, heaviness or weakness of the limbs, episodic confusion, falling, staggering, and generalized weakness. Constipation may precipitate syncopal attacks during straining. Symptoms may also worsen in the heat because of vasodilatation and volume loss due to sweating.

Symptoms of idiopathic postural tachycardia syndromes may be mistakenly attributed to postural hypotension. The most common complaints are of light-headedness, headache, and fatigue associated with postural tachycardia and palpitations, but without significant decline in blood pressure.

Impotence is a common initial symptom of autonomic dysfunction in men, often preceding other symptoms by several months or years. Bladder involvement may manifest by urinary frequency, urgency, incontinence, retention, and increased residual urine. Bowel dysfunction may lead to constipation, fecal incontinence, and diarrhea. Thermoregulatory sweating may be impaired. Pupillary abnormalities include Horner's syndrome and anisocoria. Other symptoms of dysautonomia include night blindness, nasal congestion and, sometimes, supine hypertension. Vocal abnormalities and respiratory disturbances (especially involuntary inspiratory gasps, cluster breathing, airway obstruction, and sleep apnea) sometimes occur, especially in patients with multiple system atrophy.

Syncope

Syncope refers to a sudden transient loss of consciousness due to diffuse cerebral ischemia or hypoxia. It is usually associated with flaccidity, but a generalized increase in muscle tone sometimes occurs with continuing cerebral ischemia/hypoxia, and there may be arrhythmic transient motor activity as well. Postictal confusion is usually brief (less than about 30 seconds) when it occurs at all, unlike the marked postictal confusion that often follows a convulsion. Several types of syncope have been recognized.

VASOVAGAL SYNCOPE

During vasovagal syncope there is an initial increase in heart rate, blood pressure, total peripheral resistance, and cardiac output, followed by peripheral vasodilatation, increased blood flow to the muscles, decreased heart rate, and a decrease in venous return to the heart. Blood pressure falls owing to failure to increase the heart rate and cardiac output sufficiently, a decrease in systemic vascular resistance, or both.

The vasodilatation and decline in systemic vascular resistance has been related to depressor reflexes arising from the heart, perhaps in consequence of a decrease of central blood volume.[79] Recordings from nerve fibers reveal that impulse traffic ceases in the sympathetic outflow to skeletal muscle during syncope and gradually builds up again over the following 5 minutes or so.[80]

Syncope of this sort may be precipitated by pain, fear, emotional reactions, injury, and surgical manipulation. It may occur in association with missed meals, heat, or crowds; it usually occurs while subjects are standing. Warning symptoms include weakness, sweating, pallor, nausea, yawning, sighing, hyperventilation, blurred vision, impaired external awareness, and dilatation of pupils. Lying down or squatting at this time may abort actual loss of consciousness.

SYNCOPE DUE TO ORTHOSTATIC HYPOTENSION

In patients with orthostatic hypotension due to autonomic dysfunction, there is a fall in blood pressure on standing, without adequate compensatory change in total peripheral resistance or heart rate, and syncope may result. When postural hypotension occurs because of one of the nonneurological causes discussed earlier, it may also lead to syncope if autonomically mediated compensatory mechanisms fail to limit the decline in blood pressure.

DEGLUTITION SYNCOPE

Swallowing precipitates syncope in some subjects (deglutition syncope). In such instances there may be associated esophageal disorders. The syncope has usually been attributed to atrioventricular heart block. It is presumed that the prime factor is clinical or subclinical disease of the conducting system of the heart, and that disturbances of cardiac rhythm are then triggered by reflexes originating in the esophagus. A pacemaker may prevent further episodes.

MICTURITION SYNCOPE

Micturition syncope occurs after urination, particularly when the patient has gotten up from bed at night. It may relate to sudden release of the reflex vasoconstriction elicited by a full bladder. Assumption of the upright posture, the peripheral vasodilatation resulting from the warmth of the bed, and, particularly in elderly men, straining to micturate may also contribute to the drop in blood pressure. Occasionally, syncope occurs in response to cardiac dysrhythmia induced by a full bladder before micturition.

CAROTID SINUS SYNCOPE

Carotid sinus syncope may be provoked by neckturning or a tight collar in susceptible subjects. Certain drugs have also been shown to predispose toward it,[81] especially propranolol, digitalis, and α-methyldopa. A hypersensitive carotid sinus reflex is defined by a slowing in heart rate of more than 50 percent or a decline in systolic pressure by more than 40 mmHg during carotid sinus massage.[81] However, fewer than 50 percent of patients with carotid hypersensitivity have syncope as a result. Conversely, in many patients with syncope of unidentifiable cause, the carotid sinus syndrome may have been overlooked.

SYNCOPE WITH VALSALVA MANEUVER

Vigorous coughing or straining at stool may lead to syncope due to the reduced cardiac output and the peripheral vasodilatation caused by a high intrathoracic pressure. Cerebral perfusion may also be reduced by an increase in intracranial pressure.

CARDIAC SYNCOPE

As discussed earlier, postural hypotension may have a cardiac basis. In addition, atrioventricular conduction block may lead to sudden loss of consciousness regardless of the position of the body (Adams-Stokes attacks). Further comment concerning this topic is provided in Chapter 5.

EVALUATION OF AUTONOMIC FUNCTION

Postural Change in Blood Pressure

In investigating patients with suspected autonomic dysfunction or postural hypotension, the blood pressure should be measured with the patient supine for at least 10 (preferably 20) minutes. The patient then stands up, and the blood pressure is measured again after 5 to 10 seconds, and again after 2 and 5 minutes. There is normally a small increase in pulse rate on standing, but the pulse rate may not change if there is already a high resting pulse or in patients with dysautonomia; furthermore, the change in heart rate may be blunted in the elderly. In some instances postural hypotension develops only after exercise; it is therefore worthwhile to record the postactivity blood pressure if clinically feasible. It may be necessary to record the blood pressure on a number of occasions before the diagnosis of postural hypotension can be confirmed. In other instances, prolonged tilt (for up to 60 minutes) may be required to detect abnormalities.[82]

The effect of postural change on blood pressure can be evaluated more accurately if the blood pressure is measured using an intra-arterial cannula with the patient resting quietly on a tilt-table; measurements are made continuously while the patient is supine and then at a 60° head-up tilt.

Mann and co-workers monitored ambulant intra-arterial blood pressure in six patients with autonomic failure and postural hypotension.[83] They found a consistent circadian trend in blood pressure that was the inverse of the pattern in normal subjects, with the highest pressures found at night and the lowest in the morning. Such temporal variation in blood pressure implies that physiological testing should be carried out at a standard time of day, especially if comparative studies are to be performed, and potentially harmful hypertension in response to treatment should be looked for especially during the early part of the night.

Postural Change in Heart Rate

A simple, noninvasive test of autonomic function is done by evaluating the response in heart rate to change from a recumbent to a standing position, or to 60° head-up tilt on a tilt-table. There is typically a rapid increase in heart rate that is maximal at about the 15th beat after standing, with a subsequent slowing from the initial tachycardia (i.e., a relative bradycardia) that is maximal at about the 30th beat (Fig. 8-3). This response is mediated by the vagus nerve. For testing purposes, the R-R interval at beats 15 and 30 after standing can be measured to give the 30/15

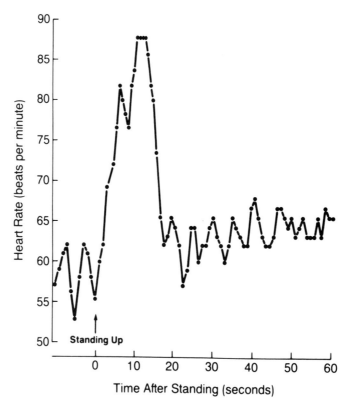

Fig. 8-3 Heart rate responses to standing in a normal subject. Immediately on standing, there is a rapid increase in heart rate that is maximal at about the 15th beat after standing.

ratio.[84] Values greater than 1.03 occur in normal subjects, whereas in diabetics with autonomic neuropathy (who typically show only a gradual increase in heart rate) values are 1.00 or less. This test does not depend on the resting heart rate and correlates well with the Valsalva ratio and the beat-to-beat variation in heart rate, described below. Recent studies suggest that the value for the 30/15 ratio declines with age in normal subjects.[85]

In some patients an excessive and sustained tachycardia develops in response to standing or head-up tilt, without significant drop in blood pressure. A prolonged tilt (for up to 60 minutes) may be necessary to elicit the abnormality.[82] The mechanisms underlying this postural tachycardia have not been clearly established.[86] The maximal increase in heart rate in response to postural tilt in normal subjects aged between 20 and 40 years was 36 per minute in men and 32 per minute in women in one study.[86]

Valsalva Maneuver

The Valsalva maneuver consists of a forced expiration maintained for at least 10 seconds (preferably 15 seconds) against a closed glottis after a full inspiration. Intrathoracic pressure should be increased by 30 to 40 mmHg. Clinically, this can be ensured by requiring the patient to blow into a mouthpiece connected to a manometer. The response can be recorded with an intra-arterial needle (Fig. 8-4), a noninvasive photoplethysmographic recording device (Finapres), or an electrocardiograph (Fig. 8-5).

The cardiovascular response is usually divided into four stages. Stage 1 is characterized by a transient increase in blood pressure at the onset of the forced expiration, reflecting the increased intrathoracic pressure. In stage 2 there is normally a gradual decrease in pulse pressure and stroke volume for several seconds due to a reduction in venous return to the heart, with an associated reflex tachycardia. Stage 3 occurs

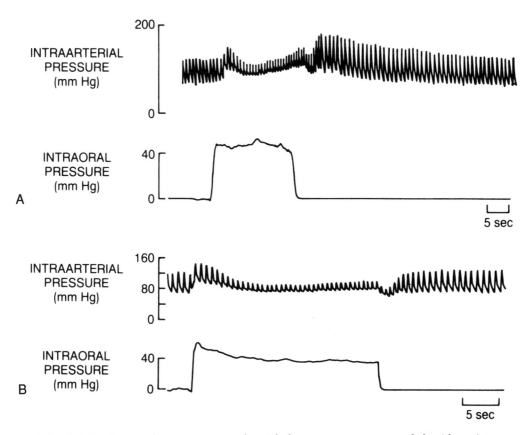

Fig. 8-4 Cardiovascular responses to the Valsalva maneuver, as recorded with an intra-arterial needle. **(A)** Normal response. **(B)** Abnormal response in a patient with Shy-Drager syndrome. (From Aminoff MJ: Electromyography in Clinical Practice. 2nd Ed. Churchill Livingstone, New York, 1987, with permission.)

when the patient releases the expiratory maneuver and is characterized by a transient fall in the blood pressure because of pooling of blood and expansion of the pulmonary vascular bed with the abrupt decline in intrathoracic pressure. In stage 4 there is an overshoot of the blood pressure above baseline value, with a compensatory bradycardia.

The Valsalva maneuver is an accurate indicator of baroreceptor reflex sensitivity. Abnormalities are found in patients with dysautonomia (Fig. 8-4) and may consist of loss of the overshoot in systolic blood pressure and compensatory bradycardia in stage 4, a fall in mean blood pressure in stage 2 to less than 50 percent of the previous resting mean pressure, and loss of the tachycardia in stage 2 or a lower heart rate in stage 2 than stage 4. However, abnormalities may also be found in patients with severe congestive heart failure and in those with cardiac lesions other than primary myocardial dysfunction.

If the response is recorded noninvasively using an electrocardiograph, the ratio of the longest R-R interval after the maneuver to the shortest R-R interval during it is determined and expressed as the Valsalva ratio. A value of 1.1 or less was arbitrarily defined by Ewing and associates as an abnormal response, 1.21 or greater as a normal response, and 1.11 to 1.20 as borderline.[87] Using such criteria, these authors found that the Valsalva maneuver was abnormal in 62 percent of diabetic patients with symptoms and signs suggestive of autonomic neuropathy. When more generous criteria for abnormality were employed, with a lower limit for normal of 1.50, the value was abnormal in 86 percent of these patients, and such an abnormality correlated well with the

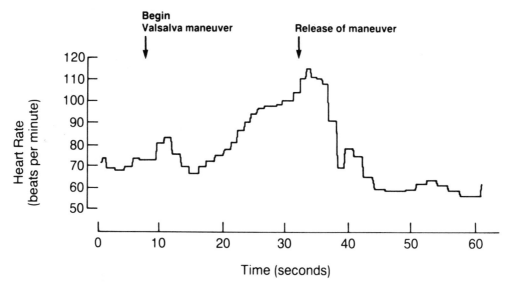

Fig. 8-5 Valsalva maneuver as recorded using an electrocardiograph or heart rate monitor in a normal subject. The tachycardia that occurs during the forced expiratory maneuver is clearly evident, as is the compensatory bradycardia that occurs when the maneuver is released.

presence of a significant postural drop in blood pressure.

Other Cardiovascular Responses

Other cardiovascular responses can also be measured noninvasively (e.g., the beat-to-beat variation in heart rate and the heart rate responses to deep breathing and sustained hand grip). Such tests of parasympathetic function appear to become abnormal more frequently and earlier than tests of sympathetic function, at least with the dysautonomia that occurs in diabetes.[84]

A particularly useful test is to measure the heart rate variation during deep breathing (Fig. 8-6). In normal subjects there is considerable heart rate variation, which is accentuated during deep breathing. This variation is reduced or absent in diabetics with autonomic neuropathy. The optimal breathing rate for this test is 6 breaths per minute (i.e., inspiration = expiration = 5 seconds). Heart rate variation scores can be calculated by measuring the difference between the minimum heart rate on inspiration and the maximum rate on expiration, taking the average from 10 breaths in and 10 breaths out. Normal subjects generally have a score greater than 9, and autonomic neu-

ropathy is probably absent if scores greater than 12 are obtained[88]; the normal range, however, may be age-dependent.[85,89,90]

An increase in heart rate and blood pressure should also occur in response to startle, such as occurs with a sudden loud noise, and to mental stress, as is produced when the patient attempts to subtract 7 serially from 100 while constantly being distracted.

Digital Blood FLow

Blood flow to a finger can be measured by conventional or photoplethysmography. A sudden inspiratory gasp causes a reflex digital vasoconstriction as a spinal reflex, and this is easily measured plethysmographically (Fig. 8-7). The response is impaired or absent in patients with a lesion of the cord or sympathetic efferent pathway, as in peripheral neuropathy. In entrapment neuropathy, such as carpal tunnel syndrome, the vasoconstrictor response may be abolished in fingers supplied by the affected nerve but not in those supplied by other nerves.[91]

Cold Pressor Test

In the cold pressor test, one hand is immersed in ice water at 4°C, and this normally produces an increase in systolic pressure of 15 mmHg or more

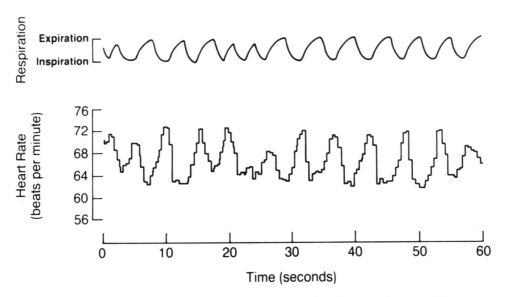

Fig. 8-6 Normal variation in heart rate that occurs in relation to deep breathing.

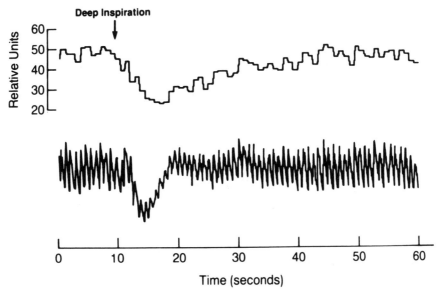

Fig. 8-7 Variation in blood volume following a deep inspiration in a normal subject, measured photoplethysmographically by means of an infrared emitter and detector placed on the pad of the index finger. The bottom trace represents the sensor output after it has been amplified by the photoplethysmographic module of a computerized autonomic testing system; it is a function of the absolute blood volume in the finger. Each peak represents a heartbeat, and the amplitude of each wave reflects blood volume in the area about the sensor. The apparent shift of the DC signal component is due to the long time constant that is necessary so that signal information is not lost. The relative voltage, representing the amplitude of each pulse, is shown in the upper trace. It can be seen from both traces that following the deep inspiration there is a reduction in digital blood flow (i.e., reduced amplitude of the waveforms in the lower trace and a corresponding decline in the upper trace).

within 1 minute. The afferent pathway involves the spinothalamic tract, and if this tract is intact, the lack of a pressor response suggests a lesion centrally or in the sympathetic efferent pathway. A normal response in a patient with an abnormal Valsalva response and intact pain and temperature sensation suggests an afferent baroreceptor lesion.

Norepinephrine Infusion

The plasma norepinephrine level can be used as an index of sympathetic activity. Perhaps of greater value, the blood pressure can be measured in response to intravenous infusion of norepinephrine at several dosage rates up to 20 μg/min.[68] In this way a dose-response curve can be constructed. In normal subjects it is usually necessary to administer 15 to 20 μg/min to increase systolic blood pressure to 40 mmHg above baseline. A similar increase in blood pressure results from doses of 5 to 10 μg/min in Shy-Drager syndrome and less than 2.5 μg/min in patients with idiopathic orthostatic hypotension.[68]

Response to Tyramine

Tyramine, an indirectly acting sympathomimetic drug, can be used to test neuronal uptake and release of norepinephrine. Bolus injections ranging from 250 to 6,000 μg are administered and blood pressure measured at 1-minute intervals. The amount of norepinephrine released into plasma by tyramine can be quantified by obtaining a blood sample shortly after the rise in blood pressure.[68]

Norepinephrine Response to Edrophonium

Intravenously administered edrophonium (10 mg) normally leads within 8 minutes to the postganglionic release of norepinephrine and thus to an increase in plasma norepinephrine levels. In patients with central dysautonomias (and intact postganglionic function), a normal response is obtained, whereas patients with more peripheral pathology have absent or attenuated responses.[92] The sensitivity and specificity of the test remains to be established.

Sweat Tests

Cutaneous blood vessels and sweat glands are supplied by sympathetic fibers intermingled in the same fascicles but of different size and conduction velocity.[14] Commonly used tests of sweating are messy and require application of heat, which is time-consuming. A heat cradle placed over the trunk is used to produce an increase of 1°C (from a resting level of 36.5° to 37.0°C) in the oral temperature over the course of 30 to 60 minutes, and the presence of sweat over selected regions of the trunk and limbs is detected by the change in color of quinizarine powder or a starch-iodide mixture that it produces. Changes in hand blood flow can also be measured with a plethysmograph. The pattern of any impairment of sweating may be helpful in suggesting the underlying cause. For example, impairment is usually distal in the limbs in patients with polyneuropathies.

The volume of sweat produced by axon-reflex stimulation either electrically (faradic sweat response) or with parasympathomimetic drugs under specified conditions indicates the state of sudomotor innervation in the tested limb. After a short latent period, sweating occurs in an area that is about 4 to 5 cm in diameter about the site of stimulation. The reflex is subserved by sympathetic postganglionic fibers; impulses pass centripetally along these fibers until they reach a branch point and then pass distally again. The receptor involved in the reflex has not been defined.[93]

Rather than detecting a sweat response by a color change, as described above, it may be necessary to quantify the volume of sweat. Recordings can then be made of the humidity change of an airstream of defined flow.[93] Using such an approach, the group at the Mayo Clinic have quantified the sudomotor response to axon reflex stimulation using electrophoresed acetylcholine to stimulate the receptors involved in the axon reflex.

The "spoon test" is a simple, nontechnical bedside test to assess sudomotor function. The curved surface of a kitchen soupspoon is drawn slowly across the skin without lifting it from the skin.[94] In patients with no sweat on the skin, pull of the spoon is reportedly smooth and unopposed, whereas if the skin is moist, the flow of the spoon is interrupted, requiring constant readjustment of the strength of pull.

Another simple technique for evaluating sudomotor function is to measure changes in skin resistance.

With sweating, there is a reduction in skin resistance. This is the so-called *galvanic skin response,* which can be elicited by painful or emotional stimuli or by deep inspiration.

Sudomotor function has also been evaluated in patients with polyneuropathies by recording the *sympathetic skin response*—that is, the change in voltage measured from the skin surface following deep inspiration or electrical stimuli applied to the skin of the wrist or ankle. Responses are recorded from a pair of electrodes placed on the palm and dorsum of the hand, or the sole and dorsum of the foot.[95]

Other Studies

RESPONSE TO LOBELINE

Intravenous lobeline induces a cough, and this response has been used as a test of the integrity of glossopharyngeal fibers.

PUPILLARY RESPONSES

Pupillary constriction with 2.5% methacholine applied locally indicates denervation supersensitivity due to interruption of postganglionic parasympathetic fibers, as in the Holmes-Adie syndrome. Local instillation of 1:1,000 epinephrine hydrochloride (1 or 2 drops) produces little or no response unless there is postganglionic sympathetic denervation, in which case marked pupillary dilatation occurs. A 4% solution of cocaine hydrochloride applied to the conjunctival sac dilates the normal pupil, but fails to do so if sympathetic innervation has been interrupted outside the CNS.

DIGITAL WRINKLING

Wrinkling of the skin of the fingers on immersion of the hands in warm water for 20 to 30 minutes is a normal phenomenon that is abolished by lesions affecting central or peripheral sympathetic pathways. It has been used as a nontechnical test of sympathetic function.

RADIOLOGICAL STUDIES

Radiological studies may be helpful in characterizing gastrointestinal and bladder function but are beyond the scope of this chapter.

DETECTION OF SYMPATHETIC RECEPTORS

An indirect measure of sympathetic autonomic function depends on the detection of "sympathetic receptors" on lymphocytes and platelets by radioligand binding techniques. In multiple system atrophy, perhaps due to reduced exposure to plasma norepinephrine, there is a marked increase in the number of α-receptors on platelets and the number of β-receptors on lymphocytes; the affinity of both α- and β-receptors appears to be normal.[96,97]

PATIENT MANAGEMENT

The initial investigative approach to patients presenting with syncope or other symptoms suggestive of postural hypotension or autonomic dysfunction is to exclude reversible causes such as hypovolemia or certain medications (see pp. 137 to 139). The history must include a detailed account of previous illnesses and drug intake. Simple laboratory investigations should include a full blood count and erythrocyte sedimentation rate as well as determination of plasma urea, electrolytes, glucose, and cortisol levels. Urinary screen for porphyrins; serum protein electrophoresis and immunopheresis; hepatic, renal, and thyroid function tests; chest radiograph; and electrocardiogram (to exclude recent cardiac infarction or cardiac ischemia, heart block, or persisting cardiac dysrhythmia) are also performed, as are serological tests for syphilis and nerve conduction studies. Neuroimaging studies may be helpful if a structural intracranial lesion is suspected. An echocardiogram and a phonocardiogram may help when evaluating patients with suspected structural lesions of the heart predisposing to syncope. In patients with symptoms of uncertain etiology in whom general medical causes have been excluded, more detailed evaluation of autonomic function in the manner suggested earlier may be helpful.

Treatment

If a specific reversible cause, such as a metabolic or endocrinological disturbance, can be recognized, it must be treated appropriately. The need for continuing with drugs likely to be responsible should be reviewed and, if feasible, treatment discontinued. Pa-

Table 8-1 Management of Postural Hypotension

Treatment of specific underlying cause or aggravating factors

    Discontinue drugs that may be responsible, if feasible

    Correct electrolyte/metabolic/hormonal disorders

    Avoid alcohol

    Eliminate conditions that favor pooling of blood or that impede venous return

    Prescribe antiarrhythmic drugs, pacemaker, or surgery for selected cardiac disorders

    Consider a cardiac pacemaker for carotid sinus hypersensitivity

Symptomatic treatment

    Nonpharmacological management

        Stand up gradually

        Eat small meals and avoid postprandial activity

        Wear waist-high elastic stockings

        Elevate the head of the bed

        Eat a liberal salt diet

    Pharmacological and other treatment

        Fludrocortisone

        Indomethacin

        Sympathomimetic drugs (phenylephrine, ephedrine, amphetamines)

        β-blocker drugs (propranolol, pindolol)

        Cardiac pacing in selected circumstances

        Experimental drug treatments:

            Vasopressin

            Dihydroergotamine

            Yohimbine

            Midodrine

            Metoclopramide

            Clonidine

            Norepinephrine (by infusion pump)

tients should be advised against using alcohol. Treatment with antiarrhythmic agents, cardiac pacemaker, or surgery may be indicated in patients with a cardiac cause of syncope or postural hypotension. Pacemaker therapy may also help patients with syncope due to carotid sinus hypersensitivity.[81]

If no specific cause can be identified, treatment should be directed to the minimization of symptoms (Table 8-1). The actual extent to which the blood pressure falls on standing, for example, is of lesser significance than the occurrence of symptoms. Patients with dysautonomia should avoid extreme heat, alcohol, large meals, rapid postural changes, and excessive straining (e.g., during micturition or defecation), each of which may exacerbate symptoms. Diuretics should be stopped, if possible, and salt intake liberalized.

When standing, patients often find it helpful to work the leg muscles, because this aids the venous return to the heart. Symptoms may also be reduced if patients stand up gradually (e.g., by first adopting the seated position and, after a short pause, getting up from this position).

Waist-high elastic stockings may be helpful in alleviating postural symptoms but are often difficult to put on (especially for elderly patients) and may be uncomfortable in hot weather. To be effective, the stockings must extend at least as high as the waist. Antigravity suits have been used in the past but are awkward, restrictive, impractical, and not generally available.

Many dysautonomic patients have a disturbance in the regulation of body fluids. In particular, there is defective sodium conservation, especially during recumbency at night, associated with, but not entirely due to, low aldosterone levels[98]; there are also abnormal posture-dependent changes in urine volume (Fig. 8-8) accompanied by an alteration in the secretion of antidiuretic hormone.[99] This leads to relative hypovolemia and postural hypotension that are worse in the morning and improve during the day. The disturbed regulation of body fluids could be due, at least in part, to diminished adrenergic activity in the renal nerves, which affects tubular reabsorption and renin release (and thus angiotensin formation). The effect of recumbency can be minimized by elevating the head of the bed by 5° to 20°, which leads to reduced renal artery pressure, thereby stimulating the renin-angiotensin system and promoting sodium retention.[2] Head-up tilt at night reduces nocturnal shifts of interstitial fluid from the legs into the circulation; furthermore, such interstitial fluid may exert hydrostatic force, opposing the tendency of blood to pool in the legs on standing.[100] Head-up tilt at night also reduces supine hypertension.

If these measures are unsuccessful, the mineralocorticoid fludrocortisone can be tried. This agent seems to exert its effect in part by temporarily increasing plasma volume and also by increasing vascular sensitivity to norepinephrine and improving the vasoconstrictor response to sympathetic stimulation.[101] Treatment is generally commenced with a daily dose of 0.1 mg, which can then be increased by 0.1 mg every 2 weeks or so until benefit occurs or there are

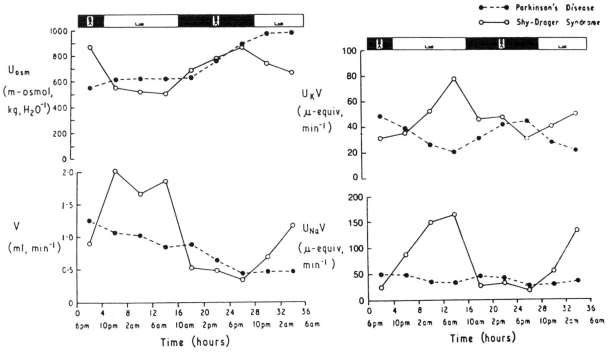

Fig. 8-8 Renal responses of five dysautonomic patients and four parkinsonian (control) subjects to fluid deprivation for 36 hours, commencing at 6 P.M. Average results are presented for urine osmolality and volume as well as potassium and sodium excretion for each successive 4-hour period. Subjects were lying down (*white bars*) during the night (10 P.M. to 10 A.M.) and up and about (*black bars*) during the day (10 A.M. to 10 P.M.). (From Wilcox CS, Aminoff MJ, Penn W: Basis of nocturnal polyuria in patients with autonomic failure. J Neurol Neurosurg Psychiatry 37:677, 1974, with permission.)

intolerable side effects. Some patients may require as much as 1.0 or 2.0 mg daily. During treatment with fludrocortisone, a positive sodium balance should be ensured, with a sodium intake of at least 150 mEq per day. Side effects include recumbent hypertension, cardiomegaly, hypokalemia, and retinopathy; coexisting diabetes mellitus may also be exacerbated.

Prostaglandin synthetase inhibitors should expand plasma volume and inhibit vasodilator prostaglandin synthesis. Indomethacin increases peripheral vascular resistance, promotes fluid retention, and may increase the sensitivity of the peripheral vasculature to norepinephrine and angiotensin II.[102] It is said to be helpful in some patients with postural hypotension,[103] especially if they are also on fludrocortisone, but in general the results with it have been disappointing despite the theoretical advantages of its use.

Dihydroergotamine is a relatively selective constrictor of peripheral veins. Its action may be mediated partially through α-adrenoreceptors, and enhanced synthesis of a vasoconstrictor prostaglandin may also be important. It is sometimes helpful for treating postural hypotension, but may cause recumbent hypertension. Although it is effective when administered intravenously, its efficacy when taken orally is more limited. Inhaled preparations may be effective.[104]

Sympathomimetic drugs that either act directly to constrict blood vessels (e.g., phenylephrine) or that have an indirect action, preventing the destruction of norepinephrine at sympathetic nerve terminals (e.g., ephedrine and amphetamines), have been used to treat postural hypotension. These drugs can sometimes be helpful, but any benefit is often mild and temporary, and they may cause severe recumbent hypertension.

Propranolol may help the postural hypotension associated with postural tachycardia and also reduces sodium excretion, leading to an increase in blood volume.[2] Furthermore, it has been said to help the hypotension of both idiopathic orthostatic hypotension and the Shy-Drager syndrome; this action has been attributed to the β-blockade correcting an imbalance of α- and β-adrenoreceptor activity in the peripheral nervous system.[105,106] Pindolol, a β-blocker with intrinsic sympathomimetic activity, has also been helpful in some instances, but more often it produces no benefit and may lead to cardiac failure.[2,107]

Two groups have reported clinical benefit and a rise in blood pressure on standing in patients with sympathetic efferent failure by cardiac pacing.[108,109] However, in a patient with more severe sympathetic involvement, Goldberg and colleagues failed to show any benefit with atrial tachypacing.[110] Bannister and associates reported a patient with selective impairment of sympathetic cardiovascular reflexes but relative sparing of cardiac parasympathetic function.[48] Because of accentuation of bradycardia and the risk of dysrhythmia with any elevation in blood pressure, it was thought that the use of pressor agents would be especially hazardous. A demand pacemaker was therefore introduced and, although it did not improve postural hypotension, it enabled blood pressure to be readily and safely controlled by drugs. Atrial tachypacing may thus prove helpful in patients with selective sympathetic autonomic neuropathy by protecting against vagal overactivity.

Vasopressin responses to upright posture are often defective in autonomic failure, and patients are hypersensitive to exogenous vasopressin. The long-term therapeutic utility of vasopressin is unclear. Wagner and Braunwald showed that a rise in blood pressure occurred after intranasal administration of posterior pituitary extract or intramuscular injection of pitressin tannate in oil in three patients with idiopathic orthostatic hypotension.[111] Kochar studied the effect of lysine vasopressin nasal spray in 10 patients with chronic orthostatic hypotension and found no significant alteration in the effect of tilt on heart rate, stroke volume, or cardiac output; there was, however, an increase in blood pressure and total peripheral resistance.[112] In five patients with chronic autonomic failure who were not receiving treatment with drugs, Mathias and associates found that the vasopressin analogue desmopressin (given intramuscularly) reduced nocturnal polyuria, raised supine blood pressure, and reduced postural drops in blood pressure.[113]

There have been a variety of other experimental

therapeutic approaches. Yohimbine, a centrally acting α2-antagonist, increases mean arterial pressure and plasma norepinephrine levels in normal subjects[114] and dysautonomic patients,[115] but its clinical utility has not been established. Midodrine is an investigational α-agonist that has been helpful in some patients with dysautonomia.[116] The use of a dopamine receptor antagonist, metoclopramide, has been suggested, since dopaminergic drugs (e.g., bromocriptine) may depress the blood pressure.[117] In a few patients with idiopathic orthostatic hypotension, the selective partial α-agonist clonidine may be helpful,[118] but it has caused profound hypotension in a patient with baroreceptor dysfunction due to irradiation of the neck. Administration of caffeine with meals may markedly reduce postprandial hypotension and is worthy of trial when symptoms are particularly troubling after meals.[110] Other investigational approaches are the use of an electromechanical device for automatic control of blood pressure by means of a norepinephrine infusion pump[119] and of erythropoietin to increase the red-cell volume.[120]

General Precautions in Management of Dysautonomic Patients

Patients may show postprandial falls in blood pressure because blood is diverted to the hepatic and splanchnic beds. Vasoactive substances may also contribute to the hypotensive response. In order to avoid or minimize this postprandial hypotension, it is helpful to eat smaller meals and to avoid excessive activity during the immediate postprandial period.

Dysautonomic patients often have low circulating catecholamine levels and denervation supersensitivity to sympathomimetic amines. Medication containing such substances should therefore be avoided, even though they are often available without prescription in over-the-counter preparations.

Patients with dysautonomia pose special problems during anesthesia. They are unable to tolerate hemodynamic stresses normally because of impaired cardiovascular reflexes. Maintenance of fluid balance is more difficult because of the abnormal manner in which they handle salt and water, and their enhanced sensitivity to volume changes influences blood pressure control.

REFERENCES

1. Schoenberger JA: Drug-induced orthostatic hypotension. Drug Saf 6:402, 1991
2. Bradshaw MJ, Edwards RTM: Postural hypotension—pathophysiology and management. Q J Med 60:643, 1986
3. Nanji AA, Freeman HJ: Postural hypotension and labile blood pressure associated with severe hypophosphatemia. Int J Cardiol 5:379, 1984
4. Blomqvist CG: Orthostatic hypotension. Hypertension 8:722, 1986
5. Schatz IJ: Orthostatic Hypotension. FA Davis, Philadelphia, 1986
6. Johnson RH, Smith AC, Spalding JMK, Wollner L: Effect of posture on blood-pressure in elderly patients. Lancet 1:731, 1965
7. Gribbin B, Pickering TG, Sleight P, Peto R: Effect of age and high blood pressure on baroreflex sensitivity in man. Circ Res 29:424, 1979
8. Minanker KL, Rowe JW, Sparrow D: Impaired cardiovascular (CV) adaptation to vasodilation in the elderly. Gerontologist 20:163, 1980
9. MacLennan WJ, Hall MRP, Timothy JI: Postural hypotension in old age: is it a disorder of the nervous system or of blood vessels? Age Ageing 9:25, 1980
10. Robinson BJ, Johnson RH, Lambie DG, Palmer KT: Do elderly patients with an excessive fall in blood pressure on standing have evidence of autonomic failure? Clin Sci 64:587, 1983
11. Swales JD: Pathophysiology of blood pressure in the elderly. Age Ageing 8:104, 1979
12. Spyer KM: Physiology of the autonomic nervous system: CNS control of the cardiovascular system. Curr Opin Neurol Neurosurg 4:528, 1991
13. Loewy AD: Anatomy of the autonomic nervous system: an overview. p. 3. In Loewy AD, Spyer KM (eds): Central Regulation of Autonomic Functions. Oxford University Press, New York, 1990
14. Wallin BG, Elam M: Microneurography and autonomic dysfunction. p. 243. In Low PA (ed): Clinical Autonomic Disorders. Little, Brown, Boston, 1993
15. Eldridge FL, Millhorn DE, Kiley JP, Waldrop TG: Stimulation by central command of locomotion, respiration and circulation during exercise. Respir Physiol 59:313, 1985
16. Nogues MA, Newman PK, Male VJ, Foster JB: Cardiovascular reflexes in syringomyelia. Brain 105:835, 1982
17. Hsu CY, Hogan EL, Wingfield W, et al: Orthostatic hypotension with brainstem tumors. Neurology 34:1137, 1984
18. Birchfield RI: Postural hypotension in Wernicke's disease. Am J Med 36:404, 1964
19. Cravioto H, Korein J, Silberman J: Wernicke's encephalopathy. Arch Neurol 4:510, 1961
20. Micieli G, Martignoni E, Cavallini A, et al: Postprandial and orthostatic hypotension in Parkinson's disease. Neurology 37:386, 1987
21. Sandroni P, Ahlskog JE, Fealey RD, Low PA: Autonomic involvement in extrapyramidal and cerebellar disorders. Clin Auton Res 1:147, 1991
22. Aminoff MJ: Other extrapyramidal disorders. p. 527. In Low PA (ed): Clinical Autonomic Disorders. Little, Brown, Boston, 1993
23. Aminoff MJ, Wilcox CS: Assessment of autonomic function in patients with a parkinsonian syndrome. Br Med J 4:80, 1971
24. Gross M, Bannister R, Godwin-Austen R: Orthostatic hypotension in Parkinson's disease. Lancet 1:174, 1972
25. Gutrecht JA: Autonomic cardiovascular reflexes in progressive supranuclear palsy. J Auton Nerv Syst 39:29, 1992
26. Aminoff MJ, Gross M: Vasoregulatory activity in patients with Huntington's chorea. J Neurol Sci 21:33, 1974
27. Sterman AB, Coyle PK, Panasci DJ, Grimson R: Disseminated abnormalities of cardiovascular autonomic functions in multiple sclerosis. Neurology 35:1665, 1985
28. Park DM, Johnson RH, Crean GP, Robinson JF: Orthostatic hypotension in bronchial carcinoma. Br Med J 3:510, 1972
29. Chiappa KH, Young RR: A case of paracarcinomatous pandysautonomia. Neurology 23:423, 1973
30. Low PA, Walsh JC, Huang CY, McLeod JG: The sympathetic nervous system in alcoholic neuropathy: a clinical and pathological study. Brain 98:357, 1975
31. Duncan G, Johnson RH, Lambie DG, Whiteside EA: Evidence of vagal neuropathy in chronic alcoholics. Lancet 2:1053, 1980
32. Ewing DJ, Winney R: Autonomic function in patients with chronic renal failure on intermittent haemodialysis. Nephron 15:424, 1975
33. Nies AS, Robertson D, Stone WJ: Hemodialysis hypotension is not the result of uremic peripheral autonomic neuropathy. J Lab Clin Med 94:395, 1979
34. McCombe PA, McLeod JG: The peripheral neuropathy of vitamin B_{12} deficiency. J Neurol Sci 66:117, 1984
35. Eisenhofer G, Lambie DG, Johnson RH, et al: Deficient catecholamine release as the basis of orthostatic hypotension in pernicious anemia. J Neurol Neurosurg Psychiatry 45:1053, 1982

36. Gadoth N, Bechar M, Kushnir M, et al: Somatosensory and autonomic neuropathy as the only manifestation of long standing leprosy. J Neurol Sci 43:471, 1979
37. Gudesblatt M, Goodman AD, Rubenstein AE, et al: Autonomic neuropathy associated with autoimmune disease. Neurology 35:261, 1985
38. Cable WJL, Kolodny EH, Adams RD: Fabry disease: impaired autonomic function. Neurology 32:498, 1982
39. Lichtenfeld P: Autonomic dysfunction in the Guillain-Barré syndrome. Am J Med 50:772, 1971
40. Tuck RR, McLeod JG: Autonomic dysfunction in Guillain-Barré syndrome. J Neurol Neurosurg Psychiatry 44:983, 1981
41. Hopkins A, Neville B, Bannister R: Autonomic neuropathy of acute onset. Lancet 1:769, 1974
42. Young RR, Asbury AK, Corbett JL, Adams RD: Pure pandysautonomia with recovery: description and discussion of diagnostic criteria. Brain 98:613, 1975
43. Colan RV, Snead OC, Oh SJ, Kashlan MB: Acute autonomic and sensory neuropathy. Ann Neurol 8: 441, 1980
44. Fagius J, Westerberg C-E, Olsson Y: Acute pandysautonomia and severe sensory deficit with poor recovery: a clinical, neurophysiological and pathological case study. J Neurol Neurosurg Psychiatry 46:725, 1983
45. Van Lieshoutt JJ, Wieling W, Van Montfrans GA, et al: Acute dysautonomia associated with Hodgkin's disease. J Neurol Neurosurg Psychiatry 49:830, 1986
46. Yahr MD, Frontera AT: Acute autonomic neuropathy: its occurrence in infectious mononucleosis. Arch Neurol 32:132, 1975
47. Edmonds ME, Jones TC, Saunders WA, Sturrock RD: Autonomic neuropathy in rheumatoid arthritis. Br Med J 2:173, 1979
48. Bannister R, Da Costa DF, Hendry WG, et al: Atrial demand pacing to protect against vagal overactivity in sympathetic autonomic neuropathy. Brain 109:345, 1986
49. Pearson J: Familial dysautonomia (a brief review). J Auton Nerv Syst 1:119, 1979
50. Dyck PJ: Neuronal atrophy and degeneration predominantly affecting peripheral sensory and autonomic neurons. p. 1065. In Dyck PJ, Thomas PK, Griffin JW, et al (eds): Peripheral Neuropathy, 3rd Ed. WB Saunders, Philadelphia, 1993
51. Brooks AP: Abnormal vascular reflexes in Charcot-Marie-Tooth disease. J Neurol Neurosurg Psychiatry 43:348, 1980
52. Rechthand E, Reife R, Kaplan JG: Hereditary neuropathy with upper motor-neuron, visual pathway, and autonomic disorders. Neurology 33:1495, 1983
53. Fraser DM, Campbell IW, Miller HC: Peripheral and autonomic neuropathy after treatment with perhexiline maleate. Br Med J 2:675, 1977
54. Hancock BW, Naysmith A: Vincristine-induced autonomic neuropathy. Br Med J 3:207, 1975
55. Kreiss K, Wegman DH, Niles CA, et al: Neurological dysfunction of the bladder in workers exposed to dimethylaminopropionitrile. JAMA 243:741, 1980
56. Keogh JP, Pestronk A, Wertheimer D, Moreland E: An epidemic of urinary retention caused by dimethylaminopropionitrile. JAMA 243:746, 1980
57. Layzer RB: Myeloneuropathy after prolonged exposure to nitrous oxide. Lancet 2:1227, 1978
58. Matikainen E, Juntunen J: Autonomic nervous system dysfunction in workers exposed to organic solvents. J Neurol Neurosurg Psychiatry 48:1021, 1985
59. Sterman AB, Panasci DJ, Sheppard RC: Autonomic-cardiovascular dysfunction accompanies sensory-motor impairment during acrylamide intoxication. Neurotoxicology 4:45, 1983
60. MacFarlane IA, Wilkinson R, Harrington JM: Severe postural hypotension following home canoe construction from polyester resins. Postgrad Med J 60:497, 1984
61. LeWitt PA: The neurotoxicity of the rat poison Vacor: a clinical study of 12 cases. N Engl J Med 302:73, 1980
62. Benowitz NL, Byrd R, Schambelan M, et al: Dihydroergotamine treatment for orthostatic hypotension from Vacor rodenticide. Ann Intern Med 92:387, 1980
53. Shy GM, Drager GA: A neurological syndrome associated with orthostatic hypotension. Arch Neurol 2: 511, 1960
64. Bradbury S, Eggleston C: Postural hypotension: a report of three cases. Am Heart J 1:73, 1925
65. Lewis P: Familial orthostatic hypotension. Brain 87: 719, 1964
66. Ziegler MG, Lake CR, Kopin IJ: The sympathetic-nervous-system defect in primary orthostatic hypotension. N Engl J Med 296:293, 1977
67. Polinsky RJ, Kopin IJ, Ebert MH, Weise V: Pharmacologic distinction of different orthostatic hypotension syndromes. Neurology 31:1, 1981
68. Polinsky RJ: Clinical autonomic neuropharmacology. Neurol Clin 8:77, 1990
69. Johnson RH, Lee G de J, Oppenheimer DR, Spalding JMK: Autonomic failure with orthostatic hypotension due to intermediolateral column degeneration: a report of two cases with autopsies. Q J Med 35:276, 1966
70. Sever PS: Plasma noradrenalin in autonomic failure. p. 155. In Bannister R (ed): Autonomic Failure. Oxford University Press, Oxford, 1983

71. Liard J-F: Cardiovascular effects of vasopressin: some recent aspects. J Cardiovasc Pharmacol 8, suppl 7: S61, 1986

72. Liard JF: Vasopressin in cardiovascular control: role of circulating vasopressin. Clin Sci 67:473, 1984

73. Puritz R, Lightman SL, Wilcox CS, et al: Blood pressure and vasopressin in progressive autonomic failure. Brain 106:503, 1983

74. Williams TDM, Lightman SL, Bannister R: Vasopressin secretion in progressive autonomic failure: evidence for defective afferent cardiovascular pathways. J Neurol Neurosurg Psychiatry 48:225, 1985

75. Johnson RH, McLellan DL, Love DR: Orthostatic hypotension and the Holmes-Adie syndrome: a study of two patients with afferent baroreceptor block. J Neurol Neurosurg Psychiatry 34:562, 1971

76. Streeten DHP, Kerr LP, Kerr CB, et al: Hyperbradykininism: a new orthostatic syndrome. Lancet 2:1048, 1972

77. Goldberg MR, Onrot J, Hollister AS, et al: Selective congenital defect in norepinephrine release as a cause of orthostatic hypotension. Clin Res 32:332A, 1984

78. Biaggioni I, Goldstein DS, Atkinson T, Robertson D: Dopamine-β-hydroxylase deficiency in humans. Neurology 40:370, 1990

79. Bergenwald L, Freyschuss U, Sjostrand T: The mechanism of orthostatic and haemorrhagic fainting. Scand J Clin Lab Invest 37:209, 1977

80. Wallin BG: New aspects of sympathetic function in man. p. 145. In Stalberg E, Young RR (eds): Clinical Neurophysiology. Butterworths, London, 1981

81. Lipsitz LA: Syncope in the elderly. Ann Intern Med 99:92, 1983

82. Low PA: Laboratory evaluation of autonomic failure. p. 169. In Low PA (ed): Clinical Autonomic Disorders. Little, Brown, Boston, 1993

83. Mann S, Altman DG, Raftery EB, Bannister R: Circadian variation of blood pressure in autonomic failure. Circulation 68:477, 1983

84. Ewing DJ, Campbell IW, Clarke BF: Assessment of cardiovascular effects in diabetic autonomic neuropathy and prognostic implications. Ann Intern Med 92(part 2):308, 1980

85. Vita G, Princi P, Calabro R, Toscano A, et al: Cardiovascular reflex tests: assessment of age-adjusted normal range. J Neurol Sci 75:263, 1986

86. Schondorf R, Low PA: Idiopathic postural tachycardia syndromes. p. 641. In Low PA (ed): Clinical Autonomic Disorders. Little, Brown, Boston, 1993

87. Ewing DJ, Campbell IW, Burt AA, Clarke BF: Vascular reflexes in diabetic autonomic neuropathy. Lancet 2:1354, 1973

88. Watkins PJ, MacKay JD: Cardiac denervation in diabetic neuropathy. Ann Intern Med 92(part 2):304, 1980

89. Smith SA: Reduced sinus arrhythmia in diabetic autonomic neuropathy: diagnostic value of an age-related normal range. Br Med J 285:1599, 1982

90. Kaijser L, Sachs C: Autonomic cardiovascular responses in old age. Clin Physiol 5:347, 1985

91. Aminoff MJ: Involvement of peripheral vasomotor fibres in carpal tunnel syndrome. J Neurol Neurosurg Psychiatry 42:649, 1979

92. Gemmill JD, Venables GS, Ewing DJ: Noradrenaline response to edrophonium in primary autonomic failure: distinction between central and peripheral damage. Lancet 1:1018, 1988

93. Low PA, Caskey PE, Tuck RR, et al: Quantitative sudomotor axon reflex test in normal and neuropathic subjects. Ann Neurol 14:573, 1983

94. Tsementzis SA, Hitchcock ER: The spoon test: a simple bedside test for assessing sudomotor autonomic failure. J Neurol Neurosurg Psychiatry 48:378, 1985

95. Shahani BT, Halperin JJ, Boulu P, Cohen J: Sympathetic skin response—a method of assessing unmyelinated axon dysfunction in peripheral neuropathies. J Neurol Neurosurg Psychiatry 47:536, 1984

96. Davies B, Sudera D, Sagnella G, et al: Increased numbers of alpha receptors in sympathetic denervation supersensitivity in man. J Clin Invest 69:779, 1982

97. Bannister R, Boylston AW, Davies IB, et al: Beta receptor numbers and thermodynamics in denervation supersensitivity. J Physiol (Lond) 319:369, 1981

98. Wilcox CS, Aminoff MJ, Slater JDH: Sodium homeostasis in patients with autonomic failure. Clin Sci Mol Med 53:321, 1977

99. Wilcox CS, Aminoff MJ, Penn W: Basis of nocturnal polyuria in patients with autonomic failure. J Neurol Neurosurg Psychiatry 37:677, 1974

100. Onrot J, Goldberg MR, Hollister AS, et al: Management of chronic orthostatic hypotension. Am J Med 80:454, 1986

101. Chobanian AV, Volicer L, Tifft CP, et al: Mineralocorticoid-induced hypertension in patients with orthostatic hypotension. N Engl J Med 301:68, 1979

102. Davies IB, Bannister R, Hensby C, Sever PS: The pressor actions of noradrenaline and angiotensin II in chronic autonomic failure treated with indomethacin. Br J Clin Pharmacol 10:223, 1980

103. Kochar MS, Itskovitz HD: Treatment of idiopathic orthostatic hypotension (Shy-Drager syndrome) with indomethacin. Lancet 1:1011, 1978

104. Biaggioni I, Zygmunt D, Haile V, Robertson D: Pressor effect of inhaled ergotamine in orthostatic hypotension. Am J Cardiol 65:89, 1990

105. Brevetti G, Chiariello M, Giudice P, et al: Effective

treatment of orthostatic hypotension by propranolol in the Shy-Drager syndrome. Am Heart J 102:938, 1981

106. Brevetti G, Chiariello M, Lavecchia G, Rengo F: Effects of propranolol in a case of orthostatic hypotension. Br Heart J 41:245, 1979

107. Davies B, Bannister R, Mathias C, Sever P: Pindolol in postural hypotension: the case for caution. Lancet 2:982, 1981

108. Moss AJ, Glaser W, Topol E: Atrial tachypacing in the treatment of a patient with primary orthostatic hypotension. N Engl J Med 302:1456, 1980

109. Kristinsson A: Programmed atrial pacing for orthostatic hypotension. Acta Med Scand 214:79, 1983

110. Goldberg MR, Robertson RM, Robertson D: Atrial tachypacing for primary orthostatic hypotension. N Engl J Med 303:885, 1980

111. Wagner HN, Braunwald E: The pressor effect of the antidiuretic principle of the posterior pituitary in orthostatic hypotension. J Clin Invest 35:1412, 1956

112. Kochar MS: Hemodynamic effects of lysine-vasopressin in orthostatic hypotension. Am J Kidney Dis 6:49, 1985

113. Mathias CJ, Fosbraey P, Da Costa DF, et al: The effect of desmopressin on nocturnal polyuria, overnight weight loss, and morning postural hypotension in patients with autonomic failure. Br Med J 293:353, 1986

114. Goldberg MR, Hollister AS, Robertson D: Influence of yohimbine on blood pressure, autonomic reflexes, and plasma catecholamines in humans. Hypertension 5:772, 1983

115. Onrot J, Goldberg MR, Biaggioni I, et al: Oral yohimbine in human autonomic failure. Neurology 37:215, 1987

116. Jankovic J, Gilden JL, Hiner BC, et al: Neurogenic orthostatic hypotension: a double-blind, placebo-controlled study with midodrine. Am J Med 95:38, 1993

117. Kuchel O, Buu NT, Gutkowska J, Genest J: Treatment of severe orthostatic hypotension by metoclopramide. Ann Intern Med 93:841, 1980

118. Robertson D, Goldberg MR, Hollister AS, et al: Clonidine raises blood pressure in severe idiopathic orthostatic hypotension. Am J Med 74:193, 1983

119. Polinsky RJ, Samaras GM, Kopin IJ: Sympathetic neural prosthesis for managing orthostatic hypotension. Lancet 1:901, 1983

120. Hoeldtke RD, Streeten DH: Treatment of orthostatic hypotension with erythropoietin. N Engl J Med 329:611, 1993

9

Neurological Complications of Cardiac Arrest

W. T. Longstreth, Jr.

Not long ago, cardiac arrest was an irreversible event that meant certain death. Respiratory arrest without cardiac arrest was not necessarily lethal, and descriptions of resuscitation from respiratory arrest using artificial ventilation may date back to biblical times.[1] But mouth-to-mouth resuscitation or other types of artificial ventilation alone are not going to save a victim of cardiac arrest. The understanding of the causes and treatment of cardiac arrest is intertwined with the study of electricity.[2] A fascinating review of the topic is contained in Jex-Blake's Goulstonian lectures presented in 1913.[3] By the middle of the eighteenth century, investigators had succeeded in producing electric shocks strong enough to kill animals. Jex-Blake described a study by Abildgaard reported in 1775 in which he was able to kill chickens with an electrical current. Abildgaard observed that the apparently dead fowl could be brought back to life again by sending a second electrical shock from breast to back. Without such treatment, the bird died.

Such observations became more pertinent by the late nineteenth and early twentieth centuries, when electricity came into widespread use in Europe and America, and when an increasing number of people were dying as a consequence of accidental electrocution. By the middle of the nineteenth century, investigators knew that electric currents caused the ventricles of experimental animals to be thrown into a state

of "Herzdelirium" or fibrillation. A series of experiments by Prevost and Battelli in dogs in 1899 established that electrical current could not only induce ventricular fibrillation but reverse it,[4] leading to Jex-Blake's conclusions[3] in 1913:

> It has been seen that in most cases death by electric shock is due to cardiac failure, the heart being thrown into fibrillary contraction. Prevost and Battelli, and others after them, have shown that the fibrillating hearts of the lower animals can be made to beat regularly and rhythmically once more by passing strong electric currents through them within a given time—a few minutes; so that the apparently dead animal is brought to life again. It is more than probable that the same treatment—a hair of the dog that bit them—could be applied with success to human beings apparently killed by electric currents, but there are two practical difficulties here. In the first place there is no experimental evidence, in the case of man, to show what voltage and what strength of current should best be employed in this method of resuscitation. In the second place, there would usually be great difficulty in providing the current at the required voltage for use on the spot and within a few minutes. Still this method is well worth further investigation and trial.

That this same mechanism might underlie other causes of sudden death was proposed in 1889 by Mac-Williams[5]:

> . . . unexpected and irretrievable cardiac failure may . . . present itself in the form of an abrupt onset of fibril-

159

lar contraction (ventricular delirium). The cardiac pump is thrown out of gear, and the last of its vital energy is dissipated in a violent and prolonged turmoil of fruitless activity in the ventricular walls.

Unfortunately, the progress made toward treatment of cardiac arrest with defibrillation was interrupted by World War I, and interest was not rekindled until the 1920s in the United States.[2] Concerned about accidental death among linemen, Consolidated Edison Company of New York City appealed to the Rockefeller Institute for help. Several investigations were initiated including in 1928 work at Johns Hopkins University by Kouwenhoven, an electrical engineer, and Langworthy, a neurologist.[6] They confirmed earlier works indicating that lower-voltage shocks induced ventricular fibrillation and higher-voltage shocks caused respiratory arrest. However, they were unable to reverse the ventricular fibrillation with various treatments. In 1930, a colleague pointed out to them the 1899 works by Provost and Battelli, which they subsequently confirmed. The treatment with electric countershock worked: "a hair of the dog that bit them." Later the Johns Hopkins investigators returned to Edison Electric Institute to have them create a portable defibrillator.

One of the defibrillators subsequently developed had paddles that had to be pushed against the chest before the current could be discharged. Investigators noted that forceful application of the paddles to the chest wall of dogs led to a rise in blood pressure while the heart was still fibrillating. This was the serendipitous observation that was to lead to closed chest compressions. The technique of mouth-to-mouth resuscitation had been perfected by Safar and colleagues.[7] Now the stage was set to treat effectively a common cause of sudden cardiac death—ventricular fibrillation. Closed chest compression and mouth-to-mouth respiration (basic life support) would keep the patient viable long enough for the portable defibrillator to be brought to the patient and applied (advanced life support). All these efforts were again interrupted, this time by World War II, and it was not until 1956 that Zoll and colleagues reported the first successful external defibrillation in humans.[8] In 1960, Kouwenhoven and co-workers reported a series of successful resuscitations with closed chest cardiac massage and external defibrillation.[9]

The decade of the 1960s found the technique of cardiopulmonary resuscitation being applied on a wide scale to patients suffering cardiac arrest inside the hospital. Several epidemiological aspects of sudden cardiac death[10,11] led in the 1970s to the application of these same techniques outside the hospital. The importance of heart disease as a cause of death was increasingly recognized. Sudden cardiac death was the presenting feature in up to one-third of people with heart disease. Finally, many people dying with heart disease, especially in the setting of myocardial infarction, were doing so outside the hospital.

One of the first prehospital emergency medical systems was developed in Belfast, Ireland.[12–14] In their 1967 report, Pantridge and Geddes describe the out-of-hospital resuscitation of a 55-year-old man who had collapsed while dancing. A bystander performed chest compressions, and personnel from the mobile unit applied cardioversion to restore spontaneous circulation.[13] Unfortunately, the patient died a week later with brain damage. This appears to be the first description of an out-of-hospital cardiac arrest occurring before the arrival of the mobile unit in which spontaneous circulation was restored. A similar emergency medical system began in Seattle, Washington, in 1970[15,16] and elsewhere in the United States. Systems rapidly proliferated, so that by the end of the decade, most cities in the United States with populations over 250,000 people had such systems. The decade of the 1980s has seen a realization that cardiopulmonary resuscitation on patients in the hospital often fails, frequently because of comorbidity. More selective application of cardiopulmonary resuscitation has become the rule rather than exception in recent years as patients, families, and physicians try to decide who is likely to benefit from this technique. Much effort has been directed to increasing the yield of successful resuscitations from out-of-hospital cardiac arrests. These efforts have been rewarded, with some systems reporting up to 30 percent of patients with out-of-hospital ventricular fibrillation surviving to be discharged from the hospital.[17] But over these decades, the realization has grown that the outcome among those in whom spontaneous circulation can be restored is often dominated by the degree of brain damage suffered during the arrest.[18,19] It is estimated that between 300,000 and 400,000 people each year in the United States experience sudden cardiac death.[20,21] With the proliferation of teams of medical personnel trained to resuscitate people from cardiac arrests both in and out of the hospital, the number of patients facing the risks of neurological sequelae can be expected to increase. Already in many regions of the country, cardiac arrest has become a leading cause of coma, along with head trauma and drug overdose.

The goal of this chapter is to discuss the neurological sequelae of cardiac arrest and address such issues as prediction of outcomes (prognostication) and alteration of outcomes (treatment). The focus is on adults, and extreme caution should be used in extrapolating to children.

OUTCOMES OF CARDIAC ARREST

To understand the outcomes of cardiac arrest, the insult must be understood. Interruption of cardiac function, as with a cardiac arrest, by definition causes insufficient blood flow to the brain leading to global brain ischemia and global brain dysfunction. The dysfunction can be transient or permanent, depending in large part upon the duration and severity of the ischemia. At the extreme, the ischemia may be complete, as in cardiac arrest where the initial electrocardiogram reveals ventricular fibrillation or asystole. With other pulseless electrocardiographic activity, such as pulseless ventricular tachycardia or electromechanical dissociation, the ischemia may be incomplete or unknown. During the resuscitation of individuals with cardiac arrest, the inability of medical personnel to detect a pulse or blood pressure does not preclude the possibility of severe hypotension, which could be detected if more sensitive means of measuring blood pressure were available. In most cardiac arrests, both incomplete and complete global brain ischemia contribute to the brain dysfunction and possible injury. For example, a patient with myocardial ischemia may have hypotension (incomplete global ischemia) preceding deterioration to ventricular fibrillation (complete global ischemia). During cardiopulmonary resuscitation and basic life support, severe hypotension can exist (incomplete brain ischemia). Finally, with restoration of spontaneous circulation, hypotension and cardiogenic shock (incomplete global ischemia) can complicate the hospital course. The duration and severity of these components of global brain ischemia probably determine the degree of brain damage and

outcome. Unfortunately, duration and severity are usually unknown.

Cardiac arrest most commonly results from a primary problem with the heart. Although the list of potential cardiac problems is long, coronary artery disease and myocardial ischemia are the most likely culprits.[22,23] Cardiac arrest can also occur secondary to other toxic and metabolic problems. With the possible exception of hypothermia and overdoses of sedative drugs, these other problems can augment the insult to the brain. This seems to be particularly true in the situation in which a respiratory arrest precedes a cardiac arrest. The respiratory arrest may occur in many settings and is often not a simple event in itself, as with drownings, decompensation of chronic lung disease, drug overdoses, hanging, strangulation, trauma, asphyxia, and carbon monoxide poisoning. In the absence of a cytotoxic agent such as carbon monoxide, the hypoxia of respiratory insufficiency can be surprisingly well tolerated by the brain.[24] However, if a cardiac arrest ensues, the consequences to the brain can be devastating.[25]

Primary neurological problems, such as focal brain ischemia, hemorrhage, or trauma, can lead to a cardiac arrest, which most commonly results from an initial respiratory arrest. Rarely will the first rhythm be ventricular fibrillation. Some neurological events can result in cardiac arrest without intervening respiratory arrest. Brain-heart interactions have been well described.[26,27] Their importance is supported by experiments in pigs.[28] When pigs were placed under psychological stress, occlusion of the left anterior descending coronary artery resulted in ventricular fibrillation. Functional blockage with cryoprobes of pathways from the frontal cortex through the posterior hypothalamus to the brainstem prevented or delayed the development of ventricular fibrillation. Such pathways may play a role in the sudden death experienced by some patients with epilepsy in whom a fatal arrhythmia is the presumed terminal event.[29–31] Evidence for a convulsion as the precipitant may be lacking in such patients.

Thomas mused on the possibility that mechanisms have evolved to assure sudden death when the end of an animal's life is near.[32] If such mechanisms exist and are triggered inappropriately, premature sudden death could result. Psychological factors may be important in triggering these responses. Richter presented an experimental model in rats of the influence of psychological factors on sudden death and proposed that deaths in humans due to hexing could represent the same phenomena. All such theories assume a strong interaction among neurological, psychological, and cardiac factors.[33]

Consequences of Global Brain Ischemia

The consequences of global brain ischemia have intrigued investigators for over a century. In 1836, Cooper, an English physician, carried out experiments on rabbits.[34] After surgically occluding both common carotid arteries, he noted that pinching of the vertebral arteries led to sudden unconsciousness. If the blood flow to the brain was not interrupted for too long, the rabbit would regain consciousness rapidly upon release of the vertebral arteries. These seminal observations were extended by Brown-Séquard, who was one of the first to introduce the concept of a rostral-caudal deterioration of brain function with global ischemia.[35] Simply put, cerebral cortical function was lost before brainstem function. The clinical stimulus for these early investigations is uncertain, given that the only examples of global brain ischemia recognized in humans at the time were conditions like beheading and hanging.

Confirmation that cerebral cortical function was lost before brainstem function with global ischemia came from additional studies in the 1940s. These studies entailed rapid inflation of a cuff about the neck of human volunteers, with interruption of blood flow to the brain. Subjects were rendered rapidly unconscious. Interestingly, the studies conducted in the United States were performed on prisoners and psychiatric patients,[36] whereas those conducted in Germany were on the investigators themselves.[37] Gastaut and Fischer-Williams reported in 1957 their study of 100 patients with syncope.[38] While recording the electroencephalogram these investigators, attempted to induce transient cardiac arrest with vagal stimulation induced by ocular compression. "When cardiac arrest lasted more than about 14 sec., one or two generalized clonic jerks appeared without affecting the E.E.G., followed by generalized tonic contraction resembling decerebrate rigidity and accompanied by complete 'flattening' of the E.E.G." More recent examples include observations made during induction of ventricular arrhythmias to test automatic implant-

able defibrillators.[39] Although the electrocerebral accompaniments of global ischemia may be more complex than suggested in the earlier studies, all studies agree that motor activity early in the course of global brain ischemia is common and not related to cerebral cortical hyperactivity. Careful video observations have also been made in patients rendered unconscious following hyperventilation, orthostasis, and the Valsalva maneuver to induce global brain ischemia.[40,41] In addition to the motor activity, various eye movement abnormalities, including downbeat nystagmus, were documented. The cerebellum, in addition to the cerebral cortex, was held to be sensitive to brief global ischemia.

Given the observations that the cerebral cortex is more sensitive than the brainstem to global ischemia, the major clinical outcomes can be anticipated.[42,43] Based on experiments of global ischemia in primates, Nemoto and colleagues proposed S-shaped curves relating the duration of ischemia with the degree of brain damage and thus with neurological deficits.[44] Hypothesizing that similarly shaped curves exist for the human brain and that for any duration of ischemia—except at extremes—damage to the cerebral cortex is greater than damage to the brainstem, Figure 9-1 can be constructed. The outcomes predicted are similar to those defined in the Glasgow Outcome Scale[45] and its modification by the Pittsburgh investigators.[46] At extreme durations of cardiac arrest, both the cerebrum and brainstem will be totally destroyed and brain death will result.[47] Such an outcome after a primary cardiac arrest, as with ventricular fibrillation or asystole, is uncommon and probably reflects the inability to resuscitate individuals whose arrest has such a long duration. In a study of 459 consecutive patients admitted to one hospital after out-of-hospital cardiac arrest and resuscitation, only about 1 percent had an outcome consistent with brain death.[19] With shorter durations of arrest, the cerebral cortex may still be entirely destroyed, but without as complete a devastation of the brainstem. Such individuals will not be brain dead in that they retain some brainstem function, but they may have evidence for forebrain failure, such as electrocerebral inactivity on the electroencephalogram.[48] Various terms have been applied to this type of brain damage, including *cortex death, neocortical death, partial brain death, death of the forebrain,* and *acute failure of forebrain with sparing of brainstem function.* Although this condi-

Outcomes

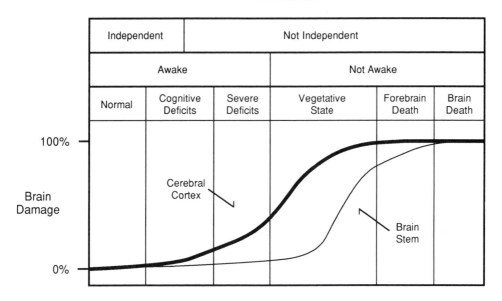

Independent	Not Independent				
Awake			Not Awake		
Normal	Cognitive Deficits	Severe Deficits	Vegetative State	Forebrain Death	Brain Death

Fig. 9-1. Hypothetical relation between duration of ischemia and brain damage, assuming that the cerebral cortex is more vulnerable to global ischemia than the brainstem.[42-44]

tion is well described after cardiac arrest, it also is unusual.

More commonly, the cerebral cortex is severely damaged but not completely destroyed. The damage is extensive enough to preclude the patient's ever regaining consciousness even though evidence of cerebral cortical activity may exist on the electroencephalogram. Evaluation of brainstem function may reveal some deficits or may be normal. Such patients are said to be in a vegetative state.[49,50] In one survey of four nursing homes in Milwaukee, Wisconsin, about 3 percent of patients were in a vegetative state.[51] In about 20 percent, the vegetative state resulted from a respiratory or cardiac arrest. The point at which a persistent vegetative state can be considered permanent has been a topic of much recent debate, with arbitrary time limits having been set anywhere from 1 month to 1 year.[52-56] Some aspects of conscious behavior may be difficult to judge, but at a minimum, vegetative patients should not follow commands or have comprehensible speech.

With a shorter duration of ischemia, the damage to the cerebral cortex is less and recovery of consciousness or awakening can occur, as evidenced by

the patient following commands or having comprehensible speech. Typically brainstem function is normal. These patients can be severely disabled because of their neurological impairments.[19] These can include spastic quadriparesis, cortical blindness, severe ataxia, bowel and bladder incontinence, and severe memory deficits. Independence in activities of daily living is not possible. In the series of 459 consecutive patients with out-of-hospital cardiac arrest, 18 (4 percent) had such an outcome, including cortical blindness in 4.[19] With still shorter duration of ischemia, less cerebral cortex is damaged and impairments relate to those parts of the brain most sensitive to ischemia, especially the hippocampus. Besides the memory impairments, the neurological findings may be unremarkable.[57-59] The memory problems can range from severe dementia to mild forgetfulness, and some of these patients may be independent in many of their activities of daily living. Positron emission tomography in such patients has suggested metabolic abnormalities in the medial temporal lobes.[60]

Finally, if the duration is brief and the resuscitation swift and effective, the brain may escape serious injury. Upon awakening, such patients almost always

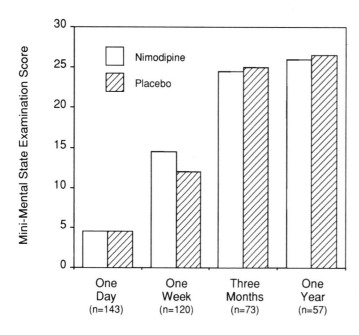

Fig. 9-2. Scores on the Mini-Mental State examination[63] at certain times after out-of-hospital cardiac arrest in patients enrolled in a randomized trial of nimodipine versus placebo. Little change occurs after 3 months. (Data from Roine and colleagues.[62])

have severe memory impairments, which clear over days. Such patients who have a complete cardiac arrest remain amnestic for the event and do not report near-death experiences.[61] Depending on the cardiac status, such patients may be able to return to their previous level of neurological function and are typically independent in their activities of daily living. Neuropsychological testing was performed on 68 long-term survivors of cardiac arrest as part of a clinical trial and showed no or mild deficits in approximately one-half at 1 year.[62] The most common deficit was in delayed memory. Changes in the Mini-Mental State examination[63] at various time after the cardiac arrest are shown in Figure 9-2. Recovery of cognitive function occurs mostly in the first 3 months after the arrest, with results at 1 year being comparable to those at 3 months after the arrest. Quality of life and the level of function have also been assessed and for many are comparable to those of similar patients who have suffered a myocardial infarction without a cardiac arrest.[64,65]

After cardiac arrest, any particular patient may pass through all of the stages described above and illustrated in Figure 9-1. At the initiation of the resuscitation, these patients may lack all evidence of brain function and, with time, move toward complete re-

covery. As with other forms of ischemic brain injury, most of the recovery occurs in the first 3 to 6 months—for example, as shown in Figure 9-2 for the Mini-Mental State Examination score. In the study from Seattle of 459 patients, 61 percent awakened after out-of-hospital cardiac arrest and about two-thirds of those awakening were left without gross neurological deficits.[19] Unfortunately, recovery can become stalled at any stage short of complete recovery, but it most commonly becomes fixed at a vegetative state.

Assessment of outcomes after cardiac arrest has most commonly involved the Glasgow Outcome Scale[45] and its modification by the Pittsburgh investigators.[46] Certain dichotomous outcomes, as in Figure 9-1, are important but vary in the ease with which they can be determined and timed. Death is clear-cut. Awakening is defined by the ability to produce comprehensible speech, follow commands, or both. The reliability of its components have been studied in detail as part of the Glasgow Coma Scale.[66] In addition, the timing of its occurrence can be determined easily, like that of death. Many legal and judicial guidelines concerning limitation of medical support address the probability of awakening. Regaining independence is of great importance to the patient and physician but lacks a uniform definition. It takes longer to achieve, it is more susceptible to the effects of comorbidity than awakening, and the timing of its occurrence can be problematic.

The pathology of global brain ischemia has been well described.[24] It confirms what is seen clinically—namely, that some cell types and some regions of the brain are more vulnerable than others. Selective neuronal necrosis occurs because neurons are more vulnerable than oligodendroglia and astrocytes, which, in turn, are more vulnerable than microglia and blood vessels. Rather than destroying all these cell types, as an infarct may do, damage after cardiac arrest may be limited to the neurons. Ischemic neurons are seen most prominently in certain layers of the cerebral cortex, parts of the hippocampus, and the Purkinje cells of the cerebellar cortex. In the neocortex, layer 3 is the most sensitive, followed by layers 5 and 6. Layers 2 and 4 are the most resistant. In the allocortex, the parts of the hippocampus most sensitive are the Sommer sector (CA_1) and the end folium (CA_3 to CA_4). The region between these two areas (CA_2) is the most resistant.[67] Evidence of selective neuronal necrosis may take hours to evolve, suggesting that processes during recirculation may be contributing to the injury.[68]

The explanation for selective vulnerability remains uncertain, but it may be a manifestation of toxicity mediated through excitatory neurotransmitters or impaired repair, as described later in this chapter (p. 174). In adults, the basal ganglia and brainstem are typically more resistant than these other brain structures, although exceptions have been described.[69,70] The gross appearance of the brain of a person autopsied following a brief comatose survival after cardiopulmonary resuscitation can look surprisingly unremarkable. Microscopic examination reveals ischemic changes as described above, but quantification of these changes is not readily available. The number of neurons that need to survive to result in the clinical outcomes described above and in Figure 9–1, except at the extremes of all or none, is unknown.

Complications

Complications estimated to occur in approximately 30 percent or more of patients following their cardiac arrest and resuscitation are seizures and myoclonus.[71–73] These tend to occur in the immediate postre-suscitation period, and long-term epilepsy is rare. Myoclonus is common and can be diffuse and multifocal.[74,75] Alternatively, the patient may have little clinical manifestation of seizure activity besides possibly eye movements, yet the electroencephalogram can show evidence of ongoing electrical seizure activity.[76,77] As discussed below, recurrent seizures and myoclonus can be especially resistant to treatment and carry a grave prognosis.

Brain swelling is common, as evidenced by results of imaging and lumbar puncture, but it rarely leads to herniation and deterioration. Exceptions are those patients in whom a respiratory arrest precedes the cardiac arrest. These patients will sometimes develop severe brain swelling, herniation, and brain death. In such circumstances, the swelling probably reflects a severely damaged brain, and treatments aimed at controlling increased pressures do not seem to affect outcomes. After cardiac arrest, patients are also at risk for numerous cardiac and general medical complications, which are beyond this discussion. All these, especially recurrent cardiac arrest and hypotension, tend to worsen the initial injury and thus the outcome.

A number of other rare complications can occur in the setting of a mixture of brain insults, sometimes including cardiac arrest. The greater the proportion of incomplete compared with complete global ischemia, the greater the risk of preferential damage to watershed regions of the brain and spinal cord. In the brain, this can result in injury between the anterior and middle cerebral artery distributions and a clinical picture of a brachial diplegia. With the upper extremities being more involved than the lower extremities, this clinical picture has been referred to as the "man-in-the-barrel" syndrome.[78] A similar watershed phenomenon in the spinal cord has been proposed to explain the paraplegia that can complicate cardiac arrest.[79,80] Emboli to the brain or spinal cord may also occur. Most commonly the emboli arise from the heart, but they may also come from bone marrow secondary to the trauma of chest compressions.[81] Interestingly, patients with focal ischemia of the cerebral cortex may have symmetrical neurological examinations upon presentation after cardiac arrest. Their examination reflects a level of function below their focal insult. If they regain function, focal abnormalities may become evident. Given such a masking capability of global brain ischemia, and given the risk that many of these patients have for sources of cardiac emboli, cerebral embolism may be missed in this setting.

Two well-described but rare complications seem to be more a function of respiratory failure mixed with cardiovascular insufficiency than simply of cardiac arrest: delayed postanoxic encephalopathy[82–84] and posthypoxic action myoclonus.[85,86] Many of the cases of delayed encephalopathy have occurred in the setting of carbon monoxide exposure. A period of improvement and return to seemingly normal function is followed by marked deterioration. Diffuse demyelination is the apparent cause of the deterioration in those who have died. Those with posthypoxic action myoclonus awaken soon after their respiratory arrest, often with normal cognitive functioning but with a severe action myoclonus. Attempts at movement are interrupted by severe myoclonic jerks. These can also be triggered by loud noises and other sensory stimuli. The pathological substrate for the condition is unknown. Treatment with valproic acid or benzodiazepines is sometimes successful. Other movement disorders, including akinetic-rigid and dystonic syndromes, have also been described, but not clearly following sole cardiac arrest with complete global brain ischemia.[87,88] Imaging and neuropathological examination reveals injury in the basal ganglia.

PREDICTING OUTCOMES OF CARDIAC ARREST

Key to making clinical decisions is information on prognosis. In those patients with a poor prognosis, the decisions may range from initiation of potentially dangerous treatments aimed at brain resuscitation to limitations in the intensity of medical support. The outcomes to be predicted include death, awakening, and independence. For the reasons discussed earlier, independence can be difficult to determine and time. Death is easily determined and timed but may relate to cardiac problems and need not reflect the degree of neurological recovery. Consequently, awakening is often used as a simple, easily determined and timed outcome for identifying important predictors. The accurate delineation of prognosis after cardiac arrest presents several challenges[89,90] and has been the topic of many reports.[18,19,91–102] Some of the major findings of these studies are summarized below.

The severity and duration of global brain ischemia are probably the most important predictors of outcome but are usually unknown or, at best, crudely estimated. The cardiac rhythm identified at the start of the resuscitation is a strong predictor of outcome. The probability of restoring a spontaneous rhythm is much higher when the initial rhythm is ventricular fibrillation rather than asystole or electromechanical dissociation.[103,104] A similar finding holds for survival and awakening. Because most patients whose initial rhythms are asystole or electromechanical dissociation cannot be resuscitated, many of the patients for whom prognostication is needed will have been resuscitated from ventricular fibrillation. Demographic factors such as age and gender are not important predictors of restoration of spontaneous circulation or survival to hospital discharge.[105,106] African Americans are more likely to have poor outcomes.[107,108] Comorbidity may be an important factor with respect to outcome and probably explains why resuscitation rates for out-of-hospital cardiac arrest in some regions of the country are better than those for in-hospital cardiac arrest.[102,109]

Physical Examination

The amount of brain dysfunction as indicated by the physical examination reflects the severity of the insult. In general, the greater the function at any particular time after the arrest, the better the eventual outcome. Nonetheless, complete loss of neurological function at the time that the resuscitation is initiated is still compatible with awakening and good recovery. The duration of arrest that is incompatible with recovery is uncertain and, as a practical matter, is often difficult to estimate. The human brain can probably not fully recover from more than 5 to 10 minutes of complete global brain ischemia, as with ventricular fibrillation or asystole.[110] Those patients with some degree of neurological function at the start of the resuscitation, such as reactive pupils or spontaneous respirations, have a better outcome than those without.[111] The physical examination performed once the patient has been stabilized with respect to cardiovascular status gives the clinician a first impression of prognosis. The less the amount of function and the longer the delay in return of function, the worse the prognosis.

As would be surmised from Figure 9-1, the finding

of persistent brainstem dysfunction suggests a poor prognosis, given that the cerebral cortex, being more sensitive, has suffered an even worse injury. Many clinical studies have supported this contention. For example, careful observations by Jørgensen and Malchow-Møller found that recovery of pupillary light reflex within 12 minutes was compatible with a good outcome, whereas its absence for more than 28 minutes predicted a poor outcome.[91,94] The pupillary light reflex has emerged as an important but not perfect prognostic factor in other studies as well. In a study from Seattle, 39 patients lacked pupillary reactivity on admission after out-of-hospital cardiac arrest and 4 (10 percent) awakened.[95] In a multicenter study by Levy and colleagues, none of the 52 patients without pupillary reactivity on an early examination regained independence, although 3 (6 percent) regained consciousness.[96] Unfortunately, as would be predicted from Figure 9-1, preservation of brainstem function does not assure a good outcome, in that the cerebral cortex may have been damaged to such a degree that awakening never occurs.

Motor function, as assessed in the Glasgow Coma Scale[66] shown in Table 9-1, is a powerful predictor in most studies. The Glasgow Coma Scale has been used by itself as a predictor of outcome[98,100,101] but is probably dominated by the motor findings. Most of these patients are intubated as part of their resuscitation, so that the verbal response cannot be assessed. Eye opening is an uncertain predictor, with some patients having spontaneous eye opening on admission and never regaining consciousness. Evaluation with the Glasgow Coma Scale in these patients should be augmented by further evaluation of brainstem function[46] to include pupillary response, corneal reflex, cough, gag, and eye movements elicited by vestibulo-ocular and cervico-ocular reflexes[112] (Table 9-1).

Agreement across clinical studies is remarkable given the diversity of populations studied and statistical methods applied. For instance, two studies examined prognostication after cardiac arrest. One study included 389 consecutive unconscious patients admitted to a single hospital in Seattle after out-of-hospital cardiac arrest with ventricular fibrillation or asystole.[95] The other was a multicenter study of 210 patients with a mixture of hypoxic-ischemic insults occurring both in and out of the hospital.[96] The studies used different multivariable techniques to identify independent early predictors of outcome, but both

Table 9-1 Aspects of the Neurological Examination Useful for Prognostication After Cardiac Arrest, Including the Glasgow Coma Scale and Other Brainstem Reflexes

Glasgow Coma Scale[a]	Other brainstem reflexes
Eye opening (E)	
4 = spontaneous	Pupillary light responses
3 = to speech	Corneal reflex
2 = to pain	Cough
1 = nil	Gag
Best motor response (M)	Spontaneous respirations
6 = obeys	
5 = localizes	**Eye movements**
4 = withdraws	Spontaneous
3 = abnormal flexion	Cervico-ocular reflex
2 = extensor response	Vestibulo-ocular reflex
1 = nil	
Verbal response (V)	
5 = oriented	
4 = confused conversation	
3 = inappropriate words	
2 = incomprehensible sounds	
1 = nil	

[a] Total score = (E + M + V), range 3 to 15
(Glasgow Coma Scale adapted from Teasdale G, Jennett B: Assessment of coma and impaired consciousness: a practical scale. Lancet 2:81, 1974, with permission.)

found that pupillary response, motor response, and eye movements were the most important predictors. The other independent predictor of outcome in the study from Seattle was the admission blood glucose (discussed below). Figure 9-3 shows a simplification of the multivariable rule from the Seattle study and its performance in predicting outcome based on information collected at the time of admission. By using this rule, the clinician can rapidly form an initial prognostic impression.

As first demonstrated by Jørgensen and Malchow-Møller[94] and subsequently confirmed by others, the longer the delay in the return of function, the worse the prognosis. For example, in the study reported by Levy and colleagues, none of the 70 patients without motor response or with posturing to painful stimuli at 3 days regained independence, although 5 (7 percent) awakened.[96] In the report by Mullie and colleagues,

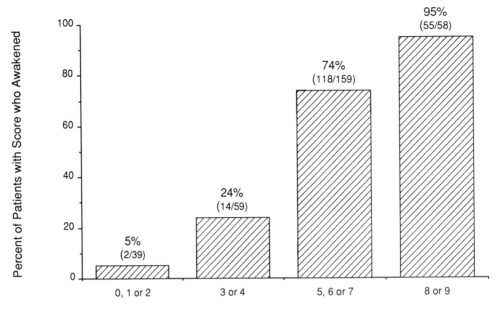

Awakening Score is sum of variables below and based on information collected on admission after out-of-hospital cardiac arrest

Motor response	0 = absent, 1 = extensor posturing, 2 = flexor posturing, 3 = nonposturing movements, 4 = withdrawal or localizing
Pupillary light response	0 = absent, 3 = present
Spontaneous eye movements	0 = absent, 1 = present
Admission blood glucose level	0 = ≥300 mg/dl, 1 = <300 mg/dl

Fig. 9-3. Performance of simple rule applied at admission to predict awakening after out-of-hospital cardiac arrest due to ventricular fibrillation or asystole. (Data from Longstreth and colleagues.[95])

a best score of 4 or less on the Glasgow Coma Scale in the first 48 hours was predictive of a poor outcome in 53 of 54 patients.[98] In the work by Edgren, a score on the Glasgow Coma Scale of 5 or less at 3 days was predictive of a poor outcome in all 45 patients.[97,99] Ultimately, the duration of unconsciousness itself becomes a predictor of the likelihood of consciousness ever returning. For example, in the study from Seattle, although overall 61 percent of the 459 patients awakened, the probability of ever awakening fell precipitously during the first 3 days after admission from out-of-hospital cardiac arrest.[19] Over 90 percent of those destined to ever awaken did so by 3 days. All those awakening after 4 days had some persistent neurological deficits, and all those awakening after 14 days had persistent severe neurological deficits.

Ancillary Tests

Although there are many potential problems with these studies,[89] a basic, unavoidable one is the reliability of the information upon which the prognosis is based.[113] Even in research settings where the question of agreement has been evaluated, it is not 100 percent. Consequently, a certain degree of random error or noise will always exist in predictive models based on the neurological examination. Laboratory tests typically have greater reliability or precision than findings on the physical examination, and several have been evaluated for their potential to predict outcome after cardiac arrest. To be clinically useful, such a test must improve upon the prediction already available from the physical examination.

Except for admission blood glucose level, routine

laboratory tests are not helpful in this regard. For example, admission values for arterial blood gas or for hematocrit are not related to outcome.[95] Admission blood glucose concentration after cardiac arrest has been shown to be associated with neurological outcome.[95,114,115] As predicted from animal experiments where a high blood glucose level preceding a cardiac arrest is associated with worse brain injury,[116] a high blood glucose level on admission after cardiac arrest was associated with a poor prognosis. In another clinical study attempting to explain this association, analyses were done of blood glucose levels determined during and immediately following out-of-hospital cardiopulmonary resuscitation.[117] The findings indicated that the blood glucose level rose during resuscitation. The rise was steepest in those in whom the efforts at resuscitation failed and was similar regardless of awakening status in those who were resuscitated and admitted to hospital. As expected, the duration of the resuscitation was longer in those destined never to regain consciousness. For them, the blood glucose level had a longer time to rise and consequently was higher on admission. The study suggested that the admission blood glucose level reflected the duration of resuscitation.

Because a small detrimental effect of glucose could not be excluded in these observational studies and because of data from experimental studies, a randomized trial in humans was performed.[118] During resuscitation of patients with out-of-hospital cardiopulmonary arrests, paramedical personnel randomized patients to receive either the standard fluid, 5 percent dextrose in water, or a glucose-free alternative (0.5 normal saline). Awakening was not related to the glucose content of the fluids that were given. Interestingly, the blood glucose levels on admission were close to those predicted by the model relating blood glucose level to duration of arrest: predicted value in those awakening was 254 mg/dl and in those not awakening, 309 mg/dl,[117] whereas observed values were 251 mg/dl and 309 mg/dl, respectively.[118] An unexpected and not easily explained finding in the clinical trial was that the relation between blood glucose level and awakening was reversed in those patients whose cardiac arrest was not due to ventricular fibrillation or asystole on a presumed cardiac basis. For these other patients, most of whom had electromechanical dissociation, a high blood glucose level on admission was associated with a favorable outcome.

Overall, these studies suggest that the admission blood glucose level after cardiac arrest depends on the duration of certain aspects of the arrest and resuscitation. Although it is an independent predictor of outcome, the blood glucose level is not a powerful as certain aspects of the physical examination, discussed earlier.[95]

Another test that is readily available in these patients is the electroencephalogram. It is useful in identifying epileptiform activity. Although a single tonic-clonic seizure may not adversely affect prognosis, recurrent seizures and myoclonic status do. The prognosis with myoclonic status epilepticus is especially poor, with none of 85 patients so affected awakening.[72–75] Such results have led some to equate myoclonic status epilepticus with an agonal phenomenon indicating severe cerebral cortical damage.[73] A classification scheme for patterns on the electroencephalogram is presented in Table 9–2.[71,94,119–121] Synek has suggested subdivisions based on amplitude, variability, reactivity, and presence of epileptiform discharges.[122] Various other modifications of the classification scheme have been proposed.[123] In addition, other specific patterns have been described, such as spindle coma, theta pattern coma, and alpha pattern coma. Electrocerebral inactivity, a burst-suppression pattern, and status epilepticus are all associated with a poor prognosis. On the other hand, alpha pattern coma is not necessarily associated with a poor prognosis.[124] Serial changes in the electroencephalogram during recovery have also been documented with return of cortical activity and movement down the stages of Table 9-2.[71,94] Part of the difficulty in assessing the prognostic utility of the electroencephalogram relates to its typically being performed early in the

Table 9-2 Classification Scheme for the Findings on Electroencephalograms Recorded After Cardiac Arrest, Based on a Number of Earlier Studies[71,94,119–121]

Grade	Findings[a]
1	Near normal with alpha dominant
2	Theta dominant
3	Delta dominant
4	Burst suppression pattern
5	Electrocerebral inactivity

[a] Scheme excludes specific patterns such as spindle coma, theta pattern coma, alpha pattern coma, and status epilepticus.

hospital course on patients who are having seizures or myoclonus or later in those who remain unconscious. The seizures and prolonged unconsciousness in themselves indicate a poor prognosis; whether the electroencephalogram provides additional prognostic information is uncertain. The role for compressed spectral analysis is also undefined.[125]

Evoked potential studies have been investigated as well. Both brainstem auditory evoked potentials and somatosensory evoked potentials can be used to confirm evidence of brainstem dysfunction and consequently a poor prognosis. Somatosensory evoked potentials are the more useful test,[126,127] with several studies showing that the absence of a short-latency cortical response is associated with a poor prognosis.[128–131] Unfortunately, the presence of such a response does not assure a good outcome. The predictive capability of the test may be improved by examination of the long-latency responses, which presumably reflect more complex cerebral cortical functions.[131] In 66 patients after cardiac arrest, good and poor outcomes were all accurately predicted using a cutoff of 118 ms for the N70 peak latency, a long-latency response.[131] These results are encouraging and need confirmation by other investigators.

Imaging of the head with computed tomography[132,133] and magnetic resonance imaging[134] may show loss of gray-white matter differentiation and evidence of swelling, but the prognostic utility of the tests is uncertain. Interestingly, evidence of swelling was more common among those who experienced respiratory failure prior to their cardiac arrest.[133] Later in the course, these studies may show atrophy in patients who remain unconscious. Functional imaging with positron emission tomography,[135,136] xenon-133 inhalation,[137] single photon emission computed tomography,[138] and magnetic resonance spectroscopy[139,140] have all been attempted, but only in a small number of patients, precluding any firm conclusions about their prognostic value.

Several cerebrospinal fluid (CSF) enzymes have been evaluated. Under normal circumstances, the activity of cytosolic enzymes in the CSF is low or undetectable. With tissue damage, these enzymes are released into the surrounding extracellular fluid and diffuse into the CSF, where they can be sampled. Several enzymes have been studied, including creatine kinase (CK), lactate dehydrogenase, adenylate kinase, and neuron-specific enolase.[141–146] Much of the work has concerned CK. The brain is rich in the BB fraction and also has mitochondrial CK.[147–149] Studies in humans[144] and animals[145] suggest that the enzymes peak in the spinal fluid 48 to 72 hours following global brain ischemia and that they correlate well with outcome: the higher the value, the greater the damage to the brain and the worse the outcome. In one series of 29 patients in whom lumbar punctures were performed 5 to 53 hours following cardiac arrest, the mean opening pressure was 183 mm of water, with a range of 110 to 260.[143] The mean total protein concentration was 40 mg/dl, and the mean glucose was 116 mg/dl. None of these variables was significantly related to awakening, unlike the CK activity in the CSF, which was significantly higher in those who never awakened (mean 120 U/L) than in those who did (mean 10 U/L).

Such enzyme tests seem to hold great promise as prognostic tools after cardiac arrest. Unlike some of the other prognostic tests, determination of CSF enzyme levels provides a quantitative rather than qualitative estimate of brain damage. In this regard, these tests could also be useful as outcome measures. Elevation of CSF enzymes is not specific to the type of injury, having been described with ischemic stroke,[150] head trauma,[151] and even placement of an intraventricular catheter.[152] Consequently caution must be exercised in interpreting results when a mixture of brain insults has occurred.

Application of Prognostic Information

These and other studies on prognostic tests raise several issues, some ethical, some legal, and some statistical.[52–56,89] Often when the prognosis for awakening is extremely poor, family members and physicians will agree that the best course of action is to limit medical support and allow the patient to die. A danger exists that the prognostic information creates a self-fulfilling prophecy. One option to avoid this possibility is to treat maximally all patients until they die of some other cause, an option unacceptable to most families and physicians. Nevertheless, support is maintained in some patients, particularly younger ones, and late awakenings have been documented. For example, in the series of 459 consecutive patients from one hospital in Seattle, the last three individuals to awaken after cardiac arrest did so at about 56, 75, and 100 days after their arrest.[19] Of note, all these patients were severely impaired and totally dependent in their activities of daily living. Similarly high morbidity has been described in other patients awakening late after cardiac arrest.[153–155] Another option in evaluating a new predictive test is to collect data without making it available to those making decisions about support; after outcomes have been determined, performance of the test can be evaluated without fear of its results having influenced decisions.[143] A final option is to require some independent "gold standard" to assess the degree of brain damage. A quantitative neuropathological examination would serve such a purpose but is currently not readily available in humans. If a treatment is being evaluated, it is essential that decisions concerning limitations of support are made in as standard a fashion as possible and without knowledge of treatment status so as to avoid biasing results.[43]

At present, a reasonable approach to prognostication after cardiac arrest involves serial neurological examinations to document baseline function and change. These examinations should include the Glasgow Coma Scale[66] and assessment of brainstem function (Table 9-1). Electroencephalograms should not be necessary except for those in whom seizure activity is suspected. If the patient is not awake by 48 to 72 hours following the arrest, additional testing may help to clarify the prognosis. The tests that seem the most useful are determination of CSF CK isoenzymes and recording of the short- and long-latency somatosensory evoked potentials. When the results of these tests are available, a meeting should be held with the patient's surrogate or family to review the results and to proffer a prognosis. If the physical examination suggests a poor prognosis—especially with persistence of posturing or no motor responses—and the results of the ancillary tests are consistent, an option of limiting medical support can be discussed. Typically, surrogates and family members insist upon limiting support. Most surrogates and family members, especially of elderly patients, strongly resist delaying decisions, especially for several months to a year, as has been suggested.[52–56,89]

These considerations raise several statistical issues as well about the confidence of predictions of outcome. The discussion by Shewmon and DeGiorgio are particularly enlightening.[89] We strive for a prognostic model with both a specificity for predicting a poor outcome and a positive predictive value of 100 percent. This goal is often claimed to have been achieved when a certain number (N) of patients have a particularly test result, and all ($N/N = 100$ percent) have a poor outcome, or alternatively none ($0/N = 0$ percent) have a good outcome. A simple rule of three ($3/N$) allows a reader to estimate the upper 95 percent confidence interval rapidly.[156] For example in one study, none of 49 patients with particular result on somatosensory evoked potentials after cardiac arrest had a good outcome.[175] We can estimate the upper 95 percent confidence interval as $3/49 = 0.06$. The lower confidence interval will be zero. We may conclude that the results are consistent with up to 6 percent of the patients with this result achieving a good outcome. If we want a prognostic model to exclude even remote possibilities of errors, huge numbers of patients followed for prolonged periods are required. Using Bayesian methodology, Shewmon demonstrated that, given N patients with a particular test result, none of whom awakened, the risk of the very next patient awakening is approximately $1/(N + 2)$.[157] Also, the risk of at least one person breaking the rule in the next $N + 1$ patients studied is around 50 percent. All of this information suggests that the search for some infallible rule is quixotic, and exceptions will probably be found if enough patients are studied.

In discussions with family members concerning issues of withdrawal of support, the inherent uncertainty should not be masked. The necessary existence of uncertainty does not preclude decisions to limit support assuming that the patient, through previously expressed opinions, or the patient's surrogate, rate a vegetative existence as worse than death. These concepts can be illustrated with decision analysis,[158–160] as in Figure 9-4, which shows a decision tree for whether to maintain or limit medical support in a patient unconscious after cardiac arrest. The tree lays out the major outcomes, their probabilities, and their values or utilities, together with definitions for the terms. Assuming awakening is assigned a utility of $100 = U_A$ and death a utility of $0 = U_D$, the utility assigned to vegetative state (U_V) becomes critical to decision making. The best decision is the one with the greatest overall utility. As shown by the calculations in the legend for Figure 9-4, the utility of full support minus the utility of limited support can be represented by:

$$100(\text{fsp}_A\text{-lsp}_A) + U_V(\text{fsp}_V\text{-lsp}_V).$$

If support is limited, death is the most likely outcome,[19] and the probabilities of awakening (lsp_A) or

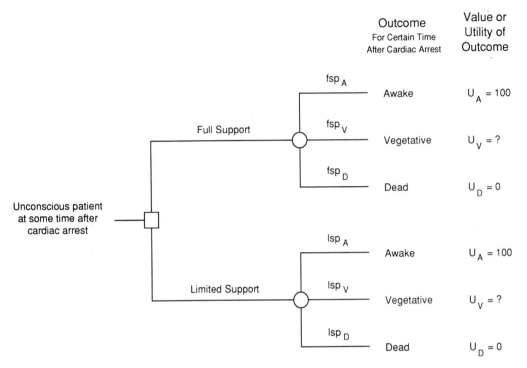

Fig. 9-4. Decision analysis on whether to maintain full support or to limit it in a patient still unconscious at some time after cardiac arrest. Abbreviations used in the figure are indicated in boldface. Probability *(p)* of awakening (A) given full support (fs), **fsp$_A$**; vegetative state (V) given full support (fs), **fsp$_V$**; death (D) given full support (fs), **fsp$_D$**; awakening (A) given limited support (ls), **lsp$_A$**; vegetative state (V) given limited support (ls), **lsp$_V$**; death (D) given limited support (ls), **lsp$_D$**. Value or utility (U) of awakening (A), **U$_A$ = 100**; of death (D), **U$_D$ = 0**; of vegetative state (V), **U$_V$ = ?**.

$$\text{Utility of full support} = (\text{fsp}_A)U_A + (\text{fsp}_V)\,U_V + (\text{fsp}_D)U_D$$
$$= 100(\text{fsp}_A) + (\text{fsp}_V)U_V$$
$$\text{Utility of limited support} = (\text{lsp}_A)U_A + (\text{lsp}_V)U_V + (\text{lsp}_D)U_D$$
$$= 100(\text{lsp}_A) + (\text{lsp}_V)U_V$$

(Utility of full support) − (utility of limited support)
$$= \{100(\text{fsp}_A) + (\text{fsp}_V)U_V)\} - \{100(\text{lsp}_A) + (\text{lsp}_V)U_V\}$$
$$= 100(\text{fsp}_A - \text{lsp}_A) + U_V(\text{fsp}_V - \text{lsp}_V)$$

If sum is greater than zero, the best decision is to maintain full support; less than zero, limit support.

being vegetative (lsp$_V$) given limited support are very small compared to the probabilities given full support (fsp$_A$ and fsp$_V$). Thus further simplification of the equation above yields a decision based on the equation: $100(\text{fsp}_A) + U_V(\text{fsp}_V)$. If this sum is greater than zero, the best decision is to maintain full support. If this sum is less than zero, the best decision is to limit support. The only way this sum can be less than zero is if the utility of being vegetative (U$_V$) is rated less than zero, namely the utility of being dead (U$_D$). Once such a rating is made, using the formula above, it is possible to see that even in the face of uncertainty, the best decision may be to limit support. The greater the negative value assigned to the vegetative state, the greater the uncertainty that is possible. How best to assign specific utilities to states worse than death presents its own challenges.

The use of decision analysis allows a quantitative

view of what most clinicians already know—namely, that decisions can be made in the face of uncertainty but that patients' or their surrogates' preferences about outcomes are important considerations. Many people would choose to give up the small chance of awakening, especially awakening with neurological deficits, rather than be trapped in a vegetative state for some length of time. The model presented is an oversimplification and can be made more comprehensive by including more outcomes and a more careful consideration of time, but the conclusion will remain the same: decisions to limit support are possible despite prognostic uncertainty. None of these considerations includes the societal view, with concerns over use of resources. Requiring prolonged support for unconscious patients will result in extensive resources being devoted to these patients.[89,136] On the contrary, considerations of resources may someday force society to mandate an extremely negative utility to the vegetative state.

ALTERATION OF OUTCOMES

Many strategies exist to reduce the brain damage from cardiac arrest. The most effective is to prevent cardiac arrest from occurring in the first place.[161] Prevention requires delineation of risk factors for cardiac arrest. Because the most common cause of cardiac arrest is atherosclerotic cardiovascular disease, the two share risk factors. With identification and control of these risk factors in recent years, the incidence of cardiac arrest may be expected to fall.

Assuming that efforts at primary prevention fail and a patient suffers a cardiac arrest, another strategy is to limit as much as possible the severity and duration of global brain ischemia. Such is the aim of what currently is the only effective treatment for brain damage following cardiac arrest—namely, cardiopulmonary resuscitation with basic and advanced life support. Brain resuscitation is the goal of cardiopulmonary resuscitation. The most treatable condition leading to cardiac arrest is ventricular fibrillation, and the necessary treatment is electrical defibrillation. Consequently, in patients with ventricular fibrillation, the outcome is determined in large part by how quickly the patient and defibrillator can be brought together.[21,162] For in-hospital arrests, this requires code teams and the availability of necessary equipment, especially in areas where arrests are known to occur more frequently, such as intensive care units,

operating suites, and the emergency room. For out-of-hospital cardiac arrest, success requires an emergency medical system capable of a rapid response and early defibrillation. Automatic defibrillators,[163,164] and even more so implantable defibrillators,[165] have led to a reduction in the time from the onset of the arrest until first defibrillatory shock. Patients with other rhythms, such as asystole and electromechanical dissociation, are less likely to have spontaneous circulation restored.[103–105] Efforts to improve the proportion resuscitated, as with high-dose epinephrine, have to date been disappointing.[166–167]

Even when resuscitation leads to restoration of a spontaneous circulation, many patients will die without ever regaining consciousness. Currently no therapeutic interventions initiated after restoration of spontaneous circulation are known to improve neurological outcomes after cardiac arrest. Efforts to identify such a treatment, namely brain resuscitation, have been great over the last several decades. Safar and colleagues have suggested that brain resuscitation includes both general brain-oriented intensive care and specific measures.[168,169] The general measures are essential and are the approach taken for any critically ill, comatose patient.[170] As mentioned, the occurrence of seizures and myoclonus tends to indicate a worse prognosis, which is not clearly improved with treatment. Brain swelling is rarely a serious problem when the mechanism of arrest is primarily cardiac, and treatments aimed at reducing swelling—such as hyperventilation, use of osmotic agents, and administration of corticosteroids—have no clear role. The efficacy of corticosteroids has not been studied in a randomized clinical trial, but in two cohort studies, one retrospective[171] and one prospective,[172] both with concurrent nonrandomized controls, outcomes were not related to their use.

It is possible that the duration and severity of complete and incomplete global brain ischemia determine the outcome, and no manner of treatment after the insult will alter the outcome. Evidence against such a nihilistic view has come from the use of experimental treatments in animal models of global brain ischemia[173] and an expanding knowledge of the brain's response to ischemia, reperfusion, and repair. Several reviews address these topics,[174–176] including attempts to distinguish complete from incomplete ischemia and global from focal ischemia.[177,178] What follows is a brief overview of this rapidly expanding field from the perspective of a clinician.

Under normal circumstances, intracellular calcium is kept quite low relative to extracellular calcium, a 10,000-fold concentration difference. During ischemia, the ability of a cell to maintain this gradient is lost, and the rise of intracellular calcium triggers a number of destructive events leading to the cell's death, including activation of calcium-dependent enzymes. Calcium can enter the cell via a number of pathways. The initial hope was that most entered through voltage-sensitive calcium channels and could be stopped with calcium entry blockers. The hypothesis has subsequently been tested in at least four randomized clinical trials of calcium entry blockers including lidoflazine,[179] nimodipine[180,181] and flunarizine.[182] In humans, none of these agents has been shown to be effective in altering outcome, although results from one study have not been presented.[182] The study of lidoflazine can be criticized for including a mixture of patients with in- and out-of-hospital cardiac arrest and for a delay in administering the study drug.[179] Similar criticisms cannot be leveled at the study of nimodipine by Roine and colleagues,[181] which has become the gold standard for such trials. It included only patients with out-of-hospital cardiac arrest with ventricular fibrillation. The treatment was initiated in the field upon restoration of spontaneous circulation. Finally, the follow-up of the patients and documentation of outcomes was superb.[62] Unfortunately, no overall benefit could be detected from the drug, although there was a suggestion that those with delayed resuscitations might have done better with nimodipine, and a multicenter European trial is promised to address this possibility.[181]

The lack of efficacy of the calcium entry blockers is better understood by realizing that calcium can also enter cells by agonist-operated channels, specifically those activated by glutamate. It is an excitatory neurotransmitter that in this setting is proposed to be an excitatory neurotoxin or excitotoxin. Glutamate acts at several receptors named for the more specific agonists that bind to them, including AMPA (alpha-amino-3-hydroxy-5-methyl-4-isoazole propionic acid) and NMDA (N-methyl-D-aspartate). The AMPA sites mediate fast synaptic transmission, opening a channel for sodium and potassium but not calcium. The NMDA channels are gated by magnesium and allow the flux of cations including calcium. Despite hopes that blockage of the NMDA sites would reduce the influx of calcium and protect the brain, experimental studies of global brain ischemia have not consistently shown benefit.[183,184]

Interestingly, the glutamate antagonists that have been most effective after global brain ischemia have blocked the AMPA sites.[185] By preventing rapid changes in sodium and potassium and thus excitatory synaptic transmission, these agents may prevent the cell from depolarizing. Without depolarization, calcium does not enter through the voltage-sensitive calcium channels. In addition, depolarization is necessary to clear magnesium from NMDA channels. Thus even in the presence of excess glutamate, if the cell is not depolarized, magnesium blocks the channel, and calcium cannot enter. Currently, none of the agents that block the AMPA receptors is available clinically.

Other methods are available to prevent cells from depolarizing. Both barbiturates and benzodiazepines do so by increasing the inhibitory effects of gamma-aminobutyric acid. Thiopental was studied in a randomized trial of humans and was not found to be effective.[186] This landmark study was the first major clinical trial to evaluate a treatment whose purpose was brain resuscitation. The lack of effect may have been related to the delay in administration of the drug. Other treatments known to reduce the metabolic demands of the cell are also available. In particular, hypothermia with even small decreases in temperature has been shown to be effective in a number of animal experiments.[187] The precise mechanism by which hypothermia confers protection is unknown, but results for both global and focal brain ischemia are consistent. However, logistical problems exist in finding an effective method to cool the brain's temperature rapidly and safely.

The sequence of events following ischemia and during reperfusion continues to be clarified. Free radicals probably play an important role in the brain injury following cardiac arrest. A number of strategies exist to deal with oxygen free radicals, including reducing their production, increasing their removal, and blocking their effects. A new class of compounds, the 21-amino steroids, has received much attention in this regard.[188,189] These steroids lack glucocorticoid activities but seem to block lipid peroxidation, one of the devastating effects of the free radicals. Exactly how nitric oxide fits into these theories of excitotoxins and free radicals remains to be fully defined.[190,191]

Finally, attention has turned in recent years to the reparative mechanisms and the possibility that some of the damage following global brain ischemia is a consequence of defective repair.[176] The production of growth factors such as nerve growth factor and insulin-like growth factor, the induction of stress proteins such as heat shock proteins, and the transcription of immediate early genes such as c-*fos* and c-*jun* are all under investigation. A better understanding of these mechanisms may lead to novel ways to improve the outcomes of patients after cardiac arrest.

In many ways, patients resuscitated from cardiac arrest represent an ideal group to evaluate treatments for brain ischemia. The condition is common, good outcomes are not rare in subgroups such as those with ventricular fibrillation, treatments can be initiated very early after restoration of spontaneous circulation, and pertinent outcomes are easily determined and timed. The randomized trials completed to date provide ample evidence of the feasibility of such studies. A factorial design seems particularly appropriate, one treatment arm being directed at calcium entry into the cell and the other aimed at free radicals. Analyses could include comparison of treatment groups for various outcomes. Because the times of occurrence of death and awakening can easily be determined, time-dependent analyses could be performed and presented, as in a recent trial of glucose-containing solutions after cardiac arrest (Fig. 9-5).

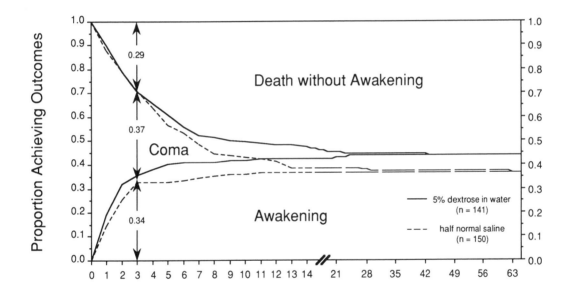

Days since Cardiopulmonary Arrest

Fig. 9-5. Example of one manner in which to present data from a clinical trial examining whether the type of fluids administered by paramedical personnel (5% dextrose in water versus 0.5 normal saline) affected outcome. The graph shows the proportion of 291 admitted patients who were all initially comatose after out-of-hospital cardiopulmonary arrest and went on to awaken or to die without awakening. Solid lines represent the experience among those who received 5% dextrose in water (*n* = 141); dashed lines, those who received 0.5 normal saline (*n* = 150). A vertical line from the horizontal axis at any particular time indicates the proportion who had awakened (from the 0.0 horizontal line to the lower pair of curves); who were still comatose (from lower to upper pair of curves); and who had died without awakening (from the upper pair of curves to the 1.0 horizontal line). For example, a vertical line at 3 days would indicate for the entire cohort that about 34 percent had awakened regardless of treatment group, that about 37 percent were still comatose (71 to 34 percent), and that the remaining 29 percent (100 to 71 percent) had died without awakening. Of the 117 patients who awakened, 15 subsequently died during hospitalization and are classified in this figure as having awakened. (From Longstreth WT Jr, Copass MK, Dennis LK, et al: Intravenous glucose after out-of-hospital cardiopulmonary arrest: a community-based randomized trial. Neurology 43:2534, 1993, with permission.)

CONCLUDING COMMENT

Neurological complications of cardiac arrest represent the consequences of an imperfect technology developed over the last 30 to 40 years. Prior to the advent of cardiopulmonary resuscitation and especially electrical defibrillation, virtually all such patients died. With the proliferation of in-hospital code teams and prehospital emergency medical systems, an increasing proportion of these patients are resuscitated. As a consequence, patients and clinicians are faced with issues of brain damage following cardiac arrest. The ability to predict outcomes has improved but will never be perfect and should not prevent physicians from working with families to make decisions about medical support. Currently, we are unable to improve the neurological outcome with treatment. Given the increasing understanding of the brain's response to ischemia, reperfusion, and repair, the expectation that an effective treatment will soon be available is not unrealistic. If so, such a treatment will find immediate use in the thousands of patients who are resuscitated from cardiac arrest each year. In the meantime, and for all time, prevention and efficient cardiopulmonary resuscitation are essential.

REFERENCES

1. Baker AB: Artificial respirations, the history of an idea. Med Hist 15:336, 1971
2. Fye WB: Ventricular fibrillation and defibrillation: historical perspectives with emphasis on the contributions of John MacWilliam, Carl Wiggers, and William Kouwenhoven. Circulation 71:858, 1985
3. Jex-Blake AJ: The Goulstonian Lectures: death by electric currents and by lightning. Br Med J 1:425, 492, 548, 601, 1913
4. Prevost J, Battelli F: La mort par les courants électrique. J Physiol Path Gen (Paris) 1:1085, 1899
5. MacWilliam JA: Cardiac failure and sudden death. Br Med J 1:6, 1889
6. Kouwenhoven WB, Langworthy OR: Cardiopulmonary resuscitation: an account of forty-five years of research. Johns Hopkins Med J 132:186, 1973
7. Safar P, Escarraga LA, Elam JO: A comparison of the mouth-to-mouth and mouth-to-airway methods of artificial respiration with the chest-pressure arm-lift methods. N Engl J Med 258:671, 1958
8. Zoll PM, Linenthal AJ, Gibbon W, et al: Termination of ventricular fibrillation in man by externally placed electric countershock. N Engl J Med 254:727, 1956
9. Kouwenhoven WB, Jude JR, Knickerbocker GG: Closed chest cardiac massage. JAMA 173:1064, 1960
10. Kuller L, Lilienfeld A, Fisher R: An epidemiological study of sudden death and unexpected deaths in adults. Medicine (Baltimore) 46:341, 1967
11. Kuller L: Sudden death in arteriosclerotic heart disease. Am J Cardiol 24:617, 1969
12. Pantridge JF, Geddes JS: Cardiac arrest after myocardial infarction. Lancet 1:807, 1966
13. Pantridge JF, Geddes JS: A mobile intensive-care unit in the management of myocardial infarction. Lancet 2:271, 1967
14. Partridge JF, Adgey AAJ: Prehospital coronary care. Am J Cardiol 24:666, 1969
15. Cobb LA, Alvarez H, Copass MK: A rapid system for out-of-hospital emergencies. Med Clin North Am 60:283, 1976
16. Cobb LA, Hallstrom AP, Thompson RG, et al: Community cardiopulmonary resuscitation. Annu Rev Med 31:453, 1980
17. Solomon NA: What are representative survival rates for out-of-hospital cardiac arrest? Insights from the New Haven (Conn) experience. Arch Intern Med 153:1218, 1993
18. Earnest MP, Yarnell PR, Merrill SL, Knapp GL: Long-term survival and neurologic status for resuscitation from out-of-hospital cardiac arrest. Neurology 30:1298, 1980
19. Longstreth WT Jr, Inui TS, Cobb LA, Copass MK: Neurologic recovery after out-of-hospital cardiac arrest. Ann Intern Med 98, part 1:588, 1983
20. Lown B: Sudden cardiac death: the major challenge confronting contemporary cardiology. Am J Cardiol 43:313, 1979
21. Eisenberg MS, Bergner L, Hallstrom AP, Cummins RO: Sudden cardiac death. Sci Am 254:37, 1986
22. Myerburg RJ, Castellanos A: Cardiovascular collapse, cardiac arrest, and sudden death. p. 237. In Wilson JD, Braunwald E, Isselbacher KJ, et al (eds): Harrison's Principles of Internal Medicine. McGraw-Hill, New York, 1991
23. Brooks R, McGovern BA, Garan H, Ruskin JN: Current treatment of patients surviving out-of-hospital cardiac arrest. JAMA 265:762, 1991
24. Graham DI: Hypoxia and vascular disorders. p. 153. In Adams JH, Duchen LW (eds): Greenfield's Neuropathology. 5th Ed. Oxford University Press, New York, 1992
25. de Courten-Myers G, Kleinholz M, Wagner KR, Myers RE: Asphyxia- compared to cardiac arrest-induced brain damage is more extensive and uniquely

involves thalamus and brainstem. Neurology 41, suppl 1:337, 1991

26. Natelson BH: Neurocardiology: an interdisciplinary area for the 80s. Arch Neurol 42:178, 1985

27. Oppenheimer SM, Cechetto DF, Hachinski VC: Cerebrogenic cardiac arrhythmias: cerebral electrocardiographic influences and their role in sudden death. Arch Neurol 47:513, 1990

28. Skinner JE, Reed JC: Blockade of frontocortical-brain stem pathway prevents ventricular fibrillation of ischemic heart. Am J Physiol 240:H156, 1981

29. Leestma JE, Kalekar MD, Teas SS, et al: Sudden unexpected death associated with seizures: analysis of 66 cases. Epilepsia 25:84, 1984

30. Dasheiff RM, Dickinson LVJ: Sudden unexpected death of epileptic patient due to cardiac arrhythmia after seizure. Arch Neurol 43:194, 1986

31. Liedholm LJ, Gudjonsson O: Cardiac arrest due to partial seizures. Neurology 42:824, 1992

32. Thomas L: Biological aspects of death. Pharos 37:83, 1974

33. Richter CP: On the phenomenon of sudden death in animals and man. Psychosom Med 19:191, 1957

34. Cooper A: Some experiments and observations on tying the carotid and vertebral arteries, and the pneumo-gastric, phenic, and sympathetic nerves. Guy's Hosp Reports 1:457, 1836

35. Brown-Séquard CE: Recherches expérimentales sur les propriétés physiologiques et les usages du sang rouge et sang noir. J Physiol (Paris) 11:119, 1858

36. Rossen R, Kabat H, Anderson JP: Acute arrest of cerebral circulation in man. Arch Neurol Psychiatry 50:510, 1943

37. Opitz E, Thorn W: Überlebenszeit und Erholungszeit des Warmblütergehirns unter dem Einfluss der Höhenanpassung. Pflügers Arch 251:369, 1949

38. Gastaut H, Fischer-Williams M: Electro-encephalographic study of syncope: its differentiation from epilepsy. Lancet 2:1018, 1957

39. Aminoff MJ, Scheinman MM, Griffin JC, Herre JM: Electrocerebral accompaniments of syncope associated with malignant ventricular arrhythmias. Ann Intern Med 108:791, 1988

40. Lempert T, Bauer M, Schmidt D: The clinical phenomenology of induced syncope. Neurology 41, suppl 1:127, 1991

41. Lempert T, von Brevern M: The eye movements of syncope. Neurology 43:A221, 1993

42. Longstreth WT Jr: Prognostic significance of neurologic examination and glycemia after cardiac arrest. Resuscitation 17:S175, 1989

43. Longstreth WT Jr, Dikmen SS: Outcomes after cardiac arrest. Ann Emerg Med 22:64, 1993

44. Nemoto EM, Bleyaert AL, Stezoski SW, et al: Global brain ischemia: a reproducible monkey model. Stroke 8:558, 1977

45. Jennett B, Teasdale G: Assessment of outcome. p. 301. In: Management of Head Injuries. FA Davis, Philadelphia, 1981

46. Brain Resuscitation Clinical Trial II Study Group: A randomized clinical trial of calcium entry blocker administration to comatose survivors of cardiac arrest: design, methods, and patient characteristics. Controlled Clin Trials 12:525, 1991

47. Walker AE: Cerebral Death. Urban & Schwarzenberg, Baltimore, 1985

48. Brierley JB, Adams JH, Graham DI, et al: Neocortical death after cardiac arrest: a clinical, neurophysiological, and neuropathological report of two cases. Lancet 2:560, 1971

49. Dougherty JH, Rawlinson DG, Levy DE, Plum F: Hypoxic-ischemic brain injury and the vegetative state: clinical and neuropathologic correlation. Neurology 31:991, 1981

50. Spudis EV: The persistent vegetative state—1990. J Neurol Sci 102:128, 1990

51. Tresch DD, Sims FH, Duthie EH, et al: Clinical characteristics of patients in the persistent vegetative state. Arch Intern Med 151:930, 1991

52. Executive Board, American Academy of Neurology: Position of the American Academy of Neurology on certain aspects of the care and management of the persistent vegetative state patient. Neurology 39:125, 1989

53. Council on Scientific Affairs and Council on Ethical and Judicial Affairs: Persistent vegetative state and the decision to withdraw or withhold life support. JAMA 263:426, 1990

54. Institute of Medical Ethics Working Party on the Ethics of Prolonging Life and Assisting Death: Withdrawal of life-support from patients in a persistent vegetative state. Lancet 337:96, 1991

55. Medical Ethics Committee: Discussion paper on treatment of patients in persistent vegetative state. British Medical Association, London, 1992

56. ANA Committee on Ethical Affairs: Persistent vegetative state: report of the American Neurological Association Committee on Ethical Affairs. Ann Neurol 33:386, 1993

57. Cummings JL, Tomiyasu U, Reed S, Benson DF: Amnesia with hippocampal lesions after cardiopulmonary arrest. Neurology 34:679, 1984

58. Volpe BT, Holtzman JD, Hirst W: Further characterization of patients with amnesia after cardiac arrest: preserved recognition memory. Neurology 36:408, 1986

59. Bertini G, Giglioli C, Giovanni F, et al: Neuropsychological outcome of survivors of out-of-hospital cardiac arrest. J Emerg Med 8:407, 1990

60. Volpe BT, Herscovitch P, Raichle ME: PET evaluation of patients with amnesia after cardiac arrest. Stroke 15:196, 1984

61. Owens JE, Cook EW, Stevenson I: Features of "near-death experience" in relation to whether or not patients were near death. Lancet 336:1175, 1990

62. Roine RO, Kajaste S, Kaste M: Neuropsychological sequence of cardiac arrest. JAMA 269:237, 1993

63. Folstein MF, Folstein SE, McHugh PR: "Mini-Mental State": a practical method for grading the cognitive state of patients for the clinician. J Psychiatr Res 12:189, 1975

64. Bergner L, Hallstrom AP, Berner M, et al: Health status of survivors of cardiac arrest and of myocardial infarction controls. Am J Public Health 75:1321, 1985

65. Ottosson J-O, Holmberg S, Ekström L: A psychiatric and neuropsychological following of CPR patients. Resuscitation 24:199, 1992

66. Teasdale G, Jennett B: Assessment of coma and impaired consciousness: a practical scale. Lancet 2:81, 1974

67. Ng T, Graham DI, Adams JH, Ford I: Changes in the hippocampus and the cerebellum resulting from hypoxic insults: frequency and distribution. Acta Neurpathol 78:438, 1989

68. Petito CK, Feldmann E, Pulsinelli WA, Plum F: Delayed hippocampal damage in humans following cardio-respiratory arrest. Neurology 37:1281, 1987

69. Janzer RC, Friede RL: Hypotensive brain stem necrosis or cardiac arrest encephalopathy. Acta Neuropathol 50:53, 1980

70. Relkin NR, Petito CK, Plum F: Coma and the vegetative state associated with thalamic injury after cardiac arrest. Ann Neurol 28:221, 1990

71. Snyder BD, Hauser WA, Loewenson RB, et al: Neurologic prognosis after cardiopulmonary arrest: III. Seizure activity. Neurology 30:1292, 1980

72. Krumholz A, Stern BJ, Weiss HD: Outcome from coma after cardiopulmonary resuscitation: relation to seizures and myoclonus. Neurology 38:401, 1988

73. Wijdicks EFM, Parisi JE, Sharbrough FW: The prognostic value of myoclonus in comatose survivors following cardiac resuscitation. Ann Neurol 34:298, 1993

74. Young GB, Gilbert JJ, Zochodne DW: The significance of myoclonic status epilepticus in postanoxic coma. Neurology 40:1843, 1990

75. Jumao-as A, Brenner RP: Myoclonic status epilepticus: a clinical and electroencephalographic study. Neurology 40:1199, 1990

76. Simon RP, Aminoff MJ: Electrographic status epilepticus in fatal anoxic coma. Ann Neurol 20:351, 1986

77. Lowenstein DH, Aminoff MJ: Clinical and EEG features of status epilepticus in comatose patients. Neurology 42:100, 1992

78. Sage JI, Van Uitert RL: Man-in-the-barrel syndrome. Neurology 36:1102, 1986

79. Gilles FH, May D: Vulnerability of human spinal cord in transient cardiac arrest. Neurology 21:833, 1971

80. Azzarelli B, Roessmann U: Diffuse "anoxic" myelopathy. Neurology 27:1049, 1977

81. Roessmann U, Zarchin LE: Cerebral bone marrow embolism after closed chest cardiac massage. Arch Neurol 36:58, 1979

82. Ginsberg MD: Delayed deterioration following hypoxia. Adv Neurol 26:21, 1979

83. Barnes MP, Newman PK: Delayed encephalopathy following cardiac arrest. Postgrad Med J 61:253, 1985

84. Hori A, Hirose G, Kataoka S, et al: Delayed postanoxic encephalopathy after strangulation: serial neuroradiological and neurochemical studies. Arch Neurol 48:871, 1991

85. Lance JW, Adams RD: The syndrome of intention and action myoclonus as a sequel to hypoxic encephalopathy. Brain 86:111, 1963

86. Fahn S: Posthypoxic action myoclonus: literature review update. Adv Neurol 43:157, 1986

87. Boylan KB, Chin JH, DeArmond SJ: Progressive dystonia following resuscitation from cardiac arrest. Neurology 40:1458, 1990

88. Bhatt MH, Obeso JA, Marsden CD: Time course of postanoxic akinetic-rigid and dystonic syndromes. Neurology 43:314, 1993

89. Shewmon DA, DeGiorgio CM: Early prognosis in anoxic coma. Neurol Clin 74:823, 1989

90. Bates D: Defining prognosis in medical coma. J Neurol Neurosurg Psychiatry 54:569, 1991

91. Jørgensen EO, Malchow-Møller A: Cerebral prognostic signs during cardiopulmonary resuscitation. Resuscitation 6:217, 1978

92. Snyder BD, Loewenson RB, Gumnit RJ, et al: Neurologic prognosis after cardiopulmonary arrest: II. Level of consciousness. Neurology 30:52, 1980

93. Snyder BD, Gumnit RJ, Leppik IE, et al: Neurologic prognosis after cardiopulmonary arrest: IV. Brain stem reflexes. Neurology 31:1092, 1981

94. Jørgensen ED, Malchow-Møller A: Natural history of global and critical brain ischemia. Resuscitation 9:133, 1981

95. Longstreth WT Jr, Diehr P, Inui TS: Prediction of awakening after out-of-hospital cardiac arrest. N Engl J Med 308:1378, 1983

96. Levy DE, Caronna JJ, Singer BH, et al: Predicting outcome from hypoxic-ischemic coma. JAMA 253: 1420, 1985
97. Edgren E, Hedstrand U, Nordin M, et al: Prediction of outcome after cardiac arrest. Crit Care Med 15:820, 1987
98. Mullie A, Verstringe P, Buylaert W, et al: Predictive value of Glasgow Coma Score for awakening after out-of-hospital cardiac arrest. Lancet 1:137, 1988
99. Edgren E: Prediction of prognosis following cardiac arrest. Acta Anaesth Belg 39, suppl 2:121, 1988
100. Edgren E: Prognostic evaluation of post-cardiac arrest patients in the intensive care. Resuscitation 17:S131, 1989
101. Niskanen M, Kari A, Nikki P, et al: Acute Physiology and Chronic Health Evaluation (APACHE II) and Glasgow Coma Scores as predictors of outcome from intensive care after cardiac arrest. Crit Care Med 19: 1465, 1991
102. Beuret P, Feihl F, Vogt P, et al: Cardiac arrest: prognostic factors and outcome at one year. Resuscitation 25:171, 1993
103. Kellerman AL, Hackman BB, Somos G: Predicting the outcome of unsuccessful prehospital advanced cardiac life support. JAMA 270:1433, 1993
104. Bonnin MJ, Pepe PE, Kimball KJ, Clark PS Jr: Distinct criteria for termination of resuscitation in the out-of-hospital setting. JAMA 270:1457, 1993
105. Longstreth WT Jr, Cobb LA, Fahrenbruch CE, Copass MK: Does age affect outcomes of out-of-hospital cardiopulmonary resuscitation? JAMA 264:2109, 1990
106. Van Hoeyweghen RJ, Bossaert LL, Mullie A, et al: Survival after out-of-hospital cardiac arrest in elderly patients: Belgian Cerebral Resuscitation Study Group. Ann Emerg Med 21:1179, 1992
107. Cowie MR, Fahrenbruch CE, Cobb LA, Hallstrom AP: Out-of-hospital cardiac arrest: racial differences in outcome in Seattle. Am J Public Health 83:955, 1993
108. Becker LB, Han BH, Meyer PM, et al: Racial differences in the incidence of cardiac arrest and subsequent survival. N Engl J Med 329:600, 1993
109. Bedell SE, Delbanco TL, Cook EF, Epstein FM: Survival after cardiopulmonary resuscitation in the hospital. N Engl J Med 309:569, 1983
110. Mullie A, van Hoeyweghen R, Quets A, et al: Influence of time intervals on outcome of CPR. Resuscitation 17, suppl:S23, 1989
111. Martens PR, Mullie A, Buylaert W, et al. Early prediction of non-survival for patients suffering cardiac arrest—a word of caution: The Belgian Cerebral Resuscitation Study Group. Intensive Care Med 18:11, 1992
112. Buettner UW, Zee DS: Vestibular testing in comatose patients. Arch Neurol 46:561, 1989
113. Rowley G, Fielding K: Reliability and accuracy of the Glasgow coma scale with experienced and inexperienced users. Lancet 337:535, 1991
114. Longstreth WT Jr, Inui TS: High blood glucose level on hospital admission and poor neurological recovery after cardiac arrest. Ann Neurol 15:58, 1984
115. Calle PA, Buylaert WA, Vanhaute OA, and the Cerebral Resuscitation Study Group: Glycemia in the post-resuscitation period. Resuscitation 17, suppl:S181, 1989
116. Myers RE, Yamaguchi M: Nervous system effects of cardiac arrest in monkeys: preservation of vision. Arch Neurol 34:65, 1977
117. Longstreth WT Jr, Diehr P, Cobb LA, et al: Neurologic outcome and blood glucose levels during out-of-hospital cardiopulmonary resuscitation. Neurology 36:1186, 1986
118. Longstreth WT Jr, Copass MK, Dennis LK, et al: Intravenous glucose after out-of-hospital cardiopulmonary arrest: a community-based randomized trial. Neurology 43:2534, 1993
119. Hockaday JM, Potts F, Epstein E, et al: Electroencephalographic changes in acute cerebral anoxia from cardiac arrest or respiratory arrest. Electroencephalogr Clin Neurophysiol 18:575, 1965
120. Prior PF: The EEG in Acute Cerebral Anoxia: Assessment of Cerebral Function and Prognosis in Patients Resuscitated after Cardiorespiratory Arrest. Excerpta Medica, Amsterdam, 1973
121. Chatrian GE: Coma, other states of altered responsiveness and brain death. p. 425. In Daly DD, Pedley TA (eds): Current Practice of Clinical Electroencephalography. 2nd Ed. Raven Press, New York, 1990
122. Synek VM: Value of a revised EEG coma scale for prognosis after cerebral anoxia and diffuse head injury. Clin Electroencephalogr 21:25, 1990
123. Scollo-Lavizzari B, Bassetti C: Prognostic value of EEG in post-anoxic coma after cardiac arrest. Eur Neurol 26:161, 1987
124. Austin EJ, Wilkus RJ, Longstreth WT Jr: Etiology and prognosis of alpha coma. Neurology 38:773, 1988
125. Young WL, Ornstein E: Compressed spectral array EEG monitoring during cardiac arrest and resuscitation. Anesthesiology 62:535, 1985
126. Goldie WD, Chiappa KH, Young RR, Brooks EB: Brainstem auditory and short-latency somatosensory evoked responses in brain death. Neurology 31:248, 1981
127. Ganji S, Peters G, Frazier E: Somatosensory and brain stem auditory evoked potential studies in nontraumatic coma. Clin Electroencephalogr 19:55, 1988
128. Brunko E, Zegers de Beyl D: Prognostic value of

early cortical somatosensory evoked potentials after resuscitation from cardiac arrest. Electroencephalogr Clin Neurophysiol 66:15, 1987

129. Karnaze D, Fisher M, Ahmadi J, Gott P: Short-latency somatosensory evoked potentials correlate with the severity of the neurological deficit and sensory abnormalities following cerebral ischemia. Electroencephalogr Clin Neurophysiol 67:147, 1987

130. Rothstein TL, Thomas EM, Sumi SM: Predicting outcome in hypoxic-ischemic coma: a prospective clinical and electrophysiologic study. Electroencephalogr Clin Neurophysiol 79:101, 1991

131. Madl C, Grimm G, Kramer L, et al: Early prediction of individual outcome after cardiopulmonary resuscitation. Lancet 341:855, 1993

132. Kjos BO, Brant-Zawadski M, Young RG: Early CT findings of global central nervous system hypoperfusion. AJR 141:1227, 1983

133. Morimoto Y, Kemmotsu O, Kitami K, et al: Acute brain swelling after out-of-hospital cardiac arrest: pathogenesis and outcome. Crit Care Med 21:104, 1993

134. Roine RO, Raininko R, Erkinjuntti T, et al: Magnetic resonance imaging findings associated with cardiac arrest. Stroke 24:1005, 1993

135. DeVolder AG, Goffinet AM, Bol A, et al: Brain glucose metabolism in postanoxic syndrome: positron emission tomographic study. Arch Neurol 47:197, 1990

136. Levy DE, Sidtis JJ, Rottenberg DA, et al: Differences in cerebral blood flow and glucose utilization in vegetative versus locked-in patients. Ann Neurol 22:673, 1987

137. Cohan SL, Mun SK, Petite J, et al: Cerebral blood flow in humans following resuscitation from cardiac arrest. Stroke 20:761, 1989

138. Roine RO, Launes J, Nikkinen P, et al: Regional cerebral blood flow after human cardiac arrest: a hexamethyl-propyleneamine oxime single photon emission computed tomographic study. Arch Neurol 48:625, 1991

139. Martin GB, Paradis NA, Helpern JA, et al: Nuclear magnetic resonance spectroscopy study of human brain after cardiac resuscitation. Stroke 22:462, 1991

140. Lechleitner P, Felber S, Birbamer G, et al: Proton magnetic resonance spectroscopy of brain after cardiac resuscitation. Lancet 340:913, 1992

141. Mullie A, Lust P, Penninckx J, et al: Monitoring of cerebrospinal fluid enzyme levels in post-ischemic encephalopathy after cardiac arrest. Crit Care Med 9:399, 1981

142. Massey TH, Goe MR: Transient creatine kinase-BB activity in serum or plasma after cardiac or respiratory arrest. Clin Chem 30:50, 1984

143. Longstreth WT Jr, Clayson KJ, Chandler WL, Sumi SM: Cerebrospinal fluid creatine kinase activity and neurologic recovery after cardiac arrest. Neurology 34:834, 1984

144. Vaagenes P, Kjekshus J, Sivertsen E, Semb G: Temporal pattern of enzyme changes in cerebrospinal fluid in patients with neurologic complications after open heart surgery. Crit Care Med 15:726, 1987

145. Vaagenes P, Safar P, Diven W, et al: Brain enzyme levels in CSF after cardiac arrest and resuscitation in dogs: markers of damage and predictors of outcome. J Cereb Blood Flow Metab 8:262, 1988

146. Kärkelä J, Bock E, Kaukinen S: CSF and serum-specific creatine kinase isoenzyme (CK-BB), neuron-specific enolase (NSE) and neural cell adhesion molecule (NCAM) as prognostic markers for hypoxic brain injury after cardiac arrest in man. J Neurol Sci 116:100, 1993

147. Chandler WL, Clayson KJ, Longstreth WT Jr, Fine JS: Creatine kinase isoenzymes in human cerebrospinal fluid and brain. Clin Chem 30:1804, 1984

148. Chandler WL, Clayson KJ, Longstreth WT Jr, et al: Mitochondrial and MB isoenzymes of creatine kinase in cerebrospinal fluid from patients with hypoxic-ischemic brain damage. Am J Clin Pathol 86:533, 1986

149. Chandler WL, Fine JS, Emery M, et al: Regional creatine kinase, adenylate kinase, and lactate dehydrogenase in normal canine brain. Stroke 19:251, 1988

150. Donnan GA, Zapf P, Doyle AE, Bladin PF: CSF enzymes in lacunar and cortical stroke. Stroke 14:266, 1983

151. Bakay RAE, Ward AA Jr: Enzymatic changes in serum and cerebrospinal fluid in neurological injury. J Neurosurg 58:27, 1983

152. Kruse A, Cesarini KG, Bach FW, Persson L: Increases of neuron-specific enolase, S-100 protein, creatine kinase and creatine kinase BB isoenzyme in CSF following intraventricular catheter implantation. Acta Neurochir 110:106, 1991

153. Yarnell PR: Neurological outcome of prolonged coma survivors of out-of-hospital cardiac arrest. Stroke 7:279, 1976

154. Rosenberg GA, Johnson SF, Brenner RP: Recovery of cognition after prolonged vegetative state. Ann Neurol 2:167, 1977

155. Andrews K: Recovery of patients after four months or more in the persistent vegetative state. Br Med J 306:1597, 1993

156. Hanley JA, Lippman-Hand A: If nothing goes wrong, is everything all right? Interpreting zero numerators. JAMA 249:1743, 1983

157. Shewmon DA: The probability of inevitability: the inherent impossibility of validating criteria for brain

death or "irreversibility" through clinical studies. Stat Med 6:535, 1987

158. Pauker SG, Kassirer JP: Decision analysis. N Engl J Med 316:250, 1987

159. Kassirer JP, Moskowitz AJ, Lan J, et al: Decision analysis: a progress report. Ann Intern Med 106:275, 1987

160. Koprowski CD, Longstreth WT Jr, Cebul RD: Clinical neuroepidemiology: III. Decisions. Arch Neurol 46:223, 1989

161. Longstreth WT Jr: Brain resuscitation after cardiopulmonary arrest. Acta Anaesth Belg 39, suppl 2:115, 1988

162. Cobb LA: Survival after cardiac arrest. p. 152. In Higgins MW, Luepker RV (eds): Trends in Coronary Heart Disease Mortality: The Influence of Medical Care. Oxford University Press, New York, 1988

163. Eisenberg MS, Copass MK, Hallstrom AP, et al: Treatment of out-of-hospital cardiac arrests with rapid defibrillation by emergency medical technicians. N Engl J Med 302:1379, 1980

164. Weaver WD, Copass MK, Hill DL, et al: Cardiac arrest treated with a new automatic external defibrillator by out-of-hospital first responders. Am J Cardiol 57:1017, 1986

165. Mirowski M, Reid PR, Mower MM: Termination of malignant ventricular arrhythmias with an implanted automatic defibrillator in human beings. N Engl J Med 303:322, 1980

166. Stiell IG, Herbert PC, Weitzman BE, et al: High-dose epinephrine in adult cardiac arrest. N Engl J Med 327:1045, 1992

167. Brown CG, Martin DR, Pepe PE, et al: A comparison of standard-dose and high-dose epinephrine in cardiac arrest outside the hospital. N Engl J Med 327:1051, 1992

168. Safar P, Bircher NG: Cardiopulmonary Cerebral Resuscitation. 3rd Ed. WB Saunders, Philadelphia, 1988

169. Safar P: Cerebral resuscitation after cardiac arrest: research initiatives and future directions. Ann Emerg Med 22:324, 1993

170. Gustafson I, Edgran E, Hulting J: Brain-oriented intensive care after resuscitation from cardiac arrest. Resuscitation 24:245, 1992

171. Grafton ST, Longstreth WT Jr: Steroids after cardiac arrest: a restrospective study with concurrent nonrandomized controls. Neurology 38:1315, 1988

172. Jastremski M, Sutton-Tyrrell K, Vaagenes P, et al: Glucocorticoid treatment does not improve neurologic recovery following cardiac arrest. JAMA 262:3427, 1989

173. Pulsinelli WA, Jaceqicz M: Animal models of brain ischemia. p. 49. In Barnett HJM, Stein BM, Mohr JP, Yatsu FM (eds): Stroke: Physiology, Diagnosis, and Management. 2nd Ed. Churchill Livingstone, New York, 1992

174. Siesjö BK: Mechanisms of ischemic brain damage. Crit Care Med 16:954, 1988

175. Meyer FB: Calcium, neuronal hyperexcitability and ischemic injury. Brain Res Rev 14:227, 1989

176. White BC, Grossman LI, Krause GS: Brain injury by global ischemia and reperfusion: a theoretical perspective on membrane damage and repair. Neurology 43:1656, 1993

177. Siesjö BK: Pathophysiology and treatment of focal cerebral ischemia: Part I. Pathophysiology. J Neurosurg 77:169, 1992

178. Siesjö BK: Pathophysiology and treatment of focal cerebral ischemia: Part II. Mechanisms of damage and treatment. J Neurosurg 77:337, 1992

179. Brain Resuscitation Clinical Trial II Study Group. A randomized clinical study of a calcium-entry blocker (lidoflazine) in the treatment of comatose survivors of cardiac arrest. N Engl J Med 324:1225, 1991

180. Forsman M, Aarseth HP, Nordy HK, et al: Effects of nimodipine on cerebral blood flow and cerebrospinal fluid pressure after cardiac arrest: correlation with neurologic outcome. Anesth Analg 68:436, 1989

181. Roine RO, Kaste M, Kinnunen A, et al: Nimodipine after resuscitation from out-of-hospital ventricular fibrillation: a placebo-controlled, double-blind, randomized trial. JAMA 264:3171, 1990

182. Schröder R: Flunarazine IV after cardiac arrest (FLUNA-Study): Study design and organizational aspects of a double-blind placebo-controlled randomized study. Resuscitation 17,suppl:S121, 1989

183. Choi DW: Possible mechanisms limiting N-methyl-D-aspartate receptor overactivation and the therapeutic efficacy of N-methy-D-aspartate antagonists. Stroke 21,suppl III:III-20, 1990

184. Buchan AM: Do NMDA antagonists prevent neuronal injury? No. Arch Neurol 49:420, 1992

185. Nellgård B, Wielock T: Postischemic blockage of AMPA but not NMDA receptors mitigates neuronal damage in the rat brain following severe cerebral ischemia. J Cereb Blood Flow Metab 12:2, 1992

186. Brain Resuscitation Clinical Trial I Study Group: Randomized clinical study of thiopental loading in comatose survivors of cardiac arrest. N Engl J Med 314:397, 1986

187. Ginsberg MD, Sternau LL, Globus MY-T, et al: Therapeutic modulation of brain temperature: relevance to ischemic brain injury. Cerebrovasc Brain Metab Rev 4:189, 1992

188. Sterz F, Safar P, Johnson DW, et al: Effects of U74006F on multifocal cerebral blood flow and metabolism after cardiac arrest in dogs. Stroke 22:889, 1991

189. Halfaer MA, Kirsch JR, Hurn PD et al: Tirilazad mesylate does not improve early cerebral-metabolic recovery following compression ischemia in dogs. Stroke 23:1479, 1992

190. Maiese K, Boniece I, DeMeo D, Wagner JA: Peptide growth factors protect against ischemia in culture by preventing nitric oxide toxicity. J Neurosci 13:3034, 1993

191. Lipton SA, Choi Y-B, Lei SZ, et al: Neuroprotective and neurodestructive effects of nitric oxide and related nitrose compounds. Ann Neurol 34:286, 1993

10

Cardiac Manifestations of Acute Neurological Lesions

Stephen Oppenheimer
John W. Norris

Recent advances in our understanding of the neurophysiology of cardiovascular control have further highlighted the importance of the central nervous system (CNS) in the production of serious cardiac malfunction. Not only has a possible mechanism been identified that explains how the brain can cause structural cardiac changes in an otherwise normal myocardium, but the importance of these mechanisms in the generation of cardiac arrhythmias has also been identified. This is of paramount importance in the understanding of sudden cardiac death, an occurrence which claims the lives of over 250,000 people a year in the United States.[1]

In the case of the commonest acute neurological lesion, stroke, the single most important cause of death during long-term follow-up is from cardiac dysfunction.[2,3] Although this has been explained by the coincidence of ischemic cardiac disease and ischemic disease of the cranial vasculature, more recent evidence suggests that this is not the entire answer. Neurological lesions themselves probably influence cardiovascular function and may thereby affect cardiac prognosis.

This chapter briefly outlines the neurophysiology and anatomy of cardiac control, discusses historical perspectives largely derived from clinical observations identifying the importance of the brain-heart interaction in patients with cerebral lesions, and elaborates on the importance of the insular cortex in neurocardiology.

THE NEUROPHYSIOLOGY AND NEUROANATOMY OF CARDIAC CONTROL

The first indication that the CNS is involved in the generation of cardiac arrhythmias arose from a series of experiments conducted during the First World War. These were directed at identifying the cause of the numerous unexpected deaths of patients undergoing surgery with chloroform anesthesia. Levy observed that the frequent ventricular premature beats that occurred in cats under light chloroform anesthesia could be blocked by cardiac sympathetic denervation and reproduced by reflex activation of the sympathetic nervous system (for example, by bleeding the animal).[4,5] These ectopic beats were often followed by ventricular fibrillation. Beattie and colleagues demonstrated that Sherringtonian decerebration abolished the arrhythmogenic effect of chloroform.[6] Removal of the cerebral cortex alone, with preservation of diencephalic structures, failed to protect against chloroform-induced cardiac arrhythmias. It was found that the optimum planes of section required to abolish chloroform-induced arrhythmogenesis lay between the superior colliculus and the posterior margin of the optic chiasm anteriorly, and through or just behind the mammillary bodies posteriorly. Using the Marchi technique, it was deduced that the lesions severed a tract arising within the hypothalamus and ending in the intermediolateral gray matter of the spinal cord, where the sympathetic preganglionic fibers originate.

The anatomy and physiology of the possible pathways involved is discussed below.

Brainstem Medullary Sites and Cardiac Control

Three vagal areas participate in cardiac control. The principal parasympathetic afferent input via the nodose ganglion is to the nucleus of the solitary tract. There are two cardiac motor efferent sources. The first is the nucleus ambiguus and the second (of lesser import) is the dorsal motor nucleus of the vagus. The nucleus of the solitary tract is situated in the dorsal medulla and extends rostrocaudally to the area postrema, which it surrounds in a V shape. Cardiac afferents project to the dorsolateral region of the nucleus of the solitary tract, with less projection to the commissural area, whereas baroreceptor input projects to the dorsolateral, medial, and commissural regions.[7,8]

Efferents from the nucleus of the solitary tract influence activity in both the nucleus ambiguus and the dorsal motor nucleus of the vagus, allowing control over cardiac parasympathetic activity.

The nucleus ambiguus is situated in the ventrolateral medullary reticular formation. Rostrally it lies dorsal to the facial nucleus and caudally it extends toward C1. The cardiomotor fibers arise from the ventrolateral division and provide efferents to the vagus nerve. This nucleus also projects to the intermediolateral cell column of the spinal cord, the parabrachial nucleus, and the nucleus of the solitary tract. In the rat, the predominant input is from this last nucleus.[9] The cardioinhibitory cells have a low basal firing rate; this activity increases with arterial baroreceptor activation, generating increasing degrees of bradycardia. Some lateralization exists in that activation of the right nucleus ambiguus principally controls the atrial rate and the left nucleus ambiguus the ventricular rate.[10]

The dorsal motor nucleus of the vagus lies in the dorsomedial region of the caudal medulla, extending as far as C1. Vagal afferents in the nodose ganglion project directly to it.[11] Some of the cells in the dorsal motor nucleus possess long dendritic fields that project to the nucleus of the solitary tract. Cardiac related cells are present in the caudolateral part of the dorsal motor nucleus in the rat.[12,13] However, it is not precisely clear to what extent this nucleus participates in cardiac function.

The principal medullary site of sympathetic cardiac control resides in the rostral ventrolateral medulla. In the rat this region extends ventrally to the medullary surface and occupies an area between the facial nucleus rostrally and the lateral reticular nucleus caudally. The area just caudal to the facial nucleus appears responsible for sympathetic cardiovascular control.[14] The medial two-thirds contain the projection cells to the intermediolateral cell column of the spinal cord from which the sympathetic preganglionic fibers originate. The principal portion of the sympathetic preganglionic output exits from the spinal cord between T1 and the upper lumbar spine.

Brainstem Supramedullary Sites and Cardiac Control

The parabrachial nucleus, which surrounds the brachium conjunctivum in the dorsolateral pons, has emerged as an important brainstem site of cardiovascular function. It serves as the second-order afferent relay for cardiovascular information from the nucleus of the solitary tract, from which it receives its principal afferent input.[15] Cardiovascular afferents are distributed to the lateral parabrachial region. From this region, efferents are distributed to the intralaminar division of the thalamus, the parvocellular portion of the nucleus ventralis posterolateralis, and other thalamic nuclei, from which projections to the sensorimotor, cingulate, infralimbic, frontal, and insular cortex are distributed. In addition, there is a direct projection to the insular cortex. The parabrachial nucleus also projects to the lateral hypothalamic area and the central nucleus of the amygdala; it also innervates brainstem vagal preganglionic sites and the intermediolateral cell column.

Other supramedullary brainstem areas which may be involved in cardiovascular control include the area postrema, the locus ceruleus, the subfornical organ, and the organum vasculosum of the lamina terminalis.

Diencephalic Sites and Cardiac Control

Substantial evidence exists to implicate the hypothalamus in cardiac control. Both anatomically and physiologically, cardiovascular afferent activity has been demonstrated for this region. Calaresu and Ciriello demonstrated that information relayed in the cat baroreceptor nerves projects to the hypothalamus bilaterally, as does the aortic depressor nerve.[16] Anatomically, there is a marked input to this region from cortical and brainstem areas intimately involved in cardiovascular control.

A variety of cardiovascular responses has been elicited on electrical stimulation of the hypothalamus. In anesthetized cats, Melville and colleagues demonstrated that bradycardia and pressor responses were specifically elicited on stimulation of the anterior hypothalamus, and that tachycardia and pressor responses were most likely to be produced by stimulation of the lateral and posterior hypothalamus.[17] However, the nature of the response to electrical stimulation may be state-dependent.

In general terms, the results of such electrical stimulation experiments suggest a division of the hypothalamus into a posteriorly located area of cardioascular sympathetic control and an anterior parasympathetic control region. Different results occur with chemical stimulation (in which case cell bodies alone are stimulated rather than a mixture of these and fibers of passage with electrical stimulation). Spencer and colleagues, using the excitatory amino acid L-glutamate, demonstrated bradycardia and depressor sites within the posterior hypothalamus, chiefly within the periventricular zone caudal to the posterior hypothalamic nucleus.[18] Glutamate stimulation of the posterior hypothalamic nucleus produced minimal bradycardia and depressor effects. Stimulation of the dorsal hypothalamic area resulted in similar responses. Using a similar technique, Gelsema and co-workers microinjected DL-homocysteic acid into various hypothalamic regions and observed the cardiovascular response.[19] Depressor responses accompanied by bradycardia were elicited from the preoptic area, the lateral hypothalamus, and the anterior hypothalamus. Increases in heart rate and blood pressure occurred from the paraventricular nucleus and an area ventral to this along the wall of the third ventricle.

Cardiac arrhythmias can be elicited on stimulation of the hypothalamus. These were first described by Beattie and co-workers.[6] Weinberg and Fuster demonstrated in paralyzed, ventilated cats that ventricular tachycardia was frequently elicited on stimulation of the posterior hypothalamus.[20] This was preceded by prolongation of the QT interval in the electrocardiogram (ECG) and marked increase in the size of the T wave. Shortening of the PR interval was also observed as well as AV dissociation. Several ectopic ventricular pacemakers may be induced by such stimulation. In similar experiments involving stimulation of the ventromedial hypothalamus, Hockman and colleagues showed that incremental intensity of stimulation increased the severity of the rhythm from sinus tachycardia to ventricular ectopy, then to ventricular tachycardia, and ultimately to ventricular fibrillation.[21] On termination of stimulation, this sequence was reversed, and the animal returned to sinus rhythm. Bilateral vagotomy had no effect on the responses. However, intravenous propranolol in the vagotomized animal abolished the effect of hypothalamic stimulation on heart rate and rhythm. This suggested that, under these circumstances, the arrhythmias were of sympathetic origin.

Other diencephalic areas that have been investigated with respect to cardiovascular changes include the thalamus and the zona incerta. In rabbits, microstimulation of the medial thalamus resulted in bradycardia achieved through cholinergic mechanisms, as this response was abolished by vagotomy or by atropine. Propranolol had no effect.[22] The principal area from which this cardiovascular response was elicitable was the mediodorsal nucleus, which has connectivity with the prefrontal cortex. Similar responses were obtained from the thalamic midline nuclei and the parafascicular region and were elicitable in the awake, chronically instrumented preparation. These mediodorsal responses were not altered by ablation of the prefrontal cortex (to which the thalamus projects), implying their generation independently of this area. Interestingly, the responses evoked in these experiments were similar to those seen in rabbits in response to environmental stresses.

Microinjection of L-glutamate into the zona incerta in rats produced a depressor response and a bradycardia that could be incompletely blocked by atropine.[23] The zona incerta is situated in the diencephalon and is bounded ventrally by the cerebral peduncle, dorsally by the medial lemniscus, laterally by the thalamus, and medially by the lateral hypothalamic area.

Many of these injections also involved the subthalamic nucleus, the ventroposterior thalamic complex, and part of the lateral hypothalamic area, so the specificity of the response to the zona incerta remains somewhat in question.

The Amygdala and Cardiac Control

Recent evidence has indicated an important role for the amygdala in the control of cardiovascular function, especially with respect to autonomic-emotional integration. The amygdala is composed of numerous subnuclei, of which the central nucleus appears to play a major role in the elaboration of autonomic responses.[24] There are profuse reciprocal connections to this region from brainstem and cortical regions involved in autonomic control.[25] Baroceptor afferent input to it has been demonstrated in the cat. Zhang and associates showed that the discharges of neurons in this region were related to the cardiac cycle and that their spontaneous firing rate could be changed by stimulation of the aortic depressor nerve and the carotid sinus nerve.[26] Similarly, in humans undergoing surgery for epilepsy, amygdaloid cells have been identified which showed correlations in their firing rate with the cardiac cycle.[27]

Reis and Oliphant demonstrated that changes in heart rate could be produced in squirrel monkeys by stimulation of the amygdala.[28] Both tachycardic and bradycardic responses were encountered, and it was concluded that each had separate representation and projection pathways. Porter and colleagues induced cardiac arrhythmias by stimulation of the feline medial amygdaloid nuclei.[29] Initially, before the arrhythmias became established, stimulation was associated with prolongation of the QT interval, ST-segment changes, and T-wave amplitude increases. These ECG changes persisted on cessation of the stimulus leading to sequential bradycardia, eventually followed by idioventricular escape rhythms and ventricular fibrillation.

Others have shown that ventricular fibrillation induced by coronary ischemia can be aborted by bilateral amygdaloid cooling, but not by similar cooling applied to adjacent areas or by unilateral cryoprobe application.[30]

Cortical Areas and Cardiac Control

Cardiovascular changes were elicited on stimulation of the cortex as early as 1875, when Schiff demonstrated that surface stimulation of the motor cortex resulted in tachycardia accompanied by, but independent of, changes in arterial blood pressure.[31] Cortical areas from which changes in heart rate have been elicited include the sigmoid cortex,[31,32] the frontal lobe and especially the medial agranular region,[33] the temporal pole,[34] and the cingulate gyrus.[34,35]

In the human, Pool and Ransohoff stimulated the rostral cingulate gyrus prior to frontal lobe resection for schizophrenia and depression.[36] Both rises and falls in heart rate and blood pressure were observed, with no evidence of chronotropic organization. Similar responses were obtained from the anterior temporal lobe and the uncus. In the rabbit, cardiovascular changes also have been elicited from the medial frontal cortex.[33] The characteristic response to such midline frontal stimulation was bradycardia associated with a decline in blood pressure. The most marked responses were obtained on stimulation of the orbitofrontal cortex. The anterior midline cortex (orbitofrontal, prelimbic, and infralimbic regions) projects to other cerebral areas involved in autonomic control, which could serve as a substrate for these responses.

In addition to alteration of cardiac chronotropicity, ECG changes indicative of repolarization abnormalities have been reported on stimulation of the feline cerebral cortex. Kenedi and Csanda evoked Q waves, alterations in size and polarity of the T wave and of the QRS complex, and elevation or depression of the ST segment on stimulation of the sigmoid gyrus and the anterior sylvian and ectosylvian gyri.[37]

The few reports of cardiac arrhythmias induced by cortical stimulation include investigations which noted the elicitation of both atrial and ventricular ectopic beats from the cat subiculum,[34] the cingulate gyrus, and the temporal pole.[36] Porter and colleagues were able to induce ventricular fibrillation after a delay of some 6 hours on stimulation of the feline hippocampus[29]; the current strength was large and the mechanism may well have involved kindled seizure activity.

The infrequent elicitation of cardiac responses from the cerebral cortex contrasts with the relative ease with which cardiac arrhythmias and ECG changes can be provoked by stimulation of the hypothalamus and certain brainstem areas.[34,38,39]

The Insular Cortex

The insular cortex is defined as that part of the cerebrum which overlies the claustrum.[40] In primates this region lies buried beneath the frontoparietal and temporal opercula. Anatomical evidence indicates widespread connectivity between the insular cortex and other areas of the brain (such as the lateral hypothalamic area, parabrachial nucleus, and the nucleus of the solitary tract) which are known to be involved in autonomic control. This would strongly suggest a role for the insula in cardiovascular function.

In a series of experiments in which extracellular recordings were made of spontaneously firing cells within the insular cortex of chloralose-anesthetized rats, Cechetto and Saper were able to demonstrate changes in firing pattern in response to a number of peripherally applied stimuli.[41] In this way a viscerotopic map of the insula was obtained. Cardiopulmonary units, sensitive to changes in blood pressure, were located posteriorly in the granular insular cortex.

By systematic exploration of the rat posterior insular cortex using phasic electrical microstimulation, tachycardia was shown to be represented in the rostral posterior insular region and bradycardia in the caudal posterior insula, with some degree of overlap.[42] On prolonged insular stimulation, a stereotyped series of ECG changes was demonstrated: progressive atrio-

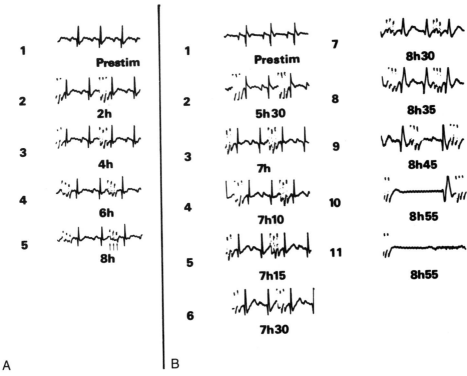

Fig. 10-1 ECG changes induced by prolonged stimulation of the insular cortex in rats. **(A)** The effects of stimulation in the frontoparietal cortex. There is little change in the ECG after 8 hours of stimulation. **(B)** The effects of prolonged stimulation within the insular cortex: progressive lengthening of the QT interval occurs, with increasing degrees of heart block, idioventricular rhythm, and finally asystole. The arrows indicate stimulation artifact, and the numbers indicate time from stimulation onset. (From Oppenheimer SM, Wilson JX, Guiraudon C, Cechetto DF: Insular cortex stimulation produces lethal cardiac arrhythmias: a mechanism of sudden death? Brain Res 550:115, 1991, with permission.)

ventricular block leading to complete heart block, interventricular block, QT-interval prolongation, ST-segment depression, ventricular ectopy, and finally death in asystole,[43] as shown in Figure 10-1. Stimulation in the adjacent piriform or frontoparietal cortex was without effect on the ECG.

Changes in the ECG were directly correlated with the presence of myocytolysis (Fig. 10-2) in the stimu-

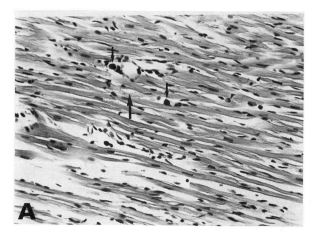

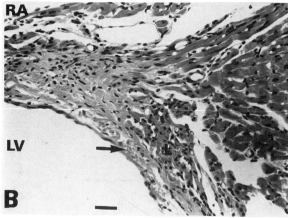

Fig. 10-2 Myocytolysis induced by insular cortex stimulation. **(A)** The effects of prolonged insular cortex stimulation on the heart (hematoxylin and eosin stain). Scattered foci of myocardial fiber necrosis are seen *(thick arrow)* in this coronal section, with surrounding areas of monocytic infiltration *(thin arrows)*. **(B)** This sagittal section (Movats stain) shows a large subendocardial hemorrhage *(thick arrow)* adjacent to the origin of the left branch of the bundle of His. The cavity of the left ventricle is designated *LV,* and of the right atrium, *RA*. The scale bar represents 50 μm. (From Oppenheimer SM, Wilson JX, Guiraudon C, Cechetto DF: Insular cortex stimulation produces lethal cardiac arrhythmias: a mechanism of sudden death? Brain Res 550:115, 1991, with permission.)

lated rats and with the demonstration of hemorrhages adjacent to the conducting system at the origin of the left branch of the bundle of His.[43] Myocytolysis represents a condition of diffuse damage to ventricular myocytes, probably on a neurogenic basis and induced by overactivation of intrinsic cardiac sympathetic nerves (see below). The presence of these changes also correlated with a significant elevation in plasma norepinephrine but not epinephrine concentrations, signifying an extra-adrenal, neural source.

These recent findings identify for the first time a site of cardiac chronotropic organization within a cortical site, from which cardiac arrhythmias can also be produced on prolonged stimulation. This suggests that the insular cortex may be of importance in cardiac regulation. Because of its profuse connectivity with the limbic system, it is suggested that the insula is involved in the modulation of cardiac rate and rhythm under conditions of emotional stress, and it may be important in the genesis of cardiac arrhythmias under these circumstances in patients with compromised hearts. In addition, when involved by acute neurological processes, such as stroke, insular activation may be involved in the ECG changes and cardiac arrhythmias documented in these circumstances, as discussed below.

STROKE AND THE HEART

The most important advances in our understanding of the way in which the heart and brain interact in neurological disease have come from clinical observations in patients with strokes. There has been extensive documentation of stroke-induced ECG changes over the past 50 years, first as occasional isolated case reports and more recently in systematic studies. One of the problems, however, with the analysis of such data is the confounding influence of associated symptomatic and asymptomatic ischemic cardiac disease. The incidence of asymptomatic coronary artery disease in patients with stroke has been investigated.[44] Coronary arteriography demonstrated coronary artery stenosis of more than 70 percent in 40 percent of patients. Nonetheless, the evidence that stroke can create cardiac lesions and result in cardiac arrhythmias even in the absence of significant coronary atherosclerosis is substantial.

The commonest cause of death after stroke is from

cardiac disturbances.[2,3] It is very likely that this represents either the effect of the cerebral lesion itself or an interaction between symptomatic or asymptomatic coronary artery lesions and the brain lesion. In addition, approximately 6 percent of patients with acute ischemic stroke die suddenly and unexpectedly during the first month of admission.[45] This is not related to the patients' neurological condition and affects not only those seriously compromised by their stroke but also those minimally limited. Consequently, understanding the mechanisms influencing cardiac prognosis may be of paramount importance in improving survival in such patients.

Stroke and the Electrocardiogram

The earliest report of the association between acute stroke and ECG changes was in 1947, when Byer and colleagues described four patients with strokes and changes initially attributed to acute myocardial infarction.[46] At least two of the patients suffered subarachnoid hemorrhage. It was decided that the ECG changes were not of ischemic cardiac origin on the basis of their development following admission, during the acute phase of the patients' illness. A few years later, Burch and colleagues investigated this phenomenon in a more structured way.[47] Among 17 patients, the commonest abnormalities developing in association with stroke onset involved primarily the repolarization phase of the ECG. Thus, prolongations of the QT interval, together with inversion or increased amplitude of the T wave and septal U waves, were the most frequent abnormalities. Such changes are illustrated in Figure 10-3. Fourteen patients had had either subarachnoid or intracerebral hemorrhage, and in this small series, uncontrolled for the incidence of associated cardiovascular disease, ECG changes were commonest following subarachnoid hemorrhage. More recent studies, albeit in small patient samples, have suggested that the incidence of repolarization changes is 5 to 17 percent after acute ischemic stroke and 60 to 70 percent after acute intracerebral or subarachnoid

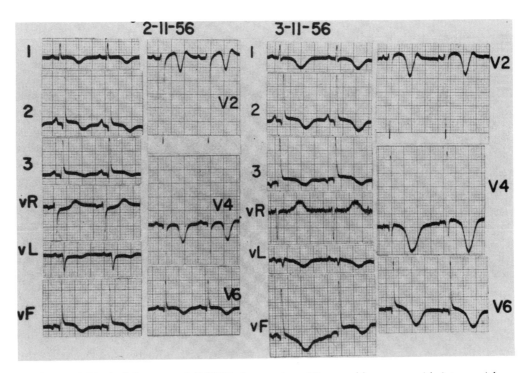

Fig. 10-3 Typical "neurogenic" ECG changes in a 55-year-old woman with intracranial hemorrhage. Autopsy revealed a normal heart. (From Cropp GJ, Manning GW: Electrocardiographic changes simulating myocardial ischemia and infarction associated with spontaneous intracranial hemorrhage. Circulation 22:25, 1960, with permission.)

hemorrhage.[48] However, the majority of these studies did not control for the incidence of concomitant ischemic cardiac disease.

A few studies have attempted to control for the association between ischemic coronary and cerebrovascular disease. The extent to which this has been successful is debatable and there is clearly a need for this work to be repeated with newer, noninvasive techniques, including thallium scintigraphy. In fact, an argument can be made for undertaking coronary angiography in all patients who have had a stroke, because the evidence suggests that such patients are at greater risk for a cardiac event than a repeated stroke.[2,3] Dimant and Grob compared ECG recordings from 100 consecutive patients with acute stroke (ischemic stroke, intracerebral hemorrhage, and subarachnoid hemorrhage) taken within 3 days of admission with those from age- and sex-matched patients admitted for carcinoma of the colon.[49] ST depression and prolongation of the QT interval were seven times more frequent in patients after acute cerebrovascular events than in the control patients; T-wave inversion and ventricular premature beats were four times more common. Although this might be taken to suggest an association between stroke and ECG changes, ischemic heart disease was three times more prevalent in the stroke group than among the controls. Moreover, it is assumed that the prevalence of asymptomatic coronary artery disease was the same in the two populations, an assumption that may not be justifiable.

Lavy and colleagues reviewed the ECGs of patients with acute ischemic stroke or intracerebral hemorrhage.[50] Patients were included in the study if they denied a history of heart disease and had a normal recording either shortly prior to or following their admission. Among 18 recruited patients with an ischemic stroke, 8 (44 percent) showed either a recent-onset "ischemia pattern" ECG or a cardiac arrhythmia (precise cardiac details were lacking); of 7 patients with intracerebral hemorrhage and no evidence of previous cardiac disease, 5 (70 percent) demonstrated the new onset of cardiac arrhythmias.

In the most detailed and largest study to date, a comparison of the ECGs of 53 patients with acute cerebrovascular disease (subarachnoid hemorrhage, intracerebral hemorrhage, and ischemic stroke) taken within 24 hours of admission was made with tracings taken on average 4 months earlier.[51] The control group comprised 63 patients matched for age and sex, admitted for nonvascular reasons, and whose previous tracings were also available. Abnormal prolongation of the QT interval not seen in previous recordings was observed in 32 percent of the stroke group and in 2 percent of the controls. New T-wave inversion was apparent in 15 percent of the stroke group and abnormal U waves in 13 percent; neither appeared as a new feature in the admission ECGs of the control group. These differences were highly significant. It seems unlikely that the new ECG findings resulted entirely from the coincidence of acute cerebrovascular and cardiac events or that the strokes in all these patients were due to a cardioembolic cause. However, concerns can be raised about this study. For example, it is not clear to what extent computed tomography (CT) was used to augment the clinical diagnosis. Moreover, comparison of ECGs with previous tracings, with a mean interval between recordings as long as 4 months, really does not preclude changes occurring prior to stroke onset, because of the length of the delay.

Stroke and Cardiac Pathology

The circumstantial evidence from the three controlled studies mentioned above implies that although ischemic coronary artery disease may contribute to the production of acute ECG changes, it is unlikely to be the only operative mechanism. However, none of the studies has been sufficiently well controlled to resolve this issue. More direct information has been gathered from autopsy studies. A high incidence of ECG changes has been noted following subarachnoid hemorrhage, and patients with such hemorrhage are often young and would not be expected to have significant ischemic heart disease. Cropp and Manning identified 29 patients who had developed ECG changes following subarachnoid hemorrhage; 8 patients died and 5 were autopsied.[52] None showed evidence of coronary artery disease or myocardial ischemia. Similar findings were noted by others.[53,54] In Goldstein's study, 8 of the 37 patients who died were autopsied.[51] All of these had elevated circulating creatine kinase (CK) levels and had died from an intracerebral hemorrhage. No evidence of an acute ischemic cardiac event was found. Again, in a series of patients with acute cerebral infarcts confirmed by autopsy, none of the patients who died and who had

ECG abnormalities showed evidence of coronary artery occlusion.[55] Connor also reported a patient who died following cerebral infarction from carotid occlusion without autopsy evidence of coronary artery stenosis.[56]

If coronary artery disease does not entirely explain the ECG changes following stroke, what else accounts for them? In 1933, Neuburger described scattering subendocardial hemorrhages in patients dying during epileptic seizures.[57] Subsequently these were observed in patients dying within a few days of onset of a stroke.[58] Greenhoot and Reichenbach noted that the cardiac pathology (termed *myocytolysis*) following stroke encompassed a wider range of changes than just subendocardial hemorrhage.[58] These included scattered foci of swollen myocytes surrounded by infiltrating monocytes; interstitial hemorrhages; and myofibrillary degeneration. Moreover, the lesions were centered on intracardiac nerves rather than blood vessels, suggesting that humoral or ischemic factors were unlikely to play a causal role.

Changes in myocardial formazan granule deposition have been observed in the tetrazolium-treated hearts of patients dying after acute cerebrovascular events.[59] These precede histological evidence of myocytolysis (Fig. 10-4). Kolin and Norris showed such changes in 89 percent of patients dying following subarachnoid hemorrhage, in 71 percent of those dying after an intracerebral hemorrhage and in 52 percent after ischemic strokes.[59] Similar abnormalities were seen in only 26 percent of hearts from control patients dying of other causes.

The mechanism of myocytolysis probably relates to excessive sympathoadrenal activation. Indeed, plasma catecholamine levels following stroke are significant elevated compared with control groups.[60] Myocytolysis may be induced by catecholamine infusion in animals or humans and is associated with pheochromocytoma.[61] Similar changes are induced by stimulation of the canine left stellate ganglion.[62] Moreover, the ECG changes following stroke may be mimicked by norepinephrine or epinephrine infusion.[63,64] Both the ECG changes and the myocardial damage following subarachnoid hemorrhage can be abolished by phentolamine and propranolol.[65] It is therefore likely that sympathoadrenal tone can be elevated by stroke producing myocardial damage evidenced by ECG and CK changes.

Stroke and Plasma Creatine Kinase Levels

It could be argued that pathological changes in the heart are seen only in patients so compromised by their stroke that they subsequently die. However, there is evidence for the occurrence of cardiac damage following acute stroke in patients who do not die. Certain enzymes are released from damaged myocardial fibers, and their presence in blood is considered a marker for cardiac damage. One such enzyme is CK. Dimant and Grob found elevated plasma CK levels in 29 percent of patients admitted following acute stroke; none of the control group had raised plasma enzyme levels.[49] The presence of increased levels correlated with an increased incidence of T-wave inversion, ST depression, and conduction defects on the ECG. Mortality was higher in those patients with stroke and elevated plasma CK levels compared with those whose levels were within the normal range. In Goldstein's study, no correlation was established between ECG abnormalities and raised plasma CK levels.[51] However, mortality was increased in those patients with the higher enzyme levels. It should be noted that neither of these studies specifically measured the cardiac isoenzyme component of the plasma total CK levels. Elevations of unfractionated CK may be due to other factors such as skeletal muscle damage, which may have contributed to the observed increases.

Norris and co-workers investigated changes in serum concentration of the cardiac isoenzyme CK-MB following stroke.[66] Elevations of this enzyme can be specifically attributed to cardiac damage. Although 44 percent of all the 230 strokes investigated were found to have raised total CK levels in the serum, the specific cardiac isoenzyme (CK-MB) was elevated in only 11 percent. Despite the total plasma CK being raised in 66 percent of control patients, no increase in the specific cardiac isoenzyme occurred except in those with obvious cardiac causes. A significant correlation was demonstrated between elevation of CK-MB and the presence of ECG changes and cardiac arrhythmias after stroke.

Following myocardial infarction, circulating levels of CK-MB rise abruptly and have reached their peak by 24 hours. However, after stroke, CK-MB levels rise more slowly and reach a peak approximately 4 days after the event.[66] This difference in pattern is

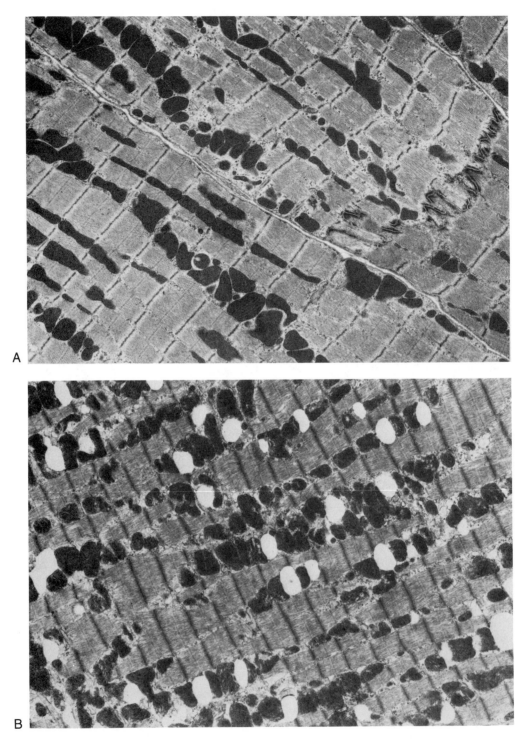

Fig. 10-4 Electron micrographs showing **(A)** normal gerbil cardiac muscle (control) and **(B)** gerbil cardiac muscle 16 hours after cerebral infarction produced by carotid ligation. Note the accumulation of fat globules due to disordered myocardial metabolism secondary to neurogenic damage. (Original magnification × 5,000.) (Courtesy of Dr. A. Kolin and Dr. A. Brezina, Department of Pathology, University of Toronto.)

further evidence against the ischemic nature of the associated cardiac injury.

Stroke and Cardiac Arrhythmias

The ECG effects described indicate changes in ventricular depolarization. This is associated with the development of cardiac arrhythmias, especially of a ventricular nature. Lavy and co-workers demonstrated a 39 percent incidence of new arrhythmias (including ventricular arrhythmias) following acute stroke in patients not known to have previous heart disease.[50] In a similar study, Goldstein found a 25 percent incidence of new arrhythmias after acute stroke, compared with an incidence of 3 percent in controls.[51] Of these cardiac arrhythmias, the commonest was atrial fibrillation (9 percent). The new onset of atrial fibrillation after hospital admission did not occur in the control group. It is conceivable—but somewhat unlikely—that the strokes in this group of patients were all caused by embolization from the heart attendant on the development of atrial fibrillation. In Goldstein's study, there was no difference in the incidence of new ventricular arrhythmias between the stroke and control groups. In a study of intracerebral hemorrhage in patients without a history of heart disease and where recent preictal ECGs were unremarkable, the incidence of ventricular arrhythmias was 10 percent.[67] This correlated with the presence of a temporoparietal hemorrhage on CT scan. In another study, in which the ECG taken within 3 days of the patients' admission was compared with ECGs taken during a similar time course in patients with carcinoma of the colon,[49] atrial fibrillation was the most common arrhythmia (21 percent); ventricular arrhythmias occurred with a frequency of 13 percent. For the control group, the figures were respectively 2 and 3 percent. No allowance was made for preexisting heart disease.

In these studies, patients were not investigated by continuous cardiac recording but by single 12-lead ECG recordings often taken at an unspecified time after stroke onset. This probably underrepresents the incidence of ventricular arrhythmias, which are often of short duration. Moreover, cardiac embolization from atrial fibrillation of recent onset may account for the apparent frequency of this arrhythmia among patients with ischemic stroke. These considerations may explain the discrepancy between the nature of the arrhythmias anticipated from the ventricular repolarization changes that occur after stroke and their observed frequency after stroke.

When data from Holter monitoring are available, the incidence of ventricular arrhythmias is higher. In one study, 60 percent of patients demonstrated ventricular arrhythmias[68]; in another, the figure was 24 percent.[67] Unfortunately, neither of these studies controlled for preexisting cardiac disease.

In studies of cardiac rhythm disturbances following subarachnoid hemorrhage, ventricular arrhythmias are exceptionally common and correlate with prolongation of the QT interval (as one might expect).[69] The overall incidence of cardiac arrhythmias reaches 98 percent in this condition, with multifocal ventricular premature beats occurring in 54 percent of patients, couplets in 40 percent, and unsustained ventricular tachycardia in 29 percent.[70] Torsades de pointes, a highly malignant form of ventricular arrhythmia that is exceptionally difficult to treat, has been reported in 4 percent of such patients.[69] No association with a history of cardiac disease has been noted. Patients with subarachnoid hemorrhage are frequently admitted to intensive care units and consequently are routinely submitted to continuous cardiac monitoring, which is likely to detect ventricular rhythm disturbances. This could account for the frequency with which ventricular arrhythmias are detected in this condition compared with strokes of other causes. In addition, atrial fibrillation is infrequently encountered after subarachnoid hemorrhage, as embolization from a cardiac source (of which the commonest is atrial fibrillation) plays no part in the etiology of this condition. However, the effects of a subarachnoid hemorrhage are seldom unifocal; vasospasm, raised intracranial pressure, and ventricular and intracerebral hemorrhages often occur and produce multiple effects in the neuraxis. This plethora of intracerebral events may well influence cardiac dynamics in a different fashion than a unifocal lesion and generate a different variety and frequency of arrhythmias.

If stroke-induced ECG effects lead to an increase in the incidence of malignant cardiac arrhythmias, this should unfavorably prejudice prognosis. A mortality of 80 percent occurs in those patients demonstrating malignant ventricular arrhythmias (tachycardia, fibrillation, asystole) compared with 23 percent in patients with strokes who do not show these changes.[51]

No other ECG parameter reflected mortality which also did not correlate with a history of ischemic heart disease. Lavy and co-workers found a mortality of 69 percent in patients with ischemic or intracerebral hemorrhagic stroke and the new onset of ECG changes (ST-segment or T-wave changes, or arrhythmias) on admission.[50] This compared with a mortality of 0 percent in patients without ECG changes.

In the case of subarachnoid hemorrhage, the presence of QT interval prolongation, ST-wave depression, or abnormal U waves is associated with the angiographic demonstration of vasospasm and a poor prognosis.[71] There appears to be no correlation with a history of cardiac disease or with the patients' neurological state.[69]

The nature of the ECG changes and the pattern of the associated pathology indicates that increased sympathoadrenal tone may be involved in the genesis of cardiac arrhythmias after stroke, but the precise mechanism is unclear. There is evidence for a specific, noradrenergic sodium channel on cardiac myocytes, whose activation depolarizes the cell membrane and predisposes to repetitive discharges.[72] This may be arrhythmogenic in itself and also could ultimately enhance calcium influx, leading to cellular damage via activation of intracellular proteases. The pathological correlate of this is probably myocytolysis. Alternatively or additionally, acute stroke may interfere with the normal patterning of activity within the cardiac sympathetic nerves. When this becomes desynchronized between the various sympathetic nerve branches and also in relation to vagal neural traffic, arrhythmias may result. Evidence for this comes from the elegant studies of Lathers (discussed below).

Other possible mechanisms of stroke-induced cardiac changes include coronary arterial vasoconstriction. There is profuse sympathetic innervation of the coronary vasculature. Coronary artery vasoconstriction has been induced by stimulating various neuraxial centers—especially the hypothalamus, central tegmental tract, and medial longitudinal fasciculus[73]—and results in changes in ST segments in the ECG. In addition, ST-segment elevation can be induced by stress in patients lacking evidence of atheromatous coronary arterial disease. This suggests that ECG changes can be evoked by limbic activation, possibly by means of the connectivity with the insular cortex (see p. 187). Such patients demonstrating coronary artery spasm have an increased incidence of sud-

den unexpected death, presumably from malignant ventricular arrhythmias.[74]

Stroke and the Insular Cortex

In animal models of stroke, myocytolysis can only be demonstrated on cardiac examination if the insular cortex is involved in the infarcted region.[75] More recently, infarction involving the insula in an animal model of stroke was associated with increased renal sympathetic nerve activity, prolongation of the QT interval (which is a frequent ECG accompaniment of acute stroke), and elevated norepinephrine levels.[76] The insular cortex is a frequent site of seizure activity. Abnormal efferent traffic from this region to brainstem sites involved in autonomic control, such as may occur during a seizure, may be arrhythmogenic. This may especially be so if anticonvulsant medication has been recently and abruptly stopped (one of the concomitants of the sudden unexpected epileptic death syndrome, as discussed below) or if the insular cortex is structurally abnormal, as from atrophy or cortical heterotopias in certain epileptics. It may therefore be that stroke alters cardiovascular tone either by directly damaging the insular cortex or by damaging interrelated adjacent areas, thereby shifting the balance toward a predominance of sympathetic activation and leading to cardiac arrhythmias by the mechanisms already outlined.

Stroke Laterality and Cardiac Effects

More than three decades ago, Penfield and colleagues stimulated the human insula and were unable to show any changes in cardiovascular parameters.[77] We recently undertook similar studies in patients undergoing temporal lobectomy for the control of intractable seizures.[78] Although changes (either increases or decreases) in blood pressure and heart rate could be obtained by stimulation of either insula, bradycardia and a reduction in blood pressure were obtained with greater frequency from the left anterior insular cortex than the right. This suggested a greater sympathetic cardiovascular representation in the right anterior insula. It is unclear whether this is true for the normal population, however, because it is unknown to what extent the responses were altered by years of anticonvulsant therapy and the effect of recurrent temporal lobe seizures on insular organization. Nevertheless, there is some circumstantial evidence to support the contention of cortical lateralization. Chapman and colleagues stimulated the temporal lobe tip in a schizophrenic patient and induced elevations in blood pressure that were greater with stimulation of the right than left temporal tip.[79] Zamrini and colleagues demonstrated that infusion of amylobarbital into the left internal carotid artery during the Wada test was associated with tachycardia, whereas the converse occurred with right internal carotid artery infusion.[80] In addition, Lane demonstrated that right hemisphere (middle cerebral artery) stroke in humans was associated with a significantly increased incidence of supraventricular tachyarrhythmias compared to similar left-sided stroke.[81]

In a rat model of stroke, we recently compared the effects of left and right middle cerebral artery occlusion on sympathetic tone.[76] Under normal circumstances during urethane anesthesia, blood pressure progressively falls; this was the case with left but not right middle cerebral artery occlusion. With right-sided occlusion, plasma norepinephrine but not epinephrine (implying a neural source) was significantly elevated and there was, compared with left-sided occlusion, a significant prolongation of the QT interval in the ECG.

Unpublished experiments from our laboratory indicate that stimulation in the frontoparietal cortex surrounding the insula actually decreases sympathoadrenal tone. This could imply an inhibitory effect of this area of surrounding cortex on the insula. This, together with the above studies, suggests that stroke involving the right frontoparietal cortex but sparing the insula may be especially arrhythmogenic in that it may augment cardiac sympathetic tone, leading to myocytolysis, changes in ECG repolarization, cardiac arrhythmias, and possibly sudden death.

EPILEPSY AND THE HEART

Epilepsy is the other major acute neurological condition associated with significant cardiac changes. Experimental consideration of the neurocardiological effects of seizures has broadened our understanding of how alterations in the relative firing patterns of various parasympathetic and sympathetic cardiac nerve branches may lead to significant cardiac arrhythmias.

Clinical study of the changes in heart rate accompanying seizures helps to explain the phenomenon of sudden unexpected death in epileptic patients.

Sinus tachycardia is the most common rhythm disturbance associated with a seizure.[82] The commonest ECG change is flattening of the T wave, which occurs in 25 percent of cases. In patients with temporal lobe seizures, tachycardias are of abrupt onset and offset, preceding or accompanying the aura and unassociated with movement.[83] This suggests that the changes in cardiac rhythm are related to the epileptic discharge. In a study of generalized seizures induced with pentylenetetrazol, tachycardia accompanied every seizure.[84] In addition, frequent atrial and ventricular ectopic rhythms were noted, and there were occasional runs of ventricular tachycardia. The ECG showed depression or elevation of the ST segment and inversion of the T wave. These findings have been confirmed in more recent studies using simultaneous ambulatory electroencephalographic (EEG)/ECG monitoring.[85] Sinus tachycardia occurring at the time of the seizure was seen in 91 percent of these recordings. Cardiac arrhythmias were identified in 52 percent of all seizures and most frequently comprised a marked beat-to-beat variation in the R-R interval accompanied by changes in P-wave shape. One patient had recurrent episodes of supraventricular tachycardia associated with seizure onset, and three had frequent ventricular extrasystoles. Sinus bradycardia was seen in only one patient.[85] In other studies, two cases of sinus arrest associated with the ictus have been reported.[86,87]

Occasionally, patients are investigated for a cardiac arrhythmia and subsequently found to have an epileptic rather than a primary cardiac cause. Walsh reported a 4-year-old boy who was repeatedly investigated for paroxysmal supraventricular tachycardia.[88] EEGs disclosed generalized spike-wave discharges statistically associated with shortening of the R-R interval and leading, on occasion, to episodes of supraventricular tachycardia. Two similar cases were investigated with intensive cardiac electrophysiological techniques without finding an intrinsic cardiac cause for the arrhythmia.[89,90] In both, a temporal lobe focus was detected on the EEG. None of these three patients responded to conventional cardiac antiarrhythmic medications; all responded well to antiepileptic medication.

Arrhythmias have also been produced by photic

stimulation. In one reported patient with secondarily generalized seizures, complete sinus arrest coincided with the onset of photically induced spike-wave activity and necessitated cardiac resuscitation procedures.[91] Sinus bradycardias and tachycardias have frequently been elicited in photosensitive epileptic patients using this technique.[92]

Sudden unexpected death is a feared complication of epilepsy. It occurs in an otherwise healthy patient in the absence of trauma, status epilepticus, aspiration, or other identifiable cause.[93–95] The cause is thought to be malignant ventricular arrhythmia. There has been one documented case of sudden cardiac collapse of an epileptic patient undergoing cardiac monitoring[96]; ventricular fibrillation of acute onset was noted, from which the patient could not be resuscitated. The incidence of sudden unexpected cardiac death in epilepsy has been estimated at between 0.05 and 0.2 percent.[93] Affected patients are usually young and have infrequent, well-controlled tonic-clonic seizures (sometimes associated with complex partial seizures) diagnosed for longer than 1 year. They are usually found dead in bed or after an otherwise typical seizure. Their anticonvulsant levels are often subtherapeutic. At autopsy, no satisfactory cause of death is found.[93–95]

The mechanism by which cortical activity leads to cardiac arrhythmia and death is suggested by the work of Lathers.[97,98] In an experimental cat model of epilepsy, increasing doses of pentylenetetrazol were injected systemically and caused increasing frequency of cortical spike activity. Recordings were made from the cardiac vagus nerve and from two different branches of the cardiac sympathetic nerve. Occasional ventricular ectopic beats occurred, together with PR-, ST-, and QT-segment changes in the ECG. As the dose of pentylenetetrazol was increased, there was an increase in cardiac arrhythmicity that corresponded with desynchronization of firing between the vagus and sympathetic nerves. The firing pattern and its desynchronization corresponded well with the increase in ictal cortical discharges. At high doses of pentylenetetrazol, the animals died either in asystole or in ventricular fibrillation. In the former case there was an abrupt cessation of all cardiac neural traffic; in the latter situation, there was a marked increase in neural discharge in one branch of the cardiac sympathetic nerve and a decrease in the other. Bursts of activity within the cardiac sympathetic nerves were synchronized with the ictal and interictal spikes. The degree of synchronization was variable and depended on the branch of the sympathetic nerve from which recordings were made. Imbalance in the firing pattern of various cardiac sympathetic nerve branches and between the sympathetic and parasympathetic systems produces inhomogeneity in cardiac depolarization and repolarization, allowing the appearance of irritable foci, reentrant circuits, and ventricular ectopic activity and ventricular fibrillation.[99]

TREATMENT

Routine prophylaxis for cardiac arrhythmias is not advocated for cerebral infarction or intracerebral hemorrhage at this time. This situation may change in the near future, once investigations have revealed which ECG features, stroke locations, and shifts in cardiac autonomic tone are strongly predictive of the occurrence of malignant cardiac arrhythmias. In the interim, ventricular tachyarrhythmias or supraventricular arrhythmias which compromise cardiac output should be treated with standard antiarrhythmic therapy once they occur. Patients whose QT interval is prolonged by such treatment or by anticonvulsants should be carefully monitored. Patients with sinus tachycardia and a normal or elevated blood pressure after subarachnoid hemorrhage should be treated with prophylactic β-blockade, as their cardiovascular sympathetic tone is probably elevated and the incidence of malignant ventricular arrhythmias is high in this condition.

CONCLUDING COMMENT

The evidence suggests overwhelmingly that cardiac arrhythmias may occur in relation to stroke and epilepsy in the absence of concomitant cardiac disease. In both human studies and experimental animal models, stroke increases sympathetic tone. Shifts in autonomic tone from parasympathetic to sympathetic predominance can induce ventricular ectopy.[100] β-Adrenergic blockers reduce the incidence of ventricular fibrillation in experimental myocardial ischemia.[101] Recently it has become possible to study noninvasively in humans the relative interactions between the parasympathetic and sympathetic nervous systems on the heart. The techniques used involve spectral analysis of the resting RR interval (using fast Fourier transforms). The presence of sustained shifts toward sympathetic dominance strongly predicts arrhythmic death after myocardial infarction. The same is likely to be true of stroke. The increased sympathetic tone may have a variety of cardiac effects: myocytolysis, direct arrhythmogenesis by an effect on sodium channels in cardiac myocytes, neurogenic vasospasm, and platelet activation within the coronary vasculature. In patients with ischemic heart disease, it is suggested that these mechanisms are compounded and may produce more severe effects. This may partly account for the ascendancy of cardiac events as the leading cause of death in such neurological conditions as stroke.

In the case of epilepsy, irregular activation of hemispheric sites of cardiac control, in association with sudden decreases in anticonvulsant levels (which have a stabilizing effect on cardiac membranes), can lead to similar shifts in autonomic balance as those seen following stroke. The consequent production of malignant cardiac arrhythmias may result in sudden cardiac death.

REFERENCES

1. Liberthson RR, Nagel EL, Hirschman JC, et al: Pathophysiological observations in prehospital ventricular fibrillation and sudden cardiac death. Circulation 49:790, 1974
2. North American Symptomatic Carotid Endarterectomy Trial Collaborators: Beneficial effect of carotid endarterectomy in symptomatic patients with high-grade stenosis. N Engl J Med 325:445, 1991
3. Hass WK, Easton JD, Adams HP, et al: A randomized trial comparing ticlopidine hydrochloride with aspirin for the prevention of stroke in high-risk patients. N Engl J Med 321:501, 1989
4. Levy AG: The exciting causes of ventricular fibrillation in animals under chloroform anaesthesia. Heart 4:319, 1913
5. Levy AG: Further remarks on ventricular extrasystoles and fibrillation under chloroform. Heart 7:105, 1919
6. Beattie J, Brow GR, Long CNH: Physiological and anatomical evidence for the existence of nerve tracts connecting the hypothalamus with spinal sympathetic centres. Proc R Soc Lond (Biol) 106:253: 1930
7. Kalia M, Mesulam MM: Brain stem projections of sensory and motor components of the vagus complex in the cat: II. Laryngeal, tracheobronchial, pulmonary, cardiac, and gastrointestinal branches. J Comp Neurol 193:467, 1980
8. Housley GD, Martin-Body RL, Dawson NJ, Sinclair JD: Brain stem projections of the glossopharyngeal nerve and its carotid sinus branch in the rat. Neuroscience 22:237, 1987
9. ter Horst GJ, Luiten PGM, Kuipers F: Descending pathways from hypothalamus to dorsal motor vagus and ambiguus nuclei in the rat. J Auton Nerv Syst 11: 59, 1984
10. Thompson ME, Felsten G, Yavorsky J, Natelson BH: Differential effect of stimulation of nucleus ambiguus on atrial and ventricular rates. Am J Physiol 253:R150, 1987
11. Shapiro RE, Miselis RR: The central organization of the vagus nerve innervating the stomach of the rat. J Comp Neurol 238:473, 1985
12. Hopkins DA: The dorsal motor nucleus of the vagus nerve and the nucleus ambiguus: structure and connections. p. 185. In Hainsworth R, McWilliam PN, Mary DASG (eds): Cardiogenic Reflexes. Oxford University Press, Oxford, 1987
13. Nosaka S, Yasunaga K, Tamai S: Vagal cardiac preganglionic neurons: distribution, cell types, and reflex discharges. Am J Physiol 243:R92, 1982
14. Gebber GL: Central determinants of sympathetic nerve discharge. p. 126. In Loewy AD, Spyer KM (eds): Central Regulation of Autonomic Functions. Oxford University Press, New York, 1990
15. Loewy AD: Central autonomic pathways. p. 88. In Loewy AD, Spyer KM (eds): Central Regulation of Autonomic Functions. Oxford University Press, New York, 1990
16. Calaresu FR, Ciriello J: Projections to the hypothalamus from buffer nerves and nucleus tractus solitarius. Am J Physiol 239:R130, 1980
17. Melville KI, Blum B, Shister HE, Silver MD: Cardiac ischemic changes and arrhythmias induced by hypothalamic stimulation. Am J Cardiol 12:781, 1963
18. Spencer SE, Sawyer WB, Loewy AD: L-Glutamate mapping of cardioreactive areas in the rat posterior hypothalamus. Brain Res 511:149, 1990
19. Gelsema AJ, Roe MJ, Calaresu FR: Neurally mediated cardiovascular responses to stimulation of cell bodies in the hypothalamus of the rat. Brain Res 482:67, 1989
20. Weinberg SJ, Fuster JM: Electrocardiographic changes produced by localized hypothalamic stimulations. Ann Intern Med 53:332, 1960
21. Hockman CH, Mauck HP, Hoff EC: ECG changes resulting from cerebral stimulation: II. A spectrum

of ventricular arrhythmias of sympathetic origin. Am Heart J 71:695, 1966

22. West CHK, Benjamin RM: Effects of stimulation of the mediodorsal nucleus and its projection cortex on heart rate in the rabbit. J Auton Nerv Syst 9:547, 1983

23. Spencer SE, Sawyer WB, Loewy AD: L-Glutamate stimulation of the zona incerta in the rat decreases heart rate and blood pressure. Brain Res 458:72, 1988

24. Price JL, Russchen FT, Amaral DG: The limbic region: II. The amygdaloid complex. p. 279. In Bjorklund A, Hökfelt T, Swanson LW (eds): Handbook of Chemical Neuroanatomy. Vol 5. Elsevier, Amsterdam, 1987

25. Yasui Y, Breder CD, Saper CB, Cechetto DF: Autonomic responses and efferent pathways from the insular cortex in the rat. J Comp Neurol 303:355, 1990

26. Zhang JX, Harper RR, Frysinger RC: Respiratory modulation of neuronal discharge in the central nucleus of the amygdala during sleep and waking states. Exp Neurol 91:193, 1986

27. Frysinger RC, Harper RM: Cardiac and respiratory correlations with unit discharge in epileptic human temporal lobe. Epilepsia 31:162, 1990

28. Reis DJ, Oliphant MC: Bradycardia and tachycardia following electrical stimulation of the amygdaloid region in monkey. J Neurophysiol 27:893, 1964

29. Porter RW, Kamikawa K, Greenhoot JH: Persistent electrocardiographic abnormalities experimentally induced by stimulation of the brain. Am Heart J 64:815, 1962

30. Carpeggiani C, Landisman C, Montaron MF, Skinner JE: Cryoblockade in limbic brain (amygdala) prevents or delays ventricular fibrillation after coronary artery occlusion in psychologically stressed pigs. Circ Res 70:600, 1992

31. Schiff M: Untersuchungen ueber die motorischen Functionen des Grosshirns. Naunyn Schmiedebergs Arch Exp Pathol Pharmakol 3:171, 1875

32. Cerevkov A: Ueber den einfluss der Gehirnhemisphaeren auf das Herz und auf das Gefassystem. Guseff, Kharkov, 1892

33. Buchanan SL, Valentine J, Powell DA: Autonomic responses are elicited by electrical stimulation of the medial but not lateral frontal cortex in rabbits. Behav Brain Res 18:51, 1985

34. MacLean P: Discussion. Physiol Rev 40, suppl 4: 114, 1960

35. Ueda H: Arrhythmias produced by cerebral stimulation. Jpn Circ J 26:225, 1962

36. Pool JL, Ransohoff J: Autonomic effects on stimulating rostral portion of cingulate gyri in man. J Neurophysiol 12:385, 1949

37. Kenedi I, Csanda E: Electrocardiographic changes in response to electrical stimulation of the cerebral cortex. Acta Physiol Acad Sci Hung 16:165, 1959

38. Allen WF: An experimentally produced premature systolic arrhythmia (pulsus bigeminus) in rabbits. Am J Physiol 98:344, 1931

39. Manning JW, Cotten M de V: Mechanism of cardiac arrhythmias induced by diencephalic stimulation. Am J Physiol 203:1120, 1962

40. Rose M: Die inselrinde des Menschen und der Tiere. J Psychol Neurol 37:467, 1928

41. Cechetto DF, Saper CB: Evidence for a viscerotopic sensory representation in the cortex and thalamus of the rat. J Comp Neurol 262:27, 1987

42. Oppenheimer SM, Cechetto DF: Cardiac chronotropic organization of the rat insular cortex. Brain Res 533:66, 1990

43. Oppenheimer SM, Wilson JX, Guiraudon C, Cechetto DF: Insular cortex stimulation produces lethal cardiac arrhythmias: a mechanism of sudden death? Brain Res 550:115, 1991

44. Hertzer NR, Young JR, Beven EG, et al: Coronary angiography in 506 patients with extracranial cerebrovascular disease. Arch Intern Med 145:849, 1985

45. Silver FL, Norris JW, Lewis AJ, Hachinski VC: Early mortality following stroke: a prospective review. Stroke 15:492, 1984

46. Byer E, Ashman R, Toth LA: Electrocardiograms with large, upright T waves and long Q-T intervals. Am Heart J 33:796, 1947

47. Burch GE, Meyers R, Abildskov JA: A new electrocardiographic pattern observed in cerebrovascular accidents. Circulation 9:719, 1954

48. Oppenheimer SM, Hachinski VC: The cardiac consequences of stroke. Neurol Clin 10:167, 1992

49. Dimant J, Grob D: Electrocardiographic changes and myocardial damage in patients with acute cerebrovascular accidents. Stroke 8:448, 1977

50. Lavy S, Yaar I, Melamed E, Stern S: The effect of acute stroke on cardiac functions as observed in an intensive stroke care unit. Stroke 5:775, 1974

51. Goldstein DS: The electrocardiogram in stroke: relationship to pathophysiological type and comparison with prior tracings. Stroke 10:253, 1979

52. Cropp GJ, Manning GW: Electrocardiographic changes simulating myocardial ischemia and infarction associated with spontaneous intracranial hemorrhage. Circulation 22:25, 1960

53. Shuster S: The electrocardiogram in subarachnoid haemorrhage. Br Heart J 22:316, 1960

54. Tobias SL, Bookatz BJ, Diamond TH: Myocardial damage and electocardiographic changes in acute cerebrovascular hemorrhage: a report of three cases and review. Heart Lung 16:521, 1987

55. Fentz V, Gormsen J: Electrocardiographic patterns in patients with cerebrovascular accidents. Circulation 25:22, 1962
56. Connor RCR: Heart damage associated with intracranial lesions. Br Med J 3:29, 1968
57. Neuberger K: Über die Herzmuskelveränderungen bei Epileptikern und ihre Beziehungen zur Angina pectoris. Frankfurt Z Pathol 46:14, 1933
58. Greenhoot JH, Reichenbach DD: Cardiac injury and subarachnoid hemorrhage: a clinical, pathological, and physiological correlation. J Neurosurg 30:521, 1969
59. Kolin A, Norris JW: Myocardial damage from acute cerebral lesions. Stroke 15:990, 1984
60. Myers MG, Norris JW, Hachinski VC, Sole MJ: Plasma norepinephrine in stroke. Stroke 12:200, 1981
61. Szakas J, Cannon A: L-Norepinephrine myocarditis. Am J Clin Pathol 30:425, 1958
62. Klouda M, Brynjolfsson G: Cardiotoxic effects of electrical stimulation of the stellate ganglia. Ann NY Acad Sci 156:271, 1969
63. Kolin A, Kvasnicka J: Pseudoinfarction pattern of the QRS complex in experimental cardiac hypoxia induced by noradrenalin. Cardiologia 43:362, 1963
64. Lepeschkin E, Marchet H, Schroeder G, et al: Effect of epinephrine and norepinephrine on the electrocardiogram of 100 normal subjects. Am J Cardiol 5:594, 1960
65. Neil-Dwyer G, Walter P, Cruickshank JM, et al: Effect of propranolol and phentolamine on myocardial necrosis after subarachnoid haemorrhage. Br Med J 2:990, 1978
66. Norris JW, Hachinski VC, Myers MG, et al: Serum cardiac enzymes in stroke. Stroke 10:548, 1979
67. Norris JW, Froggatt GM, Hachinski VC: Cardiac arrhythmias in acute stroke. Stroke 9:392, 1978
68. Rem JA, Hachinski VC, Boughner DR, Barnett HJM: Value of cardiac monitoring and echocardiography in TIA and stroke patients. Stroke 16:950, 1985
69. Di Pasquale G, Pinelli G, Andreoli A, et al: Holter detection of cardiac arrhythmias in intracranial subarachnoid hemorrhage. Am J Cardiol 59:596, 1987
70. Stober T, Anstatt T, Sen S, et al: Cardiac arrhythmias in subarachnoid haemorrhage. Acta Neurochir (Wien) 93:37, 1988
71. Cruickshank JM, Neil-Dwyer G, Brice J: Electrocardiographic changes and their prognostic significance in subarachnoid haemorrhage. J Neurol Neurosurg Psychiatry 37:755, 1974
72. Egan TM, Noble D, Noble SJ, et al: An isoprenaline activated sodium-dependent inward current in ventricular myocytes. Nature 328:634, 1987
73. Gutstein WH, Anversa P, Beghi C, et al: Coronary artery spasm in the rat induced by hypothalamic stimulation. Atherosclerosis 51:135, 1984
74. Maseri A, Severi S, De Nes M, et al: "Variant" angina: one aspect of a continuous spectrum of vasospastic myocardial ischemia. Am J Cardiol 42:1019, 1978
75. Cechetto DF, Wilson JX, Smith KE, et al: Autonomic and myocardial changes in middle cerebral artery occlusion: stroke models in the rat. Brain Res 502:296, 1989
76. Hachinski VC, Oppenheimer SM, Wilson JX, et al: Asymmetry of sympathetic consequences of experimental stroke. Arch Neurol 49:697, 1992
77. Penfield W, Rasmussen T: The Cerebral Cortex of Man. Macmillan, New York, 1957
78. Oppenheimer SM, Gelb A, Girvin JP, Hachinski VC: Cardiovascular effects of human insular cortex stimulation. Neurology 42:1727, 1992
79. Chapman WP, Livingston KE, Poppen JL: Effect upon blood pressure of electrical stimulation of the tips of temporal lobes in man. J Neurophysiol 13:65, 1950
80. Zamrini EY, Meador KJ, Loring DW, et al: Unilateral cerebral inactivation produces differential left/right heart rate responses. Neurology 40:1408, 1990
81. Lane RD, Wallace JD, Petrovsky PP, et al: Supraventricular tachycardia in patients with right hemisphere strokes. Stroke 23:362, 1992
82. Erickson TC: Cardiac activity during epileptic seizures. Arch Neurol Psychiatry 41:511, 1939
83. VanBuren JM: Some autonomic concomitants of ictal automatism. Brain 81:505, 1958
84. White PT, Grant P, Mosier J, Craig A: Changes in cerebral dynamics associated with seizures. Neurology 11:354, 1961
85. Blumhardt LD, Smith PEM, Owen L: Electrocardiographic accompaniments of temporal lobe epileptic seizures. Lancet 1:1051, 1986
86. Kiok MC, Terrence CF, Fromm GH, Lavine S: Sinus arrest in epilepsy. Neurology 36:115, 1986
87. Gilchrist JM: Arrythmogenic seizures: diagnosis by simultaneous EEG/ECG recording. Neurology 35:1503, 1985
88. Walsh GO, Masland W, Goldensohn ES: Relationship between paroxysmal atrial tachycardia and paroxysmal cerebral discharges. Bull Los Angeles Neurol Soc 37:28, 1972
89. Stephenson JBP: Electrocardiographic accompaniments of temporal lobe epileptic seizures. Lancet 1:1450, 1986
90. Pritchett ELC, McNamara JO, Gallagher JJ: Arrhythmogenic epilepsy: an hypothesis. Am Heart J 100:683, 1980
91. Ossentjuk E, Elink Sterk CJO, Storm van Leeuwen

W: Flicker-induced cardiac arrest in a patient with epilepsy. Electroencephalogr Clin Neurophysiol 20:257, 1966

92. Rabending G, Krell D: Alterations of heart rate induced by photic stimulation in healthy subjects and epileptics. Electroencephalogr Clin Neurophysiol 26:445, 1969

93. Leestma JE, Kalelkar MB, Teas SS, et al: Sudden unexpected death associated with seizures: analysis of 66 cases. Epilepsia 25:84, 1984

94. Terrence CF, Wisotzkey HM, Perper JA: Unexpected, unexplained death in epileptic patients. Neurology 25:594, 1975

95. Hirsch CS, Martin DL: Unexpected death in young epileptics. Neurology 21:682, 1971

96. Dashieff RM, Dickinson LJ: Sudden unexpected death of epileptic patient due to cardiac arrhythmia after seizure. Arch Neurol 43:194, 1986

97. Lathers CM, Schraeder PL: Autonomic dysfunction in epilepsy: characterization of autonomic cardiac neural discharge associated with pentylenetetrazol-induced epileptogenic activity. Epilepsia 23:633, 1982

98. Lathers CM, Schraeder PL, Weiner FL: Synchronization of cardiac autonomic neural discharge with epileptogenic activity: the lockstep phenomenon. Electroencephalogr Clin Neurophysiol 67:247, 1987

99. Randall WC, Kaye MP, Hageman GR, et al: Cardiac dysrhythmias in the conscious dog after surgically induced autonomic imbalance. Am J Cardiol 38:178, 1976

100. Lown B, DeSilva RA, Lenson R: Roles of psychologic stress and autonomic nervous system changes in provocation of ventricular premature complexes. Am J Cardiol 41:979, 1978

101. Anderson JL, Rodier HE, Green LS: Comparative effects of beta-adrenergic blocking drugs on experimental ventricular fibrillation threshold. Am J Cardiol 51:1196, 1983

11

Neurocutaneous Syndromes

Bruce O. Berg

The diseases usually considered in the category of neurocutaneous syndromes are characterized by their dysplastic nature and tendency to form tumors. Although the skin and central nervous system (CNS) are primarily affected, other organs systems may be involved.

Several of the diseases of this group were described during the last century, but Bielschowsky in 1914 first associated neurofibromatosis and tuberous sclerosis because of their dysplastic and neoplastic features.[1,2] Van Der Hoeve, in describing the ocular findings in these two diseases, suggested the neologism *phakomatosis* (Gr. *phakos*: lentil, mole, birthmark)—an inappropriate term—to epitomize these diseases; he later added von Hippel-Lindau disease and Sturge-Weber syndrome to this group.[3–5] In 1941 Louis-Bar reported the clinical features of a syndrome now recognized as ataxia-telangiectasia and suggested that it too belonged in this disease category.[6] During the last several decades, a variety of other disorders, all unusual and some lacking the typical features of the neurocutaneous syndromes, have been added to the group. Some of them are summarized in Table 11-1. The five most important syndromes are discussed in detail in this chapter.

Except for Sturge-Weber syndrome, these major neurocutaneous syndromes are genetically determined, although sporadic cases can occur. They are distinct clinical entities, and although there are reports of "double phakomatoses" or "overlap," reliable documentation of any combination of these diseases is rare, and such a combination occurs no more frequently than by chance.[7]

NEUROFIBROMATOSIS

Neurofibromatosis, an inherited disease transmitted as an autosomal dominant trait, is noted for its heterogeneity of clinical expression. It may involve the peripheral and central nervous systems as well as skin, bone, and the endocrine, gastrointestinal, and vascular systems. Although von Recklinghausen is credited for the initial clinical description of the disease, it had been described earlier.[8–11]

Two distinct forms of neurofibromatosis have been recognized: type 1, the most common type, is widely known as von Recklinghausen disease and is characterized by multiple hyperpigmented macules (café au lait spots) and neurofibromas; type 2 is characterized by eighth-nerve tumors, but other intracranial and intraspinal tumors are common.

The diagnosis of type 1 neurofibromatosis can be made in patients with two or more of the following clinical findings: six or more café au lait spots with a maximum diameter of more than 5 mm during prepuberty and more than 15 mm in postpubertal patients; two or more neurofibromas of any type or one plexiform neuroma; axillary or inguinal freckling; optic glioma; two or more Lisch nodules; typical bony lesions; and a first-degree relative with the dis-

Table 11-1 Selected Neurocutaneous Syndromes[a]

Disease	Clinical Features
Autosomal dominant trait	
Incontinentia pigmenti achromians (hypomelanosis of Ito)	Bilateral asymmetrical areas of hypopigmented whorls ("marbling") on different parts of body skin. Associated anomalies of CNS, eyes, teeth, skin, nails, and bone are common.
Waardenberg's syndrome (I)	Frontal patch of white hair, heterochromia iridis, lateral displacement of inner canthus, and cochlear deafness. (Deafness is not always present.)
Waardenberg's syndrome (II)	Clinical findings are the same as in type I without lateral displacement of inner canthus. Deafness is more common than in type I.
Autosomal recessive trait	
Chediak-Higashi syndrome	Rare disorder characterized by partial oculocutaneous albinism, photophobia, neurological abnormalities, and recurring infection. Giant cytoplasmic organelles are observed; there are associated immunological and bleeding disorders.
Xeroderma pigmentosum	Defect in DNA repair results in premature aging of tissues exposed to sunlight. Microcephaly, mental subnormality, ocular changes, corticospinal tract dysfunction, ataxia, and movement disorders may be present.
Rothmund-Thomson syndrome	Erythematous skin lesions in early life followed by telangiectasis, atrophy, hypo- and/or hyperpigmentation; ectodermal dysplasia. Body hair is sparse or absent. Cataracts. Short stature, hypogonadism, and skeletal abnormalities are common. Intelligence is normal.
Sjögren-Larsson syndrome	Congenital ichthyosis associated with mental subnormality and corticospinal tract dysfunction.
Rud's syndrome	Ichthyosis and hypogonadism are major features; microcephaly, sensorineural deafness, polyneuropathy, and hypoplastic teeth and nails are less frequent.
Refsum's disease	Retinal pigmentary degeneration, polyneuropathy, and ataxia are characteristic. Sensorineural deafness, anosmia, and cardiomyopathy are usually present. Abnormalities of the eyes, skin (ichthyosis), and bone are often present.
X-Linked inheritance	
Fabry-Anderson disease	A glycolipid lysosomal storage disease with wide spectrum of clinical findings. Angiokeratosis is a characteristic feature. Lancinating limb pain is often the first symptom; joint pain may resemble juvenile rheumatoid arthritis. Ocular, cardiac, and gastrointestinal symptoms may be present; cerebral vascular accidents may occur in young adults. Neuropathy. Renal disease manifests as the inability to concentrate urine, urinary frequency, polyuria, and nocturia.
Incontinentia pigmenti (Bloch-Sulzberger syndrome)	Seen almost entirely in females; it is characterized by skin lesions present during the first few weeks of life that are erythematous, macular, papular, vesicular, or bullous. Second stage skin lesions are variably verrucous, lichenoid, or keratotic; the third stage is notable for its hyperpigmentation. Abnormalities of the eyes, CNS, hair, teeth, and bone are commonly associated.

[a] Neurofibromatosis, tuberous sclerosis, von Hippel-Lindau disease, Sturge-Weber syndrome, and ataxia-telangiectasia are not included in this table because they are discussed in detail in the text.

order diagnosed by these criteria. The diagnosis of type 2 neurofibromatosis can be made if the patient has bilateral eighth-nerve masses as demonstrated by appropriate imaging techniques. The diagnosis can also be made if the patient has a first-degree relative with type 2 neurofibromatosis and either a unilateral eighth-nerve mass lesion or two of the following findings: neurofibroma, meningioma, glioma, schwannoma, or juvenile posterior subcapsular lenticular opacity.[12]

The skin changes associated with neurofibromatosis are characterized by focal or diffuse lesions (or both) that are usually present before the appearance of any neurological abnormality. They include café au lait spots, fibroma molluscum, patchy or diffuse areas of hyperpigmentation, hypopigmented spots, and angiomas.

Café au lait spots are usually present at birth. The number of spots and degree of pigmentation tend to increase during the first year of life, but after that time the number of spots remains relatively stable. These spots can appear anywhere on the body (Fig. 11-1) except probably the scalp, palms, and soles. They are typically flat, with discrete borders, and vary in size from millimeters to centimeters.[13] Crowe and associ-

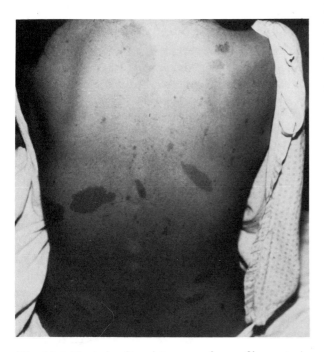

Fig. 11-1 Typical café au lait spots of neurofibromatosis, located primarily on the trunk.

ates observed that patients with six or more café au lait spots with a diameter of 1.5 cm have a presumptive diagnosis of neurofibromatosis; Crowe later reported that axillary freckling was also an important feature of the disease.[14,15] The presence of café au lait spots does not necessarily establish the diagnosis of neurofibromatosis, however, because at least 10 percent of the population have one or more hyperpigmented cutaneous macules.

Fibroma molluscum, a prominent skin lesion found in the dermis or adjacent to it, consists of discrete soft or firm papules ranging in size from a few millimeters to several centimeters. They are flat, sessile, or pedunculated and can be readily impressed into the subjacent skin. Hypopigmented spots, similar to those found in tuberous sclerosis, are sometimes present, as are discrete areas of skin hypoplasia and angiomas.

Neurofibromas can occur anywhere from the dorsal root ganglion to the terminal peripheral nerve branches and can affect any organ system. They vary in size and are more often found on the trunk than on the limbs (Fig. 11-2). Plexiform neuromas are made up of interwoven elements of tumor and connective tissue that infiltrate normal tissue. They can be superficial, involving skin and subcutaneous tissues, or deep, affecting visceral and adjacent tissues. Diffuse areas of skin hyperpigmentation may overlie the plexiform neuroma. The incidence of sarcomatous transformation of neurofibromas is generally accepted as 2 to 7 percent.[16,17]

Intracranial tumors, primarily astrocytomas, occur in neurofibromatosis and involve the cerebrum or cerebellum. There is an increased frequency of optic nerve gliomas, and other cranial nerves can be affected by neurofibromas or schwannomas. Bilateral acoustic neuromas are a characteristic feature of type 2 neurofibromatosis. Although meningiomas, both solitary and multiple, are found with increased frequency in the major type of neurofibromatosis (type 1), they are more typically observed in the type 2 disorder. Medulloblastomas, ependymomas, and hamartomas also occur more frequently in patients with neurofibromatosis than in the general population.[18]

Intraspinal tumors are single or multiple, intradural or extradural. They can be accompanied by spinal anomalies such as syringomyelia. Some intraspinal tumors assume a dumbbell shape, extending through the intervertebral foramen. They are sometimes associated with enlargement of that foramen or defect of the contiguous bone.[18]

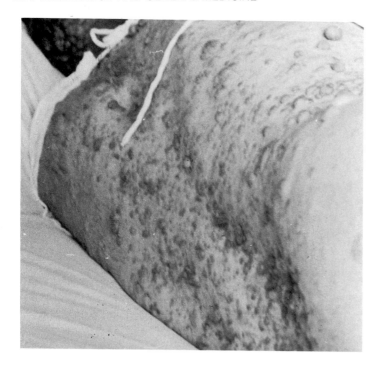

Fig. 11-2 Young adult with multiple subcutaneous neurofibromas.

Lisch nodules, a typical finding in neurofibromatosis, are melanocytic hamartomas found in the iris. Age-dependent and bilateral, they are found in about 10 percent of patients less than 6 years old, 50 percent of patients less than age 30, and almost all patients by age 50. Other ocular findings in neurofibromatosis include optic nerve gliomas (the most common CNS tumor) and congenital glaucoma. The frequency of optic gliomas in neurofibromatosis has ranged from 15 to 20 percent.[19-21] Patients usually present with symptoms of decreased visual acuity or visual field defects but may initially appear with signs and symptoms of increased intracranial pressure. The tumor mass can involve the optic chiasm or hypothalamus and rarely manifests as the diencephalic syndrome of infancy.[22] Although there is some controversy regarding the nature of the tumor, optic gliomas in children are probably congenital hamartomas, indolent and slow-growing.[23]

Congenital glaucoma, a known complication of neurofibromatosis, is commonly associated with a neurofibroma of the superior eyelid. Mechanisms of its cause include angle obstruction by neurofibromas, angle narrowing from neurofibromatous thickening of the ciliary body and choroid, fibrovascularization and synechial narrowing of the angle, and developmental anomalies of the angle.[24]

A variety of bony changes can occur in neurofibro-matosis, including a "ballooning" of the middle fossa, an enlarged sella turcica, a J-shaped sella, and abnormalities of the sphenoid wing. The optic foramina are enlarged in some patients with optic glioma; bony defects of the orbit, the area of the lambdoid sutures, and other cranial bones are not uncommon. Scoliosis is reported in 10 to 40 percent of patients, though usually it is not reported before the age of 6 years; kyphosis, anterior meningocoele, enlarged intervertebral foramina, bowing of the tibia and fibula, and bony overgrowth have also been reported. Pseudarthrosis is a characteristic feature of neurofibromatosis and usually involves the distal tibia, although other tubular bones can be affected.[25-29] The bony defects associated with neurofibromatosis are secondary to developmental abnormalities of mesenchymal tissue and are usually not the result of bone erosion by tumor.

Other features of neurofibromatosis include macrocephaly and short stature, which are reported to occur in 10 to 40 percent of patients. Mental retardation and seizures, though not necessarily related, occur in about 10 percent of patients, and 40 percent of patients have specific learning disabilities and hyperactivity.[18] Precocious puberty has been observed in patients with a hypothalamic glioma or hamartoma or in some optic chiasmal gliomas that involve the hypothalamus. It should not be presumed, however, that precocious puberty without hypothalamic involvement by mass lesion is an integral part of the disease. Hypertension can develop as a result of intimal proliferation and fibromuscular changes of the media in small renal arteries.[30]

A variety of tumors occurs more frequently than in the general population, including pheochromocytoma, leukemia, neuroblastoma, and Wilms' tumor.[18] There is an increased frequency of multiple endocrine neoplasia and medullary thyroid carcinoma. Among patients with pheochromocytomas, 4 to 23 percent have neurofibromatosis, whereas fewer than 1 percent of patients with neurofibromatosis have been found to have pheochromocytomas.[31-33]

The frequency of neurofibromatosis, inherited as an autosomal dominant trait, is about 1 in 4,000 persons for type 1 and about 1 in 50,000 persons for type 2.[12] About one-half of the cases are said to be sporadic. The risk factors of developing the varied complications of the disease are yet to be determined.[34] The gene for type 1 has been mapped to a locus on chromosome 17; for type 2 it has been localized to chromosome 22.[35]

The treatment of patients with neurofibromatosis is symptomatic. Peripheral neurofibromas are generally indolent lesions that do not require surgical removal unless they are subjected to repeated trauma or show rapid growth. On occasion, plexiform neuromas are removed for cosmetic reasons. Intracranial and intraspinal tumors are treated by appropriate surgical techniques, irradiation, or chemotherapy. Optic gliomas in children are generally thought to be hamartomas; some authors recommend that they be managed conservatively by following their growth and documenting visual function rather than by immediate surgery or irradiation therapy.[23,36,37]

TUBEROUS SCLEROSIS

Tuberous sclerosis, inherited as an autosomal dominant trait, is characterized by a wide spectrum of clinical findings including seizures, varying degrees of mental subnormality, and dysplastic and neoplastic changes of the skin, nervous system, and other organs. It was probably first described by von Recklinghausen, although Bourneville is appropriately credited for the initial clinical description of the disease.[38-41] Bourneville thought that cerebral "scleroses" and renal tumors were associated findings but paid little attention to the facial skin lesions. Vogt (1908) believed there was a typical triad of findings:

adenoma sebaceum, seizures, and mental retardation.[42]

The clinical expression of the disease depends on the patient's age and the extent of organ involvement. Seizures, the most common symptom, can appear at any time after birth. Generalized and, less commonly, partial seizures occur, and infantile spasms are often present during the first several years of life.[43] The early onset and severity of recurring seizures is correlated with mental subnormality. There is, however, notable variability of mental function in patients with tuberous sclerosis, and about one-third have normal intelligence.[44-46] Some affected children may develop normally during the first few years of life, but mental function deteriorates later in the first decade.[7]

Adenoma sebaceum, commonly considered to be the characteristic skin lesion in tuberous sclerosis, consists of angiofibromas that appear in patches or in a butterfly distribution about the nose, cheeks, and chin (Fig. 11-3). Observed in about one-half of pa-

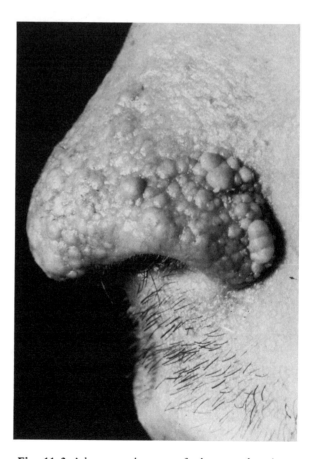

Fig. 11-3 Adenoma sebaceum of tuberous sclerosis.

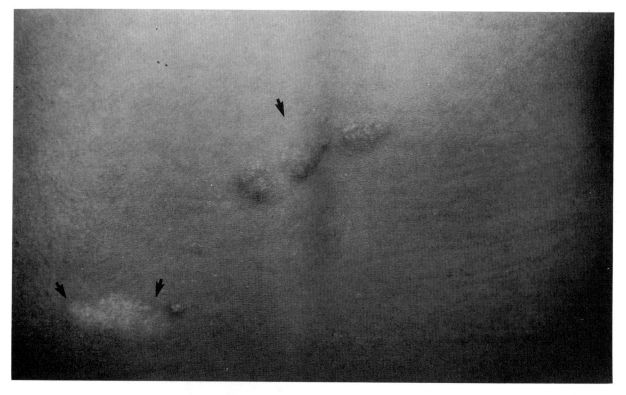

Fig. 11-4 Leaf-shaped hypopigmented macule *(left arrows)* and adjacent small fibroma *(right arrow)* commonly seen in tuberous sclerosis.

tients, they are rarely apparent at birth and are usually first observed between the ages of 1 and 4 years, tending to enlarge with time.[45–49] Hypopigmented oval (leaf-shaped) spots, present in about 90 percent of patients, vary in size from millimeters to several centimeters (Fig. 11–4). They may present at birth but become more prominent with time.[50,51] Visualization of these hypomelanotic macules is enhanced by using a Wood light, because melanin absorbs light of that frequency (360 nm), so areas deficient in melanin are accentuated.[52,53] In some patients a patch of white or gray hair precedes the appearance of hypopigmented spots.[54] Other skin changes that may occur include the shagreen patch (a "leathery" plaque usually found over the lumbosacral or gluteal area), café au lait spots, fibromas, and angiomas.

Subungual or periungual fibromas (Koenen tumors) are found in about 20 percent of patients and affect the toes more than the fingers. They are usually first noted during adolescence.[55,56] Gingival fibromas can also occur.[57]

Although retinal tumors (hamartomas) are commonly present, affected patients have few visual complaints (Fig. 11-5). These astrocytic, nodular lesions tend to calcify and may be solitary or multiple.[58,59] Gray-yellow glial patches are sometimes present. Additional ocular findings include iritic hypomelanotic spots, cataracts, and colobomas of the iris, lens, and choroid.[43]

Renal tumors are found in about one-half of patients with tuberous sclerosis and include angiomyolipomas and cystic lesions that are embedded in the renal parenchyma. These lesions are relatively benign and only rarely require surgical intervention.[60] Cardiac rhabdomyomas are found in at least one-half of patients and are solitary, multiple, or infiltrative, diffusely affecting the myocardium. Their demonstration has been notably improved with echocardiography and angiography.[61–64]

Other associated abnormalities include multicystic lung disease, which occurs almost entirely in female subjects and is manifested by dyspnea, spontaneous

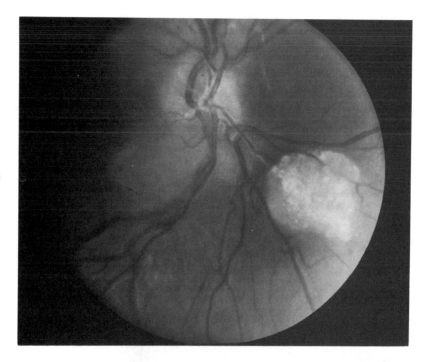

Fig. 11-5 Typical retinal (mulberry) lesion observed in tuberous sclerosis.

pneumothorax, and pulmonary hypertension.[65–67] A variety of endocrine abnormalities has been reported.[68–70]

Radiographic studies can be effectively utilized to confirm the diagnosis. Intracranial calcifications, commonly observed in the region of the foramen of Monro or the periventricular region, are present on skull radiographs in about 60 percent of affected patients. Computed tomography (CT) may demonstrate cerebral hamartomas, subependymal nodules, ventriculomegaly, and areas of diffuse demyelination (Fig. 11-6). The most reliable finding on CT head scan is the demonstration of mineralized subependymal nodules. Periventricular calcification is less specific and may not be distinguishable from toxoplasmosis, cytomegalic inclusion disease, and Fahr syndrome.[71–74]

Magnetic resonance imaging (MRI) demonstrates with great clarity not only uncalcified subependymal nodules but a marked distortion of normal cortical cytoarchitectonics (Fig. 11-7).[75]

Other typical radiographic findings include cystic rarefaction of phalanges and metacarpals, sclerotic areas of long bones, and areas of increased or decreased bony density of the skull. Those patients with pulmonary involvement may have a fine reticular infiltrate or multicystic changes on chest radiographs.

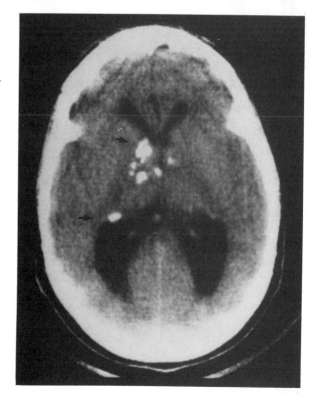

Fig. 11-6 CT scan (unenhanced axial view) of patient with tuberous sclerosis, showing calcified tubers.

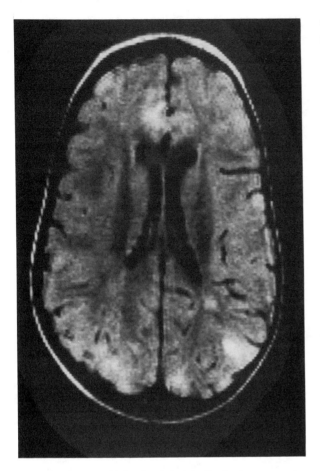

Fig. 11-7. MRI of the head (axial view), demonstrating multiple cortical and subcortical foci of increased signal intensity in tuberous sclerosis.

of cortical cytoarchitectonics. The walls of some vessels may show hyaline degeneration.[77,78]

Subependymal nodules are fibrocellular, with round or oval cells and whorls of fibrillary glial tissue. Amyloid or calcium deposits may be present within the tuber or subependymal nodule; cerebellar calcification occurs rarely.[79]

Tuberous sclerosis is inherited as an autosomal dominant trait with variable penetrance; the estimated frequency of the disease is 1 in 30,000. The reported sporadic rate, ranging from one-half to about three-fourths, is probably an overestimate, because it is likely that a diagnosis of tuberous sclerosis could be established in some of the "asymptomatic" parents of children with the disease if they were examined with current diagnostic techniques.[80,81] There is some evidence to locate the responsible gene to the long arm of chromosome 9 at q34. Other linkage studies suggesting a gene locus on chromosome 11 are as yet unconfirmed.[82–85]

Convulsive disorders are treated by administration of appropriate anticonvulsant medications; however, their control cannot be ensured. There is no specific treatment for the skin lesions unless they are subjected to frequent irritation; selected lesions can be surgically removed or treated with other dermatological measures. When the diagnosis of tuberous sclerosis is established, genetic counseling is required for all family members. Patients with tuberous sclerosis must be afforded thoughtful medical and emotional support and guidance.

Brain weight and configuration are usually normal except for the presence of cortical tubers, which may be noted anywhere in the cerebral hemisphere. Tubers are often found within the cortical gyri, though smaller nodular lesions can be observed in the region of the sulcus terminalis or basal ganglia, protruding into the ventricle. Tubers located about the foramen of Monro or the aqueduct of Sylvius may grow sufficiently to obstruct the normal circulation of cerebrospinal fluid (CSF), resulting in increased intracranial pressure.[76]

The microscopic appearance of the tuber is characterized by a decreased number of neurons with scattered large, bizarre, sometimes vacuolated "monster" neurons. Sections of cortex show proliferation of fibrillary astrocytes, demyelination, and abnormalities

VON HIPPEL-LINDAU DISEASE

Von Hippel-Lindau disease, inherited as an autosomal dominant trait, is characterized by retinal and cerebellar hemangioblastomas. Other manifestations include cysts of the pancreas, liver, and spleen as well as malignant renal tumors. There are no associated skin lesions, as are found in other neurocutaneous syndromes.

The retinal lesion was first described, though not recognized as a hemangioblastoma, by Panas and Remy in 1879.[86] Fuchs in 1882 thought the lesion was an arteriovenous malformation, and Collins in 1894 believed that it originated from capillaries and had a hereditary basis.[87,88] Von Hippel decided that the retinal lesion was a hemangioblastoma but attached

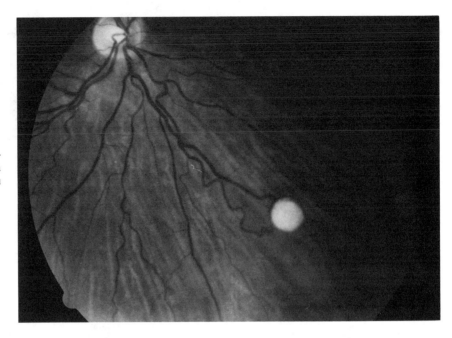

Fig. 11-8 Typical round, white-red retinal hemangioblastoma observed in von Hippel-Lindau disease.

the name of *angiomatosis retinae*."[89] In 1926, Lindau established the association of retinal and cerebellar hemangioblastomas, but he was also aware that these patients may have other lesions, including spinal cord angiomas and cystic tumors of the pancreas, kidney, and epididymis.[90]

The retinal hemangioblastoma is one of the earliest manifestations of the disorder. Though reported to occur during childhood, it is usually found initially during the third decade. The early appearance of the lesion is similar to an aneurysmal dilation of a peripheral retinal vessel; later, there are typical tortuous vessels, with an afferent arteriole and venule leading to a small, raised retinal lesion (Fig. 11-8). Some lesions are small and easily overlooked.[91–93] The retinal lesions have been divided into three categories: (1) a pinkish red vascular lesion located in the midperiphery, with visible dilated "feeder" vessels and variable exudate; (2) a pale gray lesion, with "feeder" vessels observed only on fluorescein retinal angiography; and (3) retinal lesions that are similar to diabetic microaneurysms but that are not observed to have retinal vascular connections. Patients with peripheral retinal lesions may have no significant visual impairment, but if the lesion involves the macula or optic disc, there is progressive visual loss.[94–97]

The diagnosis of cerebellar hemangioblastoma is usually first made during the third or fourth decade,

but there are rare reports of its occurrence before puberty. The initial signs and symptoms are primarily those of cerebellar dysfunction and increased intracranial pressure. Hemangioblastomas can also occur in the medulla and the spinal cord, where in about 80 percent of patients they are associated with syringomyelia.[98] Supratentorial hemangioblastomas are uncommon but have been reported in the pituitary, third ventricle, and cerebral hemispheres.

Renal lesions may be found in von Hippel-Lindau disease and include benign cysts, angiomas, and hypernephromas. Hypernephromas are common and are a prominent cause of morbidity and mortality in the disease. Benign cysts are also found in the pancreas, adrenal gland, and epididymis and are usually asymptomatic. There is an increased frequency of pheochromocytoma.

The retinal lesions are recognized by ophthalmological examination, and fluorescein retinal angiography can demonstrate the vascular characteristics of the lesion. CT and MRI delineate the structural characteristics of the cerebellar or spinal cord lesions. Intra-abdominal lesions can be demonstrated by CT and ultrasonography.

The red blood cell count may be elevated because of increased concentration of erythropoietin in the hemangioblastoma cyst fluid; the absence of polycythemia, however, does not exclude the diagnosis. Patients with CNS tumors have an elevated protein concentration in the cerebrospinal fluid. Twenty-four-hour urine collection for assay of epinephrine, norepinephrine, and vanillylmandelic acid is performed to screen for pheochromocytoma.[99–103]

The most frequent site of the tumor is the cerebellum, usually in the paramedial aspect of the cerebellar cortex, and the tumor is associated with prominent vessels. The microscopic features of the tumor are characterized by large numbers of thin-walled, closely packed blood vessels that are lined by plump endothelial cells and separated by large, pale cells incorporated into an elaborate network of reticulin fibers.[77,104–106]

Von Hippel-Lindau disease is inherited as an autosomal dominant trait with variable penetrance. There is no sex predominance. The incidence of sporadic cases is not known. The gene that causes von Hippel-Lindau disease has not been specifically identified; however, it has been localized to chromosome 3p25-26 by linkage analysis.[107–109]

Posterior fossa hemangioblastomas are treated by neurosurgical techniques to remove the cyst and associated fluid and mural nodule. Radiation therapy is of little benefit in the treatment of this tumor. Retinal hemangioblastomas are treated by a variety of methods, including laser photocoagulation and cryotherapy.

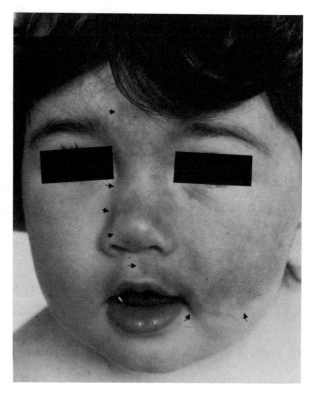

Fig. 11-9 Facial angioma (port-wine stain) of Sturge-Weber Syndrome primarily involving the left upper face *(arrows)*.

STURGE-WEBER SYNDROME

Sturge-Weber syndrome is characterized by a facial angioma (nevus, port-wine stain) associated with signs and symptoms of a leptomeningeal venous angioma. Schirmer described in 1860 a patient with a facial nevus and buphthalmos, but Sturge is credited with the first clinical description in 1879 of the syndrome in a young child who had a facial angioma, buphthalmos, and contralateral partial seizures.[110,111] He suggested that the patient had an underlying cerebral nevus, but it was not until 1897 that pathological studies confirmed his prediction.[112]

Weber subsequently described the associated intracranial calcifications noted on skull radiographs and introduced the term *encephalofacialangiomatosis,* and Van der Hoeve inappropriately suggested that the disorder was the "fourth phakomatosis."[113,114]

The facial angioma is congenital, unilateral (though it may be bilateral), and involves at least the upper face, superior eyelid, or periorbital region (Fig. 11-9). It may involve the nasopharynx, palate, lips, gingiva, and tongue. Although the facial angioma is commonly thought to conform to the sensory distribution of the first and possibly second or third divisions of the trigeminal nerve, there is reason to consider such a relation fortuitous. Rather, the distribution of the facial nevus may be determined by embryological development of the face.[115] Angiomas may also be found on the neck, trunk, or extremities. Meningeal venous angiomas may occur in the absence of any facial angioma; although secondary cerebral signs and symptoms are similar to those of the Sturge-Weber syndrome, these patients are more appropriately thought to have a separate disorder, referred to as meningeal angiomatosis.[116,117]

During early infancy, most patients with Sturge-Weber syndrome experience seizures that are primarily partial motor in type, although some patients have generalized tonic-clonic seizures. There is usually a relentless progression of severity and frequency of the convulsive disorder, and any postictal Todd paralysis often requires increasingly longer periods of time to resolve, until eventually there is a permanent hemiparesis. Other types of seizures, including infantile spasms, myoclonic seizures, and atonic attacks, occur less commonly.[118,119–121]

In earlier studies, the frequency of seizure disorders has varied from 70 to 90 percent. In a retrospective study of 102 patients evaluated between 1942 and 1986, 88 patients had one cerebral hemisphere affected and 14 patients had bilateral hemispheric involvement. Seizures occurred in 75 percent of these patients. Among 88 patients with unilateral hemispheric disease, 63 had seizures, with the mean age of seizure onset being 24 months; 13 of 14 patients with bilateral hemispheric lesions had seizure disorders, with a mean age of onset of 6 months.[122]

Hemiparesis contralateral to the facial angioma occurs in about 30 percent of patients and is sometimes apparent during infancy, before the onset of seizures. The weakness is generally exacerbated by increasingly severe recurrent seizures and may be accompanied later by hemiatrophy.[118,119] Bilateral hemipareses may be present in patients with meningeal angiomas affecting both cerebral hemispheres.

Hemisensory deficits are less frequently documented because reliable sensory examinations are difficult to carry out in the very young and in mentally subnormal patients. Homonymous hemianopia is present in about one-third of patients, and glaucoma secondary to choroidal angioma is found in about one-fourth. Other ocular findings include iritic heterochromia with the hyperpigmented iris ipsilateral to the facial angioma, optic atrophy, and strabismus.

At least 50 percent of patients are mentally subnormal, and behavioral problems are common. As seizures of early onset increase in frequency and severity, mental function and behavior often regress. In the retrospective study noted above, 25 of 88 patients with unihemispheric leptomeningeal involvement who did not have seizures were of average intelligence; 1 of 14 patients with bilateral hemispheric involvement was unaffected by seizures and that patient was of average intelligence.[122] These observations are important considerations in patient management.[118]

Electroencephalographic studies may show decreased amplitude and frequency of electrocerebral activity over the affected hemisphere. Diffuse multiple and independent spike foci are commonly present.[123]

Intracranial calcification, demonstrated on skull radiographs, is present in more than 90 percent of patients. It is rarely observed in infants but has nevertheless been reported in the neonate and is present in most patients by the end of the second decade. The calcifications, which are usually in the occipital or parieto-occipital regions, assume a linear, parallel configuration ("tram sign"). CT scans of the head demonstrate calcifications and cerebral atrophy more readily than plain radiography and may show the calcific deposits during the first few months of life.[124]

Cerebral angiography shows decreased cerebral venous drainage and dilated deep cerebral veins. About one-third of patients have a variety of vascular abnormalities including thrombotic lesions, dural venous sinus abnormalities, and arteriovenous malformations.[125–127] Positron emission tomography (PET) provides a measure of the extent of cerebral metabolic impairment, and serial PET scanning can be useful with other neuroimaging techniques to document the progression of the disease.[128]

The Sturge-Weber syndrome has no clear pattern of inheritance, although there is one report of a father and son who had a facial angioma and glaucoma.[129]

Typical pathological features include thickened, hypervascularized leptomeninges primarily involving the occipital, parietal, or temporo-occipital lobes. Meningeal vessels are small and tortuous, lending a dark, purplish blue color to the cerebral surface. These abnormal vessels rarely enter the underlying atrophic hemisphere. Calcific deposits of varying size are found in the walls of some small cerebral vessels but are primarily located in the molecular and outer pyramidal cortical layers. Although some iron associated with calcific deposits has been reported, the iron content of gray and white matter is normal, whereas calcium content is greatly increased. The pathogenesis of intracortical calcium deposition is not fully understood.[130,131]

Good management requires careful attention to every aspect of the patient's medical and emotional well-being. The seizure disorder is managed with anticonvulsant drugs. Adrenocorticotropic hormone (ACTH) may be required for patients with infantile spasms. It is not unusual for seizures to be recalcitrant to medical management; in selected cases, consideration must be given to the surgical removal of affected lobe(s) or to hemispherectomy.[121,132] Management of mental subnormality or behavioral problems requires the skilled support of the physician, psychologist, and social worker.

ATAXIA-TELANGIECTASIA

Ataxia-telangiectasia is a multisystem disease characterized by progressive cerebellar ataxia, oculocutaneous telangiectasis, proclivity to sinopulmonary infections, and immunoincompetence associated with lymphoreticular neoplasia. The disease is transmitted as an autosomal recessive trait, affecting male and female subjects equally.

Although this condition was initially described by Syllaba and Henner in 1926, Louis–Bar believed that her 1941 report of ataxia and notable cutaneous telangiectasis in a 9-year-old boy described a hitherto unrecognized disease and suggested that it was one of the phakomatoses.[133,134] Three independent reports of the disease were published in 1957: Boder and Sedgwick described the clinical features of the disease and named it ataxia-telangiectasia; Biemond described the clinical and pathological findings of the disease and emphasized the recurring sinopulmonary infections and extrapyramidal signs; Wells and Shy reported the disease as "familial choreoathetosis and cutaneous telangiectasis."[135–137]

Affected patients appear normal until the time they begin to walk independently, usually at 12 to 18 months, at which time truncal ataxia first becomes apparent. Normal motor development continues despite the ataxia, but within several years there is little question that the child is inordinately clumsy.

Abnormalities of ocular motility characterized by slow, involuntary ocular movements with erratically interspersed vertical components are common. There is a defect in the initiation of voluntary and involuntary saccades; associated eye blinking and head thrusts or jerks, consistent with congenital oculomotor apraxia, are usually present.[138,139]

Patients are generally hypotonic, and there is a paucity of muscle bulk. Stretch reflexes, usually normal in the younger child, are decreased or lost within a few years; plantar responses are nonreactive or flexor. Choreoathetosis is common in most patients and may increase in severity. There are generally no sensory abnormalities of note, although older patients may have posterior column dysfunction.

Affected patients appear rather apathetic, if not sad, but they usually have a pleasant disposition. Although dysarthria and drooling may convey the impression of dullness, mental subnormality is not a typical feature of the disease. There appears to be a "leveling off" of the acquisition of cognitive skills rather than a deterioration of mental function.[140–142]

Telangiectasias become apparent later than ataxia and are usually first observed between the ages of 3 and 5 years, though they have been observed at birth or as late as the second decade.[143] They are generally first noted in the lateral bulbar conjunctiva but gradually involve its entirety (Fig. 11-10). Exposed areas of skin are also affected, including the nasal bridge, ear, and antecubital and popliteal spaces. Telangiectasias become more prominent following exposure to sun. Progeric changes of skin and hair are common and are manifested by sclerodermoid and atrophic areas of skin and patches of gray or white hair.[144,145]

Chronic blepharitis is often present. Recurring sinopulmonary infections, affecting 90 percent of patients, usually result in chronic bronchitis or bronchiectasis. Hypogonadism is frequently present, and growth retardation is notable despite normal levels of serum growth hormone.[140]

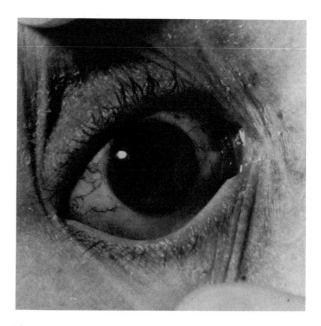

Fig. 11-10 Characteristic conjunctival telangiectasias seen in ataxia-telangiectasia.

The incidence of malignant neoplasms in patients with ataxia-telangiectasia has been reported as 10 to 15 percent. Most of these neoplasms are either lymphomas, reticulum cell sarcomas, histiocytosarcomas, or Hodgkin's disease. Other associated neoplasms include brain tumors, gastric adenocarcinomas, ovarian dysgerminomas, gonadoblastomas, cystadenofibromas, uterine leiomyomas, thyroid adenomas, and basal cell carcinomas.[146–149]

Abnormalities of both humoral and cellular immunity have been demonstrated. Most patients have absent or low levels of immunoglobulin A (IgA) and IgE; IgM and IgG_2 levels may also be decreased. Serum levels of IgM, IgG_1, and IgG_3 levels have been reported as normal or elevated.[150,151] The most consistent biochemical findings, however, are elevated serum α-fetoprotein and carcinoembryonic antigen.[150–159]

Impaired cellular immunity is common in older children as a consequence of abnormally developed or absent thymus gland, tonsils, adenoids, and lymphoid tissue. Moreover, there is an increased incidence of spontaneous or radiation-induced chromosomal breakage and rearrangement. Some observations suggest that patients with ataxia-telangiectasia have defective DNA repair mechanisms.[160–162] Chromosomal analysis for recombination involving 7p14 and 14q32 chromosome bands can be of benefit.

Pathological studies show notable cerebellar atrophy with particular involvement of Purkinje and granular cells, though basket cells may be affected as well. Neuronal degeneration of the dentate and olivary nuclei has been described, as has neuronal loss in the substantia nigra and nuclear changes in cells of the oculomotor complex and hypothalamus. In many cases of long duration, there is degeneration of the posterior columns of the spinal cord; degenerative changes of anterior horn cells have also been observed.[163–165] Bizarre dystrophic changes and nucleomegaly of satellite cells in the dorsal root ganglia and Schwann cells of peripheral nerve have been described. No characteristic vascular pathology of the nervous system has been reported.[166]

Specific treatment is not available. Patients must therefore receive vigorous supportive care, with particular attention directed to recurrent infection and pulmonary function. Attempts to improve the immunological status of patients by plasma transfusion, administration of thymosine, or fetal thymus transplants have thus far not altered the course of the disease.[165]

REFERENCES

1. Bielschowsky M: Uber tuberose Sklerose und ihre Beziehungen nur Recklinghausen Krankheit. Z Gesamte Neurol Psychiatr 26:133, 1914
2. Bielschowsky M: Entwurf eines Systems der Heredodegenerationen des Zentralnervensystems einschliesslich der Zugehoren Striatumerkrankugen. J Psychol Neurol 24:48, 1919
3. Van Der Hoeve J: Eye diseases in tuberous sclerosis of the brain and in Recklinghausen disease. Trans Ophthalmol Soc UK 43:534, 1923
4. Van Der Hoeve J: The Doyne Memorial Lecture: eye symptoms in phakomatoses. Trans Ophthalmol Soc UK 52:380, 1932
5. Van Der Hoeve J: Les phacomatoses de Bourneville, de Recklinghausen et de Von Hippel-Lindau. J Belge Neurol Psychiatr 33:752, 1933
6. Louis-Bar D: Sur un syndrome progressif comprenant des télangiectasies capillaires cutanées et conjonctivales symetriques a disposition naevoide et des troubles cérébelleux. Confin Neurol 4:32, 1941
7. Borberg A: Clinical and genetic investigations into tuberous sclerosis and Recklinghausen's neuro-fibromatosis: contributions to elucidation of interrelationship and eugenics of the syndromes. Acta Psychiatr Neurol Scand Suppl 71:3, 1951
8. Tilesius WG: Historia Pathologica Singularis Cutis Turpitudinis. Leipzig, 1793
9. Smith RW: A Treatise on the Pathology, Diagnosis and Treatment of Neuroma. Hodges & Smith, Dublin, 1849
10. Fulton JF: Robert Smith's description of generalized neurofibromatosis (1829). N Engl J Med 200:1315, 1929
11. Von Recklinghausen F: Uber die multiplen fibrome der Haut und ihre Beziehungen zu den multiplen Neuromen. Hirschwald, Berlin, 1882
12. Neurofibromatosis: National Institutes of Health: Consensus Development Conference Statement 6: No 12, 1, 1987
13. Adams RD: Neurocutaneous diseases. p. 1206. In Fitzpatrick TB, Eisen AZ, Wolff K (eds): Dermatology in General Practice. McGraw-Hill, New York, 1979
14. Crowe FW, Schull WJ, Neil JW: A Clinical, Pathological and Genetic Study of Multiple Neurofibromatosis. Charles C Thomas, Springfield, IL, 1956

15. Crowe FW: Axillary freckling as a diagnostic aid in neurofibromatosis. Ann Intern Med 61:1142, 1964

16. Canale DJ, Bebin J, Knighton RS: Neurologic manifestations of von Recklinghausen's disease of the nervous system. Confin Neurol 24:359, 1964

17. Pearce J: The central nervous system pathology in multiple neurofibromatosis. Neurology 17:691, 1967

18. Riccardi VM, Eichner JE: Neurofibromatosis—Phenotype, Natural History and Pathogenesis. Johns Hopkins University Press, Baltimore, 1986

19. Chutorian AM, Schwartz JF, Evans RA: Optic gliomas in children. Neurology 14:83, 1964

20. Lloyd LA: Gliomas of the optic nerve and chiasm in childhood. Trans Am Ophthalmol Soc 71:488, 1973

21. Lewis RA, Gerson LP, Axelson KA, et al: Von Recklinghausen neurofibromatosis: II. Incidence of optic gliomata. Ophthalmology 91:929, 1984

22. Adornato BT, Berg BO: Diencephalic syndrome in von Recklinghausen disease. Ann Neurol 2:159, 1977

23. Hoyt WF, Baghdassarian SA: Optic glioma of childhood: natural history and rationale for conservative management. Br J Ophthalmol 53:793, 1969

24. Grant WM, Walton DS: Distinctive gonioscopic findings in glaucoma due to neurofibromatosis. Arch Ophthalmol 79:127, 1968

25. Holt JF: Neurofibromatosis in children. AJR 130:615, 1978

26. Hunt JC, Pugh DG: Skeletal lesions in neurofibromatosis. Radiology 76:1, 1961

27. Taveras JM, Wood EH: Diagnostic Neuroradiology. Williams & Wilkins, Baltimore, 1964

28. Ozonoff MB: Angiography. p. 2749. In Newton TH, Potts DG (eds): Radiology of the Skull and Brain. CV Mosby, St. Louis, 1974

29. Holt JF, Wright EM: Radiologic features of neurofibromatosis. Radiology 51:647, 1948

30. Smith CJ, Hatch FE, Johnson JG, et al: Renal artery dysplasia as a cause of hypertension in neurofibromatosis. Arch Intern Med 125:1022, 1970

31. Glushien AS, Mansuy MM, Littman DS: Pheochromocytoma: its relationship to neurocutaneous syndromes. Am J Med 14:318, 1953

32. Hope DG, Mulvihill JJ: Malignancy in neurofibromatosis. Adv Neurol 29:33, 1981

33. Sipple JH: The association of pheochromocytoma with carcinoma of the thyroid. Am J Med 31:163, 1961

34. Carey JC, Lam JM, Hall BD: Penetrance and variability in neurofibromatosis: a genetic study of 60 families. Birth Defects 15:271, 1979

35. Barker D, Wright E, Nguyen K, et al: Gene for von Recklinghausen neurofibromatosis is in the pericentromeric region of chromosome 17. Science 236:110, 1987

36. Imes RK, Hoyt WF: Childhood chiasmal gliomas: update on the fate of patients in the 1969 San Francisco study. Br J Ophthalmol 70:179, 1986

37. Gould JG, Hilal SK, Chutorian AM: Efficacy of radiotherapy in optic gliomas. Pediatr Neurol 3:29, 1987

38. Von Recklinghausen F: Ein Herz von einem Neugeborenen welches mehrere Theils nach Aussen, Theils nach den Hohlen prominirende Tumoren (Myomen) trug. Verh Ges Geburtsch Monatsschr Geburts 20:1, 1862

39. Bourneville DM: Sclérose tubéreuse des circonvolutions cérébrales: idiotie et épilepsie hémiplegique. Arch Neurol (Paris) 1:81, 1880

40. Bourneville DM, Brissaud E: Encéphalite ou sclérose tubéreuse des circonvolutions cérébrales. Arch Neurol (Paris) 1:390, 1881

41. Bourneville DM, Brissaud E: Idiotie et épilepsie symptomatiques de sclérose tubéreuse ou hypertrophique. Arch Neurol (Paris) 10:29, 1900

42. Vogt H: Zur Diagnostik der tuberosen Sklerose. Z Erforsch Behandl Jugendl Schwachsinns 2:1, 1908

43. Gomez MR (ed): Tuberous Sclerosis. Raven Press, New York, 1979

44. Jeavons PM, Bower ND: Infantile spasms. p. 219. In Vinken PJ, Bruyn GW (eds): Handbook of Clinical Neurology. Vol 15. North Holland, Amsterdam, 1974

45. Pampiglione G, Moynahan EJ: The tuberous sclerosis syndrome: clinical and EEG studies in 100 children. J Neurol Neurosurg Psychiatry 39:666, 1976

46. Lagos JC, Gomez MR: Tuberous sclerosis: reappraisal of a clinical entity. Proc Mayo Clin 42:26, 1967

47. Butterworth T, Wilson M: Dermatologic aspects of tuberous sclerosis. Arch Dermatol 43:1, 1941

48. Nickel WR, Reed WB: Tuberous sclerosis. Arch Dermatol 85:209, 1962

49. Reed WB, Nickel WR, Campion G: Internal manifestations of tuberous sclerosis. Arch Dermatol 87:715, 1963

50. Chao DHC: Congenital neurocutaneous syndromes in childhood: II. Tuberous sclerosis J Pediatr 55:447, 1959

51. Gold AP, Freeman JM: Depigmented nevi: the earliest sign of tuberous sclerosis. Pediatrics 35:1003, 1965

52. Fitzpatrick TB, Szabo G, Hori Y, et al: White leaf-shaped macules: earliest visible sign of tuberous sclerosis. Arch Dermatol 98:1, 1968

53. Roth JC, Epstein CJ: Infantile spasms and hypopigmented macules: early manifestations of tuberous sclerosis. Arch Neurol 25:547, 1971

54. McWilliam RC, Stephenson JBP: Depigmented hair:

the earliest sign of tuberous sclerosis. Arch Dis Child 53:961, 1978

55. Barroeta S, Grinspan-Bozza N: Tumor de Koenen sin otras manifestaciones clinicas de epiloia. Arch Argent Dermatol 12:290, 1962

56. Kiun TP: A propos de deux cas de tumeurs de Koenen isolae. Bull Soc Fr Dermatol Syphilol 71:586, 1964

57. Papanyothou P, Verzirtzi E: Tuberous sclerosis with gingival lesions: report of a case. Oral Surg 39:578, 1975

58. Messinger HS, Clarke BW: Retinal tumors in tuberous sclerosis; review of the literature and report of a case with special attention to microscopic structure. Arch Ophthalmol 18:1, 1937

59. Walsh FB, Hoyt WF: Clinical Neuro-Ophthalmology. 3rd Ed. Williams & Wilkins, Baltimore, 1969

60. Robbins TO, Bernstein J: Renal involvement. p. 143. In Gomez MR (ed): Tuberous Sclerosis. Raven Press, New York, 1979

61. Schminke A: Kongenitale Herzhypertrophie bedingt durch diffuse Rhabdomyombildung. Beitr Pathol Anat 70:513, 1922

62. Mair DD: Cardiac manifestations. p. 155. In Gomez MR (ed): Tuberous Sclerosis. Raven Press, New York, 1979

63. Bender BL, Yunis EJ: The pathology of tuberous sclerosis. Pathol Annu 17:339, 1982

64. Konkol RJ, Walsh EP, Power T, et al: Cerebral embolism resulting from an intracardiac tumor in tuberous sclerosis. Pediatr Neurol 2:108, 1986

65. Dawson J: Pulmonary tuberous sclerosis. Q J Med 47:113, 1954

66. Dwyer JM, Hickie JB, Garvan J: Pulmonary tuberous sclerosis: report of three patients and review of the literature. Q J Med 157:115, 1971

67. Lie JT, Miller RD, Williams DE: Cystic disease of the lungs in tuberous sclerosis: clinicopathologic correlation, including body plethysmographic lung function tests. Mayo Clin Proc 55:547, 1980

68. Gutman A, Lefkowitz M: Tuberous sclerosis associated with spontaneous hypoglycemia. Br Med J 2:1065, 1959

69. Sareen K, Ruvalcaba RH, Scotvold MJ, et al: Tuberous sclerosis: clinical, endocrine and metabolic studies. Am J Dis Child 123:34, 1972

70. Hoffman WH, Perrin JCS, Hali E, et al: Acromegalic gigantism in tuberous sclerosis. J Pediatr 93:478, 1978

71. Fitz CR, Harwood-Nash DCF, Thompson JR: Neuroradiology of tuberous sclerosis in children. Radiology 110:635, 1974

72. Martin GL, Kaiserman D, Wegler D, et al: Computer assisted tomography in early diagnosis of tuberous sclerosis. JAMA 235:2323, 1976

73. Garrick R, Gomez MR, Houser OW: Demyelination of the brain in tuberous sclerosis: computed tomography evidence. Mayo Clin Proc 54:685, 1979

74. Maki Y, Enomoto T, Maruyama H, Maekawa K: Computed tomography in tuberous sclerosis: with special reference to relation between clinical manifestations and CT findings. Brain Dev 1:38, 1979

75. McMurdo SK, Moore SG, Brant-Zawadski M, et al: Magnetic imaging of intracranial tuberous sclerosis. AJNR 8:77, 1987

76. Kapp JP, Paulson GW, Odom GL: Brain tumors with tuberous sclerosis. J Neurosurg 26:191, 1967

77. Russell DS, Rubenstein LJ: Pathology of Tumours of the Nervous System. 4th Ed. Edward Arnold, London, 1977

78. Trombley IK, Mirra SS: Ultrastructure of tuberous sclerosis: cortical tubers and subependymal tumor. Ann Neurol 9:174, 1981

79. Schafer J, Berg BO: Cerebellar calcification in tuberous sclerosis. Arch Neurol 32:642, 1975

80. Bundey S, Evans K: Tuberous sclerosis: a genetic study. J Neurol Neurosurg Psychiatry 32:591, 1969

81. Berberich MS, Hall BD: Penetrance and variability in tuberous sclerosis. Birth Defects 15:297, 1979

82. Fryer AED, Chalmers A, Connor JM, et al: Evidence that the gene for tuberous sclerosis is on chromosome 9. Lancet 1:659, 1987

83. Smith M, Haines J, Trofatter J, et al: Linkage studies in tuberous sclerosis. Am J Hum Genet 41:A186, 1987

84. Haines JL, Amos JL, Attwood J, et al: Linkage heterogeneity in tuberous sclerosis. Cytogenet Cell Genet 51:1010, 1989

85. Sampson JR, Yates JRW, Pirrit LA, et al: Evidence for genetic heterogeneity in tuberous sclerosis. J Med Genet 26:511, 1989

86. Panas F, Remy DA: Anatomie Pathologique de L'Oeil. Delahaye, Paris, 1879

87. Fuchs E: Aneurysma arterio-venosum retinae. Arch Augenheilk 11:440, 1882

88. Collins ET: Intra-ocular growths: I. Two cases, brother and sister, with peculiar vascular new growth, probably retinal, affecting both eyes. Trans Ophthalmol Soc UK 14:141, 1894

89. Von Hippel E: Die anatomische Grundlage der von mir beschriebenen "sehr seltene Erkrankung der Netzhaut." Albrecht von Graefes Arch Ophthalmol 79:350, 1911

90. Lindau A: Studien uber Kleinhirncysten: Bau, Pathogenese und Beziehungen zur Angiomatosis retinae. Acta Pathol Microbiol Scand Suppl 1:1, 1926

91. Augsburger JJ, Shields JA, Goldberg RE: Classification and management of hereditary retinal angiomas. Int Ophthalmol 4:93, 1981

92. Atuk NO, McDonald T, Wood T, et al: Familial pheochromocytoma, hypercalcemia, and von Hippel-Lindau disease: a ten year study of a large family. Medicine (Baltimore) 58:209, 1979

93. Greenwald MJ, Weiss A: Ocular manifestations of the neurocutaneous syndromes. Pediatr Dermatol 2:98, 1984

94. Palmer JJ: Haemangioblastomas: a review of 81 cases. Acta Neurochir (Wien) 27:125, 1972

95. Kupersmith MJ, Berenstein A: Visual disturbances in von Hippel-Lindau disease. Ann Ophthalmol 13:195, 1981

96. Goldberg MF, Duke JR: Von Hippel-Lindau disease: case report with histopathological findings in a treated and untreated eye. Am J Ophthalmol 66:693, 1968

97. Salazar FG, Lamiell JM: Early identification of retinal angiomas in a large kindred with von Hippel-Lindau disease. Am J Ophthalmol 89:540, 1980

98. Boker DK, Wassmann H, Solymos L: Multiple spinal hemangioblastomas in a case of Lindau's disease. Surg Neurol 22:439, 1984

99. Melmon KL, Rosen SW: Lindau's disease: a review of the literature and study of a large kindred. Am J Med 36:595, 1964

100. Hardwig P, Robertson DM: von Hippel-Lindau disease: a familial, often lethal multi-system phakomatosis. Ophthalmology 91:263, 1984

101. MacMichael IM: Von Hippel-Lindau's disease of the optic disc. Trans Ophthalmol Soc UK 90:877, 1970

102. Scully RE, Galdabini JJ, McNeely BU: Case records of the Massachusetts General Hospital. N Engl J Med 298:95, 1978

103. Kramer SA, Hoffman AD, Aydin G, et al: Simple renal cysts in children. J Urol 128:1259, 1982

104. Rubenstein LJ: Tumors of the Central Nervous System. 2nd Series, Fascicle 6. Armed Forces Institute of Pathology. Washington, DC, 1972

105. Silver ML: Hereditary vascular tumors of the nervous system. JAMA 156:1053, 1954

106. Christoferson LA, Gustafson MB, Peterson AG: Von Hippel-Lindau's disease. JAMA 178:280, 1961

107. Seizinger BR, Smith DI, Filling-Katz MR, et al: Genetic flanking markers refine diagnostic criteria and provide insights into the genetics of von Hippel-Lindau disease. Proc Natl Acad Sci USA 88:2864, 1991

108. Seizinger BR, Rouleau GA, Ozelius LJ, et al: Von Hippel-Lindau disease maps to the region of chromosome 3 associated with renal cell carcinoma. Nature 332:268, 1988

109. Tory K, Brauch H, Linehan M, et al: Specific genetic change in tumors associated with von Hippel-Lindau disease. J Natl Cancer Inst 81:1097, 1989

110. Schirmer RS: Ein Fall von Telangiektasie. Albrecht von Graefes Arch Ophthalmol 7:199, 1860

111. Sturge WA: A case of partial epilepsy, apparently due to a lesion of one of the vaso-motor centres of the brain. Trans Clin Soc Lond 12:162, 1879

112. Kalischer S: Demonstration des Gehirns eines Kindes mit Telangiectasie der linksseitigen Gesichts Kopfhaut und Hirnoberflache. Berl Klin Wochenschr 34:1059, 1897

113. Weber FB: A note on the association of extensive haemangioblastomatous naevus of the skin with cerebral meningeal haemangiomas, especially cases of facial vascular naevus with contralateral hemiplegia. Proc R Soc Med 22:431, 1929

114. Van Der Hoeve J: Fourth type of phakomatosis. Arch Ophthalmol 18:679, 1937

115. Alexander GL: Sturge-Weber syndrome. p 223. In Vinken PJ, Bruyn GW (eds): Handbook of Clinical Neurology. Vol 14. North Holland, Amsterdam, 1972

116. McKusick VA: Mendelian Inheritance in Man. 10th Ed. Johns Hopkins University Press, Baltimore, 1992

117. Jacobs AH, Walton G: The incidence of birthmarks in the neonate. Pediatrics 58:218, 1976

118. Peterman AF, Hayles AB, Dockerty MB: Encephalotrigeminal angiomatosis (Sturge-Weber disease): clinical study of thirty-four cases. JAMA 167:2169, 1958

119. Chao DHC: Congenital neurocutaneous syndromes of childhood: III. Sturge-Weber disease. J Pediatr 55:635, 1959

120. Hebold O: Haemangiom der weichen Hirnhaut bei Naevus vasculosus des Gesichts. Arch Psychiatr Nervenkr 51:445, 1913

121. Hoffman HJ, Hendricks EB, Dennis M, et al: Hemispherectomy for Sturge-Weber syndrome. Childs Brain 5:223, 1979

122. Bebin EM, Gomez MR: Prognosis in Sturge-Weber disease: comparison of unihemispheric and bihemispheric involvement. J Child Neurol 3:181, 1988

123. Aminoff MJ: Electrodiagnosis in Clinical Neurology. 3rd Ed. Churchill Livingstone, New York, 1992

124. Nellhaus G, Haberlund C, Hill BJ: Sturge-Weber disease with bilateral intracranial calcifications at birth and unusual pathologic findings. Acta Neurol Scand 43:314, 1967

125. Poser CM, Taveras JM: Cerebral angiography in encephalotrigeminal angiomatosis. Radiology 68:327, 1957

126. Bentson JR, Wilson GH, Newton TH: Cerebral venous drainage pattern in Sturge-Weber syndrome. Radiology 102:111, 1971

127. Wagner EJ: CT-angiographic correlation in Sturge-Weber syndrome. J Comput Tomogr 5:324, 1981

128. Chugani HT, Mazziotta JC, Phelps ME: Sturge-Weber syndrome: a study of cerebral glucose utiliza-

tion with positron emission tomography. J Pediatr 114:244, 1989

129. Debicka A, Adamczak P: Przypadek dziedziczenia zespolu Sturge'a-Webera. Klin Oczna 81:541, 1979

130. Wachswulth N, Lowenthal A: Determination chemique d'elements mineraux dans les calcification intracerebrales de la malaidie de Sturge-Weber. Acta Neurol Psychiatr Belg 50:305, 1950

131. Tingey AH: Iron and calcium in Sturge-Weber disease. J Ment Sci 102:178, 1956

132. Rochkind S, Hoffman HJ, Hendrick EB. Sturge-Weber syndrome: natural history and prognosis. J Epilep 3, suppl: 293, 1990

133. Syllaba L, Henner K: Contribution a l'independance de l'athetose double idiopathique et congenitale. Rev Neurol (Paris) 1:541, 1926

134. Louis-Bar D: Sur un syndrome progressif comprenant des télangiectasies capillaires cutanées et conjonctivales symétriques á disposition naevoide et des troubles cérébelleux. Conf Neurol 4:32, 1941

135. Boder E, Sedgwick RP: Ataxia-telangiectasia: a familial syndrome of progressive cerebellar ataxia, oculocutaneous telangiectasia and frequent pulmonary infection: a preliminary report on 7 children, an autopsy, and a case history. Univ South Calif Med Bull 9:15, 1957

136. Biemond A: Paleocerebellar atrophy with extrapyramidal manifestations in association with bronchiectasis and telangiectasis of the conjunctiva bulbi as a familial syndrome. p. 206. In Van Bogaert L, Radermecker J (eds): Proceedings of the First International Congress of Neurological Sciences. Pergamon Press, London, 1957

137. Wells CE, Shy GM: Progressive familial choreoathetosis with cutaneous telangiectasia. J Neurol Neurosurg Psychiatry 20:98, 1957

138. Smith JL, Cogan DD: Ataxia-telangiectasia. Arch Ophthalmol 62:364, 1959

139. Baloh R, Yee RD, Boder E: Eye-movements in ataxia-telangiectasia. Neurology 28:1099, 1978

140. Sedgwick RP, Boder E: Ataxia-telangiectasia. p. 267. In Vinken PJ, Bruyn GW (eds): Handbook of Clinical Neurology. Vol 14. North Holland, Amsterdam, 1972

141. Boder E, Sedgwick RP: Ataxia-telangiectasia. p. 926. In Goldensohn ES, Appel SH (eds): Scientific Approaches to Clinical Neurology. Vol 1. Lea & Febiger, Philadelphia, 1977

142. Centerwall WR, Miller MM: Ataxia-telangiectasia and sino-pulmonary infections: a syndrome of slowly progressive deterioration in childhood. Am J Dis Child 95:385, 1958

143. McFarlin DE, Strober W, Waldmann TA: Ataxia-telangiectasia. Medicine (Baltimore) 51:281, 1972

144. Williams HE, Demis DJ, Higdon RS: Ataxia-telangiectasia: a syndrome with characteristic cutaneous manifestations. Arch Dermatol 82:937, 1960

145. Reed WB, Epstein WL, Boder E, et al: Cutaneous manifestations of ataxia-telangiectasia. JAMA 195:746, 1966

146. Aguilar MJ, Kamoshita S, Landing BH, et al: Pathological observations in ataxia-telangiectasia: a report on 5 cases. J Neuropathol Exp Neurol 27:659, 1968

147. Miller ME, Chatten J: Ovarian changes in ataxia-telangiectasia. Acta Paediatr Scand 56:559, 1967

148. Gatti RA, Good RA: Occurrence of malignancy in immunodeficiency diseases. Cancer 28:89, 1971

149. Spector BD, Filipovich AE, Perry GS, et al: Epidemiology of cancer in ataxia-telangiectasia. p. 103. In Bridges BA, Harnden D (eds): Ataxia-Telangiectasia. John Wiley & Sons, New York, 1982

150. Gatti RA, Bick M, Tam CF, et al: Ataxia-telangiectasia: a multiparameter analysis of eight families. Clin Immunol Immunopathol 23:501, 1982

151. Richkind KE, Boder E, Teplitz RL: Fetal proteins in ataxia-telangiectasia. JAMA 248:1346, 1982

152. Rosenthal IM, Markowitz AS, Medenis R: Immunologic incompetence in ataxia-telangiectasia. Am J Dis Child 110:69, 1965

153. Young RR, Austen KF, Moser HW: Abnormalities of serum gamma 1A globulin and ataxia-telangiectasia. Medicine (Baltimore) 43:423, 1964

154. Waldmann TA, McIntire KR: Serum-alpha-fetoprotein levels in patients with ataxia-telangiectasia. Lancet 2:1112, 1972

155. Sugimoto T, Sawada T, Tozawa M, et al: Plasma levels of carcinoembryonic antigen in patients with ataxia-telangiectasia. J Pediatr 92:436, 1978

156. Peterson RD, Kelly WD, Good RA: Ataxia-telangiectasia: its association with a defective thymus, immunological-deficiency disease and malignancy. Lancet 1:1189, 1964

157. Eisen AH, Karpati G, Laszlo T, et al: Immunologic deficiency in ataxia telangiectasia. N Engl J Med 272:18, 1965

158. Peterson RD, Cooper MD, Good RA: Lymphoid tissue abnormalities associated with ataxia-telangiectasia. Am J Med 41:342, 1966

159. Hecht F, Koler RD, Rigas DA, et al: Leukemia and lymphocytes in ataxia-telangiectasia. Lancet 2:1993, 1966

160. Gropp A, Flatz C: Chromosome breakage and blastic transformation of lymphocytes in ataxia-telangiectasia. Humangenetik 5:77, 1967

161. McCaw BK, Hecht F, Harnden DG, et al: Somatic rearrangement of chromosome 14 in human lymphocytes. Proc Natl Acad Sci USA 72:2071, 1975

162. Davis MM, Gatti RA, Sparkes RS: Neoplasia and chromosomal breakage in ataxia-telangiectasia: a 2:14 translocation. p. 197. In Gatti RA, Swift M (eds): Ataxia-Telangiectasia. Alan R. Liss, New York, 1985

163. Boder E: Ataxia-telangiectasia: some historic, clinical, and pathologic observations. Birth Defects 11:255, 1975

164. Sourander P, Bonnevier JO, Olsson Y: A case of ataxia-telangiectasia with lesions in the spinal cord. Acta Neurol Scand 42:354, 1966

165. Strich SJ: Pathological findings in three cases of ataxia-telangiectasia. J Neurol Neurosurg Psychiatry 29:489, 1966

166. Wara DV, Ammann AJ: Thymosine treatment of children with primary immunodeficiency disease. Transplant Proc 10:203, 1978

12

Neurological Manifestations of Hematological Disorders

G. A. B. Davies-Jones

Hematological disorders can affect the central and peripheral nervous systems in a number of different ways, producing a wide range of neurological disturbances. Some of these neurological complications are well described, but others are less clearly defined. In the present chapter, neurological aspects of each of the main groups of hematological disorders are discussed.

ANEMIA

Iron-Deficiency Anemia

Nonspecific neurological symptoms of tiredness, fatigability, weakness, poor concentration, irritability, faintness, dizziness, tinnitus, and headache are commonly associated with anemia. Occasionally, more concrete neurological syndromes arise, and a number of case reports have drawn attention to the association of benign intracranial hypertension and iron-deficiency anemia.[1,2] In some patients with iron-deficiency anemia, thrombocytosis may be marked and may be so high as to suggest a myeloproliferative disorder. The increased platelet mass may be accompanied by signs and symptoms of cerebrovascular insufficiency, either as transient cerebral ischemic attacks (TIAs) or as cerebral infarction or amaurosis fugax.[3] Profound anemia, particularly if associated

with thrombocytopenia, may produce a retinopathy comprising papilledema, cotton-wool exudates, flame-shaped hemorrhages, retinal edema, and even retinal detachment. Blindness is a rare but long-recognized complication of massive hemorrhage. Pears and Pickering described progressive fundal changes after hemorrhage.[4] The fundus was normal on the day blindness occurred, but on the following day the retinal veins were enlarged. Five days after the onset of blindness the optic disc became swollen, and within 5 weeks this had progressed to optic atrophy.

Focal neurological signs may arise from severe anemia in conjunction with severe cerebral atherosclerosis. Siekert found that reduction of the hemoglobin to 7.5 g/dl produced hemiparesis in a patient with complete occlusion of the contralateral internal carotid artery and tight stenosis of the ipsilateral carotid.[5] The symptoms resolved completely over hours as the hemoglobin was increased to 8.4 g/dl.

Transient erythroblastopenia of childhood has been noted to present with papilledema and transient hemiparesis.[6]

Vitamin B$_{12}$ Deficiency

Vitamin B$_{12}$ deficiency may result in lesions affecting the peripheral nerves, spinal cord, optic nerves, and brain. Addisonian pernicious anemia is an important cause of vitamin B_{12} deficiency, but the neurological complications may also result from vitamin B_{12} deficiency secondary to malabsorption syndromes, gastric and ileal resections, terminal ileal removal for lower urinary tract reconstruction,[7] blind loops, infestation with fish tapeworm, and dietary deficiency, particularly in vegans. It is essential to realize that all the neurological complications of vitamin B_{12} deficiency may occur with no appreciable alteration in the peripheral blood picture. There may be no anemia, and erythropoiesis may even be normoblastic. Lindenbaum and colleagues recently confirmed that neuropsychiatric disorders due to vitamin B_{12} deficiency occur commonly in the absence of anemia or macrocytosis and suggested that measurements of serum methylmalonic acid and total homocysteine both before and after treatment are useful in the diagnosis of these patients.[8]

PERIPHERAL NEUROPATHY

The frequency of peripheral neuropathy as a complication of vitamin B_{12} deficiency is difficult to determine accurately as the sensory symptoms of peripheral neuropathy may be identical to those of vitamin B_{12} myelopathy. However, the finding of muscle wasting and absent reflexes confirms the presence of neuropathy. Electrophysiological studies indicate the neuropathy to be secondary to a dying-back type of axonal degeneration, and neuropathological studies have demonstrated loss of large myelinated fibers in distal sensory nerves as well as axonal degeneration in individually teased fiber preparations.[9,10]

Parasthesias and numbness appear first in the feet and legs, accompanied by loss of reflexes, superficial sensory impairment in a stocking distribution, and impairment of vibration sense. Later there are similar sensory changes in the hands, together with wasting and weakness of the distal leg muscles.

MYELOPATHY

Demyelination followed by axonal degeneration seems to affect the most heavily myelinated fibers first, which may explain why lesions appear first in the posterior columns and later in the lateral columns. They tend first to appear in the midthoracic level. The term *subacute combined degeneration* is appropriate to describe this process in most cases because symptoms and signs usually progress over several weeks and months. However, progression may be rapid, resulting in severe clinical disability within a week or two; or it may be much more chronic, developing over a year or more.

Sensory symptoms appear first in the feet, accompanied by early and severe impairment of proprioception and vibration sense. The ankle reflexes are usually absent owing to the invariable concomitant peripheral neuropathy, but the knee reflexes become exaggerated sooner or later, and subsequently the plantar responses become extensor. Severe sensory ataxic, spastic paraparesis may be virtually the sole manifestation of vitamin B_{12} myelopathy. Bladder symptoms of urinary urgency leading to incontinence occur later.

ENCEPHALOPATHY

The pathological changes in the brain are similar to those in the spinal cord. Multiple foci or diffuse areas of demyelination in the white matter occur with little evidence of glial cell proliferation or axonal degeneration. Changes appear most marked in the corpus callosum and in the frontal and parietal white matter. A variety of symptoms occur, consisting of disorders of mood, mental slowing, poor memory, confusion, agitation, delusions, visual and auditory hallucinations, aggression, dysphasia, and incontinence. Smith and Oliver described a 53-year-old woman with peripheral neuropathy and a serum vitamin B_{12} level of 62 pg/ml due to pernicious anemia who suddenly developed extreme confusion with paranoid delusions and auditory hallucinations.[11] Within 24 hours of receiving 1,000 μg of vitamin B_{12}, her mental state improved; within a few days, she was completely normal.

Shorvon and associates assessed the neuropsychiatric state of 50 patients with megaloblastosis due to vitamin B_{12} deficiency and that of 34 patients due to folate deficiency presenting to hematologists or general physicians.[12] One-third of each group had no neuropsychiatric complications. Peripheral neuropathy was the commonest complication of vitamin B_{12} deficiency (40 percent). Eight patients (16 percent) had evidence of subacute combined degeneration of the cord and one (2 percent) had optic atrophy. Organic mental change of unspecified nature occurred in 26 percent and affective disorders in 20 percent.

Response to vitamin B_{12} therapy is variable. Healton and associates confirmed that all patients respond to some extent to treatment, and recovery was complete in virtually half.[13] The severity score was reduced by 50 percent in 91 percent of instances. Residual long-term moderate or severe neurological disabilities were observed in 6.3 percent. The degree of neurological disability remaining after treatment was related to two factors—the nature of the neurological disability and the duration of symptoms before treatment.

OPTIC NEUROPATHY

Optic neuropathy due to vitamin B_{12} deficiency is rare. Chanarin estimated an incidence of 0.3 percent in patients with pernicious anemia.[14] It is reputedly commoner in men. It may precede, coincide, or follow the anemia or the myelopathy. The characteristic visual abnormality is a centrocecal scotoma, usually appearing earlier to red than to white, which may be associated with constriction of the periphery of the visual field leading to optic atrophy. With early and adequate treatment, recovery may be complete.

EYE MOVEMENTS

Downbeat nystagmus,[15] paralysis of upward gaze,[16] and internuclear ophthalmoplegia[17] have been attributed to vitamin B_{12} deficiency and have responded to vitamin B_{12} therapy.

IMERSLUND-GRASBECK SYNDROME

Vitamin B_{12} malabsorption in the ileum has been suggested to be the underlying cause of this syndrome, which consists of megaloblastic anemia, proteinuria, and multiple neurological abnormalities. A young Saudi child with spasticity, truncal ataxia, cerebral atrophy, megaloblastic anemia, and proteinuria completely recovered following vitamin B_{12} therapy.[18]

Folate Deficiency

In the study of Shorvon and colleagues previously mentioned, affective disorders (mostly depression) and organic mental change were the most common neuropsychiatric complications of folate deficiency.[12]

Peripheral neuropathy was seen in a few, but there was no instance of optic atrophy or myelopathy. Subacute combined degeneration of the cord and optic atrophy occurred only in the patients with vitamin B_{12} deficiency. However, diet-induced folic acid deficiency and subacute combined degeneration of the spinal cord which improved significantly after treatment with folic acid has been recorded.[19]

Mental and physical retardation, hypotonia, cerebral atrophy, seizures, ataxia, and athetoid movements are associated with congenital folate malabsorption; calcification of the basal ganglia has also been reported. Allen and colleagues have associated the Kearns-Sayre syndrome—progressive external ophthalmoplegia, conduction heart block, atypical pigmentary degeneration of the retina, calcification of the basal ganglia, white matter hypodensities on cranial computed tomography (CT), and "ragged red fiber" myopathy—with low cerebrospinal fluid (CSF) folate levels.[20]

Sickle Cell Disease

Most if not all of the clinicopathological complications of sickle cell anemia (Hb SS) or of sickle C disease (Hb SC) relate to the formation of sickle cells; these cells form because of the insolubility of deoxygenated hemoglobins, and they produce vascular occlusion. In circumstances of severe anoxemia, even patients with sickle cell trait (Hb SA) may develop vaso-occlusive disease. Factors exacerbating the sickling phenomenon include hypoxia, dehydration, acidosis, and infection.

As sickling occurs in the venous circulation, central venous PO_2, not arterial PO_2 is the critical factor. There is a trace of sickling in homozygous disease even when hemoglobin is 100 percent saturated with oxygen, whereas at 65 and 50 percent oxygen saturation there is 75 and 100 percent sickling, respectively. In heterozygous disease with 40 percent hemoglobin S (Hb S), sickling starts at 40 percent saturation. The critical PO_2 is 30 mmHg for sickle cell disease and 20 to 30 mmHg for sickle cell trait.[21] In the presence of circulatory stasis or reduced cardiac output, oxygen extraction may be so high that venous PO_2 is reduced to dangerously low values despite normal arterial oxygen tension. In sickle cell trait the severity of sickling depends on the actual amount of Hb S rather than the proportions of hemoglobin A (Hb A) and Hb S. The percentage of Hb S in sickle cell trait can vary from 25 to 45 percent. In vitro studies suggest that in carriers who have a high concentration of Hb S, the risk of sickling is not much less than in patients with sickle cell disease.[22]

Portnoy and Herion established an incidence of 26 percent for neurological manifestations in their patients with sickle cell disease, cerebral infarction and hemiparesis being most common.[23] Cerebral infarction tends to occur in young children. Intracranial hemorrhage is much rarer; it tends to occur more often in adults[24] and is more commonly subarachnoid. In adults, the subarachnoid hemorrhage is usually associated with ruptured aneurysms, but in children it tends to be primary and possibly related to fibrotic endarteritis and fragmentation of the internal elastic lamina of the larger proximal intracranial arteries.[25] In an angiographic study, Stockman and colleagues found partial or complete occlusion of the internal carotid artery as well as disease of the vertebral, anterior cerebral, or middle cerebral artery in six of seven patients with sickle cell disease, and this seemed to be progressive in two.[26]

Other neurological manifestations of sickle cell disease include aphasia, cranial neuropathies,[27] radiculopathy, radiculomyelopathy from vertebral crushing as a result of successive bone infarction, paraplegia, spinal cord infarction, hypopituitarism, optic atrophy, and seizures. Hypertensive encephalopathy with intracranial bleeding complicating sickle cell disease was reported by Hamdan and colleagues in 1984.[28] Spinal cord infarction in sickle cell disease is rare, and there has been only one autopsy report of this complication.[29] Wolman and Hardy had previously described the pathological changes of spinal cord infarction in association with sickle cell trait.[30] Subcortical cerebral infarction has also been described in sickle cell trait.[31]

In contrast to homozygous sickle cell disease, cerebrovascular complications are relatively uncommon in Hb SC disease. The association of proliferative retinopathy with Hb SC disease is well known. Fabian and Peters found a significant increase in retinopathy, stupor, coma, and seizures in patients with Hb SC disease compared with matched controls.[32] Recurrent transient impairment of vision due to occlusion of major retinal vessels is an unusual manifestation of Hb SS disease. Proptosis, frontal headache, and lid edema due to infarction of the orbital bones has been described in Hb SC disease.[33]

It is important to remember that patients with sickle cell disease may develop neurological disorders unrelated to their hemoglobinopathy and so should be investigated to exclude unrelated but treatable conditions. This is illustrated by the patient of Caprioli and colleagues who developed acute monocular visual loss with no retinal or vitreous abnormalities but who had a large aneurysm of the anterior communicating artery compressing the optic nerve.[34]

Thalassemia

Chronic anemias such as thalassemia are associated with extramedullary hematopoiesis, usually in the liver, spleen, or lymph nodes. There have been a few reports of extramedullary hematopoiesis in thalassemia producing spinal cord compression and paraparesis, the hematopoietic tissue presumably arising from embryonal rests in the extradural areolar tissue of mesodermal origin. Most commonly the lesion is situated in the mid to lower dorsal region of the spinal canal, and surgical decompression plus radiotherapy is curative. Treatment with corticosteroids or repeated blood transfusions together with local radiotherapy to the tumor without surgical decompression has also been successful.[35,36] In a recent study, 20 percent of β-thalassemic patients were found to have clinical and electrophysiological findings of a predominantly motor sensorimotor neuropathy.[37]

Hereditary Spherocytosis

There has been an isolated report of two patients with hereditary spherocytosis associated with a mild spastic paraparesis for which no cause was found.[38] Although it may have been an entirely fortuitous association, the authors deliberated about a possible common mechanism for the neurological and red blood cell abnormalities. This association has not been described since.

Paroxysmal Nocturnal Hemoglobinuria

Paroxysmal nocturnal hemoglobinuria is a rare acquired hemolytic disorder that may occur de novo or in association with marrow hypoplasia. Characteristically, increased intravascular destruction of red cells occurs at night, which results in hemoglobinuria seen when the first urine is passed in the morning. One of the commonest complications of this disorder is large-vessel thrombosis, and its occurrence in the brain and portal system accounts for the death of 50 percent of patients. The cause of the thrombotic tendency is unknown. Although thrombosis has been reported in most organs, it has not been detected in the vessels of the spinal cord; most of the neurological complications of paroxysmal nocturnal hemoglobinuria relate to thrombosis of intracranial vessels. Cerebral arterial and venous thrombosis occurs, resulting in hemorrhagic infarction.[39] Barnett noted that, during the crises of paroxysmal nocturnal hemoglobinuria, an occasional patient suffers TIAs due to the hypercoagulable state induced when excess thromboplastin is released from lysing red blood cells.[40]

Kernicterus

With the virtual elimination of hemolytic disease of the newborn, kernicterus is now very uncommon. It may be produced by any hemolytic process of sufficient severity in neonates and in premature infants by "physiological jaundice." Whenever the serum unconjugated bilirubin level rises above 20 mg/dl during the first few weeks of life, kernicterus may occur. Unconjugated bilirubin is highly lipid-soluble; it enters the brain and binds to neurons, resulting in neuronal necrosis particularly in the basal nuclei and cerebellum. The neurological features include ophisthotonos, convulsions, rigidity, involuntary movements, athetosis, deafness, nystagmus, and psychotic behavior.

RARE NEUROLOGICAL SYNDROMES AND RED CELL ABNORMALITIES

The Hallervorden-Spatz syndrome of dystonia, dementia, and spasticity in childhood or adolescence been associated on one occasion with acanthocytosis.[41]

Bassen-Kornzweig disease—neuroacanthocytosis with abetalipoproteinemia—is a well-defined syndrome characterized by acanthocytosis, retinitis pigmentosa, increasing cerebellar ataxia, steatorrhea, and complete or almost complete lack of serum β-lipoproteins, with onset during childhood and recessive inheritance.

Choreo-amyotrophy-acanthocytosis is another rare neurological syndrome associated with peripheral blood acanthocytosis. The neurological features consist of adult-onset progressive choreiform movements of the limbs, lip and tongue biting, orofacial dyskinesia, high serum creatine kinase levels, peripheral neuropathy with amyotrophy, and normal serum lipoproteins. These patients may also develop features of parkinsonism.[42,43] This neurological syndrome without acanthocytosis but with chronic spherocytic hemolytic anemia was seen in two brothers by Spencer and associates.[44] At autopsy the striatum was atrophic, with iron deposition and spheroid bodies. There was degeneration of the substantia nigra and anterior horn cells of the spinal cord. These features provide an anatomical basis for the parkinsonism and motor neuron disease associated with choreo-amyotrophy-acanthocytosis.

Hardie and associates reviewed 19 cases of neuroacanthocytosis in which progressive chorea, dystonia, akinetic rigidity, orofaciolingual movements, pseudobulbar dysphagia and dysarthria, and lip and tongue biting occurred.[45] Cognitive impairment and organic personality changes occurred in over half of the cases, and more than one-third had seizures. Depressed or absent reflexes occurred in 13 and axonal neuropathy was often found electrophysiologically. The investigators emphasized that mild acanthocytosis can easily be overlooked and that scanning electronmicroscopy may be helpful. Abnormalities of membrane transport in the erythrocytes of this disorder have been described.[46]

A benign X-linked myopathy with acanthocytosis has also been described and is referred to as McLeod's syndrome.

A new progressive spinocerebellar syndrome and a sideroblastic anemia segregating together in an X-linked recessive fashion was described by Pagan and co-workers[47] and appears to be unique. The ataxia and the pyramidal signs appeared to improve with age in affected children. Linkage to phosphoglycerate kinase at band Xq13 has been described in a kindred with X-linked sideroblastic anemia and ataxia,[48] and a case of primary acquired sideroblastic anemia with a predominantly motor polyneuropathy responsive to vitamin B_6 has been documented.[49]

Triosephosphate isomerase deficiency is a rare disorder characterized by chronic hemolytic anemia, progressive neurological dysfunction, and usually an increased susceptibility to infection. The neurological features consist of a dystonic-dyskinetic syndrome, gross intention tremor and rhythmic jerky movements of the proximal parts of the limbs, generalized weakness, amyotrophy and hypotonia of the trunk and limbs, and sometimes pyramidal signs. There are electromyographic (EMG) signs of denervation with normal conduction velocities, suggestive of anterior horn cell impairment.[50] It has been suggested that low triosephosphate isomerase activity leads to a metabolic block in the glycolytic pathway and hence to an impairment of cellular energy supply.[51]

PROLIFERATIVE DISORDERS

Leukemia

The increased frequency of central nervous system (CNS) involvement in leukemia is related to the increased survival of patients. It is estimated to occur in between 2 and 4 percent of leukemic patients per month. CNS involvement is a poor prognostic sign if it is evident on presentation and even more so if it develops later.

Involvement of the CNS in leukemia is often due to infiltration with leukemic cells, but neurological complications may occur as a result of hemorrhage, infection, drug- and radiation-induced neurotoxicity, electrolyte disturbance, or impairment of cerebral circulation from leukostasis.

Leukemic cells enter the nervous system by direct seeding of circulating leukemic cells, lymphatic spread, direct invasion from overlying meninges, or from cells with hematopoietic potential lying in relationship to arachnoidal vessels.[52]

MENINGEAL LEUKEMIA

The commonest presenting symptoms of meningeal leukemia are headaches, nausea and vomiting sometimes associated with lethargy and irritability, drowsiness, coma, convulsions, and neck stiffness. Diffuse meningeal infiltration impairs the circulation of CSF and can result in obstructive or communicating hydrocephalus. Papilledema is the commonest sign, with separation of the skull sutures in young children. The leukemic deposits may compress or infiltrate the

cranial nerves or spinal nerve roots and spread between the nerve fibers. The second, third, sixth, seventh, and eight cranial nerves are the most commonly affected, but the lower cranial nerves are occasionally involved. Oculomotor palsy with pupillary sparing has been described secondary to chronic lymphocytic leukemic infiltration of the meninges.[53]

The diagnosis of meningeal leukemia is confirmed by finding leukemic cells in the CSF. Increased CSF leukocyte counts are found in approximately 90 percent of cases, and cytocentrifuge preparations enable both blast cells and mitotic figures to be identified. A study by Ricevuti and colleagues confirmed the importance of cytospin technique for discovering the disease in its early stages.[54] The CSF pressure is usually elevated, but in approximately 10 percent of cases with unequivocal clinical evidence of meningeal involvement, the CSF is normal in every respect. Reduced CSF glucose and elevated protein concentrations are frequently seen but are unreliable characteristics of meningeal disease.

Although meningeal leukemia is predominantly associated with acute lymphocytic leukemia and occasionally with acute nonlymphocytic leukemia, meningeal leukemia as the initial presentation of B-cell chronic lymphocytic leukemia has been described.[55]

More recently, it has been recognized that acute myelomonocytic leukemia accompanied by pericentric inversion of chromosome 16 is a unique subtype associated with a high incidence of CNS involvement in the form of leptomeningeal deposits and granulocytic sarcoma.

LOCALIZED LEUKEMIC DEPOSITS

Any part of the CNS may be involved by leukemic deposits. The symptoms and signs are therefore numerous and varied, and they depend on the extent of infiltration and the area of localization. The complete range of cranial nerve palsies has been described, as has hemiplegia, aphasia, hemianopia, ataxia, convulsions, and cortical blindness.[56] Blindness may also occur from leukemic infiltration of the optic nerve head.[57] I have seen three patients with mental nerve involvement that produced sensory impairment of the lower lip and painless ulceration of its buccal mucosa.

Hypothalamic and pituitary dysfunction are not uncommon, resulting in the hypothalamic obesity–somnolence syndrome, with excessive eating, headache, weight gain, somnolence, vomiting, and a change of behavior, usually to a more aggressive pattern. Histological examination of the hypothalamus in these cases shows diffuse infiltration by leukemic cells. This syndrome may also be associated with hydrocephalus, the hypothalamic pituitary dysfunction arising from the pressure effects of a distended third ventricle. Diabetes insipidus may occur alone or as part of the hypothalamic obesity syndrome.

Clinically significant spinal cord involvement is unusual in leukemia, in contrast to intracranial, especially meningeal, involvement. The clinical syndromes relating to spinal cord involvement range from a complete cord syndrome (transverse lesion of the spinal cord with paraplegia, sensory loss below the involved segment, and urinary retention) to partial cord syndromes: anterior or posterior cord syndromes or the Brown-Séquard syndrome. Back pain, frequently with root involvement, and progressive paraparesis or quadriparesis over days or weeks is another manifestation of progressive spinal cord compression from extradural deposits, usually in the thoracic area. Cervical cord, cauda equina, and conus medullaris compression occur rarely. In their review of spinal cord leukemia, Petursson and Boggs found acute myeloid leukemia to be the commonest type, followed by acute lymphoblastic and chronic myeloid leukemia, with only one instance of chronic lymphatic leukemia.[58] Cord syndromes arise from compression by extradural deposits; direct infiltration of the spinal cord and nerve roots; vascular occlusion by thrombus, leukemic cells, or a mixture of leukemic cells and thrombus; or hemorrhage. Exceptionally an acute paraneoplastic necrotizing myelopathy may occur.

Peripheral neuropathy complicating leukemia is rare. It usually results from diffuse leukemic infiltration, hemorrhage, or infarction, and it manifests by either individual or multiple nerve involvement. Proved examples of paraneoplastic neuropathy are exceptionally uncommon. Adult T cell leukemia found among subjects born in Kyushu, Japan, may be complicated by a peripheral neuropathy.[59]

CHLOROMAS

Chloromas are solid tumors of nonlymphatic leukemia. Occasionally, extramedullary chloromas occur in patients without any evidence of leukemia, which these tumors may precede by many months. Histologically, they are composed of poorly differentiated blast cells, almost invariably myeloblasts but occasionally monoblasts. Macroscopically, they have a distinctive green color that fades on exposure to light. Most occur subperiosteally, usually in the cranial and facial bones, especially the paranasal sinuses, mastoid air cells, or orbits; they are usually attached to the dura mater. More common in children than adults, they may present with ophthalmoplegia and exophthalmos if orbital in origin or facial palsy if they arise from the mastoid air cells. As a result of dural involvement, they may produce headaches, nausea, vomiting, papilledema, hemiplegia, or multiple cranial nerve palsies. They rarely invade cerebral tissue. Chloromas associated with the spinal dura mater result in spinal cord compression. Decompression together with radiotherapy or chemotherapy produces resolution of the paraplegia and disappearance of the tumor.[60] Chloromas are radiosensitive.

INTRACRANIAL HEMORRHAGE

Intracranial hemorrhage usually occurs at presentation or during relapse when the leukemic patient is unresponsive to chemotherapy. Thrombocytopenia is an almost constant concomitant of intracranial hemorrhage. It is possible, at least in some cases, that it is the result of platelet consumption due to disseminated intravascular coagulation (DIC) rather than to reduced platelet production by the bone marrow secondary to leukemic infiltration. Platelet production may also be impaired as a result of myelotoxic effects of the chemotherapy. In the absence of any other abnormality of coagulation, intracranial hemorrhage is unusual if the platelet count is greater than 20,000/mm^3. Bleeding in the CNS is usually multifocal, affecting the meninges as well as the brain or spinal cord. Characteristically, the hemorrhages vary in size from multiple petechial hemorrhages to large confluent ones. DIC is a prominent feature of promyelocytic leukemia. In other forms of leukemia, DIC is particularly marked in patients with high peripheral white cell counts, and it appears soon after the beginning of chemotherapy, presumably occurring because tissue thromboplastins are released from destroyed leukocytes.

The widespread distribution of hemorrhage in acute leukemia usually results in deep coma from the outset, rapidly progressing to death. If the bleeding is localized and not multifocal, the resultant syndromes depend on the part of the neuraxis involved. The cerebral hemispheres are most frequently implicated, particularly the white matter. Both acute and chronic subdural hematoma may occur; and cisternal, cervical, or lumbar puncture in a thrombocytopenic patient with acute leukemia may cause a spinal subdural hematoma and spinal cord or cauda equina compression.

CELLULAR HYPERVISCOSITY

The hyperviscosity syndrome embraces a symptom complex of neurological dysfunction, visual disturbances, and a hemorrhagic tendency. Marked elevation of the white cell count may produce a significant increase in whole blood viscosity. All types of leukemia, acute or chronic, may produce this syndrome, but neurological symptoms may occur more readily at lower leukocyte counts in patients with myeloid leukemia than in patients with lymphocytic leukemia. This finding is probably a reflection of the larger cell size in the myelogenous leukemias.

The signs and symptoms of cellular hyperviscosity are varied and include auditory and visual disturbances, headache, ataxia, profound lethargy, somnolence, impairment of consciousness, and TIAs (Fig. 12-1). It is important to recognize the possibility of this syndrome in patients with massively elevated white cell counts (in excess of $200 \times 10^9/L$), as treatment with leukapheresis may abolish the symptoms. It is important also to remember that blood transfusions may be hazardous in patients with high leukocyte counts because the additional red blood cells may further elevate the blood viscosity to clinically significant levels, sufficient to produce coma and even death. Hyperleukocytosis in chronic myeloid leukemia may also result in deafness.[61]

INFECTIONS

In all leukemias, but particularly in the lymphoblastic leukemia of childhood, viruses (especially mumps, measles, and varicella) are the commonest infective organisms of the CNS. Bacterial and fungal infections, especially aspergillosis, also occur. The increased incidence of CNS involvement by rare organisms or organisms that are normally nonpathogenic is contributed to by widespread use of corticosteroids, chemotherapy, and broad-spectrum antibiotics.

LEUKOENCEPHALOPATHY

Progressive multifocal leukoencephalopathy may complicate a variety of chronic diseases, including leukemias, lymphomas, carcinomas, and sarcoidosis

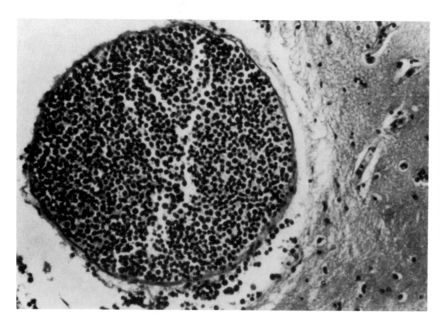

Fig. 12-1 Cellular hyperviscosity in leukemia. Virtually complete occlusion of cortical vessel with leukemic cells. (Hematoxylin and eosin. Original magnification × 504.) (From Davies-Jones GAB, Preston FE, Timperley WR: Neurological Complications in Clinical Haematology. Blackwell Scientific Publications, Oxford, 1980, with permission.)

(see Ch. 43). Another disseminated leukoencephalopathy appears in patients with acute lymphoblastic leukemia treated with cranial irradiation and intrathecal methotrexate or in those treated with craniospinal irradiation followed by intravenous methotrexate. High-dose intravenous methotrexate by itself can produce an encephalopathy. It has been suggested that, with either cranial irradiation or intrathecal methotrexate, encephalopathy develops in less than 1 percent of children and with high-dose intravenous methotrexate less than 2 percent; however, combined intravenous methotrexate and cranial irradiation or intrathecal methotrexate and cranial irradiation increases the incidence to 15 percent and 5 percent, respectively.[62]

Pathologically, the leukoencephalopathy is characterized by demyelination, axonal degeneration, gliosis, coagulation necrosis with or without fibrinoid vascular change, mineralizing microangiopathy, and calcification. The periventricular white matter seems to be preferentially involved, but the lesions may occur anywhere in the white matter of the brain and spinal cord. The clinical manifestations of this form of encephalopathy may be delayed until several months after treatment is finished. The symptoms and signs may be varied and diffuse, reflecting the disseminated neuropathological process. Clinical features include irritability, agitation, confusion, drowsiness, ataxia, dementia, hemiplegia, quadriplegia, aphasia, and hemianopia.

Cranial irradiation may produce signs of mild encephalopathy within hours of the initial dose. This usually results in somnolence but may be associated with signs of increased intracranial pressure, cranial nerve palsies, convulsions, ataxia, signs of cerebral herniation, coma, and death, especially if the patient has been given one or more injections of intrathecal chemotherapy. Cranial irradiation alone may also produce a "somnolence syndrome," which generally occurs several weeks after treatment.

Leukoencephalopathy following radiotherapy and intrathecal methotrexate may result in learning difficulties, cognitive dysfunction, and seizures in long-term survivors of childhood leukemia. Brouwers and associates showed that leukoencephalopathic patients with CT scan abnormalities of any type—calcification and cerebral atrophy—exhibited poor memory (more so for long-term retention than immediate recall) and difficulty in word finding as compared with

patients who had normal CT scans.[63] Patients with CT calcification showed greater deficits than those with cortical atrophy.

Green and colleagues studied 17 adult patients with acute lymphoblastic leukemia, assessing them by neurological examination, electroencephalography (EEG), auditory evoked potentials, CT scans, and magnetic resonance imaging (MRI).[64] They concluded that there was little evidence of major CNS sequelae to the prophylactic use of cranial irradiation and intrathecal methotrexate in adults. Only minor abnormalities were found in the neurophysiological tests, psychometry, and scans in a few of the patients.

Acute encephalopathy during induction therapy for acute lymphoblastic leukemia occurred in 21 children in the Medical Research Council UKALL VIII study and trial.[65] This was attributed to drug toxicity, probably from L-asparaginase, although vincristine may also have contributed. Convulsions (sometimes focal) and coma were the major features.

Myelomatosis

The nervous system is commonly involved in myelomatosis. The major neurological complications can be placed into four categories: (1) compression of spinal cord, cauda equina, or solitary nerve roots; (2) cranial nerve involvement; (3) intracranial myeloma; and (4) peripheral neuropathy. Pure meningeal myeloma is rare (Fig. 12-2).

SPINAL MYELOMA

The vertebrae are commonly infiltrated by myeloma cells, which may extend into the extradural space to form an extradural tumor and cause spinal cord compression. As a cause of cord compression, myeloma comes second to metastatic carcinoma in frequency. Vertebral body fragmentation and collapse may also produce neurological deficits from spinal cord and nerve root compression. Silverstein and Doniger found evidence of spinal cord compression in 22 patients and compression of the cauda equina in 5 patients among 277 cases of myelomatosis,[66] and Brenner and associates found a 16 percent incidence of spinal cord compression among similar patients.[67]

Extradural myeloma tumor may occur without local bone involvement, and intradural deposits of myeloma may arise through spread along nerve roots

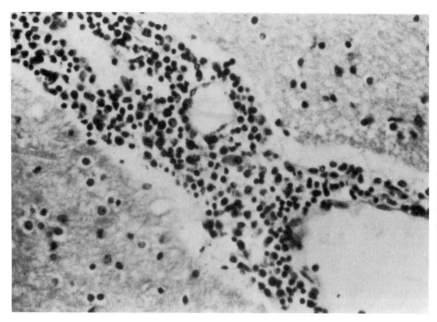

Fig. 12-2 Section of hypothalamus showing meningeal infiltration by myeloma cells. This patient had diffuse meningeal involvement by myeloma cells without parenchymatous infiltration of the brain or spinal cord. (Hematoxylin and eosin. Original magnification × 504.) (From Davies-Jones GAB, Preston FE, Timperley WR: Neurological Complications in Clinical Haematology. Blackwell Scientific Publications, Oxford, 1980, with permission.)

via intervertebral foramina. Spinal cord compression has infrequently been caused by amyloid deposits.[68] Actual infiltration of the spinal cord by myeloma cells is rare, and a paraneoplastic type of myelopathy is also an infrequent occurrence. The lower dorsal area of the spinal cord is the most commonly affected area, followed by lumbar and cauda equina involvement. Cervical cord compression is relatively rare.

The neurological symptoms develop comparatively slowly but may do so over a week or two. Usually back pain of several months' duration precedes any evidence of spinal cord compression, but occasionally the interval is a few weeks only. Syndromes typical of spinal cord or cauda equina compression occur, with sensory impairment below the lesion and a spastic or flaccid paraparesis progressing to complete paraplegia with urinary retention and incontinence.

NERVE ROOT COMPRESSION

Nerve root compression is produced by direct infiltration or compression by myeloma cells or by compression from vertebral collapse. Progressive brachialgia accompanied by sensory impairment and weakness or lumbosacral pain with sensorimotor dysfunction results.

CRANIAL MYELOMA

Cranial myeloma is rare. The predominant sites of occurrence are the region of the sella and cavernous sinus, the body of the sphenoid, and the apex of the petrous bones. Orbital myeloma is well recognized, and myeloma may present as an orbital mass with proptosis and ophthalmoplegia. Total ophthalmoplegia due to amyloid infiltration of the extraocular muscles secondary to myeloma has been described.[69] Myeloma may infiltrate the intracranial cavity from the oropharynx or paranasal sinuses. Primary plasmacytomas may originate in the cranial vault or the dura. Direct infiltration of the brain by myeloma cells is exceptionally rare, as is diffuse meningeal involvement. Bilateral optic neuritis producing painless progressive impairment of visual acuity over 12 months and bilateral central scotomas has been described in relation to IgA lambda myeloma. The optic neuritis recovered virtually to normal over 2 months, suggesting that the optic nerve involvement was unlikely to be due to infiltration and was possibly secondary to binding of IgA to myelin.[70]

Headaches and signs of raised intracranial pressure appear to be the earliest indications of intracranial myeloma. Other signs and symptoms are entirely related to the site of the lesion and can vary from a palpable lump over the skull vault to convulsions, hemiparesis, hemianopia, diabetes insipidus and hypopituitarism, cranial nerve palsies, brainstem syndromes, and symptoms of generalized cerebral impairment such as confusion, disorientation, drowsiness, and coma. The pathogenesis of the latter in the setting of myelomatosis is complicated, and undoubtedly factors such as renal failure, anemia, hypercalcemia, and hyperviscosity play a part.

Benign intracranial hypertension has been observed in three cases of IgG myeloma. None of the patients showed evidence of hyperviscosity or of intracranial myeloma.[71]

PERIPHERAL NEUROPATHY

There are four types of neuropathy secondary to myelomatosis:

1. Paraneoplastic neuropathy producing demyelination and axis cylinder degeneration
2. Ischemic neuropathy due to amyloid deposition in the vasa nervorum
3. Amyloid infiltration of the peripheral nerves (Fig. 12-3)
4. Infiltration of the peripheral nerves by myeloma tissue

Neuropathy occurring in myelomatosis results in a chronic, progressive, symmetrical sensorimotor disturbance affecting the legs first and, later and to a lesser extent, the arms. This is particularly so of the paraneoplastic variety, whereas infiltration by myeloma or amyloid tissue may produce an asymmetrical or mononeuritic picture. Although it is a complication of the established disease in diffuse myelomatosis, the paraneoplastic type of neuropathy is usually the presenting feature of a solitary, commonly sclerotic plasmacytoma. This combination has a distinct male predominance. The solitary sclerotic tumor may arise in the vertebrae, ribs, clavicles, scapulae, or long bones. The CSF protein concentration is increased, but the peripheral blood and bone marrow are normal; the erythrocyte sedimentation rate (ESR) is usually normal, and there is typically no paraprotein unless serum immunoelectrophoresis or immunofixation is performed. Localized radiotherapy to the bone lesion effectively arrests and usually alleviates the neuropathy. The outlook for survival is good.

A progressive, symmetrical sensorimotor neuropathy in patients with monoclonal gammopathy, char-

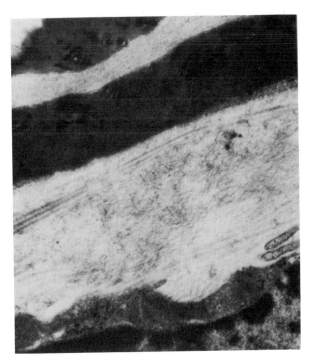

Fig. 12-3 Amyloid neuropathy in myeloma. Electron micrograph shows fibrillary deposits of amyloid adjacent to an axon. (From Davies-Jones GAB, Preston FE, Timperley WR: Neurological Complications in Clinical Haematology. Blackwell Scientific Publications, Oxford, 1980, with permission.)

acteristically osteosclerotic bone lesions, and circulating light-chain paraprotein has been described predominantly from Japan. It is sometimes called POEMS syndrome (plasma cell dyscrasia with polyneuropathy, organomegaly, endocrinopathy, monoclonal gammopathy, and skin changes). This syndrome has also been described in association with extramedullary plasmacytoma and occasionally with isolated dysproteinemia only.[72]

Osteosclerotic myeloma is a plasma cell dyscrasia characterized by sclerotic bone lesions, progressive demyelinating polyneuropathy, and bone marrow containing less than 5 percent plasma cells (in multiple myeloma the bone marrow contains more than 10 percent plasma cells). Miralles and associates suggested that the relationship between osteosclerotic myeloma and the POEMS syndrome is artificial.[73] In their study, 84 percent of patients who fulfilled the criteria for osteosclerotic myeloma had multiorgan involvement: skin change (58 percent), lymphadenopathy (42 percent), papilledema (37 percent), peripheral edema (29 percent), hepatomegaly (24 percent), splenomegaly (21 percent), and ascites (11 percent). Five patients fulfilled the criteria for the POEMS syndrome, and these patients had the same clinical outcome as those with the incomplete forms. There seemed to be no benefit in differentiating POEMS syndrome and osteosclerotic myeloma. *Plasma cell dyscrasia with polyneuropathy* is a better all-embracing term to include the variables of these two conditions.

A particularly localized form of neuropathy due to infiltration of the carpal tunnel by amyloid deposits is well recognized.

Jowitt and associates described a patient who developed polymyositis 18 months after multiple myeloma was diagnosed.[74]

NEUROLOGICAL EFFECTS OF THE METABOLIC COMPLICATIONS OF MYELOMA

Neurological complications may result from hypercalcemia, uremia, and hyperviscosity (Fig. 12-4). The hyperviscosity syndrome occurs most commonly in IgA myeloma to the extent that 25 percent of patients with this form of myeloma attending the author's hospital have at one time or another developed this complication.[75] It occurs because the IgA myeloma molecule has an inherent tendency to form high-molecular-weight polymers.

Hypercalcemia and uremia cause increasing headaches, confusion, disorientation, somnolence, stupor, coma, uremic convulsions, and myoclonic twitching. The hyperviscosity syndrome of myeloma is identical to that of Waldenström's macroglobulinemia.

NEUROLOGICAL EFFECTS OF THE IMMUNOLOGICAL COMPLICATIONS OF MYELOMA

Immunological incompetence is often a feature of myelomatosis. In the CNS, this is reflected by the development of meningitis (bacterial, viral, fungal) and cerebral abscess. Pneumococcal infection is particularly implicated, as is herpes zoster and, more rarely, cryptococcosis and toxoplasmosis. Profound septicemia may be complicated by cerebral DIC. Progressive multifocal leukoencephalopathy may also occur.

Macroglobulinemia (Waldenström's Disease)

It has been estimated that peripheral or CNS symptoms occur in 25 percent of patients with macroglobulinemia. Although peripheral neuropathy may be associated with the hyperviscosity syndrome, this is unusual; it is unlikely, therefore, that the hyperviscosity syndrome is the cause of the neuropathy in most

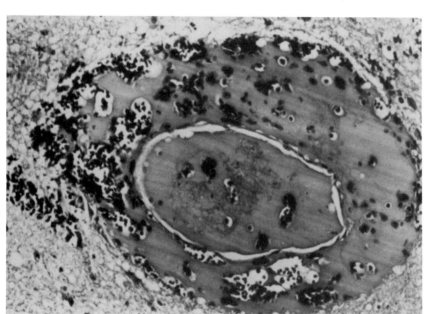

Fig. 12-4 Plugging of a cerebral vessel by hyperviscous protein with seepage into the perivascular space secondary to vessel ischemia, from a case of hyperviscosity syndrome in myeloma. (Original magnification ×504.) (From Davies-Jones GAB, Preston FE, Timperley WR: Neurological Complications in Clinical Haematology. Blackwell Scientific Publications, Oxford, 1980, with permission.)

patients with macroglobulinemia and paraproteinemia. The cause of the neuropathy is obscure but in some cases may be related to the binding of monoclonal IgM on to nerve structures. Latov and associates showed that monoclonal IgM from some patients possessed antibody activity directed against myelin antigens[76,77]; and Dellagi and colleagues, studying the binding of monoclonal IgM to human peripheral nerve in 25 patients with Waldenström's macroglobulinemia and peripheral neuropathy, found that 40 percent had antibody activity against myelin sheath.[78] Other mechanisms such as lymphocytic infiltration of the peripheral nerves, amyloidosis, and bleeding tendency have also been suggested to account for the neuropathy.

Complete unilateral ophthalmoplegia has been described as the presenting manifestation of Waldenström's macroglobunemia,[79] as has an isolated lesion of the fourth cranial nerve.[80] MRI in the latter case demonstrated an orbital apex lesion which was not biopsied. There were no other neurological lesions. Four months after initiation of treatment with prednisolone and chlorambucil, MRI revealed complete resolution of the orbital lesion, which was probably a lymphoid infiltrate.

The other neurological complications relate to hyperviscosity and bleeding tendency. Any part of the CNS may be involved, with complications presenting as strokes or other focal brain syndromes, diffuse encephalopathy, subarachnoid hemorrhage, and spinal cord symptoms from hemorrhage or infarction. Patients frequently complain of profound fatigue, lethargy, and headaches, and they develop confusion, stupor, coma, and convulsions. Visual disturbances and deafness occur and may be irreversible. Congestion, tortuosity, and segmental dilation of retinal veins occur, as do hemorrhages, exudates, and papilledema. The bleeding tendency results in spontaneous bruising, purpura, epistaxis, gastrointestinal hemorrhage, and oozing from venipuncture sites. Dramatic relief is frequently achieved by plasmapheresis. Exceptionally, Waldenström's disease is complicated by the development of primary intracerebral lymphoma.

Lymphoma

Hodgkin's disease and the non-Hodgkin's lymphomas affect the nervous system with equal frequency, but only rarely. This usually occurs by direct spread from primary nodal and extranodal sites. Occasionally, primary Hodgkin's disease and primary non-Hodgkin's lymphoma (microglioma, reticulum cell sarcoma, histiocytic lymphoma) of the CNS are seen. Although as many as 25 percent of all non-Hodgkin's lymphomas present in extranodal sites, only 1 percent or fewer present in the CNS. The neurological complications result from compression and direct invasion of the nervous system or from secondary paraneoplastic syndromes. Within the CNS, the cerebral hemispheres are the most frequent site of presentation, followed by the cerebellum and brainstem. Primary lymphomas of the spinal cord are exceptionally rare. CNS involvement occurs most commonly with lymphoblastic lymphoma, followed by diffuse undifferentiated lymphoma and diffuse histiocytic lymphoma.

SPINAL CORD AND MENINGEAL INVOLVEMENT

Spinal cord and meningeal involvement are relatively common neurological complications of the lymphomas. In one study, 38 percent of patients with systemic lymphoma and CNS involvement had spinal cord tumors.[81] Extradural deposits arise as a result of direct spread from the retroperitoneal or postmediastinal spaces via the intervertebral foramina, or by direct invasion from an affected vertebral body. The tumor often extends around the lateral aspect of the spinal cord and may encircle it completely. The dura mater usually prevents invasion of the cord itself, but the segmental arterial supply may be compressed by the tumor to produce an ischemic myelopathy. Rarely an acute necrotizing myelopathy appears as a remote paraneoplastic effect of a lymphoma. This is universally progressive. A less acute paraneoplastic myelopathy developed in a patient with pathological stage 1A Hodgkin's disease before treatment was begun; it resolved substantially with intrathecal dexamethasone.[82]

With compressive lesions, back pain, frequently worse on lying down and often associated with radicular spread, is accompanied by progressive spinal cord dysfunction, producing a spastic paraparesis, sensory impairment below the lesion, and sphincter problems resulting in incontinence. Spinal cord segments C5 to T8 are most commonly implicated, although compression of the cauda equina may occur. A Brown-Séquard syndrome secondary to extradural compression has been described. Nerve roots may be invaded by the lymphoma, causing pain and sensorimotor segmental syndromes (e.g., cervical or lumbosacral radiculopathy).

INTRACRANIAL INVOLVEMENT

Intracranial involvement usually arises from infiltration via the skull base by direct extension from involved cervical lymph nodes as well as by lymphatic spread. On rare occasions lymphoma of the skull bones has been known to spread to form an intracranial mass. Tumor is usually found extradurally but may be within the dura as a subdural mass that sometimes invades underlying brain; it may even be purely intracerebral. Typically, widespread disseminated meningeal lesions occur and characteristically produce multiple cranial nerve palsies, headaches, meningism, and papilledema. The seventh cranial nerve seems to be most commonly implicated.[83] Patients with T- and B-cell surface markers appear to be at an increased risk of cranial nerve involvement, factors also associated with increased incidence of CNS relapse. Almost all cases of lymphomatous meningitis are found in patients with diffuse non-Hodgkin's lymphoma; lymphoblastic lymphoma, diffuse histiocytic lymphoma, diffuse undifferentiated lymphoma, and diffuse lymphocytic poorly differentiated lymphoma have a high incidence of meningeal disease.

Meningeal lymphoma may have a protracted course with spontaneous remission of clinical and neuroimaging signs. A patient with spontaneous remission of a third cranial nerve palsy developed meningeal lymphoma that produced multiple lumbosacral radiculopathies a year after initial presentation. Nerve root biopsy revealed a B cell lymphoma. Serial CSF analyses over the intervening year showed occasional atypical cells that were later found to resemble closely the biopsy cell type.[84]

Intracranial deposits produce signs and symptoms of increased intracranial pressure with focal disturbances as a result of infiltration of the cerebral hemispheres, cerebellum, or brainstem. Convulsions may occur. Painful ophthalmoplegia with proptosis, together with sensory impairment of the cornea and ophthalmic division of the trigeminal nerve due to cavernous sinus infiltration, is a recognized intracranial complication and usually occurs by invasion from the ethmoid or sphenoid bones or sinuses. Intracranial deposits seem to be more often associated with histio-

cytic lymphoma and orbital deposits more commonly with lymphocytic lymphoma. Intracranial deposits are rarely seen in lymphocytic lymphoma unless leukemia has supervened.

Anterior visual system involvement in non-Hodgkin's lymphoma due to lymphomatous infiltration of the optic chiasm in one patient and bilateral optic neuropathy in another who later developed progressive multifocal leukoencephalopathy was recently reported by Zaman and associates.[85]

Younger and colleagues studied nine patients with motor neuron disease and lymphoma.[86] They described upper and lower motor neuron signs in association with lymphoma and often with paraproteinuria as well. Such signs suggestive of amyotrophic lateral sclerosis may also be accompanied by conduction block in peripheral nerves. The frequency of the paraproteinuria tentatively suggests an immunological disorder possibly induced by retroviral infection.

PARANEOPLASTIC SYNDROMES

The paraneoplastic syndromes of peripheral neuropathy, encephalomyelopathy, cerebellar cortical degeneration, polymyositis, progressive multifocal leukoencephalopathy, and an acute necrotizing myelopathy have been described in association with the lymphomas (see Ch. 21). Acute dysautonomia as the only neurological association of systemic Hodgkin's disease has been observed,[87] as has myasthenia gravis,[88] the Guillain-Barré syndrome,[89] and opsoclonus–myoclonus.[90]

OTHER NEUROLOGICAL COMPLICATIONS

Other neurological complications may occur as a result of radiotherapy or chemotherapy; opportunistic infections of the CNS due to bacteria, fungi or viruses; or from hemorrhage due to thrombocytopenia.

Burkitt's Lymphoma

Burkitt's lymphoma is associated with frequent involvement of the nervous system, the most common complications being paraplegia, cranial neuropathies, and pleocytosis of the CSF. Tumor spreads through the bones of the face, skull, and orbit and along cranial nerves. Spinal cord compression from extradural deposits again results from direct extension from the vertebral bodies or from paravertebral tumors infiltrating through the intervertebral foramina. Patients with facial tumors are likely to develop orbital involvement and ophthalmoplegia, or infiltration of the skull base to produce cranial nerve palsies and pleocytosis of the CSF. Ischemic myelopathy can result from compression of radicular arteries by retroperitoneal and retropleural tumor.

Primary Intracerebral Lymphoma

Primary CNS lymphomas are rare, accounting for about 1 percent of primary brain tumors. Although all cytological types are observed, the most common types belong to the high-grade category of non-Hodgkin's lymphoma, the majority being of B cell origin. The tumor masses are usually multicentric and ill-defined. They seem to arise in individuals given prolonged immunosuppressive therapy, patients in receipt of organ allografts, and those with inherited immunodeficiency disorders such as ataxia telangiectasia and the Wiskott-Aldrich syndrome. There is a clear association between primary cerebral non-Hodgkin's lymphoma and the HIV-associated acquired immunodeficiency syndrome (AIDS) (see Ch. 38). The incidence of these tumors is increasing and their association with AIDS only partly accounts for this.

These tumors most commonly present as discrete lesions of the cerebral cortex, corpus callosum, septum pellucidum, basal ganglia, and, to a lesser extent, the cerebellum. Bilateral cerebral involvement via the corpus callosum is a feature and presents with increasing intracranial pressure, dementia, papilledema, long tract signs, and convulsions. A case of steroid-responsive primary malignant lymphoma of the optic chiasm documented by MRI and MRI-directed stereotactic biopsy was described by Gray and colleagues,[91] and Patrick and associates described a 30-year-old woman with primary cerebral lymphoma who presented with diabetes insipidus and otherwise minimal abnormality of hypothalamic pituitary function.[92] Isolated radial nerve palsy secondary to metastasis from a primary malignant lymphoma of the brain has been described.[93] Neuroimaging displays discrete, often large tumors with bilateral hemisphere involvement in most cases, striking enhancement with contrast media, and surrounding edema. Despite the fact that these tumors are very radiosensitive, late morbidity and mortality may arise from radiation necrosis. Without biopsy confirmation, radiation necrosis is indistinguishable from recurrent tumor.[94] Cerebral radiation necrosis seems to be related to tumor dose and the bulk of residual tumor following diagnostic neurosurgery.

Primary lymphoma of the spinal cord is exceptionally rare, as is primary lymphoma of the nerve roots. The author has investigated and cared for a patient with primary lymphoma of the cauda equina (Fig. 12-5).[39]

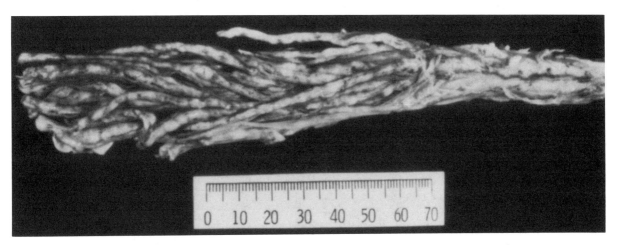

Fig. 12-5 Marked nodular thickening of the nerve roots of the cauda equina from infiltration by primary lymphoma of the CNS. (From Davies-Jones GAB, Preston FE, Timperley WR: Neurological Complications in Clinical Haematology. Blackwell Scientific Publications, Oxford, 1980, with permission.)

Peripheral neuropathy of the paraneoplastic type has been described in association with primary lymphoma of the brain.[95]

Polycythemia

An increased incidence of thrombotic and hemorrhagic complications is a well-recognized phenomenon in polycythemia, not least in the nervous system. Approximately 15 percent of patients with polycythemia die of cerebral thrombosis, 87 percent of them after repeated episodes. Thromboembolism often continues to be a major clinical problem even after hematological control has been achieved. The high incidence of thrombosis is attributed to the increased blood viscosity, reduced perfusion, vascular engorgement, atheromatous degeneration of vessel walls, and possibly to chronic DIC. Hemorrhage may be related to imperfect clot retraction, abnormal thromboplastin generation, and abnormalities of platelet count and function.

Most of the intracranial lesions are thrombotic, and they involve arteries, veins, or venous sinuses. Hemorrhage may be cerebral, extradural, subdural, or subarachnoid. Kannel and colleagues confirmed that the risk of developing cerebral infarction was proportional to the hemoglobin level.[96]

Nonspecific symptoms of fullness in the head, vertigo, tinnitus, and lack of concentration are common. More specific signs such as hemiparesis, hemianesthesia, hemianopia, and aphasia depend on the site of infarction or hemorrhage. Brainstem vascular syndromes occur, as do bulbar and pseudobulbar palsy, convulsions, and coma. Amaurosis fugax, blindness, scotomas, and transient cerebral or brainstem ischemic attacks are features as well. More rarely, signs and symptoms of a progressive cerebral lesion arise because of a subdural hematoma, an expanding intracerebral blood clot, or cerebral infarction and edema. Distention and congestion of the retinal veins, central retinal venous or arterial occlusion, and papilledema may be present. Pseudotumor cerebri has been described. Aseptic cavernous sinus thrombosis associated with internal carotid artery occlusion has been documented.[97] Treatment with repeated phlebotomies and heparin resulted in resolution of the proptosis, pain, periorbital edema, lacrimation, venous congestion, ptosis, and ophthalmoplegia, and it restored the patient's sight. The esoteric one-and-a-half

syndrome due to polycythemia was described by Lousa and associates.[98]

Spinal cord infarction is an exceptionally rare complication.[99] Chorea is another rare complication. It may be of sudden onset and tends to occur in women over 50 years old. It may resolve before any significant reduction of the red cell count but more often resolves with the correction of the polycythemia. The chorea is generalized, with predominant involvement of the face, mouth, tongue, and arms. It is not apparently related to the rare finding of a small infarct in the caudate nucleus. Some have suggested that it may result from excess dopamine presentation to the basal ganglia by the increased number of sluggishly circulating platelets.[100]

Although parasthesias are not uncommon symptoms in the extremities, peripheral neuropathy due to polycythemia is exceptionally rare. Oculomotor nerve paresis as a presenting sign of acute myeloblastic leukemia complicating polycythemia was recorded by Garfinkel and associates.[101]

Cerebellar Hemangioblastoma

Cerebellar hemangioblastoma may be associated with erythrocythemia, which arises as a response to erythropoietin secretion by the tumor. First reported by Carpenter and colleagues,[102] it was present in 18 percent of the patients in their series; more recently a similar incidence of 15 percent has been reported.[103]

The symptoms are those of increased intracranial pressure and "dizziness," with either truncal and gait ataxia or ataxia of one or the other side with nystagmus. Neck stiffness and, rarely, cerebellar fits may occur. On examination, the symmetrical or lateralized cerebellar ataxia is associated with papilledema, hemiparesis, bilateral pyramidal signs, or any combination of deficits from fifth, sixth, seventh, or eighth cranial nerve involvement. Recurrence many years after surgical treatment is typical of hemangioblastoma.

Pseudopolycythemia/Stress Polycythemia

Pseudopolycythemia is a condition in which an increased packed cell volume (hematocrit) is associated with normal red cell mass, although plasma volume may be reduced in the absence of apparent fluid loss.

It is associated with hypertension, obesity, and stress, especially in middle-aged men who are smokers. In this conditions, as in polycythemia, there is an increased risk of thromboembolism because the increased packed cell volume is associated with an increase in whole blood viscosity and reduced cerebral blood flow, which predispose to vascular occlusive episodes. In patients with a packed cell volume greater than 54 percent, regular small venisections of 100 to 250 ml are recommended to reduce the packed cell volume to around 46 percent.

Essential Thrombocythemia

Essential thrombocythemia is a rare disorder characterized more frequently by thrombotic than hemorrhagic complications. The condition is diagnosed on the basis of a persistently elevated platelet count without evidence of trauma, inflammation, hemorrhage, hyposplenism, or any other condition known to be associated with thrombocytosis.

Amaurosis fugax, transient hemiparesis or hemianesthesia, recurrent vertigo, and confusion were the characteristics of the patients studied by Preston and others.[104] Most had evidence of circulating platelet aggregates or spontaneous platelet aggregation, and three had reduced platelet survival. Considerable clinical improvement was achieved by platelet-suppressive drugs and, where appropriate, by reduction of platelet count. Jabaily and colleagues have also confirmed a high incidence of TIAs of both the anterior and posterior cerebral circulation in essential thrombocythemia.[105] The incidence of cerebral ischemia in essential thrombocythemia has been estimated to be 180 times greater than that in a control population.[106] It has been suggested that there is no correlation between the severity of the thrombocythemia and the incidence of TIAs and completed strokes,[107] but the numbers studied are insufficient to warrant this conclusion.

Myelofibrosis

Myelofibrosis is an uncommon myeloproliferative disorder arising predominantly in patients over the age of 50. It is characterized by replacement of the bone marrow by fibrous tissue associated with extramedullary hematopoiesis and marked hepatosplenomegaly. The patients are anemic, may be slightly jaundiced, and have a leukoerythroblastic blood picture. Neurological complications are very rare. Rutman and colleagues described a woman with advanced myelofibrosis who developed a left hemiparesis and left-sided agnosia.[108] At postmortem there were bilateral intracranial masses of hematopoietic tissue compressing both frontoparietal areas and arising from the meninges. Spinal cord compression and paraplegia from extramedullary hematopoiesis due to myelofibrosis is also very uncommon.[109,110]

HEMORRHAGIC DISORDERS

Hemophilia

The severity of bleeding in hemophilic patients correlates well with the factor VIII level. Severely affected hemophiliacs have factor VIII levels of less than 1 percent, and in these patients spontaneous bleeding into muscles and joints is common. With factor VIII levels of 1 to 5 percent, spontaneous bleeding may occur but is much less frequent. Excessive bleeding is precipitated by minor trauma, however. Patients with factor VIII levels greater than 10 percent can nowadays lead a normal life, and excessive blood loss occurs only after trauma and surgery.

Intracranial bleeding is the leading cause of death among hemophiliacs; in the United Kingdom between 1969 and 1974, it was responsible for 25 to 30 percent of all deaths in hemophilic patients. The incidence of intracranial hemorrhage ranges from 2.2 to 13.8 percent.[111] Bleeding tends to occur predominantly in young hemophiliacs. The most common factor associated with bleeding is trauma (53 percent), but hypertension seems to be an important factor in older patients with hemophilia. Delay in the onset of symptoms following trauma is common (50 percent), with a mean duration of 4 ± 2.2 days.[112] This long latent interval is most commonly associated with subdural hematoma. Bleeding may occur anywhere within the cranial cavity, i.e., into the subdural, extradural, or subarachnoid spaces or into the cerebral hemispheres, cerebellar hemispheres, and brainstem. The symptoms and signs depend on the site of the hemorrhage and its extent. Prognosis in intracranial hemorrhage has been considerably improved by the early use of factor VIII concentrates, and there is now no contraindication to surgical intervention provided adequate control of coagulation factors is maintained. Subdural or subarachnoid bleeding carries a better prognosis than intracerebral hemorrhage. Seizures occur in 25 percent of survivors of intracranial hemorrhage and increase the risk of further bleeding. Other sequelae include hemiparesis, aphasia, hemianopia, ataxia, and mental retardation.

Bleeding into the spinal canal is rare. With epidural hemorrhage, radicular symptoms, especially pain, are accompanied by progressive paraparesis or quadriparesis, depending on the site of the bleeding. Patients with small epidural hemorrhages and only minimal nonprogressive signs of spinal cord dysfunction may recover completely with intensive factor VIII replacement therapy alone. With signs of more severe cord compression, surgical decompression with evacuation of the clot is also necessary.

Peripheral nerve lesions are the commonest neurological complication of hemophilia. In most instances, peripheral nerve involvement occurs as a complication of intramuscular hemorrhage. The commonest intramuscular hemorrhage producing peripheral nerve damage is that into the iliac muscle, which may lead to femoral nerve palsy. Median, ulnar, and radial neuropathies may occur owing to intramuscular hemorrhage into the muscles of the arm and forearm. Nerve compression by pseudotumors (subperiosteal hemorrhages producing expanding lesions) also occurs. Duthie and colleagues found a pseudotumor of the upper third of the tibia that was causing posterior tibial nerve palsy by direct compression.[113] Severe hemophilic arthropathy of the elbow may result in ulnar nerve palsy. Intraneural hemorrhage as a cause of peripheral nerve palsy is exceptional, but Cordingley and Crawford described such a complication of the ulnar nerve in the cubital tunnel.[114] On exploration of the ulnar nerve, free blood escaped when the epineurium was divided; recovery was rapid and complete.

Von Willebrand's Disease

The bleeding complications of von Willebrand's disease are relatively mild. Spontaneous hemorrhage into joints and muscles does not occur, and acute onset of neurological dysfunction is not a feature of this disease. Nevertheless, serious hemorrhage may result from trauma, and those patients who sustain

head injuries should receive immediate factor VIII replacement therapy.

Christmas Disease

The neurological complications of Christmas disease are identical to those of hemophilia. Thus peripheral nerve compression occurs as a consequence of spontaneous intramuscular hemorrhage; intracranial hemorrhage, an important cause of death in both disorders, may occur spontaneously in severely affected patients or following trauma in less severely affected individuals. Clotting factor IX is the deficient factor requiring replacement.

Other Clotting Factor Deficiencies

Spontaneous and posttraumatic hemorrhage are features of disorders with deficiencies of other clotting factors. If any intracranial hemorrhage requires surgical removal, it must be done under cover of replacement therapy with the relevant deficient factor or with plasma or cryoprecipitate if the specific factor is not available. Similarly, replacement therapy should probably be given routinely following head injuries.

Hemorrhagic Disease of the Newborn

Intracranial hemorrhage represents the most serious complication of hemorrhagic disease of the newborn and occurs particularly after breach deliveries. Bleeding appears to occur from capillary lesions rather than major vessels, and subdural and subarachnoid hemorrhage are the most frequent form of intracranial bleeding. Intracerebral hemorrhage is rare.

Central nervous system bleeding appears to occur earlier and with greater frequency in infants born to mothers receiving anticonvulsant therapy. This is due to interference of anticonvulsant medication with vitamin K–dependent clotting factors, as discussed in Chapter 28.

Occasionally a bleeding syndrome related to vitamin K deficiency occurs in infants beyond the neonatal period, and this is associated with a greatly increased incidence of intracranial hemorrhage. Blanchet and associates described 93 infants who developed this condition between the ages of 2 weeks and 1 year.[115] Intracranial bleeding, particularly subdural and subarachnoid hemorrhage, occurred in 63 percent.

Thrombocytopenia

If platelet function is normal, satisfactory hemostasis may be achieved with a platelet count as low as 80×10^9/L. Clinically significant spontaneous hemorrhage does not usually occur if the platelet count exceeds 25×10^9/L, but below 20×10^9/L spontaneous hemorrhage is not uncommon. Cerebral, subarachnoid, and subdural hemorrhage constitutes the most serious neurological complication of thrombocytopenia. In patients with idiopathic thrombocytopenic purpura, the risk of spontaneous intracranial hemorrhage appears to be greatest during the first 2 weeks of the onset of the disorder. Severe spontaneous intracranial hemorrhage may also occur in patients with thrombocytopenia due to aplastic anemia, DIC, and acute leukemia. The risk of cerebral hemorrhage appears to be greater in DIC and leukemia than in uncomplicated idiopathic thrombocytopenic purpura, almost certainly because of other hemostatic defects present in these conditions. In aplastic anemia, bleeding becomes a much greater problem when infection supervenes, presumably because of the superimposed hemostatic defect or intravascular coagulation. In severe thrombocytopenia, although massive intracranial hemorrhage may be instantaneous and treatment of no avail, the onset of intracranial bleeding is often heralded by headaches of varying severity. In these circumstances platelet transfusion should be instituted without delay, as it also should be following head injury in patients who have significantly reduced platelet counts.

Disorders of Platelet Function

Irrespective of the platelet count, abnormal bleeding states may result from abnormalities of platelet function. Such abnormalities may be secondary to a congenital defect (as in the Bernard-Soulier syndrome, Glanzmann's thrombasthenia, or storage pool disorder) or acquired due to drugs (especially aspirin), uremia, or paraproteinemia. These disorders are rare and there is a paucity of data on intracranial hemorrhage associated with the various specific types, but

fatal cerebral hemorrhage has been described in Glanzmann's thrombasthenia.[116] In the main, bleeding due to these disorders is treated primarily with platelet transfusions. In myelomatosis or macroglobulinemia, the abnormal platelet function relates to interference by circulating paraproteins and bleeding is more readily controlled by plasmapheresis.

Disseminated Intravascular Coagulation

Disseminated intravascular coagulation is a process by which the coagulation system is activated to form either soluble or insoluble fibrin. Clotting factors and platelets are consumed and there is secondary activation of fibrinolysis. DIC results in tissue ischemia or necrosis. The clinical syndromes produced are many and varied, and they simply relate to the dysfunction of organs and tissues following vascular obstruction. They stem from the rapid release of thromboplastic substances into the circulation. The overwhelming consumption of clotting factors and platelets together with the anticoagulant properties of fibrin degradation products may also result in a bleeding tendency that can vary in severity from slight oozing at venipuncture sites, to purpura and spontaneous bruising, to massive uncontrollable gastrointestinal, genitourinary, or postoperative hemorrhage. Therefore simultaneous hemorrhage and thrombosis may occur.

Pathologically, fibrin-rich thrombi are seen in arterioles, capillaries, and venules. The brain, kidneys, gastrointestinal tract, and lungs are usually the most frequently and severely affected organs. Globules of fibrin are occasionally seen free in the circulating blood in large and small vessels, and some of these globules are large enough to obstruct the microcirculation easily. In many cases red blood cells can be forced through fine networks of fibrin strands and in this process become damaged and fragmented, resulting in *microangiopathic hemolytic anemia.*

Some of the most florid cases of DIC, particularly in young people, who usually have a vigorous fibrinolytic response, show only a hemorrhagic picture with little or no evidence of fibrin in vessels. In some instances, the hemorrhagic complication may be so marked that massive cerebral, intraventricular, or subarachnoid hemorrhages result. There are two mechanisms underlying the association of intravascular coagulation and neurological disorder. Primary

Table 12-1 Clinical Conditions Complicated by Disseminated Intravascular Coagulation

Mechanism	Clinical Condition
Tissue damage	Trauma
	Surgery
	Heat stroke
	Burns
	Dissecting aneurysm
	Neuroleptic malignant syndrome
Infection	Bacterial
	Viral
	Protozoal
	Rickettsial
Immunological disturbance	Immune complex disorders
	Allograft rejection
	Incompatible blood transfusion
Obstetrical complications	Abruptio placentae
	Amniotic fluid embolism
	Retained fetal products
	Eclampsia
Metabolic problems	Diabetic ketoacidosis
Neoplasms	Leukemia
	Mucin-secreting adenocarcinoma
Miscellaneous	Cyanotic congenital heart disease
	Cavernous hemangioma
	Shock
	Snake venoms
	Fat embolism

brain damage, by releasing powerful thromboplastins into the circulation, may precipitate DIC, and already established DIC may affect the nervous system. All patients with evidence of brain damage are at risk of developing DIC.

When DIC affects the nervous system because some other pathological process is triggering its development (Table 12-1), the symptoms and signs are related to the thrombotic and hemorrhagic complications (Fig. 12-6) as well as the primary disorder. Any part of the brain may be affected, producing focal or generalized encephalopathic manifestations or a combination of the two. It is important to realize that the symptoms and signs may fluctuate markedly with time, presumably because of the continuing deposi-

tion and lysis of fibrin, which results in intermittent obstruction of vessels and blood flow. There seems to be a level of cerebral perfusion that is sufficient to maintain the viability of neurons but nevertheless may produce marked neurological abnormalities, including coma. It should be remembered that patients may remain in coma for several days but, provided the circulation is reestablished, may then make a complete recovery.

The DIC secondary to carcinoma may result in microvascular obstruction of the brain such as to produce signs indistinguishable from metastatic deposits. Neurological complications due to DIC may antedate the clinical presentation of the underlying malignancy. In the absence of a definite metabolic, infective, paraneoplastic, or metastatic cause for an encephalopathy, especially if accompanied by fleeting and fluctuating focal neurological abnormalities, DIC should be thoroughly excluded.

With such a generalized and focal process, the neurological signs are numerous and varied, comprising confusion, disorientation, delirium, lethargy, stupor, coma, hemiparesis, aphasia, cortical blindness, focal or generalized seizures, cerebellar ataxia, and focal brainstem disease. The spinal cord may also be affected. Hershenson and associates found a subdural or epidural hematoma extending from the third cervical segment to the third dorsal segment of the spinal cord secondary to DIC that resulted from a gram-negative septicemia.[117]

Ischemic myelopathy due to DIC has been reported in a 39-year-old man with AIDS.[118] He died of diffuse encephalopathy within 9 weeks of onset of the neurological syndrome. Neuropathological examination revealed multiple, usually small, frequently hemorrhagic infarcts of various ages, with fibrin thrombi in medium and small penetrating vessels and capillaries of the brain and spinal cord, characteristic of DIC. There were no inflammatory changes.

It is important to realize that at the onset of the neurological disorder, the coagulation profile may be normal and that during pregnancy, postoperatively, following trauma, and in association with malignancy plasma fibrinogen is invariably elevated. Therefore, increased fibrinogen consumption serves only to reduce plasma fibrinogen to normal. For this reason the only laboratory evidence of DIC in this situation may be thrombocytopenia and an elevated level of fibrin degradation products. If DIC is suspected, coagula-

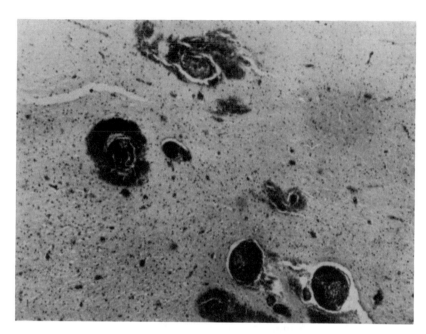

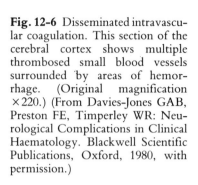

Fig. 12-6 Disseminated intravascular coagulation. This section of the cerebral cortex shows multiple thrombosed small blood vessels surrounded by areas of hemorrhage. (Original magnification ×220.) (From Davies-Jones GAB, Preston FE, Timperley WR: Neurological Complications in Clinical Haematology. Blackwell Scientific Publications, Oxford, 1980, with permission.)

tion studies should be performed at frequent intervals, and falling concentrations of the various clotting factors should be accepted as evidence of a consumptive coagulopathy.

Thrombotic Thrombocytopenic Purpura

Thrombotic thrombocytopenic purpura, a disease of unknown etiology, affects individuals of all ages but occurs most commonly between the ages of 20 and 50 years. It probably affects women more commonly than men. The outlook is poor, most patients surviving for a few weeks only, although some survive a few months with relapsing illness and fluctuating symptoms and signs. Occasionally there is complete recovery or the patient develops a more chronically relapsing form that lasts up to 12 years.[119]

The disease is characterized by thrombocytopenia, microangiopathic hemolytic anemia, neurological abnormalities, fever, and renal dysfunction. Pathologically, there is hyperplasia of endothelial and adventitial cells in arterioles, capillaries, and venules associated with platelet-rich and hyaline thrombi in these vessels, in which microaneurysms may also form. The disorder is distinguished from autoimmune (idiopathic) thrombocytopenic purpura by the presence of platelet and hyaline thrombi in small blood vessels, the predominance of neurological and renal manifestations, and the absence of circulating platelet antibodies.

Neurological features are the most frequent presenting manifestations, occurring in 60 percent of cases; during the course of the disease, 90 percent of patients at one stage or another experience neurological complications. As a result of involvement of any part of the CNS, there is an endless variety of neurological syndromes. However the more common neurological manifestations are headache, organic brain syndromes, coma, paresis, aphasia, dysarthria, syncope, vertigo, ataxia, visual symptoms, parasthesias, seizures, and cranial nerve palsies. These symptoms are typically transient and fluctuating and in some instances resemble TIAs. However, permanent neurological complications may also occur.[120] Involvement of the visual pathways commonly results in homonymous field defects, but ocular changes of exudative retinal detachment, retinal and choroidal hemorrhages, papilledema, anisocoria, and diplopia may occur. Frankel and colleagues emphasized that prolonged coma without evidence of major structural lesions in the CNS in patients with thrombotic thrombocytopenic purpura should be treated vigorously with daily repeated plasma exchange, antiplatelet drugs, corticosteroids, and vincristine, because full recovery is possible.[121]

Exceptionally, the neurological abnormalities may precede the full syndrome by months or even years. In a typical case, there may be a variety of prodromal symptoms, including fatigue, weakness, headaches, anorexia, nausea, vomiting, abdominal distress, fever, cough, hematuria, arthralgia, tachycardia, mental change, numbness, paralysis, and gastrointestinal or vaginal bleeding. At the time of presentation, the patient is usually pale, icteric, and febrile; has petechial hemorrhages in the skin; exhibits mental changes and neurological abnormalities; and has splenomegaly, hepatomegaly, lymphadenopathy, arthropathy, and some degree of hypertension and renal insufficiency.

The main laboratory abnormalities are microangiopathic hemolytic anemia, thrombocytopenia, hyperbilirubinemia, uremia, and erythroid and myeloid hyperplasia of the bone marrow with increased megakaryocytic activity. Although laboratory evidence of DIC may be present, it occurs in only a few patients.

Hemolytic-Uremic Syndrome

The hemolytic-uremic syndrome is a disease of children that is characterized by renal impairment, thrombocytopenia, and microangiopathic hemolytic anemia. Sheth and associates have confirmed that the commonest neurological manifestations are seizures, predominantly generalized tonic-clonic convulsions but occasionally focal ones.[122] Behavioral changes, diplopia, dizziness, obtundation, coma, decerebrate posturing, cerebellar ataxia, hemiparesis, hemianopia, cortical blindness, cranial nerve palsies, vitreous hemorrhages, and retinal infarction may occur. Striatal involvement due to small areas of infarction of the basal ganglia, with resultant involuntary movements, has been described.[123] The CT brain scan may show features of infarction or hemorrhage. Children who develop neurological complications seem to have an increased incidence of residual hypertension and chronic renal failure. The neuropathological features range from nonspecific changes of cerebral edema and anoxia to vascular occlusive changes.

Gaucher's Disease

An autosomal recessive disorder, Gaucher's disease is characterized by a deficiency of glucocerebrosidase and an accumulation of glucocerebroside in various organs. The adult nonneuronopathic type involves bones, liver, spleen, and lungs and characterized by hepatosplenomegaly, bony abnormalities, thrombocytopenia, and bleeding diathesis. The neuronopathic infantile type produces rapidly progressive neurological deficits beginning around 4 to 5 months of age and ending in death by the age of 2 years.

The neuronopathic juvenile and adult type has a more chronic course, with seizures and mental deterioration—which ranges from a mild memory disorder to severe dementia—being the commonest complications. The seizures may be tonic-clonic, partial complex, or myoclonic. Progressive myoclonic jerking of the face, limbs, or palate may be prominent, as may pyramidal signs, cerebellar ataxia, and cranial nerve palsies. Oculomotor apraxia has been described as the presenting sign of Gaucher's disease.[124] In addition, thrombocytopenia and prolonged prothrombin and partial thromboplastin times may cause a bleeding tendency. The patient may be anemic, and Gaucher cells may be found on bone marrow examination.

COAGULATION DISORDERS

Antiphospholipid Antibodies

Lupus anticoagulant and anticardiolipin represent separate antibodies within a group of antibodies directed against protein phospholipid complexes rather than phospholipid itself. Although lupus anticoagulant and antiphospholipin may not cause thrombosis, they are undoubtedly associated with thrombotic states; for example, in systemic lupus erythematosus the risk of thrombosis is increased two- to fivefold in subjects who have the lupus anticoagulant.[125] Venous thrombosis is most commonly seen, but arterial thrombosis undoubtedly occurs even in younger subjects without any other recognized risk factors.[126,127] In a study of 248 unselected subjects presenting with stroke and compared with hospitalized controls, evidence has been found to suggest that the presence of anticardiolipin is an independent risk factor in stroke.[128] Brey and associates found antiphospholipin in 46 percent of subjects under 50 years of age presenting with stroke or TIA compared with 8 percent in matched controls with nonthrombotic neurological disease.[129]

Sneddon's syndrome[130]—cerebral thrombosis in

association with livedo reticularis—is strongly associated with the presence of antiphospholipid antibodies, and antiphospholipid antibodies have been demonstrated in patients with central retinal artery and retinal branch occlusion,[131] retinal venous thrombosis, ischemic optic neuropathy,[132] and amaurosis fugax.[133]

Hereditary Thrombophilia

Antithrombin, protein C, and protein S deficiencies predispose to thrombosis. It is uncertain whether inherited deficiency of heparin co-factor 2, plasminogen, factor XII, or prekallikrein result in thrombosis.

Sagittal sinus and cerebral venous thrombosis have been reported in association with deficiency of antithrombin,[134] protein C,[135] and protein S.[136]

Although there are numerous reports of cerebral arterial thrombosis and infarction occurring in antithrombin,[137,138] protein C,[139] and protein S[140,141] deficiencies, the risk is extremely small compared with the risk of venous thrombosis.[142] Angiographically proven cerebral arterial occlusion has been reported in protein S deficiency but only rarely has familial thrombophilia been conclusively diagnosed by demonstrating that the deficiency persists after the acute event is over. This is particularly so regarding protein S deficiency, because as part of the acute phase response it becomes bound to a binding protein (C4bBP) which increases in amount during the acute phase and which results in an acquired reduction in free or functional protein S. Mayer and colleagues, in a case-controlled study, concluded that acquired deficiency of protein S is not a major risk factor for stroke.[143] However, in 60 patients younger than 45 years of age, Martinez and co-workers attributed ischemic stroke to deficiency of protein C in 3 men, protein S deficiency in 2 women, and antithrombin deficiency in 5 patients (3 men and 2 women).[144] All 10 patients had carotid territory infarction. With the evidence presently available, it is reasonable to conclude that a congenital or acquired deficiency of natural anticoagulants increases the risk of arterial thrombosis.

REFERENCES

1. Capriles LF: Intracranial hypertension and iron deficiency anemia. Arch Neurol 9:147, 1963
2. Parag KB, Omar MAK: Benign intracranial hypertension associated with iron deficiency anemia. S Afr Med J 63:981, 1983
3. Alexander MB: Iron deficiency anemia, thrombocytosis and cerebrovascular accident. South Med J 76: 662, 1983
4. Pears MA, Pickering GW: Changes in the fundus oculi after haemorrhage. Q J Med 29:153, 1960
5. Siekert RG: Symposium on surgical treatment of extracranial occlusive cerebrovascular disease. Proc Mayo Clin 35:473, 1960
6. Green NS, Garvin JH, Chutorian A: Transient erythroblastopenia of childhood presenting with papilledema. Clin Pediatr 25:278, 1986
7. Steiner MS, Morton RA, Marshall FF: Vitamin B_{12} deficiency in patients with ileocolic neobladders. J Urol 149:255, 1993
8. Lindenbaum J, Healton EB, Savage DG, et al: Neuropsychiatric disorders caused by cobalamin deficiency in the absence of anemia or macrocytosis. N Engl J Med 318:1720, 1988
9. Greenfield JG, Carmichael EA: The peripheral nerves in cases of subacute combined degeneration of the cord. Brain 58:483, 1935
10. McLeod JG, Walsh JC, Little JM: Sural nerve biopsy. Med J Aust 2:1092, 1960
11. Smith R, Oliver RAM: Sudden onset of psychosis in association with vitamin-B_{12} deficiency. Br Med J 3: 34, 1967
12. Shorvon SD, Carney MWP, Chanarin I, Reynolds EH: The neuropsychiatry of megaloblastic anaemia. Br Med J 281:1036, 1980
13. Healton EB, Savage DG, Brust JC, et al: Neurologic aspects of cobalamin deficiency. Medicine (Baltimore) 70:229, 1991
14. Chanarin I: Pernicious anemia and other vitamin B_{12} deficiency states. Abst World Med 44:73, 1970
15. Mayfrank L, Thoden U: Downbeat nystagmus indicates cerebellar or brain-stem lesions in vitamin B_{12} deficiency. J Neurol 233:145, 1986
16. Sandyk R: Paralysis of upward gaze as a presenting symptom of vitamin B_{12} deficiency. Eur Neurol 23: 198, 1984
17. Kandler RH, Davies-Jones GAB: Internuclear ophthalmoplegia in pernicious anemia. Br Med J 297: 1583, 1988
18. Salameh MM, Banda RW, Mohdi AA: Reversal of severe neurological abnormalities after vitamin B_{12} replacement in the Imerslund-Grasbeck syndrome. J Neurol 238:349, 1991
19. Donnelly S, Callaghan N: Subacute combined degeneration of the spinal cord due to folate deficiency in association with a psychotic illness. Ir Med J 83:73, 1990

20. Allen RJ, DiMauro S, Coulter DL, et al: Kearns–Sayre syndrome with reduced plasma and cerebrospinal fluid folate. Ann Neurol 13:679, 1983

21. Howells TH, Huntsman RG, Boys JE, Mahmood A: Anaesthesia and sickle-cell haemoglobin. Br J Anaesth 44:975, 1972

22. Dalal FY, Schmidt GB, Bennett EJ, Ramamurthy S: Sickle-cell trait: a report of a postoperative neurological complication. Br J Anaesth 46:387, 1974

23. Portnoy BA, Herion JC: Neurological manifestations in sickle-cell disease. Ann Intern Med 76:643, 1972

24. Powars D, Wilson B, Imbus C, et al: The natural history of stroke in sickle cell disease. Am J Med 65:461, 1978

25. Van Hoff J, Ritchey K, Shaywitz BA: Intracranial hemorrhage in children with sickle cell disease. Am J Dis Child 139:1120, 1985

26. Stockman JA, Nigro MA, Mishkin MM, Oski FA: Occlusion of large cerebral vessels in sickle-cell anemia. N Engl J Med 287:846, 1972

27. Asher SW: Multiple cranial neuropathies, trigeminal neuralgia, and vascular headaches in sickle cell disease, a possible common mechanism. Neurology 30:210, 1980

28. Hamdan JM, Mallou AA, Ahmad AS: Hypertension and convulsions complicating sickle cell anemia: possible role of transfusion. Ann Trop Paediatr 4:41, 1984

29. Rothman SM, Nelson JS: Spinal cord infarction in a patient with sickle cell anemia. Neurology 30:1072, 1980

30. Wolman L, Hardy AG: Spinal cord infarction associated with sickle cell trait. Paraplegia 7:282, 1969

31. Reyes MG: Subcortical cerebral infarctions in sickle cell trait. J Neurol Neurosurg Psychiatry 52:516, 1989

32. Fabian RH, Peters BH: Neurological complications of hemoglobin SC disease. Arch Neurol 41:289, 1984

33. Blank JP, Gill FM: Orbital infarction in sickle cell disease. Pediatrics 67:879, 1981

34. Caprioli J, Fagadau W, Lesser R: Acute monocular visual loss secondary to anterior communicating artery aneurysm in a patient with sickle cell disease. Ann Ophthalmol 15:873, 1983

35. Abbassioun K, Amir-Jamshidi A: Curable paraplegia due to extradural hematopoietic tissue in thalassemia. Neurosurgery 11:804, 1982

36. Abbassioun K, Amirjamshidi A, Zamanianpour M: Curable paraplegia. Neurosurgery 17:528, 1985

37. Papanastasiou DA, Papanicolaou D, Magiakou AM, et al: Peripheral neuropathy in patients with β-thalassemia. J Neurol Neurosurg Psychiatry 54:997, 1991

38. McCann SR, Jacob HS: Spinal cord disease in hereditary spherocytosis: report of two cases with a hypothesized common mechanism for neurologic and red cell abnormalities. Blood 48:259, 1976

39. Davies-Jones GAB, Preston FE, Timperley WR: Neurological Complications in Clinical Haematology. Blackwell Scientific Publications, Oxford, 1980

40. Barnett HJM: Platelet and coagulation function in relation to thromboembolic stroke. Adv Neurol 16:45, 1977

41. Swisher CN, Menkes JH, Cancill PA, Dodge PR: Coexistence of Hallervorden-Spatz disease and acanthocytosis. Trans Am Neurol Assoc 97:212, 1972

42. Spitz MC, Jankovic J, Killian JM: Familial tic disorder, parkinsonism, motor neuron disease, and acanthocytosis: a new syndrome. Neurology 35:366, 1985

43. Sakai T, Iwashita H, Kakugawa M: Neuroacanthocytosis syndrome and choreoacanthocytosis (Levine-Critchley syndrome). Neurology 35:1679, 1985

44. Spencer SE, Walker FO, Moore SA: Chorea-amyotrophy with chronic hemolytic anemia: a variant of choreo-amyotrophy with acanthocytosis. Neurology 37:645, 1987

45. Hardie RJ, Pullon HWH, Harding AE, et al: Neuroacanthocytosis: a clinical, haematological and pathological study of 19 cases. Brain 114:13, 1991

46. Kay MM, Goodman J, Lawrence C, Bosman G: Membrane channel protein abnormalities and autoantibodies in neurological disease. Brain Res Bull 24:105, 1990

47. Pagon RA, Bird TD, Detter JC, Pierce I: Hereditary sideroblastic anaemia and ataxia: an X linked recessive disorder. J Med Genet 22:267, 1985

48. Raskind WH, Wijsman E, Pagon RA, et al: X-linked sideroblastic anemia and ataxia: linkage to phosphoglycerate kinase at Xq13. Am J Hum Genet 48:335, 1991

49. Ikeda A, Shimamoto Y, Oda K, et al: A case of primary acquired sideroblastic anemia (PASA) with motor dominant polyneuropathy responsive to vitamin B6. Nippon Naika Gakkai Zasshi (J Jpn Soc Intern Med) 78:561, 1989

50. Poll-The BT, Aicardi J, Girot R, Rosa R: Neurological findings in triosephosphate isomerase deficiency. Ann Neurol 17:439, 1985

51. Eber SW, Pekrun A, Bardosi A, et al: Triosephosphate isomerase deficiency: haemolytic anaemia, myopathy with altered mitochondria and mental retardation due to a new variant with accelerated enzyme catabolism and diminished specific activity. Eur J Pediatr 150:761, 1991

52. Price RA, Johnson W: The central nervous system in childhood leukemia: I. The arachnoid. Cancer 31:520, 1973

53. Smith HP, Biller J, Kelly DL: Oculomotor palsy with pupillary sparing, coincidental aneurysm, and chronic lymphocytic leukemic meningeal infiltration. Surg Neurol 16:26, 1981

54. Ricevuti G, Savoldi F, Piccolo G, et al: Meningeal leukemia diagnosed by cytocentrifuge study of cerebrospinal fluid. Arch Neurol 43:466, 1986
55. Boogerd W, Vroom TM: Meningeal involvement as the initial symptom of B cell chronic lymphocytic leukemia. Eur Neurol 25:461, 1986
56. Ha K, Kanaya S, Ikeda T, et al: Cortical blindness in a child with acute leukemia. Acta Paediatr Scand 69: 781, 1980
57. Brown GC, Shields JA, Augsburger JJ, et al: Leukemic optic neuropathy. Int Ophthalmol 3:111, 1981
58. Petursson SE, Boggs DR: Spinal cord involvement in leukemia. Cancer 47:346, 1981
59. Okamura S, Niho Y, Mitsui T, Kikuchi M: Adult T cell leukemia and peripheral neuropathy. Acta Hematol Jpn 47:1344, 1984
60. Kellie SJ, Waters KD: Extradural chloroma with spinal compression—an unusual presentation of acute myelogenous leukemia. Aust NZ J Med 14:160, 1984
61. Williams CKO, Ogan O: Chronic myeloid leukaemia associated with impairment of hearing. Br Med J 290: 1705, 1985
62. Bleyer WA, Griffin TW: White matter necrosis, mineralizing microangiopathy and intellectual abilities in survivors of childhood leukemia associated with central nervous system irradiation and methotrexate therapy. p. 155. In Gilbert HA, Kagan AR (eds): Radiation Damage to the Nervous System. Raven Press, New York, 1980
63. Brouwers P, Riccardi R, Fedio P, Poplack DG: Long-term neuropsychologic sequelae of childhood leukemia: correlation with CT brain scan abnormalities. J Pediatr 106:723, 1985
64. Green CR, Jamal GA, Prior PF, et al: Are there any long term CNS sequelae of prophylactic intrathecal methotrexate and cranial irradiation in patients with leukemia? Communication to the Association of British Neurologists, 1987
65. Gerrard MP, Eden OB, Lilleyman JS: Acute encephalopathy during induction therapy for acute lymphoblastic leukemia. Pediatr Hematol Oncol 3:49, 1986
66. Silverstein A, Doniger DE: Neurologic complications of myelomatosis. Arch Neurol 9:534, 1963
67. Brenner B, Carter A, Tatarsky I, et al: Incidence, prognostic significance and therapeutic modalities of central nervous system involvement in multiple myeloma. Acta Haematol 68:77, 1982
68. Roslund J, Sundberg K, Tovi D: Plasma cell myeloma of thoracic vertebra with amyloid deposits. Acta Pathol Microbiol Scand 49:273, 1960
69. Raflo G, Farrell TA, Sioussat RS: Complete ophthalmoplegia secondary to amyloidosis associated with multiple myeloma. Am J Ophthalmol 92:221, 1981
70. Cox JGC, Steiger MJ, Pearce JMS: Optic neuropathy and multiple myeloma. Br J Hosp Med 39:448, 1988
71. Wasan H, Mansi JL, Benjamin S, et al: Myeloma and benign intracranial hypertension. Br Med J 304:685, 1992
72. Nakanishi T, Sobue I, Toyokura Y, et al: The Crow-Fukase syndrome: a study of 102 cases in Japan. Neurology 34:712, 1984
73. Miralles GD, O'Fallon JR, Talley NJ: Plasma-cell dyscrasia with polyneuropathy: the spectrum of POEMS syndrome. N Engl J Med 327:1919, 1992
74. Jowitt SN, Yin JA, Schady W, et al: Polymyositis in association with multiple myeloma. Br J Hosp Med 45:234, 1991
75. Preston FE, Cooke KB, Foster ME, et al: Myelomatosis and the hyperviscosity syndrome. Br J Haematol 38:517, 1978
76. Latov N, Sherman WH, Nemni R, et al: Plasma-cell dyscrasia and peripheral neuropathy with a monoclonal antibody to peripheral-nerve myelin. N Engl J Med 303:618, 1980
77. Latov N, Braun PE, Gross PB, et al: Plasma cell dyscrasia and peripheral neuropathy: identification of the myelin antigens that react with human paraproteins. Proc Natl Acad Sci USA 78:139, 1981
78. Dellagi K, Dupouey P, Brouet JC, et al: Waldenström's macroglobulinemia and peripheral neuropathy: a clinical and immunologic study of 25 patients. Blood 62:280, 1983
79. Lossos A, Averbuch-Heller L, Reches A, Abramsky O: Complete unilateral ophthalmoplegia as the presenting manifestation of Waldenström's macroglobulinemia. Neurology 40:1801, 1990
80. Moulis H, Mamus SW: Isolated trochlear nerve palsy in a patient with Waldenström's macroglobulinemia: complete recovery with combination therapy. Neurology 39:1399, 1989
81. Levitt LF, Dawson DM, Rosenthal DS, Moloney WC: CNS involvement in non-Hodgkin's lymphomas. Cancer 45:545, 1980
82. Hughes M, Ahern V, Kefford R, Boyages J: Paraneoplastic myelopathy at diagnosis in a patient with pathologic stage 1A Hodgkin disease. Cancer 70:1598, 1992
83. Cartwright RA, Boddy J, Barnard D: Association between Bell's palsy and lymphoid malignancies. Leuk Res 9:31, 1985
84. Galetta SL, Sergott RC, Wells GB, et al: Spontaneous remission of a third-nerve palsy in meningeal lymphoma. Ann Neurol 32:100, 1992
85. Zaman AG, Graham EM, Sanders MD: Anterior visual system involvement in non-Hodgkin's lymphoma. Br J Ophthalmol 77:184, 1993

86. Younger DS, Rowland LP, Latov N, et al: Lymphoma, motor neuron diseases, and amyotrophic lateral sclerosis. Ann Neurol 29:78, 1991
87. Van Lieshout JJ, Wieling W, Van Montfrans GA, et al: Acute dysautonomia associated with Hodgkin's disease. J Neurol Neurosurg Psychiatry 49:830, 1986
88. Levo Y, Kott E, Atsmon A: Association between myasthenia gravis and malignant lymphoma. Eur Neurol 13:245, 1975
89. Cros D, Harris NL, Hedley-Whyte ET: A 66-year-old man with demyelinative neuropathy and a retroperitoneal mass. N Engl J Med 323:895, 1990
90. Kay CL, Davies-Jones GAB, Singal R, Winfield DA: Paraneoplastic opsoclonus-myoclonus in Hodgkin's disease. J Neurol Neurosurg Psychiatry 59:831, 1993
91. Gray RS, Abrahams JJ, Hufnagel TJ, et al: Ghost-cell tumor of the optic chiasm: primary CNS lymphoma. J Clin Neuro Ophthalmol 9:98, 1989
92. Patrick AW, Campbell IW, Ashworth B, Gordon A: Primary cerebral lymphoma presenting with cranial diabetes insipidus. Postgrad Med J 65:771, 1989
93. Van Bolden V, Kline DG, Garcia CA, Van Bolden GD: Isolated radial nerve palsy due to metastasis from a primary malignant lymphoma of the brain. Neurosurgery 21:905, 1987
94. Merchut MP, Haberland C, Naheedy MH, Rubino FA: Long survival of primary cerebral lymphoma without progressive radiation necrosis. Neurology 35:552, 1985
95. Garofalo M, Danon MJ, Donnenfeld H, Chusid JG: Peripheral polyneuropathy associated with primary malignant lymphoma of the brain. Arch Neurol 35:50, 1978
96. Kannel WB, Gordon T, Wolf PA, McNamara PM: Hemoglobin and the risk of cerebral infarction: The Framingham Study. Stroke 3:409, 1972
97. Melamed E, Rachmilewitz EA, Reches A, Lavy S: Aseptic cavernous sinus thrombosis after internal carotid artery occlusion in polycythaemia vera. J Neurol Neurosurg Psychiatry 39:320, 1976
98. Lousa M, Gobernado JM, Gimeno A: One-and-a-half syndrome due to polycythaemia. J Neurol Neurosurg Psychiatry 46:873, 1983
99. Grunberg A, Blair JL, Rawcliffe RM: Unusual neurological symptoms in polycythaemia rubra vera. Edinb Med J 57:305, 1950
100. Edwards PD, Prosser R, Wells CEC: Chorea, polycythaemia, and cyanotic heart disease. J Neurol Neurosurg Psychiatry 38:729, 1975
101. Garfinkel D, Shoenfeld Y, Gadoth H, Pinkhas J: Oculomotor nerve paresis—presenting sign of acute myeloblastic leukemia in a patient with polycythemia vera. Haematologica 65:769, 1980
102. Carpenter G, Schwartz HG, Walker AE: Neurogenic polycythemia. Ann Intern Med 19:470, 1943
103. Constans JP, Meder F, Maiuri F, et al: Posterior fossa hemangioblastomas. Surg Neurol 25:269, 1986
104. Preston FE, Martin JF, Stewart RM, Davies-Jones GAB: Thrombocytosis, circulating platelet aggregates, and neurological dysfunction. Br Med J 2:1561, 1979
105. Jabaily J, Iland HJ, Laszlo J, et al: Neurologic manifestations of essential thrombocytopenia. Ann Intern Med 99:513, 1983
106. Lahuerta-Palacios JJ, Bornstein R, Fernandez-Debora FJ, et al: Controlled and uncontrolled thrombocytosis: its clinical role in essential thrombocythemia. Cancer 61:1207, 1988
107. Labauge R, Pagès M, Labauge P: Neurological complications of essential thrombocythemia: six cases. Rev Neurol (Paris) 147:52, 1991
108. Rutman JY, Meidinger R, Keith JI: Unusual radiologic and neurologic findings in a case of myelofibrosis with extramedullary hematopoiesis. Neurology 22:567, 1972
109. Appleby A, Batson GA, Lassman LP, Simpson CA: Spinal cord compression by extramedullary haematopoiesis in myelosclerosis. J Neurol Neurosurg Psychiatry 27:313, 1964
110. Oustwani MB, Kurtides ES, Christ M, Ciric I: Spinal cord compression with paraplegia in myelofibrosis. Arch Neurol 37:389, 1980
111. Gilchrist GS, Piepgras DG: Neurologic complications in hemophilia. Prog Pediatr Hematol Oncol 1:79, 1977
112. Eyster ME, Gill FM, Blatt PM, et al: Central nervous system bleeding in hemophiliacs. Blood 51:1179, 1978
113. Duthie RB, Matthews JM, Rizza CR, Steel WM: The Management of Musculo-skeletal Problems in the Haemophilias. Blackwell Scientific Publications, Oxford, 1972
114. Cordingley FT, Crawford GPM: Ulnar nerve palsy in a haemophiliac due to intraneural haemorrhage. Br Med J 289:18, 1984
115. Blanchet P, Tuchinda S, Hathirat P, et al: A bleeding syndrome in infants due to acquired prothrombin complex deficiency. Clin Pediatr 16:992, 1977
116. Caen J: Congenital bleeding disorders with long bleeding time and normal platelet count: I. Glanzmann's thrombasthenia. Am J Med 41:4, 1966
117. Hershenson MB, Hageman JR, Brouillette RT: Neonatal spinal cord dysfunction associated with disseminated intravascular coagulation. Dev Med Child Neurol 24:686, 1982
118. Fenelon G, Gray F, Scaravilli F, et al: Ischaemic myelopathy secondary to disseminated intravascular coagulation in AIDS. J Neurol 238:51, 1991

119. Sills RH: Thrombotic thrombocytopenic purpura (pathophysiology and clinical manifestations). Am J Pediatr Hematol Oncol 6:425, 1984
120. Ben-Yehuda D, Rose M, Michaeli Y, Éldor A: Permanent neurological complications in patients with thrombotic thrombocytopenic purpura. Am J Hematol 29:74, 1988
121. Frankel AE, Rubenstein MD, Wall RT: Thrombotic thrombocytopenic purpura: prolonged coma with recovery of neurologic function with intensive plasma exchange. Am J Hematol 10:387, 1981
122. Sheth KJ, Swick HM, Haworth N: Neurological involvement in hemolytic-uremic syndrome. Ann Neurol 19:90, 1986
123. Hue V, Leclerc F, Martinot A, et al: Striatal involvement with abnormal movements in hemolytic-uremic syndrome. Arch Fr Pediatr 49:369, 1992
124. Gross-Tsur V, Har-Even Y, Gutman I, Amir N: Oculomotor apraxia: the presenting sign of Gaucher disease. Paediatr Neurol 5:128, 1989
125. Petri M, Hochberg M, Hellman D, et al: The association of the lupus anticoagulant (LA) with thrombotic events (TE) in systemic lupus erythematosus (SLE). Clin Exp Rheumatol 8:217, 1990
126. Kushner MJ: Prospective study of anticardiolipin antibodies in stroke. Stroke 21:295, 1990
127. Levine SR, Deegan MJ, Futrell N, Welch KMA: Cerebrovascular neurologic disease associated with antiphospholipid antibodies: 48 cases. Neurology 40: 1181, 1990
128. Antiphospholipid Antibodies in Stroke Study Group: Clinical and laboratory findings in patients with antiphospholipid antibodies and cerebral ischemia. Stroke 21:1268, 1990
129. Brey RL, Hart RG, Sherman D, Tegeler CH: Antiphospholipid antibodies and cerebral ischemia in young people. Neurology 40:1190, 1990
130. Sneddon IB: Cerebrovascular lesions and livedo reticularis. Br J Dermatol 77:180, 1965
131. Kleiner RC, Najarian LV, Schatten S, et al: Vaso-occlusive retinopathy associated with antiphospholipid antibodies (lupus anticoagulant retinopathy). Ophthalmology 96:896, 1989
132. Watts MT, Greaves M, Clearkin LG, et al: Anti-phospholipid antibodies and ischaemic optic neuropathy. Lancet 335:613, 1990
133. Digre KB, Duncan FJ, Branch DW, et al: Amaurosis fugax associated with antiphospholipid antibodies. Ann Neurol 25:228, 1989
134. Lee MK, Ng SC: Cerebral venous thrombosis associated with antithrombin III deficiency: Aust NZ J Med 21:772, 1991
135. Vieregge P, Schwieder G, Kompf D: Cerebral venous thrombosis in hereditary protein C deficiency. J Neurol Neurosurg Psychiatry 52:135, 1989
136. Gros D, Coup PC, Beltran G, et al: Superior sagittal sinus thrombosis in a patient with protein S deficiency. Stroke 21:633, 1990
137. Ernerudh J, Olsson JE, von Schenck H: Antithrombin-III deficiency in ischemic stroke. Stroke 21:967, 1990
138. Shinmyoza K, Ohkatsu Y, Maruyama Y, et al: A case of congenital antithrombin III deficiency complicated by an internal carotid artery occlusion. Clin Neurol 26:162, 1986
139. Kohler J, Kasper J, Witt I, von Reutern GM: Ischemic stroke due to protein C deficiency. Stroke 21:1077, 1990
140. Davous P, Horellou MH, Conrad J, Samama M: Cerebral infarction and familial protein S deficiency. Stroke 21:1760, 1990
141. Green D, Otoya J, Oriba H, Rovner R: Protein S deficiency in middle-aged women with stroke. Neurology 42:1029, 1992
142. Greaves M: Coagulation abnormalities and cerebral infarction. J Neurol Neurosurg Psychiatry 56:433, 1993
143. Mayer SA, Sacco RL, Hurlet-Jensen A, et al: Free protein S deficiency in acute ischemic stroke: a case-control study. Stroke 24:224, 1993
144. Martinez HR, Rangel-Guerra RA, Marfil LJ: Ischemic stroke due to deficiency of coagulation inhibitors: report of 10 young adults. Stroke 24:19, 1993

13

Hepatic Encephalopathy and Other Neurological Disorders Associated with Gastrointestinal Disease

Alan H. Lockwood

The gastrointestinal system consists of many organs, each with its unique and complex structure and function. The central nervous system (CNS) is absolutely dependent on the gastrointestinal system for (1) glucose; (2) the absorption and metabolism of a variety of other nutrients, vitamins, and so on required for normal brain function; and (3) removal of toxic metabolic wastes.

Disorders of the gastrointestinal system are important contributors to morbidity and mortality in the United States. Diseases of the liver currently rank sixth as the cause of lost years of life. As liver disease, particularly cirrhosis, reaches its terminal phases, neurological impairment becomes a progressively more important problem. Diseases of the liver, particularly fulminating hepatic failure, may present to clinicians because of nervous system symptoms. Because hepatic encephalopathy is the most common nervous system disorder associated with gastrointestinal dysfunction, most of this chapter is devoted to a discussion of this disorder; other gastrointestinal disturbances are considered more briefly. Nutritional disorders are considered separately in Chapter 15.

HEPATIC ENCEPHALOPATHY

Although descriptions of what was probably hepatic encephalopathy are to be found in writings of early authors, including Galen, Hippocrates, and perhaps even Shakespeare, clear, contemporary descriptions follow Frerichs's treatise on liver disease.[1] Frerichs wrote (as translated by Murchison):

> In most cases we can distinguish two stages, that of excitement and depression . . . characterized by delirium and convulsions and . . . progressively increasing coma . . . . In most cases, the nervous system derangements appeared simultaneously with jaundice; and they usually attracted the attention of the observer sooner than the slight jaundiced tint of the conjunctivae. . . .

Frerichs noted hepatic encephalopathy is commonly first recognized by someone other than the patient or physician—that is, the "observer," who may be a family member or other associate. He further noted:

> Toward the termination of the disease the delirium and convulsions, as a general rule, gave place to stupor, which in a short time has merged into the deepest coma, from which no shaking could rouse the patient.

Frerichs was undoubtedly describing what we would now call fulminant hepatic failure. This condition, invariably fatal in Frerichs's experience, is still associated with an 85 percent mortality rate. Since Frerichs did not describe remissions or recoveries, he was probably not describing portal systemic encephalopathy. The latter condition, now the most common form of hepatic encephalopathy, probably existed at that time but was not differentiated from fulminant hepatic failure because of what must have been uniformly fatal outcomes for both conditions. The absence of specific therapies and the frequency of what were then untreatable complications, such as pneumonia and sepsis, probably inexorably and invariably caused death.

Frerichs also had excellent insight into the pathophysiological mechanisms causing encephalopathy:

> Abnormal nervous symptoms . . . must be referred to changes in the blood. I attribute the cause of the blood-intoxication to the complete arrest of the hepatic functions . . . [and] also [to] the cessation of the powerful influence which the liver exerts over the processes of metamorphosis of matter.

In a very real sense, all progress in this field consists of a refinement of this broad but accurate statement.

Portal Systemic Encephalopathy and Fulminant Hepatic Failure

Some of the current confusion in the literature on hepatic encephalopathy is the result of terminology that is poorly defined and used. The term *hepatic encephalopathy*, which is often used synonymously with *portal systemic encephalopathy*, refers to a syndrome of reversible cerebral dysfunction associated with chronic liver disease (usually cirrhosis) that is often associated with portal hypertension and shunts that divert hepatic portal blood into the systemic circulation; *chronic portal systemic encephalopathy* implies a sustained condition with a potential for reversibility and is not synonymous with chronic hepatocerebral degeneration (discussed below). Encephalopathy is, by definition, associated with *fulminant hepatic failure,* a condition in which patients with a previously normal liver develop encephalopathy within 8 weeks of the onset of their liver disease. Fulminant hepatic failure is associated with a mortality rate of about 85 percent.

Table 13-1 Features Distinguishing Fulminant Hepatic Failure from Chronic Hepatic Encephalopathy

Feature	Fulminant Hepatic Failure	Chronic Hepatic Encephalopathy
History		
Onset	Usually acute	Varies; may be insidious or subacute
Mental state	Mania may evolve to deep coma	Blunted consciousness progresses to coma
Precipitating factor	Viral infection or hepatotoxin	GI hemorrhage, exogenous protein, drugs, uremia
History of liver disease	No	Usually yes
Symptoms		
Nausea, vomiting	Common	Unusual
Abdominal pain	Common	Unusual
Signs		
Liver	Small, soft, tender	Usually large, firm, painless
Nutritional state	Normal	Cachectic
Collateral circulation	Absent	Caput medusa may be present
Ascites	Absent	May be present
Laboratory tests		
Serum transaminases	Very high	Normal or slightly high
Coagulopathy	Present	Often present

(Modified from Lockwood AH: Hepatic Encephalopathy. Butterworth-Heinemann, Boston, 1992, with permission.)

Death is often due to cerebral edema and may occur within days of the onset of the disorder. The features that differentiate fulminant hepatic failure from portal systemic encephalopathy are shown in Table 13-1.

Clinical Features

An alteration in the on–off aspect of consciousness and the content of consciousness are the hallmarks of hepatic encephalopathy. The level of consciousness is

Table 13-2 Scale for Grading Hepatic Encephalopathy

Grade	Findings
0	Normal
1	Trivial lack of awareness, short attention span, euphoria, or anxiety
2	Lethargy, disorientation, inappropriate behavior, personality changes, impaired cognition
3	Somnolence or semistupor, gross confusion, able to respond appropriately to noxious stimuli
4	Coma, no appropriate response to noxious stimuli

the basis for most grading systems, as shown in Table 13-2. There is a substantial amount of variation in the severity of these abnormalities, which may be so subtle that they are unrecognized. The onset may be slow and insidious, making early diagnosis and treatment difficult, or rapid, with progression to death within days. There may be attentional disturbances, blunting of consciousness, or, less commonly, delirious hypervigilant states. Since this is a disorder that affects the entire brain to varying degrees, all systems are affected as the clinical condition worsens.

Insight into the anatomical basis for consciousness and its two characteristic features—the on-off component and the component of content—provides a useful starting point for both a clinical description of the syndrome and consideration of the pathophysiological mechanisms that are operative. Morruzi and Magoun found that stimuli applied to the reticular formation produced an alerting response.[2] Later experimental and clinicopathological studies showed that ablation of the reticular formation, its rostral projections to the diencephalon, or the entire neocortex was each sufficient to produce coma. Patients with portal systemic encephalopathy always have abnormalities in the on–off aspect of consciousness.

The content of consciousness is also abnormal in these patients. Disorders may include defects in orientation, memory, affect, perception, attention, judgment, or cognition, which may be present in varying degrees. Mesulam and Geschwind suggested that the primary abnormality in patients whom they classified as having an acute confusional state lies in the sphere of selective attention.[3] They described an inability to

complete thought processes that can impair all of the above aspects of consciousness. Specifically, inappropriate attentional shifts to irrelevant stimuli give way to inattention as the level of consciousness declines. Lipowski differed, contending that impaired central information processing is the seminal abnormality, although he recognized disorders of attention, perception, thought processes, and memory as secondary phenomena.[4] As a consequence of disordered information processing, these patients are unable to integrate new stimuli with prior knowledge and experience, causing them to exhibit abnormalities in spatiotemporal relations and an inability to distinguish between images in dreams and true precepts. Diagnostic criteria included hallucinations, memory disorders, and a reduction in the capacity for directed or abstract thought, in addition to altered alertness and psychomotor activity.

The diagnosis may be delayed by several factors. Like many other patients with chronic problems that develop slowly, affected individuals and their families may be unaware of any deficits. Indeed, deficits are frequently detected only by formal neuropsychological testing. In patients with cirrhosis but no evidence for overt encephalopathy, as many as 70 percent will have significant impairment when tested. Visual-spatial perception is the sphere that is most frequently affected. Tests such as the Reitan Trails A and B, Block Design, and Symbol-Digit Subtests of the revised Wechsler Adult Intelligence Scale, and the Purdue Pegboard are commonly abnormal. To a large extent these deficits appear to be unrelated to the cause of cirrhosis.[5] Patients with alcohol-induced cirrhosis are more likely to have subtle memory deficits than patients with cirrhosis resulting from other causes. Ideally, patients with known or suspected cirrhosis should undergo periodic neuropsychological evaluation to detect minimal encephalopathy. Improvements in test performance typically follow conventional treatments for portal systemic encephalopathy.

The function of the cranial nerves in patients with hepatic encephalopathy is almost invariably intact unless the patient is near death, as may be the case for patients with cerebral edema complicating fulminant hepatic failure. Reliable assessment of the visual fields may be impossible (but visual evoked potentials usually indicate intact pathways). Frequently the pupils are smaller than normal, and pupillary constriction in response to light may be slower than normal. Oculovestibular responses are usually intact, and passive head moving typically produces eye movements that indicate functional integrity of the third and sixth cranial nerves. The corneal reflex is usually preserved, as are caloric responses when tested with ice water.

Motor responses may be varied, but the characteristic flapping tremor, or asterixis, is frequently encountered in patients well enough to be tested. Asterixis was originally thought to be pathognomonic for hepatic encephalopathy, but experience has shown that this still useful physical sign is associated with other metabolic causes of cerebral dysfunction, for example, uremia and structural brain lesions. Electrophysiological studies have shown that the postural lapses are associated with sudden and unexplained periods of complete electrical silence in muscles. The sign may be elicited from a variety of voluntary muscles, including arm and hand extensors, flexors of the leg, and protruders of the tongue. Increased muscle tone, hyperreflexia, and extensor plantar signs are all common and may be the source of some confusion when ruling out a structural lesion of the brain, such as an occult chronic subdural hematoma. Abnormal involuntary movements may be observed transiently as successful treatment is started.

The sensory examination may not be helpful and is probably best used to evaluate the depth of coma. Patients with liver disease may have peripheral neuropathies that may result in reflex loss or altered sensation.

Although in many cases the ultimate decision concerning the diagnosis is clinical, laboratory tests are frequently helpful. Liver function tests are usually abnormal, but derangements may not be as drastic as expected on the basis of the clinical examination. Chronic, severe liver disease may be associated with relatively normal serum enzymes and a modest level of hyperbilirubinemia. In these cases, however, hypoalbuminemia and clotting factor deficiency may be substantial and a more reliable guide to the severity of the liver disease. The arterial blood ammonia level, when done properly in the fasting state, is a useful test and provides an excellent correlation with the clinical state and the rate of ammonia uptake and metabolism by the brain.[6,7] Several precautions must be taken to ensure that the results of the test are valid. The blood *must* be arterial. Venous blood is unacceptable because of the release of ammonia by muscle made partly ischemic by a tourniquet and the unpredictable ammonia uptake by muscle itself. Because of the phenomenon of toxin hypersensitivity, discussed below, a "normal" or slightly elevated arterial ammonia level may still be compatible with encephalopathy that is severe.

Electrophysiological studies, especially electroencephalography (EEG) and perhaps visual evoked potentials, may be helpful in establishing the diagnosis and evaluating the response to therapy. Bickford and Butt described three phases in the evolution of the EEG abnormalities: a theta stage with diffuse 4- to 7-Hz waves, a triphasic stage with surface-positive maximum deflections, and a delta stage with random, nonrhythmic slowing without much bilateral synchrony.[8] Brenner's review described bursts of moderate- to high-amplitude waveforms (100 to 300 μV) with low frequencies (1.5 to 2.5 Hz) as being the most characteristic abnormality.[9] Altered visual evoked potentials suggested abnormalities in the γ-aminobutyric acid (GABA) system to Schafer and colleagues,[10,11] but the absence of similar abnormalities in patients treated with γ-vinyl-GABA,[12] a GABA-transaminase inhibitor that causes sustained increases in brain GABA levels, makes this hypothesis tenuous. However, evoked potential abnormalities are found and are helpful in some cases.

Neuroimaging studies have limited usefulness in the diagnosis of hepatic encephalopathy. They are most useful in excluding structural lesions of the brain, such as a subdural hematoma. Magnetic resonance imaging (MRI) studies have demonstrated abnormalities in the pallidum on T_1 and inversion-recovery images. The abnormality is correlated best with the blood ammonia level and may regress or disappear after a successful liver transplant.[13]

Neuropathology

The Alzheimer type II astrocyte is the neuropathological hallmark of patients with hepatic encephalopathy. Adams and Foley provided a translation of the original description in their classic paper.[14] These abnormal astrocytes are found in many locations, including the cortex and the lenticular, lateral thalamic, dentate, and red nuclei. Adams and Foley speculated that the length of coma might correlate with the severity of the abnormality. Ammonia was shown to produce the Alzheimer II transformation by Cole and associates.[15] In rats with portacaval shunt–induced hyperammonemia, Alzheimer II cells become evident after 5 weeks, a time course that parallels the development of the low blood flow and low oxygen metabolism response to chronic hyperammonemia. Ultrastructurally, these astrocytes appear to be metabolically hyperactive, and immunohistochemical staining techniques have shown increases in the activity of glutamic acid dehydrogenase and glutamine synthetase, leading Norenberg to speculate that hepatic encephalopathy is a syndrome due to astrocyte dysfunction.[16]

Pathophysiology

Improvements in the care of patients with hepatic encephalopathy have been substantial since the rather dismal account given by Frerichs.[1] These improvements have been closely linked to improvement in our understanding of the pathophysiology of the disorder. Because of the complexity of the metamorphosis of matter that attends normal hepatic function, it is no surprise that a number of hypotheses have been advanced to explain the development of hepatic encephalopathy. Suspected factors include hyperammonemia and the effects of ammonia on neural function, altered amino acid and neurotransmitter function, elevated mercaptan concentrations, high short-chain fatty acid levels, and, most recently, altered function of the GABA-benzodiazepine complex.

CEREBRAL BLOOD FLOW AND METABOLISM

Cerebral blood flow and metabolism studies in patients with hepatic coma have shown the reductions that would be expected in patients with reduced levels of consciousness.[17] Successful treatment normalizes flow and metabolism.[18,19]

Animal studies of flow and metabolism have been helpful in elucidating possible mechanisms related to ammonia intoxication. Gjedde and colleagues measured blood flow and oxygen metabolism in normal rats and in rats 4 and 8 weeks after portacaval shunting; measurements were made under baseline conditions and serially after an ammonia challenge.[20] The ammonia challenge had little effect on the control animals and in the rats at 4 weeks postoperatively, but it caused a significant reduction in flow and metabolism at 8 weeks. This increase in toxin sensitivity emerges during the same time interval that the Alzheimer II astrocyte transformation becomes apparent. These experimental data support the clinical observations and the hypothesis that toxin hypersensitivity develops as liver disease advances.[21] It is therefore possible, or even likely, that at least some of the patients seen clinically with coma and only modest or borderline elevations in the arterial ammonia concentration are in fact suffering from ammonia intoxication, in that they have a heightened sensitivity to ammonia and are comatose due to the effects of ammonia that would be innocuous in patients without prior prolonged hyperammonemia.

Animal studies using [^{14}C]deoxyglucose in portacaval-shunted rats have shown that glucose metabolism is elevated during asymptomatic hyperammonemia but that there is a considerable amount of variation in the sensitivity of various brain regions to this effect. It is least pronounced in the cortex and most marked in the basal ganglia, thalamus, and brainstem.[22] Such findings have suggested that hyperammonemia leads to a change in the metabolic anatomy of the brain, which may reflect changes in the underlying function of brain regions and suggests that many of the diverse symptoms of brain dysfunction are due to hyperammonemia.

The response of the hypothalamic satiety center is of special interest.[22] This center, like other hypothalamic regions, is sensitive to exogenous ammonia and is stimulated by relatively small amounts of ammonia delivered to the brain. Electrical stimulation of this brain region causes satiety. Thus ammonia-induced satiety may explain appetite loss and the development of cachexia in susceptible patients. Loss of muscle bulk, particularly in patients with portacaval shunts, may then facilitate the development of hyperammonemia. We have hypothesized that the effects of ammonia on the hypothalamus, the loss of skeletal muscle bulk, and the development of toxin sensitivity may be important in the emergence and perpetuation of terminal symptoms in patients with liver disease.[22]

In patients with chronic liver disease and grade 0 to 1 encephalopathy, the pattern of blood flow and glucose metabolism, as shown by positron emission tomography (PET), is abnormal even though global rates are unaffected. A more recent study in five patients with cirrhosis and minimal encephalopathy used more sophisticated statistical methods to evaluate glucose metabolism. Reductions were found in the cingulate gyrus, a part of the anterior attentional center, the frontoparietal cortex, and the cerebellum. These regions may be functionally impaired and contribute to the expression of clinical symptoms. Increases in metabolism were found in visual associative areas that may be activated to compensate for attention-mediated deficits in the processing of visual information. Further PET studies are likely to clarify the relationships between cerebral metabolism and neuropsychological test performance.

AMMONIA

Ammonia is the most completely studied of the neurotoxins implicated in the pathogenesis of hepatic encephalopathy. Early investigators thought that ammonia in blood was artifactual, produced by the breakdown of proteins as the blood stood at room temperature. However, after the perfection of suitable methodology by Conway, it was realized that ammonia is indeed present in normal blood. The beginnings of the link between ammonia and encephalopathy are best dated to the studies of Gabuzda and associates,[23] who reported the development of encephalopathy in patients treated with resins that exchanged serum sodium ions for resin-bound ammonium ions. Further studies correlated the changes in the mental status with the development of hyperammonemia and led to recommendations that ammonia-containing compounds be avoided in patients with liver disease. Later, Sherlock correlated the fasting arterial ammonia level with the severity of coma.[6] Subsequently, a number of publications and reviews supported and strengthened this correlation.[7,24,25] The evidence that supports the ammonia hypothesis can be summarized briefly. First, there is a good correlation between the degree of hyperammonemia and the depth of coma, and glutamine and α-ketoglutaramate (metabolites of ammonia) are elevated in the brain and cerebrospinal fluid (CSF) of patients with hepatic encephalopathy. Second, patients with encephalopathy have higher rates of ammonia uptake and metabolic trapping by the brain than do nonencephalopathic controls. Third, ammonia reproducibly precipitates episodes of coma, along with compounds that form ammonia in the gastrointestinal tract, such as blood from hemorrhage or protein meals. Fourth and finally, the most effective

treatments for hepatic encephalopathy—in fact, all proven treatments—act to reduce blood ammonia levels.

Ammonia is a gas that is highly soluble in water, where it forms a weakly basic solution that, at physiological pH values, contains 1 to 2 percent ammonia gas, with the remainder present as ammonium ions. Ammonia is normally produced in the gastrointestinal tract and carried to the liver by the hepatic portal vein (Fig. 13-1). In the liver, ammonia is converted to urea by the enzymes of the urea cycle, and the urea is excreted by the kidneys. A portion of the urea enters the gastrointestinal tract and is hydrolyzed to form ammonia in an enterohepatic circulation of nitrogen. In the rest of the body, ammonia is taken up by skeletal muscle to form glutamine, which is then transported to the liver, where the amide nitrogen is used in urea synthesis. Ammonia is released by skeletal muscle and the kidney. About 7 percent of the ammonia in the systemic circulation is trapped by the brain. Liver disease leads to the shunting of ammonia-rich blood from the portal into the systemic circulation.

Cerebral ammonia metabolism studies have been facilitated by the use of the cyclotron-produced radioactive isotope ^{13}N, which is easily made into [^{13}N]ammonia.

Quantitative studies of ammonia metabolism have been performed by Lockwood and associates[7] using [^{13}N]ammonia. These studies showed that about 1 mol of ammonia is removed from the systemic circulation each day by the various body organs. Somewhat surprisingly, skeletal muscle was found to be a major organ in ammonia homeostasis. In patients with end-to-side portacaval shunts, skeletal muscle becomes the single most important organ for maintaining ammonia homeostasis. Studies using [^{13}N]ammonia have shown that the blood-brain barrier is highly permeable to ammonia, despite the fact that it is highly ionized at physiological pH values and that the permeability of the barrier to ammonia is such that, at normal blood flow and pH values, about half of the ammonia presented to the brain is extracted by the brain and metabolically trapped.

Two studies of cerebral ammonia metabolism have shown that the rate of ammonia uptake and metabolic trapping is disproportionately high in patients with hyperammonemia and cirrhosis.[7,26] This is probably due to an increase of the permeability–surface area

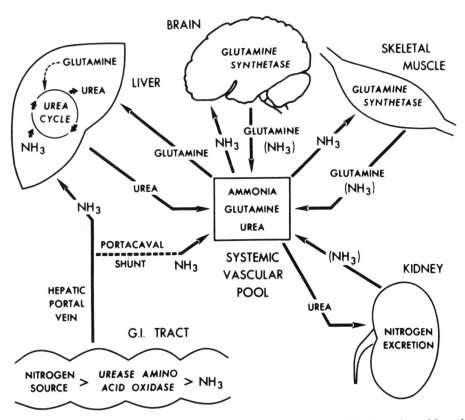

Fig. 13-1 Human ammonia metabolism. Most ammonia is formed in the colon, although other organs make a contribution as well. Ammonia in the hepatic portal vein is normally detoxified by the enzymes of the urea cycle in the liver. Portal-systemic shunts cause excessive amounts of ammonia and probably other toxins to enter the systemic circulation and reach the brain. About 7 percent of the ammonia in the systemic circulation is taken up and metabolized by the brain. Skeletal muscle is also an important organ for ammonia homeostasis, taking up ammonia and converting it to glutamine, which is subsequently converted to urea in the liver. Recent data suggest a complex interaction between hyperammonemia, its effects on cerebral satiety centers, and the development of cachexia. (From Lockwood AH, McDonald JM, Reiman RE, et al: The dynamics of ammonia metabolism in man: effects of liver disease and hyperammonemia. J Clin Invest 63:449, 1979, with permission.)

product of the blood-brain barrier to ammonia.[26] The increase in the ease with which ammonia in the arterial blood gains access to the brain may explain why some patients with minimal hyperammonemia become symptomatic. The time course for the development of this abnormality is not known, but this disturbance of blood-brain barrier may explain why patients with liver disease appear to be increasingly sensitive to factors that precipitate encephalopathy.

The mechanisms by which ammonia affects brain function are unresolved. Virtually every aspect of neuronal function appears to be affected by ammonia. In addition to affecting glucose metabolism, ammonia affects brain energy metabolism, disrupts amino acids profiles in the brain (particularly that of glutamate), and alters the physiology of neural membranes by affecting the chloride pump, producing a reversible depolarizing shift in the inhibitory postsynaptic potential toward the resting potential. The subject is reviewed in detail elsewhere.[25]

ABNORMALITIES OF NEUROTRANSMISSION

Neurotransmitters and their role in normal brain function are among the most important characteristics that differentiate brain from other organs, and abnormalities of neurotransmitter function are proved or implied in a variety of diseases ranging from parkinsonism to schizophrenia. It is therefore not surprising that neurotransmitter abnormalities have been proposed as being of potential importance in the pathogenesis of hepatic encephalopathy.

Glutamate was the first of the amino acid transmitters to be implicated, and this led to unsuccessful attempts to treat patients with glutamic acid infusions.[27,28] Hindfelt and associates observed small reductions in brain glutamate levels in animals challenged with ammonia.[29] The anatomical locus of the depleted glutamate could not be determined from that study. Glutaminase inhibition and reduced hippocampal glutamate release have also been suggested.

Parker and associates produced ammonia intoxication in animals and measured normal acetylcholine levels in the brain.[30] They concluded that this transmitter is not affected in hepatic coma.

Biogenic amines and false neurotransmitters, notably octopamine, have been the source of considerable interest since Fischer and Baldessarini proposed the false neurotransmitter hypothesis in 1971.[31] They found that octopamine and phenylethanolamine were present in increased quantities in the brains and hearts of animals after a two-stage ligation of the hepatic artery. Octopamine is a low-potency transmitter and, due to competition at postsynaptic receptor sites, it may displace true transmitters, causing a reduction in the functional activity of the system and encephalopathy. These and similar observations were buttressed by uncontrolled trials suggesting that some patients awoke in a near-miraculous fashion after the administration of levodopa. These observations were combined with new and existing data on the plasma amino acid profile associated with liver disease to produce a new hypothesis. This hypothesis stated that the ratio of the sum of the concentrations of valine, leucine, and isoleucine divided by the sum of the phenylalanine and tyrosine concentration is a useful predictor and index of the severity of encephalopathy, and that normalization of the ratio by the infusion of amino acid mixtures rich in the branched-chain amino acids of the numerator is therapeutic. A subsequent refinement of the hypothesis suggested that the high brain glutamine level acts as the driving force behind the uptake of the deleterious aromatic amino acids.

The hypothesis was supported by uncontrolled clinical trials of branched-chain amino acids.[32,33]

Controlled trials were disappointing. Michel and associates found levodopa to be ineffective[34]; and although Morgan and colleagues found bromocriptine therapy to be associated with an improvement in blood flow,[35] this treatment has not been tried on any scale, presumably due to the results of the levodopa study. Two of the controlled studies of branched-chain amino acids showed no effect,[36,37] one showed worsening,[38] and a fourth reported improved survival and cerebral function.[39] In all of these studies it was reported that the amino acid ratio was improved, but there was no correlation with EEG or clinical improvement. Thus the potential benefit of this therapy is not defined.

In addition to the disappointing results of the branched-chain amino acid trials, the false neurotransmitter hypothesis has been weakened on other grounds. Zieve and Olsen injected octopamine directly into the brains of animals at concentrations 20,000 times those encountered in life, with no effect on behavior.[40] Similarly, monoamine oxidase inhibition and imipramine therapy both lead to increases in brain octopamine without the induction of encephalopathy.[41]

GABA-BENZODIAZEPINE COMPLEX

The hypothesis that excessive GABAergic tone causes hepatic encephalopathy has generated a great deal of attention. Normally, the brain is protected from numerous compounds in the blood, including GABA, by the impermeable blood-brain barrier. According to this hypothesis, excess GABA is produced in the gastrointestinal tract and enters the brain through a damaged, or permeable, blood-brain barrier. The GABA then binds to GABA receptors, which are present in excess numbers, and the increased inhibitory tone is expressed as coma.

The normal GABA system is complex. The GABA receptor itself is a complicated molecule, with at least five specific components: a GABA recognition site, a GABA-modulin, a chloride ion channel, a benzodiazepine-binding protein, and a protein that couples the GABA-recognition and ion channels. There are further complexities: GABA autoreceptors—GABA-sensitive sites on GABA terminals—bind GABA but inhibit GABA release. There are also GABA-sensitive sites in the nervous system that have no direct GABA input. This array of unpredictable interactions gives the system the potential for multiple actions that cause significant problems in the interpretation of pharmacological studies of GABA actions in the brain.[42]

Experimental evaluation of the GABA hypothesis has made it less credible. Improved analytical methods have shown that early reports of elevated blood GABA levels were erroneous, GABA probably does not cross the blood-brain barrier to any appreciable extent,[43] GABA levels in the brains of patients who have died in hepatic encephalopathy are normal,[44] and inhibition of GABA transaminase (which increases brain GABA levels) does not cause encephalopathy.[45] As interest in GABA has waned, more attention has been directed to the benzodiazepines.

Patients with cirrhosis have a heightened sensitivity to this class of drugs, suggesting to some that they, or an endogenous ligand with benzodiazepine activity, may cause hepatic encephalopathy. Reports of near-miraculous recovery after the administration of the benzodiazepine antagonist flumazenil (RO 15-1788 or Anexate), has increased interest in the benzodiazepines. While there is no reason to doubt the validity of these anecdotal reports and open trials, the evidence that these responders had not taken benzodiazepines is often incomplete. Although there are reports of elevated levels of endogenous benzodiazepines in some comatose patients, the levels are lower than those associated with anxiolytic activity in normal subjects. Benzodiazepine receptors are present in normal numbers and exhibit normal kinetics in the brains of patients with fatal hepatic encephalopathy.[46] Controlled trials of flumazenil[47,48] have shown that more patients responded in the flumazenil group than in the control group, but there was no good evidence for the presence of a benzodiazepine in the responders. The action of this drug may therefore relate in part to its general ability to activate the brain rather than simply to the displacement of a benzodiazepine. Among patients who improve after flumazenil, complete recovery is unusual, suggesting that any benzodiazepine effect is probably augmented by other pathophysiological mechanisms.

MERCAPTANS

Mercaptans are thio alcohols, containing -SH groups, in contrast to the -OH groups in conventional alcohols. Because of the -SH group, these compounds are malodorous and are responsible for the fetor hepaticus that is occasionally encountered in patients with hepatic encephalopathy.

Methanethiol is the principal mercaptan in humans and is formed by the catabolism of methionine in the gastrointestinal system. Methanethiol levels are elevated in the blood and end-tidal air samples of patients with hepatic encephalopathy,[49,50] and levels have been correlated with the severity of the encephalopathy. Mercaptans are capable of precipitating coma in animals when given by injection or inhalation.[51] Mercaptans also appear to act in a synergistic fashion with other toxins, notably ammonia and fatty acids, to produce coma in animals.[52] For example, mercaptan administered at a subcoma dose in combination with either of the other test compounds, also at a subcoma dosage, produces unconsciousness.[52]

Mardini and associates have challenged the mercaptan hypothesis.[53] They used improved methodology for the measurement of mercaptan levels and found that, although the levels were indeed elevated in encephalopathic patients, the correlation between concentration and the severity of symptoms was poor. They also described problems of producing coma in animals with reliability, even when doses sufficient to produce blood levels ten times those seen in patients were used. These data and conclusions may not take the synergism hypothesis into account, and there may be substantial differences in the dose-response relation in humans and animals, even if the toxin-hypersensitization hypothesis is taken into account.

SHORT-CHAIN FATTY ACIDS

Abnormalities in short-chain fatty acid concentrations affect a variety of metabolic reactions or processes directly or indirectly in a fashion that may cause or contribute to the development of encephalopathy. Hird and Weidemann[54] reported uncoupling of oxidative phosphorylation; Derr and Zieve[55] reported inhibition of hepatic urea formation; and Ansevin[56] presented evidence that short-chain fatty acids may alter the mitochondrial respiratory state and state-control mechanisms. Coma has been produced in animals by the intraperitoneal injection of short- and medium-chain fatty acids. Muto reported elevations in hexanoic and valeric acid blood levels in patients in hepatic coma,[57] leading to speculation that these substances may produce coma alone or by acting synergistically with other toxins. Deficiency of medium-chain acylcoenzyme A (CoA) dehydrogenase appears to be a common condition that may present as coma and often mimics other conditions, such as Reye's syndrome[58]; the coma appears to depend on the action of fatty acids on the brain, lending further support to the hypothesis that fatty acids may be important in the pathogenesis of hepatic encephalopathy.

SUMMARY

A variety of compounds have been implicated in the pathogenesis of the encephalopathy associated with portal-systemic shunting of blood and fulminant hepatic failure. A similarly large number of experimental models has been used to study these conditions. It is not presently possible to create a unifying hypothesis that explains all aspects of this encephalopathy, but certain general comments can be made. First, ammonia is probably of central importance in the pathogenesis of portal systemic encephalopathy. Second, the actions of ammonia appear to be affected by the development of toxin hypersensitivity and synergism with other toxins. Third, endogenous benzodiazepine ligands may contribute to the development of the disorder. Fourth, many models of liver disease are most appropriately considered as models of fulminant hepatic failure, and the mechanisms causing brain dysfunction in this disorder are poorly understood, as is witnessed by the poor therapies available to treat this condition.

Therapy

The management of liver failure accompanied by neurological disturbances may be complex because many patients have a variety of complicating problems, including severe infections, abnormalities of renal function, cardiovascular collapse, hemorrhagic disorders due to ruptured varices, hypersplenism, or clotting factor deficiencies. Thus it is unusual to encounter patients with relatively uncomplicated hepatic encephalopathy.

In planning therapy, it is critical to differentiate patients with fulminant hepatic failure, for whom there is little in the way of proved specific therapy other than general support, from patients with portal systemic encephalopathy, for whom there are a number of proved, highly effective treatment regimens. In

evaluating the results of the many reported therapies for encephalopathy associated with liver disease, it is critical to remember that mere inclusion in a therapeutic trial is likely to be beneficial because investigators are then better able to control diet, alcohol consumption, and other precipitating factors that are critical to the success of treatment. Because of this, open trials of almost any therapy for portal systemic encephalopathy are likely to be associated with improvement in clinical and laboratory measures designed to evaluate a response to therapy.

Success in treating fulminant hepatic failure depends on maintaining the patient until hepatic regeneration occurs or until transplantation can be accomplished if the patient is a suitable candidate. Many therapeutic strategies have been tried for this disorder, with little success, including various methods designed to remove unspecified toxins from blood by exchange transfusion, dialysis, or use of various purification columns. Perfusion through cadaver and xenograft livers has also been tried. In the terminal phases of the disease, coma with physical signs indicative of cerebral edema may be present. In these individuals intracranial pressure monitoring, corticosteroid therapy, and use of osmotic diuretics may provide transient benefit but are not clearly helpful. This dismal situation reflects the lack of understanding of the basic mechanisms responsible for the encephalopathy. A mortality rate of 85 present can be expected.

Most of the therapies that are clearly effective in the treatment of portal systemic encephalopathy are believed to work by influencing ammonia metabolism. These therapies are considered in some detail.

GENERAL MEASURES

Because much of the body burden of ammonia is due to the action of urease and amino acid oxidases in the colon, a variety of successful measures designed to reduce colonic ammonia production have been evaluated. Much of the ammonia formed in the colon is derived from protein, and control of protein is therefore critical. This control can be achieved by several means, each of which should be considered. Dietary protein must be monitored and controlled. During acute exacerbations, complete elimination of dietary protein may be required. Bleeding in the gastrointestinal tract must be controlled as quickly as possible, and elimination of blood must be facilitated by the judicious use of purgatives and enemas. These measures should be considered in every patient, especially when a history of constipation is obtained. Constipation maximizes the dwell-time for nitrogenous compounds in the colon and thereby the potential for conversion to ammonia. More aggressive measures such as surgery to remove or bypass the colon have been evaluated, but the morbidity and mortality of the surgery are high and obscure any possible therapeutic benefit.

In patients with chronic liver disease, it is important to maintain adequate nutrition to optimize hepatic regeneration and prevent the development of cachexia. This may be an indication for the use of the branched-chain amino acid mixtures that have been developed for both intravenous and oral use, but further evaluation of this approach is required. Uribe and associates compared various diets, including 40 g of meat protein plus neomycin, 40 g of vegetable protein without neomycin, and 80 g of vegetable protein without neomycin.[59] Both vegetable protein diets were found to be superior to the diet containing meat protein plus neomycin. However, two patients receiving the vegetable protein diet had episodes of hypoglycemia, and most patients found it difficult to eat the large volumes of food required to ingest 80 g of vegetable protein. These forms of therapy may work by reducing dietary methionine and its subsequent conversion to methanethiol and ammonia and by the cathartic effect of the fiber in diets that are high in vegetable protein.

LACTULOSE

Lactulose, a synthetic disaccharide, is currently the mainstay in the treatment of portal systemic encephalopathy and has largely replaced neomycin, as it is not associated with renal toxicity or ototoxicity. Effective lactulose therapy is associated with reductions in the arterial ammonia concentration that are paralleled by normalization of the EEG and improvements in mental status. Its therapeutic efficacy is therefore thought to be related to its effect on ammonia, but the manner in which this occurs has been determined only recently.

The history of lactulose is of considerable interest. It was first given to patients with the expectation that it would acidify the colon, leading to repopulation of

the colon with bacteria that did not contain urease. It was hoped that this situation, in turn, would lead to reduction in the ammonia concentration and to clinical improvement. Although the treated patients did improve, the mechanism involved has only recently been clarified.

Several double-blind trials were subsequently performed (with crossover to placebo given in the form of sorbitol to reproduce the cathartic effect of lactulose). Elkington and colleagues administered the treatment sequence to seven patients with chronic encephalopathy and observed clinical improvement, reductions in ammonia, and improved EEGs during lactulose therapy in five.[60] In all seven patients, lactulose was judged to be effective in the prevention or reduction in severity of exacerbations of encephalopathy. Sorbitol was without any discernible effect. The most definitive study, however, did not appear for almost another decade.[61] In that multicenter trial, 33 patients with chronic encephalopathy were treated in a double-blind fashion with neomycin plus sorbitol or with lactulose. Dietary protein was kept at about 40 g/d. Lactulose was effective in 90 percent of patients and neomycin-sorbitol in 83 percent. The investigators suggested that some patients appeared to respond preferentially to one form of therapy or the other, but they were unable to explain the observation. They concluded that lactulose was effective and potentially less toxic than neomycin when chronic therapy is required. Lactulose has also been shown to be effective in the management of acute portal systemic encephalopathy.

The dose of lactulose varies from patient to patient, but 20 to 30 g four times daily is a typical, effective regimen. The dose should be adjusted until two to three bowel movements per day are produced without unacceptable side effects. Patients presenting with coma require more aggressive initial therapy, with hourly doses of 20 to 30 g of lactulose until a catharsis is produced, after which the dose is reduced. Adverse reactions most commonly include abdominal bloating and diarrhea. These symptoms are dose-related, and adjustments in the therapeutic regimen usually allow continuation of therapy. Care must be taken to prevent diarrhea and secondary electrolyte abnormalities. Patients with liver disease may be more susceptible to the development of central pontine myelinolysis than other patients when hyponatremia is corrected too rapidly. This complication must be avoided.

The mechanism of action of lactulose has only recently been elucidated. Initially it was believed that the mechanism centered on the acidification of the colonic contents by the hydrolysis of lactulose. This theory has been challenged by Wrong and associates, who failed to document any increase in the ammonium excreted. They subsequently speculated that lactulose served as a substrate for ammonia-fixing reactions or suppressed deamidation reactions.[62] Weber and colleagues have recently reported that the nitrogen content of the bacterial and soluble fractions of feces increased to 165 and 135 percent of control, respectively, after the administration of lactulose, supporting the nitrogen-fixation theory.[63] They also found that during neomycin therapy, the bacterial nitrogen content fell by 28 percent, presumably because bacteria are killed by the drug. The urea production rate during neomycin therapy was significantly reduced by 23 percent, again presumably because urease-containing bacteria are killed and the enterohepatic circulation of ammonia is reduced. This study is important in confirming the presumed mechanisms of the two most important drugs for managing hyperammonemia of portal systemic encephalopathy.

NEOMYCIN

Although the efficacy of neomycin was widely accepted, proof of its utility did not come until the same cooperative study that proved the efficacy of lactulose.[61] Neomycin is also clearly effective in the management of acute encephalopathy. For this condition, the usual dose ranges between 4 and 12 g/d in divided doses, whereas chronic therapy is usually accomplished with 2 to 3 g/d. When chronic neomycin therapy is required, monitoring of drug levels and otological and renal function is mandatory to detect early toxicity.

LACTITOL

Another synthetic disaccharide, lactitol, has been reported to be as effective as lactulose in the treatment of acute portal systemic encephalopathy[64] and chronic encephalopathy.[65] It remains to be seen whether this drug will find widespread acceptance.

Clinical Course, Complications, Conclusions

Patients with fulminant hepatic failure have an 80 to 85 percent expected mortality rate, and treatment has been of little help. The ultimate prognosis depends on the severity of the liver disease, the presence of complications, and in some cases the availability of livers for transplantation.

Patients with portal systemic encephalopathy fare much better than do patients with fulminant hepatic failure. Most patients with relatively uncomplicated encephalopathy can be expected to make full recoveries, at least after the initial episode. Again, complications and the nature of the precipitating factor have an impact on survival.

Severe hepatic coma carries a substantial risk of death or permanent neurological disability. Levy and colleagues encountered 51 patients with hepatic coma in their prospective analysis of nontraumatic coma of at least 6 hours' duration.[66] In that group, 49 percent showed no sign of recovery over the first year after diagnosis, whereas 27 percent regained the ability to live independently and made a good neurological recovery. Among the remainder, 2 percent developed a persistent vegetative state, 14 percent were left with severe disability, and 8 percent remained with moderate disability over a 1-year period. These patients probably represent a worst-case group because of the requirement for very deep and prolonged coma that had to be satisfied prior to enrollment in the study. Orlandi and associates studied a less severely affected population and reported a mortality rate of 6.1 percent for patients with grade 1 encephalopathy, rising to 27 percent in patients with grade 2 or higher.[67] An identifiable precipitating factor and a short duration were favorable indicators, whereas hyperbilirubinemia, prolongation of the prothrombin time, ascites, or cachexia predicted an unfavorable outcome.

OTHER NEUROLOGICAL DISORDERS ASSOCIATED WITH LIVER DISEASE

Chronic Non-Wilsonian Hepatocerebral Degeneration

Chronic non-Wilsonian hepatocerebral degeneration is similar to the neurological disorders that occur in Wilson's disease. It was described by Victor and co-workers in 1965 and in their opinion represents the consequence of prolonged exposure to the metabolic toxins that cause encephalopathy.[68] They reported 27 cases, including 17 with autopsies. Well-defined episodes of hepatic coma were evident in 23 of the 27 patients, and 12 patients had surgical portacaval shunts, including 1 patient shunted in the absence of definable liver disease. All patients had hyperammonemia or abnormal ammonia tolerance tests. The clinical constellation included dementia of varied severity, dysarthria and other evidence for cerebellar dysfunction, and movement disorders that included choreoathetosis and tremor during sustained posture (stated specifically as not being asterixis). Diffuse rigidity, positive grasp reflexes, nystagmus, and other types of tremor were less common. Pathological examination of the brain showed polymicrocavitary degeneration of layers 5 and 6 of the cerebral cortex, underlying white matter, basal ganglia, and cerebellum. Other stigmata of hepatic encephalopathy were present as well, including Alzheimer II astrocytosis. Three patients had spinal cord abnormalities.

Diverse CNS Disorders

Signs of myelopathy may appear without other stigmata of hepatocerebral degeneration.[69,70] These patients are typically similar to those with hepatocerebral degeneration of the non-Wilsonian type. They have chronic or episodic encephalopathy and frequently portacaval shunts. Spastic paraparesis usually persists after the resolution of other symptoms of encephalopathy, characteristically worsening after subsequent episodes of encephalopathy. Pathologically, polymicrocavitary degeneration of the corticospinal tracts and loss of Betz cells are observed. The diagnosis may be difficult to make in early or mild cases because the clinical spectrum of abnormal muscle tone, hyperreflexia, and extensor plantar responses that are typically seen in uncomplicated portal systemic encephalopathy may blend indistinguishably with the signs of hepatic myelopathy.

Marchiafava-Bignami syndrome and central pontine myelinolysis were once believed to be complications of alcoholism and were most commonly encountered in patients with liver disease. The former syndrome, which is discussed in Chapter 30, remains of undefined etiology, but pontine myelinolysis now clearly seems to be a complication of excessively rapid correction of hyponatremia.[71] Sterns and colleagues have reported eight patients with central pontine myelinolysis whose hyponatremia had been corrected at a rate in excess of 12 mEq sodium/L/d; in contrast, none of 60 patients whose hyponatremia (less than 116 mEq/L) was corrected more slowly developed evidence of demyelination.[72] It is still not clear whether liver disease is a predisposing factor. Hyponatremia is common in patients with hepatic encephalopathy, and severe electrolyte abnormalities may be encountered in patients with unsupervised use of lactulose, but correction of hyponatremia at appropriate rates should prevent the development of this disabling and occasionally fatal disorder. Further discussion of central pontine myelinolysis can be found in Chapters 17 and 30.

REYE'S SYNDROME AND RELATED DISORDERS

Reye's syndrome was first described in 1963[73] and has been the subject of numerous reports and investigations since then. The syndrome is almost exclusively confined to children, although rare reports of adults with the disorder have been published. Prodromal symptoms are usually those of a viral illness and include malaise, cough, rhinorrhea, and other nonspecific symptoms. Following a suspected association between the use of aspirin and the subsequent development of the syndrome, numerous epidemiological studies have conclusively established that there is an increased risk for the development of Reye's syndrome after aspirin use, and it has been recommended that salicylates be avoided, particularly for varicella and influenza-like syndromes, in children. After a latent period of variable duration, there is rapid neurological deterioration characterized by nausea, vomiting, delirium, convulsions, and coma. Severely affected children develop alterations in muscle tone that may be followed by decorticate posturing. Central herniation may ensue as a result of generalized severe brain edema. The liver is often palpably enlarged.

Laboratory tests are valuable in supporting the diagnosis. Hypoglycemia is common and may be profound. Marked elevations of hepatic transaminases are the rule, and prolongation of the prothrombin time is common. Hyperammonemia is characteristic and may be severe. Increases in plasma fatty acid levels have been reported and implicated in the pathogenesis of the disorder.

Therapy of Reye's syndrome is supportive. Initial reports of success in the use of exchange transfusions to control hyperammonemia have been tempered by more recent studies showing no benefit from this form of therapy. Patients with proved or suspected Reye's syndrome do benefit from intensive care and support, with maintenance of blood glucose levels and the use of corticosteroids and osmotic diuretics for the control of cerebral edema.

Initial reports suggested a mortality rate of approximately 80 percent. More recently, the mortality rate has declined considerably, probably because less severe forms of the disorder are now correctly diagnosed and other conditions simulating it are correctly distinguished. In addition, the prevalence of the syndrome seems to be declining, perhaps because of recognition of its relation to the use of aspirin, although other factors cannot be excluded. Pathologically this disorder is associated with fatty infiltration of the liver and other viscera.

There have been several reports of a disorder similar to Reye's syndrome in children who may have had siblings with sudden infant death syndrome.[58] These patients may present with coma, profound hypoglycemia, hyperammonemia, hepatic enlargement with fatty infiltration, and low serum carnitine levels. Investigation of affected individuals has revealed the presence of a medium–chain acyl-CoA dehydrogenase deficiency. This enzyme, normally present in mitochondria, is essential to the metabolism of fatty acids during the process of shortening the chain length and the production of acetyl-CoA and short-chain acyl-CoA. The metabolic block leads to the excretion of medium–chain acylcarnitines (e.g., octanoylcarnitine) formed by the action of carnitine octanoyltransferase, and thus to carnitine deficiency. These non-toxic acylcarnitines can be detected by fast atom bombardment–mass spectroscopy. The carnitine deficiency may give rise to symptoms of proximal muscle weakness, mimicking a myopathy. The administration of oral carnitine appears to prevent the disorder effectively. Because carnitine is excreted in breast milk, maternal therapy protects affected infants.

It is likely that many patients with previously diagnosed Reye's syndrome or sudden infant death syndrome may have had this disorder, which appears to be quite common. Therefore it is prudent to evaluate families and children at risk by screening patients for the presence of urinary acylcarnitines.

OTHER ENCEPHALOPATHIES ASSOCIATED WITH HYPERAMMONEMIA

The Krebs-Henselite or urea cycle is the most important metabolic pathway for ammonia homeostasis and the elimination of this toxic metabolite. The enzymes for the complete cycle are found in the liver: only a partial cycle exists in the brain. Enzymatic deficiencies produce symptoms that are almost always confined to the perinatal or early childhood periods. There are five steps in the cycle, and defects have been described in each. Deficiency states include the following: (1) carbamylphosphate synthetase deficiency and ornithine transcarbamylase deficiency, both of which present as hyperammonemia; (2) arginosuccinic aciduria, which is probably the most common of the disorders and which exists in three clinically and genetically distinct forms, all of which result from arginosuccinate lyase deficiency; (3) citrullinemia, secondary to arginosuccinic acid synthetase deficiency; and (4) hyperargininemia, resulting from arginase deficiency. Most of these diseases are characterized by mental retardation, seizures, lethargy, nausea, and vomiting. Many of the symptoms are attributable to a failure to detoxify ammonia. Attacks can be precipitated or exacerbated by protein meals.

Treatment strategies generally include limiting dietary protein, spreading total daily protein intake over extended periods of time, exchange transfusion, dialysis, and the use of ketoacid analogue therapy.[74,75] A definitive diagnosis cannot be made on clinical criteria alone: tissue sampling and measurement of specific enzymatic activities are required.

An increase in the awareness of urea cycle deficiency states has led to more widespread measurement of blood ammonia levels in infants with relatively nonspecific symptoms. Goldberg and colleagues described 12 hyperammonemic infants presenting over a 12-month period with severe fetal bradycardia or who required prolonged resuscitation.[76] Five of the seven survivors were left with severe neurological deficits. A prompt response to the aggressive treatment of hyperammonemia by exchange transfusion and peritoneal dialysis has been reported in a group of patients with hyperammonemia of undetermined etiology.[75] Normal development in survivors supports the need for these aggressive forms of therapy.

Hyperammonemia has also been encountered in patients who have had urinary diversion procedures, typically ureterosigmoidostomies, with coexisting liver disease. The ammonia is formed when the diverted urine is infected with organisms that contain urease. The urea formed in the diverted urine escapes detoxification because of the liver disease and produces symptomatic hyperammonemia. A single patient with hyperammonemia and normal liver function has been described.[77] Hyperammonemia has also been associated with high-dose salicylate therapy,[78] valproic acid administration, and parenteral hyperalimentation.

PANCREATIC ENCEPHALOPATHY

Acute pancreatitis is a relatively common entity that is usually not associated with neurological abnormalities. There have been a number of reports linking acute pancreatitis with a transient encephalopathy,[79–83] but it remains unclear if this encephalopathy is a distinct nosological entity. Many of the reports are of single cases, and none of the reported series contains more than 20 patients. The symptoms described (agitation, anxiety, clouding of consciousness, and coma) are those that are seen in any metabolic encephalopathy. In many of the reported cases it is not possible to exclude liver failure or an electrolyte disorder as the cause of the encephalopathy.

In a few cases where neuropathological examinations are reported, findings such as capillary necrosis and subependymal gliosis do not clearly describe a defined entity. Balart and Ferrante alluded to this fact by mentioning fat embolism, intravascular coagulation, hyperosmolarity, and hypoxia as events that could be contributory factors in the development of a syndrome that includes neurological dysfunction and pancreatitis.[83] The CSF lipase concentration is reportedly increased in patients with pancreatitis and accompanying encephalopathy, as compared with levels in the CSF of patients with pancreatitis without

encephalopathy.[79] One patient reportedly improved on treatment with aprotinin (Trasylol),[82] but reports of successful therapy in single cases must be interpreted cautiously.

WILSON'S DISEASE (HEPATOLENTICULAR DEGENERATION)

Wilson's disease is a rare autosomal recessive disease of copper metabolism. The primary genetic defect remains unknown; therefore there are occasional patients in whom the diagnosis is difficult. Usually the diagnosis can be made easily when Wilson's disease is suspected.

Many patients with Wilson's disease present with a neurological syndrome characterized by the following: alterations in the personality that may range from emotional lability to progressive dementia; movement disorders including tremors of the hand, head, or whole body, dystonia, and rigidity; and occasionally epileptic seizures. At the time that neurological disease becomes manifest, a Kayser-Fleischer ring, due to deposition of copper in Descemet's membrane of the cornea, is seen in virtually every case.

Other patients present with hepatic disease, ranging from cirrhosis to acute fulminant hepatic necrosis. Hemolytic anemia and various renal abnormalities including failure to acidify the urine, reduced glomerular and tubular function, aminoaciduria, glycosuria, hypercalciuria, and hypophosphaturia (which may, in turn, cause skeletal abnormalities) also occur.

The diversity of the presenting signs and symptoms and the rarity of the disease often lead to a delay in making the diagnosis when Wilson's disease is not considered.[84] Hepatic and neurological manifestations commonly occur together but may occur in isolation. The disease presents usually by the end of the second decade of life. Typically, when hepatic manifestations predominate, the disease presents somewhat earlier than it does when neurological symptoms predominate.

Although the basic enzymatic defect is not known, the manifestations of the disease have been attributed to the toxic effects of excessive copper accumulation by various organs, including the brain, liver, and kidneys. The excess in copper results, in turn, from a failure to excrete normal amounts of copper in the bile.

The diagnosis of Wilson's disease is based on the characteristic clinical manifestations and confirmatory laboratory tests for abnormalities of copper metabolism. Although the Kayser-Fleischer ring is characteristic of the disease, it may be very difficult to detect, even when careful slit-lamp examinations are performed. The presence of the Kayser-Fleischer ring was once thought to be pathognomonic for Wilson's disease but has also been described in a small number of patients with biliary cirrhosis and other forms of intrahepatic cholestasis. The mechanism for this abnormality probably centers on a failure to excrete copper via the bile, leading to secondary increases in copper stores in the liver and elsewhere in the body. In these cases the ceruloplasmin is almost invariably elevated. By contrast, in Wilson's disease the serum ceruloplasmin is low (less than 20 mg/dl and commonly less than 10 mg/dl), although about 5 percent of patients with Wilson's disease have normal ceruloplasmin levels. The reasons for this finding are not clear but may relate to the effects of estrogens and chronic liver disease on ceruloplasmin levels. Some asymptomatic carriers have ceruloplasmin levels below the lower limit of normal. The concentration of unbound copper is elevated in the blood, which leads to excessive copper excretion in the urine (more than 100 μg/24 h). Patients with biliary cirrhosis may also have increased urinary copper excretion. Additional tests that are sometimes necessary include liver biopsy for the measurement of liver copper levels and copper metabolism studies using radioactive ^{64}Cu or ^{67}Cu. (^{67}Cu is more expensive but is needed for longer-duration studies because of its longer half-life). The performance and interpretation of these studies may be complex. Abnormalities depend on demonstrating alterations in copper metabolism as indicated by a decrease in the rate of copper incorporation into ceruloplasmin, an altered hepatic copper uptake, or prolonged copper turnover.[84]

Prior to beginning therapy, it is essential that the diagnosis be established beyond any reasonable doubt because therapy itself has hazards and must be continued for life. Treatment leaches copper out of Descemet's membrane and the liver, causing the Kayser-Fleischer ring to fade or disappear and the hepatic copper stores to become normal. The neurological and hepatic manifestations of the disease disappear, which may lead to confusion about the diagnosis. Because the disease is inherited in an autosomal recessive manner, it is important to evaluate other family members to detect asymptomatic homozygotes, so that therapy can be started before neurological or hepatic damage appears. Moreover, appropriate genetic counseling can be offered to heterozygotes and patients with the disease who are as yet asymptomatic. This task has been aided by recent reports describing the use of DNA markers to identify presymptomatic patients.[85]

Treatment is with a low-copper diet, which is difficult because of the ubiquity of copper, and with a chelating agent such as penicillamine. This drug, which must be continued for life, has side effects that include fever, rash, bone marrow suppression, autoimmune and immune complex disorders, nephrotic syndrome, optic neuropathy, and loss of taste. Doses required range between 1 and 2 g/d in divided doses. Pyridoxine should be given concurrently to prevent symptoms of deficiency. There are some patients who are unable to tolerate penicillamine even with the concurrent use of corticosteroids. Oral zinc therapy may be effective in these patients.[86] Administration of 25 mg of elemental zinc as zinc acetate every 4 hours during the day plus a 50-mg dose at bedtime, combined with no food intake 1 hour before or after zinc ingestion, has been successful in inducing a negative or at least a neutral copper balance in a limited number of patients.[86]

PORPHYRIA

The porphyrias are a group of disorders characterized by abnormalities of porphyrin metabolism that lead to neurological or cutaneous manifestations or both. Three forms of hepatic porphyria produce neurological symptoms: acute intermittent porphyria, hereditary coproporphyria, and variegate porphyria. The latter two forms have cutaneous as well as neurological manifestations.

The porphyrias are the clinical expression of one of many possible abnormalities in the metabolic pathway that converts glycine and succinyl-CoA to heme. The pathway requires pyridoxal phosphate. The critical enzyme is δ-aminolevulinic acid (δ-ALA) synthetase, a mitochondrial enzyme that is rate-limiting for heme synthesis in the liver. The pathway is controlled by the effects of heme on δ-ALA synthetase.

Acute intermittent porphyria is the most common and important of these disorders to the neurologist. It results from an inherited partial deficiency of porphobilinogen deaminase and is diagnosed by the excretion of excess δ-ALA and porphobilinogen in the urine. Hereditary coproporphyria occurs because of a deficiency of coproporphyrinogen oxidase; there is excessive excretion of δ-ALA, porphobilinogen, uroporphyrin, and coproporphyrin in the urine and coproporphyrin in the feces. Variegate porphyria is due to a partial deficiency of protoporphyrin oxidase and is characterized by excess excretion of δ-ALA, porphobilinogen, uroporphyrin, and coproporphyrin in the urine and excess coproporphyrin and protoporphyrin in the feces and plasma.

Clinically, all of these disorders have similar neurological presentations. Abdominal pain is the most common complaint and probably results from an underlying autonomic neuropathy and dilatation of the bowel. Other evidence of autonomic dysfunction may be encountered, including tachycardia. Peripheral neuropathy is common and may develop acutely, causing confusion with the Guillain-Barré syndrome. The neuropathy may become severe enough to require respiratory support. Nonspecific symptoms such as mood swings and back or extremity pain may have been present long before an acute attack. CNS manifestations are also common and include behavioral abnormalities, seizures, and other signs that are probably secondary to focal demyelination, such as aphasia, hemiparesis, and visual field abnormalities.

Treatment is mainly symptomatic. Treatment of an acute attack should include the administration of a high-carbohydrate diet, prevention and treatment of water and electrolyte disorders that may result from inappropriate antidiuretic hormone production, ventilatory support if required, general supportive measures aimed at relief of pain, and suppression of symptoms of bowel distention and autonomic insufficiency.

Long-term management of the porphyrias consists of genetic counseling and the avoidance of drugs that precipitate acute attacks. The drugs to be avoided include all barbiturates, phenytoin (a problem when patients have epileptic seizures), meprobamate, griseofulvin, sulfonamides, and others.

WHIPPLE'S DISEASE

Whipple's disease is a multisystem illness of presumed infectious etiology. Clinically, it is characterized by malabsorption with steatorrhea, arthralgia and nondeforming arthritis, lymphadenopathy, and—in rare instances—neurological involvement. Although Whipple's disease is uncommon, its incidence may be increasing, and it should be suspected in patients with acquired immunodeficiency syndrome (AIDS) who exhibit findings characteristic of the disorder.

The diagnosis is usually made by jejunal biopsy, which reveals numerous macrophages laden with periodic acid-Schiff (PAS)-positive granules. Electron microscopic examination of involved tissue demonstrates bacilli within macrophages, but organisms have not been identified by culture.

Neurological involvement is rare, and asymptomatic involvement of the nervous system may be present.[87-89] Dementia is the most common neurological feature. Other neurological manifestations include visual impairment, papilledema, supranuclear ophthalmoplegia, seizures, myoclonus, cerebellar ataxia, and a depressed level of consciousness. Oculomasticatory myorhythmia may be a movement disorder that is unique to patients with Whipple's disease.[90] PAS-positive cells have been found in the CSF and the brain parenchyma at the time of biopsy or postmortem examination.[88] Even if the typical PAS-positive cells are not found in the CSF, the spinal fluid may be abnormal, with an increased protein concentration and lymphocytic pleocytosis; in other instances, however, it is completely normal. Computed tomography and presumably MRI of the brain may show focal abnormalities.

The treatment of Whipple's disease involves antimicrobial drugs. Penicillin G, tetracycline, or ampicillin may be used. Corticosteroids may benefit patients who are seriously ill. Improvement may be noted after 4 to 6 weeks of treatment. The total duration of therapy should be governed in part by the clinical response, but indefinite periods of treatment are usually required.

REFERENCES

1. Frerichs FT: A Clinical Treatise on Liver Disease 1858. Translated by C. Murcheson. William Wood, New York, 1879

2. Moruzzi G, Magoun HW: Brai stem reticular formation and activation of the EEG. Electroencephalogr Clin Neurophysiol 1:455, 1949

3. Mesulam MM, Geschwind N: Disordered mental states in the postoperative period. Urol Clin North Am 3:199, 1976

4. Lipowski ZJ: Organic brain syndromes: a reformulation. Compr Psychiatry 19:309, 1978

5. Tarter RE, Hegedus AM, Van Thiel DH, et al: Neurobehavioral correlates of cholestatic and hepatocellular disease: differentiation according to disease-specific characteristics and severity of the identified cerebral dysfunction. Int J Neurosci 32:901, 1987

6. Sherlock S: Pathogenesis and management of hepatic coma. Am J Med 24:805, 1958

7. Lockwood AH, McDonald JM, Reiman RE, et al: The dynamics of ammonia metabolism in man: effects of liver disease and hyperammonia. J Clin Invest 63:449, 1979

8. Bickford RG, Butt HR: Hepatic coma: the electroencephalographic pattern. J Clin Invest 34:790, 1955

9. Brenner RP: The electroencephalogram in altered states of consciousness. Neurol Clin 3:615, 1985

10. Schafer DF, Pappas SC, Brody LE: Visual evoked potentials in a rabbit model of hepatic encephalopathy: I. Sequential changes and comparisons with drug-induced coma. Gastroenterology 86:540, 1984

11. Pappas CS, Ferenci P, Schafer DF, Jones EA: Visual evoked potentials in a rabbit model of hepatic encephalopathy: II. Comparison of hyperammonemic encephalopathy, postictal coma, and coma induced by synergistic neurotoxins. Gastroenterology 86:546, 1984

12. Hammond EJ, Wilder BJ: Effect of gamma-vinyl GABA on human pattern evoked visual potentials. Neurology 35:1801, 1985

13. Kulisevsky J, Pujol J, Balanzo C, et al: Pallidal hyperintensity on magnetic resonance imaging in cirrhotic patients: clinical correlations. Hepatology 16:1382, 1992

14. Adams RD, Foley JS: The neurological disorder associated with liver disease. Res Publ Assoc Res Nerv Ment Dis 32:198, 1953

15. Cole M, Rutherford RB, Smith FO: Experimental ammonia encephalopathy in the primate. Arch Neurol 26:130, 1972

16. Norenberg MD: A light and electron microscopic study of experimental portal-systemic (ammonia) encephalopathy: progression and reversal of the disorder. Lab Invest 36:618, 1977

17. Posner JB, Plum F: The toxic effects of carbon dioxide and acetazolamide in hepatic encephalopathy. J Clin Invest 39:1246, 1960

18. James IM, Garassini M: Effect of lactulose on cerebral metabolism in patients with chronic portosystemic encephalopathy. Gut 12:702, 1971

19. Morgan MY, Jakobovits AW, James IM, Sherlock S: Successful use of bromocriptine in the treatment of chronic hepatic encephalopathy. Gastroenterology 78:663, 1980

20. Gjedde A, Lockwood AH, Duffy TE, Plum F: Cerebral blood flow and metabolism in chronically hyperammonemic rats: effect of an acute ammonia challenge. Ann Neurol 3:325, 1978

21. Walker C, Schenker S: Pathogenesis of hepatic encephalopathy with special reference to the role of ammonia. Am J Clin Nutr 23:619, 1970

22. Lockwood AH, Ginsberg MD, Rhoades HM, Gutierrez MT: Cerebral glucose metabolism after portacaval shunting in the rat: patterns of metabolism and implications for the pathogenesis of hepatic encephalopathy. J Clin Invest 78:86, 1986

23. Gabuzda G Jr, Phillips GB, Davidson CS: Reversible toxic manifestations in patients with cirrhosis of the liver given cation-exchange resins. N Engl J Med 246:124, 1952

24. Cooper AJL, Plum F: Biochemistry and physiology of brain ammonia. Physiol Rev 67:440, 1987

25. Lockwood AH: Hepatic Encephalopathy. Boston, Butterworth-Heinemann, 1992

26. Lockwood AH, Yap EWH, Wong W-H: Cerebral ammonia metabolism in patients with severe liver disease and minimal hepatic encephalopathy. J Cereb Blood Flow Metab 11:337, 1991

27. Webster LT Jr, Davidson CS: The effect of sodium glutamate on hepatic coma. J Clin Invest 35:191, 1956

28. McDermott WR Jr, Wareham J, Riddell AG: Treatment of hepatic coma with L-glutamic acid. N Engl J Med 253:1093, 1955

29. Hindfelt B, Plum F, Duffy TE: Effect of acute ammonia intoxication on cerebral metabolism in rats with portacaval shunts. J Clin Invest 59:386, 1977

30. Parker TH, Roberts RK, Vorhees CV, et al: The effect of acute and subacute ammonia intoxication on regional cerebral acetylcholine levels in rats. Biochem Med 18:235, 1977

31. Fischer JE, Baldessarini RJ: False neurotransmitters and hepatic failure. Lancet 2:75, 1971

32. Fischer JE, Yoshimura N, Aguirre A, et al: Plasma amino acids in patients with hepatic encephalopathy: effects of amino acid infusions. Am J Surg 127:40, 1974

33. Fischer JE, Rosen HM, Ebeid AM, et al: The effect of normalization of plasma amino acids on hepatic encephalopathy in man. Surgery 80:77, 1976

34. Michel H, Solere M, Granier P, et al: Treatment of cirrhotic hepatic encephalopathy with L-dopa: a controlled trial. Gastroenterology 79:207, 1980

35. Morgan MY, Jakobovits AW, James IM, Sherlock S: Successful use of bromocriptine in the treatment of

chronic hepatic encephalopathy. Gastroenterology 78: 663, 1980

36. Michel H, Pomier-Layrargues G, Aubin JP, et al: Treatment of hepatic encephalopathy by infusion of a modified amino acid solution: results of a controlled study in 47 cirrhotic patients. p. 301. In Capocassia L, Fischer JE, Rossi-Fanella F (eds): Hepatic Encephalopathy in Chronic Liver Failure. Plenum, New York, 1984

37. Eriksson LS, Person A, Wahren J: Branched chain amino acids in the treatment of chronic hepatic encephalopathy. Gut 23:801, 1983

38. Wahren J, Denis J, Desurmont P, et al: Is intravenous administration of branched chain amino acids effective in the treatment of hepatic encephalopathy? A multicenter study. Hepatology 3:475, 1983

39. Cerra FB, Cheung NK, Fischer JE, et al: Disease-specific amino acid infusion (FO80) in hepatic encephalopathy: a prospective, randomized, double-blind, controlled trial. J Parenter Enter Nutr 9:288, 1985

40. Zieve L, Olsen RL: Can hepatic coma be caused by a reduction of brain noradrenaline or dopamine? Gut 18: 688, 1977

41. Harmar AJ, Horn AS: Octopamine in mammalian brain: rapid post mortem increase and effects of drugs. J Neurochem 26:987, 1976

42. Enna SJ: Commentary: GABA receptor pharmacology: functional considerations. Biochem Pharmacol 30: 907, 1981

43. Knudsen GM, Poulsen HE, Paulson OB: Blood-brain barrier permeability in galactosamine-induced hepatic encephalopathy: no evidence for increased GABA-transport. J Hepatol 6:187, 1988

44. Lavoie J, Giguere JF, Pomier Layrargues GP, Butterworth RF: Amino acid changes in autopsied brain tissue from cirrhotic patients with hepatic encephalopathy. J Neurochem 49:692, 1987

45. Schechter PJ, Hanke NFJ, Groves J, et al: Biochemical and clinical effects of γ-vinyl GABA in patients with epilepsy. Neurology 34:182, 1984

46. Butterworth RF, Lavoie J, Giguere JF, Pomier Layrargues G: Affinities and densities of high-affinity ^{3}H-muscimol (GABA-A) binding sites and of central benzodiazepine receptors are unchanged in autopsied brain tissue from cirrhotic patients with hepatic encephalopathy. Hepatology 8:1084, 1988

47. van der Rijt CCD, Schalm SW, Mulstee J, Stijnen T: Flumazenil therapy for hepatic encephalopathy: a double-blind crossover study. Hepatology 10:590, 1989

48. Pomier Layrargues G, Giguere JF, Lavoie J, et al: Efficacy of RO 15-1788 in cirrhotic patients with hepatic coma: results of a randomized double-blind placebo-controlled crossover trial. Hepatology 16:122A, 1992

49. McClain CJ, Zieve L, Doizaki WM, et al: Blood meth-anethiol in alcoholic liver disease with and without hepatic encephalopathy. Gut 21:318, 1980

50. Chen S, Zieve L, Mahadevan V: Mercaptans and dimethyl sulfide in the breath of patients with cirrhosis of the liver. J Lab Clin Med 75:628, 1970

51. Zieve L, Doizaki WM: Brain and blood methanethiol and ammonia concentrations in experimental hepatic coma and coma due to injections of various combinations of these substances. Gastroenterology 79:1070, 1980

52. Zieve L, Doizaki WM, Zieve FJ: Synergism between mercaptans and ammonia or fatty acids in the production of coma: a possible role for mercaptans in the pathogenesis of hepatic coma. J Lab Clin Med 83:16, 1974

53. Mardini HA, Bartlett K, Record CO: Blood and brain concentrations of mercaptans in hepatic and methanethiol induced coma. Gut 25:284, 1984

54. Hird FGR, Weidemann MJ: Oxidative phosphorylation accompanying oxidation of short-chain fatty acids in rat liver mitochondria. Biochem J 98:378, 1966

55. Derr RF, Zieve L: Effect of fatty acids on the disposition of ammonia. J Pharmacol Exp Ther 197:675, 1976

56. Ansevin CF: Reye syndrome: serum-induced alterations in brain mitochondrial functions are blocked by fatty-acid-free albumin. Neurology 30:160, 1980

57. Muto YI: Clinical study on the relationship of short chain fatty acids and hepatic encephalopathy. Jpn J Gastroenterol 63:19, 1966

58. Roe CR, Millington DS, Maltby DA, Kinnebrew P: Recognition of medium-chain acyl-CoA dehydrogenase deficiency in asymptomatic siblings of children dying of sudden infant death or Reye-like syndromes. J Pediatr 108:13, 1986

59. Uribe M, Marquez MA, Ramos GG, et al: Treatment of chronic portal-systemic encephalopathy with vegetable and animal protein diets: a controlled crossover study. Dig Dis Sci 27:1109, 1982

60. Elkington SG, Floch MH, Conn HO: Lactulose in the treatment of chronic portal-systemic encephalopathy: a double-blind clinical trial. N Engl J Med 281:408, 1969

61. Conn HO, Leevy CM, Vlahcevic ZR, et al: Comparison of lactulose and neomycin in the treatment of chronic portal-systemic encephalopathy: a double blind controlled trial. Gastroenterology 72:573, 1977

62. Vince A, Killingley M, Wrong OM: Effects of lactulose on ammonia in a fecal incubation system. Gastroenterology 74:544, 1978

63. Weber FL, Banwell JG, Fresard KM, Cummings JH: Nitrogen in fecal bacterial, fiber, and soluble fractions of patients with cirrhosis; effects of lactulose and lactulose plus neomycin. J Lab Clin Med 110:259, 1987

64. Heredia D, Caballeria J, Arroyo V, et al: Lactitol versus

lactulose in the treatment of acute portal systemic encephalopathy (PSE). J Hepatol 4:293, 1987

65. Morgan MY, Hawley KE, Stambick D: Lactitol versus lactulose in the treatment of chronic hepatic encephalopathy. J Hepatol 4:236, 1987

66. Levy DE, Bates D, Caronna JJ, et al: Prognosis in nontraumatic coma. Ann Intern Med 94:293, 1981

67. Orlandi F, Freddara U, Candelaresi MT, et al: Comparison between neomycin and lactulose in 173 patients with hepatic encephalopathy. Dig Dis Sci 26:498, 1981

68. Victor M, Adams RD, Cole M: The acquired (non-Wilsonian) type of chronic hepatocerebral degeneration. Medicine (Baltimore) 44:345, 1965

69. Pant SS, Rebeiz JJ, Richardson EP Jr: Spastic paraparesis following portacaval shunts. Neurology 18:135, 1968

70. Bechar M, Freud M, Kott E, et al: Hepatic cirrhosis with post-shunt myelopathy. J Neurol Sci 11:101, 1970

71. Kleinschmidt-DeMasters BK, Norenberg MD: Rapid correction of hyponatremia causes demyelination: relation to central pontine myelinolysis. Science 216:1068, 1981

72. Sterns RH, Riggs JE, Schochet SS Jr: Osmotic demyelination syndrome following correction of hyponatremia. N Engl J Med 314:1535, 1986

73. Reye RDK, Morgan G, Baral J: Encephalopathy and fatty degeneration of the viscera: a disease entity in childhood. Lancet 2:749, 1963

74. Batshaw M, Brusilow S, Walter M: Treatment of carbamylphosphate synthetase deficiency with keto-analogues of essential amino acids. N Engl J Med 292:1985, 1975

75. Ballard RA, Vinocur B, Reynolds JW, et al: Transient hyperammonemia of the preterm infant. N Engl J Med 299:920, 1978

76. Goldberg RN, Cabal LA, Sinatra FR, et al: Hyperammonemia associated with perinatal asphyxia. Pediatrics 64:336, 1979

77. Drayna CJ, Titcomb CP, Varma RR, Soergel KH: Hyperammonemic encephalopathy caused by infection in a neurogenic bladder. N Engl J Med 304:766, 1981

78. Makela A-L, Lang H, Korpela P: Toxic encephalopathy with hyperammonaemia during high-dose salicylate therapy. Acta Neurol Scand 61:146, 1980

79. Estrada RV, Moreno J, Martinez E, et al: Pancreatic encephalopathy. Acta Neurol Scand 59:135, 1979

80. Sjaastad O, Gjessing L, Ritland S, et al: Chronic relapsing pancreatitis, encephalopathy with disturbance of consciousness, and CSF amino acid aberration. J Neurol 220:83, 1979

81. Rothermich NO, von Hamm E: Pancreatic encephalopathy. J Clin Endocrinol 1:872, 1941

82. Sharf B, Bental E: Pancreatic encephalopathy. J Neurol Neurosurg Psychiatry 34:357, 1971

83. Balart LA, Ferrante WA: Pathophysiology of acute and chronic pancreatitis. Arch Intern Med 142:113, 1982

84. Sternlieb I: Diagnosis of Wilson's disease. Gastroenterology 74:787, 1978

85. Farrer LA, Bowcock AM, Helbert JM et al: Predictive testing for Wilson's disease using tightly linked and flanking DNA markers. Neurology 41:992, 1991

86. Brewer GJ, Hill GM, Prasad AS, et al: Oral zinc therapy for Wilson's disease. Ann Intern Med 99:314, 1983

87. Schochet SS, Lampert PW: Granulomatous encephalitis in Whipple's disease: electron microscopic observations. Acta Neuropathol (Berl) 13:1, 1969

88. Halperin JJ, Landis DMD, Kleinman GM: Whipple disease of the nervous system. Neurology 32:612, 1982

89. Stoupel N, Monseu G, Pardoe A, et al: Encephalitis with myoclonus in Whipple's disease. J Neurol Neurosurg Psychiatry 32:338, 1969

90. Schwartz MA, Selhorst JB, Ochs AL, et al: Oculomasticatory myorhythmia: a unique movement disorder occurring in Whipple's disease. Ann Neurol 20:677, 1986

14

Disturbances of Gastrointestinal Motility and the Nervous System

Michael Camilleri

The nervous system modulates normal gut function through the extrinsic neural supply and the enteric nervous system of the gastrointestinal tract. Disorders of the nervous system affecting gastrointestinal tract function are manifested primarily as abnormalities in motor rather than absorptive or secretory functions or other digestive processes. This chapter will review the normal neural-gut interactions, common clinical manifestations of gut dysmotility encountered in neurological disorders, and gastrointestinal functions as responses to assess extrinsic autonomic control of viscera. Finally, the main features in the diagnosis and treatment of neurological diseases affecting the gut will be discussed.

INTERACTIONS BETWEEN THE EXTRINSIC NERVOUS SYSTEM AND THE GUT

Normal motility and transit through the gastrointestinal tract result from an intricately balanced series of control mechanisms (Fig. 14-1): the electrical and contractile properties of the smooth muscle cell; control by the intrinsic nervous system through chemical transmitters such as acetylcholine, biogenic amines, gastrointestinal neuropeptides, and nitric oxide; and regulatory extrinsic pathways (sympathetic and parasympathetic nervous systems). The neuropeptides may act as circulating hormones or at the site of their release (paracrine).

The electrical properties of gut smooth muscle result from transmembrane fluxes of ions; as in other excitable tissues, these fluxes alter the membrane potential and result in muscle contraction. In some parts of the digestive tract, such as stomach and small bowel, a contraction occurs once a threshold potential is exceeded by a spike potential. In other regions (e.g., internal anal sphincter), no such spike occurs, but contractions are nevertheless observed and associated with altered basal electrical rhythm. Infiltrative or degenerative processes that affect the excitability of the smooth muscle cells of the gut are typically manifestations of myopathic disorders and prevent normal contractions, resulting in gastrointestinal dysmotility.

In the mammalian digestive tract, the intrinsic (or enteric) nervous system contains about 100 million neurons, approximately the number present in the spinal cord. This integrative system is organized in ganglionated plexuses (Fig. 14-2), and is separate

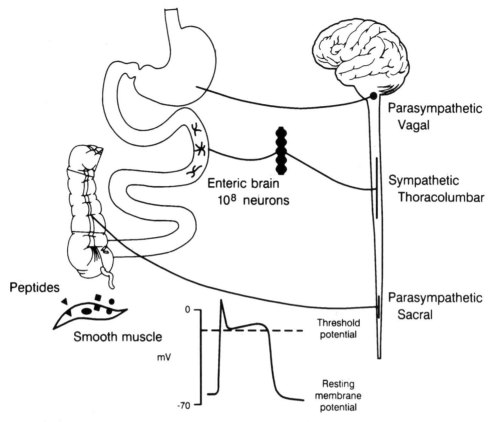

Fig. 14-1 Control of gut motility: interactions between extrinsic neural pathways and the intrinsic nervous system ("enteric brain") modulate contractions of gastrointestinal smooth muscle. Interactions between transmitters (e.g., peptides and amines) and receptors alter muscle membrane potentials by stimulating bidirectional ion fluxes. In turn, membrane characteristics dictate whether or not the muscle cell contracts. (From Camilleri M, Phillips SF: Disorders of small intestinal motility. Gastroenterol Clin North Am 18:405, 1989, by permission of Mayo Foundation.)

from the sympathetic and parasympathetic portions of the autonomic nervous system. It has several components: sensory mechanoreceptors and chemoreceptors, interneurons that process sensory input and control effector (motor and sensory) units, and effector motor neurons involved in motor function of the gut. Preprogrammed neural circuits serve to integrate motor function within and between different regions and thereby control the coordinated functions of the entire gastrointestinal tract, such as the peristaltic reflex and probably the interdigestive migrating motor complex (Fig. 14-3). The synaptic pathways in the gut wall are capable of autonomous adjustment in response to sensory input. They can also be modulated by the extrinsic nervous system so that excita-

tion results from the activity of vagal preganglionic fibers, and inhibition from sympathetic activity.

The vagus is composed of preganglionic cholinergic fibers that synapse with preprogrammed circuits in the ganglionated enteric plexuses. These enteric neurons include myenteric cholinergic neurons that, in turn, excite smooth muscle cells to produce contraction, or surface epithelial cells to absorb or secrete fluids and electrolytes. Since there is a great disparity between the limited number of extrinsic nerve fibers and the millions of enteric plexus neurons, it is currently believed that motor or secretory programmed circuits are controlled by command vagal preganglionic or sympathetic postganglionic fibers. Thus, there are approximately 40,000 preganglionic vagal

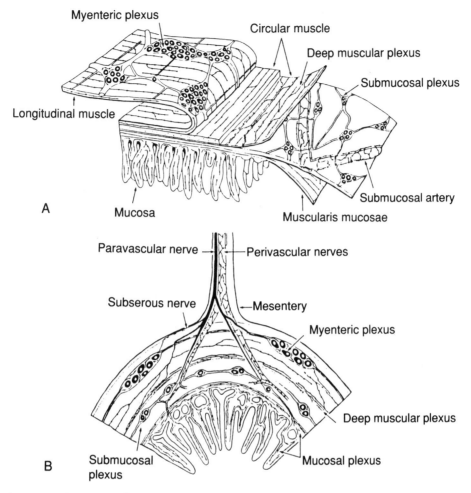

Fig. 14-2 The enteric plexuses in whole mounts of intestine **(A)** and in transverse section **(B).** (From Furness JB, Bornstein JC, Smith TK: The normal structure of gastrointestinal innervation. J Gastroenterol Hepatol 1:1, 1990, with permission.)

fibers (many of which are afferent, not efferent) at the level of the diaphragm; in contrast, 100 million neurons populate the enteric nervous system. The sympathetic supply inactivates neural circuits that generate motor activity while allowing intrinsic inhibitory innervation by the enteric nerves. Extrinsic vagal fibers also synapse with nonadrenergic inhibitory intramural neurons in the gut, which produce transmitters such as nitric oxide, vasoactive intestinal peptide, and somatostatin. Loss of the sympathetic inhibitory supply ("the brake") results in excessive or uncoordinated phasic pressure activity in the gut.

The extrinsic innervation of the gut consists of the parasympathetic vagal and sacral (S2, S3, and S4)

nerves and the sympathetic outflow from the intermediolateral column of the spinal cord between the fifth thoracic and upper lumbar levels. The sympathetic nerves synapse in the prevertebral celiac, superior mesenteric, and inferior mesenteric ganglia; sympathetic fibers follow the respective arterial trunks.

Extrinsic nerves are intimately involved in the control of the striated muscle portions of the esophagus and the external anal sphincter. Although the smooth muscle portion of the gut can function fairly normally without the extrinsic nerves, the latter modulate the intrinsic neural circuits, integrate activity in widely separated regions of the gastrointestinal tract, and appear to influence greater control in certain regions

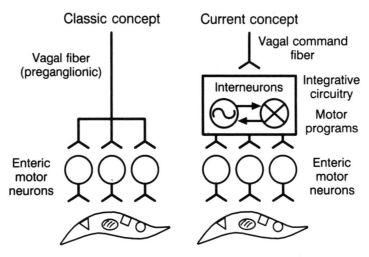

Fig. 14-3 Classic and current concepts of interaction between extrinsic and enteric plexuses. According to the classic concept, preganglionic cholinergic fibers synapse with a small number of enteric neurons; according to the current concept, vagal command fibers synapse with preprogrammed circuits with "hard-wired" functions. (Modified from Wood JD, Wingate DL: Gastrointestinal Neurophysiology, Unit 20. In: The UTP Slide Lecture Series. Milner Fenwick, Timonium, MD, 1987, with permission.)

(e.g., the stomach and distal portion of the colon) than in others (such as the small bowel).

COMMON GASTROINTESTINAL SYMPTOMS IN NEUROLOGICAL DISORDERS

Dysphagia

Dysphagia is the sensation of difficult swallowing. Neurological disorders typically result in oropharyngeal dysfunction or transfer dysphagia, in which there is an inability to propel the food bolus from the mouth to the esophagus or initiate the swallow.[1] This is encountered in diseases of the pharyngeal skeletal muscles such as occurs with lower motor neuron (e.g., bulbar polio) or muscle diseases. Dysphagia may also result from esophageal smooth muscle disorders, typically in progressive systemic sclerosis. Peristalsis is abnormal, with incoordination during early stages or reduced amplitude of contractions during later stages of the disease. There is also evidence that idiopathic achalasia or cardiospasm is associated with abnormal vagal nuclei or efferent fibers. It re-

sults in failure of the lower esophageal sphincter to relax fully on deglutition; this functional obstruction sets up a common cavity effect within the esophagus, resulting in simultaneous esophageal contractions.

Dysphagia that is restricted to solids suggests that a mechanical cause or narrowed lumen fails to allow the bolus to pass through the esophagus. Dysphagia restricted primarily to liquids is suggestive of oropharyngeal disease or achalasia; neuromuscular dysphagia typically results in dysphagia to both liquids and solids.

Physical examination shows evidence of the coexisting neurological disease, such as abnormal palatal or pharyngeal movements or a brisk jaw jerk, suggesting pseudobulbar palsy. Barium videofluoroscopy is an essential part of the evaluation; pharyngoesophageal motility studies, preferably using solid-state pressure transducers, complement the diagnosis. Re-education of the swallowing process is feasible in many patients, often in a program that incorporates speech therapy. Nutritional support and prevention of bronchial aspiration are predominant considerations in planning therapy for those with more severe dysphagia not responding to these conservative measures.

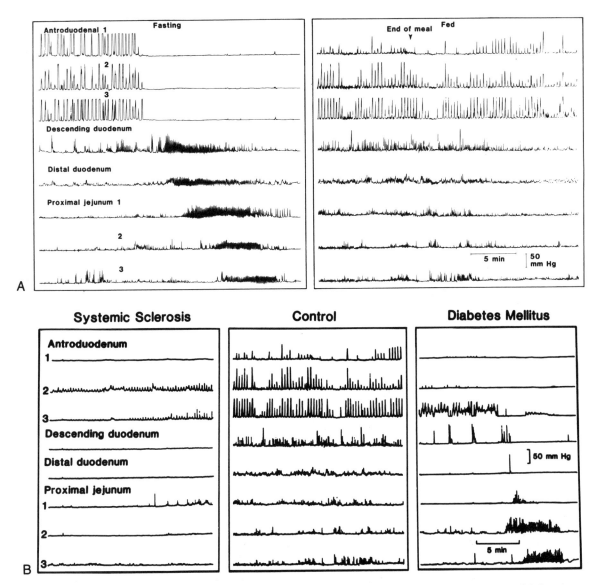

Fig. 14-4 (A) Tracing showing normal upper gastrointestinal motility in the fasting and fed states. The fasting tracing shows phase III of the interdigestive migrating motor complex. **(B)** Manometric tracings showing the myopathic pattern of intestinal pseudo-obstruction due to systemic sclerosis (*left panel*). Note the low amplitude of phasic pressure activity compared to control (*middle panel*). A manometric example of neuropathic intestinal pseudo-obstruction in diabetes mellitus. Note the absence of antral contractions and persistence of cyclical fasting-type motility in the postprandial period (*right panel*). (**A** from Malagelada J-R, Camilleri M, Stanghellini V: Manometric Diagnosis of Gastrointestinal Motility Disorders. Thieme, New York, 1986, by permission of Mayo Foundation. **B** from Camilleri M: Medical treatment of chronic intestinal pseudo-obstruction. Pract Gastroenterol 15:10, 1991, with permission.)

Gastroparesis

Gastric motor dysfunction resulting in delayed gastric emptying is a common gastrointestinal manifestation of autonomic neuropathies such as that associated with diabetes mellitus.[2,3] Symptoms range from vague postprandial abdominal discomfort to recurrent postprandial emesis, resulting in weight loss and malnutrition. Iatrogenic gastroparesis is induced by surgical vagotomy and by numerous medications, most commonly narcotic analgesics and tricyclic antidepressants. There may be a succussion splash on physical examination. It is essential to exclude gastric outlet obstruction by a barium study or gastroscopy. Scintigraphic gastric emptying tests confirm the impaired emptying of solids from the stomach; they may be extended over time to assess small bowel transit too.[4] Gastric stasis may result from abnormal motility of the stomach or small bowel,[5] and studies of pressure profiles by manometry or solid-state pressure transducers placed in the distal stomach and small bowel can help to identify abnormality of motor function (Fig. 14-4A), differentiate neuropathic from myopathic processes (Fig. 14-4B),[6] and exclude mechanical obstruction that may have been missed on previous radiographic studies of the small bowel.[7]

Prokinetic agents and use of a more easily digestible diet (low in fat and fiber) may be beneficial in the treatment of gastroparesis. Rarely, a feeding gastrostomy with a percutaneously placed tube is required. In patients with previous gastric surgery, a total gastrectomy with esophago-Roux-Y-jejunostomy may be necessary.

Chronic Intestinal Pseudo-obstruction

Chronic intestinal pseudo-obstruction is a syndrome characterized by nausea, vomiting, early satiety, abdominal discomfort, weight loss, and altered bowel movements suggestive of intestinal obstruction in the absence of a mechanical cause. These symptoms are the consequence of abnormal intestinal motility rather than mechanical obstruction. The syndrome may result from a number of neurological diseases extrinsic to the gut (e.g., disorders at any level of the neural axis), from dysfunction of neurons in the myenteric plexus,[2] or from degeneration of gut smooth muscle in familial or sporadic hollow visceral

Table 14-1 Causes of Chronic Intestinal Pseudo-Obstruction

	Myopathic	Neuropathic
Infiltrative	Progressive systemic sclerosis (PSS)	Early PSS
	Amyloidosis	Amyloidosis
Familial	Familial visceral myopathies (autosomal dominant or recessive)	Familial visceral neuropathies
General neurological diseases	Myotonic and other dystrophies	Diabetes mellitus Porphyria Heavy metal poisoning Brainstem tumor Parkinson's disease Multiple sclerosis Spinal cord transection
Infectious		Chagas' disease Cytomegalovirus
Drug-induced		Tricyclic antidepressants Narcotic bowel syndrome
Neoplastic		Paraneoplastic (bronchial small cell carcinoma or carcinoid)
Idiopathic	Hollow visceral myopathy	Chronic intestinal pseudo-obstruction (possibly myenteric plexopathy)

myopathy (Table 14-1). The pathophysiology of these diseases can be broadly subdivided into myopathic (e.g., infiltrative amyloidosis, hollow visceral myopathy, or muscular dystrophies) and neuropathic processes (Table 14-1).

The patient's accompanying clinical features may suggest an underlying disease process: these features include postural dizziness, difficulties in visual accommodation in bright lights, and sweating abnormalities suggestive of an autonomic neuropathy; alternatively, the occurrence of urinary symptoms such as recurrent urinary infections and problems with bladder voiding suggest genitourinary involvement by a generalized visceral neuromyopathic disorder, and accompanying peripheral sensory or motor symptoms suggest an associated peripheral neuropathy. Patients should be questioned about the use of phenothiazines, antihypertensive agents such as clonidine, tricyclic antidepressants that have anticholinergic effects, and calcium channel blockers. The physical examination should pay particular attention to evaluation of pupillary reflexes to light and accommodation, measurement of the blood pressure and pulse with the patient lying and standing, and a search for abdominal distention or a succussion splash.

Plain radiographs and barium studies are often nonspecific; dilatation of the small intestine is found in about 60 percent of patients with chronic idiopathic intestinal pseudo-obstruction,[8] but it is probably more frequent in myopathic disorders. Contrast studies of the small bowel and important in ruling out mechanical obstruction but rarely lead to an etiologic diagnosis. Motility studies (Fig. 14-4) help to differentiate myopathic and neuropathic processes and may also suggest the presence of mechanical obstruction, even in the presence of an underlying neuromuscular disorder.[7] When the motility tracing is suggestive of a neuropathic process, assessment of autonomic function and radiological and serological tests should be performed to identify the cause of the autonomic neuropathy or cerebrospinal disease (see below).

The goals of treatment of chronic intestinal pseudo-obstruction include the restoration of hydration and nutrition, stimulation of normal intestinal propulsion, and suppression of bacterial overgrowth. Specific medications are discussed below.

Constipation

Constipation is a common complaint and may be perceived by the patient as infrequent, incomplete evacuation or excessively hard stools. Most causes of constipation are easily identifiable and partially correctable, such as lack of exercise (which may be important in inactive patients with neurological disorders such as parkinsonism or paraplegia). Other factors contributing to constipation are inadequate intake of fiber in the diet, lack of rectal sensation, and neglect of the urge to defecate. After excluding or correcting these causes, constipation may be due to obstructing lesions that are identified by barium ra-

diographic studies or colonoscopy, altered colonic motility, or disordered defecation.[9]

Continence of stools requires maintenance of the acute angle between the rectum and anal canal, and normal function of the anal sphincters. The puborectalis muscle serves to maintain the acute anorectal angle; during defecation (Fig. 14-5), relaxation of the pelvic floor, including the puborectalis, results in straightening of the rectoanal angle, with descent of the pelvic floor and facilitation of the passage of stool. As the stool volume in the sigmoid colon increases, contractions are stimulated and move stool into the rectum, thereby inducing inhibition of the internal anal sphincter. This defecatory reflex function can be tested by inflating a balloon in the rectum and measuring the resting anal sphincter tone, which should be reduced on inflation of the rectal balloon, the so-called rectoanal inhibitory reflex. Increases in the intra-abdominal and intrarectal pressures induced by straining cause reflex relaxation of the external and internal anal sphincters and the puborectalis muscles. This causes the pelvic floor to descend, and the fecal bolus is then expelled.[9]

Patients use the term *constipation* to describe a variety of disturbances: a careful history can contribute significantly to understanding the cause. For example, the need of enemas or finger evacuation to expel the stool from the lower rectum suggests a disturbance of the pelvic floor or anorectum. The coexistence of incontinence and lack of rectal sensation suggests a pudendal neuropathy and is common among patients with diabetic neuropathy. The presence of blood in the stool necessitates further tests to exclude colonic mucosal lesions, such as polyps, or perianal conditions, such as hemorrhoids.

Anatomical abnormalities such as tumors, megacolon, megarectum, volvulus, occult mucosal prolapse, and rectoceles can be effectively excluded by barium enema, including defecation proctography if clinically indicated. Exclusion of these disorders, which are amenable to surgical treatment, is essential in all patients, even if there is an underlying neurological disorder that could contribute to constipation.

Colonic transit studies using radiopaque markers[10] or radioscintigraphy[11] will detect abnormally prolonged transit; however, pelvic floor dysfunction may result in outlet obstruction and secondarily prolonged colonic transit. Hence, anorectal manometry, evaluation of rectal emptying (e.g., by testing the

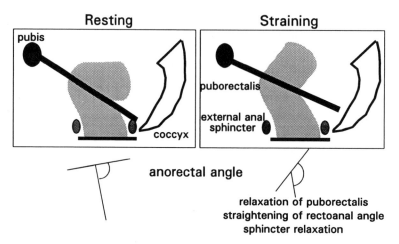

Fig. 14-5 Schema showing normal alterations of pelvic floor, rectoanal angle, and sphincters during defecation. (From Camilleri M: Four patients with intractable constipation. Gastrointest Dis Today 2:7, 1993, with permission.)

ability to expel a balloon), and rectal sensation, as well as measurements of the anorectal angle during defecation proctography in selected cases, are useful in assessing patients with disorders of defecation. These principles are reviewed elsewhere.[9,12] Rarely, sphincter electromyography (EMG) or estimation of pudendal nerve terminal motor latency may be needed to demonstrate sphincter or pelvic floor denervation. Recent studies have used ultrasonography to assess physical defects in the anal sphincters. These are typically identified in multiparous patients with incontinence.

Most constipated patients respond well to fiber, bulking agents, or stool softeners. Slow colonic transit occurs frequently in wheelchair- or bed-bound patients and may require the addition of stimulant cathartics or prokinetic medications such as cisapride. Patients with spinal cord injuries will usually respond to a combination of bulk laxatives and scheduled enemas daily or on alternate days. In patients with paraplegia, computer-assisted sacral anterior root stimulation can be used to evoke a coordinated sequence of sigmoid and rectal contractions and sphincter relaxation, thereby simulating the dynamic events occurring during defecation.[13] It has been shown to reduce the interval between defecations and the time taken to defecate. A dorsal rhizotomy must be performed to avoid general stimulation of autonomic responses. Surgery (e.g., colostomy or subtotal colectomy with ileorectostomy) is reserved for patients with intracta-

ble colonic inertia or local correction of abnormalities resulting from the chronic constipation, such as rectal prolapse, rectocele, or painful perianal conditions (e.g., anal fissure). In severe cases, patients with disorders of defecation have been treated with biofeedback with some success.[14]

Fecal Incontinence

Major incontinence with loss of formed stool is frequently due to progressive neurological damage to the pelvic nerves. This results in denervation of the pelvic floor musculature and the external and internal anal sphincters.[9] Stretching of the pudendal nerves with repetitive prolonged straining may complicate disorders of colonic transit and, hence, may be secondary to a primary disease process that causes delayed colonic transit. Incontinence occurring only at night suggests internal anal sphincter dysfunction (e.g., progressive systemic sclerosis); stress incontinence during coughing, sneezing, or laughing suggests loss of external sphincter control, typically from the pudendal nerve or S2, S3, and S4 root lesions.

In evaluating such patients, it is important first to exclude overflow incontinence due to fecal impaction. Similarly, overuse of laxatives or other medications, such as magnesium-containing antacids, may result in reversible incontinence. Among patients with weakness of rectal and anal musculature, there may be little that can be achieved with medical or biofeedback therapy. A colostomy may be more manageable. It is important to exclude mucosal prolapse in association with incontinence; surgical correction of the prolapse may at least temporarily improve continence by permitting better function of the external sphincter.[15]

Examination of the incontinent patient should include inspection of the anus with and without straining to detect rectal prolapse; a digital rectal examination to exclude impaction or mucosal disease; and proctoscopy and barium enema or colonoscopy to exclude mucosal lesions. If these fail to identify the cause of incontinence, further tests may be necessary: anorectal manometry, assessment of rectal sensation and the ability to expel a balloon from the rectum, and assessment of anorectal angle and defecating proctogram will assess the defecation process. EMG of the external anal sphincter and puborectalis muscle and pudendal nerve conduction studies (terminal motor latency) are seldom necessary.

Initial treatment of patients with denervation-induced incontinence includes care of the perianal skin and use of incontinence pads. Biofeedback training is rarely helpful. Recent data suggest that magnetoelectric stimulation may be used to assess the function of lumbosacral motor roots and hence determine which patients have sufficient residual innervation to be likely to respond to biofeedback training.[14]

EXTRINSIC NEUROLOGICAL DISORDERS CAUSING GUT DYSMOTILITY

It is possible to distinguish disorders that affect the gut muscle ("myopathic disorders"), those involving the myenteric plexus, and diseases of the extrinsic pathways that supply the gut. Some diseases affect both intrinsic and extrinsic neural control.[16] This review concentrates on diseases of extrinsic neural control and smooth muscle. Diseases affecting the enteric nervous system are reviewed elsewhere.[17]

Brain Diseases

CEREBROVASCULAR ACCIDENT

Dysphagia may result from cranial nerve involvement and may cause malnutrition or aspiration pneumonia. Videofluoroscopy of the pharynx and upper esophagus typically shows transfer dysphagia or tracheal aspiration. Colonic pseudo-obstruction occurs rarely.[18] Placement of a percutaneous endoscopic gastrostomy is usually the most effective method to provide nutrition without interfering with rehabilitation; feedings can be given in the form of boluses or by infusion at night. Not infrequently, patients eventually recover some degree of oropharyngeal coordination; the gastrostomy tube can be removed when oral intake is shown to be sufficient to maintain caloric requirements.

PARKINSONISM

Patients with Parkinson's disease or progressive supranuclear palsy may have oropharyngeal dysfunction with impaired swallowing.[19] Shy-Drager syndrome or multiple system atrophy is considered below. Patients may have mild to moderate malnutrition; moderate dysphagia may be diagnosed by videofluoroscopy. In the absence of severe malnutrition or significant aspiration, conservative treatment with attention to the consistency of food (thickened liquids) and ensuring adequate caloric content of meals will suffice. Feeding through a percutaneous gastrostomy is an appropriate alternative for severe dysphagia.

Constipation is common in patients with parkinsonism[19] and may be the result of slow colonic transit or of pelvic floor[20] or anal sphincter dysfunction.[21] Gastrointestinal hypomotility, generalized hypokinesia, associated autonomic dysfunction, and the effects of various anticholinergic and dopamine agonist medications may all play a role. The bioavailability of other medications can be altered considerably by the effects of parkinsonism on gut transit and delivery of medications to the small bowel for absorption.

HEAD INJURY

Immediately following moderate to severe head injury, most patients develop transient delays in gastric emptying. The underlying mechanism is unknown, although a correlation exists between the severity of injury, increased intracranial pressure, and severity of the gastric stasis. These patients are frequently intolerant of enteral feeding and require parenteral nutrition to meet their increased metabolic demands. In practice, enteral nutrition can often be reintroduced within 2 to 3 weeks as the gastric stasis resolves.[22]

AUTONOMIC EPILEPSY AND MIGRAINE

Autonomic epilepsy and migraine are infrequent causes of upper abdominal symptoms such as nausea and vomiting. Treatment is of the underlying neurological disorder.

AMYOTROPHIC LATERAL SCLEROSIS

Patients with amyotrophic lateral sclerosis (ALS) and progressive bulbar palsy have predominant weakness of the muscles supplied by the glossopharyngeal and vagus nerves.[23] Dysphagia is a frequent complaint, and patients may have respiratory difficulty while eating as a result of aspiration or respiratory muscle fatigue. Rarely, patients with vagal dysfunction will show features of a chronic intestinal pseudo-obstruction syndrome.[24]

Physical examination shows the cranial nerve palsies and muscle fasciculations. An exaggerated jaw jerk may be present in ALS. Videofluoroscopic barium swallow of liquids and solids evaluates swallowing, determines whether aspiration occurs, and guides decisions on the route to use for nutritional support (oral feeding or a percutaneous gastrostomy). Cervical esophagostomy or cricopharyngeal myotomy has been performed in selected cases for significant cricopharyngeal muscle dysfunction.

POSTPOLIO DYSPHAGIA

Patients with postpolio syndrome frequently have dysphagia and aspiration, especially if there was bulbar involvement during the initial attack. Videofluoroscopy is useful for screening and monitoring progression of disease. Attention to the position of the patient's head during swallowing and alteration of food consistency to a semisolid state can decrease the incidence of choking and aspiration.[25]

BRAINSTEM TUMORS

Brainstem lesions can present with isolated gastrointestinal motor dysfunction. In the absence of increased intracranial pressure, such symptoms are probably the result of a direct mass effect in the brainstem, with distortion of the vomiting center on the floor of the fourth ventricle. Motor dysfunction is typically evident on manometric or radionuclide studies of the stomach and small bowel.[26] Although vomiting is the most common symptom, colonic or anorectal dysfunction has also been described.[27] The presence of more widespread autonomic dysfunction, particularly if preganglionic sympathetic nerves are involved, necessitates a search for a structural lesion in the central nervous system.

Autonomic System Degenerations

PANDYSAUTONOMIAS OR SELECTIVE DYSAUTONOMIAS

Pandysautonomias are characterized by preganglionic or postganglionic lesions affecting both the sympathetic and parasympathetic nervous systems. Vomiting, paralytic ileus, constipation, or a chronic pseudo-obstruction syndrome have been reported in acute, subacute, or congenital pandysautonomia.[28] Motor disturbances have been substantiated in the esophagus, stomach, and small bowel. Selective cholinergic dysautonomia may also impair upper and lower gastrointestinal motor activity. This picture usually follows a viral infection such as infectious mononucleosis.[29]

IDIOPATHIC ORTHOSTATIC HYPOTENSION

Idiopathic orthostatic hypotension is sometimes associated with motor dysfunction of the gut, such as esophageal dysmotility, gastric stasis, alteration in bowel movements, and fecal incontinence.[30,31] Cardiovascular and sudomotor abnormalities usually precede gut involvement. The precise site of the lesion causing the gut dysmotility is unknown.

SHY-DRAGER SYNDROME

In the original description by Shy and Drager, constipation and fecal incontinence were included among the classic features of the disorder named after them.[32] Other reports have documented substantial reduction in fasting and postprandial antral and small bowel motility. Abnormal esophageal motility was demonstrated by videofluoroscopy and by the occurrence of frequent, simultaneous, low-amplitude peristaltic waves during esophageal manometry.[30]

Spinal Cord Lesions

SPINAL CORD INJURY

Ileus is a frequent finding soon after spinal cord injury, but it is rarely prolonged. In the chronic phase after injury, disorders of upper gastrointestinal motility are uncommon, whereas colonic and anorectal dysfunction are common. The latter probably result from interruption of supraspinal control of the sacral parasympathetic supply to the colon, pelvic floor, and anal sphincters.[33,34] There is a decrease in colonic compliance and an absence of postprandial colonic motor and myoelectric activity in patients with thoracic spinal cord injury.[35]

The loss of voluntary control of defecation may be the most significant disturbance in patients who rely on reflex rectal stimulation for stool evacuation. Loss of control of the external anal sphincter, with resulting fecal incontinence, is the most common gastrointestinal problem in patients with spinal cord injury.

The usual management for irregular bowel function is a combination of bulking agents and scheduled enemas. Computerized stimulation of the sacral anterior roots has been proposed as a method to restore normal function to the pelvic colon and anorectal sphincters[13]; however, relatively few patients have been treated by this means on a long-term basis.

MULTIPLE SCLEROSIS

Severe constipation frequently accompanies urinary bladder dysfunction in patients with advanced multiple sclerosis.[36] In one study, colonic transit of radiopaque markers was prolonged in 14 of 16 patients with multiple sclerosis and urinary bladder involvement; 10 patients also had evidence of fecal incontinence, and 5 had spontaneous rectal contractions. The studies performed to date have not been sufficiently detailed to assess the extent to which such symptoms relate to sympathetic and parasympathetic denervation. Pelvic colonic dysfunction is probably due to impaired function of the supraspinal or descending pathways that control the sacral parasympathetic outflow. Further studies are needed to address the mechanism of impaired gut transit in multiple sclerosis, which, as with spinal cord injury, results in motility disturbances more frequently in the lower than in the upper gut.[37]

Peripheral Neuropathy

ACUTE PERIPHERAL NEUROPATHY

Autonomic dysfunction associated with certain acute viral infections may result in nausea, vomiting, abdominal cramps, constipation, or a clinical picture of pseudo-obstruction. In the Guillain-Barré syndrome, visceral involvement may include gastric distention or adynamic ileus. Persistent gastrointestinal motor disturbances may also occur in association with herpes zoster, Epstein-Barr virus infection, or botulism B. The site of the neurological lesion is uncertain. Cytomegalovirus has been identified in myenteric plexus in some patients with chronic intestinal pseudo-obstruction.[38] Selective cholinergic dysautonomia (with associated gastrointestinal dysfunction) has been reported to develop within a week of the onset of infectious mononucleosis.[29] Diarrhea induced by human immunodeficiency virus (HIV) may be another manifestation of autonomic dysfunction (see below), but the data require confirmation.

CHRONIC PERIPHERAL NEUROPATHY

Chronic peripheral neuropathy is the most commonly encountered extrinsic neurological disorder that results in gastrointestinal motor dysfunction.

Diabetes Mellitus

Diabetic autonomic neuropathy of the gut has been studied extensively and has been reviewed elsewhere.[39] In patients with type I diabetes seen at university medical centers, gastrointestinal symptoms, particularly constipation, are very common.[40] However, a recent questionnaire-based Finnish study in a randomly selected population suggests that the occurrence and spectrum of gastrointestinal symptoms in middle-aged subjects with insulin- and non-insulin-dependent diabetes mellitus do not differ from those of the general population.[41] Gastric emptying of digestible or nondigestible solids is abnormal in patients with diabetes mellitus and gastrointestinal symptoms ("gastroparesis"). Studies in humans have demonstrated a paucity of distal antral contractions during fasting and postprandially; small bowel motility may also be abnormal.[5] These features are consistent with an "autovagotomy," a concept originally proposed in studies of gastric secretion.[42]

Constipation is a frequent, although often unreported, symptom in patients with diabetes. Colonic motor dysfunction is associated with constipation.[43] Streptozotocin-treated rats develop abnormal colonic compliance and selective deficiencies of certain neurotransmitters (e.g., calcitonin gene-related peptide) in the myenteric plexus. However, there are no mechanistic data to explain this frequent symptom in patients with diabetes. In contrast, diarrhea or fecal incontinence (or both) may result from several mechanisms (reviewed in detail elsewhere[44]): dysfunction of the anorectal sphincter or abnormal rectal sensation, osmotic diarrhea from bacterial overgrowth due to small bowel stasis, or rapid transit from uncoordinated small bowel motor activity. Rarely, an associated gluten-sensitive enteropathy or pancreatic exocrine insufficiency is present. These associated conditions should be sought, since they are potentially reversible.

Histopathological studies of the vagus nerve have revealed a reduction in the number of unmyelinated axons; surviving axons are usually of small caliber. In patients with diabetic diarrhea, there are giant sympathetic neurons and dendritic swelling of the postganglionic neurons in prevertebral and paravertebral sympathetic ganglia as well as reduced fiber density in the splanchnic nerves.[45,46]

Peripheral cholinergic agonists (such as metoclopramide, bethanechol, and cisapride) and α_2-adrenergic agonists (such as clonidine) have been used respectively to treat gastric stasis and diarrhea secondary to diabetic gut neuropathy.[47] Available therapeutic options have resulted in only transient relief. Erythromycin (administered intravenously) is useful during the acute phase, but few patients tolerate it beyond 2 weeks.[48] Pancreas transplantation is reported to restore normal gastric emptying in patients with diabetic gastroparesis.[49] Long-term results are not yet available, however, and we have certainly observed persistent gastric stasis in patients with an autonomic neuropathy that preceded the pancreas transplant.

Paraneoplastic Neuropathy

Autonomic neuropathy and gastrointestinal symptoms have been reported in association with small cell carcinoma of the lung or pulmonary carcinoid.[50] In the largest published series, all seven patients suffered constipation, six had gastroparesis, four had esophageal dysmotility suggestive of spasm or achalasia, and two had other evidence of autonomic neuropathy that affected bladder and blood pressure control.[50] Our group has recently detected a circulating IgG antibody directed against enteric neuronal nuclei,[51] suggesting that the enteric plexus is the major target of this paraneoplastic phenomenon. However, several patients have also had evidence of extrinsic visceral neuropathies.[50,52] suggesting a more extensive neuropathological process. The chest x-ray is frequently normal in these patients; a chest CT scan is therefore indicated when the syndrome is suspected, typically in middle-aged smokers with recent onset of nausea, vomiting, or feeding intolerance.

Amyloid Neuropathy

Amyloid neuropathy may lead to constipation,[53] diarrhea, and steatorrhea. Patients have uncoordinated nonpropagated contractions in the small bowel.[29] These features are similar to the intestinal myoelectric disturbances observed in animals subjected to ganglionectomy.[54] Familial amyloidosis may also affect the gut.

Manometric studies and monitoring of the acute effects of cholinomimetic agents can distinguish between neuropathic (uncoordinated but normal-amplitude pressure activity) and myopathic (low-amplitude pressure activity) types of amyloid gastroenteropathy.[53] These strategies may identify patients (i.e., those with the neuropathic variant) who are more likely to respond to prokinetic agents.

Chronic Sensory and Autonomic Neuropathy of Unknown Cause

This is a rare, nonfamilial form of slowly progressive neuropathy that affects a number of autonomic functions.[55] Patients may exhibit only a chronic autonomic disturbance (e.g., abnormal sudomotor, vasomotor, or gastrointestinal function) for many years before peripheral sensory symptoms develop. Autonomic dysfunction is probably responsible for functional gastrointestinal motor disorders when these develop prior to the onset of more obvious features of dysautonomia. This may account for a subset of patients who present with features suggesting the irritable bowel syndrome.[16]

Other investigators have reported familial cases of intestinal pseudo-obstruction with degeneration of the myenteric plexus and evidence of sensory or motor neuropathies affecting peripheral or cranial nerves.[17]

Porphyria

Acute intermittent porphyria and hereditary coproporphyria frequently present with abdominal pain, nausea, vomiting, and constipation.[56,57] Porphyric polyneuropathy may lead to dilatation and impaired motor function in any part of the intestinal tract, presumably because of autonomic dysfunction. Effects of porphyria on the enteric nervous system have not been described.

Human Immunodeficiency Virus Infection

It is well known that neurological disease may manifest at any phase of HIV infection. Chronic diarrhea may result from increased extrinsic parasympathetic activity to the gut[58] or damage to adrenergic fibers within the enteric plexuses.[59] Further studies are needed to characterize these abnormalities; it is, of course, important to exclude gut infections or infestations in patients with HIV seropositivity and diarrhea.

GENERAL MUSCULAR DISEASES CAUSING GUT DYSMOTILITY

At an advanced stage, progressive systemic sclerosis and amyloidosis result in an infiltrative replacement of smooth muscle cells in the digestive tract. Rarely, Duchenne dystrophy[60] and polymyositis or dermatomyositis[61-63] have been associated with gastroparesis. There are a number of case or family reports of chronic intestinal pseudo-obstruction, sometimes in association with an external ophthalmoplegia, secondary to a mitochondrial myopathy.[64-66] Patients with myotonic dystrophy may have megacolon[67]; anal sphincter dysfunction also occurs and is consistent with an expression of myopa-

thy, muscular atrophy, and neural abnormalities.[68] The myopathic nature of these disorders is reflected by the low-amplitude contractions at affected levels of the gut.[69-71] Myopathic disorders may be complicated by bacterial overgrowth; pneumatosis cystoides intestinalis and spontaneous pneumoperitoneum sometimes occur in progressive systemic sclerosis. However, it is worth noting that the latter disorder affects the gut from the distal two-thirds of the esophagus to the anorectum; thus, it may present with dysphagia (which may also be due to reflux esophagitis and stricture), gastric stasis, intestinal pseudo-obstruction, steatorrhea due to bacterial overgrowth, constipation, incontinence (particularly at night, due to involvement of the internal anal sphincter), and rectal prolapse.[15]

Treatment includes restoration of nutrition (which may necessitate total parenteral nutrition), suppression of bacterial overgrowth, and treatment of complications such as gastroesophageal reflux (with an H_2-receptor antagonist or proton pump inhibitor) or esophageal strictures (by endoscopic dilatation). Colonic dilatation and intractable constipation may necessitate subtotal colectomy with ileorectostomy. Prokinetics are rarely effective[72] but should at least be tried. There is preliminary evidence to suggest that the somatostatin analog octreotide improves symptoms in the short term and may suppress bacterial overgrowth.[73]

IDENTIFICATION OF EXTRINSIC NEUROLOGICAL DISEASE IN PATIENTS WITH GASTROINTESTINAL SYMPTOMS SUGGESTIVE OF A MOTILITY DISORDER

Patients with lesions at virtually any level of the nervous system may have symptoms of gastrointestinal motor dysfunction. Therefore, a strategy is necessary in the diagnostic evaluation of disordered gastrointestinal function (Fig. 14-6). It is here that there is a convergence of the paths of the neurologist and gastroenterologist. Patients should undergo further testing, particularly if they have clinical features suggestive of autonomic or peripheral nerve dysfunction or a known underlying neuromuscular disorder.

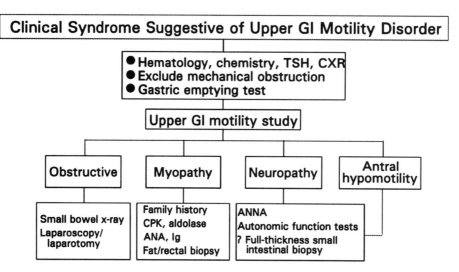

Fig. 14-6 Algorithm for the investigation of patients with suspected gastrointestinal (GI) dysmotility. TSH, thyroid-stimulating hormone; CXR, chest radiograph; CPK, creatine kinase; ANA, antinuclear antibodies; Ig, immunoglobulin; ANNA, antineuronal enteric antibodies. (From Camilleri M: Study of human gastroduodenojejunal motility: applied physiology in clinical practice. Dig Dis Sci 38:785, 1993, with permission.)

It is essential to record the use of all medications that influence gut motility.

Gastrointestinal motility and transit measurements help the clinician to confirm the disturbance in the motor function of the gut and to distinguish between neuropathic and myopathic disorders. Tests of autonomic function (discussed in Ch. 8) are useful for identifying the extent of involvement and localizing the anatomical level of the disturbance in extrinsic neural control. There is generally good agreement between abnormalities of abdominal vagal function, including the plasma pancreatic polypeptide response

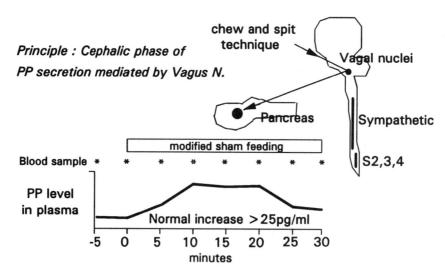

Fig. 14-7 Assessment of abdominal vagal function by the plasma pancreatic polypeptide (PP) response to modified sham feeding by chewing and spitting a bacon-and-cheese toasted sandwich.

to modified sham feeding (Fig. 14-7) and cardiovagal dysfunction in patients with diabetes.[74] When a defect of the sympathetic nervous system has been identified by conventional tests, the effect of intravenous administration of edrophonium on plasma norepinephrine levels may provide further assessment of the integrity of postganglionic sympathetic nerves, many of which supply the digestive tract.[75,76]

Once visceral autonomic neuropathy is identified, further tests are needed to identify any occult causes of the neuropathy; examples include lung tumors (computed tomography of the chest), porphyria (uroporphyrinogen-1-synthase and coproporphyrinogen oxidase in erythrocytes), or amyloidosis (special protein studies in blood and urine, fat or rectal biopsy). Imaging of the brain and spinal cord is needed when autonomic tests indicate a central lesion, as when a thermoregulatory sweat test is abnormal but tests of postganglionic nerves (e.g., the quantitative sudomotor axon reflex test, or plasma norepinephrine response to edrophonium) are normal.[52]

MANAGEMENT

The principles of management of any gastrointestinal motility disorder are restoration of hydration and nutrition by the oral, enteral, or parenteral route; suppression of bacterial overgrowth (e.g., with oral tetracycline); use of prokinetic agents or stimulant laxatives; and resection of localized disease.

The prokinetic effects of metoclopramide (a peripheral cholinergic agonist and dopamine D2 antagonist) are limited to the esophagus and stomach. Its clinical efficacy is restricted by the relatively high frequency of side effects, and especially of changes in affect, extrapyramidal disorders, and hyperprolactinemia (which may result in altered menstrual function and galactorrhea).

Bethanechol (10 to 25 mg, 4 times daily) is a cholinergic agonist that is not specific for the gastrointestinal tract. It is helpful only in mild cases of gastroparesis and is now seldom used; it is sometimes prescribed in combination with metoclopramide.

A substituted benzamide, cisapride, is a general prokinetic with proven short-term efficacy in stimulating transit and motor function at all levels of the gastrointestinal tract. It is a serotonin type 4 receptor agonist and cholinergic agonist. It is generally a very safe medication that is at least as efficacious as metoclopramide. Cisapride also stimulates colonic transit in some paraplegic patients and is a useful adjunct to stool softening and increasing the fiber content of the diet in those patients. The response of neuropathic chronic intestinal pseudo-obstruction to prokinetic agents may vary depending on whether the pathophysiological process is neuropathic or myopathic and whether the neuropathy stems from the enteric plexus or an extrinsic neuropathy.[77] Our recent data suggest that extrinsic vagal and general sympathetic dysfunction are predictors of poor response to cisapride.[78]

Erythromycin, a macrolide antibiotic, stimulates smooth muscle motilin receptors in the gastrointestinal tract. It has a role in relieving acute gastric stasis but is of little benefit beyond 2 weeks of treatment.[48]

Octreotide's efficacy has been tested only in patients with systemic sclerosis.[63] Preliminary data suggest that it does not usually induce normally propagated activity in the small bowel, but it may help clear residue by virtue of the intensity of contractions and increased duration of the migrating complex that it induces in the small bowel.[79]

In patients with a neurological cause of constipation, it is important to ensure adequate hydration. Osmotic laxatives (e.g., milk of magnesia tablets, 2 tablets three times daily, or lactulose, 10 to 20 ml up to four times per day) may be helpful, as may increasing bulk (as with a high-fiber diet, ispaghula, or psyllium), and a stimulant laxative. Cisapride may be an alternative to the stimulant laxatives. If such a regime does not work, scheduled enemas every 1 to 2 days are necessary. Sacral anterior root stimulation is worthy of further research and trials in patients with disturbances in the neural control of the process of defecation.

The role of surgery for motility disorders due to neurological disease is restricted to those patients with intractable colonic or rectal symptoms, particularly incontinence. There is no good rationale for vagotomy or for partial or total gastrectomy in patients with chronic neuropathies causing gastric stasis. In patients with severe colonic inertia, subtotal colectomy with ileorectostomy is usually successful, but this treatment has been used only rarely in patients with neurological or muscle disease. Surgery for local complications of severe constipation may be necessary, as in patients with rectal intussusception or prolapse.

CONCLUDING COMMENT

Gastrointestinal motor abnormalities result when extrinsic nerves are disturbed and are unable to modulate the motor functions of the digestive tract, which depend on the enteric nervous system and the automaticity of the smooth muscles. Disorders at all anatomical levels of the extrinsic neural control system and degenerations of gut smooth muscle have been reported in association with gut motor dysfunction and illustrate the important role of the nervous system in the etiology of gastrointestinal symptoms. Although much emphasis in the literature is laid on dysphagia and constipation in neurological disorders, more recent studies have highlighted incontinence, vomiting, and abdominal distention in the symptomatology of such patients. Strategies that evaluate the physiological functions of the digestive tract and the function of the extrinsic neural control are available and aid in the selection of rational therapies for patients, including physical and biofeedback training (e.g., for dysphagia or incontinence), prokinetic agents (for neuropathic forms of gastroparesis, intestinal pseudo-obstruction, or slow-transit colonic disorders), and nutritional support using the enteral or parenteral route. Electrical or magnetic stimulation of lumbar sacral roots provides an exciting new method of attempting to alleviate certain symptoms, such as constipation in paraplegics.

REFERENCES

1. Nelson JB, Richter JE: Upper esophageal motility disorders. Gastroenterol Clin North Am 18:195, 1989
2. Colemont L, Camilleri M: Chronic intestinal pseudo-obstruction: diagnosis and treatment. Mayo Clin Proc 64:60, 1989
3. Read NW, Houghton LA: Physiology of gastric emptying and pathophysiology of gastroparesis. Gastroenterol Clin North Am 18:359, 1989
4. Camilleri M, Zinsmeister AR, Greydanus MP, et al: Towards a less costly but accurate test of gastric emptying and small bowel transit. Dig Dis Sci 36:609, 1991
5. Camilleri M, Malagelada J-R: Abnormal intestinal motility in diabetics with gastroparesis. Eur J Clin Invest 14:420, 1984
6. Camilleri M: Medical treatment of chronic intestinal pseudo-obstruction. Practical Gastroenterol 15:10, 1991
7. Frank JW, Sarr MG, Camilleri M: Use of gastroduodenal manometry to differentiate mechanical and functional intestinal obstruction: an analysis of clinical outcome. Am J Gastroenterol 89:339, 1994
8. Stanghellini V, Camilleri M, Malagelada J-R: Chronic idiopathic intestinal pseudo-obstruction: clinical and intestinal manometric findings. Gut 28:5, 1987
9. Pemberton JH, Phillips SF: Constipation and diarrhea. p. 39. In Moody FG (ed): Surgical Treatment of Digestive Diseases. 2nd Ed. Year Book Medical Publishers, Chicago, 1990
10. Metcalf AM, Phillips SF, Zinsmeister AR, et al: Simplified assessment of segmental colonic transit. Gastroenterology 92:40, 1987
11. Stivland T, Camilleri M, Vassallo M, et al: Scintigraphic measurement of regional gut transit in idiopathic constipation. Gastroenterology 101:107, 1991
12. Wald A: Colonic transit and anorectal manometry in chronic idiopathic constipation. Arch Intern Med 146:1713, 1986
13. MacDonagh RP, Sun WM, Smallwood R, et al: Control of defecation in patients with spinal injuries by stimulation of sacral anterior nerve roots. Br Med J 300:1494, 1990
14. Bielefeldt K, Enck P, Wienbeck M: Diagnosis and treatment of fecal incontinence. Dig Dis 8:179, 1990
15. Leighton JA, Valdovinos MA, Pemberton JH, et al: Anorectal dysfunction and rectal prolapse in progressive systemic sclerosis. Dis Colon Rectum 36:182, 1993
16. Camilleri M, Fealey RD: Idiopathic autonomic denervation in eight patients presenting with functional gastrointestinal disease: a causal association? Dig Dis Sci 35:609, 1990
17. Krishnamurthy S, Schuffler MD: Pathology of neuromuscular disorders of the small intestine and colon. Gastroenterology 93:610, 1987
18. Reynolds BJ, Eliasson SG: Colonic pseudoobstruction in patients with stroke. Ann Neurol 1:305, 1977
19. Edwards LL, Pfeiffer RF, Quigley EMM, et al: Gastrointestinal symptoms in Parkinson's disease. Mov Disord 6:151, 1991
20. Kupsky WJ, Grimes MM, Sweeting J, et al: Parkinson's disease and megacolon: concentric hyaline inclusions (Lewy bodies) in enteric ganglion cells. Neurology 37:1253, 1987
21. Mathers SE, Kempster PA, Law PJ, et al: Anal sphincter dysfunction in Parkinson's disease. Arch Neurol 46:1061, 1989
22. Ott L, Young B, Phillips R, et al: Altered gastric emptying in the head-injured patient: relationship to feeding intolerance. J Neurosurg 74:738, 1991
23. Hillel AD, Miller RM: Management of bulbar symptoms in amyotrophic lateral sclerosis. Adv Exp Med Biol 209:201, 1987

24. Camilleri M, Balm RK, Low PA: Autonomic dysfunction in patients with chronic intestinal pseudo-obstruction. Clin Auton Res 3:95, 1993
25. Sonies BC, Dalakas MC: Dysphagia in patients with the post-polio syndrome. N Engl J Med 324:1162, 1991
26. Wood JR, Camilleri M, Low PA, Malagelada J-R: Brainstem tumor presenting as an upper gut motility disorder. Gastroenterology 89:1411, 1985
27. Weber J, Denis P, Mihout B, et al: Effect of brain-stem lesion on colonic and anorectal motility: study of three patients. Dig Dis Sci 30:419, 1985
28. Camilleri M: Disorders of gastrointestinal motility in neurologic diseases. Mayo Clin Proc 65:825, 1990
29. Vassallo M, Camilleri M, Caron BL, Low PA: Gastrointestinal motor dysfunction in acquired selective cholinergic dysautonomia associated with infectious mononucleosis. Gastroenterology 100:252, 1991
30. Camilleri M, Malagelada J-R, Stanghellini V, et al: Gastrointestinal motility disturbances in patients with orthostatic hypotension. Gastroenterology 88:1852, 1985
31. Thatcher BS, Achkar E, Fouad FM, et al: Altered gastroesophageal motility in patients with idiopathic orthostatic hypotension. Cleve Clin J Med 54:77, 1987
32. Shy GM, Drager GA: A neurological syndrome associated with orthostatic hypotension: a clinical-pathologic study. Arch Neurol 2:511, 1960
33. Stone JM, Nino-Murcia M, Wolfe VA, Perkash I: Chronic gastrointestinal problems in spinal cord injury patients: a prospective analysis. Am J Gastroenterol 85:114, 1990
34. Sun WM, Read NW, Donnelly TC: Anorectal function in incontinent patients with cerebrospinal disease. Gastroenterology 99:1372, 1990
35. Meshkinpour H, Nowroozi F, Glick ME: Colonic compliance in patients with spinal cord injury. Arch Phys Med Rehabil 64:111, 1983
36. Weber J, Grise P, Roquebert M, et al: Radiopaque markers transit and anorectal manometry in 16 patients with multiple sclerosis and urinary bladder dysfunction. Dis Colon Rectum 30:95, 1987
37. Caruana BJ, Wald A, Hinds JP, Eidelman BH: Anorectal sensory and motor function in neurogenic fecal incontinence. Comparison between multiple sclerosis and diabetes mellitus. Gastroenterology 100:465, 1991
38. Sonsino E, Mouy R, Foucaud P, et al: Intestinal pseudo-obstruction related to cytomegalovirus infection of the myenteric plexus. N Engl J Med 311:196, 1984
39. von der Ohe M, Camilleri M, Zimmerman BR: Management of diabetic enteropathy. Endocrinologist 3:400, 1993
40. Feldman M, Schiller LR: Disorders of gastrointestinal motility associated with diabetes mellitus. Ann Intern Med 98:378, 1983
41. Janatuinen E, Pikkarainen P, Laakso M, Pyorala K: Gastrointestinal symptoms in middle-aged diabetic patients. Scand J Gastroenterol 28:427, 1993
42. Feldman M, Corbett DB, Ramsey EJ, et al: Abnormal gastric function in long-standing insulin-dependent diabetic patients. Gastroenterology 77:127, 1979
43. Battle WM, Snape WJ Jr, Alavi A, et al: Colonic dysfunction in diabetes mellitus. Gastroenterology 79:1217, 1980
44. Valdovinos MA, Camilleri M, Zimmerman BR: Chronic diarrhea in diabetes mellitus: mechanisms and an approach to diagnosis and treatment. Mayo Clin Proc 68:691, 1993
45. Duchen LW, Anjorin A, Watkins PJ, Mackay JD: Pathology of autonomic neuropathy in diabetes mellitus. Ann Intern Med 92:301, 1980
46. Low PA, Walsh JC, Huang CY, McLeod JG: The sympathetic nervous system in diabetic neuropathy: a clinical and pathological study. Brain 98:341, 1975
47. Camilleri M: A guide to the treatment of GI motility disorders. Drug Ther 21:15, 1991
48. Camilleri M: The current role of erythromycin in the clinical management of gastric emptying disorders. Am J Gastroenterol 88:169, 1993
49. Murat A, Vecchierini MF, Lucas B, et al: Amélioration de la neuropathie périphérique et de la vidange gastrique après transplantation simultanée rénale et pancréatique. Diabete Metab 16:419, 1990
50. Chinn JS, Schuffler MD: Paraneoplastic visceral neuropathy is a cause of severe gastrointestinal motor dysfunction in patients with lung cancer. Gastroenterology 92:1345, 1987
51. Lennon VA, Sas DF, Busk MF, et al: Enteric neuronal autoantibodies in pseudoobstruction with small-cell lung carcinoma. Gastroenterology 100:137, 1991
52. Sodhi N, Camilleri M, Camoriano JK, et al: Autonomic function and motility in intestinal pseudoobstruction caused by paraneoplastic syndrome. Dig Dis Sci 34:1937, 1989
53. Battle WM, Rubin MR, Cohen S, Snape WJ Jr: Gastrointestinal-motility dysfunction in amyloidosis. N Engl J Med 301:24, 1979
54. Marlett JA, Code CF: Effects of celiac and superior mesenteric ganglionectomy on interdigestive myoelectric complex in dogs. Am J Physiol 237:E432, 1979
55. Okajima T, Yamamura S, Hamada K, et al: Chronic sensory and autonomic neuropathy. Neurology 33:1061, 1983
56. Berlin L, Cotton R: Gastro-intestinal manifestations of porphyria. Am J Dig Dis 17:110, 1950
57. Stein JA, Tschudy DP: Acute intermittent porphyria. Medicine (Baltimore) 49:1, 1970
58. Coker RJ, Horner P, Bleasdale-Barr K, et al: Increased

gut parasympathetic activity and chronic diarrhoea in a patient with the acquired immunodeficiency syndrome. Clin Auton Res 2:295, 1992

59. Griffin GE, Miller A, Batman P, et al: Damage to jejunal intrinsic autonomic nerves in HIV infection. AIDS 2:379, 1988

60. Barohn RJ, Levine EJ, Olson JO, Mendell JR: Gastric hypomotility in Duchenne's muscular dystrophy. N Engl J Med 319:15, 1988

61. Malkinson FD, Rothman S: Changes in the gastrointestinal tract in scleroderma and other diffuse connective tissue disorders. Am J Gastroenterol 26:414, 1956

62. Feldman F, Marshak RH: Dermatomyositis with significant involvement of the gastrointestinal tract. Am J Roentgenol 90:746, 1963

63. Horowitz M, McNeil JD, Maddern GJ, et al: Abnormalities of gastric and esophageal emptying in polymyositis and dermatomyositis. Gastroenterology 90:434, 1986

64. Cervera R, Bruix J, Bayes A, et al: Chronic intestinal pseudoobstuction and ophthalmoplegia in a patient with mitrochondrial myopathy. Gut 29:544, 1988

65. Lowsky R, Davidson G, Wolman S, et al: Familial visceral myopathy associated with a mitochondrial myopathy. Gut 34:279, 1993

66. Li V, Hostein J, Romero NB, et al: Chronic intestinal pseudoobstruction with myopathy and ophthalmoplegia. Dig Dis Sci 37:456, 1992

67. Yoshida MM, Krishnamurthy S, Wattchow DA, et al: Megacolon in myotonic dystrophy caused by a degenerative neuropathy of the myenteric plexus. Gastroenterology 95:820, 1988

68. Eckardt VF, Nix W: The anal sphincter in patients with myotonic muscular dystrophy. Gastroenterology 100:424, 1991

69. Greydanus MP, Camilleri M: Abnormal postcibal antral and small bowel motility due to neuropathy or myopathy in systemic sclerosis. Gastroenterology 96:110, 1989

70. Cohen S, Fisher R, Lipshutz W, et al: The pathogenesis of esophageal dysfunction in scleroderma and Raynaud's disease. J Clin Invest 51:2663, 1972

71. Battle WM, Snape WJ Jr, Wright S, et al: Abnormal colonic motility in progressive systemic sclerosis. Ann Intern Med 94:749, 1981

72. Horowitz M, Maddern GJ, Maddox A, et al: Effects of cisapride on gastric and esophageal emptying in progressive systemic sclerosis. Gastroenterology 93:311, 1987

73. Soudah HC, Hasler WL, Owyang C: Effect of octreotide on intestinal motility and bacterial overgrowth in scleroderma. N Engl J Med 325:1461, 1991

74. Buysschaert M, Donckier J, Dive A, et al: Gastric acid and pancreatic polypeptide responses to sham feeding are impaired in diabetic subjects with autonomic neuropathy. Diabetes 34:1181, 1985

75. Leveston SA, Shah SD, Cryer PE: Cholinergic stimulation of norepinephrine release in man: evidence of a sympathetic postganglionic axonal lesion in diabetic adrenergic neuropathy. J Clin Invest 64:374, 1979

76. Gemmill JD, Venables GS, Ewing DJ: Noradrenaline response to edrophonium in primary autonomic failure: distinction between central and peripheral damage. Lancet 1:1018, 1988

77. Hyman PE, DiLorenzo C, McAdams L, et al: Predicting the clinical response to cisapride in children with chronic intestinal pseudo-obstruction. Am J Gastroenterol 88:832, 1993

78. Camilleri M, Balm RK, Zinsmeister AR: Influence of neurologic dysfunction on response to cisapride in adults with chronic intestinal pseudo-obstruction. Gastroenterology 104:A486, 1993

79. Haruma K, Camilleri M: Octreotide provocative test in antroduodenojejunal manometry: a pilot study. Gastroenterology 104:A518, 1993

15

Nutritional Disorders of the Nervous System

Elliott L. Mancall

Nutritional disorders of the nervous system, although changing to some extent in character and distribution over the years, remain remarkably common. Affecting individuals from birth—or before—to old age, such disorders are of universal concern. Widely recognized in the urban United States, particularly in the nutritionally depleted adult alcoholic population,[1] nervous system diseases due to dietary deprivation appear under circumstances as diverse as famine, extreme poverty, incarceration in prisoner-of-war camps, intestinal malabsorption due to disorders such as sprue or to major gastrointestinal surgery including gastric plication, administration of metabolic antagonists such as isonicotinic acid hydrazide (INH), anorexia nervosa, and food fads, especially among adolescents.

As a general rule, affections of the nervous system due to nutritional depletion present in a symmetrical distribution, both clinically and pathologically, and in a stereotyped and thus readily identified fashion. The precise factor(s) underlying development of such neurological disease has been well established in only some instances, for example, the Wernicke-Korsakoff syndrome. Often the exact nutrient lacking cannot be defined with certainty, and it is not unlikely that a combination of dietary defects may be necessary for a given disease to develop. The complex interrelation between total caloric intake, relative balance of carbo-hydrate/protein/fat in the diet, and lack of one or more specific nutrients appears important under some circumstances; extreme caloric deprivation alone may not be a sufficient explanation for these disorders. At times, totally unanticipated factors—for example, autoimmune mechanisms, as documented for pernicious anemia, or inherent genetic defects, as have been suggested in the Wernicke-Korsakoff syndrome—may be of fundamental pathogenetic significance. Difficulties encountered in establishing a clear-cut dietary history and practical problems in the documentation of deficiencies of, for example, isolated vitamins in the clinical laboratory, add yet more complications to the assessment of nutritional disorders as a whole. Finally, our understanding of these disorders is impeded by the fact that data derived from animal investigations cannot always be translated successfully to naturally occurring disease in the human.

In view of the lack of precision related to establishing the pathogenesis of many of these disorders, no classification can be entirely satisfactory. Because most clearly defined nutritional diseases reflect depletion of a vitamin or vitamins (most commonly the group B vitamins), the presentation of these disorders that follows adheres to an outline based on specific vitamins whenever possible. The ambiguities and uncertainties of such an approach cannot, however, be ignored. Perhaps not surprisingly, many of these disorders occur in combination with one another, rendering any classification still more arbitrary and incomplete.

RETINOL (VITAMIN A, β-CAROTENE)

A *deficiency* of vitamin A is remarkably common in parts of the world, such as Southeast Asia, Africa, and the Middle East, where extreme poverty and nutritional depletion are endemic.[2] Hypovitaminosis A leads most importantly to a variety of ophthalmic disorders, loosely grouped under the rubric "xerophthalmia."[3] An early manifestation of such depletion is *night blindness,* reflecting the importance of retinol in the production of rhodopsin (visual purple). Following light absorption in the rods, retinol is released from rhodopsin and is available for recycling, with continuous regeneration of rhodopsin. The rods, which are present in the more peripheral portions of the retina but not in the macula, and which subserve vision in conditions of low illumination, utilize rhodopsin as their primary chemical photoreceptor. A defect in vitamin A leads directly to deficient rod performance and thus to night blindness. The potential additive or potentiating role of protein malnutrition (e.g., kwashiorkor) remains insufficiently explored.

A continuing severe deficiency of vitamin A results in progressive changes in both the conjunctiva and cornea. Corneal ulceration and keratomalacia lead ultimately to irreversible corneal damage and blindness.

Hypovitaminosis A has also been implicated, albeit rarely, in the development of pseudotumor cerebri during infancy[4] (see below).

Recommended daily allowances of vitamin A are 4,000 USP units in female subjects and 5,000 in male subjects; both parenteral and oral preparations of retinol are available for management of documented hypovitaminosis A, but great care must be used to avoid toxicity when administering this agent chronically.

An *excess* of vitamin A results from a diversity of factors, including ingestion of carotene-rich polar bear liver or excessive amounts of vitamin A itself, ingested either because it is a food fad or as treatment for a host of dermatological conditions. A daily intake of as little as 7.5 mg retinol over time may produce toxic manifestations; acute hypervitaminosis A may follow the ingestion of 500 mg retinol in the adult,

less in infants and children. Such an excess is among the identified causes of the syndrome of *pseudotumor cerebri* (benign intracranial hypertension), a disorder characterized by generalized brain swelling associated with clinical features of increased intracranial pressure. Patients experience headache and at times slowed intellectual function; examination reveals papilledema, enlargement of the physiological blind spot, and, on occasion, nonspecific sixth nerve palsies. The cerebrospinal fluid (CSF) pressure is elevated, but the spinal fluid itself is otherwise normal. Computed tomography (CT) scanning or magnetic resonance imaging (MRI) demonstrates diffuse brain swelling with symmetrically placed ventricles, which may be small, normal, or, uncommonly, mildly enlarged. This condition represents a major threat, particularly to vision, because consecutive ("secondary") optic atrophy may lead to progressive visual loss. Every effort must be made to prevent this complication by reducing the intracranial pressure. Therapeutic measures include the use of diuretics, corticosteroid preparations such as dexamethasone, repeated lumbar punctures, or a surgically established subarachnoid-extracranial shunt. Surgical cranial decompression should be avoided if possible, and rarely requires serious consideration.

B COMPLEX OF VITAMINS

A number of factors in the B group of vitamins are of clinical importance with regard to neurological disease. These vitamins include thiamine (vitamin B_1), niacin (nicotinic acid), pyridoxine (vitamin B_6), and cobalamin (vitamin B_{12}). Although each is considered separately below, in many instances deficiencies of these and other vitamins occur in combination and may lead to complex clinical disturbances.

THIAMINE (VITAMIN B_1)

Thiamine pyrophosphate, or cocarboxylase, functions as a cofactor in intermediary carbohydrate metabolism. It serves as a coenzyme in the decarboxylation of α-keto acids, that is, α-ketoglutaric acid and pyruvate dehydrogenase; it also acts as a cofactor to the enzyme transketolase in the hexose monophosphate shunt. Deficiency of thiamine in animals results in accumulation of lactic acid and reduction in oxygen uptake, especially in the brainstem, and depression of transketolase activity, again most strikingly in the brainstem.[5-8] Such observations are intriguing in light of the known predilection of the lesions of Wernicke's encephalopathy for brainstem structures.

In developed countries, thiamine deficiency in humans has been studied particularly in chronic alcoholics.[9] In this context, alcohol plays a secondary role, essentially serving to displace food in the diet. For the most part, observations in alcoholics appear readily transposed to those in nutritionally depleted nonalcoholics. Such discrepancies as do exist may well be explained on the basis of multiple vitamin deficiencies and varying ethnic and regional dietary habits and susceptibilities.

Two disorders that appear most clearly related to thiamine deficiency are nutritional polyneuropathy and the Wernicke-Korsakoff syndrome. Two others, cortical cerebellar degeneration ("alcoholic cerebellar degeneration") and nutritional amblyopia, are probably not related to thiamine deficiency alone but nevertheless seem intimately related to thiamine lack and are considered here as well.

Nutritional Polyneuropathy

Nutritional polyneuropathy (neuritic or dry beriberi, alcoholic neuropathy)[10] is the most common of all nutritional disorders of the nervous system. Whether it relates to isolated deficiency of thiamine or more accurately reflects deficiencies of multiple vitamins in the B group, including pyridoxine and pantothenic acid, remains unsettled. It is clear, however, that thiamine deficiency plays a dominant role in the pathogenesis of polyneuropathy in both the alcoholic and nonalcoholic population.

Clinically, nutritional polyneuropathy presents as a largely symmetrical, mixed sensorimotor neuropathy. The onset of symptoms is usually insidious and progression is slow, but evolution is occasionally rapid. The lower extremities tend to be involved earlier and more severely than the upper extremities, and in many cases the arms appear to be spared. The distal portions of the limbs are characteristically affected more than the proximal segments. Complaints include numbness or tingling paresthesias distally in the limbs, frequently accompanied by pain. Although it is usually dull and aching in quality, the pain is some-

times sharp and lancinating, reminiscent of the pain of tabes dorsalis. (At times it is sufficiently severe to warrant the appellation *pseudotabes*.) Cramps in the feet and calves are common. Patients may complain of severe burning pain in the feet ("burning feet syndrome") and often experience prominent and at times disabling dysesthetic sensations that are so uncomfortable that simple weight-bearing may become impossible.

Examination demonstrates variable weakness, at times amounting to virtual paralysis of the legs. Footdrop with a resultant steppage gait is frequent, and the distal muscles atrophy. The muscles may be tender to palpation, especially in acute cases. The tendon reflexes are reduced or lost. Sensory examination demonstrates reduction or loss of vibratory sense, particularly at the ankles. Proprioception may be impaired, at times profoundly. Reduction of cutaneous sensation generally takes the form of a distal impairment of pain and light touch in a glove-and-stocking distribution; thermal sensibility is reduced in a corresponding manner. The hypalgesic areas are not crisply defined, the border between normal and abnormal portions of the limbs tending to be indistinct (in contrast to the sharply delineated glove-and-stocking sensory loss found in the patient with a conversion reaction). Not all sensory modalities are involved to an equal degree, the severity and extent of loss exhibiting considerable variability from patient to patient.

Signs and symptoms of dysfunction of the autonomic nervous system are sometimes encountered as well, including vocal cord paralysis with hoarseness, dysphagia, pupillary abnormalities, and hypotension. Hyperhidrosis of the hands and feet is common.

Examination of the CSF usually demonstrates at most only a mild increase in protein content. Electrophysiological studies reveal findings suggestive of an axonal polyneuropathy, but there may also be features of superimposed compressive mononeuropathies. Pathologically, the primary change is segmental demyelination associated with axonal degeneration, affecting particularly the distal portion of the peripheral nerves. Changes in the sympathetic nervous system may also occur. In long-standing cases, retrograde changes may be found within the spinal cord, including chromatolytic changes in the anterior horn cells and secondary (ascending) degeneration in the posterior columns.

Restoration of a well balanced diet with supplemental vitamins of the B group, especially thiamine, is the keystone of therapy. The parenteral use of vitamin preparations is advisable in the early stages of treatment. Although the minimum daily requirement of thiamine in the adult is only approximately 1 mg, injections of 50 to 100 mg daily may be utilized early in therapy, with 50 to 100 mg subsequently taken by mouth several times daily. Symptomatic management includes the use of analgesics, amitriptyline (25 to 50 mg or more at bedtime), or carbamazepine (up to 800 mg or more per day as required) for relief of pain. Sympathetic block may be necessary in instances of severe and intractable burning. Unfortunately, recovery tends to be slow and incomplete; residual and at times severe sensory and motor alterations are common, even in individuals who maintain a normal dietary intake with vitamin supplementation.

Wernicke-Korsakoff Syndrome

Although Wernicke's encephalopathy and Korsakoff's syndrome are traditionally looked on as two distinct entities, they are best regarded as representing simply two aspects of the same disease, separable chronologically into acute (Wernicke's encephalopathy) and chronic (Korsakoff's syndrome) phases.[11] Considerable evidence has accumulated to support the notion that these two disorders are indeed intimately linked. Thus the typical mental changes of Korsakoff's syndrome may be present from the earliest stages of acute Wernicke's encephalopathy or may emerge during the treatment of that disorder as other clinical manifestations recede. Furthermore, examination of patients with classic Korsakoff's psychosis often reveals residual features of previous, perhaps unrecognized, Wernicke's encephalopathy, such as nystagmus and truncal ataxia. Finally, both the nature and the distribution of the pathological changes appear identical in the two conditions, such differences as do exist being accounted for by differences in the chronology of the lesions rather than reflecting a fundamental difference in kind.

There can be little doubt as to the central role of acquired thiamine deficiency in the pathogenesis of this disorder. Such deficiency is found most commonly, though certainly not invariably, on a background of long-standing dietary insufficiency conditioned by the excessive use of alcohol, at least in western society. Thiamine deficiency associated with Wernicke-Korsakoff syndrome has also been recorded in patients on dialysis[12] as well as in those with acquired immunodeficiency syndrome (AIDS), hyperemesis gravidarum, carcinoma treated with the chemotherapeutic agent fluoropyrimidine dexifluridine,[13] and following gastroplasty performed for management of obesity. The possibility of an inherent predisposition to Wernicke's encephalopathy, reflecting a genetically determined error in transketolase, has been suggested as of significance in at least some instances of the disease.[14–17]

WERNICKE'S ENCEPHALOPATHY

Wernicke's disease, or encephalopathy, is an acute or subacutely evolving disorder. Appearing on a background of chronic and severe undernutrition, it is frequently preceded by some additional metabolic stress related, for example, to serious trauma or infection. A carbohydrate load is the immediate precipitating factor in some patients. Characteristic clinical features of this disorder include the following.

1. *Abnormal mental status.* Some patients appear apathetic and listless, with a short attention span, little spontaneity of speech, mental confusion, and excessive drowsiness. Coma is rare. Other patients have perceptual distortions, hallucinations, agitation, confusion, and other clinical features reminiscent of delirium tremens. Finally, some exhibit features of an amnestic dementia (i.e., of the typical mental alteration of Korsakoff's syndrome) with an otherwise clear sensorium.

2. *Ophthalmoplegia.* Ocular palsies are a hallmark of Wernicke's encephalopathy. Bilateral sixth nerve palsies are most common, but virtually any pattern of restricted ocular motility may be found, including conjugate gaze palsies and internuclear ophthalmoplegia. Diplopia is characteristically experienced and, in fact, often represents the first subjective manifestation of the disease. Involvement of the pupils is rare.

3. *Nystagmus.* Nystagmus is typically encountered in both the horizontal and vertical planes. In the presence of severe abducens palsies, however, nystagmus may be lacking in the abducting eye, becoming apparent only in the course of treatment as the ophthalmoplegia itself subsides.

4. *Ataxia.* Patients with Wernicke's encephalopathy typically evidence an ataxia of trunk and gait, at times associated with severe truncal titubation. Only modest ataxia is observed with the heel-to-knee test, and the arms tend to be involved little if at all. In some patients ataxia is minimal, being evident only with attempts at tandem walking.

Autonomic changes such as postural hypotension and altered cardiac function may also be encountered in Wernicke's encephalopathy, although not with sufficient frequency to be considered characteristic of the disease. True beriberi heart disease is infrequent, but sudden death may occur as a manifestation of acute cardiovascular collapse, so-called shoshin beriberi.[18]

The clinical course of Wernicke's encephalopathy is dramatically altered by the administration of thiamine.[11] Within hours of the parenteral administration of 25 to 50 mg thiamine, the ophthalmoplegia improves, and ocular palsies generally disappear entirely within several days. Nystagmus similarly improves but less dramatically, and most patients are left with permanent horizontal nystagmus of modest amplitude. The truncal ataxia also improves, but again rather slowly and often incompletely; one-half of the patients continue to exhibit at least mild residual ataxia. In contrast, improvement in the mental status is less predictable. Patients with a quiet confusional state or delirium tend to improve over a period of weeks; all too often, however, memory impairment, the hallmark of Korsakoff's syndrome, appears in the course of recovery and may persist thereafter. After initial management with parenteral thiamine in doses of 50 to 100 mg, patients are maintained on an oral dosage at 50 to 100 mg three or four times daily.

The pathological alterations of Wernicke's encephalopathy are found in a remarkably stereotyped distribution, predominantly involving brainstem and hypothalamus. The characteristic lesion is one of subtotal tissue necrosis involving neurons, axons, and myelin to variable degrees. Lesions are typically found centrally disposed in the mammillary bodies, along the walls of the third ventricle, in the medial dorsal nucleus of the thalamus, in the periaqueductal gray matter of the mesencephalon, in the floor of the fourth ventricle, and in the superior cerebellar vermis. Within the lesions there is a glial response that is chronologically appropriate to the age of the destructive lesions. Inflammatory changes are lacking. In some cases fresh hemorrhages are found (responsible at least in part for the name Wernicke himself gave to this disease, i.e., *polioencephalitis hemorrhagica superioris*). It is probable that these hemorrhagic changes are secondary rather than primary events. Vascular proliferation is occasionally encountered. In terms of clinicopathological correlation, it is likely that the ophthalmoplegias are caused by lesions in the periaqueductal gray matter and pontine tegmentum, nystagmus by lesions typically involving the vestibular complex at the pontomedullary junction, and truncal ataxia by lesions in the superior cerebellar vermis. The alterations in attention, cognition, and memory are probably caused by lesions in the mammillary bodies and medial and posterior thalamus.

KORSAKOFF'S SYNDROME

Korsakoff's syndrome or psychosis, the chronic form of the Wernicke-Korsakoff syndrome, is characterized primarily by an amnestic dementia, that is, a profound disorder of memory with relative preservation of cognitive abilities per se. The core of the defect appears to be an impairment of the ability to acquire new information (i.e., to establish new memories); thus anterograde amnesia results. Patients with Korsakoff's psychosis also typically have some degree of retrograde amnesia, extending backward over a variable period of time before onset of the disease. Memories of events in the more remote past are often retained, but commonly in chronological disarray. The most striking impairment is without doubt the inability to learn newly presented information. Confabulation, probably representing, in large part, suggestibility on the part of the patient, is frequently encountered in Korsakoff's syndrome, but not invariably so. Because confabulation also occurs in other states of mental incapacity, it cannot be looked on as specific or in any way pathognomonic of Korsakoff's syndrome. The degree to which conscious mechanisms enter into confabulation under any circumstances remains unclear.

Although the primary defect in Korsakoff's syndrome centers about memory, other cognitive impairment may be found, although usually of lesser severity. Thus, defects may be evident in visual and verbal abstracting ability, shifting mental sets, and concept formation, which are functions in which memory does not play a major role. Additionally, the behavior of many patients with Korsakoff's syndrome is abnormal, being characterized by apathy, disinterest, and listlessness, although without a clear defect in attention or vigilance.

On careful examination, most patients with Korsakoff's syndrome show other clinical features of the Wernicke-Korsakoff syndrome, including horizontal nystagmus and variable gait ataxia. Not unexpectedly, many also demonstrate features of an associated nutritional polyneuropathy.

The outlook for patients with established Korsakoff's syndrome is discouraging. Only a relatively small proportion of these individuals recover memory function to any significant degree, although many evidence at least modest return, permitting them to function to a limited extent in society. One would anticipate that if vigorous therapy with thiamine were to be instituted during the acute phase of the disease (i.e., early in the course of Wernicke's encephalopathy) there would be a greater chance of either avoiding or appreciably lessening the ultimate memory defect; unfortunately, this has not been well documented. It is clear, however, that with continuing administration of thiamine in oral dosages of 50 to 100 mg three or four times daily over a period of many months, some patients who originally show little or no improvement may demonstrate gradual and at times remarkably complete functional recovery.

The neuropathological changes in Korsakoff's syndrome are essentially identical in distribution and histological character to those of Wernicke's encephalopathy. The only noteworthy difference is that of a more chronic (i.e., astrocytic) form of glial reaction, in keeping with the more protracted clinical course. In terms of the anatomical substrate for the memory defect, the lesions in the mammillary bodies and thalamus appear to be of particular importance. The studies of Victor and associates have clearly demonstrated that the lesions in the medial dorsal and perhaps posterior nuclei of the thalamus are central to the memory defect.[11] In a large series of pathologically documented cases, they were able to demonstrate lesions invariably in the thalamus in patients with Korsakoff's syndrome, whereas lesions in the mammillary bodies were not consistently observed. Although cortical atrophy is a commonplace observation in the brains of chronic alcoholics, it is doubtful that cortical pathology plays a significant role in producing the mental changes of classic Korsakoff's syndrome.

Cortical Cerebellar Degeneration

Cortical cerebellar degeneration, or "alcoholic cerebellar degeneration," appears intimately linked to Wernicke's encephalopathy. Although a primary role for thiamine deficiency has not been convincingly established, this disorder is clearly of nutritional origin, and its close association with Wernicke's disease warrants its inclusion here.

Cortical cerebellar degeneration is a relatively frequent complication of chronic alcoholism and is the most common of the acquired cerebellar degenerations.[19,20] Usually beginning in midlife and almost always on a background of long-standing and excessive ethanol abuse and chronic nutritional depletion, the onset of the disease is commonly marked by complaints of disordered gait or truncal stability. The gait disability worsens in subacute fashion for a period of several weeks or months or even longer, but it ultimately stabilizes, usually when patients become abstinent and improve their nutritional status. At times the disorder evolves in an episodic manner, seemingly in relation to severe systemic illness.

Examination demonstrates that the primary defect is referable to the gait and stance. Truncal instability is common, and a wide-based ataxia of gait with ataxia of individual leg movements is characteristic. The patient is unable to make rapid postural adjustments and walks in tandem fashion only with difficulty. At times the ataxia is so severe that the patient cannot stand unaided, even on a wide base; most patients require at least some support for either standing or walking. In contrast to the severe affection of the lower extremities, the arms are affected little if at all. There may be ocular dysmetria, but other features suggestive of cerebellar dysfunction are either minimal or entirely lacking: dysarthria, when present, tends to be mild, and nystagmus is uncommon. Features of other neurological disorders, particularly those of Wernicke's encephalopathy and nutritional polyneuropathy, are often present.

Following stabilization, patients may show modest improvement as their nutrition improves, especially if supplemental vitamins are taken. However, a significant cerebellar deficit invariably remains and persists for years thereafter.

Pathological changes predominate in, and may be confined to, the anterior and superior portions of the cerebellar vermis and hemispheres. Occasional lesions are also found elsewhere in the cerebellar cortex. In almost all cases the lingula, central lobule, and culmen and adjacent declive are affected in the vermis, whereas in the hemispheres it is the more anterior portion of the anterior lobes that is most commonly affected. Within these areas, all neurocellular elements are destroyed, although to variable degrees; the Purkinje cells appear to be especially vulnerable. Secondary changes may be found in the cerebellar white matter, deep cerebellar nuclei, and related brainstem nuclei, such as the olivary complex. The typical histological features of Wernicke's encephalopathy are conjoined in many cases.

Well-documented cases of a similar form of cerebellar degeneration occurring in conditions of severe nutritional depletion unrelated to the abuse of alcohol have been reported,[21] suggesting that "alcoholic" cerebellar degeneration is in fact of nutritional origin. The appearance of similar clinical and pathological features in the course of Wernicke's encephalopathy, and the occurrence of characteristic features of Wernicke's encephalopathy in otherwise straightforward instances of cerebellar degeneration, suggest that the two disorders are closely linked. It is therefore tempting to ascribe the cerebellar disease also to thiamine deficiency, but this cannot be stated with certainty at this time. The significance of the reportedly low CSF levels of thiamine in certain inherited ataxias, and specifically in olivopontocerebellar atrophy and Friedreich's ataxia,[22] remains unclear in this respect.

The transient cerebellar syndrome encountered as an evanescent ataxia of gait in acute alcoholic intoxication (or rarely in withdrawal states) is not associated with any fixed cerebellar lesions. The cerebellar dysfunction that occurs in these circumstances presumably reflects a reversible biochemical lesion that conceivably also relates to thiamine deficiency, although this relationship remains to be established.

Nutritional Amblyopia

Nutritional amblyopia (deficiency amblyopia, nutritional retrobulbar neuritis, tobacco-alcohol amblyopia) appears most frequently in the chronically malnourished alcoholic and appears firmly established as a deficiency disorder of the B group of vitamins.[23] As its name implies, it is characterized primarily by defective vision. Its onset is insidious and its course

progressive. Initial impairment of the ability to read small print or to distinguish colors leads eventually to serious impairment of visual acuity, but with few (if any) other subjective ocular complaints. Examination typically demonstrates a bilateral and fairly symmetrical loss of visual acuity, with bilateral central, cecocentral, or paracentral scotomas. Peripheral fields are unaffected. Funduscopic examination is generally unrevealing, although in advanced stages there may be mild optic atrophy. Signs of other disorders of nutritional origin (e.g., polyneuropathy or the Wernicke-Korsakoff syndrome) may be found. The salient pathological changes are found in the optic nerves, chiasm, and tracts in a position that corresponds to the location of the papillomacular bundles. Transsynaptic degeneration is sometimes seen in the nerve cells of the lateral geniculate body, and in severe cases there may be loss of ganglion cells in the macular region of the retina. The primary site of involvement, however, is the conducting pathways themselves, in contrast to the amblyopia of methyl alcohol toxicity, which is due to primary degeneration of the retinal nerve cells.

This disorder is encountered worldwide among undernourished alcoholics, in conditions of naturally occurring famine, and among incarcerated groups of people. Although there is widespread agreement that deficiency of group B vitamins is important in the pathogenesis of nutritional amblyopia,[24,25] it does not necessarily imply a central role for thiamine alone; a similar syndrome may appear in patients with deficiency of vitamin B_{12} and perhaps of riboflavin. Despite the term *tobacco-alcohol amblyopia* traditionally applied to this condition, it is unlikely that either tobacco or ethyl alcohol plays a significant role as directly toxic agents. Dramatic improvement in vision, with complete return to normal acuity and fields, follows the timely introduction of treatment with group B vitamins, even if the patient continues to smoke and consume ethanol as before. If the disease is not recognized early and treated promptly, the visual changes become irreversible, with permanent blindness and optic atrophy.

Subacute Necrotizing Encephalomyelopathy (Leigh's Disease)

The relation of subacute necrotizing encephalopathy of childhood to Wernicke's disease itself remains unclear. Inherited as an autosomal recessive trait, Leigh's disease typically develops within the first 2 years of life.[26] An adult form has been described. It is characterized by weakness, hypotonia, intellectual deterioration, seizures, deafness, optic atrophy and blindness, irregular respirations, ataxia, abnormal eye movements, vomiting, and nystagmus. The disease is usually fatal within several months, but occasional patients have pursued a much more chronic course. Clinically, it thus bears no obvious relation to Wernicke's encephalopathy. However, lesions reminiscent of Wernicke's disease are found in the thalamus and brainstem; necrotic lesions may also be found in the optic nerves and posterior columns of the spinal cord. The mammillary bodies are infrequently involved.

In view of this pathological resemblance to Wernicke's encephalopathy, the possibility that Leigh's disease relates to thiamine deficiency[27,28] must be considered, particularly in light of the observation of elevated blood pyruvate and lactate levels[29] and of lactic acidosis,[30] suggesting a defect in pyruvate decarboxylation in at least some cases. Pincus and colleagues have observed an absence of thiamine triphosphate in the brain of a patient dying of this disorder and noted the presence in blood, urine, and CSF of a factor inhibiting the conversion of thiamine pyrophosphate to thiamine triphosphate (and therefore inhibiting the action of thiamine pyrophosphate–ATP phosphotransferase).[31,32] Reduction in thiamine triphosphate content has been documented in other cases as well, and temporary benefit has been noted following the administration of thiamine in large amounts in at least some instances. It therefore seems that thiamine has some role in the pathogenesis of this obscure disorder, although a simple dietary lack of thiamine does not appear to be of significance.

NIACIN (NICOTINIC ACID)

A deficiency of nicotinic acid or of its metabolic amino acid precursor tryptophan is widely accepted as the cause of *pellagra*. Relatively uncommon today, pellagra is occasionally encountered as a neuropathological curiosity in chronic alcoholics. It is not rare, however, in institutionalized mentally retarded or demented patients. In its fully developed clinical form, pellagra comprises a host of symptoms referable to the gastrointestinal tract (anorexia, nausea, vomiting, diarrhea), skin, and nervous system. Both central and peripheral nervous systems may be affected. Evidence of involvement of the central nervous system (CNS) includes irritability, insomnia, depression, mania, confusion, intellectual deterioration, and memory impairment. Extrapyramidal or cerebellar deficits may develop, and the optic nerves may be involved. The appearance of a polyneuropathy, generally of mild to moderate degree, indicates peripheral involvement. The clinical features are typical of most metabolic polyneuropathies and include tenderness of nerve trunks and muscles, cramps, distal weakness of the limbs, depressed tendon reflexes, and distal impairment of cutaneous sensibility. Loss of proprioception and vibratory sense may reflect either the neuropathy or an associated myelopathy whose presence is suggested by the occasional appearance of extensor plantar responses. The corneal reflexes may be decreased and the pupillary light reflexes impaired.

Pathological changes in pellagra are found in the cerebrum, spinal cord, and peripheral nerves and roots. Chromatolytic changes in neurons (the "central neuritis" of Adolph Meyer) are encountered, involving most prominently the large Betz cells of the motor cortex; a similar neuronal change may be found ubiquitously throughout the central gray matter. Degenerative changes are found symmetrically in the posterior and lateral columns of the spinal cord. The peripheral nerves show a patchy loss of myelin and axons.

Although it is widely held that all the clinical manifestations of pellagra are due to niacin deficiency, the neurological changes are remarkably resistant to treatment with niacin alone, even when 25 mg is administered intravenously twice daily. Deficiency of other vitamins such as thiamine may be important, particularly in the pathogenesis of the polyneuropathy. Furthermore, Victor and Adams have demonstrated the appearance of the typical neuronal changes of pellagra in experimental pyridoxine deficiency.[33] It is therefore possible that the full clinical syndrome of pellagra reflects deficiency of several vitamins in the B group.

A reversible syndrome of niacin deficiency termed *nicotinic acid deficiency encephalopathy* has also been described,[34] predominantly although not exclusively[35] in the literature of the 1940s. This poorly understood syndrome appears to involve particularly the elderly.

It is characterized by mental confusion, stupor, cogwheel rigidity, and the appearance of primitive reflexes (e.g., forced grasping). The exact nature of this disorder has never been clarified, and there are reservations as to its relation to nicotinic acid deficiency as such, since most affected patients appear to have experienced much broader nutritional defects.

Finally, a relation of nicotinic acid deficiency to Hartnup's disease is suggested by the similarity of the clinical picture of this infantile, recessively inherited familial disorder to pellagra. A genetically determined defect in intestinal transport of the nicotinic acid precursor tryptophan (and other amino acids) and reported benefit from the administration of nicotinic acid are features of Hartnup's disease that support the notion of such a relation.

PYRIDOXINE (VITAMIN B₆)

Neurological disorders reflecting both pyridoxine deficiency and pyridoxine excess have been recognized. Pyridoxine is a water-soluble vitamin that is converted by the enzymes pyridoxal kinase and pyridoxine phosphate oxidase to its active form, pyridoxal phosphate, a coenzyme involved in a number of decarboxylation and transamination reactions.

Excessive intake of pyridoxine may saturate either of these enzyme systems, with a resultant accumulation of (inactive) pyridoxine, which occupies binding sites on the appropriate apoenzymes and thus acts as a competitive inhibitor for pyridoxal phosphate. In essence, an excess or overdose of pyridoxine leads to a deficiency of pyridoxal phosphate.

Deficiency of dietary pyridoxine causes a mixed distal symmetrical polyneuropathy. The lack of pyridoxal phosphate functioning as a coenzyme for serine palmityltransferase (as required for the synthesis of sphingomyelin) or amino acid decarboxylase, or both, may be responsible for the polyneuropathy. Polyneuropathy due to pyridoxine deficiency is found in patients treated for tuberculosis with isonicotinic acid hydrazide (INH),[36] an agent that inhibits pyridoxine phosphorylation. Patients treated with INH commonly describe numbness and tingling in the limbs, particularly involving the lower extremities, together with tenderness in the calves and pain (often burning) distally in the limbs. Examination demonstrates reflex loss, impairment of superficial sensa-tion, and weakness in the lower extremities, with little, if any, affection of the arms. At times, INH neuropathy is extraordinary severe, especially in seriously malnourished tubercular patients and particularly in those who are also chronic alcoholics. This finding suggests the likelihood of multiple nutritional deficiencies acting synergistically to produce a devastating neuropathy. Of additional interest in this connection is the observation that the typical central features of pellagra may appear in patients receiving INH, along with the classic dermatological and intestinal manifestations of the naturally occurring disease.[37]

Neuropathy caused by INH may be prevented by the concomitant administration of pyridoxine. Although the minimum daily requirement of pyridoxine is only approximately 2 mg in adults, 50 mg/d or more may be required for successful therapy in the deficiency states.

A predominantly sensory neuropathy or neuronopathy has also been recognized as a result of *pyridoxine abuse.*[38,39] Female subjects are affected almost exclusively, perhaps reflecting the widespread use of pyridoxine in the management of premenstrual symptoms. All exhibit symmetrical and distal sensory loss; vibratory and position sense may be markedly impaired, and sensory ataxia is often prominent. The legs are usually more severely involved than the arms, reflecting the fact that the disorder is primarily a distal axonopathy. Muscle weakness has been described in a few patients. The Achilles reflexes are invariably lost. Electrophysiological studies demonstrate absent or severely reduced sensory nerve action potentials, with mild slowing of sensory nerve conduction velocities. Compound muscle action potential amplitudes and motor nerve conduction velocities are normal. Improvement occurs following discontinuation of pyridoxine. Complete recovery may occur in patients with a mild neuropathy who had been taking only low doses of the vitamin.

During infancy, pyridoxine deficiency results in seizures, excessive irritability, tremulousness, and poor psychomotor development. This disorder appears due to an inherited metabolic defect transmitted in an autosomal recessive manner. The seizures presumably result from depletion of γ-amino butyric acid (GABA), the normal conversion of glutamic acid being thwarted by the absence of the coenzyme pyridoxal phosphate, acting in concert with the apoenzyme glutamic acid decarboxylase. The administration of pyridoxine arrests seizures and may also foster normal development.

COBALAMIN (VITAMIN B₁₂)

As is well known, pernicious anemia, which is characterized by malabsorption of vitamin B_{12}, reflects a lack of intrinsic factor associated with gastric atrophy and gastric achlorhydria. It may have an autoimmune basis, as suggested by the fact that many patients with pernicious anemia have antibodies against gastric parietal cells as well as antithyroid antibodies; immunoglobulin G (IgG) antibodies against intrinsic factor itself may also be demonstrated. Further supporting the notion of autoimmune causation is the association of pernicious anemia with myasthenia gravis, a disorder of known autoimmune cause.[40] Vitamin B_{12} malabsorption and deficiency may also occur under a number of other circumstances, including fish tapeworm infestation, celiac disease, sprue, gastric malignancy, chronic gastritis, thyrotoxicosis, myxedema, an extreme vegetarian diet, chronic pancreatic insufficiency, and following gastrectomy or gastrojejunostomy. Whatever its cause, vitamin B_{12} deficiency may lead to serious disease involving both central and peripheral nervous systems, although the precise pathophysiological mechanisms remain unclear.

The most widely recognized CNS disorder resulting from vitamin B_{12} deficiency is *subacute combined degeneration of the spinal cord,* often erroneously referred to as posterolateral sclerosis or combined system disease. Clinically it presents with tingling paresthesias involving the feet, subsequently associated with weakness and stiffness of the legs and a spastic gait. As the disease progresses, the upper extremities come to be involved. Loss of vibratory sense, particularly in the feet, and impairment of proprioception with a resultant sensory ataxia are characteristic features. Hyperreflexia and extensor plantar responses may give way to areflexia as an associated polyneuropathy appears. Signs of a hypertonic bladder are frequent. On occasion, segmental impairment of cutaneous sensibility is observed over the torso.

In addition to such features of myelopathy, many patients with subacute combined degeneration develop impairment of vision, reflecting involvement of the optic nerves; altered visual evoked potentials are common.[41] Primary optic atrophy may appear. Central or cecocentral scotomas may be documented with visual field examination. A variety of mental changes may also be seen, ranging from depression to paranoid states, and, most importantly, progressive dementia with impairment of both memory and cognitive function.

Pathologically, the earliest changes within the spinal cord are in the posterior columns of the thoracic cord; these changes are characterized by patchy, eventually confluent areas of myelin swelling and degeneration, ultimately with loss of axons.[42] As the disease progresses, patchy demyelination appears in the lateral columns and sometimes spreads to involve the white matter of the cord in its entirety. The process extends to the cervical cord as the disease evolves. Demyelination may be encountered in the cerebral white matter—presumably accounting for the psychological changes found in the disease—and in the optic nerves.

Disease of the peripheral nervous system is observed in vitamin B_{12} deficiency as well,[43–45] but the frequency of polyneuropathy is not clear. Clinical criteria alone may be insufficient to establish a diagnosis in that complaints of numbness or paresthesias, which are typical symptoms of a sensory neuropathy, are also encountered in patients with disease of the posterior columns. In addition to loss of posterior column sensibility attributable to myelopathy, however, some patients exhibit a distal impairment of cutaneous sensibility in a glove-and-stocking distribution. This sensory change, coupled with loss of tendon reflexes in the legs, may be taken as evidence of polyneuropathy appearing either independently of or superimposed on the myelopathy. There is also abundant electrophysiological evidence of polyneuropathy occurring in pernicious anemia.[46] A decrease in distal sensory nerve conduction velocity is characteristic and is in keeping with the observation of Greenfield and Carmichael of a reduction in the number and diameters of myelinated axons in the distal portion of peripheral nerves in patients with subacute combined degeneration.[47] In general, the electrophysiological features in these patients are suggestive of a mixed demyelinating and axonal neuropathy; reversal of such abnormalities occurs to a variable extent with vitamin B_{12} treatment. Electrophysiological evidence of subclinical polyneuropathy may also be found in patients with vitamin B_{12} deficiency.

Vitamin B_{12} deficiency, marginal or overt, has recently been implicated as a possible cofactor in the pathogenesis of cognitive alterations in patients with human immunodeficiency virus (HIV-1) infection,[48,49] although the evidence for such a relationship is not compelling.[50] Vitamin B_{12} deficiency has also been noted in some cases of multiple sclerosis and documented by depressed levels in both blood and CSF and elevation of plasma homocysteine and R-binder capacity.[51,52] There is anecdotal evidence of clinical improvement in some patients with multiple sclerosis treated with vitamin B_{12} supplements.

Features of both central and peripheral nervous system disease similar to those encountered in classic subacute combined degeneration with associated polyneuropathy may occur as a reflection of deficiency in R-binder protein,[53] one of the two carriers responsible for extracellular transport of vitamin B_{12} in plasma. Attention has been drawn to the appearance of subacute combined degeneration in a patient with an abnormal plasma B_{12}-binding protein, with *high* serum vitamin B_{12} levels.[54]

In patients with neurological dysfunction secondary to deficiency of vitamin B_{12}, therapy must be prompt and aggressive. At the outset, 1,000 μg cyanocobalamin should be administered intramuscularly daily. This dose should be continued on a daily basis, or at least several times weekly, for several months, while the patient's neurological progress is monitored. Subsequently, 1,000 μg cyanocobalamin should be given intramuscularly every 2 weeks indefinitely to patients with pernicious anemia.

CALCIFEROL (VITAMIN D)

The exact role of vitamin D in neuromuscular function is unclear. This nutrient appears to be involved in muscle metabolism and contractility by virtue of action either on the Ca^{2+}-dependent myosin adenosine triphosphatase (ATPase) system or directly on the phospholipid component of the sarcolemmal membrane. A deficiency in vitamin D has been held responsible at least in part for the weakness, fatigability, and muscular atrophy encountered in patients with hyperparathyroidism and renal tubular acidosis,[55] and minor changes in muscle have been encountered histologically in patients with parathyroid disease.[56] Intestinal malabsorption or dietary insuffi-

ciency may lead to vitamin D deficiency, with resultant hypocalcemia, osteomalacia, muscle weakness, and tetany; again, minor myopathic features may be noted histologically.

Hearing loss has also been reported as a reflection of hypovitaminosis D.[57] Of particular interest is the often unappreciated development of hypovitaminosis D with hypocalcemia in the course of prolonged use of anticonvulsants,[58–60] including phenytoin, phenobarbital, and carbamazepine. A depression of vitamin D levels is not invariable, however, even in the presence of significant hypocalcemia.[61,62]

TOCOPHEROL (VITAMIN E)

There has been growing awareness of the role of acquired vitamin E deficiency in the production of neurological dysfunction in both children and adults.[63–65] The exact role of vitamin E in the nervous system is not known, although it appears important in maintaining the integrity of biological membranes and has antioxidant properties.

On a background of chronic fat malabsorption—as occurs for example in cholestatic liver disease, cystic fibrosis, or celiac disease—a deficiency of vitamin E results in a remarkable constellation of neurological abnormalities referable to both the central and peripheral nervous systems.[66–74] Features of both spinocerebellar degeneration and polyneuropathy have been recognized clinically, including progressive gait ataxia, incoordination of the limbs, ophthalmoplegia, dysarthria, extensor plantar responses, loss of reflexes in the legs, limb weakness, and marked impairment of vibratory and position sense. The occurrence of seizures has been recorded,[75] and there may be involvement of the autonomic nervous system. Vitamin E deficiency has also been documented in several instances of infantile motor neuron disease (Werdnig-Hoffman disease),[76] although without demonstrable intestinal malabsorption. When the typical clinical features of vitamin E deficiency are associated with retinitis pigmentosa, acanthocytosis, and abetalipoproteinemia, the rubric *Bassen-Kornzweig syndrome* is employed.[77]

A lack of tocopherol has been demonstrated in peripheral nerves in vitamin E–deficient patients.[78] Electrophysiological studies demonstrate reduced sensory action potentials and at least mild abnormalities of peripheral sensory conduction velocity, reverting to normal after treatment with vitamin E.[79] Somatosensory evoked potentials exhibit a central delay in conduction, in keeping with pathological changes in the posterior columns, and there may be a prolonged P100 latency in visual evoked potentials.

Pathological studies demonstrate loss of large-caliber myelinated axons in the peripheral nerves; accumulation of lipid pigment in nerve cells bodies in the dorsal root ganglia, anterior horns, and brainstem motor nuclei; degenerative changes in the cerebellar cortex; and, most strikingly, degeneration of the posterior columns and, to a lesser extent, the spinocerebellar tracts. There is remarkable plate- or disc-like swelling of axons in the posterior columns, in Clarke's column, and in the cuneate nuclei of the brainstem. Such axonal swelling, referred to as *neuroaxonal dystrophy,* is also found in experimental vitamin E deficiency. Similar disc-like swellings of axons are found in Hallervorden-Spatz disease, but no definite alteration of vitamin E absorption has been documented in that disorder; furthermore, the vitamin E deficiency disorders fail to demonstrate deposition of iron in the basal ganglia, which is the hallmark of Hallervorden-Spatz disease.

Variable improvement in the clinical and electrophysiological manifestations of vitamin E deficiency has been observed following the administration of tocopherol either orally or, perhaps preferably, parenterally. It has been noted that intramuscular injection of 50 to 100 mg of vitamin E, given every 3 to 7 days for up to 44 months, may arrest the evolution of the neurological disease but not necessarily reverse the clinical symptomatology.[80]

Chronic oxygen neurotoxicity, perhaps in association with a loss of calcium homeostasis, may be a pathogenetic factor of possible significance in degenerative diseases of the nervous system such as Parkinson's disease, Huntington's disease, amyotrophic lateral sclerosis, and Alzheimer's disease.[81,82] The recent demonstration of a genetically determined deficiency of superoxide dismutase,[83] an enzyme that detoxifies oxygen free radicals, in familial instances of amyotrophic lateral sclerosis underscores the potential importance of this concept. As a corollary, the antioxidant properties of α-tocopherol and of ascorbic acid and β-carotene as free radical scavengers have prompted their consideration as therapeutic agents in such degenerative disorders. There is, however, disagree-

ment as to the actual tissue level of these agents, particularly tocopherol, at least in Parkinson's disease.[84] Moreover, in preliminary studies, any benefit from the use of these antioxidants appears conjectural at best.

OTHER DISORDERS FOR WHICH A NUTRITIONAL DEFECT HAS BEEN SUGGESTED

Marchiafava-Bignami Disease

Marchiafava-Bignami disease, or primary degeneration of the corpus callosum, is a rare disorder encountered largely, although not exclusively, in nutritionally depleted chronic alcoholics.[20,85] Originally thought to appear particularly in middle-aged or elderly men of Italian descent addicted to drinking crude red wine, it is clear that the most important factor underlying its appearance is actually chronic and severe nutritional depletion. Characteristic changes of the disease have been noted in association with disorders of clearly recognized nutritional origin such as Wernicke's encephalopathy and pellagra; in several well-documented, pathologically verified instances, there has been no history of alcohol ingestion.[86] It is unfortunately not possible to define more precisely the specific nutritional defect in this disease, although it has been suggested that thiamine deficiency is of primary importance.

The clinical features of Marchiafava-Bignami disease, which are nonspecific, include a variety of psychiatric symptoms, dementia, aphasia, seizures, heightened muscle tone, tremor, paralysis, stupor, and coma. The course of the disease may be measured in terms of months, occasionally years. Although progressive in an overall sense, patients have occasionally exhibited clinical plateaus or even frank remissions in their clinical course. The fundamental pathological change is a symmetrical degeneration of the myelin sheaths in the midzone of the corpus callosum, with relatively good preservation of axons and without appreciable inflammatory changes. Such degenerative changes are not confined to the corpus callosum; similar changes may be found in the anterior commissure, symmetrically disposed in the cerebral white matter, the optic chiasm, or the middle cerebellar peduncles. Although once looked on as a neuropathological curiosity not diagnosable during life, the lesions may be readily identified with CT scanning or MRI.

Central Pontine Myelinolysis

First described in 1959[87] but reported in large numbers since, central pontine myelinolysis is characterized clinically by a rapidly evolving flaccid quadriplegia with bulbar paralysis; pathologically it is identified by demyelination confined for the most part to the basal portion of the mid and upper pons and symmetrically distributed about the midline. Consciousness is preserved, and patients may be able to communicate by moving the eyelids, the only motor activity remaining in extreme cases; the term *locked-in syndrome* is appropriately applied to cases of this sort. The course of the disease is rapid, patients generally dying within 3 weeks of the onset.

Although originally looked on as nutritional in origin, it has become apparent that many if not most cases of central pontine myelinolysis are in fact due to overly vigorous correction of the hyponatremia frequently encountered in the neglected malnourished alcoholic,[88-90] as discussed in detail in Chapters 17 and 30. It has been suggested that an osmotic shift may be more important in producing demyelination than the serum level of sodium per se.[91] It is unclear if chronic nutritional depletion plays a specific role in the pathogenesis.

Jamaican Neuropathy

In 1897 Strachan described a group of patients in Jamaica who presented with numbness and burning in the limbs, girdle pains, impaired vision and hearing, muscle weakness and wasting, hyporeflexia, and sensory ataxia in association with a mucocutaneous lesion such as angular stomatitis and glossitis.[92] Virtually identical cases were subsequently reported in a variety of circumstances of nutritional depletion.[93] The clinical features are predominantly those of a sensory neuropathy. Pathological alterations have been described in the peripheral nerves, posterior columns, spinocerebellar tracts, and optic nerves. Similar clinical features occurring in association with spasticity were later described by Denny-Brown[94] and Cruickshank.[95] In the spastic form of the disease, severe degeneration of both the pyramidal tracts and posterior columns of the spinal cord has been documented, with involvement of the spinocerebellar and spinothalamic pathways in some cases. It is unclear whether the neuropathic disorder of Strachan and the myelopathic variety of Cruickshank represent different entities or simply different manifestations of the same process. The designation *Jamaican neuropathy* is often applied indiscriminately to all such instances. Those disorders characterized by myelopathic features, i.e., spasticity, are, however, sometimes referred to as *tropical spastic paraparesis;* in the latter group, antibody titers to the human T lymphotrophic retrovirus HTLV-I have been repeatedly documented,[96-98] and it is presumed on this basis that viral infection plays a major role in pathogenesis. Whether nutritional depletion plays any role in either form of the disease remains unclear at present. The use of clioquinol has been implicated in the development of subacute myeloptic neuropathy (SMON), a similar disorder occurring most commonly in Japan.

HYPERALIMENTATION

Parenteral hyperalimentation utilizing a central venous catheter, generally placed in a jugular vein, is widely used in the management of chronic nutritional depletion at all ages. A number of neurological disorders appear in such patients,[99] reflecting either mechanical or metabolic problems. Complications attributed to mechanical factors, with or without sepsis, include infected subdural collections, cerebral air embolization,[100] cortical vein thrombosis,[101] pseudotumor cerebri,[102] and—in infants—communicating hydrocephalus.[103-105] Metabolic alterations are generally held responsible for a variety of encephalopathic, neuropathic, or myopathic manifestations, virtually all of which are reversible when the underlying metabolic defect is identified and treated appropriately. Encephalopathy is attributed most commonly to hypophosphatemia[106,107] or hyperammonemia[108]; hyperosmolarity has also been implicated and appears to be of particular importance in experimental models of the disorder.[109,110] Biotin deficiency has been described.[111] Patients receiving prolonged parenteral nutrition without thiamine supplementation are at risk for developing an acute and fatal encephalopathy resembling Wernicke's disease.[112]

Severe hypophosphatemia has also been blamed for the appearance of a peripheral neuropathy[113] characterized by weakness, areflexia, and paresthesias and sensory impairment. Ataxias, cranial nerve palsies, ophthalmoplegia, blurred vision, and respiratory failure have all been described. At times the clinical evolution of this disorder is sufficiently acute to suggest a diagnosis of Guillain-Barré syndrome.[114,115] Chromium[116] and linolenic acid[117] deficiency have been documented in individual cases. Selenium deficiency has been associated with a reversible myopathy,[118,119] evidenced by proximal muscle weakness and tenderness and an elevated creatine kinase level.

The possible role of vitamin D deficiency in the production not only of osteomalacia but also of some of these neurological disorders remains to be explored.

REFERENCES

1. Victor M, Adams RD: On the etiology of the alcoholic neurologic diseases: with special reference to the role of nutrition. Am J Clin Nutr 9:379, 1961
2. Roels OA: Vitamin A physiology. JAMA 214:1097, 1970
3. Goodman DS: Vitamin A and retinoids in health and disease. N Engl J Med 310:1023, 1984
4. Kasarskis EJ, Bass NH: Benign intracranial hypertension induced by deficiency of vitamin A during infancy. Neurology 32:1292, 1982
5. Dreyfus PM, Victor M: Effects of thiamine deficiency on the central nervous system. Am J Clin Nutr 9:414, 1961
6. Dreyfus PM: The quantitative histochemical distribution of thiamine in normal rat brain. J Neurochem 4:183, 1959
7. Dreyfus PM: The quantitative histochemical distribution of thiamine in deficient rat brain. J Neurochem 8:139, 1961
8. Jubb KV, Saunders LZ, Coats HV: Thiamine deficiency encephalopathy in cats. J Comp Pathol 66:217, 1956
9. Victor M: Alcohol and nutritional diseases of the nervous system. JAMA 167:65, 1958
10. Hornabrook RW: Alcoholic neuropathy. Am J Clin Nutr 9:398, 1961
11. Victor M, Adams RD, Collins GH: The Wernicke-Korsakoff Syndrome. FA Davis, Philadelphia, 1971
12. Jagadha V, Deck JHN, Halliday WC, Smyth HS: Wernicke's encephalopathy in patients on peritoneal dialysis or hemodialysis. Ann Neurol 21:78, 1987
13. Heier MS, Fossa SD: Wernicke-Korsakoff-like syndrome in patients with colorectal carcinoma treated with high-dose doxifluridine (5'-dFUrd). Acta Neurol Scand 73:449, 1986
14. Leigh D, McBurney A, McIlwain H: Erythrocyte transketolase activity in the Wernicke-Korsakoff syndrome. Br J Psychiatry 139:153, 1981
15. Leigh D, McBurney A, McIlwain H: Wernicke-Korsakoff syndrome in monozygotic twins: a biochemical pecularity. Br J Psychiatry 139:156, 1981
16. Nixon PF: Is there a genetic component to the pathogenesis of the Wernicke-Korsakoff syndrome? Alcohol Alcohol 19:219, 1984
17. Mukherjee AB, Ghazanfari A, Svoronos S, et al: Transketolase abnormality in tolazamide-induced Wernicke's encephalopathy. Neurology 36:1508, 1986
18. Wolf PL, Levin MB: Shoshin beriberi. N Engl J Med 262:1302, 1960
19. Victor M, Adams RD, Mancall EL: A restricted form of cerebellar cortical degeneration occurring in alcoholic patients. Arch Neurol 1:579, 1959
20. Mancall EL: Some unusual neurologic diseases complicating chronic alcoholism. Am J Clin Nutr 9:404, 1961
21. Mancall EL, McEntee WJ: Alteration of the cerebellar cortex in nutritional encephalopathy. Neurology 15:303, 1965
22. Pedraza OL, Botez MI: Thiamine status in inherited degenerative ataxias. J Neurol Neurosurg Psychiatry 55:136, 1992
23. Victor M, Mancall EL, Dreyfus PM: Deficiency amblyopia in the alcoholic patient: a clinicopathological study. Arch Ophthalmol 64:1, 1960
24. Carroll FD: The etiology and treatment of tobacco-alcohol amblyopia. Am J Ophthalmol 27:713, 847 (two parts), 1944
25. Victor M: Tobacco-alcohol amblyopia: a critique of current concepts of this disorder, with special reference to the role of nutritional deficiency in its causation. Arch Ophthalmol 70:313, 1963
26. Leigh D: Subacute necrotizing encephalomyelopathy in an infant. J Neurol Neurosurg Psychiatry 14:216, 1951
27. Greenhouse AH, Schneck SA: Subacute necrotizing encephalomyelopathy: a reappraisal of the thiamine deficiency hypothesis. Neurology 18:1, 1968
28. Wyatt DT, Noetzel MJ, Hillman RE: Infantile beriberi presenting as subacute necrotizing encephalomyelopathy. J Pediatr 110:888, 1987
29. Hommes FA, Polman HA, Reerink JD: Leigh's encephalomyelopathy: an inborn error of gluconeogenesis. Arch Dis Child 43:423, 1968
30. Worsley HE, Brookfield RW, Elwood JS, et al: Lactic

acidosis with necrotizing encephalopathy in two sibs. Arch Dis Child 40:492, 1965

31. Pincus JH, Itokawa Y, Cooper JR: Enzyme inhibiting factor in subacute necrotizing encephalomyelopathy. Neurology 19:841, 1969

32. Cooper JR, Pincus JH: Thiamine triphosphate deficiency in Leigh's disease (subacute necrotizing encephalomyelopathy). In Hommes FA, Van den Berg CT (eds): Inborn Errors of Metabolism. Academic Press, New York, 1973

33. Victor M, Adams RD: The neuropathology of experimental vitamin B_6 deficiency in monkeys. Am J Clin Nutr 4:346, 1956

34. Jolliffe N, Bowman KM, Rosenblum LA, Fein HD: Nicotinic acid deficiency and encephalopathy. JAMA 114:307, 1940

35. Lishman WA: Cerebral disorders in alcoholism: syndromes of impairment. Brain 104:1, 1981

36. Blakemore WF: Isoniazid. p. 476. In Spencer PS, Schaumburg HH (eds): Experimental and Clinical Neurotoxicology. Williams & Wilkins, Baltimore, 1980

37. Ishii N, Nishihara Y: Pellagra encephalopathy among tuberculous patients: its relation to isoniazid therapy. J Neurol Neurosurg Psychiatry 48:628, 1985

38. Parry GJ, Bredesen DE: Sensory neuropathy with low-dose pyridoxine. Neurology 35:1466, 1985

39. Dalton K, Dalton MJT: Characteristics of pyridoxine overdose neuropathy syndrome. Acta Neurol Scand 76:8, 1987

40. Blecher TE, Williams ER: Simultaneous myasthenia gravis and pernicious anemia: a case report with organ antibody studies. Postgrad Med J 43:122, 1967

41. Troncoso J, Mancall EL, Schatz NJ: Visual evoked responses in pernicious anemia. Arch Neurol 36:168, 1979

42. Pant SS, Asbury AK, Richardson EP Jr: The myelopathy of pernicious anemia: a neuropathological reappraisal. Acta Neurol Scand 44, suppl 35:1, 1968

43. Mayer RF: Peripheral nerve function in vitamin B_{12} deficiency. Arch Neurol 13:355, 1965

44. Cox-Klazinga M, Endtz LJ: Peripheral nerve involvement in pernicious anaemia. J Neurol Sci 45:367, 1980

45. McCombe PA, McLeod JG: The peripheral neuropathy of vitamin B_{12} deficiency. J Neurol Sci 66:117, 1984

46. Fine EJ, Hallett M: Neurophysiological study of subacute combined degeneration. J Neurol Sci 45:331, 1980

47. Greenfield JG, Carmichael EA: The peripheral nerves in cases of subacute combined degeneration of the cord. Brain 58:483, 1935

48. Beach RS, Morgan R, Wilkie F, et al: Plasma vitamin B_{12} level as a potential cofactor in studies of human immunodeficiency virus type 1–related cognitive changes. Arch Neurol 49:501, 1992

49. Herbert V: Vitamin B_{12} deficiency neuropsychiatric damage in acquired immunodeficiency syndrome. Arch Neurol 50:569, 1993

50. Robertson KR, Stern RA, Hall CD, et al: Vitamin B_{12} deficiency and nervous system disease in HIV infection. Arch Neurol 50:807, 1993

51. Reynolds EH, Bottiglieri T, Laundy M, et al: Vitamin B_{12} metabolism in multiple sclerosis. Arch Neurol 49:649, 1992

52. Reynolds EH: Multiple sclerosis and vitamin B_{12} metabolism. J Neurol Neurosurg Psychiatry 55:339, 1992

53. Sigal SH, Hall CA, Antel JP: Plasma R binder deficiency and neurologic disease. N Engl J Med 317:1330, 1987

54. Reynolds EH, Bottiglieri T, Laundy M, et al: Subacute combined degeneration with high serum vitamin B_{12} level and abnormal vitamin B_{12} binding protein: new cause of an old syndrome. Arch Neurol 50:739, 1993

55. Vicale CT: The diagnostic features of a muscular syndrome resulting from hyperparathyroidism, osteomalacia owing to renal tubular acidosis, and perhaps to related disorders of calcium metabolism. Trans Am Neurol Assoc 74:143, 1949

56. Snowdon JA, Macfie AC, Pearce JB: Hypocalcaemic myopathy with paranoid psychosis. J Neurol Neurosurg Psychiatry 39:48, 1976

57. Irwin J: Hearing loss and calciferol deficiency. J Laryngol Otol 100:1245, 1986

58. Davie MWJ, Emberson CE, Lawson DEM, et al: Low plasma 25-hydroxyvitamin D and serum calcium levels in institutionalized epileptic subjects: associated risk factors, consequences and response to treatment with vitamin D. Q J Med 52:79, 1983

59. Rajantie J, Lamberg-Allardt C, Wilska M: Does carbamazepine treatment lead to a need of extra vitamin D in some mentally retarded children? Acta Paediatr Scand 73:325, 1984

60. Gough H, Goggin T, Bissessar A, et al: A comparative study of the relative influence of different anticonvulsant drugs, UV exposure and diet on vitamin D and calcium metabolism in out-patients with epilepsy. Q J Med 59:569, 1986

61. William C, Netzloff M, Folkerts L, et al: Vitamin D metabolism and anticonvulsant therapy: effect of sunshine on incidence of osteomalacia. South Med J 77:834, 1984

62. Weinstein RS, Bryce GF, Sappington LJ, et al: Decreased serum ionized calcium and normal vitamin D

metabolic levels with anticonvulsant drug treatment. J Clin Endocrinol Metab 58:1003, 1984

63. Bieri JG, Corash L, Hubbard VS: Medical uses of vitamin E. N Engl J Med 308:1063, 1983

64. Muller DPR, Lloyd JK, Wolff OH: Vitamin E and neurological function. Lancet 1:225, 1983

65. Satya-Murti S, Howard L, Krohel G, Wolf B: The spectrum of neurologic disorder from vitamin E deficiency. Neurology 36:917, 1986

66. Rosenblum JL, Keating JP, Prensky AL, Nelson JS: A progressive neurologic syndrome in children with chronic liver disease. N Engl J Med 304:503, 1981

67. Guggenheim MA, Ringel SP, Silverman A, Grabert BE: Progressive neuromuscular disease in children with chronic cholestasis and vitamin E deficiency: diagnosis and treatment with alpha tocopherol. J Pediatr 100:51, 1982

68. Werlin SL, Harb JM, Swick H, Blank E: Neuromuscular dysfunction and ultrastructural pathology in children with chronic cholestasis and vitamin E deficiency. Ann Neurol 13:291, 1983

69. Sokol RJ, Guggenheim MA, Iannaccone ST, et al: Improved neurologic function after long-term correction of vitamin E deficiency in children with chronic cholestasis. N Engl J Med 313:1580, 1985

70. Weder B, Meienberg O, Wildi E, Meier C: Neurologic disorder of vitamin E deficiency in acquired intestinal malabsorption. Neurology 34:1561, 1984

71. Harding AE, Muller DPR, Thomas PK, Willison HJ: Spinocerebellar degeneration secondary to chronic intestinal malabsorption: a vitamin E deficiency syndrome. Ann Neurol 12:419, 1982

72. Harding AE, Matthews S, Jones S, et al: Spinocerebellar degeneration associated with a selective defect of vitamin E absorption. N Engl J Med 313:32, 1985

73. Landrieu P, Selva J, Alvarez F, et al: Peripheral nerve involvement in children with chronic cholestasis and vitamin E deficiency: a clinical, electrophysiological and morphological study. Neuropediatrics 16:194, 1985

74. Davidai G, Zakaria T, Goldstein R, et al: Hypovitaminosis E induced neuropathy in exocrine pancreatic failure. Arch Dis Child 61:901, 1986

75. Ogumekan AO: Vitamin E deficiency and seizures in animals and man. Can J Neurol Sci 6:43, 1979

76. Shapira Y, Amit R, Rachmilewitz E: Vitamin E deficiency in Werdnig-Hoffman disease. Ann Neurol 10:266, 1981

77. Sobrevilla LA, Goodman ML, Kane CA: Demyelinating central nervous system disease, macular atrophy and acanthocytosis (Bassen-Kornzweig syndrome). Am J Med 37:821, 1964

78. Traber MG, Sokol RJ, Ringel SP, et al: Lack of tocopherol in peripheral nerves of vitamin E-deficient patients with peripheral neuropathy. N Engl J Med 317:262, 1987

79. Brin MF, Pedley TA, Lovelace RE, et al: Electrophysiologic features of abetalipoproteinemia: functional consequences of vitamin E deficiency. Neurology 36:669, 1986

80. Perlmutter DH, Gross P, Jones HR, et al: Intramuscular vitamin E repletion in children with chronic cholestasis. Am J Dis Child 141:170, 1987

81. Jesberger JA, Richardson JS: Oxygen free radicals and brain dysfunction. Int J Neurosci 57:1, 1991

82. Tangney CC, Tanner CM: Vitamin E and PD. Neurology 43:634, 1993

83. Rosen DR, Siddique T, Patterson D, et al: Mutations in Cu/Zn superoxide dismutase gene are associated with familial amyotrophic lateral sclerosis. Nature 362:59, 1993

84. Dexter DT, Ward RJ, Wells FR, et al: Alpha-tocopherol levels in brain are not altered in Parkinson's disease. Ann Neurol 32:591, 1992

85. Marchiafava E: Degeneration of the brain in chronic alcoholism. Proc R Soc Med 26:1151, 1933

86. Kosaka K, Aoki M, Kawasaki N, et al: A non-alcoholic Japanese patient with Wernicke's encephalopathy and Marchiafava-Bignami disease. Clin Neuropathol 3:231, 1984

87. Adams RD, Victor M, Mancall EL: Central pontine myelinolysis: a hitherto undescribed disease occurring in alcoholic and malnourished patients. Arch Neurol Psychiatry 81:154, 1959

88. Laureno R: Pontine and extrapontine myelinolysis following rapid correction of experimental hyponatremia. Trans Am Neurol Assoc 106:98, 1981

89. Laureno R: Central pontine myelinolysis following rapid correction of hyponatremia. Ann Neurol 13:232, 1983

90. Ayus JC, Krothapalli RK, Arieff AI: Treatment of symptomatic hyponatremia and its relation to brain damage. N Engl J Med 317:1190, 1987

91. McKee AC, Winkelman MD, Banker BQ: Central pontine myelinolysis in severely burned patients: relationship to serum hyperosmolality. Neurology 38:1211, 1988

92. Strachan H: On a form of multiple neuritis prevalent in the West Indies. Practitioner 59:477, 1897

93. Fisher M: Residual neuropathological changes in Canadians held prisoners of war by the Japanese. Can Serv Med J 11:157, 1955

94. Denny-Brown D: Neurological conditions resulting from prolonged and severe dietary restriction. Medicine (Baltimore) 26:41, 1947

95. Cruickshank EK: Neuromuscular disease in relation to nutrition. Fed Proc 20, suppl 7:345, 1961

96. Osame M, Matsumoto T, Usuku K, et al: Chronic progressive myelopathy associated with elevated antibodies to human T-lymphotropic virus type I and adult T-cell leukemialike cells. Ann Neurol 21:117, 1987

97. Vernant JC, Maurs L, Gessian A, et al: Endemic tropical spastic paraparesis associated with human T-lymphotropic virus type I: a clinical and seroepidemiological study of 25 cases. Ann Neurol 21:123, 1987

98. Brew BJ, Price RW: Another retroviral disease of the nervous system: chronic progressive myelopathy due to HTLV-I. N Engl J Med 318:1195, 1988

99. Wolfe BM, Ryder MA, Nishikawa RA, et al: Complications of parenteral nutrition. Am J Surg 152:93, 1986

100. Hwang TL, Fremaux R, Sears ES, et al: Confirmation of cerebral air embolism with computerized tomography. Ann Neurol 13:214, 1983

101. Souter RG, Mitchell A: Spreading cortical venous thrombosis due to infusion of hyperosmolar solution into the internal jugular vein. Br Med J 285:935, 1982

102. Saxena VK, Heilpern J, Murphy SF: Pseudotumor cerebri: a complication of parenteral hyperalimentation. JAMA 235:2124, 1976

103. Haar FL, Miller CA: Hydrocephalus resulting from superior vena cava thrombosis in an infant. J Neurosurg 42:597, 1975

104. Stewart DR, Johnson DG, Myers GG: Hydrocephalus as a complication of jugular catheterization during total parenteral nutrition. J Pediatr Surg 10:771, 1975

105. Puljic S, Newman LJ, Heitlinger L, et al: Radiography of hydrocephalus after total parenteral nutrition. Neuroradiology 16:76, 1978

106. Silvis SE, DiBartolomeo AG, Aaker HM: Hypophosphatemia and neurological changes secondary to oral caloric intake: a variant of hyperalimentation syndrome. Am J Gastroenterol 73:215, 1980

107. Baughman FA Jr, Papp JP: Wernicke's encephalopathy with intravenous hyperalimentation: remarks on similarities between Wernicke's encephalopathy and the phosphate depletion syndrome. Mt Sinai J Med 43:48, 1976

108. Grazer RE, Sutton JM, Friedstrom S, McBarron FD: Hyperammonemic encephalopathy due to essential amino acid hyperalimentation. Arch Intern Med 144:2278, 1984

109. Derr R, Zieve L: Intracellular distribution of phosphate in the underfed rat developing weakness and coma following total parenteral nutrition. J Nutr 106:1398, 1976

110. Derr RF, Zieve L: Weakness, neuropathy and coma following total parenteral nutrition in underfed or starved rats: relationship to blood hyperosmolarity and brain water loss. J Lab Clin Med 92:521, 1978

111. Kien CL, Kohler E, Goodman SI, et al: Biotin-responsive in vivo carboxylase deficiency in two siblings with secretory diarrhea receiving total parenteral nutrition. J Pediatr 99:546, 1981

112. Vortmeyer AO, Hagel C, Laas R: Haemorrhagic thiamine deficient encephalopathy following prolonged parenteral nutrition. J Neurol Neurosurg Psychiatry 55:826, 1992

113. Yagnik P, Singh N, Burns R: Peripheral neuropathy with hypophosphatemia in a patient receiving intravenous hyperalimentation. South Med J 78:1381, 1985

114. Furlan AJ, Hanson M, Cooperman A, Farmer RG: Acute areflexic paralysis: association with hyperalimentation and hypophosphatemia. Arch Neurol 32:706, 1975

115. Weintraub MI: Hypophosphatemia mimicking acute Guillain-Barré-Strohl syndrome: a complication of parenteral hyperalimentation. JAMA 235:1040, 1976

116. Jeejeebhoy KN, Chu RC, Marliss EB, et al: Chromium deficiency, glucose intolerance, and neuropathy reversed by chromium supplementation, in a patient receiving long-term total parenteral nutrition. Am J Clin Nutr 30:531, 1977

117. Holman RT, Johnson SB, Hatch TF: A case of human linolenic acid deficiency involving neurological abnormalities. Am J Clin Nutr 35:617, 1982

118. Kien CL, Ganther HE: Manifestations of chronic selenium deficiency in a child receiving total parenteral nutrition. Am J Clin Nutr 37:319, 1983

119. Brown MR, Cohen HJ, Lyons JM, et al: Proximal muscle weakness and selenium deficiency associated with long term parenteral nutrition. Am J Clin Nutr 43:549, 1986

16

Neurological Complications of Renal Failure

Neil H. Raskin

The natural history of renal failure and its clinical manifestations has changed since the advent of dialysis programs and kidney transplantation. New neurological syndromes have been defined as a consequence of both increased longevity and the complications of therapy. This chapter summarizes current views of the neurological features of uremia and the neurological complications of dialysis and renal transplantation. Neurological complications of renal carcinoma are not discussed, and paraneoplastic syndromes of the nervous system are reviewed in Chapter 21.

UREMIC ENCEPHALOPATHY

The neurological consequences of uremia are similar in many ways to the effects of other metabolic and toxic disorders on the central nervous system (CNS). There is an aggregation of signs of neural dysfunction, comprising sensorial clouding, dysarthria, gait ataxia, asterixis, action tremor, multifocal myoclonus, and seizures. One or more of these signs may predominate, and their fluctuation from day to day, or sometimes from hour to hour, is characteristic of metabolic encephalopathy.[1]

The clinical features of uremic encephalopathy do not correlate well with any single laboratory abnormality but appear to be related in many patients to the rate of development of renal failure. Thus, stupor and coma are not uncommon in acute renal failure, whereas the CNS may be deranged to a lesser degree in chronic renal failure, despite greater degrees of azotemia.

Alterations of alertness and awareness of the environment are the earliest and most reliable indications of uremic encephalopathy.[2] Initially patients report that their ability to concentrate is impaired; they appear to be fatigued, preoccupied, and apathetic. These symptoms usually wax and wane so that episodes of good performance often occur, but they are short-lived. As the disorder progresses, obtundation becomes more apparent, so that shouting or prodding may be necessary to elicit responses, some of which may be incorrect or inappropriate. The patient's attention span is diminished, so that the ability to subtract 7 from 100 serially may be impaired. There may be perceptual errors, such as misidentification of people and objects; and defective recall and mild confusion become evident. Illusions and misperceptions may progress to frank visual hallucinations. Patients are usually agitated at this point and often recognize, at least at the outset, that they are hallucinating. Thus, a delirium may result from uremia and is indistinguishable from a sedative withdrawal state or an intoxication with psychotropic drugs.

Asterixis

Tremulousness usually appears before asterixis is evident and may be a more sensitive index of encephalopathy.[3] The tremor is coarse and irregular, absent at rest, and most evident in the fingers of the outstretched hands. It becomes more apparent during the elicitation of asterixis.

Asterixis is nearly always present once sensorial clouding appears; it is a sensitive, early, reliable indication of uremic encephalopathy. First described by Adams and Foley in patients with portal-systemic encephalopathy,[4] asterixis is now known to be a nonspecific sign of metabolic cerebral disruption.[5] It is most effectively elicited by having the patient hold the upper limbs outstretched in fixed hyperextension at the elbow and wrist, with fingers spread apart.[6] After a latency of up to 30 seconds, there appear at irregular intervals side-to-side movements of the fingers, flexion-extension ("flapping") of the fingers at the metacarpophalangeal joints, and flexion-extension at the wrist. These movements are rapid and arrhythmic, and the flexion phase is more rapid than that of extension. When intravenous devices or restraints preclude testing the upper limbs, it is useful to attempt to elicit asterixis in the lower limbs. The recumbent patient dorsiflexes the foot with the leg extended and elevated; sudden downward jerking of the foot with a slower return to the original downflexed position occurs, as in the upper limbs. The limbs are affected bilaterally but asynchronously. Flapping may be elicited in the face by forceful eyelid closure, strong retraction of the corners of the mouth, pursing of the lips, or protrusion of the tongue. Some degree of voluntary muscle control is necessary to demonstrate asterixis by the aforementioned maneuvers; once stupor or coma supervenes, it is best elicited at the hip joints.[7] With the patient lying supine, the examiner grasps both feet at the ankles and moves the feet upward toward the patient's body so that the thighs are flexed and abducted (Fig. 16-1). Rapid, irregular abduction-adduction movements at the hips signify a positive test.

Electromyography (EMG) performed during asterixis shows periods of complete electrical silence in wrist flexors and extensors during downward flapping movements, which is followed by a compensatory muscle contraction as the extensors restore the limb's posture.[3] This momentary period of electrical

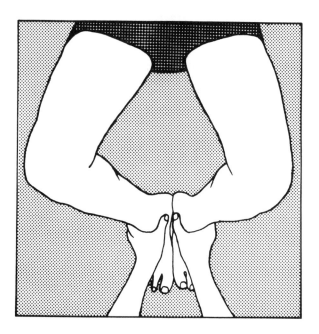

Fig. 16-1 Technique for eliciting asterixis in the stuporous or comatose patient. (Modified from Noda S, Ito H, Umezaki H, Minato S: Hip flexion-abduction to elicit asterixis in unresponsive patients. Ann Neurol 18:96, 1985, with permission.)

silence is not accompanied by electroencephalographic (EEG) changes. The jerky movement of asterixis is temporally related to the offset, rather than the onset, of EMG silence.[8]

It is widely held that asterixis is not an involuntary movement disorder; rather, it is said to be a failure to maintain a sustained posture (*asterixis* is derived from the Greek *a sterigma*: "without support"). However, the author has observed that many of these patients, when tested with their upper limbs supinated, display flapping movements at the wrists *against* gravity; thus, asterixis, as Shahani and Young[9] have suggested, is probably a disorder of the central mechanisms underlying sustained muscle contraction, a "negative" form of myoclonus. This conclusion is supported by the additional observation (unpublished) that many patients with illnesses that result in myoclonus also display asterixis.

Myoclonus

Multifocal myoclonus is a gross twitching of muscles that is sudden, arrhythmic, and asymmetrical, involving muscles first at one locus, then another, affecting chiefly the facial and proximal limb musculature.[10,11] It commonly occurs in uremia and in the encephalopathies that accompany pulmonary insufficiency, hyperosmolar states, and penicillin intoxication; it is a strong indication of a severe metabolic disturbance and usually does not appear until stupor has supervened. This form of myoclonus probably signifies cortical irritability; in fact, at times it is difficult to distinguish from a multifocal seizure disorder. However, the muscle twitching is usually not reflected by EEG spike discharges.[1] An unusual form of myoclonus that occurs primarily during willed movements may also occur[12]; bilateral EEG spike discharges occurred concurrent with uremic action myoclonus in one carefully studied case.[13] Intravenous benzodiazepine drugs abolished the involuntary movements in three treated patients.[12,13]

Asterixis and multifocal myoclonus may be so intense in uremia that muscles appear to fasciculate, giving rise to the term *uremic twitching*. Twitching is often widely distributed and may involve the perioral or lingual musculature in severe cases. On the other hand, grosser movements of the limb musculature may also result from myoclonus and simulate chorea or ballismus.[14]

Uremic twitching has been linked to the alterations in cerebral phosphate metabolism that occur in uremia; Harrison and co-workers found that the occurrence of twitching correlated better with phosphate levels in the cerebrospinal fluid (CSF) than in serum in experimental canine uremic encephalopathy.[15,16] Large intravenous doses of phosphate resulted in twitching with a delay that correlated with the time of elevation of CSF phosphate. Moreover, intracisternal injection of phosphate caused profound twitching. In a clinical account of 17 uremic patients, it was noted that although ratios of CSF to serum phosphate were widely dispersed and not significantly different from those in control patients, the 5 patients with twitching had CSF phosphate levels above 3.8 mg/dl. None of the other 12 uremic patients achieved levels greater than 3.3 mg/dl, and twitching was not evident in any of them.[17] Much more must be known about cerebral phosphate metabolism in uremia to clarify its pathophysiological role.

Motor Abnormalities

During the early stages of uremia, patients are usually clumsy when walking and performing fine

movements of the limbs. Paratonia, snouting, and grasp reflexes may be elicited, probably caused by depression of frontal lobe inhibitory mechanisms.[18] As brainstem function becomes less efficient, limb tone becomes altered. In uremia, extensor muscle tone is usually heightened and is sometimes asymmetrical, unlike the flaccidity that characterizes sedative-induced coma; the stretch reflexes are often hyperactive, and ankle clonus and extensor plantar responses may be elicited. With progression of the illness, muscle tone increases further, so that opisthotonos or decorticate posturing of the limbs may appear.[19]

Most uremic patients are diffusely weak (asthenic) and commonly display focal motor signs such as stretch-reflex asymmetry and hemiparesis. Hemiparesis was manifested by 10 of 45 patients studied by Plum and Posner[1]; it often cleared soon after hemodialysis, or it shifted sides during the course of the illness. Hyperkalemia may attend acute renal failure and result in the appearance of flaccid quadriparesis that simulates an acute motor polyneuropathy.

Electroencephalography

The EEG often shows slow background activity and an excess of theta and delta waves, usually frontal in location, perhaps reflecting the decreased cerebral metabolic rate that occurs eventually in all metabolic encephalopathies. Bilateral spike-wave complexes were seen in 14 percent of patients on a chronic hemodialysis program, none of whom had experienced a seizure.[20] As the uremic state progresses, the EEG becomes slower and correlates best with retained nitrogenous compounds, but there is no clear relation between the EEG and a specific serological biochemical abnormality. Similarly, there are delays of visual, auditory, and somatosensory evoked cerebral potentials.[21] Secondary hyperparathyroidism may play a role in generating some of the slowing seen on the EEG; parathyroidectomy prevents EEG slowing in canine renal failure, whereas the administration of parathyroid hormone further slows the EEG.[22]

Convulsions

In acute renal failure, convulsions occurred in 5 of 13 cases reported by Locke and associates.[23] The seizures occurred between the eighth and eleventh days of renal failure and were frequently multiple. They often developed as a terminal event in patients with varying degrees of obtundation. In chronic renal failure, convulsions are usually a late manifestation, nowadays occurring in about 10 percent of patients.[2] Convulsions also occur in association with hemodialysis as part of the *dysequilibrium syndrome*, which is discussed below. There is little evidence that water intoxication or hypertension is the primary cause of uremic seizures. Whereas convulsions are relatively uncommon in other metabolic encephalopathies, the curious admixture of clinical signs of cerebral depression and signs of cerebral excitation is distinctive of uremic encephalopathy.

In the older literature on uremic encephalopathy, convulsions were believed to occur far more often than is reported currently. This misapprehension may have been the result of a failure to differentiate hypertensive encephalopathy from uremia, conditions that sometimes coexist. The presence of hypertensive retinopathy with papilledema is a major sign that distinguishes the two conditions; furthermore, fleeting focal signs of cerebral dysfunction, such as aphasia and cortical blindness, are far more common in hypertensive brain disease than in uremia.

TREATMENT OF UREMIC CONVULSIONS

The pharmacokinetics of anticonvulsant drugs are altered in uremic patients; for example, plasma levels of phenytoin are about 25 percent of those shown by controls for identical dosages.[24] The volume of distribution of drugs is larger in uremia, which is the major reason that plasma levels are lower.[25] In the case of phenytoin, there is also an increased rate of conversion to hydroxylated derivatives by the liver.[26] However, these factors are offset by *higher* plasma levels of free, unbound phenytoin because of the decreased protein binding of drugs that attends renal failure[27]; because the rate of diffusion into brain of anticonvulsant drugs is proportional to the free drug concentration,[28] the latter is the determinant regarding anticonvulsant benefit. Because the free fraction of phenytoin is increased by a factor approximately equal to the factor lowering the plasma concentration of the drug (bound plus unbound fractions), ordinary dosages suffice despite low plasma levels. However, these mechanisms are unbalanced in occasional patients; the author has seen three patients who required

1000 mg/d of phenytoin for adequate anticonvulsant protection, but plasma levels never exceeded 1 mg/L. These principles also apply to valproic acid metabolism,[29] but plasma levels of phenobarbital are unaffected by renal insufficiency.[30]

Meningeal Signs and Cerebrospinal Fluid

Nuchal rigidity, CSF pleocytosis, and alteration of the blood-CSF barrier have all occurred in uremic encephalopathy. In one series, almost one-third of the uremic patients examined had nuchal rigidity and Kernig's sign; about one-half of these patients were shown also to have CSF pleocytosis.[31] In another series, about 10 percent of the uremic patients studied had more than 5 leukocytes per cubic millimeter (range 7 to 600) in the CSF. Pleocytosis bore no relation to the degree of azotemia.[32] Schreiner and Maher found that 30 of 52 uremic patients had CSF protein levels greater than 60 mg/dl; 19 exceeded 80 mg/dl, and 11 were over 100 mg/dl.[32] Elevations of CSF protein may be reduced to the normal range during the immediate postdialysis period.[17] The increments in CSF protein content relate to an alteration in the permeability properties of capillary endothelial cells in brain, adjacent to the CSF, which have tight intercellular junctions.[33]

Pathophysiology of Uremic Encephalopathy

A variety of pathological changes in brain were reported in early studies of uremia. An extensive survey by Olsen indicated that these changes are probably nonspecific and not necessarily related to the uremic state.[34] Neuronal degeneration and necrosis of the granular cell layer of the cerebellar cortex are found often, probably resulting from preterminal hypoxia. Areas of focal demyelination and necrosis are occasionally seen and are probably due to small infarcts resulting from coexisting hypertensive cerebrovascular disease. The water content of uremic brain is normal[34,35]; thus, cerebral edema is not a uremic concomitant.

The cerebral utilization of oxygen declines in uremic encephalopathy, as it does in other metabolic encephalopathies,[36,37] but the correlation between the degree of sensorial clouding and depression of the cerebral oxygen consumption is poor in uremic patients. Levels of cerebral high-energy phosphates are normal, whereas glycolysis and energy utilization are reduced.[38] The basis for reduced brain metabolism in uremia is interference with synaptic transmission, which results in both diminished functional activity and decreased cerebral oxygen consumption because of the reduced neuronal interaction. Thus, in the stuporous states associated with metabolic diseases, the depression of both cerebral metabolic rate and cerebral function, although generally correlated, are probably independent reflections of a general impairment of neuronal processes.

Several mechanisms limit the entry of organic acids into CSF and brain.[39] Organic acids that share a common transport mechanism in the renal tubule are relatively excluded from brain because of poor lipid solubility and binding to plasma proteins. In addition, there is an active transport system in the choroid plexus[40] (an "intracranial proximal renal tubule") that can remove these organic acids from CSF and from the extracellular fluid of brain. These organic acids are neurotoxic, evoking convulsions and myoclonic jerks when given intracisternally or intracortically in low concentration. Uremic encephalopathy may be caused by the accumulation of toxic organic acids, which overwhelm the mechanisms for excluding such compounds from the CNS. Furthermore, a nonspecific increase in cerebral membrane permeability occurs in the uremic animal,[41] one consequence of which is the greater entry into brain of organic acids. The rapid clearing of uremic encephalopathy with dialysis favors the hypothesis that a variety of small, water-soluble molecules are responsible for the encephalopathy.

Many additional biochemical abnormalities have been detected in uremia, but the large number of biological depressants in uremic serum make it difficult to determine their individual significance. For example, many enzyme activities are altered.[42] The systemic acidosis that attends the uremic state is not reflected within the CNS.[43] Membrane "pumps" for both Na-K ATPase and the calcium ion are altered.[44,45] The calcium pump alteration is probably caused by the accumulation of parathyroid hormone and leads to an increase in brain calcium of about 50 percent.[46] Because of these findings and others, it has been speculated that parathyroid hormone is a uremic toxin,[47] but the fact that the hormone is not dialyzable limits interest in this possibility.

UREMIC NEUROPATHY

Neuropathy is the commonest neurological consequence of uremia, occurring in at least 60 percent of patients who begin dialysis for chronic renal failure.[48] It is a distal, symmetrical, mixed sensorimotor polyneuropathy, affecting the lower limbs to a greater extent than the upper limbs. It is clinically indistinguishable from such other neuropathies as those associated with chronic alcohol abuse, diabetes mellitus, and systemic lupus erythematosus. The rate of progression, severity, and prominence of motor or sensory signs are variable. Men are affected far more frequently than women. Serological biochemical abnormalities do not correlate well with this or any other neurological manifestation of the uremic state; the chronicity and severity of renal failure appear to be more important to the development of neuropathy.

The earliest signs of neuropathy are impaired vibratory sensation in the lower limbs[49] and loss of the tendon reflexes, first the Achilles and then the patellar responses.[19] The neuropathy usually evolves over several months but on occasion follows a fulminant course. In some patients an acute disabling flaccid quadriplegia develops.[50] In others, distal weakness, muscle atrophy, and sensory loss progress over several months, plateau, and then remain stationary despite worsening of the renal failure. The factors that determine these differences in the clinical course of the neuropathy are unclear.

Burning feet reportedly occurred in 7 percent of patients in early series[51]; nowadays this symptom is far less common, probably because of the widespread practice of prescribing the B vitamins for these patients. Over 40 percent of patients report dysesthesia; unpleasant tingling, band-like constrictions, swelling sensations, and tender distal limbs are described by many patients with early uremic neuropathy. *Muscle cramps* of the distal limbs also occur commonly[52] and have been held to herald peripheral nerve involvement; however, many patients with such cramps have no other manifestations of neuropathy. Cramps occur more often in acute uremia and probably reflect either shifts of fluid into muscle or the effects of retained uremic toxins on the muscle membrane.

The *restless legs syndrome* occurs in over 40 percent of patients with varying degrees of renal failure,[52] often accompanied by other signs and symptoms of neuropathy, such as distal dysesthesia or slowing of nerve conduction velocity; it has also been held to herald peripheral nerve involvement. The syndrome comprises creeping, crawling, prickling, pruritic sensations deep within the lower limbs that are worse in the evening and are relieved by movement of the limbs.[53,54] These unpleasant sensations are usually localized to the legs but occasionally occur in the thighs, feet, and upper limbs. Because peripheral neuropathies of assorted cause appear to give rise to the syndrome, sensory input from dysesthetic limbs may well serve as the inciting stimulus of this syndrome; however, Walters and Hening have put forth evidence that spontaneous central sensory interneuronal activity is an alternate possibility.[55] Effective treatment for the restless legs syndrome is now at hand; bedtime doses of clonazepam, bromocriptine, levodopa, or the opioids (propoxyphene or codeine) have all been shown to suppress it.[55,56]

Rapidly advancing *visual loss* may occur over several days, accompanied by reduced pupillary light reactions and edema of the optic discs, presumably reflecting an optic neuropathy. Prompt hemodialysis and corticosteroid therapy can restore vision in most patients.[57]

Effect of Treatment of Renal Failure

In most patients on long-term dialysis, the neuropathy either stabilizes or improves slowly.[58] Patients with mild neuropathy often recover completely with dialysis, but those with severe neuropathy rarely recover even after several years of dialysis. Neuropathy occasionally appears or worsens during the initial weeks of dialysis, a development that is usually interpreted as an indication to increase dialysis time. In recent years the appearance of neuropathy in patients on chronic hemodialysis has become rare,[59] as the result of earlier treatment, more intensive dialysis, and, more importantly, technical improvements in (and thinner) dialysis membranes.

Successful renal transplantation has a clear-cut, predictable, beneficial effect on uremic neuropathy. Progressive improvement usually occurs over 6 to 12 months, often with complete recovery, even in patients who had severe neuropathy before transplantation.[60,61] Recovery may take place biphasically, with an early rapid phase and a later slow phase. Enhanced motor and sensory nerve conduction velocities occur within *days* of renal transplantation.[62]

Electrophysiological Studies

Slowed nerve conduction is a frequent occurrence in uremic patients without other symptoms or signs of neuropathy. In patients with moderate renal failure not requiring dialysis, the serum creatinine elevation correlates with the decreased velocity of motor nerve conduction.[63] Clinical neuropathy appears in patients whose renal function has deteriorated most markedly and whose conduction velocities have slowed the most.[63] Slowing is generalized, involving both motor and sensory fibers in proximal and distal segments of the upper and lower limbs.[64] It has also been shown that late responses (H reflex and F response) become abnormally delayed, more so in the lower limbs, early in the course of renal failure when standard nerve conduction studies are normal.[65] Asbury has observed that the mechanisms accounting for slowed nerve conduction and for neuropathy may be disparate[48]; slowed nerve conduction occurs when creatinine clearance falls below 10 percent of normal[64] and is evident throughout the peripheral nervous system, with slowing often being greater in proximal segments. Once established, slowed nerve conduction is little affected by chronic dialysis. By contrast, neuropathy develops unpredictably, affects the lower limbs distally, and is improved or stabilized by dialysis.

Pathology

The original description of uremic neuropathy as a primary axonal degeneration with secondary segmental demyelination has been corroborated,[66,67] although some would argue that a predominantly demyelinative neuropathy may occur.[68] The segmental loss of myelin appears to be consequent to an abnormality in the axon cylinder, which probably reflects metabolic failure of the perikaryon. All fiber sizes, both myelinated and unmyelinated, are affected, although the largest and most distal fibers are selectively vulnerable. Segmental demyelination occurs in fibers about to undergo breakdown, although nerve fibers degenerating rapidly probably bypass the demyelinative phase.[48] The pathological findings are not specific for uremia; they are not easily distinguishable from those of alcoholic neuropathy, another axonal degeneration that is more severe in the distal aspects of the neuron.

Pathophysiology

The observation that uremic neuropathy improves with dialysis has led most observers to conclude that neuropathy results from the accumulation of dialyzable metabolites. Scribner and colleagues proposed that these substances might be in the "middle molecule" range (molecular weight 500 to 2,000)[69]; compounds of this size cross dialysis membranes much more slowly than smaller molecules such as creatinine and urea, removal of which are the usual measures of chemical control of uremia. Thus, one could achieve chemical control of uremia, using the standard clinical assessments, while failing to remove the putative toxins.

The early hemodialysis experience supports the middle molecule hypothesis. Formerly, dialysis membranes at least 300-μm thick were used, and these cleared middle molecules poorly. Furthermore, increasing dialysis time has a much larger effect on the removal of middle molecules than small molecules.[70] When thinner membranes and longer dialysis time became commonplace, severe neuropathy became much less common. These changes in dialysis technique probably had a large effect on the reduction of middle molecule concentrations relative to those of small molecules. Moreover, peritoneal dialysis is not associated with neuropathy despite greater retention of urea and creatinine, suggesting that the peritoneal membrane is selectively permeable to toxic molecules. Babb and associates have reviewed the data both supporting and refuting the middle molecule hypothesis[70]; the weight of evidence supports the validity of the hypothesis, but convincing supportive studies are lacking.

How a dialyzable toxin might produce neuropathy is of some interest. Inhibition of the metabolism of several B vitamins and the occurrence of nutritional deficiencies have been considered, but no fresh insights have been gained.[14] The elevation of plasma myoinositol levels that occurs in uremic patients led to speculation that this compound bears on the problem of neuropathy.[71] However, early reports that hypermyoinositolemia slowed nerve conduction in animals[72] could not be replicated.[73] Others have found no evidence that myoinositol serves as a uremic neurotoxin.[74,75] Similarly, elevated levels of parathyroid hormone (despite the nondialyzability of the hormone) have been regarded as neurotoxic,[76] but the findings in a study of uremic patients following parathyroidectomy are discordant with this hypothesis.[77] On the other hand, a proximal myopathy may also occur in uremic patients,[78] one major cause of which is secondary hyperparathyroidism.[79]

AUTONOMIC DYSFUNCTION

Several symptoms are commonly reported by uremic patients that probably indicate disordered autonomic function; they include orthostatic lightheadedness, impotence, diarrhea, and excessive perspiration.[80] Direct testing of autonomic responsiveness has shown abnormal responsiveness to the Valsalva maneuver, defective heart rate response to atropine, and reduced baroreceptor sensitivity.[81,82] Hemodialysis-induced hypotension appears to be caused by reduced baroreceptor activity.[80] Whether these alterations are centrally or peripherally mediated remains to be determined.

NEUROLOGICAL COMPLICATIONS OF DIALYSIS

Dialysis prevents terminal uremia but it permits the persistence of an attenuated uremic state that is attended by subtle cognitive alterations.[83,84] Although dialysis stabilizes or prevents uremic encephalopathy and neuropathy, it also causes other neurological disturbances that are found predominantly in dialyzed uremic patients.

Neuropathy from Arteriovenous Fistulas and Amyloid Deposition

The placement of an arteriovenous (A-V) shunt in a limb is requisite for hemodialysis but may disturb peripheral nerve function distal to it. Peripheral nerves in uremic patients appear to be unusually resistant to ischemia.[85] Nevertheless, many A-V shunts result in the "stealing" of blood from the distal limb, producing an ischemic neuropathy characterized by continuous, distal burning pain and, less often, motor dysfunction.[86–88]

The carpal tunnel syndrome may also occur because of the increased venous pressure in the distal limb that is produced by an A-V shunt, leading to increased extravascular volume within the carpal tunnel and thus accounting for median nerve compression.[89] Another operant mechanism is thickening of the synovia of flexor tendons within the carpal tunnel because of a granulomatous reaction with amyloid deposition. This latter mechanism seldom occurs within the first 5 years of dialysis but thereafter becomes increasingly common. The protein constituent of the amyloid has been identified as B_2-microglobulin.[90] Amyloid deposition occasionally occurs epidurally, causing spinal cord compression.[91]

Dysequilibrium Syndrome

A host of neurological problems may arise during or after hemodialysis or peritoneal dialysis, including headache, nausea, muscle cramps, irritability, agitation, delirium, obtundation, and convulsions.[92,93] The more serious neurological sequelae were seen frequently during the 1960s, when patients with advanced uremia were dialyzed aggressively; nowadays, with patients entering dialysis programs early in the course of renal failure and with shortened dialysis times, they are far less common but continue to occur.

Although the syndrome appears most often during the early phases of a rapid hemodialysis program, it may also occur following routine maintenance dialysis. Symptoms usually appear toward the end of a dialysis run, sometimes 8 to 24 hours later, and subside over several hours. When a delirium appears, it usually persists for several days.[94,95] Many patients manifest *exophthalmos* and *increased intraocular pressure* at the height of the syndrome,[96] conditions that, if present, are helpful in the differential diagnosis. The other clinical correlates of the syndrome include increased intracranial pressure, papilledema, and generalized slowing of the EEG.[97,98]

Headache is the commonest symptom reported by patients undergoing dialysis, occurring in about 70 percent of cases.[99] In many patients with preexisting migraine, headaches identical to their spontaneous ones develop during or after hemodialysis. Other patients without prior headache disorders experience headache only in association with dialysis. Headache is usually diffuse and throbbing in quality, similar to the headache that results from uremia per se.

The preponderance of evidence points to shifts of water into the brain as the cause of the dysequilibrium syndrome.[100,101] It was originally postulated that the rapid reduction in blood urea could not be paralleled by brain urea because of the influence of the blood-brain barrier. This effect was believed to produce an osmotic gradient between blood and brain, causing movement of water into brain and resulting in encephalopathy, increased intracranial pressure, and cerebral edema. This hypothesis became known as the "reverse urea effect," and the unequal effects of dialysis on tissue and blood solutes, resulting in an osmotic gradient, underlie the naming of this disorder, the "dysequilibrium" syndrome. Experimental models of dysequilibrium have shown that an osmotic gradient between brain and blood is not created by the movement of urea alone; however, the principle of the hypothesis has been supported by the demonstration that unidentified osmotically active substances ("idiogenic osmoles") are present in brain in the dialyzed uremic animal (and not in the dialyzed nonuremic animal), creating an osmotic gradient between brain and blood that results in shifts of water into brain.[98] Arieff and co-workers have shown that a decrease in the intracellular pH of cerebral cortex attends experimental dysequilibrium, reflecting an increased production of organic acids[102]; the latter are osmotically active solutes that may account for the osmotic gradient.

Wernicke's Encephalopathy

Because thiamine is a water-soluble vitamin that might be expected to pass through dialysis membranes with ease, it may seem surprising that evidence of thiamine deficiency does not appear more often in patients undergoing chronic dialysis. However, Wernicke's encephalopathy has occurred in a child and others on chronic dialysis who did not receive regular thiamine supplementation.[103,104] A report of five cases diagnosed by autopsy made the point that ophthalmoplegia was evident in only one of them.[105]

Data pertaining to vitamin turnover in dialyzed patients are surprisingly sparse. In general, dialysis does not remove more thiamine than would normally be excreted in the urine.[106] There is no consistent change in the plasma levels of the B vitamins before and after hemodialysis, but occasional patients have shown 40 percent decrements in thiamine levels.[107] Vitamin levels in the dialysate are generally too low to be measured. Firm plasma protein binding of vitamins may account for these findings. Individual differences in protein binding or in the tissue turnover of thiamine may explain the occasional appearance of Wernicke's disease among dialyzed patients. B-vitamin supplementation is necessary for all of these patients.

Dialysis Dementia

A distinctive, progressive, usually fatal encephalopathy may occur in patients who are chronically dialyzed for periods that exceed 1 year (Figs. 16-2 and 16-3).[108-111] The first symptom is usually a stammering hesitancy of speech that eventually progresses to speech arrest. The speech disorder is intensified during and immediately after dialysis and at first may be seen only during these periods. A thought disorder is usually evident, and there is a consistent EEG abnormality (Fig. 16-4),[112] with bursts of high-voltage slowing and spikes in the frontal leads. As the disorder progresses, speech becomes more dysarthric and aphasic; dementia and myoclonic jerks usually become apparent (Table 16-1) at this time. The other elements of the encephalopathy include hallucinations, delusional thinking, convulsions, asterixis, and, occasionally, focal neurological abnormalities. Early in the course, diazepam is effective in lessening

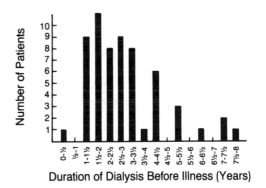

Fig. 16-3 Duration of dialysis prior to onset of symptoms in 60 patients with dialysis dementia. The mean is 2.5 years. (Modified from Chui HC, Damasio AR: Progressive dialysis encephalopathy ("dialysis dementia"). J Neurol 222: 145, 1980, with permission.)

myoclonus and seizures and in improving speech; it becomes less effective later. The CSF is nonrevealing. Increased dialysis time and renal transplantation have not altered the course of the disease. Without treatment, death usually occurs 6 to 9 months after the onset of symptoms (Fig. 16-5). No distinctive abnormalities have been found in brain at autopsy.[2,108,113] Whereas profound undialyzed uremic encephalopathy, especially in infants less than 1 year of age, can resemble dialysis dementia,[114-116] it is not clear whether such cases should be included under this rubric.

Table 16-1 Dialysis Dementia: Analysis of 42 Patients

Feature	Totals
Age at onset (years)	21–68 (average 45)
Months on hemodialysis at onset	9–84 (average 37)
Duration of illness until death (months)	1–15 (average 6)
Sex	21 M, 21 F
Incidence of symptoms (%)	
Dementia	98
Speech impairment	95
Myoclonus	81
Seizures	57
Behavioral abnormalities	52
Gait disorder	17
Tremor	7

(Modified from Lederman RJ, Henry CE: Progressive dialysis encephalopathy. Ann Neurol 4:199, 1978, with permission.)

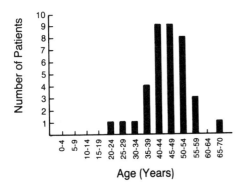

Fig. 16-2 Age distribution of 37 patients with dialysis dementia. The median age is 46 years. (Modified from Chui HC, Damasio AR: Progressive dialysis encephalopathy ("dialysis dementia"). J Neurol 222:145, 1980, with permission.)

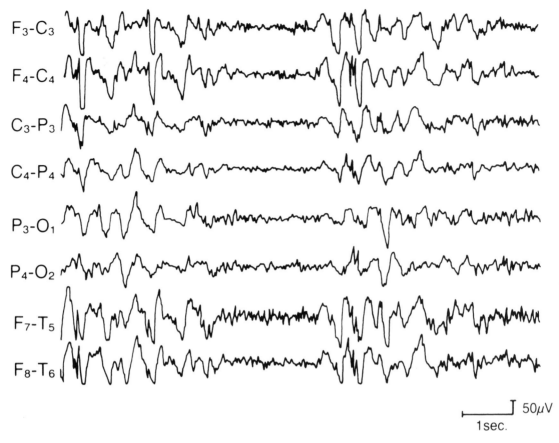

Fig. 16-4 Bilateral spike-wave complexes in dialysis dementia. (Modified from Hughes JR, Schreeder MT: EEG in dialysis encephalopathy. Neurology 30:1148, 1980, with permission.)

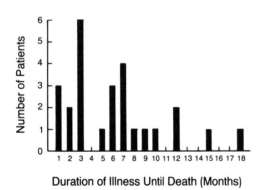

Fig. 16-5 Duration of dialysis dementia until death in 26 patients. The mean is 6 months. (Modified from Chui HC, Damasio AR: Progressive dialysis encephalopathy ("dialysis dementia"). J Neurol 222:145, 1980, with permission.)

PATHOPHYSIOLOGY

The marked geographical variation in the incidence of dialysis dementia throughout the world suggested that an environmental neurotoxin was its cause. Aluminum was incriminated when levels were found to be high in the cerebral gray matter of patients who died from this condition.[117–119] Municipal water supplies heavily contaminated with aluminum have been linked to the appearance of the syndrome in epidemiological studies.[120] Any aluminum present in the dialysate is readily transferred to the patient during dialysis because aluminum is tightly bound to plasma protein, maintaining a gradient from dialysate to plasma; the binding also precludes the removal of aluminum from the patient during dialysis.[121] Persuasive evidence that aluminum was the agent responsible for dialysis dementia was registered when the disease was largely eliminated by removing aluminum from the water used for the dialysate.[122] However, the disease has not quite vanished; another source of aluminum is the orally administered phosphate-binding gels that are given to uremic patients.[123] Remission of the disease may occur when aluminum is removed from the diet, from the dialysate, or from patients by chelation with deferoxamine.[124–126] The neurotoxicity of aluminum may stem from inhibition of an enzyme (dihydropteridine reductase) that is essential for the maintenance of the normal brain levels of tetrahydrobiopterin that are required for the synthesis of specific neurotransmitters.[127]

Aluminum Metabolism

Compared to a daily aluminum intake of a few milligrams in food, dialyzed patients ingest gram amounts as aluminum hydroxide. Only a small fraction of it is absorbed, but considerable aluminum accumulation results. Whereas normal plasma aluminum levels are 6 ± 3 μg/L, dialyzed patients receiving oral aluminum gels (undergoing dialysis with aluminum-free dialysate) have plasma aluminum levels of 55 ± 28 μg/L.[128] Plasma levels under 100 μg/L are believed to be unlikely to result in encephalopathy in dialyzed patients; those with levels between 100 and 200 μg/L are monitored closely; and at levels above 200 μg/L, treatment with deferoxamine may be recommended.[127] However, plasma levels correlate imperfectly with brain levels of aluminum; several patients with dialysis dementia have had plasma aluminum levels below 100 μg/L.[125] Nevertheless, plasma levels provide a reasonable indication of tissue aluminum; bone aluminum determinations provide a better index of the body's accumulation of the element but are far more difficult to obtain. CSF aluminum is normal in patients with dialysis dementia; therefore such measurement is not useful diagnostically.[109]

In chronic renal failure alone, without dialysis, aluminum stores are often markedly increased by mechanisms that are not clear. The inability to excrete aluminum normally absorbed from food sources cannot alone account for the amount of aluminum retained.[119,129] Parathyroid hormone can augment aluminum absorption from the gut, suggesting that the secondary hyperparathyroidism that occurs in uremic patients could result in enhanced aluminum absorption.[130,131] However, parathyroidectomy has not affected the course of dialysis dementia.[119] Following restoration of normal renal function by transplantation, plasma aluminum normalizes within a few weeks, but brain levels remain high for years.[125]

Deferoxamine

Deferoxamine is a chelating agent that binds aluminum with greater affinity than that of the proteins to which aluminum is bound in plasma. The aluminum-deferoxamine complex has a molecular weight of 600 and is easily removed from body fluids by dialysis.[132,133] The aluminum mobilized by deferoxamine administration is an index of total body aluminum, so that this agent has utility in diagnosis[134] as well as in therapy. It is given intravenously, 40 mg/kg, during the last 30 minutes of a dialysis session, and a positive result is obtained if the plasma aluminum, assayed in a specimen obtained 48 hours later, increases by more than 100 μg/L[125]; other investigators use an increment of 200 μg/L[109] as the criterion for a positive test.

Deferoxamine is the mainstay of treatment for dialysis dementia; several protocols for its administration have been proposed. The usual dose is 4 to 6 g/wk, 1 to 2 g given intravenously during the last 2 hours of each dialysis session. For improvement to be seen in dialysis dementia, a year of treatment may be required.[109] Many cases of dialysis dementia have been stabilized or improved by deferoxamine.[133,135] How long treatment must be continued has not yet been determined.

COMPLICATIONS OF TRANSPLANTATION

The major sequelae of transplantation are those related to the abnormal immune state that exists in allograft recipients. This abnormal state may result in the development of brain tumors and unusual infections of the nervous system.

Brain Tumors

The risk that lymphoma will occur after a transplant is about 35 times higher than normal; this increased risk depends almost entirely on the increased incidence of primary lymphoma (formerly known as reticulum cell sarcoma) in brain.[136–139] Prior to the advent of cyclosporine, the average interval to the development of lymphoma was 3 to 6 years[139]; patients receiving cyclosporine, presumably because of more intense immunosuppression, have had a much shorter interval prior to the development of lymphoma, averaging 3 to 6 months.[140,141]

Primary brain lymphoma produces a clinical syndrome that includes increased intracranial pressure, rapidly evolving focal neurological signs, or both. Convulsions are relatively uncommon. Most of these tumors are situated within the deep central structures of the hemisphere periventricularly; involvement of the corpus callosum and fornix and subependymal spread are characteristic. The computed tomography (CT) scan usually shows a mass much larger than is suggested by the clinical findings; there are usually isodense and hypodense areas, with striking enhancement following the administration of contrast material. One-third of these tumors are multifocal.[142] Most tumor-afflicted patients die within a few weeks to months after diagnosis, although a few patients are responsive to corticosteroids and radiotherapy. Primary brain lymphoma that arises in the nonimmunocompromised patient has a far better prognosis and is usually radiosensitive.[143]

Lymphomas occur with greater frequency in allograft recipients receiving immunosuppressant therapy than in immunosuppressed patients who have not received a transplant. This finding suggests that factors in addition to drug-induced immune deficiency are important.

Infections of the Central Nervous System

Systemic fungal infections are found at autopsy in about 45 percent of allograft recipients; brain abscess formation occurs in about one-third.[144] In nearly all of these cases, the primary source of infection is the lung. Chest x-ray examination and fever are therefore important diagnostic aids in differentiating fungal brain abscess from brain tumor in transplant patients. *Aspergillus* has a unique predilection for dissemination to brain and accounts for most fungal brain abscesses; *Candida* is the second common offending fungus, and *Nocardia* and *Histoplasma* account for the rest.

The clinical syndrome resulting from fungal brain abscess is usually a delirium accompanied by seizures and focal neurological signs.[145] The CT scan often shows low absorption areas with minimal or no enhancement and little mass effect.[146] The CSF is often unrevealing.[147] Brain biopsy may be the only reliable way to establish a diagnosis.

Cryptococcal meningitis is particularly common in transplant patients,[148] but cerebral infarction is their commonest neurological affliction.[149] Progressive multifocal leukoencephalopathy,[150] central pontine myelinolysis,[151] and toxoplasmosis[152] also occur in these patients.

Further details concerning fungal infections involving the CNS are provided in Chapter 40.

REFERENCES

1. Plum F, Posner JB: Multifocal, diffuse, and metabolic brain diseases causing stupor or coma. p. 177. In: The Diagnosis of Stupor and Coma. 3rd Ed. FA Davis, Philadelphia, 1980
2. Tyler HR, Tyler KL: Neurologic complications. p. 311. In Eknoyan G, Knochel JP (eds): The Systemic Consequences of Renal Failure. Grune & Stratton, Orlando, FL, 1984
3. Leavitt S, Tyler HR: Studies in asterixis. Arch Neurol 10:360, 1964
4. Adams RD, Foley JM: The neurologic changes in the more common types of severe liver disease. Trans Am Neurol Assoc 74:217, 1949
5. Conn HO: Asterixis in non-hepatic disorders. Am J Med 29:647, 1960
6. Adams RD, Foley JM: The neurological disorder associated with liver disease. Res Publ Assoc Res Nerv Ment Dis 32:198, 1953
7. Noda S, Ito H, Umezaki H, Minato S: Hip flexion-abduction to elicit asterixis in unresponsive patients. Ann Neurol 18:96, 1985
8. Ugawa Y, Genba K, Shimpo T, Mannen T: Onset and offset of electromyographic (EMG) silence in asterixis. J Neurol Neurosurg Psychiatry 53:260, 1990
9. Shahani BT, Young RR: Asterixis—a disorder of the neural mechanisms underlying sustained muscle contraction. p. 301. In Shahani M (ed): The Motor System: Neurophysiology and Muscle Mechanisms. Elsevier, New York, 1976
10. Halliday AM: The electrophysiologic study of myoclonus in man. Brain 90:241, 1967
11. Chadwick D, Hallett M, Harris R, et al: Clinical, bio-

chemical and physiological factors distinguishing myoclonus responsive to 5-hydroxytryptophan, tryptophan plus a monoamine oxidase inhibitor, and clonazepam. Brain 100:455, 1977

12. Chadwick D, French AT: Uraemic myoclonus: an example of reticular reflex myoclonus? J Neurol Neurosurg Psychiatry 42:52, 1979
13. Stark RJ: Reversible myoclonus with uraemia. Br Med J 282:1119, 1981
14. Raskin NH, Fishman RA: Neurologic disorders in renal failure. N Engl J Med 294:143 and 204 (two parts), 1976
15. Harrison TR, Mason MF, Resnik H: Observations on the mechanism of muscular twitchings in uremia. J Clin Invest 15:463, 1936
16. Harrison TR, Mason MF: The pathogenesis of the uremic syndrome. Medicine (Baltimore) 16:1, 1937
17. Freeman RB, Sheff MF, Maher JF, et al: The blood–cerebrospinal fluid barrier in uremia. Ann Intern Med 56:233, 1962
18. Cooper JD, Lazarowitz VC, Arieff AI: Neurodiagnostic abnormalities in patients with acute renal failure: evidence for neurotoxicity of parathyroid hormone. J Clin Invest 61:1448, 1978
19. Tyler HR: Neurologic disorders in renal failure. Am J Med 44:734, 1968
20. Hughes JR: Correlations between EEG and chemical changes in uremia. Electroencephalogr Clin Neurophysiol 48:583, 1980
21. Komosuoglu SS, Mehta R, Jones LA, Harding GFA: Brainstem auditory evoked potentials in chronic renal failure and maintenance hemodialysis. Neurology 35:419, 1985
22. Luria AR: Frontal lobe syndrome. p. 725. In Vinken PJ, Bruyn GW (eds): Handbook of Clinical Neurology. Vol 2. North Holland, Amsterdam, 1969
23. Locke S, Merrill JP, Tyler HR: Neurologic complications of uremia. Arch Intern Med 108:519, 1961
24. Letteri JM, Mellk H, Louis S, et al: Diphenylhydantoin metabolism in uremia. N Engl J Med 285:648, 1971
25. Burgess ED, Friel PN, Blair AD, Raisys VA: Serum phenytoin concentrations in uremia. Ann Intern Med 94:59, 1981
26. Borga O, Hoppel C, Odar-Cederlöf I, Garle M: Plasma levels and renal excretion of phenytoin and its metabolites in patients with renal failure. Clin Pharmacol Ther 26:306, 1979
27. Campion DS: Decreased drug binding by serum albumin during renal failure. Toxicol Appl Pharmacol 25:391, 1973
28. Martin BK: Potential effect of the plasma proteins on drug distribution. Nature 207:274, 1965
29. Brewster D, Muir NC: Valproate plasma protein binding in the uremic condition. Clin Pharmacol Ther 27:76, 1980
30. Fabre J, de Freudenreich J, Duckert A, et al: Influence of renal insufficiency on the excretion of chloroquine, phenobarbital, phenothiazines, and methacycline. Helv Med Acta 33:307, 1966
31. Madonick MJ, Berke K, Schiffer I: Pleocytosis and meningeal signs in uremia: report on sixty-two cases. Arch Neurol Psychiatry 64:431, 1950
32. Schreiner G, Maher JF: Uremia: Biochemistry, Pathogenesis and Treatment. Charles C Thomas, Springfield, IL, 1961
33. Sterrett PR, Thompson AM, Chapman AL, et al: The effects of hyperosmolarity on the blood-brain barrier: a morphological and physiological correlation. Brain Res 77:281, 1974
34. Olsen S: The brain in uremia. Acta Psychiatr Neurol Scand Suppl 156:1, 1961
35. Fishman RA, Raskin NH: Experimental uremic encephalopathy: permeability and electrolyte metabolism of brain and other tissues. Arch Neurol 17:10, 1967
36. Scheinberg P: Effects of uremia on cerebral blood flow and metabolism. Neurology 4:101, 1954
37. Heyman A, Patterson JL Jr, Jones RW Jr: Cerebral circulation and metabolism in uremia. Circulation 3:558, 1951
38. Van den Noort S, Ekel RE, Brine KL, et al: Brain metabolism in experimental uremia. Arch Intern Med 126:831, 1970
39. Fishman RA: Blood-brain and CSF barriers to penicillin and related organic acids. Arch Neurol 15:113, 1966
40. Cserr HF: Physiology of the choroid plexus. Physiol Rev 51:273, 1971
41. Fishman RA, Raskin NH: Experimental uremic encephalopathy: permeability, ion exchange, and brain "spaces." Trans Am Neurol Assoc 90:71, 1965
42. Hicks JM, Young DS, Wootton IDP: The effect of uraemic blood constituents on certain cerebral enzymes. Clin Chim Acta 9:228, 1964
43. Posner JB, Swanson AG, Plum F: Acid-base balance in cerebrospinal fluid. Arch Neurol 12:479, 1965
44. Fraser CL, Sarnacki P, Arieff AI: Abnormal sodium transport in synaptosomes from brain of uremic rats. J Clin Invest 75:2014, 1985
45. Fraser CL, Sarnacki P, Arieff AI: Calcium transport abnormality in uremic rat brain synaptosomes. J Clin Invest 76:1789, 1985
46. Arieff AI, Massry S: Calcium metabolism of brain in acute renal failure. J Clin Invest 53:387, 1974

47. Massry SG: Current status of the role of parathyroid hormone in uremic toxicity. Contrib Nephrol 49:1, 1985

48. Asbury AK: Uremic neuropathy. p. 1811. In Dyck PJ, Thomas PK, Lambert EH, Bunge R (eds): Peripheral Neuropathy. 2nd Ed. WB Saunders, Philadelphia, 1984

49. Nielsen VK: The peripheral nerve function in chronic renal failure: IV. An analysis of the vibratory perception threshold. Acta Med Scand 191:287, 1972

50. Ropper AH: Accelerated neuropathy of renal failure. Arch Neurol 50:536, 1993

51. Nielsen VK: The peripheral nerve function in chronic renal failure: II. Intercorrelation of clinical symptoms and signs and clinical grading of neuropathy. Acta Med Scand 190:113, 1971

52. Nielsen VK: The peripheral nerve function in chronic renal failure: I. Clinical symptoms and signs. Acta Med Scand 190:105, 1971

53. Ekbom KA: Restless legs syndrome. Neurology 10:868, 1960

54. Callaghan N: Restless legs syndrome in uremic neuropathy. Neurology 16:359, 1966

55. Walters AS, Hening W: Clinical presentation and neuropharmacology of restless legs syndrome. Clin Neuropharmacol 10:225, 1987

56. Guilleminault C, Cetel M, Philip P: Dopaminergic treatment of restless legs and rebound phenomenon. Neurology 43:445, 1993

57. Knox DL, Hanneken AM, Hollows FC, et al: Uremic optic neuropathy. Arch Ophthalmol 106:50, 1988

58. Nielsen VK: The peripheral nerve function in chronic renal failure: VII. Longitudinal course during terminal renal failure and regular hemodialysis. Acta Med Scand 195:155, 1974

59. Manis T, Friedman EA: Dialytic therapy for irreversible uremia. N Engl J Med 301:1260 and 1321 (two parts), 1979

60. Bolton CF, Baltzan MA, Baltzan RB: Effects of renal transplantation on uremic neuropathy. N Engl J Med 284:1170, 1971

61. Nielsen VK: The peripheral nerve function in chronic renal failure: VIII. Recovery after renal transplantation: clinical aspects. Acta Med Scand 195:163, 1974

62. Oh SJ, Clements RS Jr, Lee YW, Diethelm AG: Rapid improvement in nerve conduction velocity following renal transplantation. Ann Neurol 4:369, 1978

63. Jebsen RH, Tenckhoff H, Honet JC: Natural history of uremic polyneuropathy and effects of dialysis. N Engl J Med 277:327, 1967

64. Nielsen VK: The peripheral nerve function in chronic renal failure: VI. The relationship between sensory and motor nerve conduction and kidney function, azotemia, age, sex and clinical neuropathy. Acta Med Scand 194:455, 1973

65. Ackil AA, Shahani BT, Young RR, Rubin NE: Late response and sural conduction studies. Arch Neurol 38:482, 1981

66. Dyck PJ, Johnson WJ, Lambert EH, et al: Segmental demyelination secondary to axonal degeneration in uremic neuropathy. Mayo Clin Proc 46:400, 1971

67. Forno L, Alston W: Uremic polyneuropathy. Acta Neurol Scand 43:640, 1967

68. Said G, Bondier L, Selva J, et al: Different patterns of uremic polyneuropathy: clinicopathologic study. Neurology 33:567, 1983

69. Scribner BH, Farrell PC, Miltutinovic J, et al: Evolution of the middle molecule hypothesis. p. 190. In: Proceedings of the Fifth International Congress of Nephrology, Vol 3, 1972

70. Babb AL, Ahmad S, Bergström J, Scribner BH: The middle molecule hypothesis in perspective. Am J Kidney Dis 1:46, 1981

71. Clements RS Jr, De Jesus PV Jr, Winegrad AI: Raised plasma-myoinositol levels in uraemia and experimental neuropathy. Lancet 1:1137, 1973

72. De Jesus PV Jr, Clements RS Jr, Winegrad AI: Hypermyoinositolemic polyneuropathy in rats. J Neurol Sci 21:237, 1974

73. Jeffreys JGR, Palmano KP, Sharma AK, Thomas PK: Influence of dietary myoinositol on nerve conduction and inositol phospholipids in normal and diabetic rats. J Neurol Neurosurg Psychiatry 41:333, 1978

74. Reznek RH, Salway JG, Thomas PK: Plasma myoinositol concentration in uraemic neuropathy. Lancet 1:675, 1977

75. Blumberg A, Esslen E, Burgi W: Myoinositol—a uremic neurotoxin? Nephron 21:186, 1978

76. Avram MM, Feinfeld DA, Huatuco AH: Search for the uremic toxin: decreased motor-nerve conduction velocity and elevated parathyroid hormone in uremia. N Engl J Med 298:1000, 1978

77. Giulio SD, Chkoff N, Lhoste F, et al: Parathormone as a nerve poison in uremia. N Engl J Med 299:1134, 1978

78. Lazaro RP, Kirshner HS: Proximal muscle weakness in uremia: case report and review of the literature. Arch Neurol 37:555, 1980

79. Patten BM: Neuromuscular complications. p. 281. In Eknoyan G, Knochel JP (eds): The Systemic Consequences of Renal Failure. Grune & Stratton, Orlando, FL, 1984

80. Zucchelli P, Sturani A, Zuccala A, et al: Dysfunction of the autonomic nervous system in patients with end-stage renal failure. Contrib Nephrol 45:69, 1985

81. Campese VM, Romoff MS, Levitan D, et al: Mechanisms of autonomic nervous system dysfunction in uremia. Kidney Int 20:246, 1981

82. Campese VM, Procci WR, Levitan D, et al: Autonomic nervous system dysfunction and impotence in uremia. Am J Nephrol 2:140, 1982

83. Osberg JW, Meares GJ, McKee DC, Burnett GB: Intellectual functioning in renal failure and chronic dialysis. J Chronic Dis 35:445, 1982

84. English A, Savage RD, Britton PG, et al: Intellectual impairment in chronic renal failure. Br Med J 1:888, 1978

85. Castaigne P, Cathala HP, Beaussart-Boulenge L, Petrover M: Effect of ischaemia on peripheral nerve function in patients with chronic renal failure undergoing dialysis treatment. J Neurol Neurosurg Psychiatry 35:631, 1972

86. Bolton CF, Driedger AA, Lindsay RM: Ischaemic neuropathy in uraemic patients caused by bovine arteriovenous shunt. J Neurol Neurosurg Psychiatry 42:810, 1979

87. Wilbourn AJ, Furlan AJ, Hulley W, Ruschhaupt W: Ischemic monomelic neuropathy. Neurology 33:447, 1983

88. Wytrzes L, Markley HG, Fisher M, Alfred H: Brachial neuropathy after brachial artery-antecubital vein shunts for chronic hemodialysis. Neurology 37:1398, 1987

89. Warren DJ, Otieno LS: Carpal tunnel syndrome in patients on intermittent haemodialysis. Postgrad Med J 51:450, 1975

90. Ullian ME, Hammond WS, Alfrey AC, et al: Beta-2-microglobulin-associated amyloidosis in chronic hemodialysis patients with carpal tunnel syndrome. Medicine (Baltimore) 68:107, 1989

91. Allain TJ, Stevens PE, Bridges LR, Phillips ME: Dialysis myelopathy: quadriparesis due to extradural amyloid of β_2 microglobulin origin. Br Med J 296:752, 1988

92. Peterson H, Swanson AG: Acute encephalopathy occurring during hemodialysis. Arch Intern Med 113:877, 1964

93. Kennedy AC, Linton AL, Luke RG, et al: The pathogenesis and prevention of cerebral dysfunction during dialysis. Lancet 1:790, 1964

94. Tyler HR: Neurological complications of dialysis, transplantation, and other forms of treatment in chronic uremia. Neurology 15:1081, 1965

95. Glick ID, Goldfield MD, Kovnat PJ: Recognition and management of psychosis associated with hemodialysis. Calif Med 119:56, 1973

96. Sitprija V, Holmes JH: Preliminary observations on the changes in intracranial pressure and intraocular pressure during hemodialysis. Trans Am Soc Artif Intern Organs 8:300, 1962

97. Hampers CL, Doak PB, Callaghan MN, et al: The electroencephalogram and spinal fluid during hemodialysis. Arch Intern Med 118:340, 1966

98. Arieff AI, Massry SG, Barrientos A, et al: Brain water and electrolyte metabolism in uremia: effects of slow and rapid hemodialysis. Kidney Int 4:177, 1973

99. Bana DS, Yap AU, Graham JR: Headache during hemodialysis. Headache 12:1, 1972

100. Arieff AI, Lazarowitz VC, Guisado R: Experimental dialysis disequilibrium syndrome: prevention with glycerol. Kidney Int 14:270, 1978

101. Wakim KG: The pathophysiology of the dialysis disequilibrium syndrome. Mayo Clin Proc 44:406, 1969

102. Arieff AI, Guisado R, Massry SG, Lazarowitz VC: Central nervous system pH in uremia and the effects of hemodialysis. J Clin Invest 58:306, 1977

103. Faris AA: Wernicke's encephalopathy in uremia. Neurology 22:1293, 1972

104. Lopez RI, Collins GK: Wernicke's encephalopathy: a complication of chronic hemodialysis. Arch Neurol 18:248, 1968

105. Jagadha V, Deck JHN, Halliday WC, Smyth HS: Wernicke's encephalopathy in patients on peritoneal dialysis or hemodialysis. Ann Neurol 21:78, 1987

106. Debari VA, Frank O, Baker H, Needle MA: Water soluble vitamins in granulocytes, erythrocytes and plasma obtained from chronic hemodialysis patients. Am J Clin Nutr 39:410, 1984

107. Lasker N, Harvey A, Baker H: Vitamin levels in hemodialysis and intermittent peritoneal dialysis. Trans Am Soc Artif Intern Organs 9:51, 1963

108. Alfrey AC, Mishell JM, Burks J, et al: Syndrome of dyspraxia and multifocal seizures associated with chronic hemodialysis. Trans Am Soc Artif Intern Organs 18:257, 1972

109. Alfrey AC: Neurologic manifestations of renal diseases. p. 1483. In Asbury AK, McKhann GM, McDonald WI (eds): Diseases of the Nervous System. WB Saunders, Philadelphia, 1986

110. Chui HC, Damasio AR: Progressive dialysis encephalopathy ("dialysis dementia"). J Neurol 222:145, 1980

111. Lederman RJ, Henry CE: Progressive dialysis encephalopathy. Ann Neurol 4:199, 1978

112. Hughes JR, Schreeder MT: EEG in dialysis encephalopathy. Neurology 30:1148, 1980

113. Burks JS, Alfrey AC, Huddleston J, et al: A fatal encephalopathy in chronic hemodialysis patients. Lancet 1:764, 1976

114. Rotundo A, Nevins TE, Lipton M, et al: Progressive

encephalopathy in children with chronic renal insufficiency in infancy. Kidney Int 21:486, 1982

115. Foley CM, Polinsky MS, Gruskin AB, et al: Encephalopathy in infants and children with chronic renal disease. Arch Neurol 38:656, 1981

116. Etheridge WB, O'Neill WM Jr: The "dialysis encephalopathy syndrome" without dialysis. Clin Nephrol 10:250, 1978

117. Alfrey AC, LeGendre GR, Kaehny WD: The dialysis encephalopathy syndrome: possible aluminum intoxication. N Engl J Med 294:184, 1976

118. McDermott JR, Smith AI, Ward MK, et al: Brain-aluminium concentration in dialysis encephalopathy. Lancet 1:901, 1978

119. Alfrey AC: Aluminum metabolism in uremia. Neurotoxicology 1:43, 1980

120. Report from the registration committee of the European dialysis and transplant association: Dialysis dementia in Europe. Lancet 2:190, 1980

121. Kaehny WD, Alfrey AC, Holman RE, Shorr WJ: Aluminum transfer during hemodialysis. Kidney Int 12:361, 1977

122. Davison AM, Walker GS, Oli H, Lewins AM: Water supply aluminium concentration, dialysis dementia, and effect of reverse-osmosis water treatment. Lancet 2:785, 1982

123. Salusky IB, Foley J, Nelson P, Goodman WG: Aluminum accumulation during treatment with aluminum hydroxide and dialysis in children and young adults with chronic renal disease. N Engl J Med 324:527, 1991

124. Milne FJ, Sharf B, Bell P, Meyers AM: The effect of low aluminum water and desferrioxamine on the outcome of dialysis encephalopathy. Clin Nephrol 20:202, 1983

125. Van de Vyver FL, Silva FJE, D'Haese PC, et al: Aluminum toxicity in dialysis patients. Contrib Nephrol 55:198, 1987

126. Sideman S, Manor D: The dialysis dementia syndrome and aluminum intoxication. Nephron 31:1, 1982

127. Altmann P, Al-Salihi F, Butter K, et al: Serum aluminum levels and erythrocyte dihydropteridine reductase activity in patients on hemodialysis. N Engl J Med 317:80, 1987

128. Alfrey AC: Aluminum. Adv Clin Chem 23:69, 1983

129. Arieff AI, Cooper JD, Armstrong D, Lazarowitz VC: Dementia, renal failure, and brain aluminum. Ann Intern Med 90:741, 1979

130. Mayor GH, Remedi RF, Sprague SM, Lovell KL: Central nervous system manifestations of oral aluminum: effect of parathyroid hormone. Neurotoxicology 1:33, 1980

131. Slatopolsky E: The interaction of parathyroid hormone and aluminum in renal osteodystrophy. Kidney Int 31:842, 1987

132. Molitoris BA, Alfrey PS, Miller NL, et al: Efficacy of intramuscular and intraperitoneal deferoxamine for aluminum chelation. Kidney Int 31:986, 1987

133. Swartz RD: Deferoxamine and aluminum removal. Am J Kidney Dis 6:358, 1985

134. Milliner DS, Nebeker HG, Ott SM, et al: Use of the deferoxamine infusion test in the diagnosis of aluminum-related osteodystrophy. Ann Intern Med 101:775, 1984

135. Sprague SM, Corwin HL, Wilson RS, et al: Encephalopathy in chronic renal failure responsive to deferoxamine therapy. Arch Intern Med 146:2063, 1986

136. Hoover R, Fraumeni JF Jr: Risk of cancer in renal-transplant recipients. Lancet 2:55, 1973

137. Schneck SA, Penn I: De novo brain tumours in renal-transplant recipients. Lancet 1:983, 1971

138. Schneck SA, Penn I: Cerebral neoplasms associated with renal transplantation. Arch Neurol 22:226, 1970

139. Penn I: Depressed immunity and the development of cancer. Clin Exp Immunol 46:459, 1981

140. Cleary ML, Warnke R, Sklar J: Monoclonality of lymphoproliferative lesions in cardiac transplant recipients: clonal analysis based on immunoglobulin-gene rearrangements. N Engl J Med 310:477, 1984

141. Starzl TE, Nalesnik MA, Porter KA, et al: Reversibility of lymphomas and lymphoproliferative lesions developing under cyclosporin-steroid therapy. Lancet 1:583, 1984

142. Spillane JA, Kendall BE, Moseley IF: Cerebral lymphoma: clinical-radiological correlation. J Neurol Neurosurg Psychiatry 45:199, 1982

143. Schaumburg HH, Plank CR, Adams RD: The reticulum cell sarcoma–microglioma group of brain tumours: a consideration of their clinical features and therapy. Brain 95:199, 1972

144. Rifkind D, Marchioro TL, Schneck SA, et al: Systemic fungal infections complicating renal transplantation and immunosuppressive therapy: clinical, microbiologic, neurologic and pathologic features. Am J Med 43:28, 1967

145. Beal MF, O'Carroll CP, Kleinman GM, Grossman RI: Aspergillosis of the nervous system. Neurology 32:473, 1982

146. Enzmann DR, Brant-Zawadzki M, Britt RH: CT of central nervous system infections in immunocompromised patients. AJNR 1:239, 1980

147. Carbone P, Sabesin SM, Sidransky H, et al: Secondary aspergillosis. Ann Intern Med 60:556, 1964

148. Schröter GPJ, Temple DR, Husberg BS, et al: Cryp-

tococcosis after renal transplantation: report of ten cases. Surgery 79:268, 1976

149. Adams HP Jr, Dawson G, Coffman TJ, Corry RJ: Stroke in renal transplant recipients. Arch Neurol 43: 113, 1986

150. McCormick WF, Schochet SS Jr, Sarles HE, Calverley JR: Progressive multifocal leukoencephalopathy in renal transplant recipients. Arch Intern Med 136:829, 1976

151. Schneck SA: Neuropathological features of human organ transplantation: II. Central pontine myelinolysis and neuroaxonal dystrophy. J Neuropathol Exp Neurol 25:18, 1966

152. Townsend JJ, Wolinsky JS, Baringer JR, et al: Acquired toxoplasmosis: a neglected cause of treatable nervous system disease. Arch Neurol 32:335, 1975

17

Neurological Manifestations of Electrolyte Disturbances

Jack E. Riggs

Electrolyte disturbances are encountered frequently in clinical practice and are associated with a variety of characteristic central or peripheral (including muscle) neurological manifestations.[1] Since electrolyte disturbances are secondary processes, effective management requires identification and treatment of the primary disorder in addition to correction of the electrolyte abnormality. The neurological consequences of electrolyte disorders are usually functional rather than structural, and the clinical neurological manifestations of these disorders are therefore usually reversible with appropriate therapy. The neurological manifestations of abnormalities of serum sodium, potassium, calcium, and magnesium are reviewed in this chapter.

SODIUM

Extracellular fluid volume is directly dependent upon total body sodium, the principal osmotic component of that fluid compartment. In general, most patients with hyponatremia are hypo-osmolar, and those with hypernatremia are hyperosmolar. The neurological manifestations of sodium abnormalities, whether hyponatremia or hypernatremia, usually involve the central rather than the peripheral nervous system and reflect respectively hypo-osmolarity and hyperosmolarity. Because of the brain's ability to adapt to changes in serum osmolarity, the propensity of hyponatremia or hypernatremia to produce neurological symptoms depends upon the rapidity with which the sodium disturbance develops.[1]

Hyponatremia

Although relatively infrequent, hyponatremia with normal osmolarity (pseudohyponatremia) typically occurs in the setting of hyperlipidemia or hyperproteinemia. Hyponatremia with hyperosmolarity usually occurs in the setting of hyperglycemia. Hyponatremia is most often associated with hypo-osmolarity and is usually separated into three categories depending upon whether the extracellular fluid volume is decreased, normal, or increased. *Hypo-osmolar hyponatremia with hypovolemia* results from renal loss (e.g., after diuretic usage or with mineralocorticoid deficiency, salt-losing nephropathy, and osmotic diuresis) or extrarenal loss (e.g., by vomiting, diarrhea, and third-space losses) of sodium. *Hypo-osmolar hyponatremia with normovolemia* (no edema) results from conditions such as the syndrome of inappropriate secretion of antidiuretic hormone (SIADH), glucocorticoid deficiency, hypothyroidism, or stress and in response to various drugs (including carbamazepine and many psychotropic agents). *Hypo-osmolar hypona-*

tremia with excess extracellular fluid (edema) occurs in conditions such as cirrhosis, cardiac failure, nephrotic syndrome, and acute or chronic renal failure. The separation of hypo-osmolar hyponatremia into these three categories based on the extracellular fluid volume status has therapeutic implications. In normovolemic and hypervolemic hypo-osmolar hyponatremia, the fundamental principle of therapy is water restriction, whereas in hypovolemic hypo-osmolar hyponatremia the basis of therapy is replacement of water and sodium (generally with isotonic saline).[2]

Among hospitalized patients, hyponatremia occurs with an incidence of about 1.0 percent and a prevalence of about 2.5 percent.[3] The seriousness of hyponatremia cannot be overemphasized. Hyponatremic patients have an overall mortality rate 7 to 60 times that of hospitalized patients without hyponatremia.[3,4] However, the increased mortality associated with hyponatremia may reflect the seriousness of underlying disorders rather than the hyponatremia per se.[1]

Neurological symptoms related to hyponatremia are seen much more frequently in patients with acute rather than chronic hyponatremia.[5–7] For example, a serum sodium concentration of 130 mEq/L may produce neurological symptoms if it developed rapidly, whereas a serum sodium concentration of 115 mEq/L may be asymptomatic if it developed slowly. An alteration in mental status is the most common neurological manifestation of hyponatremia and may range from mild confusion to coma. The encephalopathy is associated with nonspecific generalized slowing on the electroencephalogram. The occurrence of convulsions in the setting of acute hyponatremia (typically with a serum sodium concentration less than 115 mEq/L) is ominous and portends a mortality rate of more than 50 percent. The occurrence of seizures in patients with acute hyponatremia represents a medical emergency and necessitates rapid but only partial correction of the serum sodium concentration. Control of hyponatremic seizures has been described with the use of 3% saline (4 to 6 ml/kg), which acutely raised serum sodium 3 to 5 mEq/L.[8] Occasionally focal neurological signs and symptoms are seen in the setting of hyponatremia; they include hemiparesis, monoparesis, ataxia, nystagmus, tremor, rigidity, aphasia, and unilateral corticospinal tract signs. These focal abnormalities usually represent aggravation of an underlying structural lesion and remit with resolution of the hyponatremia. Although occasional muscle twitches and fasciculations may be seen in acute hyponatremia, muscle symptoms other than cramps are not common.[9] The central nervous system (CNS) manifestations of acute hyponatremia may be related to the cerebral edema that occurs in this setting.[10] Details regarding the factors that mitigate hyponatremic osmotic brain swelling are not fully understood.[11] However, sustained hyponatremia is associated with large reductions in the brain's content of intracellular organic osmolytes.[12]

The use or restriction of fluids may have profound effects on the eventual outcome of patients with hyponatremia and acute neurological disease.

SUBARACHNOID HEMORRHAGE AND UNSELECTED INTRACRANIAL DISEASE

Hyponatremia frequently develops in patients with subarachnoid hemorrhage due to ruptured saccular aneurysms and is usually attributed to SIADH. Clinicians often manage these patients by instituting some degree of fluid restriction. This measure is not entirely unwarranted, since patients with subarachnoid hemorrhage may do somewhat better when fluid is restricted early in their course.[13] In a retrospective study of 134 consecutive patients from The Netherlands, 44 patients developed hyponatremia between the second and tenth days following aneurysmal subarachnoid hemorrhage.[14] Hyponatremia was defined as a serum sodium level below 135 mEq/L on at least 2 consecutive days. Of the 44 hyponatremic patients, 25 fulfilled the laboratory criteria for SIADH. Cerebral infarction, defined as a focal neurological deficit with or without computed tomographic (CT) confirmation or a deterioration in the level of consciousness with CT confirmation of ischemic changes, occurred in 46 of the 134 patients. Of the cerebral infarcts, 27 occurred in the 44 hyponatremic patients (61.4 percent), but only 19 occurred in the 90 normonatremic patients (21.1 percent). Of the 44 hyponatremic patients, 26 were fluid-restricted; of these, 21 developed infarcts (80.8 percent). Of the 18 hyponatremic patients who were not fluid-restricted, only 6 developed infarcts (33.3 percent). Of the 25 patients who fulfilled the laboratory criteria for SIADH, 17 were fluid-restricted; of these, 15 developed infarcts (88.2 percent). Thus, fluid restriction in hyponatremia following subarachnoid hemorrhage, particularly in those thought to have SIADH, appears to increase markedly the risk of cerebral infarction.

Some insight has been gained into the basis for this apparent hazard of fluid restriction in patients with subarachnoid hemorrhage who develop hyponatremia. In a study of 12 unselected neurosurgical patients with intracranial disease who fulfilled the laboratory criteria for SIADH, 10 had significant decreases in their total blood volume.[15] Because absence of hypovolemia is considered one of the criteria for making the diagnosis of SIADH,[16] the finding of decreased blood volume in patients with hyponatremia and intracranial disease suggests that these patients do not have true SIADH. In a prospective study of 21 patients with aneurysmal subarachnoid hemorrhage, plasma volume decreased by more than 10 percent in 11 of the patients.[17] Serum sodium decreased in 9 of the 21 patients. Plasma volume decreased by more than 10 percent in 6 of 9 patients with hyponatremia and in 5 of 12 patients with normal serum sodium. Of the 9 patients with hyponatremia, 8 had a negative sodium balance, whereas only 4 of the 12 patients with normal serum sodium had a negative sodium balance. Finally, 10 of the 12 patients with a negative sodium balance had a decrease in plasma volume of more than 10 percent. Hyponatremia following aneurysmal subarachnoid hemorrhage thus appears to be related to salt-wasting, as was originally suggested,[18] and not to SIADH. Fluid restriction instituted to correct hyponatremia attributed to presumed SIADH in such patients appears to exacerbate an already volume-depleted state and subjects the patient to an even greater risk of ischemic cerebral damage from vasospasm. Hypervolemic therapy prevents volume depletion but not hyponatremia in patients with subarachnoid hemorrhage.[19]

CENTRAL PONTINE MYELINOLYSIS (OSMOTIC MYELINOLYSIS)

Central pontine myelinolysis was recognized as a distinct clinical entity in 1959.[20] Four cases occurring on a background of alcoholism and malnutrition were described. The pathological features of the disorder consist of symmetrical noninflammatory demyelination in the base of the pons, with relative sparing of neurons and axons. The classic clinical presentation is with pseudobulbar palsy and associated spastic

quadriparesis. Following the original description, many additional cases were reported in rapid succession, suggesting that central pontine myelinolysis is not a rare disorder. Many cases were not associated with alcoholism or malnutrition. By 1964, the relatively high frequency of small subclinical lesions (Fig. 17-1) was noted,[21] and this was validated by subsequent reports.[22–24]

Aleu and Terry, in 1963, suggested that central pontine myelinolysis must be related to some recently introduced factor(s).[25] In that same year, the initial suggestion was made that an "electrolyte imbalance may be a contributing factor" in its development.[26] In 1969 the interesting observation was reported that the acute quadriparesis of central pontine myelinolysis developed only in hospitalized patients who were being hydrated.[27] From an analysis of 12 cases of acute central pontine myelinolysis, Leslie and associates in 1980 noted that there had been a recent rapid rise of serum sodium in each patient.[28] They suggested that central pontine myelinolysis "is an iatrogenic disorder that in most cases is caused by a rapid correction of serum sodium rather than by hyponatremia per se."[28] The factors that led to the appearance of the disorder during the 1950s were the introduction of diuretics, the liberal use of intravenous fluids, and the ability to measure rapidly the serum electrolytes.[1]

Sterns and colleagues, in a review of their experience, noted neurological complications in eight patients whose serum sodium had been corrected by more than 12 mEq/L/d.[29] Conversely, patients with hyponatremia that was corrected more slowly made uncomplicated recoveries. In a review of the literature, these authors found 80 patients with severe hyponatremia (serum sodium less than 106 mEq/L), and in 51 of these enough detail was reported to determine a maximal rate of correction of serum sodium. In the 39 patients who were corrected rapidly (more than 12 mEq/L/d), 22 (58 percent) had some type of neurological complication and 14 were suspected of having central pontine myelinolysis. Among the 13 patients whose hyponatremia was corrected slowly (less than 12 mEq/L/d), none experienced a neurological complication.

Concerning the optimal rate of correction of hyponatremia, even advocates of rapid correction agree that large increases in serum sodium concentration can result in cerebral demyelination.[30] Because

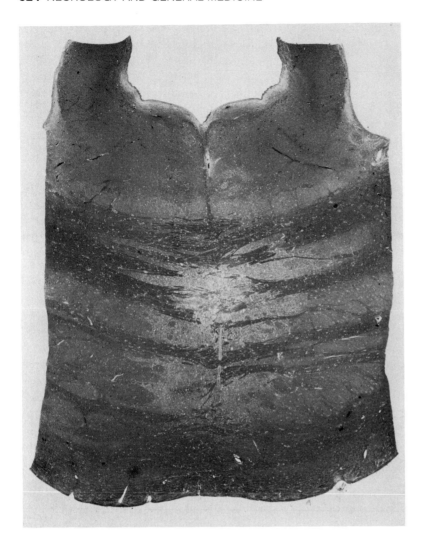

Fig. 17-1 Macrosection of the pons demonstrating central demyelination, an incidental finding of subclinical central pontine myelinolysis in a patient with a history of electrolyte abnormalities and diuretic use. (Luxol-fast blue.)

chronic hyponatremia is less likely to produce neurological symptoms and rapid correction of chronic hyponatremia is more likely to produce neurological injury in experimental models,[31] a judicious approach to the correction of chronic hyponatremia is urged. There is no justification for using hypertonic saline to treat relatively asymptomatic hyponatremia or to correct hyponatremia rapidly to levels above 120 to 125 mEq/L in symptomatic patients.

Animal models of central pontine myelinolysis have now been developed in the dog and the rat.[32–34] In both animals, demyelination follows rapid correction of sustained vasopressin-induced hyponatremia with hypertonic saline. The label *osmotic myelinolysis* has been suggested in preference to *central pontine myelinolysis* because of the well-recognized occurrence of extrapontine myelinolysis.[35] The myelinolysis occurs in areas of the brain characterized by an extensive admixture and apposition of gray and white matter. Although the pathogenesis of osmotic myelinolysis remains undefined, the topography of oligodendrocytes may play a role. Oligodendrocytes in these vulnerable areas are predominantly located within adjacent gray matter rather than within the white matter bundles (Fig. 17-2). Since gray matter is much more vascular than white matter, oligodendrocytes in this location may be more vulnerable to serum osmotic shifts.[35]

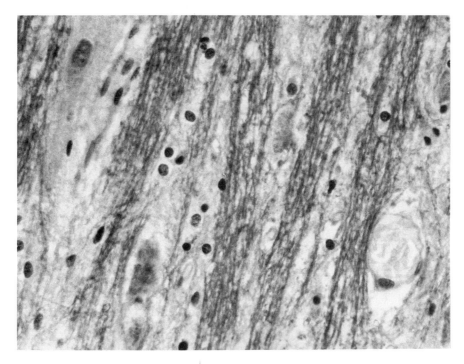

Fig. 17-2 Gray and white matter bundles in normal human pons. Note that most oligodendrocytes (small cells with dark nuclei) are within gray matter rather than within the white matter bundles. (Hematoxylin and eosin × 640.)

Hypernatremia

Symptoms due to hypernatremia are usually referable to the CNS and are most often seen with serum sodium concentrations above 160 mEq/L.[1] Hypernatremia is most frequently encountered in the very young or the very old. In infants, fluid loss due to gastroenteritis is a common cause. In the elderly, dehydration resulting from an inability to obtain water because of debilitation is the most frequent cause. Diabetes insipidus rarely presents with severe hypernatremia unless the patient is also denied access to water. Structural lesions (e.g., gliomas and metastatic tumors) in the hypothalamic thirst center are an uncommon cause of hypernatremia in patients with neurological disease.

Alteration of mental status is a frequent manifestation of hypernatremia and ranges from lethargy to coma.[6,36] Pathological studies suggest that osmotic forces present during the development of hypernatremia, particularly when acute, may produce shrinkage of brain parenchyma. This may result in parenchymal hemorrhages or tearing of bridging veins, producing subdural hematomas or subarachnoid hemorrhage. An initial mortality rate of 20 percent and an incidence of permanent brain damage of more than 33 percent have been noted in children with severe hypernatremia.[37] Seizures frequently occur in the setting of hypernatremia and paradoxically may be more frequent during rehydration.[38] The seizures may be related to either the focal hemorrhages that occur during the development of hypernatremia or the cerebral edema that may develop during the rehydration phase of treatment. Rigidity, tremor, myoclonus, asterixis, and chorea have been associated with hypernatremia.[39] Neuromuscular manifestations of hypernatremia are much less frequent. Rhabdomyolysis has been reported.[8,40–42] Episodic muscle weakness may occur in patients with essential hypernatremia.[43,44]

POTASSIUM

In contrast to sodium, the neurological manifestations of potassium disturbance, whether hypokalemia or hyperkalemia, rarely involve the CNS.[1] About 98 percent of total body potassium is located intracellularly; 60 percent of intracellular potassium is within muscle. This may account in part for the predominance of muscular symptoms in disorders producing hypokalemia or hyperkalemia.

Hypokalemia

Hypokalemia is the most frequent electrolyte disorder encountered in clinical practice. It is produced by a variety of mechanisms, including inadequate potassium intake or excessive renal or gastrointestinal potassium loss. Symptoms of hypokalemia are typically muscular.[6,9,45] Serum potassium concentrations of 3.0 to 3.5 mEq/L may be associated with mild muscle weakness, myalgia, and easy fatigability. Serum potassium concentrations of 2.5 to 3.0 mEq/L are associated with the development of clinically significant muscle weakness, particularly of the proximal limb muscles. The cranial musculature is characteristically spared in hypokalemia-induced muscle weakness. When the serum potassium level falls below 2.5 mEq/L, and usually below 2.0 mEq/L, structural muscle damage, including rhabdomyolysis and myoglobinuria, may occur.[46–48] In the setting of hypokalemia, serum hyperosmolality may be a predictor of rhabdomyolysis.[48] Muscle biopsy typically demonstrates segmental muscle necrosis, degeneration, and vacuoles.[49] Complete recovery following adequate potassium replacement is the rule.

Tetany occurs in some patients with hypokalemia, particularly when associated with alkalosis.[1] Hypokalemia may mask the tetany of hypocalcemia. Paradoxically, tetany may occur during the treatment of hypokalemia in patients who are also hypocalcemic.

Cerebral symptoms in hypokalemia are distinctly unusual.[1] Reference to symptoms such as lethargy, apathy, drowsiness, confusion, irritability, delirium, and coma in hypokalemia is rare,[50,51] suggesting that an associated acid–base disturbance may have been responsible for these encephalopathic symptoms.

Hyperkalemia

The cardiac toxicity of hyperkalemia essentially precludes the appearance of significant neurological manifestations.[1] Most patients develop serious cardiac abnormalities such as ventricular fibrillation or asystole before the appearance of neurological symptoms.[6,52]

Chronic potassium homeostasis is dependent upon renal mechanisms. Acute potassium regulation is dependent on extrarenal hormonal mechanisms primarily involving insulin, aldosterone, and epinephrine. Clinically important etiologies of hyperkalemia include renal failure, adrenal insufficiency (Addison's disease), and acidosis with or without insulin deficiency. Cerebral symptoms due to hyperkalemia must be uncommon, as they do not occur in hyperkalemic periodic paralysis.[53] The cerebral symptoms (nervousness and lethargy) that frequently occur in Addison's disease are probably related to the associated hyponatremia or acidosis. The most frequent neurological manifestation of hyperkalemia is the development of muscle weakness,[6,9,49,52] which occurs most often in the setting of chronic adrenal insufficiency.[54] However, profound muscle weakness is rarely reported with hyperkalemia.[55]

CALCIUM

Plasma calcium stabilizes excitable membranes in muscle and nervous tissue. Disorders of calcium would therefore be expected to produce neurological manifestations.[1] The coordinated interactions of parathyroid hormone, cholecalciferol, and probably calcitonin regulate intestinal calcium absorption, renal calcium reabsorption, and bone resorption to control closely the plasma calcium concentration.[56,57]

Hypercalcemia

Malignant neoplasms and hyperparathyroidism account for 70 to 80 percent of cases of hypercalcemia.[57] The neoplasms most frequently associated with hypercalcemia are breast cancer, lung cancer, and multiple myeloma. Although most instances of hypercalcemia in the setting of malignancy are due to osteolytic skeletal metastases, some carcinomas, particularly of the lung, are associated with elevated levels of parathyroid hormone. Single adenomas of the parathyroid gland account for 75 percent of cases of primary hyperparathyroidism. Because patients with malignant neoplasms often have several mechanisms of neurological injury, the incidence of neurological manifestations in hyperparathyroidism (which is at least 40 percent) represents a reasonable incidence of the neurological manifestations of hypercalcemia.[58,59] Alterations in mental status are common in hypercalcemia (particularly with serum calcium concentrations of more than 14 mg/dl) and generally consist of progressive lethargy, confusion, and ultimately coma. These reversible symptoms are directly related to the degree of hypercalcemia and require immediate therapy. Headache, elevated cerebrospinal fluid protein concentration, and, rarely, convulsions also occur in patients with hypercalcemia.[6] Hyperparathyroidism has also rarely been associated with severe CNS dysfunction, including ataxia, internuclear ophthalmoplegia, corticospinal tract dysfunction, dysarthria, and dysphagia.[60] Hypercalcemia has been associated with apnea in children.[61]

Hypercalcemia produces reduced neuromuscular excitability and may cause muscle weakness. Easy fatigability and muscle weakness are more common in hyperparathyroidism[62,63] than in other hypercalcemic conditions. The clinical features of hyperparathyroid myopathy include proximal, though seldom disabling, muscle weakness and wasting with preserved or even brisk reflexes and mild nonspecific myopathic features on electromyogram and muscle biopsy.[62–65] The pathogenesis of hyperparathyroid myopathy remains undefined, although hypercalcemia, vitamin D deficiency, chronic phosphate deficiency, or neuropathic influences may play a role.[49] Hyperparathyroid myopathy is similar to the vitamin D deficiency myopathy that can occur with uremia, phenytoin therapy, and osteomalacia. The carpal tunnel syndrome has occasionally been associated with hyperparathyroidism.[66]

Hypocalcemia

Hypocalcemia is relatively rare except in neonates and patients with renal failure. Severe acute hypocalcemia is most frequently encountered following thyroid or parathyroid surgery. Hypocalcemia is also a common complication of acute pancreatitis. The neurological manifestations of hypoparathyroidism resulting from primary, secondary, or pseudohypoparathyroidism (parathyroid hormone–resistant syndromes) largely reflect hypocalcemia. The most common CNS manifestations are seizures (which may be focal or generalized) and alterations of mental function.[67–72] The latter symptoms include irritability,

anxiety, agitation, confusion, delirium, delusions, hallucinations, psychosis, depression, mental dullness, mental retardation, and dementia. Chorea and parkinsonism are seen with increased frequency in patients with chronic hypocalcemia. Although a causal relation has not been established, the regularity with which calcification of the basal ganglia is seen in patients with chronic hypoparathyroidism[73–75] seems more than coincidental. Some patients with chronic hypoparathyroidism may have quite extensive brain calcification and associated neurological symptoms.[76] Less frequent CNS manifestations of hypoparathyroidism are pseudotumor cerebri and myelopathy due to overgrowth of the vertebral lamina.

Tetany is the most frequently recognized symptom of hypocalcemia referable to the peripheral nervous system.[49] It originates in the peripheral nerve axon and is due to spontaneous, irregular, repetitive nerve action potentials. When the ionized calcium concentration reaches a low enough level, the peripheral nerve membrane may spontaneously discharge at the normal resting membrane potential. Latent tetany may be unmasked clinically by hyperventilation or ischemia (Trousseau test). The first symptom of tetany is tingling that initially occurs periorally and distally in the limbs and then spreads proximally. This is followed by a feeling of muscle spasm that has an initial distribution similar to that of the early sensory complaints and becomes increasingly severe as it spreads proximally. Finally, muscles may go into tonic spasms, commencing distally (carpopedal spasm). Laryngeal stridor may ultimately develop.[77] Opisthotonos may occur if spasms involve the trunk.

Elevated serum creatine kinase levels have been reported in patients with hypoparathyroidism, although clinical and morphological evidence of myopathy has been scant.

Hypoparathyroidism has been associated with the Kearns-Sayre syndrome and muscle phosphorylase deficiency (perhaps related to a failure of calcium to activate phosphorylase kinase).

MAGNESIUM

Less than 2 percent of total body magnesium is located within the extracellular fluid compartment. Although magnesium has an intracellular-extracellular distribution similar to that of potassium, most of the intracellular magnesium is bound and not exchangeable with the extracellular fluid. In fact, intracellular free magnesium is rigidly regulated despite wide variations in extracellular magnesium concentrations. The teleological basis for this situation relates to the critical role of magnesium in intracellular metabolism. Magnesium is required for activation of a wide range of intracellular enzymes. Additionally, extracellular magnesium exerts significant effects on synaptic transmission in the central and peripheral nervous systems.[78]

Hypomagnesemia

Because magnesium is predominantly an intracellular electrolyte, the finding of hypomagnesemia (which occurs in about 10 percent of hospitalized patients) does not always accurately reflect magnesium depletion.[79] Important mechanisms of hypomagnesemia and magnesium depletion include decreased intake (as in starvation), decreased intestinal absorption (as in malabsorption syndromes such as nontropical sprue), and increased renal loss (as with diuretic usage, chronic alcoholism, diabetic acidosis, and renal tubular acidosis).

The neurological manifestations of hypomagnesemia are essentially hyperirritability with agitation, confusion, convulsions, tremor, myoclonus, hyperreflexia, Chvostek's sign, and tetany.[80,81] These signs and symptoms typically occur with serum magnesium concentrations of less than 0.8 mEq/L. When convulsions occur, parenteral administration of magnesium salts is required. However, renal function should be assessed before administering parenteral magnesium. When magnesium is being given by slow intravenous bolus, calcium gluconate should be available to counteract transient hypermagnesemia, which may cause apnea as a result of respiratory muscle paralysis. The neurological manifestations of hypomagnesemia are similar to those of hypocalcemia, which is not surprising, since hypocalcemia often accompanies hypomagnesemia.[82] The hypocalcemia or hypomagnesemia is produced or exaggerated in some instances by a hypomagnesemia-induced decrease in parathyroid hormone or end-organ resistance to the action of parathyroid hormone.[83] This leads to an important therapeutic point—it is necessary to evaluate magnesium in a hypocalcemic patient who fails to respond to calcium supplementation. Conversely, in magnesium-deficient patients who are normocalcemic but have symptoms suggestive of hypocalcemia,[84] calcium may still be responsible for the symptoms because normocalcemic hypomagnesemic patients may have decreased serum ionized calcium concentrations.[85] Hypomagnesemia develops frequently with cisplatin use. In that setting, only patients who are also hypocalcemic develop tetany with carpopedal spasm.[86] Muscle weakness develops in some patients with hypomagnesemia, although coexistent hypokalemia or hypophosphatemia may contribute.[49] In the dog and rat, a necrotizing myopathy has been induced by chronic magnesium depletion.[87,88] Chronic hypomagnesemia has been associated with a cardioskeletal mitochondrial myopathy.[89]

Hypermagnesemia

Symptomatic hypermagnesemia is uncommon in clinical practice and is typically encountered in the setting of excessive magnesium intake in conjunction with impaired renal function. In contrast to hypomagnesemia, the neurological manifestations of hypermagnesemia are characterized by nervous system depression. Loss of deep tendon reflexes is an early sign of hypermagnesemia and occurs at serum magnesium concentrations of 5 to 6 mEq/L. At serum magnesium concentrations of 8 to 10 mEq/L, CNS depression is said to occur, with lethargy and confusion being the most common neurological manifestations.[90–92] However, in human subjects in whom the serum magnesium concentration was increased to 15 mEq/L, no CNS depression occurred, although there was slowing of the electroencephalogram.[93] The predominant neurological manifestation of severe hypermagnesemia is muscle weakness or paralysis,[49] due to a blockade of neuromuscular transmission.[94] Untreated, this weakness, which can involve respiratory muscles, may result in respiratory insufficiency, with subsequent hypoxia, hypercarbia, coma, and ultimately death.

REFERENCES

1. Riggs JE: Neurologic manifestations of fluid and electrolyte disturbances. Neurol Clin 7:509, 1989
2. Rossi NF, Schrier RW: Hyponatremic states. p. 461. In Maxwell MH, Kleeman CR, Narins RG (eds): Clinical

Disorders of Fluid and Electrolyte Metabolism. 4th Ed. McGraw-Hill, New York, 1987

3. Anderson RJ, Chung HM, Kluge R, Schrier RW: Hyponatremia: a prospective analysis of its epidemiology and the pathogenetic role of vasopressin. Ann Intern Med 102:164, 1985

4. Tierney WM, Martin DK, Greenlee MC, et al: The prognosis of hyponatremia at hospital admission. J Gen Intern Med 1:380, 1986

5. Arieff AI, Guisado R: Effects on the central nervous system of hypernatremic and hyponatremic states. Kidney Int 10:104, 1976

6. Epstein FH: Signs and symptoms of electrolyte disorders. p. 499. In Maxwell MH, Kleeman CR (eds): Clinical Disorders of Fluid and Electrolyte Metabolism. 3rd Ed. McGraw-Hill, New York, 1979

7. Daggett P, Deanfield J, Moss F: Neurological aspects of hyponatremia. Postgrad Med J 58:737, 1982

8. Sarnaik AP, Meert K, Hackbarth R, Fleischmann L: Management of hyponatremic seizures in children with hypertonic saline: a safe and effective strategy. Crit Care Med 19:758, 1991

9. Corbett AJ: Electrolyte disorders affecting muscle. Semin Neurol 3:248, 1983

10. Arieff AI, Llach F, Massry SG: Neurological manifestations and morbidity of hyponatremia: correlation with brain water and electrolytes. Medicine (Baltimore) 55: 121, 1976

11. Melton JE, Patlak CS, Pettigrew KD, Cserr HF: Volume regulatory loss of Na, Cl, and K from rat brain during acute hyponatremia. Am J Physiol 252:F661, 1987

12. Verbalis JG, Gullans SR: Hyponatremia causes large sustained reductions in brain content of multiple organic osmolytes in rats. Brain Res 567:274, 1991

13. Nibbelink DW, Torner JC, Burmeister LF: Fluid restriction in combination with antifibrinolytic therapy. p. 307. In Sahs AL, Nibbelink DW, Torner JC (eds): Aneurysmal Subarachnoid Hemorrhage: Report of the Cooperative Study. Urban & Schwarzenberg, Baltimore, 1981

14. Wijdicks EFM, Vermeulen M, Hijdra A, van Gijn J: Hyponatremia and cerebral infarction in patients with ruptured intracranial aneurysms: is fluid restriction harmful? Ann Neurol 17:137, 1985

15. Nelson PB, Seif SM, Maroon JC, Robinson AG: Hyponatremia in intracranial disease: perhaps not the syndrome of inappropriate secretion of antidiuretic hormone (SIADH). J Neurosurg 55:938, 1981

16. Goldberg M: Hyponatremia. Med Clin North Am 65: 251, 1981

17. Wijdicks EFM, Vermeulen M, ten Haaf JA, et al: Volume depletion and natriuresis in patients with a ruptured intracranial aneurysm. Ann Neurol 18:211, 1985

18. Peters JP, Welt LG, Sims EAH, et al: A salt-wasting syndrome associated with cerebral disease. Trans Assoc Am Physicians 63:57, 1950

19. Diringer MN, Wu KC, Verbalis JG, Hanley DF: Hypervolemic therapy prevents volume contraction but not hyponatremia following subarachnoid hemorrhage. Ann Neurol 31:543, 1992

20. Adams RD, Victor M, Mancall EL: Central pontine myelinolysis: a hitherto undescribed disease occurring in alcoholic and malnourished patients. Arch Neurol Psychiatry 81:154, 1959

21. Chason JL, Landers JW, Gonzales JE: Central pontine myelinolysis. J Neurol Neurosurg Psychiatry 27:317, 1964

22. Shurtliff LF, Ajax ET, Englert E, D'Agostino AN: Central pontine myelinolysis and cirrhosis of the liver: a report of four cases. Am J Clin Pathol 46:239, 1966

23. Mathews T, Moossy J: Central pontine myelinolysis: lesion evolution and pathogenesis. J Neuropathol Exp Neurol 34:77, 1975

24. Endo Y, Oda M, Hara M: Central pontine myelinolysis, a study of 37 cases in 1,000 consecutive autopsies. Acta Neuropathol (Berl) 53:145, 1981

25. Aleu FP, Terry RD: Central pontine myelinolysis: a report of two cases. Arch Pathol 76:140, 1963

26. Berry K, Olszewski J: Central pontine myelinolysis: a case report. Neurology 13:531, 1963

27. Paguirigan A, Lefken EB: Central pontine myelinolysis. Neurology 19:1007, 1969

28. Leslie KO, Robertson AS, Norenberg MD: Central pontine myelinolysis: an osmotic gradient pathogenesis. J Neuropathol Exp Neurol 39:370, 1980

29. Sterns RH, Riggs JE, Schochet SS: Osmotic demyelination syndrome following correction of hyponatremia. N Engl J Med 314:1535, 1986

30. Ayus JC, Krothapalli RK, Arieff AI: Treatment of symptomatic hyponatremia and its relation to brain damage: a prospective study. N Engl J Med 317:1190, 1987

31. Norenberg MD, Papendick RE: Chronicity of hyponatremia as a factor in experimental myelinolysis. Ann Neurol 15:544, 1984

32. Laureno R: Central pontine myelinolysis following rapid correction of hyponatremia. Ann Neurol 13:232, 1983

33. Kleinschmidt-DeMasters BK, Norenberg MD: Neuropathologic observations in electrolyte-induced myelinolysis in the rat. J Neuropathol Exp Neurol 41:67, 1982

34. Verbalis JG, Martinez AJ, Drutarosky MD: Neurological and neuropathological sequelae of correction of chronic hyponatremia. Kidney Int 39:1274, 1991

35. Riggs JE, Schochet SS: Osmotic stress, osmotic my-

elinolysis, and oligodendrocyte topography. Arch Pathol Lab Med 113:1386, 1989

36. Arieff AI: Central nervous system manifestations of disordered sodium metabolism. Clin Endocrinol Metab 13:269, 1984

37. Morris-Jones PH, Houston IB, Evans RC: Prognosis of the neurological complications of acute hypernatraemia. Lancet 2:1385, 1967

38. Hogan GR, Dodge PR, Gill SR, et al: The incidence of seizures after rehydration of hypernatremic rabbits with intravenous or ad libitum oral fluids. Pediatr Res 18:340, 1983

39. Sparacio RR, Anziska B, Schutta HS: Hypernatremia and chorea: a report of two cases. Neurology 26:46, 1976

40. Ulvila JM, Nessan VJ: Hypernatremia with myoglobinuria. Am J Med Sci 265:79, 1973

41. Kung AWC, Pun KK, Lam KSL, Yeung RTT: Rhabdomyolysis associated with cranial diabetes insipidus. Postgrad Med J 67:912, 1991

42. Abramovici MI, Singhal PC, Trachtman H: Hypernatremia and rhabdomyolysis. J Med 23:17, 1992

43. Maddy JA, Winternitz WW: Hypothalamic syndrome with hypernatremia and muscular paralysis. Am J Med 51:394, 1971

44. Alford FP, Scoggins BA, Wharton C: Symptomatic normovolemic essential hypernatremia: a clinical and physiologic study. Am J Med 54:359, 1973

45. Raymond KH, Kunau RT: Hypokalemic states. p. 519. In Maxwell MH, Kleeman CR, Narins RG (eds): Clinical Disorders of Fluid and Electrolyte Metabolism. 4th Ed. McGraw-Hill, New York, 1987

46. Knochel JP: Rhabdomyolysis and effects of potassium deficiency on muscle structure and function. Cardiovasc Med 3:247, 1978

47. Knochel JP: Neuromuscular manifestations of electrolyte disorders. Am J Med 72:521, 1982

48. Singhal PC, Abramovici M, Venkatesan J, Mattana J: Hypokalemia and rhabdomyolysis. Miner Electrolyte Metab 17:335, 1991

49. Layzer RB: Neuromuscular Manifestations of Systemic Disease. FA Davis, Philadelphia, 1985

50. Elman R, Shatz BA, Keating RE, Weichselbaum TE: Intracellular and extracellular potassium deficits in surgical patients. Ann Surg 136:111, 1952

51. Mitchell W, Feldman F: Neuropsychiatric aspects of hypokalemia. Can Med Assoc J 98:49, 1968

52. DeFronzo RA: Hyperkalemic states. p. 547. In Maxwell MH, Kleeman CR, Narins RG (eds): Clinical Disorders of Fluid and Electrolyte Metabolism. 4th Ed. McGraw-Hill, New York, 1987

53. Riggs JE: The periodic paralyses. Neurol Clin 6:485, 1988

54. Pollen RH, Williams RH: Hyperkalemic neuromyopathy in Addison's disease. N Engl J Med 263:273, 1960

55. Freeman SJ, Fale AD: Muscular paralysis and ventilatory failure caused by hyperkalemia. Br J Anaesth 70:226, 1993

56. Marx SJ, Bourdeau JE: Calcium metabolism. p. 207. In Maxwell MH, Kleeman CR, Narins RG (eds): Clinical Disorders of Fluid and Electrolyte Metabolism. 4th Ed. McGraw-Hill, New York, 1987

57. Benabe JE, Martinez-Maldonado M: Disorders of calcium metabolism. p. 759. In Maxwell MH, Kleeman CR, Narins RG (eds): Clinical Disorders of Fluid and Electrolyte Metabolism. 4th Ed. McGraw-Hill, New York, 1987

58. Karpati G, Frame B: Neuropsychiatric disorders in primary hyperparathyroidism: clinical analysis with review of the literature. Arch Neurol 10:387, 1964

59. Hensen RA: The neurological aspects of hypercalcemia: with special reference to primary hyperparathyroidism. J R Coll Physicians Lond 1:41, 1966

60. Patten BM, Page M: Severe neurological disease associated with hyperparathyroidism. Ann Neurol 15:453, 1984

61. Kooh S-W, Binet A: Hypercalcemia in infants presenting with apnea. Can Med Assoc J 143:509, 1990

62. Frame B, Heinze EG, Block MA, Manson GA: Myopathy in primary hyperparathyroidism: observations in three patients. Ann Intern Med 68:1022, 1968

63. Patten BM, Bilezikian JP, Mallette LE, et al: Neuromuscular disease in primary hyperparathyroidism. Ann Intern Med 80:182, 1974

64. Bischoff A, Esslen E: Myopathy with primary hyperparathyroidism. Neurology 15:64, 1965

65. Cholod EJ, Haust MD, Hudson AJ, Lewis FN: Myopathy in primary familial hyperparathyroidism: clinical and morphologic studies. Am J Med 48:700, 1970

66. Palma G: Carpal tunnel syndrome and hyperparathyroidism. Ann Neurol 14:592, 1983

67. Gotta H: Tetany and epilepsy. Arch Neurol Psychiatry 66:714, 1951

68. Sugar O: Central neurological complications of hyperparathyroidism. Arch Neurol Psychiatry 70:86, 1953

69. Frame B, Carter S: Pseudohypoparathyroidism: clinical picture and relation to convulsive seizures. Neurology 5:297, 1955

70. Rose GA, Vas CJ: Neurological complications and electroencephalographic changes in hypoparathyroidism. Acta Neurol Scand 42:537, 1966

71. Fonseca OA, Calverly JR: Neurological manifestations of hypoparathyroidism. Arch Intern Med 120:202, 1967

72. Shu-lian Y, Chang-hua W, Ying-kun F: Neurologic and psychiatric manifestations in hypoparathyroidism: clinical analysis of 71 cases. Chin Med J 97:267, 1984

73. Sachs C, Sjoberg HE, Ericson K: Basal ganglia calcifications on CT: relation to hypoparathyroidism. Neurology 32:779, 1982

74. Illum F, Dupont E: Prevalences of CT-detected calcification in the basal ganglia in idiopathic hypoparathyroidism and pseudohypoparathyroidism. Neuroradiology 27:32, 1985

75. Bhimani S, Sarwar M, Virapongse C, et al: Computed tomography of cerebrovascular calcifications in postsurgical hypoparathyroidism. J Comput Assist Tomogr 9:121, 1985

76. Cheek JC, Riggs JE, Lilly RL: Extensive brain calcification and progressive dysarthria and dysphagia associated with chronic hypoparathyroidism. Arch Neurol 47:1038, 1990

77. Sharief N, Matthew DJ, Dillon MJ: Hypocalcemic stridor in children. How often is it missed? Clin Pediatr 30:51, 1991

78. Quamme GA, Dirks JH: Magnesium metabolism. p. 297. In Maxwell MH, Kleeman CR, Narins RG (eds): Clinical Disorders of Fluid and Electrolyte Metabolism. 4th Ed. McGraw-Hill, New York, 1987

79. Brautbar N, Massry SG: Hypomagnesemia and hypermagnesemia. p. 831. In Maxwell MH, Kleeman GR, Narins RG (eds): Clinical Disorders of Fluid and Electrolyte Metabolism. 4th Ed. McGraw-Hill, New York, 1987

80. Fishman RA: Neurological aspects of magnesium metabolism. Arch Neurol 12:562, 1965

81. Shils ME: Experimental human magnesium depletion. Medicine (Baltimore) 48:61, 1969

82. Flink EB: Magnesium deficiency: etiology and clinical spectrum. Acta Med Scand Suppl 647:125, 1981

83. Rude RK, Oldham SB, Singer FR: Functional hypoparathyroidism and parathyroid hormone end-organ resistance in human magnesium deficiency. Clin Endocrinol 5:209, 1976

84. Wacker WEC, Moore FD, Ulmer DD, Vallee BL: Normocalcemic magnesium deficiency tetany. JAMA 180:161, 1962

85. Zimmet P, Breidahl HD, Nayler WG: Plasma ionized calcium in hypomagnesaemia. Br Med J 1:622, 1968

86. Hayes FA, Green AA, Senzer N, Pratt CB: Tetany: a complication of cis-dichlorodiammineplatinum (II) therapy. Cancer Treat Rep 63:547, 1979

87. Cronin RE, Ferguson ER, Shannon WA, Knochel JP: Skeletal muscle injury after magnesium depletion in the dog. Am J Physiol 243:F113, 1982

88. Robeson BL, Martin WG, Friedman MH: A biochemical and ultrastructural study of skeletal muscle from rats fed a magnesium-deficit diet. J Nutr 110:2078, 1980

89. Riggs JE, Klingberg WG, Flink EB, et al: Cardioskeletal mitochondrial myopathy associated with chronic hypomagnesemia. Neurology 42:128, 1992

90. Stevens AR, Wolff HG: Magnesium intoxication: absorption from the intact gastrointestinal tract. Arch Neurol Psychiatry 63:749, 1950

91. Randall RE, Cohen MD, Spray CC, Rossmeisl EC: Hypermagnesemia in renal failure: etiology and toxic manifestations. Ann Intern Med 61:73, 1964

92. Alfrey AC, Terman DS, Brettschneider L: Hypermagnesemia after renal homotransplantation. Ann Intern Med 73:367, 1970

93. Somjen G, Hilmy M, Stephen CR: Failure to anesthetize human subjects by intravenous administration of magnesium sulfate. J Pharmacol Exp Ther 154:652, 1966

94. Swift TR: Weakness from magnesium-containing cathartics: electrophysiologic studies. Muscle Nerve 2: 295, 1979

18

Thyroid Disease and the Nervous System

William K. Abend
H. Richard Tyler

Neurological dysfunction associated with diseases of the thyroid gland usually results from hormonal imbalance or from what are presumed to be immune mechanisms associated with thyroid disease. The hormonal disturbance may lead to a new neurological disorder, exacerbate an antecedent neurological deficit, or enhance a subclinical disease. Direct compromise of structures by enlargement of the thyroid gland occasionally causes neurological disorders. Rarely, central mass effects or increased intracranial pressure relate to pituitary enlargement secondary to thyroid failure, intracranial metastases from thyroid carcinoma, or associated pseudotumor cerebri. The effects of thyroid disease on the development of the nervous system and hormone imbalance resulting from neural disorders are not discussed here.

THYROTOXICOSIS AND GRAVES' DISEASE

Mental Changes

Most patients with thyrotoxicosis do not have a significant mental disorder. They may experience nonspecific symptoms, however, that are attributable to concern and apprehension regarding the primary disease. More specific difficulties may include insomnia, poor concentration, and decreased attention span. Acquaintances often describe irritability, capriciousness, and emotional lability. These problems usually resolve if the patient is returned to a euthyroid state.

Individual case reports have suggested an infrequent association between thyrotoxicosis and many types of mental disorder. For some, a postulated relation is based on anecdotal evidence. In other situations, however, a causal relation is suggested by the temporal correspondence, by resolution of the neurological deficit with treatment of the thyroid condition, and by a direct relation between the degree of hormonal imbalance and the severity of the neurological disease. The mechanism for these effects is not known. One factor may be deranged brain sodium and potassium exchange, which has been demonstrated in dysthyroid rats.[1] In addition, thyroid hormone receptors in the brain[2] could mediate the mental changes, but it is not clear to what degree these receptors are active in the adult. We are not aware of any substantial data indicating the presence of antibodies against neural tissue in patients with thyrotoxicosis.

Agitated delirium, with confusion, restlessness, and hyperkinesia,[3,4] is rare but does occur. "Apathetic hyperthyroidism," a state in which elderly thyrotoxic patients become lethargic and depressed, has also been described.[5] A variety of psychometric abnormalities has been found.[6] These abnormalities may well be caused by the thyrotoxicosis, since they generally resolve with successful treatment of the thyroid disorder. However, these conditions may occur with either high or only mildly elevated thyroid hormone levels, which could mean that the neurological deficit is not caused solely by the elevated thyroid hormone level but, rather, by some other associated chemical imbalance.

The syndrome of "thyroid storm" is now rare but may be seen in thyrotoxic patients who are untreated or who develop a new, acute medical disorder. In addition to the typical manifestations of thyrotoxicosis, the patient may have fever, tachycardia, cardiac failure and arrhythmias, and vomiting and diarrhea, with resulting electrolyte abnormalities. There is confusion and agitation. In the late stages, there may be stupor or coma accompanied by pyramidal dysfunction,[7] bulbar signs,[8] or convulsions. Therapy for thyroid storm usually includes the use of hydration, cooling, antithyroid medication, iodine, β-blocking agents, and dexamethasone. If this regimen does not alleviate severe neurological effects, plasmapheresis may be useful.[7]

Psychiatric illnesses associated with thyrotoxicosis are usually affective in nature and may be of a psychotic type. Depression,[9] mania,[10] and bipolar illnesses[11] have been described. In assessing these reports, it is important to recall that lithium therapy itself may mask thyrotoxicosis or produce hypothyroidism.[12] Schizophrenia has also been reported in association with thyrotoxicosis,[13] and treatment of thyrotoxicosis may improve the psychiatric condition.[14]

Several studies have been directed at determining the incidence of subclinical thyroid disorders in patients with psychiatric diseases. The results of various series have differed, with some showing no clear association and others showing surprisingly high rates of hyper- or hypothyroidism.[15–17] In these studies, no systematic attempt was made to determine the effect on the psychiatric condition of correcting the thyroid abnormality.

Seizure Disorders, Sleep Disturbance, Electroencephalographic Abnormalities

Hyperthyroidism may cause exacerbations of an existing seizure disorder. More interesting is the occurrence of seizures that are secondary to the thyrotoxic state.[18] This phenomenon is generally considered to be rare, although one study reported generalized and focal seizures in 10 percent of thyrotoxic patients.[19] The disorder becomes quiescent on return to a euthyroid state.[20] The reason for this increased seizure risk is not clear. Cerebral oxygen consumption is not clearly affected by hyperthyroidism.[21] The fact that administering thyroid hormone to animals lowers the threshold to induce seizures[22] suggests that it is the thyroxine itself that underlies the seizures and not some other accompanying factor. One report has described a mentally retarded patient in whom seizures occurred for the first time when a hypothyroid state was rapidly corrected with thyroxine.[23] The use of propranolol and other β-blocking agents to treat the hyperthyroidism may cause seizures.[20]

Electroencephalographic (EEG) abnormalities may occur in association with thyrotoxicosis.[24–26] Typical abnormal findings include slow activity,[18] increased alpha frequency and beta activity,[24] and increased voltage of the response to intermittent photic stimulation.[25] These EEG effects have been induced in normal humans by the administration of thyroxine.[27] A more unusual abnormality, seen in some cases of thyrotoxic encephalopathy, is the presence of triphasic delta waves.[28] Rarely, focal slowing is seen.[18] One study found no correlation between the degree of thyroid abnormality and the EEG findings,[18] whereas another did.[26] Nevertheless, the EEG findings can be helpful for assessing response to treatment. The abnormalities are generally reversible if a euthyroid state is attained[18]; they return with poor thyroid control.[26] In some cases there may be only partial resolution even with good thyroid control.[26]

Although sleep disturbances are more common in hypothyroidism (see below), thyrotoxic patients may have insomnia. Physiological sleep cycles may be disturbed, with shortening of stages III and IV.[26] Rarely, a goiter causes airway obstruction,[29] and it has been suggested that secondary sleep apnea may result.[30]

Headaches

Headaches may occur in patients with hyperthyroidism and may be migrainous or muscular in character. Migraine phenomena can also improve with the onset of hyperthyroidism, but this is unusual. "Fullness of the head" and tinnitus are described occasionally and could be related to exophthalmos, muscle contraction, or vascular mechanisms. It has been proposed that intracranial pressure may be raised in hyperthyroidism,[31] but this has not been investigated systematically. Pseudotumor cerebri has been found in association with thyrotoxicosis,[32] but this is even more unusual than the association with hypothyroidism, discussed below.

Disorders of the Cranial Nerve Systems

Orbital congestion is a component of Graves' disease but can appear with little other indication of this disease. We agree with the suggestion that the condition is better referred to as *dysthyroid orbitopathy* than Graves' ophthalmopathy.[33]

Pathologically, the orbital tissues other than the globe are edematous and infiltrated with lymphocytes and plasmacytes. The cause is not known, but it does not appear to result from hyperthyroidism, as it is seen in patients with Graves' disease who are euthyroid or hypothyroid. In hyperthyroid patients with Graves' disease, the severity of the orbitopathy does not correlate with the circulating level of thyroid hormone.[34,35] Additionally, orbitopathy is not seen with hyperthyroidism due to other causes, such as thyroid adenoma. Antibodies to orbital tissue have been found in patients with orbitopathy,[36] but it is not known whether these play a primary role in the disorder.

Clinically, the orbitopathy may precede other signs of Graves' disease, occur concomitantly with the hyperthyroidism, develop after treatment of the hyperthyroidism,[37] or even appear in patients who have developed hypothyroidism.[38,39] Orbital congestion is present, with discomfort, a sensation of orbital fullness, conjunctival hyperemia, chemosis, and edema of the eyelids. The extraocular muscles may become massively enlarged, resulting in proptosis and the possibility of exposure keratopathy. It can usually be distinguished from the other causes of proptosis with computed tomography (CT) and magnetic resonance imaging (MRI) of the orbit, which show muscle enlargement without enlargement of the tendons.[40] It is usually bilateral but can be highly asymmetrical. There is a "staring" appearance, and diplopia is frequently present.[41] Eye movements are often limited, vertical diplopia is common, and there may be progression to total external ophthalmoplegia. The ophthalmoparesis is usually attributed to mechanical impairment of movement rather than a neural lesion,[40] but the degree of eye muscle paresis does not always correlate with the severity of the orbitopathy.[42] The orbitopathy may improve with treatment of the thyroid condition.[43] If proptosis is accompanied by a significant extraocular movement disorder, treatment with corticosteroids can be considered but is controversial. When corticosteroids are used, treatment should probably be limited to several weeks and discontinued earlier than planned if no definite benefit is apparent. Extraocular muscle surgery is occasionally employed[44] once the patient is euthyroid and the eye condition is stable.

It is important to evaluate patients for the appearance of *dysthyroid optic neuropathy,* an uncommon but treatable complication of orbitopathy.[45] It generally occurs in the presence of prominent dysthyroid orbitopathy. Distinct visual symptoms and signs may appear rapidly, but the importance of monitoring patients for subtle visual disturbances has been emphasized.[46] The incidence of optic neuropathy among patients with orbitopathy was 8.6 percent in one study.[46] Many patients did not notice or comment upon mild disturbances. The two most common visual findings were color defects and abnormal visual evoked responses. A variety of visual field defects appeared before central acuity was disturbed. Possible etiologies for the neuropathy are optic nerve infiltration and compression of the optic nerve by enlarged ocular muscles. Most authorities feel that treatment should be started rapidly. Therapeutic approaches have included treatment with corticosteroids,[47] corticosteroids combined with cyclosporine,[48] radiation,[49] and orbital decompression.[50] These approaches have been compared,[45] and there appears to be a role for each. In some situations, it may be necessary to combine treatment modalities or use them in rapid succession. The differential diagnosis for each of the components of dysthyroid orbitopathy has been discussed elsewhere.[33]

One of the most common signs of hyperthyroidism is eyelid retraction. It may occur in the absence of exophthalmos and, in different situations, may be the result of contracture of the levator palpebrae superioris muscle[51] or of sympathetic overactivity[52] causing increased tone in Müller's muscle. Eyelid retraction may manifest in several ways. With downward eye movement, the lids seem to lag, leaving a larger than normal portion of the sclera visible (von Graefe's sign). Dalrymple's sign refers to retraction of the upper and lower lids and the resulting widened palpebral fissure.[53] The patient may have a staring expression with infrequent blinking (Stellwag's sign) and may not contract the frontalis muscle when looking upward (Joffroy's sign). The overactivity of the sympathetic system may also cause exophthalmos, and the patient may then have decreased ability to converge (Möbius' sign). Attempts to treat lid retraction have included sympatholytic medication and a variety of surgical procedures.[54,55]

Dysphagia, dysarthria, and weakness of the neck flexors can result from a coexisting myasthenic or myopathic condition.

Motor Disorders

Anxiety and fidgetiness are common in thyrotoxicosis. Rarely, true chorea or choreoathetosis appears,[56,57] and it is not always symmetrical. Paroxysmal kinesogenic choreoathetosis has been observed in a patient with iatrogenic hyperthyroidism.[58] The movement disorder usually resolves completely with the use of antithyroid medications and reduction of the adrenergic effects of thyroid hormone by β-blocking agents or reserpine. Adventitious movements recur if hyperthyroidism redevelops.[57] The disorder has been attributed to enhanced catecholamine receptor sensitivity,[57] which is caused by elevated thyroid hormone levels. We are not aware of attempts to treat the choreoathetosis with sympatholytic agents in the absence of antithyroid medications. Treatment with haloperidol has been successful,[59] suggesting that the disorder may result from enhanced striatal dopaminergic sensitivity.[60]

Tremor is frequently seen in thyrotoxicosis, especially in the outstretched hands, protruded tongue, and eyelids. The tremor has the characteristics of an exaggerated physiological tremor. It is rapid (8 to 12 Hz), persists during movement, and is absent at rest.

The amplitude of the tremor is related to the speed of muscle contraction,[61] which itself correlates with the level of thyroid hormone.[62,63] It probably results from elevated β-adrenergic activity, because it is reduced by β-adrenergic blockade.[63,64] Electromyographic (EMG) recordings reveal simultaneous bursts of activity in agonist and antagonist muscles. The segmental stretch reflex may play a role in producing the tremor by producing rhythmic motor outflow at a frequency that enhances the mechanical resonant properties of the limb.[65] Rare cases of coexisting parkinsonism and thyrotoxicosis probably represent the coincidence of two common illnesses.[66] Both hyper- and hypothyroidism may be more difficult to detect in the presence of parkinsonism when the dysthyroid symptoms include slowness, sweating, weight loss, or cognitive changes. The possibility of hyperthyroidism should also be considered when parkinsonian patients develop dyskinetic effects of levodopa therapy.[67]

Brisk reflexes are common, possibly secondary to pyramidal disease (see below) or to the heightened velocity of muscle contraction and shortened relaxation time.[62]

There have been reports of states resembling *amyotrophic lateral sclerosis,* with muscle wasting, hyperactive tendon reflexes, and extensor plantar responses.[3,68] We have never encountered such clinical changes, but case reports continue to appear. In some cases there is no neurological response to treatment of the thyroid disorder, possibly because these situations represent a chance concurrence of two illnesses.[68]

Among a series of patients with amyotrophic lateral sclerosis, a large number had a personal or family history of thyroid disease or abnormal thyroid antibody levels; however, it was concluded that the two illnesses were either unrelated or that both resulted from an altered immune state.[69] In another series, no thyroid abnormality was found.[70] It may be relevant to note in this regard that there are also reports of thyrotoxicosis associated only with myopathy,[71,72] peripheral nerve disease,[73] or pyramidal tract disease[74]; some of the reported patients improved neurologically with thyroid treatment. In one case report, it was suggested that a combination of these thyrotoxic effects may have served to mimic amyotrophic lateral sclerosis.[75] The electrodiagnostic studies obtained in this case revealed evidence of denervation and sensorimotor neuropathy, and the patient improved with thyroid treatment.

Myopathy

Muscle weakness is common with hyperthyroidism. It tends to be slowly progressive, is usually proximal and most prevalent at the shoulder girdle and hip flexors, and may be accompanied by prominent atrophy.[76,77] The severity of the muscle weakness does not necessarily correlate with the level of thyroid hormone. Some patients presenting with severe muscle weakness may have only mild thyrotoxicosis. Fasciculations may be noted. "Spasms"[78] and myokymia[79] are infrequent.

The serum creatine kinase (CK) concentration is usually normal or mildly reduced,[80] except that rhabdomyolysis may occur in thyroid storm.[81] An EMG often reveals brief, low-amplitude, polyphasic motor unit action potentials. Fibrillations and fasciculations may be detected.[82] The motor unit abnormalities probably denote muscle fiber atrophy. However, repetitive motor nerve stimulation may show an edrophonium-responsive decrement in the size of the compound muscle action potentials and posttetanic effects of a type denoting either a postsynaptic or presynaptic neuromuscular junction disorder,[83] so that a component of the motor unit abnormalities may be due to abnormal neuromuscular transmission. Muscle biopsy may be normal or reveal occasional small or necrotic muscle fibers[76] and increased numbers of type II fibers. On the basis of an electrophysiological study of biopsied intercostal muscle of thyrotoxic patients, it has been suggested that muscle weakness is due to reduced membrane excitability.[84]

Even this complication of thyrotoxicosis may improve with the use of propranolol.[85] The disorder slowly resolves after a euthyroid state is reached. Widespread bulbar weakness, which may occur, appears not to be due to concomitant myasthenia gravis; it responds to treatment of the thyroid condition.[76,86]

There are reports of thyrotoxicosis appearing in patients with myotonic dystrophy.[87] Prominent weakness was noted and resolved with treatment of the thyroid condition. Although thyroid function is usually normal in myotonic dystrophy, there is a report of a series of patients with myotonic dystrophy who were euthyroid but had an increased incidence of palpable thyroid gland abnormalities and a decreased thyrotropin (TSH) response to thyrotropin-releasing hormone.[88]

Myasthenia Gravis

An association between thyroid disease and myasthenia gravis is well recognized. There may also be a history of pernicious anemia, rheumatoid arthritis, or systemic lupus erythematosus. The thyroid disease is often of an autoimmune form.[89,90]

Approximately 5 percent of patients with myasthenia gravis also have hyperthyroidism, though the incidence of myasthenia in hyperthyroid patients is considerably lower.[91] If myasthenia develops, it usually occurs before or along with the onset of hyperthyroidism.[76,92]

In general there are no unusual characteristics of either disorder when the two appear in the same patient. Treatment of the thyroid condition does not have a predictable effect on the myasthenia. There have been reports of striking seesaw effects, with increased severity of the myasthenia after thyroid treatment,[93] but this is unusual.[94] Rarely, there is improvement of the myasthenia after treatment of the thyroid condition,[95] possibly because thyrotoxicosis reduces the magnitude of miniature end-plate potentials.[96] There have been reports of thyrotoxic, myasthenic patients in whom testing by repetitive nerve stimulation suggested the presence of either a disorder such as the Lambert-Eaton myasthenic syndrome or both pre- and postsynaptic disturbances of neuromuscular transmission.[97,98]

Distinguishing ophthalmoplegia due to myasthenia gravis from thyrotoxic orbitopathy may be difficult, and the two may coexist.[99] Signs of orbital congestion or abnormal forced ductions suggest the presence of orbitopathy. The presence of ptosis or weakness of the orbicularis oculi muscle points toward myasthenia gravis. Trials with anticholinesterases may not be helpful, since a normal result can be obtained with myasthenia and improvement may occur in the presence of orbitopathy. CT evidence of orbitopathy is helpful, though one patient apparently had myasthenia and orbitopathy in the same muscle.[100]

Thyrotoxic Periodic Paralysis

Patients with hyperthyroidism may experience secondary hypokalemic periodic paralysis. The attacks of weakness and provoking factors of thyrotoxic and familial periodic paralysis are similar. Attacks usually involve the limb musculature and spare the bulbar and ocular muscles; they often occur during sleeping, last for several hours, and seem to be provoked by heavy exercise or meals containing excessive carbohydrates. Most patients with this disorder are Asian. Two recent reports have discussed the experience of North American medical centers and compared it with the experience among Asian populations.[101,102] The American groups included almost no Asians, but did include Hispanics, American Indians, blacks, and whites.[101,102] The incidence rate in one American population was 0.1 to 0.2 percent, which is about one-tenth the Asian rate.[101] In Asians, the thyrotoxic state usually appears before or around the time of onset of periodic paralysis. In the American experience, the clinical features of hyperthyroidism were often subtle. The well-known male prevalence in Asians was also found in non-Asians.

Patients with thyrotoxic and primary forms of periodic paralysis usually have an abnormality of the compound muscle action potential even when no clinical weakness is present.[103] After exercise the action potential exhibits an abnormal increase in magnitude, followed by a very gradual decline. In one case the abnormality resolved when a euthyroid state was achieved.[104]

In most cases the attacks will stop when a euthyroid state is reached. If hypothyroidism occurs, excessive thyroid replacement therapy may allow further attacks to occur.[102] Patients who are still at risk of having attacks should avoid precipitating factors. Propranolol will decrease the number of attacks in most patients. Potassium supplements during attacks are helpful. The value of acetazolamide or potassium supplements between attacks is unproved.[102]

Neuropathy

Reports of a distal sensorimotor polyneuropathy associated with hyperthyroidism (Basedow's paraplegia) appear infrequently. Patients with varying degrees of symmetrical lower extremity changes, with reduction of reflexes, sensory loss, and weakness but no sphincter dysfunction are described. Slowing of nerve conduction velocity has been found in some patients,[73] and an association with Guillain-Barré syndrome has been suggested.[105] Other reports have emphasized the presence of an axonal neuropathy.[106] Patients may improve with thyroid hormone treatment.[73,75]

HYPOTHYROIDISM

Mental Changes

In contrast to hyperthyroidism, many patients with hypothyroidism have alterations of mental status. Patients describe a sense of slowness, decreased concentration, and poor attention, often accompanied by somnolence and lethargy. These symptoms can be difficult to distinguish from those of depression, which may coexist. It is controversial whether the depression that can occur in association with myxedema is a direct result of the lack of thyroid hormone or is unmasked by the deficiency. Hypothyroidism with circulating thyroid antibodies secondary to the use of lithium in the treatment of affective illness further complicates the study of these relations.[107]

Florid psychiatric syndromes are common in severe untreated myxedema. Asher coined the colorful term "myxedema madness"[108] to describe the symptoms, which include irritability, suspiciousness, hallucinations, delirium, and psychosis.[109] The disorder improves with thyroid hormone treatment.[110]

Dementia can occur and must be distinguished from depression.[111] Patients with dementia are often somnolent and abulic. Speech and thought processes are greatly slowed. Studies of thyroid function should be obtained in demented patients, as the effects of hypofunction are reversible.[112] There does not appear to be an increased incidence of thyroid abnormalities in sporadic Alzheimer's disease,[113] but there may be in familial cases.[114]

Several reports have been directed at determining the incidence of psychiatric disorders that result from subclinical hypothyroidism detected by laboratory tests. In one study of patients in a psychogeriatric hospital, there was no statistically significant increase in the incidence of abnormal thyroid function tests.[15] However, other reports have suggested an increased incidence of subclinical hypothyroidism in depressed patients,[16,115] and there may be improvement with thyroid replacement therapy.[116] It has been suggested that thyroid studies should be obtained in any depressed patient who does not respond favorably to antidepressant drugs.[117] Thyroid function abnormalities appear to be common in patients with rapidly cycling bipolar illness,[11] and this may be important when planning treatment of the psychiatric illness.[118]

The thyrotropin–releasing hormone test may be particularly useful.[115,116]

Myxedema coma is an umbrella term referring to the clinical state of patients with severe myxedema who develop hypothermia, bradycardia, hypotension, and respiratory failure. A metabolic disorder supervenes, with abnormal electrolytes or hypoglycemia. In this setting, coma and seizures occur and may prove fatal.[119]

The mortality of myxedema coma is significant.[120] Neuropathological studies show only cerebral edema, with or without diffuse neuronal changes. It is important to ensure the maintenance of respiratory function and blood pressure. Continuous electrocardiographic (ECG) monitoring is desirable because a major cause of death is cardiac arrhythmia. Hyponatremia can be treated with fluid restriction, though in rare cases more aggressive therapy is required. Treatment is usually with thyroid hormone and gluco- and mineralocorticoids.[121]

Seizures, Sleep Disturbance, EEG Abnormalities

There is a high incidence of seizures in patients with hypothyroidism.[122] In one series, about 20 percent of the patients had seizures or syncope.[123] Return to euthyroidism facilitates control. The EEG characteristically shows mild slowing[124] and reduced photic driving.[125] With severe hypothyroidism, the EEG may show little voltage change and superficially appear "flat." When chemical evidence of a thyroid disorder in an epileptic patient is obtained, it is important to bear in mind that some anticonvulsant drugs alter thyroid hormone levels, though they do not usually affect the clinical thyroid status.[126]

Both obstructive and central sleep apnea may occur in the presence of hypothyroidism.[127,128] The obstructive form may respond to thyroid hormone replacement therapy.[129]

Disorders of the Cranial Nerve Systems

Cranial nerve involvement is unusual in hypothyroidism. Disturbed visual acuity, together with optic atrophy and central scotoma, may occur. Visual evoked potentials may be abnormal and respond to treatment.[130] Uveitis has been reported.[131] In primary hypothyroidism, enlargement of the pituitary gland may cause deterioration of vision by compressing the optic chiasm,[132] and hormone treatment may lead to visual improvement by reducing pituitary size.[133] Papilledema can result from pseudotumor cerebri, which may appear when hypothyroidism is treated by hormone replacement.[134] A facial pain syndrome and Bell's palsy may occur in hypothyroidism.[135] Subjective hearing loss and tinnitus may be reported,[136] and there is a report of improvement with thyroid treatment.[137] However, one recent study found no statistical evidence of decreased hearing in 15 hypothyroid patients as compared with controls, no histological abnormalities, and no improvement in hearing after thyroid treatment.[138] The degree of hypothyroidism in these patients was not stated. Vestibular dysfunction is uncommon.[139] Hypothyroidism is associated with a reduced sense of taste.[140] A large survey of patients with disturbances of smell or taste revealed that 14 had no certain etiology but were taking levothyroxine.[141] These patients had an increased incidence of a burning sensation in the mouth and a subjective decrease in taste sensitivity but a higher score than others on their ability to identify tastes. Vocal changes appear to result from local myxedematous changes in the larynx and vocal cords rather than neuronal disease.[142]

Motor Disorders

Cerebellar ataxia (myxedema staggers) is seen in 5 to 10 percent of patients.[72,143] A typical cerebellar gait disturbance appears. Cell loss in the cerebellum has been detected and is most apparent at the anterior superior vermis.[144] The problem is often reversible with thyroid treatment.

Reflexes are often slow or "hung up" (Woltman's sign). This is most apparent at the ankle and is a reflection of slowed muscle contraction and relaxation times.[62,145] Clinically, this slowness correlates with the degree of hypothyroidism[62] and improves with treatment.

A report has suggested an increased incidence of hypothyroidism in parkinsonism and pointed out that parkinsonism may mimic clinical signs of hypothyroidism.[146] There has been interest in the possibility that levodopa therapy may cause hypothyroidism because the human thyrotropin-releasing hormone response is reduced by levodopa,[147] but there is no clear alteration in thyroxine level.[146,148]

Myopathy

Many patients with hypothyroidism have proximal weakness that is usually mild but may be severe and associated with atrophy.[149,150] Muscle stiffness, cramps, and pain occur,[151] and polymyositis may be simulated.[152] There is usually good resolution with thyroid hormone therapy.

Circulating CK levels are increased, and only the muscle isozyme level is affected.[153] However, this cannot be used as an indication of a myopathy in the presence of hypothyroidism. There is often an increase in the enzyme level in myxedema that appears to result from decreased enzyme turnover[154] and decreased clearance.[155] The EMG examination of proximal muscles commonly reveals findings consistent with the presence of a myopathic condition even when no clear weakness is present. The mean duration and amplitude of motor unit action potentials is decreased, and there is a tendency toward increased polyphasia, but there is usually no abnormal spontaneous activity.[150] Muscle biopsy may reveal few abnormalities even when prominent weakness is present. Type II fibers may be atrophic, may be decreased in number, and may contain increased numbers of central nuclei; excessive glycogen accumulation may be found.[156] One patient with hypothyroidism also had rhabdomyolysis and secondary renal failure.[157]

Muscle enlargement in the limbs and tongue may occur with hypothyroidism (Hoffmann's syndrome). Occurring gradually and resulting in a "muscle bound" appearance, it is more common in children (Kocher-Debré-Semelaigne syndrome) than in adults.[77,149] Patients with this disorder commonly have muscular aches and cramps, dysarthria, slow movement, and slow relaxation that becomes worse in the cold. It does not appear to be a form of myotonia because there is slowness of contraction, no percussion myotonia, no improvement with exercise, and no EMG activity indicative of myotonia. The muscles may become progressively more contracted with exercise, so that a patient is able to start walking but then becomes progressively less capable of moving. The cause of the enlargement is not known. There is no clear increase in size of the muscle fibers nor any other associated pathological finding.[158] The

hypertrophy may result from the prolongation of activity when the muscle is used. Improvement occurs with treatment of the thyroid condition.[159]

It is common in hypothyroidism for percussion of muscle to cause a slow, prolonged, electrically silent, local mounding called myoedema,[160] which may be the result of abnormal calcium mechanisms.[161] There have been rare reports of patients with myotonic dystrophy who developed hypothyroidism.[162]

Myasthenia Gravis

Patients with hypothyroidism and myasthenia gravis are occasionally encountered. In one series of patients with myasthenia, there were more patients with hypothyroidism than thyrotoxicosis,[94] but it is generally believed that hyperthyroidism is the more common association. Some hypothyroid myasthenic patients may be in a hypothyroid phase of a primary thyrotoxic disorder[95] and therefore are not representative of an authentic association. Two patients with hypothyroidism and weakness were reported to have electrodiagnostic findings indicative of the myasthenic syndrome.[163] For this reason it may be useful for patients with hypothyroidism and clinical myasthenia to undergo appropriate electrophysiological studies in order to characterize fully any defect in neuromuscular transmission. The weakness may improve with thyroid hormone replacement.[98]

Peripheral Nervous System

Mono- and polyneuropathies may result from myxedema. The most common mononeuropathy is the *carpal tunnel syndrome*,[164] which may appear in as many as 10 percent of hypothyroid patients.[165] It is commonly bilateral but may be subclinical on one side. Pathologically, both axonal and myelin loss are found in the median nerve at the level of the carpal tunnel. Entrapment may be the result of acid mucopolysaccharides in the tissues surrounding the nerve.[166] The syndrome resolves slowly if a euthyroid state is reached,[164] so that surgical release is not usually required.

By comparison with thyrotoxicosis, there is more substantial information indicating an occasional association of polyneuropathy with hypothyroidism.[143] There may be paresthesias, lancinating pain, and sensorimotor involvement, often with reduced knee and ankle reflexes and mildly impaired vibration and position sense.[167] In some patients, a severe neuropathy develops.[166] In others, only electrodiagnostic abnormalities are found, but abnormal nerve conduction velocity must be interpreted with caution if there is a reduced core temperature.[167] Some electrophysiological and histological studies have suggested that segmental demyelination occurs,[166] while others have shown evidence of axonal loss.[168] A tendency to affect only large myelinated fibers has been noted.[169] Gradual improvement may occur with treatment of the thyroid disorder.[168]

There are interesting reports concerning the effects of hypothyroidism on respiratory function.[170] Patients may have dyspnea and exercise limitation, and the results of pulmonary studies may indicate diaphragmatic weakness. Improvement occurs with endocrine treatment. Different reports have attributed the dysfunction to phrenic nerve pathology and to a myopathy. Perhaps an associated neuromuscular junction disorder is also involved.

Cerebrospinal Fluid and Intracranial Pressure

A summary of the physiology of thyrotropin, thyrotropin-releasing hormone, and thyroid hormones in the cerebrospinal fluid (CSF) is available elsewhere.[171] Free thyroxine level and thyroxine transport in the serum and CSF are nearly the same in normal subjects, and the CSF thyroxine level is decreased in hypothyroidism and increased in hyperthyroidism.[172,173] The CSF protein concentration is often elevated in hypothyroidism and rarely may exceed 300 mg/dl.[174] Elevations in gamma globulin and CSF pressure may also be found.[175] The CSF protein level is usually normal in thyrotoxicosis but is occasionally reduced.[176]

There are rare reports of pseudotumor cerebri occurring in association with hypothyroidism. It occurs in children during a period several weeks after initiation of thyroid hormone replacement for primary or hypothalamic hypothyroidism.[134] The cause is unknown. In one adult patient, both pseudotumor and hypothyroidism were present, though replacement therapy had not been started; because the pseudotumor condition was not affected by hormone replacement, it was suggested that the case represented a chance association.[177] Empty sella syndrome may also be found in these circumstances.[134]

NONHORMONAL DISEASE

Papillary-follicular thyroid carcinoma may metastasize to cranial or vertebral bone, meninges, or CNS parenchyma. Studies of patients with thyroid cancer have shown incidences of cranial-spinal involvement of about 1 percent or less.[178,179] Brain involvement has appeared from a matter of months to two or more decades after the original diagnosis. Typical signs of cranial or spinal cord involvement appear. Metastases to brain parenchyma may occur in the apparent absence of other metastatic disease.[179] However, it has been our impression that involvement of the cranial bone and meninges is much more common than parenchymal metastases and that lung involvement almost always accompanies brain involvement. Brain lesions may follow a benign clinical course for a long period. A case of paraneoplastic opsoclonus-myoclonus syndrome in an adult with metastatic medullary thyroid carcinoma has been described.[180]

An interesting association of Hashimoto's thyroiditis and encephalopathy has been described.[181] Patients have the subacute onset of confusion and altered consciousness, seizures, myoclonus, and tremor; focal deficits may occur. The disorder has a relapsing course, and is associated with EEG slowing and a high CSF protein concentration. Patients have usually been euthyroid or nearly so, but have a high thyroid cytoplasmic antibody, antithyroglobulin titer, or thyroid microsomal titer. Treatment with corticosteroids may be helpful. It is theorized that the thyroiditis is accompanied by a cerebral vasculitis or an autoimmune encephalitis.

Enlargement of the thyroid gland from any cause may lead to a compressive neuropathy. Phrenic nerve involvement occurs and can be bilateral.[182] Compression by a thyroid cancer or goiter may cause dysphagia or produce a Bernard-Horner syndrome by involvement of the cervical sympathetic chain.[183] Recurrent laryngeal nerve injury can occur with benign thyroid disease but should always raise suspicion of neoplasia. Injury to one or both of these nerves is the most common complication of surgery on the thyroid gland, but its incidence has been reduced with careful exposure of the nerve and the use of electrophysiological monitoring techniques. Paralysis appearing immediately after surgery may warrant reexploration, with possible reconstruction. Paralysis occurring several days postoperatively may not improve and has been attributed to the effects of local edema. Injury produces hoarseness and, if bilateral, respiratory compromise. Spontaneous recovery from surgical injury occurs frequently.

REFERENCES

1. Raskin NH, Fishman RA: Effects of thyroid on permeability, composition and electrolyte metabolism of brain and other tissues. Arch Neurol 14:21, 1966
2. Thompson CC, Weinberger C, Lebo R, Evans RM: Identification of a novel thyroid hormone receptor expressed in the mammalian central nervous system. Science 237:1610, 1987
3. Logothetis J: Neurologic and muscular manifestations of hyperthyroidism. Arch Neurol 5:533, 1961
4. Bursten B: Psychoses associated with thyrotoxicosis. Arch Gen Psychiatry 4:267, 1961
5. Thomas FB, Mazzaferri EL, Skillman TG: Apathetic thyrotoxicosis: a distinctive clinical and laboratory entity. Ann Intern Med 72:679, 1970
6. Zeitlhofer J, Saletu B, Stary J, Ahmadi R: Cerebral function in hyperthyroid patients: psychopathology, psychometric variables, central arousal and time perception before and after thyreostatic therapy. Neuropsychobiology 11:89, 1984
7. Newcomer J, Haire W, Hartman CR: Coma and thyrotoxicosis. Ann Neurol 14:689, 1983
8. Laurent LPE: Acute thyrotoxic bulbar palsy. Lancet 1:87, 1944
9. Kathol RG, Turner R, Delahunt J: Depression and anxiety associated with hyperthyroidism: response to antithyroid therapy. Psychosomatics 27:501, 1986
10. Parker PE, Walter-Ryan WG, Pittman CS, Folks DG: Lithium treatment of hyperthyroidism and mania. J Clin Psychiatry 47:264, 1986
11. Bauer MS, Whybrow PC: The effect of changing thyroid function on cyclic affective illness in a human subject. Am J Psychiatry 143:633, 1986
12. Norris MS, Matthew RJ, Webb WW: Delirium associated with lithium-induced hypothyroidism: a case report. Am J Psychiatry 140:355, 1983
13. Sandler AP, Thompson J, Putney D: Symptomatic thyroiditis and schizophrenia in a six-year-old girl. J Clin Psychiatry 45:36, 1984
14. Lazarus A, Jaffe R: Resolution of thyroid-induced schizophreniform disorder following subtotal thyroidectomy: case report. Gen Hosp Psychiatry 8:29, 1986
15. Tappy L, Randin JP, Schwed P, et al: Prevalence of thyroid disorders in psychogeriatric inpatients: a possible relationship of hypothyroidism with neurotic depression but not with dementia. J Am Geriatr Soc 35:526, 1987
16. Sternbach HA, Gold MS, Pottash AC, Extein I: Thyroid failure and protirelin (thyrotropin-releasing hormone) test abnormalities in depressed outpatients. JAMA 249:1618, 1983
17. Spratt DI, Pont A, Miller MB, et al: Hyperthyroxinemia in patients with acute psychiatric disorders. Am J Med 73:41, 1982
18. Skanse B, Nyman G: Thyrotoxicosis as a cause of cerebral dysrhythmia and convulsive seizures. Acta Endocrinol (Copenh) 22:246, 1956
19. Jabbari B, Huott AD: Seizures in thyrotoxicosis. Epilepsia 21:91, 1980
20. Smith DL, Looney TJ: Seizures secondary to thyrotoxicosis and high-dosage propranolol therapy. Arch Neurol 40:457, 1983
21. Sokoloff L, Wechsler R, Mangold R, et al: Cerebral blood flow and oxygen consumption in hyperthyroidism before and after treatment. J Clin Invest 32:202, 1953
22. Seyfried TN, Glaser GH, Yu RK: Thyroid hormone influence on the susceptibility of mice to audiogenic seizures. Science 205:598, 1979
23. Sundaram MB, Hill A, Lowry N: Thyroxine-induced petit mal status epilepticus. Neurology 35:1792, 1985
24. Ross DA, Schwab RS: The cortical alpha rhythm in thyroid disorders. Endocrinology 25:75, 1939
25. Wilson W, Johnson J: Thyroid hormone and brain function: I. The EEG in hyperthyroidism with observations on the effect of age, sex, and reserpine in the production of abnormalities. Electroencephalogr Clin Neurophysiol 16:321, 1964
26. Zander Olsen P, Stoler M, Siersbaek-Nielsen K, et al: Electroencephalographic findings in hyperthyroidism. Electroencephalogr Clin Neurophysiol 32:171, 1972
27. Wilson W, Johnson J: Thyroid hormone and brain function: II. Changes in photically elicited EEG responses following the administration of triiodothyronine to normal subjects. Electroencephalogr Clin Neurophysiol 16:329, 1964
28. Scherokman BJ: Triphasic delta waves in a patient with acute hyperthyroidism. Arch Neurol 37:731, 1980
29. Shambaugh GE, Seed R, Korn A: Airway obstruction in substernal goiter. J Chronic Dis 26:737, 1973
30. Stafford N, Youngs R, Waldron J, et al: Obstructive sleep apnoea in association with retrosternal goiter and acromegaly. J Laryngol Otol 100:861, 1986

31. Stern BJ, Gruen R, Koeppel J, et al: Recurrent thyrotoxicosis and papilledema in a patient with communicating hydrocephalus. Arch Neurol 41:65, 1984
32. Dickman MS, Somasundaram M, Brzozowski L: Pseudotumor cerebri and hyperthyroidism. NY State J Med 80:1118, 1980
33. Dresner SC, Kennerdell JS: Dysthyroid orbitopathy. Neurology 35:1628, 1985
34. Brain R, Turnball HM: Exophthalmic ophthalmoplegia. Q J Med 31:293, 1938
35. McGill DA, Asper S: Endocrine exophthalmos. N Engl J Med 267:133, 1962
36. Kendall-Taylor P, Perros P: Circulating retrobulbar antibodies in Graves' ophthalmopathy. Acta Endocrinol (Copenh) 121, suppl 2:31, 1989
37. Gorman CA: Temporal relationship between onset of Graves' ophthalmopathy and diagnosis of thyrotoxicosis. Mayo Clin Proc 58:515, 1983
38. Solomon DH, Chopra IJ, Chopra U, Smith FJ: Identification of subgroups of euthyroid Graves' ophthalmopathy. N Engl J Med 296:181, 1977
39. Spoor TC, Kennerdell JS: Thyrotropin-releasing hormone test and the diagnosis of dysthyroid ophthalmopathy. Ann Ophthalmol 13:443, 1981
40. Trokel SL, Jakobiec FA: Correlation of CT scanning and pathologic features of ophthalmic Graves' disease. Ophthalmology 88:553, 1981
41. Feldon SE, Unsold R: Graves' ophthalmopathy evaluated by infrared eye-movement recordings. Arch Ophthalmol 100:324, 1982
42. Brain R: Pathogenesis and treatment of endocrine exophthalmos. Lancet 1:109, 1959
43. Prummel MF, Wiersinga WM, Mourits MP, et al: Amelioration of eye changes of Graves' ophthalmopathy by achieving euthyroidism. Acta Endocrinol (Copenh) 121, suppl 2:185, 1989
44. Evans D, Kennerdell JS: Extraocular muscle surgery for dysthyroid myopathy. Am J Ophthalmol 95:767, 1983
45. Trobe JD, Glaser JS, Laflamme P: Dysthyroid optic neuropathy. Arch Ophthalmol 96:1199, 1978
46. Neigel JM, Rootman J, Belkin RI, et al. Dysthyroid optic neuropathy. The crowded orbital apex syndrome. Ophthalmology 95:1515, 1988
47. Klingele TG, Hart WM, Burde RM: Management of dysthyroid optic neuropathy. Ophthalmologica 174:327, 1977
48. Prummel MF, Mourits MP, Berghout A, et al: Prednisone and cyclosporine in the treatment of Graves' ophthalmopathy. N Engl J Med 321:1353, 1989
49. Ravin JG, Sisson JC, Knapp WT: Orbital radiation for the ocular changes of Graves' disease. Am J Ophthalmol 79:285, 1975
50. Hallin ES, Feldon SE, Luttrell J: Graves' ophthalmopathy: III. Effect of transantral orbital decompression on optic neuropathy. Br J Ophthalmol 72:683, 1988
51. Pochin E: The mechanism of lid retraction in Graves' disease. Clin Sci 4:91, 1939
52. Emlen W, Segal DS, Mandell AJ: Thyroid state: effects on pre- and postsynaptic central noradrenergic mechanisms. Science 175:79, 1972
53. Cohen MM, Lessell S: Retraction of the lower eyelid. Neurology 29:386, 1979
54. Leone CR: The management of ophthalmic Graves' disease. Ophthalmology 91:770, 1984
55. Putterman AM: Surgical treatment of dysthyroid eyelid retraction and orbital fat herniation. Otolaryngol Clin North Am 13:39, 1980
56. Dhar SK, Nair CP: Choreoathetosis and thyrotoxicosis. Ann Intern Med 80:426, 1974
57. Heffron W, Eaton RP: Thyrotoxicosis presenting as choreoathetosis. Ann Intern Med 73:425, 1970
58. Drake ME: Paroxysmal kinesigenic choreoathetosis in hyperthyroidism. Postgrad Med J 63:1089, 1987
59. Klawans H, Shenker D, Weiner W: Observations on the dopaminergic nature of hyperthyroid chorea. Adv Neurol 1:543, 1973
60. Weiner W, Klawans H: Hyperthyroid chorea. p. 279. In Vinken P, Bruyn G (eds): Handbook of Clinical Neurology. Vol 27. North Holland, New York, 1976
61. Marsden CD, Meadows JC, Lange GW: Effect of speed of muscle contraction on physiological tremor in normal subjects and in patients with thyrotoxicosis and myxoedema. J Neurol Neurosurg Psychiatry 33:776, 1970
62. Lawson J: The free Achilles reflex in hypothyroidism and hyperthyroidism. N Engl J Med 259:761, 1958
63. Marsden CD, Gimlette TM, McAllister RG, et al: Effect of beta-adrenergic blockade on finger tremor and Achilles reflex time in anxious and thyrotoxic patients. Acta Endocrinol (Copenh) 57:353, 1968
64. Young RR, Growdon JH, Shahani BT: Beta-adrenergic mechanisms in action tremor. N Engl J Med 293:950, 1975
65. Hagbarth K-E, Young RR: Participation of the stretch reflex in human physiological tremor. Brain 102:509, 1979
66. Bartels E, Rohart R: The relationship of hyperthyroidism and parkinsonism. Arch Intern Med 101:562, 1958
67. Caradoc-Davies TH: Resolution of dyskinesia and the "on-off" phenomenon in thyrotoxic patients with Parkinson's disease after antithyroid treatment. Br Med J 293:38, 1986
68. McMenamin J, Croxson M: Motor neurone disease and hyperthyroid Graves' disease: a chance association? J Neurol Neurosurg Psychiatry 43:46, 1980

69. Appel SH, Stockton-Appel V, Stewart SS, Kerman RH: Amyotrophic lateral sclerosis: associated clinical disorders and immunological evaluations. Arch Neurol 43:234, 1986
70. Kiessling WR: Thyroid function in 44 patients with amyotrophic lateral sclerosis. Arch Neurol 39:241, 1982
71. Engel AG: Neuromuscular manifestations of Graves' disease. Mayo Clin Proc 47:919, 1972
72. Swanson JW, Kelly JJ Jr, McConahey WM: Neurologic aspects of thyroid dysfunction. Mayo Clin Proc 56:504, 181
73. Feibel JH, Campa JF: Thyrotoxic neuropathy (Basedow's paraplegia). J Neurol Neurosurg Psychiatry 39:491, 1976
74. Garcia CA, Fleming RH: Reversible corticospinal tract disease due to hyperthyroidism. Arch Neurol 34:647, 1977
75. Fisher M, Mateer JE, Ullrich I, Gutrecht JA: Pyramidal tract deficits and polyneuropathy in hyperthyroidism: combination clinically mimicking amyotrophic lateral sclerosis. Am J Med 78:1041, 1985
76. Ramsay I: Thyroid Disease and Muscle Dysfunction. Year Book, Chicago, 1974
77. Adams RD, Rosman NP: Neuromuscular disorders. In Werner SC, Ingbar SH (eds): The Thyroid. 4th Ed. Harper & Row, New York, 1978
78. Alting van Geusau RB, Howeller DH: Reversible muscle spasms in hyperthyroidism. J Neurol Neurosurg Psychiatry 49:1322, 1986
79. Harman JB, Richardson AT: Generalized myokymia in thyrotoxicosis: report of a case. Lancet 1:473, 1954
80. Graig F, Smith J: Serum creatine phosphokinase activity in altered thyroid states. J Clin Endocrinol 25:723, 1965
81. Bennett WR, Huston DP: Rhabdomyolysis in thyroid storm. Am J Med 77:733, 1984
82. Puvanendran K, Cheah J, Naganathan N, Wong PK: Thyrotoxic myopathy: a clinical and quantitative analytic electromyographic study. J Neurol Sci 42:441, 1979
83. Puvanendran K, Cheah J, Naganathan N, et al: Neuromuscular transmission in thyrotoxicosis. J Neurol Sci 43:47, 1979
84. Gruener R, Stern LZ, Payne C, Hannapel L: Hyperthyroid myopathy: intracellular electrophysiological measurements in biopsied human intercostal muscle. J Neurol Sci 24:339, 1975
85. Pimstone N, Marine N, Pimstone B: Beta-adrenergic blockade in thyrotoxic myopathy. Lancet 2:1219, 1968
86. Kammer GM, Hamilton CR: Acue bulbar muscle dysfunction and hyperthyroidism: a study of four cases and review of the literature. Am J Med 56:464, 1974
87. Okuno T, Mori K, Furomi K, et al: Myotonic dystrophy and hyperthyroidism. Neurology 31:91, 1981
88. Steinbeck KS, Carter JN: Thyroid abnormalities in patients with myotonic dystrophy. Clin Endocrinol 17:449, 1982
89. Drachman DB: Myasthenia gravis and the thyroid gland. N Engl J Med 266:330, 1962
90. Engel AG: Thyroid function and myasthenia gravis. Arch Neurol 4:663, 1961
91. Ohno M, Hamada N, Yamakawa J, et al: Myasthenia gravis associated with Graves' disease in Japan. Jpn J Med 26:2, 1987
92. Kiessling WR, Pflughaupt KW, Ricker K, et al: Thyroid function and circulating antithyroid antibodies in myasthenia gravis. Neurology 31:771, 1981
93. Silver S, Osserman KE: Hyperthyroidism and myasthenia gravis. J Mt Sinai Hosp 24:1214, 1957
94. Sahay BM, Blendis LM, Greene R: Relation between myasthenia gravis and thyroid disease. Br Med J 1:762, 1965
95. Feinberg WD, Underdahl LO, Eaton LM: Myasthenia gravis and myxedema. Mayo Clin Proc 32:299, 1957
96. Hofmann WW, Denys E: Effects of thyroid hormone at the neuromuscular junction. Am J Physiol 223:283, 1972
97. Mori M, Takamori M: Hyperthyroidism and myasthenia gravis with features of Eaton-Lambert syndrome. Neurology 26:882, 1976
98. Norris FH Jr: Neuromuscular transmission in thyroid disease. Ann Intern Med 64:81, 1966
99. Czernobilsky J, Ziegler R: Graves' ophthalmopathy, ocular myasthenia gravis and Hashimoto's thyroiditis. Isr J Med Sci 21:377, 1985
100. Spoor TC, Martinez AJ, Kennerdell JS, Mark LE: Dysthyroid and myasthenic myopathy of the medial rectus: a clinical pathologic report. Neurology 30:939, 1980
101. Kelley DE, Gharib H, Kennedy FP, et al: Thyrotoxic periodic paralysis: report of 10 cases and review of electromyographic findings. Arch Intern Med 149:2597, 1989
102. Ober KP: Thyrotoxic periodic paralysis in the United States: report of 7 cases and review of the literature. Medicine (Baltimore) 71:109, 1992
103. McManis PG, Lambert EH, Daube JR: The exercise test in periodic paralysis. Muscle Nerve 9:704, 1986
104. Jackson CE, Barohn RJ: Improvement of the exercise test after therapy in thyrotoxic periodic paralysis. Muscle Nerve 15:1069, 1992
105. Bronsky D, Kaganiec GI, Waldstein SS: An associa-

tion between the Guillain-Barré syndrome and hyperthyroidism. Am J Med Sci 247:196, 1964

106. Ludin HP, Spiess H, Koenig MP: Neuromuscular dysfunction associated with thyrotoxicosis. Eur Neurol 2:269, 1969

107. Calabrese JR, Gulledge AD, Hahn K, et al: Autoimmune thyroiditis in manic-depressive patients treated with lithium. Am J Psychiatry 142:1318, 1985

108. Asher R: Myxoedematous madness. Br Med J 2:555, 1949

109. Norris MS, Mathew RJ, Webb WW: Delirium associated with lithium-induced hypothyroidism. Am J Psychiatry 140:355, 1983

110. Cook DM, Boyle PJ: Rapid reversal of myxedema madness with triiodothyronine. Ann Intern Med 104:893, 1986

111. Peabody CA, Thornton JE, Tinklenberg JR: Progressive dementia associated with thyroid disease. J Clin Psychiatry 47:100, 1986

112. Larson EB, Reifler BV, Featherstone HJ, English DR: Dementia in elderly outpatients: a prospective study. Ann Intern Med 100:417, 1984

113. Yoshimasu F, Kokmen E, Hay ID, et al: The association between Alzheimer's disease and thyroid disease in Rochester, Minnesota. Neurology 41:1745, 1991

114. Ewins DL, Rossor MN, Butler J, et al: Association between autoimmune thyroid disease and familial Alzheimer's disease. Clin Endocrinol 35:93, 1991

115. Gold MS, Pottash ALC, Extein I: Hypothyroidism and depression. JAMA 245:1919, 1981

116. Targum SD, Greenberg RD, Harmon RL, et al: Thyroid hormone and the TRH stimulation test in refractory depression. J Clin Psychiatry 45:345, 1984

117. Des Lauriers A, Baruch P, Vindreau C, et al: Depressions resistent aux traitements antidepresseurs tricycliques et hypothyroidie. Ann Med Interne (Paris) 138:119, 1987

118. Extein I, Pottash AL, Gold MS: Does subclinical hypothyroidism predispose to tricyclic-induced rapid mood cycles? J Clin Psychiatry 43:290, 1982

119. Nickel SN, Frame B: Nervous and muscular systems in myxedema. J Clin Dis 14:570, 1961

120. Blum M: Myxedema coma. Am J Med Sci 264:432, 1972

121. McConahey WM: Diagnosing and treating myxedema coma. Geriatrics 33:61, 1978

122. Evans EC: Neurologic complications of myxedema: convulsions. Ann Intern Med 52:434, 1960

123. Millichap JG: Metabolic and endocrine factors. p. 311. In Vinken PJ, Bruyn GW (eds): Handbook of Clinical Neurology. Vol 15. North Holland, Amsterdam, 1974

124. Barlow JS: Intrinsic and induced EEG rhythms in se-

vere hypothyroidism secondary to panhypopituitarism: a case report. Electroencephalogr Clin Neurophysiol 22:266, 1967

125. Lansing RW, Trunnel JB: Electroencephalographic changes accompanying thyroid deficiency in man. J Clin Endocrinol Metab 23:470, 1963

126. Gadoth N, Kushnir M, Bechar M: Hypothyroidism and phenytoin intoxication. Ann Intern Med 103:640, 1985

127. Rajagopal KR, Abbrecht PH, Derderian SS, et al: Obstructive sleep apnea in hypothyroidism. Ann Intern Med 101:491, 1984

128. Millman RP, Bevilacqua J, Peterson DD, Pack AI: Central sleep apnea in hypothyroidism. Am Rev Respir Dis 127:504, 1983

129. McNamara ME, Southwick SM, Fogel BS: Sleep apnea and hypothyroidism presenting as depression in two patients. J Clin Psychiatry 48:164, 1987

130. Ladenson PW, Stakes JW, Ridgeway EC: Reversible alteration of the visual evoked potential in hypothyroidism. Am J Med 77:1010, 1984

131. Cantor LB, Weber JC, Schlaegel TF: Thyroid dysfunction and uveitis. Ann Ophthalmol 14:515, 1982

132. Yamamoto K, Saito K, Takai T, et al: Visual field defects and pituitary enlargement in primary hypothyroidism. J Clin Endocrinol Metab 57:283, 1983

133. Lecky BR, Williams TD, Lightman SL, et al: Myxoedema presenting with chiasmal compression: resolution after thyroxine replacement. Lancet 1:1347, 1987

134. Van Dop C, Conte FA, Koch TK, et al: Pseudotumor cerebri associated with initiation of levothyroxine therapy for juvenile hypothyroidism. N Engl J Med 308:1076, 1983

135. Watts FB: Atypical facial neuralgia in the hypothyroid state. Ann Intern Med 35:186, 1951

136. Van't Hoff W, Stuart DW: Deafness in myxoedema. Q J Med 48:361, 1979

137. Ritter RN: Reversible hearing loss in human hypothyroidism and correlated changes in the chick inner ear. Laryngoscope 70:393, 1960

138. Parving A: Hearing problems and hormonal disturbances in the elderly. Acta Otolaryngol Suppl (Stockh) 476:44, 1991

139. Bhatia PL, Gupta OP, Agrawal MK, Mishr SK: Audiological and vestibular function tests in hypothyroidism. Laryngoscope 87:2082, 1977

140. McConnell RJ, Menendez CE, Smith FR, et al: Defects of taste and smell in patients with hypothyroidism. Am J Med 59:354, 1975

141. Deems DA, Doty RL, Settle RG, et al: Smell and taste disorders: a study of 750 patients from the University of Pennsylvania Smell and Taste Center. Arch Otolaryngol Head Neck Surg 117:519, 1991

142. Ritter FN: The effects of hypothyroidism upon the ear, nose and throat: a clinical and experimental study. Laryngoscope 77:1427, 1967

143. Cremer GM, Goldstein NP, Paris J: Myxedema and ataxia. Neurology 19:37, 1969

144. Rosman NP: Neurological muscular aspects of thyroid dysfunction in childhood. Pediatr Clin North Am 23:575, 1976

145. Lambert EH, Underdahl LO, Beckett S, Mederos LO: A study of the ankle jerk in myxedema. J Clin Endocrinol 11:1186, 1951

146. Berger JR, Kelley RE: Thyroid function in Parkinson disease. Neurology 31:93, 1981

147. Spaulding SW, Burrow GN, Donabedian R, van Woert M: L-dopa suppression of thyrotropin-releasing hormone response in man. J Clin Endocrinol Metab 35:182, 1972

148. Wingert TD, Hershman JM: Sinemet and thyroid function in Parkinson disease. Neurology 29:1073, 1979

149. Norris FH Jr, Panner BJ: Hypothyroid myopathy: clinical, electromyographical, and ultrastructural observations. Arch Neurol 14:574, 1966

150. Rao SN, Katiyar BC, Nair KRP, Misra S: Neuromuscular status in hypothyroidism. Acta Neurol Scand 61:167, 1980

151. Margolis J, Margolis DA: Severe muscle spasms: an unusual manifestation of hypothyroidism. South Med J 74:1551, 1981

152. Hochberg MC, Koppes GM, Edwards CQ, et al: Hypothyroidism presenting as a polymyositis-like syndrome. Arthritis Rheum 19:1363, 1976

153. Goto I: Serum creatine phosphokinase isozymes in hypothyroidism, convulsion, myocardial infarction and other diseases. Clin Chim Acta 52:27, 1974

154. Doran GR, Wilkinson JH: Serum creatine kinase and adenylate kinase in thyroid disease. Clin Chim Acta 35:115, 1971

155. Karlsberg RP, Roberts R: Effect of altered thyroid function on plasma creatine kinase clearance in the dog. Am J Physiol 235:E614, 1978

156. McKeran RO, Slavin G, Ward P, et al: Hypothyroid myopathy. J Pathol 132:35, 1980

157. Halverson PB, Kozin F, Ryan LM, Sulaiman AR: Rhabdomyolysis and renal failure in hypothyroidism. Ann Intern Med 91:57, 1979

158. Afifi A, Najjar SS, Mire-Salman J, Bergman RA: The myopathy of the Kocher-Debré-Semelaigne syndrome. J Neurol Sci 22:445, 1974

159. Klein I, Parker M, Shebert R, et al: Hypothyroidism presenting as muscle stiffness and pseudohypertrophy: Hoffman's syndrome. Am J Med 70:891, 1981

160. Salick AI, Pearson CM: Electrical silence of myoedema. Neurology 17:899, 1967

161. Mizusawa H, Takagi A, Sugita H, Toyokura Y: Mounding phenomenon: an experimental study in vitro. Neurology 33:90, 1983

162. Brumlick J, Maier RJ: Myxedema and myotonic dystrophy. Arch Intern Med 129:120, 1972

163. Takamori M, Gutmann L, Crosby TW, Martin JD: Myasthenic syndromes in hypothyroidism: electrophysiological study of neuromuscular transmission and muscle contraction in two patients. Arch Neurol 26:326, 1972

164. Purnell DC, Daly DD, Lipscomb PR, et al: Carpal tunnel syndrome associated with myxedema. Arch Intern Med 108:751, 1961

165. Gelberman RH, Aronson D, Weisman MH: Carpal-tunnel syndrome: results of a prospective trial of steroid injection and splinting. J Bone Joint Surg [Am] 62:1181, 1980

166. Dyck PJ, Lambert EH: Polyneuropathy associated with hypothyroidism. J Neuropathol Exp Neurol 29:631, 1970

167. Abbott RJ, O'Malley BP: Responses to temperature in primary hypothyroidism. J Neurol Neurosurg Psychiatry 54:188, 1991

168. Nemni R, Bottacchi E, Fazio R, et al: Polyneuropathy in hypothyroidism: clinical, electrophysiological and morphological findings in four cases. J Neurol Neurosurg Psychiatry 50:1454, 1987

169. Pollard JD, McLeod JG, Honnibal TG, Verheijden MA: Hypothyroid polyneuropathy: clinical, electrophysiological and nerve biopsy findings in two cases. J Neurol Sci 53:461, 1982

170. Martinez FJ, Bermudez-Gomez M, Celli BR: Hypothyroidism: a reversible cause of diaphragmatic dysfunction. Chest 96:1059, 1989

171. Wood JH: Physiological neurochemistry of cerebrospinal fluid. p. 415. In Lajtha A (ed): Handbook of Neurochemistry. Vol 1. 2nd Ed. Plenum Press, New York, 1982

172. Hagen GA, Elliott WJ: Transport of thyroid hormones in serum and cerebrospinal fluid. J Clin Endocrinol Metab 37:415, 1973

173. Hansen JM, Siersbaek-Nielsen K: Cerebrospinal fluid thyroxine. J Clin Endocrinol Metab 29:1023, 1969

174. Bronsky D, Shrifter H, De La Huerge J, et al: Cerebrospinal fluid proteins in myxedema with special reference to electrophoretic partition. J Clin Endocrinol Metab 18:470, 1958

175. Bloomer HA, Papadopoulos NM, McLane JE: Cerebrospinal fluid gamma globulin concentration in myxedema. J Clin Endocrinol Metab 20:869, 1960

176. Thompson WO, Alexander B: Exophthalmic goiter: the protein content of the cerebrospinal fluid. Arch Intern Med 45:122, 1930

177. Press OW, Ladenson PW: Pseudotumor cerebri and hypothyroidism. Arch Intern Med 143:167, 1983

178. McConahey WM, Hay ID, Woolner LB, et al: Papillary thyroid cancer treated at the Mayo Clinic, 1946 through 1970: initial manifestations, pathologic findings, therapy, and outcome. Mayo Clin Proc 61:978, 1986

179. Parker LN, Wu S-Y, Kim DD, et al: Recurrence of papillary thyroid carcinoma presenting as a focal neurologic deficit. Arch Intern Med 146:1985, 1986

180. Dropcho E, Payne R: Paraneoplastic opsoclonus-myoclonus: association with medullary thyroid carcinoma and review of the literature. Arch Neurol 43:410, 1986

181. Shaw PJ, Walls TJ, Newman MK, et al: Hashimoto's encephalopathy: a steroid-responsive disorder associated with high anti-thyroid antibody titers—report of 5 cases. Neurology 41:228, 1991

182. Manning PB, Thompson NW: Bilateral phrenic nerve palsy associated with benign thyroid goiter. Acta Chir Scand 155:429, 1989

183. Lowry SR, Shinton RA, Jamieson G, Manche A: Benign multinodular goitre and reversible Horner's syndrome. Br Med J 296:529, 1988

19

Diabetes and the Nervous System

Anthony J. Windebank
Kathleen M. McEvoy

Diabetes is a systemic disorder of energy metabolism. The central feature of the disease is hyperglycemia secondary to lack of insulin, cellular resistance to the effects of insulin, or a combination of both. It was recognized many years ago that there are several different forms of diabetes. The presently accepted classification system was proposed by the National Diabetes Data Group (NDDG)[1] and is summarized in Table 19-1. The criteria for diagnosis are set out in detail elsewhere.[1] For adults, the major criteria are a fasting blood sugar greater than 140 mg/dl on two occasions or a blood sugar greater than 200 mg/dl at two time points: one at 30, 60, or 90 minutes and one at 120 minutes after a 75-g oral glucose load. For the purposes of this review, patients with either insulin- or non-insulin-dependent diabetes mellitus (IDDM and NIDDM) will be considered. In general, the complications of the two types of diabetes are similar. The best evidence suggests that the incidence of complications increases with duration of disease and severity of hyperglycemia.[2] It also appears that other complications are associated with neurological complications; a patient with retinopathy and nephropathy is more likely to have neuropathy than a patient without these complications.[2] This suggests a common underlying mechanism for these complications. Diabetes is associated primarily with disorders of the peripheral nervous system, including the cranial nerves. Consideration will also be given to the central nervous system (CNS) complications. Retinopathy will not be reviewed.

PERIPHERAL NERVOUS SYSTEM COMPLICATIONS

The incidence of neuropathic complications in the diabetic population is not clearly known.[3] In studies with more than 100 patients, the incidence varies from 10 to 50 percent. There are two major reasons for this wide variability: bias in the selection of diabetic patients and lack of consistent criteria for the definition of peripheral neuropathy. Most studies have used patients attending diabetic clinics as the denominator in incidence or prevalence studies. It is probable that these patients have more severe diabetes or more complications than the general population of diabetics. The difficulty in defining minimal criteria for the diagnosis of neuropathy has been reviewed recently.[4–6] Authors have used criteria as variable as loss of vibration perception and reflexes in the distal lower limbs,[2] abnormalities of nerve conduction,[7] and pathological abnormalities in sural nerve.[8] Gilliatt

Table 19-1 Classification of Diabetes Mellitus

Insulin-dependent diabetes mellitus (IDDM, type I)
    Usually young, thin patients; absolute insulin deficiency; ketosis-prone

Non-insulin-dependent diabetes mellitus (NIDDM, type II)
    Usually older obese patients; relative insulin lack and tissue resistance to insulin effects; not ketosis-prone; often have positive family history

Diabetes mellitus associated with other conditions (secondary diabetes)
    Hyperglycemia associated with other hormonal, metabolic, or genetic disorders (e.g., acromegaly)

Impaired glucose tolerance (IGT)
    Hyperglycemia that is not of sufficient degree to meet the criteria for diabetes mellitus

Gestational diabetes mellitus (GDM)
    Hyperglycemia associated with pregnancy and meeting the criteria for diagnosis of diabetes mellitus, resolves after parturition

and Willison proposed that symptoms severe enough to prompt the patient to seek medical help should be the minimum criterion.[9] The criteria set out by Dyck and colleagues use a combination of abnormalities on clinical examination, electrophysiological evaluation, special sensory testing, or pathological studies.[6] A combination of two abnormalities defines neuropathy. This type of definition is essential for clinical trials. For the clinician, the definition used by Gilliatt and Willison is appropriate.[9]

Three issues will provide the focus of this review. The first concerns diagnosis. In the diabetic patient who presents with new symptoms, it is important to determine whether these symptoms are due to neuropathy. This may be evident if the presentation involves numbness and burning in the feet. However, in the patient who presents with diarrhea due to autonomic neuropathy or chest pain due to thoracic radiculopathy, the diagnosis may require careful consideration to avoid extensive evaluation for visceral causes of the symptoms. The second diagnostic issue concerns the diabetic patient who presents with neuropathy. Because the manifestations of diabetic neuropathy are protean, it is important to exclude other causes of peripheral neuropathy that might be treated differently or have a different prognosis. Awareness of the different patterns of neuropathy complicating

diabetes and the differential diagnosis allows for a more directed evaluation. The third issue, which is most important for patients, is treatment. Virtually all forms of diabetic neuropathy can be treated. In many cases this involves symptomatic treatment. Rational approaches to symptomatic treatment can be developed that should offer relief to the most troublesome symptoms.

Pathogenesis of Diabetic Neuropathy

METABOLIC HYPOTHESES

The cellular events linking hyperglycemia and insulin deficiency to the development of peripheral neuropathy are not completely known. However, there have been major advances in the understanding of the pathological changes that occur. Two recent reviews have detailed the historical development of our understanding of the pathogenesis of diabetic neuropathy.[10,11] From the early studies of Woltman and Wilder until the 1950s, it was believed that large or small blood vessel pathology might underlie the neuropathy.[12] In the 1960s, with increasing recognition of the many cellular metabolic abnormalities accompanying the diabetic state, several hypotheses were proposed.[10] These included the accumulation of sorbitol[13] and decrease of myoinositol[14] in neural tissue. In normal tissue, glucose enters the cell and is phosphorylated by hexokinase to form glucose-6-phosphate, which is then metabolized by the glycolytic pathway. Under aerobic conditions, the products of glycolysis enter the Krebs cycle to generate energy by way of the electron transport chain. Glucose entry into peripheral nerve tissue is not insulin-dependent.[15] Therefore when hyperglycemia occurs, intracellular glucose rises and hexokinase may be saturated. Glucose is shunted to the polyol pathway by way of aldose reductase, which has a much lower affinity for glucose than hexokinase (Fig. 19-1).[16]

Sorbitol accumulation is also associated with myoinositol depletion which, in turn, is related to alterations in Na^+/K^+ ATPase activity.[17] Greene and colleagues have suggested that this leads to disruption of membrane contact between Schwann cells and axons immediately adjacent to the node of Ranvier (axoglial dysjunction). The alteration of Na^+/K^+ ATPase activity and paranodal structure were associated with

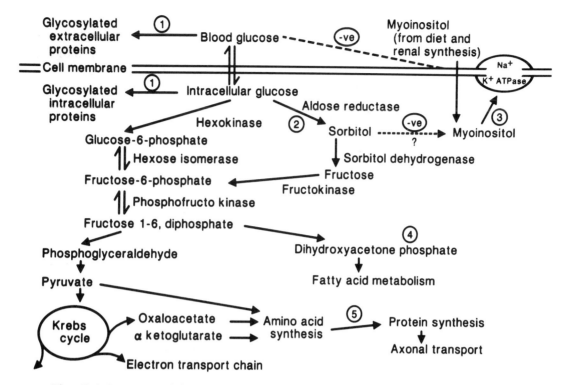

Fig. 19-1 Summary of the metabolic fate of glucose in diabetic nerve and the relation of those pathways to the various "metabolic" theories of the pathogenesis of diabetic neuropathy. Excess glucose levels lead to nonenzymatic glycosylation (1) of blood (e.g., glycosylated hemoglobin), extracellular matrix (especially collagen), and intracellular proteins. This occurs in the protein of peripheral nerve. When excess intracellular glucose is present, it is shunted by way of aldose reductase into sorbitol and fructose production (2). Because of cellular impermeability and low tissue fructokinase levels, there is an intracellular accumulation of these metabolites, which may cause damage by osmotic or other mechanisms.[13] Myoinositol (3) is taken in from the diet and synthesized in the kidneys. The compound is maintained in peripheral nerve cells at about 100 times the serum level by a sodium- and energy-dependent uptake system. High glucose levels inhibit this uptake. High sorbitol levels may also, by some other unknown mechanism, decrease myoinositol levels.[16] Myoinositol is a precursor of the phosphoinositides, which are important in membrane control phenomena. Decreased myoinositol content correlates with a defect in Na^+/K^+ ATPase activity,[17] which may lead to changes in the conduction properties of excitable cells. Alterations in diketone metabolism (4) were considered but could not be correlated with neuropathy. Amino acid synthesis (5) and amino acid uptake by neurons[20] is altered in diabetes, and this may underlie the decreased protein synthesis and changes in slow axonal transport of structural proteins observed in diabetic rats.[19]

nerve conduction slowing in a genetic animal model of diabetes.[18]

The interrelationship of this with other metabolic alterations accompanying the hyperglycemic state is summarized in Figure 19-1.[19,20] There is no doubt that all of these metabolic alterations have been well documented in peripheral nervous system tissue. From that point, arguments concerning causation be-

come more tenuous (Fig. 19-2). Most of these metabolic alterations have been studied in animal models of diabetes, either chemically induced (alloxan or streptozotocin) or genetically determined. Although these animals do develop mild structural neuropathy and some slowing of nerve conduction velocity early in the course of their hyperglycemia, it is not clear how well they represent the human disease. The second type of study has involved the use of human autopsy or biopsy material. Frequently, this utilizes nerve tissue with advanced disease. It is therefore difficult to compare the metabolic activity of disease specimens with controls because the population of cells is quite different. Studies that have tried to correlate pathological alterations with levels of various metabolites have not produced clear correlations between biochemical and pathological abnormality.[8,21] This may relate in part to the cells in which the changes are taking place. There are undoubtedly pathological changes affecting both axon and Schwann cell in human diabetic nerve. It is possible that the biochemical abnormality is prominent in one cell (e.g., the neuron or axon) and that in pathological material the variability present due to loss of axons overshadows the measurable metabolic change. Studies that utilize tissue early in the course of disease or before clinically overt disease has developed are likely to be most rewarding.[22] The implications of various treatment approaches upon interpretation of these hypotheses will be discussed below.

VASCULAR AND HYPOXIC HYPOTHESES

Any theory of the pathogenesis of diabetic neuropathy must take into account the association of diabetic complications. In two large studies[2,23] and many subsequent smaller studies, it has been noted that patients with neuropathy are more likely to have retinopathy and nephropathy than patients without neuropathy. In all of these studies the trend is consistent, so that common mechanisms should underlie the pathological changes. This might be a common metabolic change or type of cell damage (Fig. 19-2) to which the eye, kidney, and nerve are more susceptible, or it might be an organ-specific process of cell injury. In the retina and kidney there is compelling evidence that microvascular changes are integral to the pathological process. Recently, two lines of evidence have suggested that this may be the case in the peripheral nervous system. The first line comes from animal studies in which endoneurial hypoxia has been demonstrated. Microelectrode studies[24] have shown that hypoxia develops in the sciatic nerve after induction of diabetes by streptozotocin. This hypoxia is due to changes in capillary blood flow and is accompanied by biochemical changes[25] that can be simulated by hypoxia in nondiabetic animals.[26] Similar changes have been demonstrated in diabetic human nerve.[27] These hypoxic changes have also been correlated with physiological abnormalities in human nerve.[28] This suggests that the degree of hypoxia is sufficient to cause metabolic changes in cellular energy metabolism. These changes are partially compensated for by high substrate levels of glucose. This shift toward anaerobic or glycolytic metabolism (Fig. 19-3) in the presence of excess glucose would then explain the observation that diabetic nerve is resistant to conduction

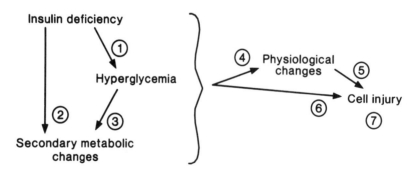

Fig. 19-2 Elements that must be present in the pathogenesis of diabetic neuropathy. Insulin deficiency leads to hyperglycemia *(1)* and secondary changes in many metabolic pathways *(2,3)*. These events lead to physiological changes *(4)*, for example, slowing of motor nerve conduction velocity. These changes may be the forerunners *(5)* or consequences of cell injury *(6)*. The immediate cell injury may be to capillary endothelial cells, neurons, axons, or Schwann cells. Animal models have concentrated on steps 1 through 4. Studies in patients with advanced disease have investigated established pathology *(7)*.

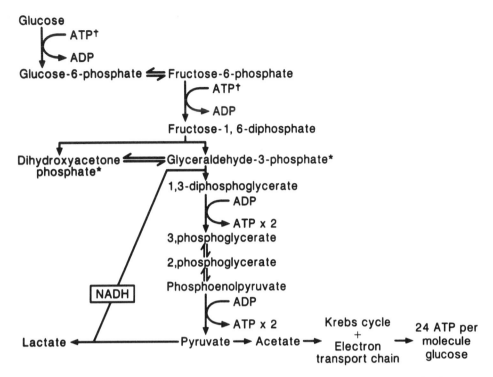

Fig. 19-3 Embden-Meyerhof pathway of glycolysis by which glucose is metabolized to two phosphorylated 3-carbon molecules (⋆) at the expense of two molecules of ATP (†). Glyceraldehyde-3-phosphate can then be metabolized to pyruvate, generating two molecules of ATP per 3-carbon unit for net ATP production of 2 mol ATP/mol glucose. If pyruvate is not utilized in the Krebs cycle, lactate is formed. The electron transport chain, which generates ATP from the reduction products of the Krebs cycle, is down-regulated if oxygen is not available. This condition, in turn, reduces flux through the Krebs cycle. It is proposed that if substrate levels (glucose) are high, the cell can meet its energy demands with anaerobic (glycolytic) metabolism provided that lactate can be removed. This system is much less efficient than oxidative metabolism, which would yield an extra 24 mol ATP/mol glucose. However, it would render the cell less susceptible to hypoxic or ischemic injury.

block produced by experimental ischemia.[29] The biochemical changes and some of the electrophysiological changes in diabetic animal nerves can be prevented by environmental oxygen supplementation.[30,31] These observations strongly suggest a link between the development of hypoxia and early metabolic and physiological changes in experimental diabetes.

The demonstration of significant microvascular changes in human diabetic nerve[32] is an indication that these experimental alterations may be relevant to the human disease. Extensive morphometric studies in autopsy[33] and biopsy material[34] have shown that the major pathological change is multifocal axonal loss identical to that seen in experimental models of microvascular ischemia of nerve.[35] The autopsy stud-

ies have identified nerve fiber pathology at different levels from proximal to distal in the sciatic nerve. This demonstrates that focal lesions at the level of the sciatic nerve may appear as diffuse fiber loss distally because of the intermingling of fibers and because of additions of new lesions along the distal course of the nerve (Fig. 19-4). It has been argued that a similar distribution of fiber loss may be seen in neuropathy of nonvascular etiology.[36]

The fiber loss is associated with an increased number of closed capillaries in diabetic sural nerves. In turn, the number of closed capillaries correlates with an index of pathology that quantitates both fiber loss and fiber abnormality.[37] The vessel changes include thickening of basement membrane and increase in the

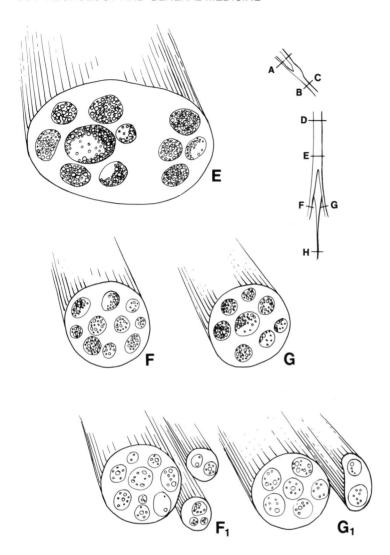

Fig. 19-4 Spatial distribution of myelinated fiber loss in diabetic polyneuropathy. From proximal to distal sites, multifocal fiber loss begins in the sciatic nerve **(E)**. At a more distal level—proximal tibial **(F)** and peroneal **(G)** nerves—there is a greater fiber loss, and additional new multifocal regions of damage are added. At an even more distal level of tibial **(F₁)** and peroneal **(G₁)** nerves, fiber loss has continued to increase, with new regions showing. These changes are consistent with multifocal ischemic injury along the length of nerves. (From Dyck PJ, Karnes JL, O'Brien P, et al: The spatial distribution of fiber loss in diabetic polyneuropathy suggests ischemia. Ann Neurol 19: 440, 1986, with permission).

number and size of capillary endothelial cells, with a reciprocal decrease in the capillary luminal area (Fig. 19-5).[38]

These studies indicate that the capillary endothelial cells or other vascular components bear the initial brunt of the injury. Changes in axons and Schwann cells are then secondary to these vascular alterations. The pathogenesis of the vascular changes, although not understood, is presumably the same as that in other tissues that suffer the complications of diabetes. One plausible theory involves the formation of advanced glycosylation end products. When proteins are exposed chronically to high levels of glucose, a process of nonenzymatic glycosylation occurs. This process alters the interaction between proteins and

may have effects both inside and outside the cell. Extracellular matrix proteins are particularly involved, and this may be the mechanism of basement membrane thickening. The process has been implicated in microvascular changes associated with hyperglycemia.[39] Such a mechanism would link the experimental observations of hypoxia with the beneficial effect of improved glycemic control on nerve function (discussed below). The mechanism by which hypoxia produces cell damage in the peripheral nerve is also unknown. The role of oxygen free radical production and reduction in levels of nitric oxide has been investigated in model systems, but no clear conclusions have been reached.[40,41]

Further evidence that vascular changes may be

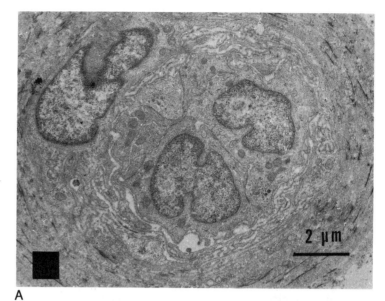

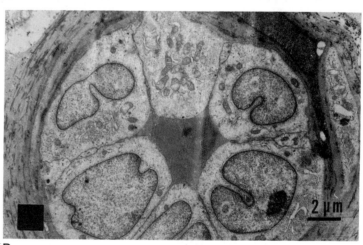

Fig. 19-5 (A) Capillary from diabetic has closed lumen. **(B)** Capillary from a diabetic demonstrating an increased number of endothelial cells and nuclei. The cells appear to be hypertrophied. The lumen has a small caliber. (Original magnifications: **A** ×4,600; **B** ×7,700). (From Yasuda H, Dyck PJ: Abnormalities of endoneurial microvessels and sural nerve pathology in diabetic neuropathy. Neurology 37:20, 1987, with permission.)

more important than primary metabolic changes has come from studies in which diabetics with early or mild neuropathy have undergone sural nerve biopsy. Nerve pathology has not correlated with either increased levels of sorbitol or decreased levels of myoinositol in this nerve tissue.[8,22]

If vascular changes and hypoxia do relate directly to hyperglycemia, then control of blood glucose concentration is the ideal primary therapy for prevention of neurological complications. The success of various treatment modalities and their relevance to the understanding of the pathogenesis of the neuropathy is discussed in the section dealing with treatment, below.

Classification of Diabetic Neuropathy

One of the major issues that has not been satisfactorily addressed concerns the classification of different clinical presentations for patients with diabetes and neuropathy. There is no doubt that patients with diabetes may present their neuropathic symptoms in different ways, but it is not clear whether this represents a continuous spectrum of disease or separate disease entities. A brief classification is presented in Table 19-2. This type of classification stresses predominant clinical forms of neuropathy and is similar to that proposed by Dyck and colleagues[4] and Thomas and

Table 19-2 Classification of Diabetic Neuropathy

Symmetrical distal neuropathy
   Small fiber predominant (painful or anesthetic)
   Large fiber predominant (ataxic or pseudotabetic)
   Autonomic neuropathy
Asymmetrical neuropathy
   Cranial neuropathies (especially third-nerve palsy)
   Plexopathies (including amyotrophy)
   Mono- and polyradiculopathies
   Increased susceptibility to pressure palsy

Eliasson.[42] It classifies on the basis of localization and fiber type of neuropathic abnormality. It is preferable to the complex descriptive type of classification used by Ellenberg[43] and others. If a single mechanism is shown to underlie all types of diabetic neuropathy, the value of classification systems will be less.

Classification provides a framework for differential diagnosis. In approaching a diabetic patient with neuropathy, it is useful to know whether the type of neuropathy is compatible with a diabetic etiology; the less a particular pattern is associated with diabetes, the more vigorously an alternative explanation should be sought. The other value of classification is that it may help in offering prognosis to the individual patient. Indolently progressive, distal symmetrical neuropathy will remit rarely. The subacute, asymmetrical, proximal neuropathies, on the other hand, usually reach a plateau of maximum deficit and then improve spontaneously.

Evaluation of Diabetic Neuropathy

Accurate evaluation is important for diagnostic purposes, for serial observation of patients, and for use in research protocols. This should involve both qualitative and quantitative approaches to the assessment of symptoms and deficit.

EVALUATION OF SYMPTOMS

Some form of structured inquiry about symptoms is essential for following the diabetic patient. Symptom inquiry will be the major source of serial evaluation for most patients. It is therefore necessary to ask about the presence of specific symptoms that may not be volunteered in the setting of a busy diabetic clinic.

Specific inquiry should be made about motor, sensory, and autonomic symptoms. At least the symptoms summarized in Table 19-3 should be sought. This type of structured history has been formalized into detailed computer-scored questionnaires for research purposes.[44] In the diabetic clinic, a less structured checklist following the guidelines set out in Table 19-3 can be used to evaluate and record symptoms quickly. Particular attention should be paid to symptoms that are not usually volunteered either because of embarrassment or because the patient believes they are trivial. Systematic approaches to symptom inquiry have been of benefit in clinical trials.[6,44]

EVALUATION OF MOTOR DEFICIT

Different approaches to the evaluation of motor deficit have been reviewed recently.[6,45] Three types of evaluation can be used apart from purely descriptive recording: functional timed tests, clinical scoring of muscle strength, and mechanical strength measurements. Functional tests such as the ability to stand or walk a defined distance without support are relatively insensitive in terms of defining extent or distribution of motor deficit. They are also not specific for weakness, because defects in coordination or sensation can also impair overall function. Mechanical, isometric strength tests will be of increasing value in clinical trials in the future; however, they are not useful for individual patient management. Mechanical measurement is time-consuming if performed with adequate safeguards to ensure reproducibility. In our laboratory, testing of eight muscle pairs requires approximately 1 hour.

The most practical approach is the scored clinical examination. The physician examines a panel of muscles. A numerical grade is then assigned to the muscle strength. This grade is related to the examiner's opinion of what should be normal for that muscle in the individual patient. Two muscle-strength grading systems have been widely used.[46,47] In the Medical Research Council (MRC) system, a numerical grade is assigned to a described state of muscle power, whereas in the other system an examiner estimates the degree of weakness and assigns a numerical grade (Table 19-4). This scored clinical evaluation is useful for both sequential observation in single patients and for clinical trials.

Table 19-3 Symptom Inquiry in Diabetes Mellitus

System	Common Discriptors
Sensory	
Negative symptoms	Numbness, deadness, "cotton wool feeling," "walking on stilts," "feels like I am wearing gloves," loss of balance (especially with eyes closed), loss of dexterity, inability to find or identify objects in pocket or purse, painless injuries, ulcers
Positive symptoms	Burning, prickling, pain, supersensitivity to light touch, stabbing, electric shock, tearing, tight, band-like
Focal symptoms	Depend on severity and distribution
Motor	
Distal weakness	Impaired fine coordination of hands, inability to turn keys or open jars, toe scuffing, tripping, foot slapping
Proximal weakness	Difficulty with stairs, inability to rise from chair or floor, falls due to knee "giving," difficulty working with or raising arms above the shoulder
Focal weakness	Depends on severity and distribution
Autonomic	
Sudomotor	Loss of sweating, excessive sweating in defined areas, gustatory sweating, dry skin
Cardiovascular	Postural light-headedness, fainting, micturition syncope, cough syncope, exertional syncope
Pupillary	Usually asymptomatic, poor dark adaptation, intolerance of bright light
Sexual	Impotence, loss of ejaculation, retrograde ejaculation, loss of ability to reach sexual climax
Bladder	Urgency, incontinence, dribbling, hesitancy
Bowels	Vomiting (especially of retained food), diarrhea, nocturnal diarrhea, constipation

Table 19-4 Comparison of the Mayo and MRC Grading Systems[a]

Description of Muscle Strength	Mayo Grade[47]	MRC Grade[46]
Normal power	0	5
Mild weakness (25% loss)	−1	—
Active but weak movement against gravity and resistance	—	4
Active movement against gravity but no resistance	—	3
Moderate weakness (50% loss)	−2	—
Active movement with gravity eliminated	—	2
Severe weakness (75% loss)	−3	—
Flicker of contraction	—	1
No contraction	−4	0

[a] Both systems have been in use for more than 70 years and have been subdivided to give greater sensitivity.
(From Windebank AJ: Clinical evaluation of motor function. p. 100. In Dyck PJ, Thomas PK, Asbury AK, et al (eds): Diabetic Neuropathy. WB Saunders, Philadelphia, 1987, with permission.)

Loss of reflexes correlates with both sensory loss and motor loss. Loss of reflexes has little functional significance, but observation of reflex changes is helpful in securing the anatomical diagnosis and in serial observations in individual patients.

EVALUATION OF SENSATION

Sensory loss must be defined in terms of extent, distribution, and modality involved. In the clinical examination, there is always a compromise between completeness and time required for the examination. The patient's cooperation and alertness are essential, and the experienced examiner knows that a reliable sensory examination must be obtained quickly, before the patient becomes bored and inattentive. For this reason, if a focal deficit is suspected, that should be defined first. If a generalized distal abnormality is suspected or a screening examination is undertaken, the examiner should use defined points on all four extremities.[48] The dorsum of the digit just proximal to the nail provides an area of skin that is not usually subject to trauma and is therefore less prone to callus formation. A survey of sensory function might include assessment of threshold for vibration, light touch, joint position, and pin sensation. Evaluation of threshold is probably more reproducible than subjective assessment by the patient of the strength of stimulus. The examiner can vary the intensity of vibration and assess whether the threshold at which the patient perceives vibration is normal. For focal sensory loss, mapping is best done with pin, touch, and temperature sensation.

Quantitation of sensory deficit using automated or computer-assisted techniques[49] has the most value in studying populations of patients either for the purpose of defining natural history of disease or response to treatment in a clinical trial.

AUTONOMIC FUNCTION

A detailed discussion of autonomic function testing is beyond the scope of this review but is considered in Chapter 8. Increasingly sophisticated methods are becoming available to assess all modalities of autonomic function.[50] Certain bedside and office tests of autonomic function are simple and reproducible.

Orthostatic hypotension can be evaluated by measuring blood pressure in the supine, sitting, and standing positions. The blood pressure should be recorded after the subject has been in the position for 1 minute. A fall in systolic pressure of more than 20 percent is considered by us to be abnormal. Others consider a fall in the absolute value of the systolic pressure by 25 or 30 mmHg or of the diastolic pressure by 10 mmHg on standing to be abnormal. If there is a fall in blood pressure associated with assuming the erect position, heart rate should also be recorded. If the sympathetic input to the heart is intact, a reflex tachycardia should accompany the fall of the blood pressure. A fall in blood pressure accompanied by an increase in heart rate might be due to volume depletion secondary to hyperglycemia, dehydration, or diuretic use. If the pulse rate does not increase, sympathetic denervation should be suspected. A fixed tachycardia which does not slow in response to the Valsalva maneuver may indicate loss of parasympathetic vagal innervation to the heart.

Abnormalities of sweating cannot be quantitated in the office, although dry skin may be one indicator of loss of sudomotor function. The thermoregulatory sweat test measures distribution of sweating in response to heating the body core temperature by 1°C. If combined with sudomotor axon reflex testing, it can determine whether sweating loss is due to central or peripheral autonomic failure.[50]

Electrophysiological Testing

Nerve conduction studies and electromyography (needle electrode examination of muscle) may aid in the clinical evaluation or study of diabetic patients in several ways: confirmation of the clinical diagnosis of neuropathy, identification of a pattern of electrophysiological changes characteristic of diabetes, monitoring of progression or remission of disease, and detection of asymptomatic cases.

In general, electrophysiological studies are not required to make a diagnosis of peripheral neuropathy. This can be made on a clinical basis in most cases. In some patients, however, the diagnosis may not be completely clear clinically. In the patient with purely autonomic symptoms and signs, electrophysiological demonstration of generalized neuropathy may help by demonstrating that the peripheral nervous system is involved in a neuropathic process. In the patient with pain alone, particularly localized pain from truncal radiculopathy or lancinating distal limb pain, the electrophysiological studies again may add information by showing generalized nerve involvement. It should be noted that distal burning pain and hypalgesia may be produced by relatively pure small-fiber (unmyelinated and slowly conducting myelinated C fibers) involvement that would be undetected by standard electrophysiological testing. Such selective small-fiber loss is uncommon in diabetes even when the clinical picture is suggestive. This is different from hereditary neuropathies, in which a single class of fibers may be affected almost exclusively.

Electrophysiological studies cannot specifically diagnose diabetic neuropathy. There is no pattern of change that is pathognomonic of the condition. However, there are patterns that are suggestive of diabetic neuropathy. These may be summarized briefly. In very mild or asymptomatic cases, the only changes may be distal slowing of conduction. This is usually not uniform, some nerves being more affected than others, with focal areas of slowing, particularly at common compression sites. In cases of clinically overt neuropathy, there is virtually always a mixture of changes suggesting both demyelination and axonal degeneration. As the neuropathy progressively worsens, the findings of axonal degeneration predominate:

decreased amplitude of compound muscle action potential (CMAP) and sensory nerve action potential (SNAP), relative preservation of proximal conduction velocities, and evidence of fibrillation potentials and motor unit remodeling on needle examination. Careful examination of multiple nerves usually shows a multifocal pattern of involvement rather than a completely diffuse symmetrical pattern.[51] In clinically focal cases of neuropathy, there are electrophysiological signs of more widespread involvement. For example, in patients presenting with a monoradiculopathy, particularly of the truncal (thoracic or upper lumbar) type, the needle examination shows diffuse change in paraspinal muscles characteristic of polyradiculopathy. In patients with signs of single entrapment neuropathy, there are often more diffuse changes, with slowing of conduction across multiple entrapment points.

SIGNIFICANCE OF CHANGES IN CONDUCTION VELOCITY

For purposes of patient management, it is not necessary to use electrophysiological testing to monitor progression or remission of neuropathic changes; this can be done comprehensively and efficiently by clinical examination. In clinical trials, however, electrophysiological testing is an important part of objective monitoring, although it has probably been overemphasized in the past.[7] Exclusive reliance on electrophysiological changes is not appropriate, but the studies are an important adjunct to assessment of symptoms and other special tests of sensation and autonomic function.

Electrophysiological abnormalities are frequently present in completely asymptomatic individual diabetics. These observations are of interest in population studies, in clinical trials, and in trying to understand the pathogenesis of diabetic neuropathy. However, it is unknown whether minor degrees of conduction slowing are signs of impending clinical neuropathy. If they are and if effective treatment becomes available, then screening for these early changes may become very important in clinical management.

When neuropathy is established, there is a general relationship between degree of structural change and abnormalities in nerve conduction, as is true for any form of peripheral neuropathy. However, early in the course of human diabetes as well as in animal models, reversible changes in conduction velocity occur. It is not clear whether these represent acute metabolic changes and are unrelated to the later development of structural neuropathy, whether they are the forerunners of later structural changes, or whether they represent markers of early but readily reversible structural change. There is some evidence in favor of each viewpoint. Reversibility can be accomplished in humans by the establishment of glycemic control[52–54] and prevented from developing in animals by administration of insulin, dietary supplementation with myoinositol, or use of aldose reductase inhibitors that prevent sorbitol increase in nerve.[55] The conduction changes may be mimicked acutely by glucose infusion into rats, and the degree of change correlates with change in nerve fiber geometry (shrinkage), presumably produced by acute osmotic changes.[56,57] There is also some evidence, however, that these conduction changes may represent early and reversible structural changes at the node of Ranvier.[58] Brismar and colleagues propose that in the diabetic BB rat, early conduction changes correlate with a readily reversible myoinositol-related defect in Na^+/K^+ ATPase.[58] This defect then progresses to "axoglial" dysjunction, in which the terminal loops of myelin adjacent to the node begin to strip away. They suggest that this is less reversible and represents the first stage in demyelination.

Clinical Patterns of Diabetic Neuropathy

A recent population-based cohort study showed that, overall, about two-thirds of diabetic patients have some variety of neuropathy.[59] This included 66 percent of patients with type I (IDDM) and 59 percent of patients with type II (NIDDM) diabetes. Approximately half of the patients had symmetrical polyneuropathy, one-fourth had carpal tunnel syndrome, and the remainder had various forms of autonomic or other neuropathy. Symptoms of the symmetrical polyneuropathy occurred in 15 percent of IDDM and 13 percent of NIDDM patients. Severe and functionally limiting neuropathy was seen in only 6 percent of IDDM and 1 percent of NIDDM patients. Although carpal tunnel syndrome was diagnosed electrophysiologically in one-quarter of the patients, only 7.7 percent had symptoms.

As discussed earlier, there is a continuing debate

about the discrete or continuous nature of diabetic neuropathic disorders. Whatever the truth, there are syndromes of neuropathy that are characteristic of diabetes.

DISTAL SYMMETRICAL NEUROPATHY

This is the most common form of diabetic neuropathy.[59] In the diabetic patient with distal symmetrical neuropathy, symptoms usually being insidiously and may be positive or negative. Negative symptoms in the feet may be described in a variety of ways (Table 19-3). If nociceptive fibers are involved, loss of feeling may not be noticed and the patient may present with painless injury. An object may become lodged in the shoe and erode through the skin with normal walking and weight bearing. Painless ulcers may develop over pressure points, most commonly under the metatarsal heads. However, any areas of skin subjected to constant friction may ulcerate. This is almost always seen in association with significant atherosclerosis of large vessels or impaired circulation in the skin. Another presentation for painless neuropathy is with the Charcot joint. The patient complains of progressive ankle and foot deformity with relatively little pain. Radiographs show disorganization and collapse of the ankle joint. This presentation may occur when the signs of neuropathy are otherwise minimal.

In the patient with more involvement of large sensory fibers, the negative symptoms may include loss of balance, especially at night or with the eyes closed.

Positive symptoms also vary according to the class of sensory fibers involved. Small-fiber involvement produces burning and stinging sensations that are almost constant. Involvement of larger fibers tends to produce a tight, band-like feeling around the extremity or an electrical tingling sensation. These symptoms are often similar to those described by patients with lesions in the posterior columns of the cord.

The first step in evaluating these symptoms in a diabetic patient is to confirm the presence of neuropathy by clinical examination. In most cases, distal symmetrical sensory loss is apparent. Among patients who complain only of distal burning, the loss of distal pain sensation may be subtle. If distal symmetrical neuropathy progresses, motor involvement becomes clinically apparent. It begins distally with weakness of toe dorsiflexion and intrinsic hand muscles. This

weakness may gradually progress to involve the leg muscles, but it is very rare for weakness to occur proximal to the knee or elbow. Diminution of deep tendon reflexes tends to parallel the sensory loss.

Electrophysiological studies are virtually always abnormal in this group of patients.[59] Nerve conduction velocities are usually slowed, with the most prominent changes observed distally. There may be areas of partial conduction block, particularly at common pressure points.[51] The changes in sensory conduction are usually more prominent than the motor conduction changes. However, even in patients with signs and symptoms that are purely sensory, slowing of motor nerve conduction velocity is common. Needle electrode examination of muscle shows distal changes indicative of chronic partial denervation with reinnervation. The degree of electrophysiological change does relate approximately to the severity of the physical signs, but the quality of the symptoms does not appear to relate to the electrophysiological abnormalities. In patients with distal burning and pain as the only symptoms, there are usually some of the electrophysiological changes described above. By contrast, patients with hereditary selective small-fiber neuropathy may present with distal ulceration, Charcot joints, or painful feet and have little electrophysiological change[60,61] because standard tests only measure conduction in the larger sensory or motor fibers. These electrophysiological observations support the hypothesis that symmetrical diabetic neuropathy is a pathologically homogeneous process and that its different symptom complexes represent points in the spectrum of abnormality.

Investigations for other causes of neuropathy are normal. The cerebrospinal fluid (CSF) protein may be normal or modestly elevated (less than 80 mg/dl). In the established diabetic, there is rarely any confusion about the diagnosis of this type of neuropathy. The factors summarized in Table 19-5 suggest other etiologies for neuropathy in patients with diabetes.

The major diagnostic difficulty concerns the patient who presents with neuropathy and is found to have minimal or borderline diabetes mellitus. This problem occurs only in the type II diabetic. If the clinical presentation of the neuropathy is appropriate for diabetes, no other cause is found, and the patient meets the diagnostic criteria for diabetes outlined earlier, it is probable that the diabetes and neuropathy are related. If the first two conditions are met and the pa-

Table 19-5 Clinical Features Suggesting a Nondiabetic Etiology for Neuropathy in Diabetic Patients

Clinical Features	Consider
Family history of neuropathy, painful feet	Hereditary motor and sensory neuropathy (HMSN)
Abrupt onset	Inflammatory neuropathy
Pes cavus and hammertoes	HMSN
Monoclonal gammopathy in serum	Primary systemic amyloidosis
	Myeloma
	Lymphoma
	Monoclonal gammopathy-associated neuropathy
CSF protein >100 mg/dl	Inflammatory neuropathy
Elevated ESR, positive rheumatoid factor, antinuclear antibody, etc.	Inflammatory neuropathy Necrotizing angiopathy as part of collagen vascular disease

tient does not meet the blood sugar requirements but has an elevated glycosylated hemoglobin level, it is also likely that the neuropathy is secondary to diabetes. The elevated level of glycohemoglobin suggests that significant hyperglycemia has been present even though it has not been observed in periodic blood sugar measurements. Finally, if the first two conditions are met but the patient does not have a sufficiently elevated blood glucose concentration and has a normal glycosylated hemoglobin, the diagnosis should be left open and the patient observed periodically.

AUTONOMIC NEUROPATHY

In most patients with diabetes and peripheral neuropathy, some degree of autonomic neuropathy can be detected by using special testing methods.[62] In some cases the autonomic abnormalities may be asymptomatic. However, if carefully questioned, many patients with diabetes and distal symmetrical neuropathy have some of the symptoms described below. When severe autonomic neuropathy is present, it has an adverse effect on survival.[63]

Pupil Abnormalities

Pupil abnormalities are seen commonly but are usually asymptomatic. Although some patients may complain of accommodation difficulty, this usually relates to changes in lens and ocular hydration rather than autonomic neuropathy. The variation in hydration depends acutely on changes in blood sugar. When autonomic neuropathy is present, pupil size usually decreases and response to light or accommodation is lost. In extreme cases this may mimic the Argyll-Robertson pupil of tabes.[64]

Sudomotor Function

Sudomotor function is almost universally affected in diabetics with neuropathy.[50] This loss of sweating capacity is usually asymptomatic. In severe cases, loss of thermoregulation may occur. Occasionally, compensatory hyperhidrosis or gustatory sweating in areas of retained sudomotor function is reported. It is possible that loss of sweat secretion contributes to skin ulceration, but this has not been studied.

Cardiovascular Abnormalities

Cardiovascular abnormalities may produce very significant symptoms of orthostatic hypotension. In the older patient, these symptoms may be vague and potentiated by diuretics. In other patients the symptoms of orthostatic hypotension may be confused with those of hypoglycemia. The recording of lying and standing blood pressures and pulse rates should be a routine part of the neurological examination of diabetics. More extensive testing methods are available[50] but not usually necessary for clinical purposes. If the blood pressure falls upon standing and there is no compensatory rise in pulse rate and if the patient is not on medications affecting heart rate, an autonomic neuropathy is likely. If the blood pressure fall is accompanied by an increased heart rate, volume depletion should be suspected.

Gastrointestinal Function

Gastrointestinal function may be affected in a variety of ways; the most common are gastroparesis and diarrhea. Any part of the gastrointestinal tract can exhibit reduced motility,[50] but this is usually asymptomatic. Gastroparesis may be asymptomatic, but it may also present acutely with nausea and vomiting or with chronic vomiting. The vomiting is characterized by the presence of food eaten more than 12 hours previously.

Diabetic diarrhea probably results from disordered motility of the small intestine. Significant abnormalities of intestinal motility occur in diabetic subjects. Disordered motility alone is not the only cause of the diarrhea; other factors—such as metabolic alteration, vascular changes, altered hormonal control, and increased susceptibility to infection—also play a role. Decreased motility with secondary bacterial overgrowth produces diarrhea that responds to treatment with tetracycline. The clinical features of the diarrhea are characteristic. It is usually explosive and frequently occurs at night, which may lead to nocturnal incontinence. It is usually painless, watery, and very rarely bloody. Periods of diarrhea are interspersed with periods of resistant constipation. An obstructing bowel lesion must be ruled out with contrast studies and proctoscopy before the diagnosis of diabetic complications can be made confidently. During the contrast studies, the radiologist can also make estimates of transit time through the stomach and intestines and observe gastric dilatation if present.

Diabetic Bladder Disease

Diabetic bladder disease is usually asymptomatic until recurrent urinary tract infections occur. These may precipitate or potentiate renal failure. Loss of afferent information from nerves in the detrusor muscle leads to progressive bladder enlargement.[65]

Impairment of Sexual Function

Impairment of sexual function has been studied only in men. This bias, although in part cultural, is also due to the relative ease with which penile erectile impotence is recognized by the patient and studied by the investigator. Mechanisms for studying disorders of the physiology of female sexual response have not generally been applied to diabetics. There is some evidence that diabetic women with autonomic neuropathy are less prone to sexual dysfunction than men.[66] In diabetic men with autonomic involvement, erectile impotence or ejaculatory failure is common. Evaluation of this problem is complex and involves psychological considerations. The techniques available to study the physiology of erection are discussed in Chapter 27.

Insensitivity to Hypoglycemia

Insensitivity to hypoglycemia may occur. The physiological response to hypoglycemia involves epinephrine release and increased sympathetic activity, which produce the characteristic symptoms of hypoglycemia. Since epinephrine release is mediated by the splanchnic nerves, this response may be lost in patients with autonomic neuropathy. This leads to attenuation of both the symptoms of and physiological compensation for hypoglycemia.

SUBACUTE SYMMETRICAL NEUROPATHIES

The neuropathic syndromes described above begin insidiously and usually progress slowly without remission. The types of neuropathy discussed in the following section have an acute or subacute onset. After a period of progression, there is a period of stability and then gradual improvement. This temporal profile is more characteristic of the focal neuropathies but is occasionally seen in the distinctive syndromes described below.

ACUTE PAINFUL NEUROPATHY WITH WEIGHT LOSS

This syndrome was first described by Ellenberg[67] and then more clearly delineated in neurological terms by Archer and colleagues.[68] All of the cases described by these workers were male, whereas we have observed the syndrome in patients of either sex. The cardinal features are weight loss and severe pain, often accompanied by depression and impotence. There appear to be two circumstances in which this syndrome occurs. The first involves a profound weight loss over a fairly short period of time. This loss may exceed 50 percent of original body weight, and may occur spontaneously due to uncontrolled diabetes or intentionally as part of the management of diabetes. Once the pain begins, the patient becomes anorectic and depressed, which accelerates the weight loss. In the second circumstance, the patient has had uncontrolled hyperglycemia for a prolonged period, either because the diabetes was undiagnosed or the disease was recognized but poorly controlled. Within 1 to 2 weeks of instituting tight control, the painful neuropathic symptoms begin. We have seen examples of this occurring in patients who have started treatment with continuous insulin infusion pumps.

In either circumstance, there is the rapid onset of severe, superficial pain which is usually described as burning, stinging, or like an electric shock. This pain may begin distally in the limbs and spread proximally or, in some cases, begin proximally in the anterior thighs. The pain is worse with weight bearing, and the patient cannot bear to have the skin touched by clothes or bed coverings. In our experience and in the patients described by Archer and co-workers[68] sensory loss on examination was minimal and there was no weakness. Ellenberg described weakness in his cases,[67] but it is not clear whether this was neuropathic weakness or generalized weakness secondary to cachexia and pain. Improvement begins after the patient starts to regain weight, which is often helped by the use of antidepressants. In those individuals in whom the pain began after institution of good control, some relief can be obtained by relaxing the glycemic control and then gradually reinstituting normoglycemia.

The association of this syndrome with either weight loss or institution of good control suggests that metabolic changes may trigger the symptoms. Low[25] has suggested that the nerve fibers are hypoxic, but with increased substrate levels of glucose, they can maintain energy supplies using anaerobic, glycolytic respiration (see p. 352). If the substrate is depleted either by institution of control or complete depletion of body stores (severe cachexia), the nerve fiber becomes unable to maintain energy metabolism.

Complete resolution of symptoms is the rule, but it usually occurs over 6 to 24 months, suggesting that axonal regeneration is a factor.

HYPOGLYCEMIC NEUROPATHY

It remains controversial whether damage to the peripheral nervous system occurs as a result of hypoglycemia. Early accounts of diabetic neuropathy included descriptions of "insulin neuritis."[69–71] Cases were described in which neuropathic symptoms began or worsened following institution of insulin therapy. These almost certainly represent the syndrome described above rather than a true hypoglycemia-induced neuropathy.

Case reports have suggested the development of neuromuscular symptoms in nondiabetic cases of hyperinsulinemia and consequent hypoglycemia. This resulted from insulinoma[72,73] or insulin shock therapy for schizophrenia.[74] The evidence from animal studies is not definite. There is some evidence that severe, prolonged hypoglycemia may result in neuronal or axonal damage.[75] It is not clear whether this is clinically relevant in diabetic patients.

FOCAL AND MULTIFOCAL NEUROPATHY

Two types of focal neuropathy are seen in diabetic patients: those occurring spontaneously in nerves and those occurring as a result of nerves crossing common pressure points. The spontaneously occurring neuropathies characteristically occur at the level of root, plexus, or individual nerve. The underlying pathology in these cases is clearly vascular.

DIABETIC RADICULOPATHY AND POLYRADICULOPATHY

Radiculopathy may be the presenting feature of diabetes, but more commonly it occurs in the context of long-standing disease. It is very uncommon in patients below the age of 40 years. Monoradiculopathies may occur at any spinal level and therefore may be confused with a compressive root lesion. Clinical features help to differentiate between compressive and diabetic root lesions. Location of the symptoms and character of the pain are the most useful items. Pain is the prominent symptom and begins acutely or subacutely. It occurs most frequently on the trunk and is unilateral. Burning and supersensitivity of the skin are the most common features of the pain, but it may be of a deep, aching character. Although pain is severe, sensory loss is minimal or absent on examination and weakness is not usually apparent in the trunk muscles. Characteristically, thoracic and upper lumbar roots are involved. If L3 and L4 are affected, the pain begins in the anterior thigh and is followed quite rapidly by weakness of quadriceps and other muscles. Some cases cannot be resolved on a clinical basis and the electrophysiological features may then be helpful. In the diabetic, the symptoms and signs may be entirely at one root level, but the electrophysiological changes are more diffuse. Typically, fibrillation potentials are found at multiple levels in the paraspinal muscles. The electrophysiological changes of polyneuropathy may not be present.[76] If there is diagnostic uncertainty, imaging may be required to exclude a mass lesion.

Because of the common occurrence of this problem in the thoracic and lumbar region, the differential diagnosis may include a visceral cause for the pain. In the chest, cardiac or pleural disease may be suspected. Significant weight loss occurs in more than 50 percent of cases,[77] and a search for malignancy may be initiated.

The prognosis for recovery from these symptoms is excellent. The pain usually reaches a maximum within weeks of onset, persists for several months, and then gradually resolves completely.

A small number of patients develop recurrent diabetic radiculopathy at different spinal levels. Episodes may be separated by months or years. Multiple levels may be involved coincidentally in the form of a polyradiculopathy. Symptoms may begin in one limb, with focal pain that spreads to involve different dermatomes; it is then followed over days or weeks by weakness in corresponding myotomes. The symptoms in one root level may be stable or even improving as another root becomes involved. This sequence may then spread from one leg to the other and rarely to the cervical levels, producing arm pain and weakness. Progression may occur over many months, with one limb improving as another becomes involved. The ultimate prognosis for some degree of recovery is good, but improvement may be prolonged over many years because of the severity of involvement (unpublished observation, AJW).

The differential diagnosis includes chronic inflammatory demyelinating polyradiculoneuropathy, Lyme disease, malignant infiltration (especially by lymphoma), acquired immunodeficiency syndrome (AIDS), and sarcoidosis. Electrophysiological features may help to separate diabetic polyradiculopathy from chronic inflammatory demyelinating polyradiculoneuropathy. The diabetic process has the features of an axonal lesion, often without slowing of conduction, and the evidence of polyneuropathy may be minimal or absent.

Examination of the CSF may be very helpful and is mandatory in the differential diagnosis set out above. The protein concentration is modestly elevated (50 to 150 mg/dl) in the diabetic patients. In chronic inflammatory demyelinating polyradiculoneuropathy, it may be much higher (100 to 4,000 mg/dl). Pleocytosis is usually not present in either case.

The presence of cells in the CSF raises the question of lymphoma, sarcoid, AIDS, or Lyme disease. In the latter three cases the cells are usually polyclonal. The last two can be readily distinguished by serology. Infiltration of roots by lymphoma should be suspected if surface markers suggest a monoclonal cell line in the CSF. Infiltration of roots by other malignant cells would be confirmed by cytological identification in the CSF.

PLEXOPATHY

Plexopathy overlaps in clinical presentation with diabetic radiculopathy and polyradiculopathy. The terms *diabetic amyotrophy*,[78] *diabetic myelopathy*,[79] *diabetic femoral neuropathy*,[80,81] and more recently *proximal motor neuropathy*[77] have all been used to describe this syndrome. The preferred terms are *proximal motor neuropathy* or *radiculoplexopathy*.

The characteristic syndrome of diabetic plexopathy begins rapidly over days to a few weeks, typically in older patients. The initial symptom is pain in the anterior thigh followed by buckling of the knee due to quadriceps weakness. Maximum deficit is usually reached in a few weeks; the deficit is then stable for weeks to months and improves over months to years. Some degree of improvement is universal and usually functional recovery is good. Neurological examination shows weakness and often severe atrophy of the quadriceps muscle. There may be accompanying weakness of any of the muscles innervated by the lumbar or sacral plexus. The most commonly affected muscles are those supplied by the L3 and L4 roots. Sensory loss is minimal; typically, small patchy areas of hypesthesia or hyperpathia over the anterior thigh are observed. The knee reflex is reduced or absent.

Extensive investigations are not usually necessary. The differential diagnosis during the progressive phase may lead to a suspicion of malignant infiltration of the plexus, especially in the older patient who has accompanying weight loss. Computed tomography (CT) scanning through the plexus and a period of clinical observation resolve this question. If the CSF is examined, it is usually normal. Electromyography shows involvement of muscles beyond those that are clinically weak. Evidence of distal peripheral neuropathy may or may not be present.[76,82] It has been suggested that patients with accompanying distal neuropathy tend to have more severe diabetes and a more indolent clinical course of the proximal motor neuropathy.[82]

CRANIAL NEUROPATHY

The occurrence of isolated third and sixth nerve palsies is well recognized as a complication of diabetes. Trigeminal neuropathy and trigeminal neuralgia do not appear to be more common in diabetics.

Oculomotor palsy is characterized by rapid onset over hours to days accompanied by pain in the forehead. Examination shows typical third nerve palsy with ptosis but sparing of the pupillary reflex. The differential diagnosis includes compressive lesions, especially aneurysms and meningiomas, which usually produce early loss of the pupillary reflex. Intrinsic brainstem lesions in the region of the third-nerve nucleus and medial longitudinal fasciculus may produce oculomotor paralysis with pupil sparing. Complete recovery is the rule. The underlying pathology is a vascular lesion in the third nerve that spares the more circumferentially placed pupillomotor fibers.[77]

COMPRESSION NEUROPATHIES

All clinicians who see diabetic patients believe that the incidence of compression neuropathies (carpal tunnel syndrome, ulnar neuropathy at the elbow, and peroneal neuropathy at the fibular head) is higher in diabetics than in the population at large. One population study has demonstrated this to be the case for median neuropathy at the wrist.[59] Management of compression neuropathy in the diabetic is similar to that in the nondiabetic except that surgical decompression should be contemplated only when the nerve entrapment is clearly producing a significant deficit. Transposition of the ulnar nerve is virtually never indicated in the diabetic patient.

Treatment of Diabetic Neuropathy

Treatment can be broadly divided into those therapies aimed at correcting the underlying pathogenetic mechanism and those that help relieve symptoms. Both are important. Most cases of diabetic neuropathy are treatable to some extent; a nihilistic approach to therapy is not appropriate.

CONTROL OF BLOOD GLUCOSE LEVEL

The role of normalizing blood sugar concentration in the control of diabetic complications is not fully elucidated. However, there is increasing evidence that the probability of developing microvascular complications, including neuropathy, is reduced by good control. This been difficult to prove because of the lack of good animal models, the difficulty in normalizing blood sugar in diabetic patients, and the lack of well-defined endpoints.[7,83] However, two major studies have strongly suggested that normalization of blood glucose levels has a major effect in preventing microvascular complications, including neuropathy.[23,84] Both studies involved randomization of IDDM patients between conventional insulin therapy and a multiple injection regimen[23,84] or continuous subcutaneous insulin infusion pumps.[84] In both studies there was an unequivocal benefit of near normoglycemia. The physician must therefore provide diabetic patients with access to the best methods of obtaining glycemic control.

ALDOSE REDUCTASE INHIBITION

The possible role of abnormal accumulation of alcohol sugars in the pathogenesis of diabetic neuropathy is discussed on page 350. Drugs that inhibit aldose reductase can reduce this accumulation in animal models and human diabetic nerves.[17,22,85] In spite of extensive clinical studies, it is not clear that these drugs influence the course of symptomatic diabetic neuropathy.[86–91] The role of supplementary dietary intake of myoinositol is similarly unclear at the present time.[92]

SYMPTOMATIC TREATMENT

Physical Approaches

In patients with distal symmetrical neuropathy, pain and anesthesia are the most troubling features. Anesthesia predisposes the ischemic limb to ulceration and infection. Proper footwear is essential, and the diabetic with an anesthetic foot must be instructed in foot care. The inside of shoes should be inspected three times each day to ensure that stones or other sharp objects are not producing perforation. Any suggestion of blistering due to pressure from shoes must be corrected immediately. Any signs of local infection should be treated aggressively by medical and surgical means. Cessation of weight bearing is usually necessary to ensure healing of plantar ulcers. The painful foot may be helped by alternating hot and cold soaks, especially before retiring to bed. To avoid burns, water temperature should be checked by thermometer or by someone with normal sensation. Soaks should not exceed 10 minutes to avoid the complication of immersion foot.

In patients with compression neuropathy, education in the avoidance of repeated trauma is important. Crossing of the legs and leaning on the elbows may be the cause of symptoms and should be avoided. Nocturnal splinting may help the patient with carpal tunnel syndrome. Attention to the avoidance of intraoperative pressure or traction trauma to nerves is particularly important in the diabetic.

Patients with focal neuropathies should receive aggressive physical therapy. The prognosis for recovery from radiculopathies and plexopathies is excellent. The weakness may be profound and recovery slow, so that avoidance of pressure injury to skin or joint contractures requires the help of the skilled physiotherapist.

Pharmacological Approaches

The major symptom requiring treatment in the patient with neuropathy is pain. The mechanisms important in modulating pain are multifactorial (Fig. 19-6). There is good evidence that the major generator of pain in peripheral neuropathy is the distal end of the damaged fiber.[93] It is not clear whether distal degeneration or regenerative sprouting is the most important component. Ectopic impulses may be generated by unstable distal membranes or possibly by ephaptic transmission from demyelinated adjacent fibers.

The character of the pain is important in determining appropriate medication. The lancinating or lightning pains of some patients respond dramatically to treatment with carbamazepine. Such pains often occur in one area repetitively and then move to a different area. Carbamazepine can be started at 100 mg three times daily and then gradually increased to 200 mg three times daily. Starting at the lower dose avoids nausea. It is rare for doses greater than 200 mg three times daily to be required. The usual precautions against marrow suppression should be observed. Carbamazepine is thought to act by increasing membrane stability. Phenytoin has been tried in many cases and is occasionally helpful.

Burning, steady pain is more likely to respond to treatment with antidepressants, although their mechanism of action is unknown. They appear to help at lower doses than those required for treating depression, and they may work in patients who are not depressed. It is likely, therefore, that the mode of action is central but independent of the antidepressant effect. The use of a combination of antidepressants and major tranquilizers has been advocated in the past. In this author's experience the tranquilizer does not help, and the risk of tardive dyskinesia is not therefore justified. The antidepressant used most frequently is amitriptyline. If the anticholinergic side effects are not well tolerated, doxepin is an alternative. It is impor-

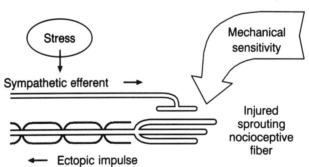

Fig. 19-6 Mechanisms that may be involved in pain generation. Pain correlates best with the pathological change of axonal degeneration. It is suggested that an ectopic impulse arises in the injured end of a nociceptive fiber because of membrane instability. Rate of ectopic generation is increased by mechanical factors or situations increasing sympathetic activity. Ephaptic transmission may play a role, but this has not been demonstrated in the diabetic.

tant to explain the anticholinergic side effects so that the patient will persist in taking the drug for a reasonable trial. To avoid these side effects it is important to start with a very low dose of amitriptyline and increase it gradually. Sedative side effects can be an advantage if the entire daily dose is taken about 1 hour before retiring. Some patients require as little as 12.5 mg of amitriptyline daily to reduce symptoms. It has been suggested that higher doses may cause the therapeutic effect to be lost.

In order to reduce the sympathetic drive that may be potentiating pain, α-adrenergic receptor blocking agents have been used. Drugs such as phenoxybenzamine may be tried cautiously in the diabetic. The major dose-limiting side effect is usually postural hypotension. The diabetic who often has a component of autonomic neuropathy is particularly prone to this side effect. Other agents, such as mexilitine, which improve peripheral nerve blood flow, benefit occasional patients.

Simple analgesics have an important role. Because of the chronic nature of the problem, narcotics should be avoided. Drugs with prostaglandin inhibiting activity, such as aspirin, have been suggested. Unfortunately, as with all of the drugs discussed above, there have been no carefully controlled trials of efficacy.

Attentive listening and sympathetic counseling are very important parts of the physician's therapeutic role.

CENTRAL NERVOUS SYSTEM COMPLICATIONS

In addition to the well-recognized peripheral nervous system complications of diabetes mellitus, some derangements of CNS function are commonly encountered in diabetics. Most of these result from the severe metabolic abnormalities that may develop during the course of the disease and attempts at its control (e.g., diabetic ketoacidosis or hypoglycemia) or from the increase in cerebrovascular disease known to afflict diabetics.

Metabolic Derangements

DIABETIC KETOACIDOSIS

Diabetic ketoacidosis, once the most common cause of diabetic death (74 percent of deaths due to diabetes prior to insulin therapy), is still a major cause of morbidity (up to 14 percent of diabetic hospitalizations) and mortality (9 to 10 percent of deaths due to diabetes yearly).[94] It is characterized by hyperglycemia (usually more than 400 mg/dl), dehydration, and metabolic acidosis (blood pH less than 7.2) due to the presence of ketone bodies (acetoacetate and β-hydroxybutyrate) in blood and urine.

It develops acutely or subacutely over a period of days as a result of hypoinsulinism often due to cessation of administration or due to increased need during physical or emotional stress. Up to 30 percent of new cases of diabetes present with diabetic ketoacidosis. This lack of insulin coupled with the effect of counterregulatory hormones, especially glucagon, causes impaired entry of glucose into target tissues and augmented glucose production via glycogenolysis and gluconeogenesis, leading to hyperglycemia. In addition, hepatic fatty acid catabolism is increased, leading to ketosis.

These metabolic derangements produce the typical clinical syndrome of dehydration due to osmotic diuresis, with thirst, polyuria, anorexia, and fatigue. Only about 10 percent of patients with diabetic ketoacidosis progress to frank coma, but most show some alteration of consciousness. Focal neurological findings or seizures are not common.[95]

The pathophysiological mechanisms leading to stupor and coma are not adequately understood and appear to be complex and multifactorial. Most authors seem to agree that serum hyperosmolality is a major contributing factor. Many other possible mechanisms have been suggested, including acidosis, alterations in cerebral blood flow, disseminated intravascular coagulation, toxicity by lysolecithins and free fatty acids, hypoxia, and a defect in brain carbohydrate metabolism.

Serum hyperosmolality provides a driving force for water efflux from brain cells. The resultant shrinkage of cells is counteracted in part by slow inward diffusion of certain osmotically active agents (such as sodium or glucose) into brain tissue, and also by production of "idiogenic osmoles," which are as yet unidentified osmotically active particles that contribute to the osmotic pressure of brain cells but are not measurable as part of the usual osmotically active agents.[96] They are believed to arise at least in part from production of free amino acids such as glutamine, glutamate, and aspartate, and from dissociation of free intracellular cations, potassium in particular.

Clearly such changes in intracellular constituents would have significant effects on cellular excitability in addition to providing osmotic stabilization, and this could play a role in the development of encephalopathy in diabetic ketoacidosis.

It is also possible that hyperosmolality disrupts the blood-brain barrier by shrinking endothelial cells[97] and loosening tight junctions, thereby altering the brain's internal environment and perhaps contributing to an encephalopathy. Although hyperosmolality itself may produce brain dysfunction, its successful treatment may trigger an even more profound disorder, cerebral edema, which is discussed below.

Acidosis itself is usually not a cause of encephalopathy in most cases of diabetic ketoacidosis because the respiratory compensation induced by the metabolic acidosis reduces CSF as well as serum CO_2, and the blood-brain barrier protects the brain from acid metabolites. Thus the pH of the CSF is maintained near normal in the face of significant systemic acidosis.[98,99] There is no correlation between the state of consciousness and the serum pH. In severe and protracted cases of diabetic ketoacidosis, the pH of the CSF may fall and stupor or coma may result.[98] Furthermore, during treatment of systemic acidosis with bicarbonate, a transient acidification of CSF may occur because increased CO_2 in blood is transported into the CSF more rapidly than the bicarbonate.[98,99] This produces a mild, transient depression in the level of consciousness.[98]

There is poor correlation between the level of consciousness and the level of ketone bodies in blood or CSF in diabetic ketoacidosis.[99] Although infusion of acetoacetate into experimental animals may cause coma, β-hydroxybutyrate, the major abnormal anion in diabetic ketoacidosis, does not produce encephalopathy.[100]

Despite reduced arterial PCO_2, dehydration, and sometimes hypotension, cerebral blood flow has been shown to be normal or even greater than normal in comatose ketoacidotic patients.[101] There may thus be impaired regulation of cerebral blood flow, but clearly hypoperfusion cannot be the cause of the alteration in consciousness in diabetic ketoacidosis.

Pathological evidence of disseminated intravascular coagulation (DIC) has been found in several cases of fatal diabetic ketoacidosis, with premortem documentation of disturbance of fibrinolytic and coagulation mechanisms in some instances.[102] It has been suggested that DIC may be a major factor contributing to the encephalopathy of diabetic coma, but clinical evidence of this entity seldom develops during diabetic ketoacidosis, and other autopsy studies have failed to find pathological support for this concept. There is one reported case of nonketotic diabetic coma with clinical and laboratory evidence of DIC that responded to anticoagulant therapy.[103]

Another possible contribution to CNS dysfunction in diabetic ketoacidosis might come from the toxic effects of elevated levels of lysolecithins and nonesterified fatty acids, analogous to their putative toxic effects in Reye's syndrome and acute pancreatitis.[104] It is also possible that in the setting of grossly deranged carbohydrate and lipid metabolism in diabetic ketoacidosis, a primary defect in cerebral carbohydrate metabolism underlies the encephalopathy.

Complications of Therapy for Diabetic Ketoacidosis

Various other complicating factors may serve to contribute to the degree of CNS dysfunction, either initially or during the course of therapy, including electrolyte disorders, thrombotic phenomena, and infection.

Hypokalemia and hypophosphatemia frequently develop with insulin and fluid replacement, and although the theoretical CNS sequelae of hypophosphatemia have not been clearly demonstrated to occur in diabetic ketoacidosis,[105] it is prudent to replace deficits. Hyponatremia may develop with overly rapid correction of hyperosmolality, especially in cases of inappropriate antidiuretic hormone (ADH) secretion.[106]

Thromboembolic disorders can complicate the course of diabetic ketoacidosis, contributing to the degree of stupor or coma. They are precipitated by the increased blood viscosity due to dehydration and by the increased platelet adhesiveness and decreased fibrinolytic activity that occur in these patients.[107] Complications such as myocardial, cerebral, or mesenteric infarction are important causes of death in ketoacidotic patients.[107]

Infection may be difficult to recognize because some degree of hypothermia is common in diabetic ketoacidosis and may mask a fever, and because a leukocytosis is commonly seen even in the absence of infection. Signs of meningitis, however, would not be masked.

Hypoxemia may be a contributing factor to CNS depression in certain circumstances, such as severe diabetic ketoacidosis with respiratory depression, and during vigorous fluid replacement with crystalloids when some degree of pulmonary edema or adult respiratory distress syndrome may develop.[108] In addition, there may be a shift to the left of the hemoglobin-oxygen dissociation curve due to depressed levels of 2,3 diphosphoglycerate in red cells.[109]

Cerebral edema may develop during otherwise successful treatment for diabetic ketoacidosis—an occurrence more common in young patients and almost uniformly fatal once it is clinically apparent.[106] The typical setting is that of apparently good response to insulin and fluid therapy, with correction of the acidosis and improvement in hyperglycemia. Sudden neurological deterioration may be heralded by headache and confusion, but it soon progresses until there is markedly increased intracranial pressure with herniation. Pathological examination reveals massive cerebral edema. Rapid, aggressive therapy with mannitol has salvaged a few patients, but these have had severe neurological sequelae.[110]

Serial measurements of CSF pressure[111] or CT scans[112] have shown that some degree of elevated intracranial pressure or brain swelling is common during the course of therapy for diabetic ketoacidosis in both children and adults. In one series, there was a correlation between the degree of increased pressure and transient depression in consciousness.[111] In other cases the swelling appeared to be asymptomatic.[112]

The pathogenesis of this cerebral edema is not clearly understood. Osmotic dysequilibrium is thought to develop between brain and blood as a result of rapid correction or overcorrection of serum osmolality.[113] It may be exacerbated by production of "idiogenic osmoles,"[96] by activation of the sodium-hydrogen ion transport system,[114] or by serum hyponatremia. Alterations in the cerebral capillary blood-brain barrier may play a role in edema formation.[115] In some cases arterial thrombosis may precipitate the event.[116]

Because the mechanism by which cerebral edema is produced is unclear, it is necessary to reduce the risk by empirical observations. There appears to be some benefit to slow fluid replacement (over 36 hours), initially with normal saline and, once the plasma glucose level is less than 300 mg/dl, with a glucose-containing medium.[113] There is controversy concerning the appropriate amount of insulin to use, but in general good results have been found with the newer "low-dose" regimens (10 U/h).[105]

Although cerebral edema has occurred even in cases where fluid and insulin were administered very cautiously,[117] it appears that the risk is greater if fluids are replaced at a rate above 4 L/m²/d and if hyponatremia develops.[106]

NONKETOTIC HYPEROSMOLAR COMA

Hyperglycemia with hyperosmolality may occur in diabetics without significant ketosis and commonly leads to progressive mental obtundation, or nonketotic hyperosmolar coma. This is most commonly encountered in elderly diabetics with mild disease or as a first manifestation of the disease. It can be seen in young type I diabetics as well, and indeed the same patient may develop diabetic ketoacidosis or nonketotic hyperosmolar coma on different occasions.

The metabolic derangement progresses gradually over several days to weeks, with hyperglycemia, osmotic diuresis, and dehydration, eventually leading to extremely high serum glucose levels (often greater than 800 mg/dl) and serum osmolality (greater than 350 mOsm/kg). Virtually all patients with nonketotic hyperosmolar coma show some degree of renal dysfunction,[113] which potentiates the development of hyperglycemia. There is no significant associated ketoacidosis. The small amount of insulin activity present in these patients is believed to be sufficient to prevent hepatic activation of ketogenesis.[118]

Many patients with nonketotic hyperosmolar coma do show some degree of metabolic acidosis,[119] due to either lactic acidosis or an unidentified anion. Some have small amounts of ketoacids present; indeed, rather than two pathophysiologically distinct entities, diabetic ketoacidosis and nonketotic hyperosmolar coma probably represent extremes of a continuum, the metabolic result of decreased or absent insulin effect and increased glucagon effect.

A large proportion of cases of nonketotic hyperosmolar coma are accompanied by serious medical conditions, which in some cases may have triggered the metabolic changes. These include gram-negative pneumonia, myocardial infarction, stroke, gastrointestinal hemorrhage, gram-negative sepsis, pulmonary embolism, uremia, and pancreatitis.[119,120] These illnesses may contribute to the inadequate hydration and lack of recognition of symptoms during progression of the syndrome and are the major reasons for the generally high mortality rate of 40 to 50 percent associated with this condition.[94,119]

Nonketotic hyperosmolar coma has also been reported in association with corticosteroid therapy,[121] thiazide diuretics,[122] renal dialysis,[123] severe burns,[124] and heat stroke,[125] or without clear precipitating or associated factors.

Progressive lethargy leading to unresponsiveness is the most common reason for seeking medical attention,[119] but a number of other neurological symptoms and signs may be the presenting feature of nonketotic hyperosmolar coma. Seizures and focal neurological deficits are quite common in this condition, unlike diabetic ketoacidosis.[95] Focal[126,127] and generalized seizures may occur,[113] and stroke-like syndromes are common, sometimes with radiological evidence for cerebral infarction.[119,126,128] A flapping tremor of the upper extremities,[129] hemichoreoathetosis,[130,131] hallucinations,[129] and hemianopia[132] have also been reported. A patient who died with nonketotic hyperosmolar coma developed lateral pontine and extrapontine myelinolysis, presumably due to the rapid increase in serum osmolality.[133]

Alterations in level of consciousness are more prevalent in nonketotic hyperosmolar coma than in diabetic ketoacidosis. In one series, 30 of 34 patients had decreased levels of consciousness,[119] reflecting both the higher serum osmolalities (due to glucose and sodium) and the compounding effects of associated medical illness on the encephalopathy.

Despite the very high serum osmolalities reached, with serum glucose sometimes surpassing 2,000 mg/dl and osmolality greater than 450 mOsm/kg, treatment with insulin and fluids has only rarely resulted in cerebral edema such as is encountered in diabetic ketoacidosis. Arieff described five cases,[113] all of which involved rapid lowering of plasma glucose to below 300 mg/dl in the first 24 hours of therapy. This situation, he believed, produces an accumulation of "idiogenic osmoles" within the brain, thereby producing cerebral edema.[95,113] Little or no insulin appears to be required to correct the hyperglycemia of nonketotic hyperosmolar coma once fluid replacement is undertaken.[134]

Lactic acidosis is more common in diabetics than in the general population, but accurate figures on its incidence are not available.[94] In one study, 50 percent of the reported cases of idiopathic lactic acidosis occurred in diabetics.[135] The reason for this association is not clear, but vascular disease and congestive heart failure predisposing to tissue ischemia may be responsible. In past years, prior to its discontinued use, administration of the biguanide oral hypoglycemic agent phenformin was associated with an increased incidence of lactic acidosis.

Treatment should be directed to reversing the underlying cause of lactic acid accumulation wherever possible and to correcting severe acidemia, which sometimes requires very large amounts of sodium bicarbonate.[136] It has been suggested that bicarbonate treatment may worsen lactate levels by increasing lactate production.[137]

HYPOGLYCEMIA

Hypoglycemia may occur in a large number of different conditions, but excessive doses of insulin for the treatment of diabetes are the most common cause of severe hypoglycemic coma. In addition, early diabetics or diabetics with renal insufficiency may show spontaneous mild postprandial hypoglycemia,[138] and both insulin and oral hypoglycemic agents may produce hypoglycemia of varying severity with a corresponding range of neurological symptoms and signs.

Diabetics may not only be more prone to develop hypoglycemia but may also be particularly sensitive to it, for there is evidence that chronically high blood glucose produces a reduction in the number and activity of glucose carriers in the blood-brain barrier, so that glucose transport into the brain is even lower at a given low plasma glucose level.[139] Clinically, this correlates with the "hypoglycemic" symptoms that occur despite blood glucose levels in the normal range in diabetics after rapid reduction from hyperglycemia. Intensively treated diabetics with tight control seem to be at greater risk for both severe and symptomatic hypoglycemia. One study has shown that the epinephrine and other counterregulatory responses were delayed and diminished in these patients, while electroencephalographic changes compatible with hypoglycemia were more commonly seen than in poorly controlled or nondiabetic patients with similar blood glucose levels.

The metabolic alterations underlying the brain dysfunction and pathological changes that occur in hypoglycemia are not completely understood. Many comparisons have been drawn between anoxic and hypoglycemic damage.[140,141] Notable differences include the profound functional changes in brain activity early in hypoglycemia, with alterations in consciousness despite relative maintenance of cerebral blood flow, oxygen utilization, and high energy phosphate stores, as well as the remarkable capacity for recovery even after prolonged hypoglycemic coma. It appears that energy failure is not the cause of the alteration in consciousness in hypoglycemic patients, but rather that some other aspect of glucose metabolism is rapidly impaired despite high energy stores. The ongoing oxidative metabolism suggests that other substrates are being utilized, such as endogenous glycogen, and this may contribute to the capacity for recovery.

Striking similarities have been noted between the pathological changes in anoxia, status epilepticus, and hypoglycemia with respect to the nature and distribution of cell changes.[140] All exhibit "selective neuronal vulnerability," with damage mainly in certain layers of the cerebral cortex, areas of the hippocampus, parts of the striatum, and the cerebellum.[141] Some differences exist both on a subcellular level and in topographical distribution between hypoglycemia and anoxia or status epilepticus, but the similarities are so great as to suggest a common pathophysiological mechanism in all three cases. A great deal of evidence has been gathered implicating increased intracellular calcium and excitatory neurotransmitters as possible mediators of this selective cellular injury, and intracellular acidosis and toxic free radical formation may also be involved.[142,143]

If strict control is attempted, an occasional "insulin reaction" is unavoidable. Diabetics are familiar with the typical symptoms of the "sympathetic" phase of hypoglycemia, which usually occurs at plasma glucose levels of less than 40 to 50 mg/dl. This phase includes dizziness, weakness, tremor, and palpitations due to epinephrine release.[144] Such warning signs may be absent in diabetics with autonomic dysfunction[145] or may be neglected because of intervening "neuroglycopenic" symptoms affecting behavior and judgment. One study showed nocturnal hypoglycemia in 22 of 39 poorly controlled diabetics; it lasted more than 3 hours in 17 patients.[146] Although

family members reported daytime behavioral abnormalities, only 6 patients were aware of hypoglycemia. Recurrent nocturnal hypoglycemia has produced the clinical picture of dementia,[146,147] which reversed with appropriate treatment. In other patients, repeated or prolonged hypoglycemic attacks may produce dementia and irreversible pathological changes.[148,149]

The neurological effects of hypoglycemia have been described as progressing in a reverse phylogenetic order,[150] with the cerebral hemispheres affected first and most commonly and patients subsequently progressing to diencephalic, mesencephalic, and finally medullary phases of dysfunction. Such a neat topographical progression is not often borne out in clinical experience; instead, different areas of the brain appear to be most affected in different attacks. Four forms of acute metabolic encephalopathy have been described in hypoglycemia: (1) delirium, either quiet or manic; (2) multifocal brainstem dysfunction with neurogenic hyperventilation and decerebrate spasms but with preserved oculocephalic and oculovestibular responses; (3) stroke-like events with or without coma, with focal deficits that may shift from one side to the other, tend to resolve, and may occur without evidence for underlying vascular or other pathology[144,151]; and (4) seizures, single or multiple, which may be the only manifestation of hypoglycemia. Hypothermia is common and may be a clue to the presence of hypoglycemia.[140,152]

Although there is not a tight correlation between plasma glucose levels and neurological symptoms,[144] confusion and behavioral changes generally appear at levels below 30 to 40 mg/dl, with stupor and seizures occurring as the level drops further, and profound coma with levels below 10 mg/dl.[153]

In milder cases, hypoglycemic symptoms are quickly reversed by oral or intravenous glucose. In some cases, however, coma may persist despite restitution of normoglycemia, for reasons that are not clear. In general, complete recovery is the rule, even after an hour or more of coma. There may be some residual focal neurological signs after recovery[144] and repeated severe attacks are known to produce cognitive decline.[148,149]

In addition to the behavioral changes, alterations in consciousness, and focal hemispheric and brainstem signs described above, hypoglycemia has also been reported to cause recurrent or persistent choreoathetosis[154] (presumably reflecting susceptibility of the basal ganglia to hypoglycemia) and recurrent focal neurological deficits in the distribution of a stenosed atherosclerotic vessel[155] (probably reflecting disruption of borderline perfusion and substrate delivery in the normoglycemic state).

Cerebrovascular Disease

Stroke is two to six times more common in diabetics than in nondiabetics and is involved in about 25 percent of diabetic deaths.[156] While much of this increase in stroke is probably attributable to an increase in cerebral atherosclerosis,[157] other factors are probably also important. Hypertension is common in diabetics and, in addition to contributing to atherosclerosis, also promotes both intracranial small vessel disease and heart disease, which can lead to lacunar and embolic infarction, respectively. Atherosclerotic heart disease and congestive heart failure are more common in diabetics than nondiabetics.[158] Metabolic and hematological abnormalities occurring in diabetes may aggravate the damage resulting from any of these ischemic insults. Hemorrhagic stroke is not increased in diabetes and may actually be less frequent.[159–161]

It was believed until recently that cerebrovascular disease and stroke were not more common in diabetics than in the general population.[159,162] Large autopsy studies, however, have shown an increase in encephalomalacia (cerebral infarcts) in diabetics, with 1.5 to 2.0 times the incidence of infarcts,[159,163] particularly in small, deep, and infratentorial areas, suggesting small vessel disease. The increase over nondiabetics was more apparent in subjects less than 60 years of age. Hypertension did not account for all of the increased incidence of encephalomalacia in diabetics.[159] Furthermore, in all of these studies, hemorrhagic stroke was found to be less frequent in diabetics than in nondiabetics, which would not be expected if hypertension were the only pathogenetic influence.

HYPERTENSION AND ARTERIOLOSCLEROSIS

Hypertension is known to be a major risk factor for cerebral infarction. It contributes to the pathogenesis of lacunar and atherothrombotic infarction and also to that of cardioembolic brain infarcts as a result of

related heart disease and atrial fibrillation. Hypertension is 1.5 to 3 times more common in diabetics than in the general population. One-half of diabetics have a medical history of hypertension, and it is controlled in only 30 to 50 percent.[164]

Arteriolosclerosis is associated with hypertension. It is characterized by thickening of the arteriolar wall ("hyaline degeneration") and in some cases permeation of plasma into the wall, rendering it an amorphous mass ("fibrinoid necrosis").[165] This process appears to be physiologically related to aging but is accelerated by hypertension and is also increased in diabetic tissue, where it may be seen even in the absence of hypertension.[165] In brain it has been found to be increased in proportion to the increased frequency of hypertension in diabetics.[163]

The clinical correlate of arteriolosclerosis is infarction, particularly of deep structures supplied by end-arterioles—so-called lacunar infarction. Intraparenchymal hemorrhage, another common consequence of hypertensive small vessel disease, is actually reduced in diabetics, as noted above. One study found arteriolar necrosis, which may be the lesion more likely to lead to hypertensive hemorrhages, to be significantly less common in diabetics than in nondiabetics of equivalent hypertensive status.[159] It has been suggested that some specific diabetic changes protect the arterioles from hypertensive damage. Large vessel atherosclerosis is also promoted by hypertension.

ATHEROSCLEROSIS

Atherosclerosis is known to be more common in diabetics, to be more severe at an earlier age, and to involve smaller vessels than in nondiabetics.[162,165] The vessels of the lower extremities, the heart, and the brain are all affected. Comparison of atherosclerosis in the circle of Willis as a function of sex, age, and diabetic status showed striking increases in the frequency and severity of atherosclerosis in diabetes, especially in women who, by the fourth decade, surpassed diabetic men in this regard.[157] These data were not corrected for the presence of hypertension, which is more common in diabetics and certainly contributes to this increase in atherosclerosis.

The epidemiology of vascular disease in diabetics is thoroughly discussed and documented in West's book on the subject.[166] In those with onset of diabetes before 40 years of age, the influence of duration of diabetes on severity of vascular disease is striking, with very few patients free of significant disease after 20 years of diabetes. Autopsy studies have provided much data but are not necessarily representative of the population as a whole. Population studies have confirmed the excess of atherosclerosis in diabetes[158,160,161] and have shown that the usual measurable associated risk factors cannot account for the total increase in symptomatic arteriosclerotic disease in diabetics.

STROKE IN DIABETICS

Determining in an individual patient whether a stroke has occurred (and, if so, its pathogenesis) is difficult. This leads to methodological problems in epidemiological studies of stroke and diabetes. Although CT scans are a major help in distinguishing hemorrhagic events, they are usually negative in acute ischemic stroke. The best criterion for determining that a stroke has occurred is a neurologist's clinical evaluation at the time of the acute events. An attempt should be made to determine the subtype of ischemic stroke: large vessel occlusive disease due to atherothrombosis, lacunar infarction due to arteriolar disease, or embolic stroke due to cardiac disease. Diabetes and related conditions may contribute to each of these.

The increased incidence of stroke in diabetics has now been well documented in epidemiological studies.[158,160,161] That diabetes itself represents a separate independent risk factor in addition to associated factors such as hypertension, hyperlipidemia, and obesity has been disputed.

Although one study showed no increased risk of stroke in normotensive diabetics,[167] this same study did find an increased risk of stroke in hypertensive diabetics as compared to hypertensive nondiabetics. Furthermore, a number of large prospective studies, including the Honolulu Heart Program, the Gothenburg cohort study, and The Framingham Study have found diabetes to provide a separate risk for stroke, independent of associated risk factors.[158,160,161]

The relative risk for stroke due to diabetes itself is about twice normal.[158,160] Even high-normal serum glucose levels in those not carrying a diagnosis of diabetes is associated with an increased risk of stroke.[160] Including all risk factors, the relative risk

for stroke in diabetics is higher in women[158] and may be as high as 13-fold in the younger age groups.[161]

In addition to increased frequency of stroke in diabetes, the resulting impairment tends to be greater and survival poorer in diabetic as compared to nondiabetic stroke patients. In a study of patients with peripheral vascular disease, the incidence of stroke with permanent neurological deficit was twice as high in diabetics as in nondiabetics with equivalent atherosclerotic cerebrovascular disease as determined by noninvasive tests.[168] Nondiabetics, however, had more transient ischemic attacks (TIAs), and the total number of ischemic events in the two groups was equivalent. This suggests that diabetics are more prone to irreversible destruction of ischemic brain tissue. In another study, diabetic patients followed for 5 years after their first stroke or TIA showed only a 20 percent 5-year survival, compared with 40 percent in matched or random nondiabetic stroke patients.[169]

Thus, diabetes provides an independent risk for ischemic stroke, separate from other risk factors. In addition, it appears to increase the morbidity and mortality following stroke. This may be mediated in part by an increase in severity of atherosclerosis in diabetics. It is possible that some risk factors serve to increase atherosclerosis in diabetics even beyond the increase that would be expected on the basis of known associated risk factors such as hypertension, hyperlipidemia, and obesity. Possibilities include an atherogenic effect of hyperglycemia itself or of insulin, alterations in blood coagulability and viscosity, possible effects of microvascular disease on arterial walls, or a genetic predisposition to enhanced atherogenesis in diabetics.

It is the clinical impact of cerebrovascular disease rather than severity of atherosclerosis that is measured in epidemiological studies. Although the rate of stroke may reflect an actual increase in vascular disease per se, it may also reflect an increased tendency to stroke on the basis of blood or tissue factors. Certain features common in diabetes may serve to enhance the rate of atherogenesis, promote thrombosis, or reduce the ability of brain tissue to tolerate an ischemic insult.

Hyperglycemia, for example, has been shown to be associated with an increased morbidity after stroke, and in animals to enhance the extent and degree of brain damage from controlled degrees of cerebral ischemia.[170] This has been shown to result from intracellular lactic acidosis in tissue receiving a trickle of flow rich in glucose.[143] Because hyperglycemia is common following stroke even in patients not previously diagnosed as diabetic,[171] it clearly may aggravate the morbidity due to stroke; indeed, stroke and TIA have been shown to occur more frequently in diabetics with poor control.[167] Hyperglycemia may act in another way to promote stroke in that it may promote atherogenesis,[172] although the epidemiological data correlating the two are controversial.[166,173,174]

Alterations in platelet adhesiveness, coagulation factors, and fibrinolytic activity have been documented in diabetics.[175] Through their relation to endothelial cell function, these factors may be involved in the pathogenesis of atherosclerosis.[176] Clearly they may also lead to the thrombotic complications of diabetes.[116,162] A prospective study showed a significantly increased risk of arterial occlusion in diabetic men, with increased spontaneous platelet aggregation or abnormalities in fibrinogen or von Willebrand's factor.[177]

Alterations in vasomotor reactive, perhaps reflecting cerebral microangiopathy, have been demonstrated in the cerebral vasculature of diabetics.[178] Glycosylation of hemoglobin results in impaired oxygen delivery by shifting the oxygen-hemoglobin dissociation curve to the left.[109] Both these factors would serve to reduce the reserve available to protect the diabetic brain from anoxic-ischemic insult and so might increase the risk and morbidity of stroke.

Thus diabetes, with its associated metabolic and vascular abnormalities, greatly increases the risk of ischemic stroke. Some of the abnormalities may be unmodifiable, but a significant part of this increased risk may be amenable to treatment, with good control of hyperglycemia and hypertension.[166,174]

Other CNS Abnormalities in Diabetes

The most common CNS abnormalities in diabetics result from cerebrovascular disease and metabolic derangement as described above. Whether there are in addition primary abnormalities of the CNS inherent to diabetes is less clear.

A number of autopsy studies have documented spinal cord lesions in diabetics.[179] Many show degeneration of the posterior columns, which probably is secondary to disease of the dorsal root ganglia or the peripheral nerves.[180] Corticospinal tract degeneration has been related to lesions higher in the nervous system.[181] Some authors believe that diabetic myelopathy exists as a distinct entity.[182]

The existence of a primary diabetic encephalopathy is similarly unclear. Several reports document slowing of conduction velocity in brainstem auditory or somatosensory evoked potentials,[183–186] but it is possible that this is due to ischemic microvascular damage. Overall there is no convincing clinical or pathological evidence to suggest brain dysfunction or lesions that could not be explained on the basis of previous metabolic or vascular insults.[149,165,179]

Some of the peripheral complications of diabetes can lead indirectly to alterations in brain function. Autonomic neuropathy may produce syncope from orthostatic hypotension. Generalized cerebral hypoperfusion and decreased levels of consciousness may occur with a painless myocardial infarction.[187] Uremic encephalopathy should be considered in a diabetic with nephropathy.

Other CNS changes reported in diabetes include abnormal hypothalamic regulation of growth hormone in poorly controlled diabetes,[188] focal seizures with isolated hypomagnesemia,[189] and pituitary insufficiency.[190] The prevalence of migraine is reported to be lower in diabetics,[191] and it has been suggested that the diminished vasodilatory capacity in diabetic brain may be protective.[192] Diabetics may be at increased risk to develop neuroleptic-induced tardive dyskinesia.[193–195]

Certain other neurological entities are well known to be associated with secondary diabetes, including Friedreich's ataxia and myotonic dystrophy. An increased prevalence of diabetes has also been shown in Huntington's disease.[196] A large proportion of patients with stiff-man syndrome are diabetic, probably on the basis of the anti–islet cell antibodies that are strongly associated with this condition.[197]

Although it has been commonly held that diabetics are more prone to infection, presumably on the basis of impaired neutrophil function, epidemiological data do not confirm a significant increase in infection in diabetics other than bacteriuria.[198,199] Certain unusual infections, however, are seen essentially only in diabetics.[198] Rhinocerebral mucor is the only one affecting the CNS. This fungal infection of the nose and orbit may invade the brain, with neurological sequelae, or it may invade to produce peripheral facial weakness.[200] It is more common in acidotic patients but may occur in any diabetic.[201]

Although the greatest impact of diabetes is on the peripheral nervous system, there are significant effects on central neurological function, mediated by vascular disease and metabolic derangements. Neurological disease in a diabetic should be viewed with this in mind.

REFERENCES

1. National Diabetes Data Group: Classification and diagnosis of diabetes mellitus and other categories of glucose intolerance. Diabetes 28:1039, 1979
2. Pirart J: Diabetes mellitus and its degenerative complications: a prospective study of 4,400 patients observed between 1947 and 1973. Diabetes Care 1:168, 1978
3. Melton LJ, Dyck PJ: Epidemiology. p. 27. In Dyck PJ, Thomas PK, Asbury AK, et al (eds): Diabetic Neuropathy. WB Saunders, Philadelphia, 1987
4. Dyck PJ, Karnes J, O'Brien PC: Diagnosis, staging, and classification of diabetic neuropathy and associations with other complications. p. 36. In Dyck PJ, Thomas PK, Asbury AK, et al (eds): Diabetic Neuropathy. WB Saunders, Philadelphia, 1987
5. Dyck PJ, Kratz KM, Lehman KA, et al: The Rochester Diabetic Neuropathy Study: design, criteria for types of neuropathy, selection bias, and reproducibility of neuropathic tests. Neurology 41:799, 1991
6. Dyck PJ, Karnes JL, O'Brien PC, et al: The Rochester Diabetic Neuropathy Study: reassessment of tests and criteria for diagnosis and staged severity. Neurology 42:1164, 1992
7. Windebank AJ: Diabetic control and peripheral neuropathy. Mayo Clin Proc 58:344, 1983
8. Dyck PJ, Sherman WR, Hallcher LM, et al: Human diabetic endoneurial sorbitol, fructose, and myo-inositol related to sural nerve morphometry. Ann Neurol 8:590, 1980
9. Gilliatt RW, Willison RG: Peripheral nerve conduction in diabetic neuropathy. J Neurol Neurosurg Psychiatry 25:11, 1962
10. Harati Y: Diabetic peripheral neuropathies. Ann Intern Med 107:546, 1987
11. Thomas PK, Tomlinson DR: Diabetic and hypoglycemic neuropathy. p. 1219. In Dyck PJ, Thomas PK, Griffin JW, et al (eds): Peripheral Neuropathy. 3rd Ed. WB Saunders, Philadelphia, 1993
12. Woltman HW, Wilder RM: Diabetes mellitus: pathological changes in the spinal cord and peripheral nerves. Arch Intern Med 44:576, 1929
13. Gabbay KH, Merola LO, Field RA: Sorbitol pathway: presence in nerve and cord with substrate accumulation in diabetes. Science 151:209, 1966
14. Greene DA, Lattimer SA, Sima AA: Sorbitol, phosphoinositides, and sodium-potassium-ATPase in the pathogenesis of diabetic complications. N Engl J Med 316:599, 1987
15. Greene DA, Winegrade AI: In vitro studies of the substrates for energy production and the effects of insulin on glucose utilization in the neural components of peripheral nerve. Diabetes 28:878, 1979
16. Finegold D, Lattimer SA, Nolle S, et al: Polyol pathway activity and myo-inositol metabolism: a suggested relationship in the pathogenesis of diabetic neuropathy. Diabetes 32:988, 1983
17. Greene DA: A sodium-pump defect in diabetic peripheral nerve corrected by sorbinil administration: relationship to myo-inositol metabolism and nerve conduction slowing. Metabolism 35:60, 1986
18. Greene DA, Chakrabarti S, Lattimer SA, Sima AA: Role of sorbitol accumulation and myo-inositol depletion in paranodal swelling of large myelinated nerve fibers in the insulin-deficient spontaneously diabetic bio-breeding rat: reversal by insulin replacement, an aldose reductase inhibitor, and myo-inositol. J Clin Invest 79:1479, 1987
19. Sidenius P, Jakobsen J: Reversibility and preventability of the decrease in slow axonal transport velocity in experimental diabetes. Diabetes 31:689, 1982
20. Thomas PK, Wright DW, Tzebelikos E: Amino acid uptake by dorsal root ganglia from streptozotocin-diabetic rats. J Neurol Neurosurg Psychiatry 47:912, 1984
21. Mayhew JA, Gillon KR, Hawthorne JN: Free and lipid inositol, sorbitol and sugars in sciatic nerve obtained post-mortem from diabetic patients and control subjects. Diabetologia 24:13, 1983
22. Dyck PJ, Zimmerman BR, Vilen TH, et al: Nerve glucose, fructose, sorbitol, *myo*-inositol, and fiber degeneration and regeneration in diabetic neuropathy. N Engl J Med 319:542, 1988
23. The Diabetes Control and Complications Trial Research Group: The effect of intensive treatment of diabetes on the development and progression of long-term complications in insulin-dependent diabetes mellitus. N Engl J Med 329:977, 1993
24. Tuck RR, Schmelzer JD, Low PA: Endoneurial blood flow and oxygen tension in the sciatic nerves of rats with experimental diabetic neuropathy. Brain 107:935, 1984
25. Low PA: Recent advances in the pathogenesis of diabetic neuropathy. Muscle Nerve 10:121, 1987

26. Low PA, Schmelzer JD, Ward KK, Yao JK: Experimental chronic hypoxic neuropathy: relevance to diabetic neuropathy. Am J Physiol 250:E94, 1986

27. Newrick PG, Wilson AJ, Jakubowski J, et al: Sural nerve oxygen tension in diabetes. Br Med J 293:1053, 1986

28. Young MJ, Veves A, Walker MG, Boulton AJ: Correlations between nerve function and tissue oxygenation in diabetic patients: further clues to the aetiology of diabetic neuropathy? Diabetologia 325:1146, 1992

29. Low PA, Ward K, Schmelzer JD, Brimijoin S: Ischemic conduction failure and energy metabolism in experimental diabetic neuropathy. Am J Physiol 248:E457, 1985

30. Low PA, Tuck RR, Dyck PJ, et al: Prevention of some electrophysiologic and biochemical abnormalities with oxygen supplementation in experimental diabetic neuropathy. Proc Natl Acad Sci USA 81:6894, 1984

31. Yao JK, Low PA: Improvement of endoneurial lipid abnormalities in experimental diabetic neuropathy by oxygen modification. Brain Res 362:362, 1986

32. Johnson PC, Doll SC, Cromey DW: Pathogenesis of diabetic neuropathy. Ann Neurol 19:450, 1986

33. Dyck PJ, Karnes JL, O'Brien P, et al: The spatial distribution of fiber loss in diabetic polyneuropathy suggests ischemia. Ann Neurol 19:440, 1986

34. Dyck PJ, Lais A, Karnes JL, et al: Fiber loss is primary and multifocal in sural nerves in diabetic polyneuropathy. Ann Neurol 19:425, 1986

35. Nukada H, Dyck PJ: Microsphere embolization of nerve capillaries and fiber degeneration. Am J Pathol 115:275, 1984

36. Thomas PK: A critical assessment of vascular factors in the causation of diabetic polyneuropathy. Diabet Med 10:62S, 1993

37. Dyck PJ, Hansen S, Karnes J, et al: Capillary number and percentage closed in human diabetic sural nerve. Proc Natl Acad Sci USA 82:2513, 1985

38. Yasuda H, Dyck PJ: Abnormalities of endoneurial microvessels and sural nerve pathology in diabetic neuropathy. Neurology 37:20, 1987

39. Brownlee M, Cerami A, Vlassara H: Advanced products of nonenzymatic glycosylation and the pathogenesis of diabetic vascular disease. Diabetes Metab Rev 4:437, 1988

40. Low PA, Nickander KK: Oxygen free radical effects in sciatic nerve in experimental diabetes. Diabetes 40:873, 1991

41. McVeigh G, Brennan G, Johnston GD, Hayes R: Impaired endothelium dependent and independent responses in non-insulin dependent diabetes mellitus. Diabetologia 35:771, 1991

42. Thomas PK, Eliasson SG: Diabetic neuropathy. p. 1773. In Dyck PJ, Thomas PK, Lambert EH, Bunge R (eds): Peripheral Neuropathy. 2nd Ed. WB Saunders, Philadelphia, 1984

43. Ellenberg M: Diabetic neuropathy: clinical aspects. Metabolism 25:1627, 1976

44. Dyck PJ, Karnes J, O'Brien PC, Swanson CJ: Neuropathy Symptom Profile in health, motor neuron disease, diabetic neuropathy, and amyloidosis. Neurology 36:1300, 1986

45. Windebank AJ: Clinical evaluation of motor function. p. 100. In Dyck PJ, Thomas PK, Asbury AK, et al (eds): Diabetic Neuropathy. WB Saunders, Philadelphia, 1987

46. Medical Research Council: Aids to the Examination of the Peripheral Nervous System. Memorandum No. 45. Her Majesty's Stationery Office, London, 1976

47. Aronson AE, Auger RG, Bastron JA, et al: Clinical Examinations in Neurology. 5th Ed. WB Saunders, Philadelphia, 1981

48. Ahlskog JE, Aksamit AJ, Aronson AE, et al: Clinical Examinations in Neurology. 6th Ed. p. 255. Mosby-Year Book, St Louis, MO, 1991

49. Dyck PJ, Karnes J, O'Brien PC: Detection thresholds of cutaneous sensation. p. 107. In Dyck PJ, Thomas PK, Asbury AK, et al (eds): Diabetic Neuropathy. WB Saunders, Philadelphia, 1987

50. Low PA: Quantitation of autonomic responses. p. 729. In Dyck PJ, Thomas PK, Griffin JW, et al (eds): Peripheral Neuropathy. 3rd Ed. WB Saunders, Philadelphia, 1993

51. Daube JR: Electrophysiological testing in diabetic neuropathy. p. 162. In Dyck PJ, Thomas PK, Asbury AK, et al (eds): Diabetic Neuropathy. WB Saunders, Philadelphia, 1987

52. Gregersen G: Variations in motor conduction velocity produced by acute changes of the metabolic state in diabetic patients. Diabetologia 4:273, 1968

53. Ward JD, Barnes CG, Fisher DJ, et al: Improvement in nerve conduction following treatment in newly diagnosed diabetics. Lancet 1:428, 1971

54. Terkildsen AB, Christensen NJ: Reversible nervous abnormalities in juvenile diabetics with recently diagnosed diabetes. Diabetologia 7:113, 1971

55. Kikkawa R, Hatanaka I, Yasuda H, et al: Prevention of peripheral nerve dysfunction by an aldose reductase inhibitor in streptozotocin-diabetic rats. Metabolism 33:212, 1984

56. Jakobsen J: Early and preventable changes of peripheral nerve structure and function in insulin-deficient diabetic rats. J Neurol Neurosurg Psychiatry 42:509, 1979

57. Dyck PJ, Lambert EH, Windebank AJ, et al: Acute hyperosmolar hyperglycemia causes axonal shrinkage and reduced nerve conduction velocity. Exp Neurol 71:507, 1981

58. Brismar T, Sima AA, Greene DA: Reversible and irreversible nodal dysfunction in diabetic neuropathy. Ann Neurol 21:504, 1987

59. Dyck PJ, Kratz KM, Karnes JL, et al: The prevalence by staged severity of various types of diabetic neuropathy, retinopathy, and nephropathy in a population-based cohort: The Rochester Diabetic Neuropathy Study. Neurology 43:817, 1993

60. Dyck PJ, Low PA, Stevens JC: "Burning feet" as the only manifestation of dominantly inherited sensory neuropathy. Mayo Clin Proc 58:426, 1983

61. Dyck PJ: Neuronal atrophy and degeneration predominantly affecting peripheral sensory and autonomic neurons. p. 1557. In Dyck PJ, Thomas PK, Lambert EH, Bunge R (eds): Peripheral Neuropathy. 2nd Ed. WB Saunders, Philadelphia, 1984

62. Ewing DJ, Clarke BF: Diabetic autonomic neuropathy: a clinical viewpoint. p. 66. In Dyck PJ, Thomas PK, Asbury AK, et al (eds): Diabetic Neuropathy. WB Saunders, Philadelphia, 1987

63. Ewing DJ, Campbell IW, Clarke BF: The natural history of diabetic autonomic neuropathy. Q J Med 49:95, 1980

64. Smith MD: Diabetic neuropathy with Argyll-Robertson pupils: report on two cases. Glasg Med J 30:181, 1949

65. Bradley WE: Diagnosis of urinary bladder dysfunction in diabetes mellitus. Ann Intern Med 92:323, 1980

66. Tyrer G, Steel JM, Ewing DJ, et al: Sexual responsiveness in diabetic women. Diabetologia 24:166, 1983

67. Ellenberg M: Diabetic neuropathic cachexia. Diabetes 23:418, 1974

68. Archer AG, Watkins PJ, Thomas PK, et al: The natural history of acute painful neuropathy in diabetes mellitus. J Neurol Neurosurg Psychiatry 46:491, 1983

69. Caravati CM: Insulin neuritis: a case report. Va Med Monthly 59:745, 1933

70. Jordan WR: Neuritic manifestations in diabetes mellitus. Arch Intern Med 57:307, 1936

71. Rundles RW: Diabetic neuropathy: general review with report of 125 cases. Medicine (Baltimore) 24:111, 1945

72. Lambert EH, Mulder DW, Bastron JA: Regeneration of peripheral nerves with hyperinsulin neuronopathy: report of case. Neurology 10:851, 1960

73. Jaspan JB, Wollman RL, Bernstein L, Rubenstein AH: Hypoglycemic peripheral neuropathy in association with insulinoma: implication of glucopenia rather than hyperinsulinism. Case report and literature review. Medicine (Baltimore) 61:33, 1982

74. Ziegler DK: Minor neurologic signs and symptoms following insulin coma therapy. J Nerv Ment Dis 120:75, 1954

75. Jakobsen J, Sidenius P: Hypoglycemic neuropathy. p. 94. In Dyck PJ, Thomas PK, Asbury AK, et al (eds): Diabetic Neuropathy. WB Saunders, Philadelphia, 1987

76. Bastron JA, Thomas JE: Diabetic polyradiculopathy: clinical and electromyographic findings in 105 patients. Mayo Clin Proc 56:725, 1981

77. Asbury AK: Focal and multifocal neuropathies of diabetes. p. 45. In Dyck PJ, Thomas PK, Asbury AK, et al (eds): Diabetic Neuropathy. WB Saunders, Philadelphia, 1987

78. Garland HT: Diabetic amyotrophy. Br Med J 2:1287, 1955

79. Garland HT, Taverner D: Diabetic myelopathy. Br Med J 1:1405, 1953

80. Goodman JI: Femoral neuropathy in relation to diabetes mellitus: report of 17 cases. Diabetes 3:266, 1954

81. Calverley JR, Mulder DW: Femoral neuropathy. Neurology 10:963, 1960

82. Subramony SH, Wilbourn AJ: Diabetic proximal neuropathy. Clinical and electromyographic studies. J Neurol Sci 53:293, 1982

83. Greene DA: Glycemic control. p. 177. In Dyck PJ, Thomas PK, Asbury AK, et al (eds): Diabetic Neuropathy. WB Saunders, Philadelphia, 1987

84. Dahl-Jorgensen K, Brinchmann-Hansen O, Hanssen KF, et al: Effect of near normoglycaemia for two years on progression of early diabetic retinopathy, nephropathy, and neuropathy: the Oslo study. Br Med J 293:1195, 1986

85. Willars GB, Tomlinson DR, Robinson JP: Studies of sorbinil on axonal transport in streptozotocin-diabetic rats. Metabolism 35:66, 1986

86. Zimmerman BR: Aldose reductase inhibitors. p. 190. In Dyck PJ, Thomas PK, Asbury AK, et al (eds): Diabetic Neuropathy. WB Saunders, Philadelphia, 1987

87. Hotta N, Kakuta H, Ando F, Sakamoto N: Current progress in clinical trials of aldose reductase inhibitors in Japan. Exp Eye Res 50:625, 1990

88. Tomlinson DR, Willars GB, Carrington AL: Aldose reductase inhibitors and diabetic complications. Pharmacol Ther 54:151, 1992

89. Krans HM: Recent clinical experience with aldose reductase inhibitors. J Diabetes Complications 6:39, 1992

90. Greene DA: Effects of aldose reductase inhibitors on the progression of nerve fiber damage in diabetic neuropathy. J Diabetes Complications 6:35, 1992

91. Sorbinil Retinopathy Trial Research Group: The sorbinil retinopathy trial: neuropathy results. Neurology 43:1141, 1993

92. Gregersen G: Myo-inositol supplementation. p. 188. In Dyck PJ, Thomas PK, Asbury AK, et al (eds): Diabetic Neuropathy. WB Saunders, Philadelphia, 1987

93. Thomas PK, Scadding JW: Treatment of pain in diabetic neuropathy. p. 216. In Dyck PJ, Thomas PK, Asbury AK, et al (eds): Diabetic Neuropathy. WB Saunders, Philadelphia, 1987

94. Fishbein HA: Diabetic ketoacidosis, hyperosmotic nonketotic coma, lactic acidosis, and hypoglycemia. p. XII-1. In National Diabetes Data Group (ed): Diabetes in America. US Department of Health and Human Services, NIH Publication 85-1468, Bethesda, MD, 1985

95. Winegrad AI, Morrison AD: Diabetic ketoacidosis, nonketotic hyperosmolar coma, and lactic acidosis. p. 1025. In DeGroot LJ (ed): Endocrinology. Vol 2. Grune & Stratton, Orlando, FL, 1979

96. Arieff AI, Kleeman CR: Studies on mechanisms of cerebral edema in diabetic comas: effects of hyperglycemia and rapid lowering of plasma glucose in normal rabbits. J Clin Invest 52:571, 1973

97. Rapoport SI, Fredericks WR, Ohno K, Pettigrew KD: Quantitative aspects of reversible osmotic opening of the blood-brain barrier. Am J Physiol 238:R421, 1980

98. Posner JB, Plum F: Spinal fluid pH and neurologic symptoms in systemic acidosis. N Engl J Med 277:605, 1967

99. Oman JL Jr, Marliss EB, Aoki TT, et al: The cerebrospinal fluid in diabetic ketoacidosis. N Engl J Med 284:283, 1971

100. Schneider R, Droller H: The relative importance of ketosis and acidosis in the production of diabetic coma. Q J Exp Physiol 28:323, 1938

101. Kety SS, Polis BD, Nadler CS, Schmidt DF: The blood flow and oxygen consumption of the human brain in diabetic acidosis and coma. J Clin Invest 27:500, 1948

102. Timperley WR, Preston FE, Ward JD: Cerebral intravascular coagulation in diabetic ketoacidosis. Lancet 1:952, 1974

103. Nicholson G, Tomkin GH: Successful treatment of disseminated intravascular coagulopathy complicating diabetic coma. Br Med J 4:450, 1974

104. Shaw W: Possible role of lysolecithins and nonesterified fatty acids in the pathogenesis of Reye's syndrome, sudden infant death syndrome, acute pancreatitis, and diabetic ketoacidosis. Clin Chem 31:1109, 1985

105. Foster DW, McGarry JD: The metabolic derangements and treatment of diabetic ketoacidosis. N Engl J Med 309:159, 1983

106. Duck SC, Weldon VV, Pagliara AS, Haymond MW: Cerebral edema complicating therapy for diabetic ketoacidosis. Diabetes 25:111, 1976

107. Keller U: Diabetic ketoacidosis: current views on pathogenesis and treatment. Diabetologia 29:71, 1986

108. Fein IA, Rachow EC, Sprung CL, Grodman R: Relation of colloid osmotic pressure to arterial hypoxemia and cerebral edema during crystalloid volume loading of patients with diabetic ketoacidosis. Ann Intern Med 96:570, 1982

109. Ditzel J: Oxygen transport impairment in diabetes. Diabetes 25:832, 1976

110. Lufkin EG, Reagan TJ, Doan DH, Yanagihara T: Acute cerebral dysfunction in diabetic ketoacidosis: survival followed by panhypopituitarism. Metabolism 26:363, 1977

111. Clements RS Jr, Blumenthal SA, Morrison AD, Winegrad AI: Increased cerebrospinal-fluid pressure during treatment of diabetic ketosis. Lancet 2:671, 1971

112. Krane EJ, Rockoff MA, Wallman JK, Wolfsdorf JI: Subclinical brain swelling in children during treatment of diabetic ketoacidosis. N Engl J Med 312:1147, 1985

113. Arieff AI: Cerebral edema complicating nonketotic hyperosmolar coma. Miner Electrolyte Metab 12:383, 1986

114. Van der Meulen JA, Klip A, Grinstein S: Possible mechanism for cerebral oedema in diabetic ketoacidosis. Lancet 2:306, 1987

115. Winegrad AI, Kern EF, Simmons DA: Cerebral edema in diabetic ketoacidosis. N Engl J Med 312:1184, 1985

116. Kanter RK, Oliphant M, Zimmerman JJ, Stuart MJ: Arterial thrombosis causing cerebral edema in association with diabetic ketoacidosis. Crit Care Med 15:175, 1987

117. Garre M, Boles JM, Garo B, Mabin D: Cerebral oedema in diabetic ketoacidosis: do we use too much insulin? Lancet 1:220, 1986

118. Zierler KL, Rabinowitz D: Roles of insulin and growth hormone, based on studies of forearm metabolism in man. Medicine (Baltimore) 42:385, 1963

119. Arieff AI, Carroll HJ: Nonketotic hyperosmolar coma with hyperglycemia: clinical features, pathophysiology, renal function, acid-base balance, plasma-cerebrospinal fluid equilibria and the effects of therapy in 37 cases. Medicine (Baltimore) 51:73, 1972

120. Asplund K, Eriksson S, Hagg E, et al: Hyperosmolar non-ketotic coma in diabetic stroke patients. Acta Med Scand 212:407, 1982

121. Boyer MH: Hyperosmolar anacidotic coma in association with glucocorticoid therapy. JAMA 202:1007, 1967

122. McCurdy DK: Hyperosmolar hyperglycemic nonketotic diabetic coma. Med Clin North Am 54:683, 1970

123. Potter DJ: Death as a result of hyperglycemia without

ketosis—a complication of hemodialysis. Ann Intern Med 64:399, 1966

124. Rosenberg SA, Brief DK, Kinney JM, et al: The syndrome of dehydration, coma, and severe hyperglycemia without ketosis in patients convalescing from burns. N Engl J Med 272:931, 1965

125. Monteleone JA, Keefe DM: Transient hyperglycemia and aketotic hyperosmolar acidosis with heat stroke. Pediatrics 44:737, 1969

126. Singh BM, Strobos RJ: Epilepsia partialis continua associated with nonketotic hyperglycemia: clinical and biochemical profile of 21 patients. Ann Neurol 8: 155, 1980

127. Grant C, Warlow C: Focal epilepsy in diabetic nonketotic hyperglycaemia. Br Med J 290:1204, 1985

128. Park BE, Meacham WF, Netsky MG: Nonketotic hyperglycemic hyperosmolar coma: report of neurosurgical cases with a review of mechanisms and treatment. J Neurosurg 44:409, 1976

129. Mahon WA, Holland J, Urowitz MB: Hyperosmolar, non-ketotic diabetic coma. Can Med Assoc J 99:1090, 1968

130. Rector WG Jr, Herlong HF, Moses H: Nonketotic hyperglycemia appearing as choreoathetosis or ballism. Arch Intern Med 142:154, 1982

131. Sanfield JA, Finkel J, Lewis S, Rosen SG: Alternating choreoathetosis associated with uncontrolled diabetes mellitus and basal ganglia calcification. Diabetes Care 9:100, 1986

132. Agarwal AP, Parkes WE: Hyperosmolary non-ketoacidotic coma in diabetes. J Ir Med Assoc 61:323, 1968

133. McComb RD, Pfeiffer RF, Casey JH, et al: Lateral pontine and extrapontine myelinolysis associated with hypernatremia and hyperglycemia. Clin Neuropathol 8:284, 1989

134. Sacks HS, Shahshahani M, Kitabchi AE, et al: Similar responsiveness of diabetic ketoacidosis to low-dose insulin by intramuscular injection and albumin-free infusion. Ann Intern Med 90:36, 1979

135. Oliva PB: Lactic acidosis. Am J Med 48:209, 1970

136. Richardson RMA, Kunau RT: Disorders of acid-base balance. p. 824. In Stein JH (ed): Internal Medicine. 2nd Ed. Little, Brown, Boston, 1987

137. Parke R, Arieff AI: Lactic acidosis: current concepts. Clin Endocrinol Metab 12:339, 1983

138. Block MB, Rubenstein AH: Spontaneous hypoglycemia in diabetic patients with renal insufficiency. JAMA 213:1863, 1970

139. Gjedde A, Crone C: Blood-brain glucose transfer: repression in chronic hyperglycemia. Science 214:456, 1981

140. McCandless DW, Abel MS: Hypoglycemia and cerebral energy metabolism. p. 27. In McCandless DW (ed): Cerebral Energy Metabolism and Metabolic Encephalopathy. Plenum Press, New York, 1985

141. Simon RP, Meldrum BS, Schmidley JW, et al: Mechanisms of selective vulnerability: hypoglycemia. p. 13. In Raichle ME, Powers WJ (eds): Cerebrovascular Diseases. Raven Press, New York, 1987

142. Wieloch T: Neurochemical correlates to selective neuronal vulnerability. p. 69. In Kogure K, Hossmann KA, Siesjo BK, Welch FA (eds): Progress in Brain Research. Vol 63. Elsevier, Amsterdam, 1985

143. Siesjo B, Smith M, Warner DS: Acidosis and ischemic brain damage. p. 83. In Raichle ME, Powers WJ (eds): Cerebrovascular Diseases. Raven Press, New York, 1987

144. Malouf R, Brust JC: Hypoglycemia: causes, neurological manifestations, and outcome. Ann Neurol 17: 421, 1985

145. Hoeldtke RD, Boden G, Shuman CR, Owen OE: Reduced epinephrine secretion and hypoglycemia unawareness in diabetic autonomic neuropathy. Ann Intern Med 96:459, 1982

146. Gale EA, Tattersall RB: Unrecognised nocturnal hypoglycaemia in insulin-treated diabetics. Lancet 1: 1049, 1979

147. Ramasamy R: Unrecognised nocturnal hypoglycaemia masquerading as senile dementia. Postgrad Med J 59:575, 1983

148. Bale RN: Brain damage in diabetes mellitus. Br J Psychiatry 122:337, 1973

149. Skenazy JA, Bigler ED: Neuropsychological findings in diabetes mellitus. J Clin Psychol 40:246, 1984

150. Himwich EW, Frostig JP, Fazekas JF, Hadidian Z: The mechanism of the symptoms of insulin hypoglycemia. Am J Psychiatry 96:371, 1939

151. Wallis WE, Donaldson I, Scott RS, Wilson J: Hypoglycemia masquerading as cerebrovascular disease (hypoglycemic hemiplegia). Ann Neurol 18:510, 1985

152. Carter WP Jr: Hypothermia: a sign of hypoglycemia. J Am Coll Emer Rm Phys 5:594, 1976

153. Morris JC, Ferrendelli JA: Metabolic encephalopathy. p. 314. In Pearlman AL, Collins RC (eds): Neurologic Pathophysiology. 3rd Ed. Oxford University Press, New York, 1984

154. Hefter H, Mayer P, Benecke R: Persistent chorea after recurrent hypoglycemia: a case report. Eur Neurol 33: 244, 1993

155. Portnoy HD: Transient "ischemic" attacks produced by carotid stenosis and hypoglycemia. Neurology 15: 830, 1965

156. Kuller LH, Dorman JS, Wolf PA: Cerebrovascular disease and diabetes. p. XVIII-1. In National Diabetes Data Group (eds): Diabetes in America. U.S. Department of Health and Human Services, NIH Publication 85:1468, Bethesda, MD, 1985

157. Flora GC, Baker AB, Loewenson RB, Klassen AC: A comparative study of cerebral atherosclerosis in males and females. Circulation 38:859, 1968

158. Kannel WB, McGee DL: Diabetes and cardiovascular disease: The Framingham Study. JAMA 241:2035, 1979

159. Aronson SM: Intracranial vascular lesions in patients with diabetes mellitus. J Neuropathol Exp Neurol 32: 183, 1973

160. Abbott RD, Donahue RP, MacMahon SW, et al: Diabetes and the risk of stroke: The Honolulu Heart Program. JAMA 257:949, 1987

161. Lindegard B, Hillbom M: Associations between brain infarction, diabetes and alcoholism: observations from the Gothenburg population cohort study. Acta Neurol Scand 75:195, 1987

162. Ross Russell RW: Less common varieties of cerebral vascular disease. p. 368. In Ross Russell RW (ed): Vascular Disease of the Central Nervous System. 2nd Ed. Churchill Livingstone, Edinburgh, 1983

163. Alex M, Baron EK, Coldenberg S, Blumenthal HT: An autopsy study of cerebrovascular accident in diabetes mellitus. Circulation 25:663, 1962

164. Horan MJ: Diabetes and hypertension. p. XVII-1. In National Diabetes Data Group (eds): Diabetes in America. US Department of Health and Human Services, NIH Publication 85-1468, Bethesda, MD, 1985

165. Okazaki H: Fundamentals of Neuropathology. Igaku-Shoin, New York, 1983

166. West KM: Epidemiology of Diabetes and Its Vascular Lesions. Elsevier, New York, 1978

167. Roehmholdt ME, Palumbo PJ, Whisnant JP, Elveback LR: Transient ischemic attack and stroke in a community-based diabetic cohort. Mayo Clin Proc 58:56, 1983

168. Weinberger J, Biscarra V, Weisberg MK, Jacobson JH: Factors contributing to stroke in patients with atherosclerotic disease of the great vessels: the role of diabetes. Stroke 14:709, 1983

169. Asplund K, Hagg E, Helmers C, et al: The natural history of stroke in diabetic patients. Acta Med Scand 207:417, 1980

170. Pulsinelli WA, Levy DE, Sigsbee B, et al: Increased damage after ischemic stroke in patients with hyperglycemia with or without established diabetes mellitus. Am J Med 74:540, 1983

171. Samanta A, Blandford RL, Burden AC, Castleden CM: Glucose tolerance following strokes in the elderly. Age Ageing 15:111, 1986

172. Keen H, Jarrett RJ, Fuller JH, McCartney P: Hyperglycemia and arterial disease. Diabetes 30:49, 1981

173. West KM, Ahuja MM, Bennett PH, et al: The role of circulating glucose and triglyceride concentrations and their interactions with other "risk factors" as determinants of arterial disease in nine diabetic population samples from the WHO multinational study. Diabetes Care 6:361, 1983

174. Feingold KR, Siperstein MD: Diabetic vascular disease. Adv Intern Med 31:309, 1986

175. Chakrabarti R, Meade TW: Clotting factors, platelet function, and fibrinolytic activity in diabetics and in a comparison group: WHO Multinational Group. Diabetologia 12:283, 1976

176. Colwell JA, Winocour PD, Lopes-Virella M, Halushka PV: New concepts about the pathogenesis of atherosclerosis in diabetes mellitus. Am J Med 75:67, 1983

177. Breddin HK, Krzywanek HJ, Althoff P, et al: Spontaneous platelet aggregation and coagulation parameters as risk factors for arterial occlusions in diabetics: results of the PARD-study. Int Angiol 5:181, 1986

178. Tooke JE: The microcirculation in diabetes. Diabet Med 4:189, 1987

179. DeJong RN: The neurologic manifestations of diabetes mellitus. p. 99. In Vinken PJ, Bruyn GW (eds): Handbook of Clinical Neurology. Vol 27. North-Holland, Amsterdam, 1976

180. Ohnishi A, Harada M, Tateishi J, et al: Segmental demyelination and remyelination in lumbar and spinal roots of patients dying with diabetes mellitus. Ann Neurol 13:541, 1983

181. Olsson Y, Säve-Söderbergh J, Sourander P, Angervall L: A patho-anatomical study of the central and peripheral nervous system in diabetes of early onset and long duration. Pathol Eur 3:62, 1968

182. Giladi N, Turezkite T, Harel D: Myelopathy as a complication of diabetes mellitus. Isr J Med Sci 27: 316, 1991

183. Martini A, Comacchio F, Fedele D, et al: Auditory brainstem evoked responses in the clinical evaluation and follow-up of insulin-dependent diabetic subjects. Acta Otolaryngol 103:620, 1987

184. Buller N, Shvili Y, Laurian N, et al: Delayed brainstem auditory evoked responses in diabetic patients. J Laryngol Otol 102:857, 1988

185. Dejgaard A, Gade A, Larsson H, et al: Evidence for diabetic encephalopathy. Diabet Med 8:162, 1991

186. Nakamura R, Noritake M, Hosoda Y, et al: Somatosensory conduction delay in central and peripheral nervous system of diabetic patients. Diabetes Care 15: 532, 1992

187. Faerman I, Faccio E, Milei J, et al: Autonomic neuropathy and painless myocardial infarction in diabetic patients: histologic evidence of their relationship. Diabetes 26:1147, 1977

188. Molitch ME, Hou SH: Neuroendocrine alterations in systemic disease. Clin Endocrinol Metab 12:825, 1983

189. Matthey F, Gelder CM, Schon FE: Isolated hypomagnesaemia presenting as focal seizures in diabetes mellitus. Br Med J 293:1409, 1986
190. Laidler P, Pieterse AS, Pounder DJ: Diabetes mellitus and hypopituitarism. Forensic Sci Int 18:169, 1981
191. Burn WK, Machin D, Waters WE: Prevalance of migraine in patients with diabetes. Br Med J 289:1579, 1984
192. Dandona P, James IM, Beckett AG: Prevalence of migraine in patients with diabetes. Br Med J 290:467, 1985
193. Ganzini L, Heintz RT, Hoffman WF, Casey DE: The prevalence of tardive dyskinesia in neuroleptic-treated diabetics: a controlled study. Arch Gen Psychiatry 48:259, 1991
194. Ganzini L, Casey DE, Hoffman WF, Heintz RT: Tardive dyskinesia and diabetes mellitus. Psychopharmacol Bull 28:281, 1992
195. Woerner MG, Saltz BL, Kane JM, et al: Diabetes and development of tardive dyskinesia. Am J Psychiatry 150:966, 1993
196. Farrer LA: Diabetes mellitus in Huntington disease. Clin Genet 27:62, 1985
197. McEvoy KM: Stiffman syndrome. p. 197. In Pascuzzi R (ed): Seminars in Neurology: Disorders of Muscle Stiffness. Thieme Medical Publishers, New York, 1991
198. Wheat LJ: Infection and diabetes mellitus. Diabetes Care 3:187, 1980
199. Kaslow RA: Infections in diabetics. p. XIX-1. In National Diabetes Data Group (eds): Diabetes in America. U.S. Department of Health and Human Services, NIH Publication 85-1468, Bethesda, MD, 1985
200. Rogers WD Jr: Facial paralysis and epistaxis in a diabetic: a typical presentation for rhinocerebral mucormycosis. Ann Emerg Med 13:560, 1984
201. Anderson NE, Ali MR, Simpson IJ: Rhinocerebral mucormycosis complicating poorly controlled diabetes mellitus: case report. NZ Med J 96:521, 1983

20

Other Endocrinopathies and the Nervous System

Hyman M. Schipper
Gary M. Abrams

The endocrine and nervous systems are richly interrelated on many levels. In recent years, it has become increasingly evident that the nervous system plays a critical role in regulating the normal physiological activity of the endocrine glands. Conversely, systemic metabolic events, which are characteristically influenced by a variety of endocrine secretions (including some originating from neurons), have profound effects on central and peripheral nervous system function. Thus, neurological disorders may result in endocrine dysfunction and endocrine diseases are the source of many neurological symptoms.

Most neurological complications of endocrine disease that present in a general medical setting undoubtedly relate to diabetes mellitus and thyroid disorders. These topics have been addressed in previous chapters. There are certainly numerous ways in which other endocrine disturbances will lead to neurological symptoms or modulate the presentation of various neuropathological entities. In addition, frequently used therapeutic agents (e.g., oral contraceptives and corticosteroids) can also present neurological problems. The following discussion reviews some of the more common endocrinopathies that might require evaluation or assessment by a neurologist and examines the influence of selected hormones on neurological disorders.

PITUITARY GLAND

The pituitary gland is located in the bony sella turcica at the base of the skull. The sella turcica sits within the sphenoid bone, separated from the intracranial cavity by a reflection of toughened dura, the diaphragma sella. In humans, the gland has two divisions: the anterior lobe, or adenohypophysis, and the posterior lobe, or neurohypophysis. The pituitary stalk, which passes through the diaphragma sella, provides a direct neural and vascular link to the pituitary from the hypothalamus. The pituitary is derived embryologically from Rathke's pouch, which gives rise to the adenohypophysis. Within the pars distalis of the adenohypophysis, clusters of hormone-secreting cells are organized around sinusoids. The neurohypophysis arises from an outpouching of the ventral diencephalon that joins the adenohypophysis. This structure is composed largely of axons and terminals projecting from neurosecretory neurons in the supraoptic and paraventricular nuclei of the hypothalamus. The neurohypophysis is essentially a neural structure. The adenohypophysis has insignificant, if any, direct innervation by the brain. It is nonetheless influenced by the brain via the neurovascular network of the pituitary stalk. This elegant neuroendocrine system enables the hypothalamus to exert direct control over the secretory activity of the adenohypophysis.[1]

Endocrine disturbances of the pituitary may arise from insufficient or excessive secretion of one or more of the clinically important pituitary hormones. Hypothalamic modulation of pituitary secretion is important, and changes in pituitary secretory activity may sometimes reflect disorders of the hypothalamus or its afferent pathways in the central nervous system (CNS). Hypothalamic amenorrhea, for example, is a disorder of the CNS that presents with abnormalities in cyclic gonadotropin secretion and subsequent ovarian dysfunction.[2]

Clinical pituitary disease may produce symptoms that result from a direct metabolic effect of a pituitary hormone or may reflect changes in the activity of a target endocrine system. Thus, hypersecretion of growth hormone primarily presents with clinical symptoms of bone or connective tissue changes related to the metabolic effects of the hormone or growth factors stimulated by it. On the other hand, the predominant clinical symptoms of thyrotropin deficiency are indirectly expressed by hypothyroidism rather than through systemic effects of thyrotropin. Interactions between the brain, pituitary, and an endocrine target hormone can often present puzzling diagnostic problems. On many occasions, the abnormality of the hypothalamic-pituitary-endocrine organ axis can be identified by dynamic evaluation of the axis with selected stimulation or inhibition tests. Major advances in the effectiveness of these tests is in large part due to the explosion in neuroendocrinology that accompanied the isolation and characterization of the initial hypothalamic releasing factors.[3] Detailed description of the many neuroendocrine and systemic influences on the pituitary is beyond the scope of this chapter; clinicians, however, are increasingly required to consider the role that hypothalamic secretory neurons and their extrahypothalamic connections play in both normal and abnormal pituitary activity.

Prolactin Disorders

Prolactin is a protein hormone synthesized and secreted by the lactotrope, which usually corresponds to a subgroup of acidophilic or chromophobic cells in the anterior pituitary. Prolactin secretion is primarily under tonic inhibition by prolactin inhibitory factor. The major inhibitory factor has been identified as dopamine, which is secreted by neurons in the tuberoinfundibular region of the hypothalamus.[4] The identity of prolactin-releasing factor is unknown, although thyrotropin-releasing factor is a potent stimulator of prolactin release.[5] Clinically, any disorder that pharmacologically or structurally interrupts the hypothalamic dopaminergic projection to the portal capillary system leads to hyperprolactinemia. Loss of dopaminergic inhibition leading to hyperprolactinemia may be an important indicator of hypothalamic disease.

Prolactin promotes lactation via its action on mammary tissue.[6] Hypogonadism is commonly associated with hyperprolactinemia due to inhibition of cyclic gonadotropin secretion and direct suppression of ovarian or testicular function.[7] The prolactin-secreting adenoma, or prolactinoma, is the most commonly identified secretory adenoma of the pituitary and is also the most common cause of clinically significant hyperprolactinemia.[8] In women, this tumor often presents as a microadenoma (less than 10 mm in diameter), with symptoms of amenorrhea and galactorrhea. In men, the endocrine effects (impotence, infertility, and, rarely, galactorrhea) are relatively silent, and prolactin-secreting tumors more commonly present as macroadenomas (more than 10 mm in diameter). These larger tumors may cause headaches, visual field deficits, and ocular motility problems, which are typical of many large intrasellar lesions.[9]

Several random prolactin levels of more than 200 ng/ml virtually establish the diagnosis of a prolactinoma. More modest elevations of prolactin may also be consistent with the presence of a prolactinoma, but consideration of other causes of hyperprolactinemia (e.g., hypothalamic disorders, dopamine-altering drugs, or hypothyroidism) becomes important. Neuroimaging of the sellar region with computed tomography (CT) scanning and magnetic resonance imaging (MRI) is excellent and often establishes the diagnosis.[10]

Treatment of hyperprolactinemia is effectively accomplished with dopaminergic agonists, most notably the ergot derivatives.[11] Bromocriptine normalizes prolactin levels in more than 80 percent of patients with hyperprolactinemia, including those with prolactinomas. Most of these patients have restoration of normal gonadal function with cessation of galactorrhea. In patients with prolactinomas, bromocriptine will decrease tumor size and can be utilized for long-term management of macroprolactinomas.[12] A nonergot dopaminergic agonist, CV 205-502, has advantages over bromocriptine and is undergoing clinical trial.[13]

Transsphenoidal adenomectomy is also an effective treatment for prolactinomas. The highest success rates are seen in patients with microprolactinomas or tumors accompanied by moderately elevated serum prolactin levels.[10] Long-term follow-up of patients treated with surgery suggests a recurrence rate of at least 20 percent in 5 years.[10,14] Radiotherapy offers an effective therapeutic option in individuals with larger tumors who cannot tolerate pharmacotherapy or surgery.[15]

Growth Hormone Disorders

Growth hormone is secreted by the somatotropes of the anterior pituitary. Histologically, these cells classically appear eosinophilic and may be precisely identified using immunohistochemical techniques. Growth hormone promotes linear growth and plays an important role in metabolism via its anabolic and diabetogenic effects. Neurochemical control of its secretion is complex, with the major releasing and inhibitory factors being growth hormone releasing factor and somatostatin, respectively. Growth hormone is predominantly secreted at night and is influenced by age and sleep.[16]

Acromegaly or excessive growth typically results from hypersecretion of growth hormone by a pituitary adenoma.[17] In young patients without epiphyseal closure, gigantism occurs. In adults, the characteristic features of acromegaly include enlargement of the skull, jaw, feet, and hands. Muscle weakness is often present, and laboratory studies are most consistent with a myopathy.[18] Symptoms suggestive of peripheral neuropathy may occur and carpal tunnel syndrome secondary to hypertrophy of the transverse carpal ligament has been described.[19] Other common clinical features include hyperhidrosis, carbohydrate intolerance, and hypogonadism. The diagnosis of acromegaly is most easily established by demonstrating sustained elevation of growth hormone levels that cannot be suppressed by glucose and elevation of plasma insulin-like growth factor I.[20] Neuroimaging studies are very useful, and adenomas secreting growth hormone frequently present as lesions larger than prolactinomas. Surgical removal is recommended when possible; the cure rate is highest for microadenomas.[10] Pharmacotherapy with dopaminergic agonists has been successful, and the use of somatostatin analogues such as octreotide has been useful in the control of growth hormone secretion and tumor growth.[21] Radiotherapy can be effective and may be used as a primary treatment or as an adjunct to surgery.[22]

Hypersecretion of growth hormone has been reported in association with the diencephalic syndrome of infancy.[23] This disorder is seen in children and is characterized by profound emaciation. The etiology appears to be destruction of the anterior hypothalamus or disconnection of the anterior hypothalamus from selected caudal projections emanating from the brainstem. Paradoxical responses of growth hormone to stimuli such as glucose are also a feature of this disorder.[24] Similar paradoxical growth hormone responses are seen late in Huntington's disease, with profound emaciation.[25]

Adrenocorticotropin Disorders

Adrenocorticotropin (ACTH) is a 39-amino-acid peptide derived from a large precursor molecule (proopiomelanocortin), which also gives rise to β-endorphin and β-lipotropin.[26] ACTH is secreted by the basophilic corticotropes of the anterior pituitary.

Cushing's disease results from hypersecretion of ACTH by a pituitary adenoma. These tumors usually present as small lesions with prominent systemic symptoms including centripetal obesity, hypertension, diabetes, amenorrhea, hirsutism, acne, and osteoporosis. Differential diagnosis includes other causes of Cushing's syndrome such as adrenal adenomas and ectopic ACTH production by neoplasia.[27] The ACTH-secreting adenoma may be difficult to detect even by MRI with gadolinium enhancement, and measures such as differential response to corticotropin-releasing hormone and petrosal sinus sampling for ACTH may be necessary to establish a pituitary source.[20,28,29] Transspenoidal adenomectomy appears to be the therapy of choice.[10,30] Nelson's syndrome refers to a condition in which a rather aggressive ACTH-secreting adenoma enlarges after bilateral adrenalectomy for treatment of Cushing's syndrome.[31] Presumably this occurs due to loss of corticosteroid inhibition.

Hypopituitarism

Impaired secretion of pituitary hormones results from disorders of the hypothalamus or intrinsic pathological processes in the pituitary. Absence of individual hormones may be secondary to isolated releasing factor deficiencies. Multiple hormones may be lost when destructive processes affect the hypothalamus or there are diffuse lesions of the pituitary as seen with ischemic damage.[32] Hypersecretion of a pituitary hormone may accompany deficiency of other hormones in patients with large secretory adenomas. In general, the triad of diabetes insipidus, hyperprolactinemia, and one or more pituitary hormone deficiencies is indicative of hypothalamic disorder or a destructive process involving the hypothalamic pituitary stalk. Diabetes insipidus does not commonly occur with pituitary adenomas. Modest hyperprolactinemia (up to 150 ng/ml) is consistent with hypothalamic disconnection from the pituitary and may be seen with large destructive processes of the pituitary involving the stalk. Deficiencies in gonadotropins or growth hormone secretion are the most common pituitary abnormalities in both hypothalamic disorders and pituitary diseases. Thyrotropin and ACTH deficiencies occur less frequently. In most cases, a careful history, imaging, and endocrine assessment will be necessary to establish a diagnosis with accuracy.

The symptoms of hypopituitarism reflect the extensiveness of trophic hormone deficiency. Age of onset is critical for the expression of growth hormone deficiency; growth failure occurs during childhood. ACTH deficiency leads to less profound manifestations of hypoadrenalism than intrinsic adrenal failure owing to the relative preservation of mineralocorticoid secretion. Hypothyroidism due to thyrotropin deficiency may not be as severe as when it is encountered in primary hypothyroidism. Prolactin deficiency is usually unrecognized. Nevertheless, all the features of systemic gonadal, adrenal, or thyroid failure may be seen with hypopituitarism. CNS manifestations include apathy, dementia, and affective disorders and probably represent a combined effect of multiendocrine deficiency. Treatment depends on the clinical situation and may be directed at either restoration of pituitary function or replacement of systemic endocrine hormones.

POSTERIOR PITUITARY

Diabetes Insipidus

Diabetes insipidus is characterized by excessive water loss due to the inability of the kidney to reabsorb water and concentrate urine. It may evolve from a variety of problems leading to deficiency in vasopressin secretion or from partial or complete lack of renal responsiveness to the action of vasopressin. This latter condition is termed *nephrogenic diabetes insipidus* and occurs as a congenital condition or, more commonly, as an acquired disease of the renal tubules. Uncompensated diabetes insipidus may result in hypertonic dehydration. Neurological manifestations include mental status changes ranging from irritability to coma, often accompanied by hyperthermia and hypotension.

The major causes of diabetes insipidus are idiopathic, tumors or granulomatous disease of the hypothalamic-pituitary region, head trauma, and neurosurgical interruption of the neurohypophyseal tract. Vasopressin is synthesized by magnocellular secretory neurons in the supraoptic and paraventricular nuclei of the hypothalamus and transported to the posterior pituitary.[33] Acquired diabetes insipidus, which accounts for most cases encountered by neurologists, is characterized by damage to these neurosecretory neurons. Simple removal of the posterior pituitary may not be sufficient. Transient diabetes insipidus commonly occurs in association with trauma or surgery.

The diagnosis of diabetes insipidus is based on the demonstration of an inability to concentrate urine and conserve water and on the effectiveness of vasopressin in reversing the situation. The most practical tests for clinical diagnosis rely on observation of urine and plasma osmolality in the face of dehydration. The differential diagnostic and therapeutic considerations in diabetes insipidus have been reviewed extensively.[34] Direct measurement of plasma vasopressin by radioimmunoassay is available, although it is not widely utilized clinically.[35] MRI of the pituitary reveals a "bright spot" in the region of the posterior pituitary on T_1 images. This hyperintense signal may be absent or displaced in diabetes insipidus.[36]

Treatment has been markedly improved with the introduction of desmopressin.[37] This long-acting vasopressin analogue is nearly devoid of vasoconstrictor activity and can be conveniently administered by nasal instillation. A parenteral preparation is also available. Side effects are uncommon. In postoperative situations, diabetes insipidus may occur immediately or transiently, and rapid, short-acting, antidiuresis is often necessary. Aqueous vasopressin in typical dosages up to 5 U subcutaneously continues to remain particularly useful in neurosurgery. Fortunately, most patients with diabetes insipidus have preserved thirst mechanisms and can self-modulate fluid intake and water balance. The usual therapeutic goal is to eliminate nocturia and reduce daytime polyuria.

Syndrome of Inappropriate Antidiuretic Hormone Secretion

Inappropriate secretion of vasopressin occurs in a variety of neurological or systemic conditions. The criteria for the diagnosis of the syndrome of inappropriate antidiuretic hormone secretion (SIADH) were initially described by Bartter and Schwartz.[38] These are (1) hyponatremia with low plasma osmolality; (2) elevated urinary sodium excretion; (3) absence of volume depletion or edema; and (4) normal renal, hepatic, and adrenal function. In general, structural diseases directly involving the hypothalamus are not associated with SIADH. SIADH may be seen with intracranial trauma, tumors, or infections that lead to changes in osmolality or volume-sensing mechanisms. The number of systemic disorders associated with SIADH is extensive. With certain malignancies, vasopressin may be produced ectopically. Drugs are also a common cause of SIADH, and it is likely that several act directly on neural and chemical control systems for vasopressin-secreting neurons. The neurological manifestations of SIADH are those of hyponatremia (i.e., diffuse encephalopathy and seizures).

Management of SIADH depends on the etiology and the severity of the induced hyponatremia and reduced plasma osmolality. In most cases, fluid restriction is the cornerstone of treatment. In severe or resistant cases, careful forced water diuresis and sodium replacement may be necessary. Rapid correction of hyponatremia has been reported to be associated with CNS demyelination and should be avoided.[39] The use of agents such as demeclocycline to induce nephrogenic diabetes insipidus has been advocated for se-

vere, chronic SIADH.[40] Lithium has been reported to be effective in selected cases.[41]

PARATHYROID GLANDS

The parathyroid glands are two paired endodermal structures that are embryologically derived from the third and fourth branchial pouches. The principal parenchymal cells of the parathyroid glands are the chief cells, which are responsible for the synthesis and secretion of parathyroid hormone. The biology of parathyroid hormone has been extensively studied and represents a prototype for the production of endocrine polypeptide hormones.[42] Secretion of parathyroid hormone is primarily regulated by the concentration of ionized calcium in extracellular fluid. Bone and kidney are the major target organs for the hormone. In bone, it (1) stimulates the activity of osteocytes and osteoclasts, (2) inhibits osteoblast function, and (3) stimulates the differentiation of precursor cells to osteoclasts. In the kidney, parathyroid hormone decreases the tubular resorption of phosphate and increases calcium reabsorption in the distal nephron. Parathyroid function affects the nervous system primarily via changes in calcium levels. There is some evidence to suggest that the hormone may have direct effects on the brain microvasculature.[43] Calcitonin, a polypeptide hormone secreted by the parafollicular cells of the thyroid, inhibits some effects of parathyroid hormone under certain physiological conditions. Other factors, such as vitamin D, also play an important role in calcium and phosphate homeostasis, and the clinical symptoms associated with parathyroid dysfunction are the expression of many factors that influence the complex regulation of mineral metabolism.

Hyperparathyroidism

The neurological manifestations of hyperparathyroidism reflect the important and diverse effects of calcium and phosphorus on nerve and muscle. Primary hyperparathyroidism is most commonly due to oversecretion of parathyroid hormone by a solitary adenoma of the parathyroid glands. The classic but now rare clinical presentation is a combination of renal lithiasis, osteitis, and peptic ulcer disease. Recent studies have shown that neurological or neuromuscular symptoms are not common in patients with mild disease.[44] The definitive diagnosis of hyperparathyroidism is based on the demonstration of hypercalcemia in association with abnormal parathyroid function. Laboratory evaluation will usually reveal hypercalcemia and hypophosphatemia accompanied by elevated levels of immunoreactive parathyroid hormone. In situations in which the disorder is mild or asymptomatic, management is controversial. The diagnosis may be difficult to establish and requires full consideration of the many causes of hypercalcemia. Hypercalcemia associated with cancer, with or without ectopic production of parathyroid hormone, may pose a major challenge in differential diagnosis.

Subjective complaints of weakness and fatigue are perhaps the most common symptoms seen in primary hyperparathyroidism.[45] Mental status changes are frequently noted, including decreased recent memory, irritability, depression, and psychosis.[46] The severity of symptoms does not appear to be directly related to the degree of hypercalcemia, although symptoms respond to normalization of the serum calcium level.

Patients with primary hyperparathyroidism can occasionally present with frank muscle weakness, fatigability, and muscle atrophy.[45] The proximal musculature of the lower extremities is most often affected, and deep tendon reflexes are normal or hyperactive. Electromyographic studies have revealed short-duration, low-amplitude, motor unit action potentials in some patients, and high-amplitude, long-duration, polyphasic potentials in others. Muscle biopsies are abnormal and most show some evidence of neuropathic disease. The severity of muscle weakness is not readily correlated with serum calcium levels but appears to be closely related to the duration of illness. Symptoms usually improve following removal of a parathyroid adenoma.[47] Patients with secondary hyperparathyroidism also have a neuropathic type of neuromuscular disease, which closely resembles that found in primary hyperparathyroidism.[48]

Hypoparathyroidism

Hypoparathyroidism may be due to either decreased secretion or lack of peripheral action of parathyroid hormone. The serum calcium level is low and hyperphosphatemia is present. Deficiency of the hormone is most often seen postoperatively following thyroidectomy; less commonly, it occurs idiopathically. There are a variety of pseudohypoparathyroid states characterized by peripheral resistance to the hormone, for example, because of circulating antagonist to its action, abnormal receptors for it, or abnormal receptor-linked enzymatic activity.[49] Common clinical features of hypoparathyroidism and pseudohypoparathyroidism include mental deficiency, cataracts, tetany, and seizures in approximately 40 to 50 percent of patients.[49,50] The neurological manifestations of hypoparathyroidism are predominantly related to the effects of hypocalcemia on the nervous system.

Hypocalcemia produces varied alterations in mental status, ranging from dementia to frank psychosis.[51,52] Mental retardation is a common feature of familial hypoparathyroidism and pseudohypoparathyroidism.[50]

Convulsions are a well-recognized sign of hypocalcemia, regardless of etiology. However, most patients with hypocalcemia and tetany do not have epilepsy. Seizures are usually generalized. The electroencephalogram (EEG) shows generalized abnormalities, but they are nonspecific.[52] The CNS irritability and EEG changes revert to normal with correction of the serum calcium. Anticonvulsants are usually not effective.

Intracranial calcifications are a common feature of hypoparathyroid states. They occur predominantly in the basal ganglia, although other regions may be involved.[53] This finding is usually not associated with symptoms, but choreoathetosis, tremor, and parkinsonism have been reported.[54]

Increased intracranial pressure with papilledema has been reported on many occasions in patients with hypoparathyroidism.[51] These reports are consistent with the inclusion of hypoparathyroidism as a cause of pseudotumor cerebri. Increased intracranial pressure is reversed with correction of the serum calcium.

Hypocalcemia produces enhanced neuromuscular excitability and tetany, depending on the severity of metabolic derangement. Neurological examination may reveal Chvostek's or Trousseau's sign, yet the tendon reflexes are often depressed. Symptoms range from muscle pain and paresthesias to carpopedal spasms or laryngeal stridor. The autonomic nervous system may similarly be affected by hypocalcemia. Electrocardiographic changes including prolongation of the Q-T interval, and T wave changes are characteristic.[55] Clinically significant autonomic dysfunction is rare.

ADRENAL GLANDS

The adrenals are paired glands that adhere to the upper poles of the kidneys. The adrenal medulla is a derivative of neuroectoderm and is enveloped by the mesodermal adrenal cortex. The adrenal medulla is composed almost entirely of the histologically distinct chromaffin cells, which secrete catecholamines, predominantly epinephrine, into the circulation. The three-zoned adrenal cortex is concerned with the biosynthesis and secretion of mineralocorticoids, corticosteroids, progestogens, estrogens, and androgens. Aldosterone, the principal mineralocorticoid, is synthesized in the zona glomerulosa; the other steroids are secreted by the zona fasciculata and zona reticularis. These two inner zones of the adrenal cortex are primarily controlled by ACTH from the pituitary. Innervation of the adrenal medulla and cortex integrates the critical activity of the adrenal gland with the neural, metabolic, and endocrine systems, coordinating complex physiological processes such as stress responses or energy homeostasis.

Pheochromocytoma

Pheochromocytoma is a rare catecholamine-producing tumor derived from adrenal medullary cells. It presents with a variety of paroxysmal symptoms related to excess secretion of catecholamines. The tumor may occur familially, alone or as part of the multiple endocrine adenoma syndromes. The association of pheochromocytomas with neurofibromatosis and von Hippel–Lindau disease has been recognized.[56] The most common presentation is paroxysmal or sustained hypertension with episodic headache, palpitations, or hyperhidrosis. "Anxiety" and related somatic symptomatology are common. Seizures have been reported in 5 percent of cases.[57] The broad range of symptoms produced by pheochromocytomas makes it an important differential diagnostic consideration in many paroxysmal neurological disorders. The clinical features of this disorder have been reviewed elsewhere.[58]

Cushing's Syndrome

The term *Cushing's syndrome* designates any disorder resulting from excessive amounts of circulating adrenal corticosteroids. Traditionally, *Cushing's disease* refers to hypersecretion of ACTH by the pituitary, leading to this syndrome. The clinical features of Cushing's syndrome include obesity, facial plethora, hirsutism, menstrual disorders, and hypertension. Common neurological symptoms are muscle weakness and changes in mental status. The muscle weakness is most prominent in the lower extremities, consistent with a myopathic process.[59] The mental status changes are variable, ranging from emotional lability and irritability to frank psychosis and affective disorders.

The differential diagnosis of Cushing's syndrome is primarily based upon the suppressibility of the hypercortisolism. An initial evaluation might include (1) the overnight dexamethasone suppression test and (2) a 24-hour urine collection for free cortisol. If both these tests are normal, Cushing's syndrome can usually be excluded. If Cushing's syndrome is present, a series of suppression tests may be needed to clarify the etiology of the adrenal hyperactivity—that is, to determine whether it relates to adrenal tumor, ectopic ACTH syndrome, or Cushing's disease. The etiology of Cushing's syndrome can be very difficult to establish. Obesity and depression, two common clinical conditions, may pose problems with interpretation of the various tests necessary for confirming the diagnosis. Other confounding factors include the effect of anticonvulsant drugs on cortisol metabolism.

Treatment has been reconsidered in recent years but is always directed at inhibition of excess steroid production.[60] Ketoconazole, an inhibitor of adrenal steroid synthesis, has been useful in managing the hypercortisolism of Cushing's syndrome.[60] When bilateral adrenalectomy is required, Nelson's syndrome may arise.[30] The success of transsphenoidal adenomectomy for treatment of Cushing's disease has helped reduce the risk of Nelson's syndrome.

Hyperaldosteronism

Primary aldosteronism most commonly occurs in association with an aldosterone-secreting adenoma of the adrenal. The clinical presentation is with hypertension and hypokalemia. Neurological symptoms are secondary to hypokalemia and alkalosis; they may include paresthesias, tetany, or muscle paralysis.[61] Secondary aldosteronism is due to stimulation of the zona glomerulosa by extra-adrenal influences. Bartter's syndrome is a rare disorder characterized by hyperreninemia, hyperaldosteronism, hypokalemic alkalosis, normal blood pressure, and absence of edema. The finding of increased urinary prostaglandins has led to treatment of this disorder with prostaglandin inhibitors. This treatment has been reported to cause pseudotumor cerebri.[62]

Addison's Disease

Adrenal insufficiency may result from pituitary or adrenal failure or, more commonly, iatrogenically from withdrawal of exogenous steroids. Chronic adrenal insufficiency commonly occurs as an autoimmune disorder, occasionally associated with other autoimmune diseases such as myasthenia gravis.[63] The cardinal signs and symptoms are weakness, fatigue, anorexia and weight loss, hyperpigmentation, and electrolyte disturbances. CNS manifestations are common. Mental status changes are frequent and varied. EEG abnormalities are seen commonly, although seizures are unusual.[64] Increased intracranial pressure with or without overt cerebral edema may occur.[65] Treatment with glucocorticoids and mineralocorticoids reverses the symptoms. In secondary adrenal insufficiency due to hypopituitarism, symptoms are usually not as severe, and treatment with mineralocorticoids is not necessary.

SEX HORMONES AND NEUROLOGICAL DISEASE

Estrogens, progestins, and androgens are secreted directly from ovaries, testes, and adrenal glands, but they are also derived via enzyme-mediated conversions from prohormones in brain and other extraglandular tissues. Approximately 98 percent of the circulating sex hormone pool is protein-bound and functionally inert. The remaining "free" fraction is highly lipophilic and readily penetrates the blood-brain barrier and neuronal cell membranes. Within the cytoplasm or nucleus of the target cells, sex hormones form complexes with specific receptor proteins.[66] Subsequent binding of these complexes to

chromatin acceptor sites promotes selective gene transcription. In neurons, sex steroids induce the synthesis of enzymes and structural proteins concerned with cell membrane function, energy metabolism, hormonal sensitivity, and neurotransmission.[67]

The many actions of gonadal hormones within the CNS are essential to the sexual differentiation of the brain, control of the brain-pituitary-gonadal axis, and the establishment of normal patterns of sexual and aggressive behavior. Hormonal fluctuations associated with (1) specific phases of the menstrual cycle, (2) pregnancy, (3) the menopause, and (4) exposure to exogenous sex hormones may induce or modify a host of neurological and neuropsychiatric disorders.

Migraine

Approximately 60 percent of women with migraine experience perimenstrual exacerbations of their headaches (catamenial migraine).[68,69] The late luteal phase decline in plasma estradiol appears to play an important role in the precipitation of catamenial migraine.[70–72] The frequency or severity (or both) of migraine attacks often diminishes with gestation, particularly in patients whose headaches are linked to the menstrual cycle.[73,74] The absence of rhythmic estrogen "withdrawal" characteristic of the pregnant state is felt to be responsible for the reduction in migraine activity. Indeed, many women whose headaches are attenuated by pregnancy experience relapses at the time of parturition, when sex hormone levels fall precipitously.[75] In some patients, migraine arises de novo or appears to worsen during gestation.[76]

An association between migraine and "the pill" is frequently encountered in general and neurological practices. Women often exhibit new-onset or exacerbation of migraine while taking oral contraceptives. Attacks tend to become manifest during the first few cycles (particularly on placebo days in consonance with the estrogen withdrawal hypothesis) and usually but not invariably resolve upon discontinuation of the medication.[69,77] A qualitative change in the pattern of migraine is noted in some patients. For example, a migraineur may develop a focal prodrome for the first time while taking oral contraceptives. Women in this category may be at high risk for infarction in regions reflecting the distribution of their auras.[78,79] Amelioration of migraine following exposure to oral contraceptives is observed in a few women. Psychological factors, such as the diminished fear of accidental pregnancy, may in part contribute to the improvement.[79]

The pathophysiology of estrogen-related migraine is incompletely understood. Estrogens may act directly on vascular smooth muscle as well as modulate the activity of vasoactive substances at the neurovascular junction. In addition, by altering central prostaglandin, serotonin, opioid, or prolactin metabolism,[80] premenstrual changes in circulating estrogens may activate vasoregulatory elements in the brainstem or hypothalamus which, in turn, may trigger symptomatic alterations in cerebrovascular tone.[81]

First-line therapy for menstrual migraine should include the standard pharmacological, dietary, and psychological modalities employed in the general migraine population. Refractory cases of severe catamenial migraine may benefit from late luteal phase therapy with prostaglandin inhibitors and mild diuretics.[82] Various hormonal interventions in catamenial migraine have been largely unsuccessful and often complicated by unpleasant side effects. Oral contraceptives usually exacerbate migraine and probably should not be used in the treatment of this disorder. The use of estrogen implants has yielded contradictory results.[72,83] The risk-benefit ratio accruing to long-term estrogen therapy must be carefully assessed before such treatment can be advocated for this relatively benign condition. Paradoxically, the antiestrogen tamoxifen may alleviate catamenial migraine in some patients. This effect may be due in part to inhibition of calcium uptake or prostaglandin E synthesis in these subjects.[84] In two anecdotal reports,[85,86] danazol, a testosterone derivative used in the management of endometriosis, completely aborted premenstrual migraine for the duration of treatment.

Stroke

"The pill" has been implicated as a significant risk factor in thromboembolic cerebral infarction, subarachnoid hemorrhage, and cerebral venous thrombosis. In 1969, American[87] and British[88] case-control studies reported, respectively, a 19- and 6-fold increased risk of ischemic stroke in young women related to the use of oral contraceptives. Hypertension, migraine, and age greater than 35 years were associated but independent risk factors for cerebral infarction in patients taking oral contraceptives.[89,90] Ciga-

rette smoking by women on "the pill" was found to increase further the likelihood of hemorrhagic but not thromboembolic stroke.[79] Ingestion of lower-dose (30 μg) estrogen preparations appears to be responsible for a recent decline in rates of thromboembolic disease among users of oral contraceptives.[91–93] Progestins may also contribute to the danger of cerebral infarction by promoting hypertension, hypercoagulability, and adverse serum lipoprotein levels.[94,95]

Ischemic strokes in users of oral contraceptives have been localized to the carotid (usually the middle cerebral artery or its deep penetrating branches) and vertebrobasilar distributions.[79] There is usually no radiological or pathological evidence of disseminated vascular disease in young women with oral contraceptive-related stroke.[96] Cerebral thromboembolism resulting from estrogen-induced hypercoagulability is a likely etiology for such strokes. Estrogen increases plasma levels of fibrinogen and clotting factors VII, VIII, IX, X, and XII. The steroid also enhances platelet aggregation and suppresses antithrombin III activity and the fibrinolytic system.[97] Elam and associates have reported an increased prevalence of mitral valve prolapse among users of oral contraceptives with ischemic stroke.[98] The combination of a fixed valvular anomaly and an estrogen-related hypercoagulable state may render patients particularly vulnerable to thromboembolic complications. Sex hormone–induced hypercoagulability is also thought to play an important role in the pathogenesis of cerebral venous thrombosis complicating pregnancy, the puerperium, and use of oral contraceptives.[99] In contrast, postmenopausal estrogen replacement has a beneficial effect on lipoprotein profiles and confers protection against cardiovascular and cerebrovascular disease.[100–102] Finally, there is some evidence implicating a primary immune-mediated vasculitis in the pathogenesis of oral contraceptive–related stroke.[103,104]

In a study by the Royal College of General Practitioners, the relative risk for subarachnoid hemorrhage in former users, current users, or subjects who had ever used oral contraceptives was 4.5, 3.2, and 4.0, respectively.[105] Cigarette smoking and age greater than 35 years further increased the risk of subarachnoid hemorrhage in this population. Female sex hormones may predispose to bleeding from both aneurysms and arteriovenous malformations, although this hypothesis is controversial.[96] By analogy to their effects on endometrial spiral arteries, fluctuating sex hormone levels may compromise the integrity of cerebral arterial walls, rendering them more susceptible to rupture.[106] Rarely, subarachnoid hemorrhage is secondary to cyclic bleeding from hormone-sensitive ectopic endometriomas of the spinal canal.[107]

Epilepsy

Normal reproductive processes may be disrupted by seizure disorders and their therapies. Abnormal limbic discharges may be responsible for the hyposexuality[108,109] and increased prevalence of hypogonadotropic hypogonadism and polycystic ovary syndrome[110] noted in patients with temporal lobe epilepsy. Anticonvulsant therapy in women of childbearing age may result in failure of oral contraceptives and in teratogenicity,[111,112] as discussed in Chapter 28.

Conversely, the course of epilepsy and its management may be greatly influenced by specific phases of the reproductive cycle and exposure to steroid contraceptives. A variety of seizure disorders have been documented to worsen premenstrually (catamenial epilepsy) and during pregnancy.[113,114] Data amassed from human[115] and animal[116,117] studies suggest that estrogens and progestins have epileptogenic and anticonvulsant properties, respectively. Conceivably, a rising estrogen-progesterone ratio during the late luteal phase triggers catamenial seizure activity. Furthermore, the markedly elevated estrogen:progesterone ratio characteristic of the polycystic ovary syndrome may, in part, contribute to the relatively frequent association of this reproductive disorder with temporal lobe epilepsy. Exposure to oral contraceptives consisting of estrogen-progestin combinations does not appear to alter seizure frequencies significantly.[118,119] Progesterone suppositories may actually improve seizure control in some patients.[120]

With respect to gestational epilepsy, factors such as maternal sleep deprivation, stress, and inadequate anticonvulsant levels are probably more important than direct hormonal epileptogenesis. During pregnancy, serum levels of phenytoin, phenobarbital, and valproic acid may decrease by 30 to 40 percent of pregestational levels, with a lesser decline in carbamazepine. Primidone levels are reportedly stable during pregnancy, but the concentration of primidone-derived phenobarbital is reduced.[121] Decreased drug compliance, bioavailability, and protein binding, as well as an increased volume of distribution and metabolic clearance are factors contributing to the fall in anticonvulsant levels during pregnancy.[121] The influences of the menstrual cycle and of oral contraceptive preparations on anticonvulsant disposition appear to be of minor clinical significance.[122]

Movement Disorders

CHOREA

Rarely, pregnancy and steroid contraceptive therapy are complicated by the acute or subacute development of choreiform movements of the face and extremities associated with limb hypotonia and pendular reflexes. Fever, dysarthria, and neuropsychiatric symptoms may complete the clinical picture. Gestational and oral contraceptive-related chorea have a close association with previous rheumatic fever.[96] In fact, clinical, epidemiological, and pathological evidence suggests that altered hormonal patterns characteristic of pregnancy and ingestion of oral contraceptives may "unmask" latent chorea by modulating the activity of basal ganglia previously damaged by rheumatic or hypoxic encephalopathy.[81] In most cases, chorea gravidarum and oral contraceptive-related dyskinesias resolve completely by the end of pregnancy or following discontinuation of the medication, respectively. As many as 20 percent of women experience recurrences of chorea with subsequent pregnancies.[123] Patients with chorea gravidarum are at increased risk of later developing oral contraceptive-related dyskinesias,[124] and vice versa.[125]

In patients with suspected chorea gravidarum, appropriate clinical and laboratory investigations may be required to exclude other causes of chorea, such as acute rheumatic fever, systemic lupus erythematosus, hyperthyroidism, and Wilson's disease. Chorea gravidarum is usually self-limited, and abortion or premature delivery is rarely indicated. Judicious use of neuroleptics or other medications may afford symptomatic relief in severe cases. Women with a history of gestational or oral contraceptive-induced chorea should probably minimize further exposure to any estrogen-containing medications.

PARKINSONISM

Data concerning the effects of estrogen on patients with parkinsonism are contradictory. There are anecdotal reports of clinical deterioration in idiopathic and neuroleptic-induced parkinsonism following exposure to exogenous estrogen.[126] Furthermore, premenopausal women are reportedly more susceptible to drug-induced parkinsonism than men of similar age. These observations argue for a potentially antidopaminergic role of estrogen in this condition. Yet in a study of premenopausal women with idiopathic Parkinson's disease, Quinn and Marsden reported symptom exacerbations premenstrually, when estrogen titers are falling,[127] favoring a stimulatory influence of estrogen on striatal dopamine. There is evidence for both pro- and antidopaminergic effects of estradiol in various rodent models of striatal dysfunction (reviewed elsewhere[81]). Variations in methodology, multimodal dose-response relations, and species, age, and sex differences may account for these conflicting observations.[128,129]

OTHER MOVEMENT DISORDERS

A broad spectrum of movement disturbances appear to be influenced by changes in the sex steroid milieu. Included are cases of posthypoxic[130] and hereditary[131] myoclonus, dominantly inherited myoclonic dystonia,[132] tardive dyskinesia,[133] a pyramidal-extrapyramidal syndrome,[134] hemiballismus, ill-defined tremors and drop attacks,[79] familial episodic ataxia,[135] Gilles de la Tourette's syndrome,[136] and the neuroleptic malignant syndrome.[136,137] In patients with Wilson's disease, estrogens may raise serum ceruloplasmin levels into the normal range, and this may result in delay in diagnosis.[81]

Nervous System Neoplasms

MENINGIOMAS

Sex steroids may play an important role in the biology of meningiomas. These tumors occur more frequently in women than in men[138,139] and are rarely diagnosed before puberty or during the senium, corresponding to the time of maximal gonadal activity.[140] Meningiomas have been documented clinically and radiologically to undergo relatively rapid expansion during pregnancy, followed by spontaneous regression postpartum.[81,141] Some women suffer exacerbations of symptoms in the luteal phase of the menstrual cycle.[142]

Numerous laboratories have demonstrated the presence of progestin- and, to a lesser extent, estrogen- and androgen-binding proteins in a significant number of human meningioma specimens.[81] These observations suggest that progestins and possibly other gonadal steroids may directly modify the growth and differentiation of these tumors. In an early study, the antiestrogen tamoxifen did not appreciably affect tumor size or neurological status in patients with inoperable meningiomas.[143] On the other hand, the antiprogestin RU486 has recently been reported to induce stabilization or regression of meningiomas in a cohort of patients, suggesting that antiprogesterone therapy may be useful in the management of these tumors.[144] However, the effects of progestins and RU486 on meningioma growth in vitro are contradictory,[145–147] and patients chronically treated with RU486 may require glucocorticoid replacement to counteract the antiglucocorticoid effects of this agent.[148]

GLIOMAS

There are rare reports of astrocytomas enlarging during pregnancy, only to shrink spontaneously in the puerperium.[149] As in the case of meningiomas, certain human gliomas may selectively bind estrogens, progestins, and androgens. Some of these tumors may also contain enzymes (e.g., 17 β-oxidoreductase and aromatase) that catalyze steroid hormone interconversions.[81,150] The origin of putative steroid receptors in glial cell tumors is obscure, although significant numbers of normal astrocytes in certain brain regions possess estrogen receptors.[151] In one study of human astrocytomas, a possible correlation was observed between grade of malignancy (possibly dedifferentiation) and the presence of hormone binding.[152] If substantiated, the detection of steroid-binding proteins in tumor biopsy specimens could provide important prognostic information. In a recent anecdotal report, high-dose tamoxifen therapy may have resulted in stabilization of a recurrent astrocytoma previously treated with surgery and radiation.[153] Human oligodendrogliomas have also been reported to contain sex steroid receptors and may therefore be subject to hormonal manipulations.[154]

OTHER TUMORS

Responsiveness to sex hormones has been reported in cases of acoustic neuromas,[155] pituitary adenomas,[156] and breast metastases to the nervous system.[157,158]

Sex steroid receptors have also been reported in hemangioblastomas, anaplastic ependymomas, and malignant lymphomas, suggesting that the natural history of these neoplasms may be influenced by sex hormones and their antagonists.[159]

Peripheral Nerve Disorders

PORPHYRIAS

The porphyrias are characterized by the excessive production of porphyrins and porphyrin precursors resulting from specific enzymatic defects in the heme biosynthetic pathway. Neurological manifestations, when present, include sensorimotor and autonomic neuropathies, seizures, and neuropsychiatric symptoms. Estradiol and other steroids with a 5-β configuration induce the enzyme δ-aminolevulinic acid synthase and may thereby precipitate porphyric crises.[160,161] Oral contraceptives increase urinary excretion of this enzyme in normal individuals, and it has been suggested that asymptomatic relatives of patients with porphyria should avoid "the pill."[162] In many women with acute intermittent porphyria, cyclic attacks of variable severity may occur during the late luteal phase or, less commonly, at ovulation.[163] Paradoxically, some patients exhibit prolonged remissions following suppression of ovarian cyclicity with oral contraceptives.[81] Chronic administration of agonists of gonadotropin-releasing hormone—for example, D-His or leuprolide—also suppresses pituitary-ovarian function and in one case[164] resulted in complete remission of severe premenstrual porphyria for the duration of therapy. D-His, unlike sex steroids, does not appear to induce porphyrin accumulation in chick embryo hepatic cell culture[164] and may provide a rational approach to the management of catamenial porphyria.

OTHER NEUROMUSCULAR DISORDERS

Endogenous and administered sex hormones may influence the natural history of Bell's palsy, recurrent brachial plexopathy, endometriotic sciatica, and the carpal tunnel syndrome.[81] Abnormally high estrogen levels have been reported in male patients with amyotrophic lateral sclerosis, Kugelberg-Welander disease, bulbospinal muscular atrophy of the Kennedy-Alter-Sung type, Duchenne muscular dystrophy, and the Crow-Fukase syndrome (polyneuropathy associated with plasma cell dyscrasias, anasarca, and altered skin pigmentation).[81,165] It is unclear whether the hyperestrogenemia plays any significant role in the pathogenesis of these neuromuscular disorders.

Neuropsychiatric Disorders

PREMENSTRUAL SYNDROME

The premenstrual syndrome occurs in approximately 30 percent of women during their reproductive years. Common neuropsychiatric symptoms of this disorder include headache, fatigue, depression, irritability, increased thirst or appetite, and craving for sweet or salty foods.[166] Symptoms typically begin toward the end of the luteal phase of the cycle and usually, but not invariably, resolve with the onset of flow. The pathophysiology of this disorder remains obscure. An increased luteal phase estrogen:progesterone ratio, hyperprolactinemia, disturbances of the renin-angiotensin-aldosterone axis, hypothyroidism, and abnormal secretion of opioid peptides are among the etiologies considered for this enigmatic condition.[166] Numerous hormonal and nonhormonal therapies—including natural progesterone, oral contraceptives, bromocriptine, gonadotropin-releasing hormone agonists, diuretics, prostaglandin inhibitors, vitamin B_6, and lithium—are prescribed for the management of premenstrual syndrome. However, with the possible exception of the agonists of gonadotropin-releasing hormone, none has proved to be unequivocally effective.[166] In a double-blind crossover trial,[167] induction of "artificial menopause" with an agonist of gonadotropin-releasing hormone (D-Trp-Pro-NEt-Gn-RH, 50 μg/d subcutaneously) relieved both physical and neuropsychiatric symptoms in eight women with rigorously defined premenstrual syndrome. Although the authors reported no side effects (except for hot flashes in one patient), prolonged hypoestrogenemia resulting from the long-term use of these agents may predispose to osteoporosis. Such therapy should probably be reserved for patients with truly incapacitating symptoms, and low-dose estrogen replacement may have to be considered when the duration of treatment exceeds several months.

DEPRESSION AND PSYCHOSIS

Depression and other major affective disorders may surface in relation to the menstrual cycle, the puerperium, and menopause. In patients with postmenopausal depression, mood elevation and anxiolysis often occur promptly in response to estrogen replacement.[67] Paradoxically, oral contraceptives may precipitate depression in susceptible individuals.[168] Estrogen has also been implicated in the pathogenesis of anorexia nervosa in view of the high preponderance of this condition in women and the potent anorexic effects of estrogen in animals.[169]

Psychotic disorders characterized by extreme agitation, hallucinations, paranoid delusions, incoherent speech, and mood lability may arise during the postpartum period[170] or may recur consistently during the late luteal phase of the cycle. Such disorders may be refractory to conventional therapies (neuroleptics, lithium, electroconvulsive treatment) but may respond dramatically to specific hormonal interventions, including the use of oral contraceptives,[171] intramuscular progesterone,[172] and danazol.[173] "Menopause" induced by agonists of gonadotropin-releasing hormone may also be of considerable benefit in the management of cyclical psychosis.

Other Neurological Disorders

SLEEP DISORDERS

Estrogen and progestin replacement may shorten mean sleep latencies and extend the duration of REM periods, thereby improving sleep in hypogonadal women.[174–176] Progestins may also provide stimulatory drive to brainstem respiratory centers in subjects with central sleep apnea and thereby ameliorate hypoventilation.[177]

CEREBRAL INJURY

Progesterone has been shown to suppress posttraumatic cerebral edema and intracranial hypertension in rodents. This progestational effect has been attributed to reduction in blood-brain barrier permeability and inhibition of CSF production by the choroid plexus.[178–180] Estrogens, by contrast, appear to enhance cerebral endothelial cell permeability and posttraumatic brain edema in female rats.[181,182] Estrogenic attenuation of the blood-brain barrier may also

play a role in the pathogenesis of pseudotumor cerebri in humans and explain the robust female predilection for this disorder.[181]

REFERENCES

1. Green JD, Harris GW: Neurovascular link between neurohypophysis and adenohypophysis. J Endocrinol 5:136, 1947
2. Barnea ER, Naftolin F, Tolis G, De Cherney A: Hypothalamic amenorrhea syndromes. p. 147. In Givens JR (ed): The Hypothalamus. Year Book, Chicago, 1984
3. Guillemin R: Peptides in the brain: the new endocrinology of the neuron. Science 202:390, 1978
4. Gibbs DM, Neill JD: Dopamine levels in hypophysial stalk blood in the rat are sufficient to inhibit prolactin secretion in vivo. Endocrinology 102:1895, 1978
5. Jacobs LS, Snyder PJ, Utiger RD, Daughaday WH: Prolactin response to thyrotropin releasing hormone in normal subjects. J Clin Endocrinol Metab 36:1069, 1973
6. Kleinberg DL, Noel GL, Frantz AG: Galactorrhea: a study of 235 cases, including 48 with pituitary tumors. N Engl J Med 296:589, 1977
7. Evans WS, Thorner MO: Mechanisms for hypogonadism in hyperprolactinemia. Semin Reprod Endocrinol 2:9, 1984
8. Nabarro JDN: Pituitary prolactinomas. Clin Endocrinol 17:129, 1982
9. Braunstein GD: Diagnosis. p. 244. In Melmed S (moderator). Pituitary tumors secreting growth hormone and prolactin. Ann Intern Med 105:238, 1986
10. Post KD, Muraszko K: Management of pituitary tumors. Neurol Clin 4:801, 1986
11. Vance ML, Evans WS, Thorner MO: Drugs five years later: bromocriptine. Ann Intern Med 100:78, 1984
12. Molitch ME, Elton RL, Blackwell RE, et al: Bromocriptine as primary therapy for prolactin-secreting macroadenomas: results of a prospective multicenter study. J Clin Endocrinol Metab 60:698, 1985
13. Vance ML, Cragun JR, Reimnitz C, et al: CV 205-502 treatment of hyperprolactinemia. J Clin Endocrinol Metab 68:336, 1989
14. Serri O, Rasio E, Beauregard H, et al: Recurrence of hyperprolactinemia after selective transsphenoidal adenomectomy in women with prolactinoma. N Engl J Med 309:280, 1983
15. Sheline GE, Grossman A, Jones AE: Radiation therapy for prolactinomas. p. 93. In Black PM, Zervas NT, Ridgeway EC (eds): Secretory tumors of the Pituitary Gland. Raven Press, New York, 1984

16. Casanueva FF: Physiology of growth hormone secretion and action. Endocrinol Metab Clin North Am 21:483, 1992

17. Melmed S: Acromegaly. N Engl J Med 322:966, 1990

18. Khaleeli AA, Levy RD, Edwards RHT, et al: The neuromuscular features of acromegaly: a clinical and pathological study. J Neurol Neurosurg Psychiatry 47:1009, 1984

19. Schiller F, Kolb F: Carpal tunnel syndrome in acromegaly. Neurology 4:271, 1954

20. Klibanski A, Zervas NT: Diagnosis and management of hormone-secreting pituitary adenomas. N Engl J Med 324:822, 1991

21. Lamberts SW, Uitterlinden P, Verschoor L, et al: Long-term treatment of acromegaly with the somatostatin analogue SMS 201-995. N Engl J Med 313:1576, 1985

22. Eastman RC, Gorden P, Glatstein E, Roth J: Radiation therapy of acromegaly. Endocrinol Metab Clin North Am 21:693, 1992

23. Burr IM, Slonim AE, Danish RK, et al: Diencephalic syndrome revisited. J Pediatr 88:439, 1976

24. Drop SL, Guyda HJ, Colle E: Inappropriate growth hormone release in the diencephalic syndrome of childhood: case report and 4 year endocrinological follow-up. Clin Endocrinol 13:181, 1980

25. Podolsky S, Leopold NA: Growth hormone abnormalities in Huntington's chorea: effect of L-dopa administration. J Clin Endocrinol Metab 39:36, 1974

26. Eipper BA, Mains RE: Structure and biosynthesis of pro-adrenocorticotropin/endorphin and related peptides. Endocr Rev 1:1, 1980

27. Carpenter PC: Cushing's syndrome: update of diagnosis and management. Mayo Clin Proc 61:49, 1986

28. Loriaux DL, Nieman L: Corticotropin releasing hormone testing in pituitary disease. Endocrinol Metab Clin North Am 20:363, 1991

29. Oldfield EH, Chrousos GP, Schulte HM, et al: Preoperative lateralization of ACTH-secreting pituitary micradenomas by bilateral and simultaneous inferior petrosal venous sinus sampling. N Engl J Med 312:100, 1985

30. Styne DM, Grumbach MM, Kaplan SL, et al: Treatment of Cushing's disease in childhood and adolescence by transsphenoidal microadenomectomy. N Engl J Med 310:889, 1984

31. Moore TJ, Dluhy RG, Williams GH, Cain JP: Nelson's syndrome: frequency, prognosis, and effect of prior pituitary irradiation. Ann Intern Med 85:731, 1976

32. Kovacs K: Necrosis of anterior pituitary in humans. Neuroendocrinology 4:170, 201, 1969

33. Silverman AJ, Zimmerman EA: Magnocellular neurosecretory system. Annu Rev Neurosci 6:357, 1983

34. Moses AM: Clinical and laboratory features of central and nephrogenic diabetes insipidus and primary polydipsia. p. 115. In Reichlin S (ed): The Neurohypophysis. Plenum, New York, 1984

35. Zerbe RL, Robertson GL: A comparison of plasma vasopressin measurements with a standard indirect test in the differential diagnosis of polyuria. N Engl J Med 305:1539, 1981

36. Scotti G, Triulzi F, Chiumello G, Dinatale B: New imaging techniques in endocrinology: magnetic resonance of the pituitary gland and sella turcica. Acta Paediatr Scand Suppl 356:5, 1989

37. Robinson AG: DDAVP in the treatment of central diabetes insipidus. N Engl J Med 294:507, 1976

38. Bartter F, Schwartz WB: The syndrome of inappropriate secretion of antidiuretic hormone. Am J Med 42:790, 1967

39. Sterns RH, Riggs JE, Schochet SS: Osmotic demyelination syndrome following correction of hyponatremia. N Engl J Med 314:1535, 1986

40. Forrest JN, Cox M, Hong C, et al: Superiority of demeclocycline over lithium in the treatment of chronic syndrome of inappropriate secretion of antidiuretic hormone. N Engl J Med 298:173, 1978

41. White MG, Fetner CD: Treatment of the syndrome of inappropriate secretion of antidiuretic hormone with lithium carbonate. N Engl J Med 292:390, 1975

42. Habener JF, Potts JT: Biosynthesis of parathyroid hormone. N Engl J Med 299:580 and 635, 1978

43. Huang M, Hanley DA, Rorstad OP: Parathyroid hormone stimulates adenylate cyclase in rat cerebral microvessels. Life Sci 32:1009, 1983

44. Turken SA, Cafferty M, Silverberg SJ, et al: Neuromuscular involvement in mild, asymptomatic primary hyperparathyroidism. Am J Med 87:553, 1989

45. Mallette LE, Bilezikian JP, Heath DA, Auerbach GD: Primary hyperparathyroidism: clinical and biochemical features. Medicine (Baltimore) 53:127, 1974

46. Alarcon RD, Franceschini JA: Hyperparathyroidism and paranoid psychosis: case report and review of the literature. Br J Psychiatry 145:477, 1984

47. Patten BM, Bilezikian JP, Mallette LE, et al: Neuromuscular disease in primary hyperparathyroidism. Ann Intern Med 80:182, 1974

48. Mallette LE, Patten BM, Engel WK: Neuromuscular disease in secondary hyperparathyroidism. Ann Intern Med 82:474, 1975

49. Nusynowitz ML, Frame B, Kolb FO: The spectrum of the hypoparathyroid states. Medicine (Baltimore) 55:105, 1976

50. Frame B, Carter S: Pseudohypoparathyroidism. Neurology 5:297, 1955

51. Sugar O: Central neurological complications of hypoparathyroidism. Arch Neurol Psychiatry 70:86, 1953

52. Simpson JA: The neurological manifestations of idiopathic hypoparathyroidism. Brain 75:76, 1952

53. Illum F, Dupont E: Prevalences of CT-detected calcification in the basal ganglia in idiopathic hypoparathyroidism and pseudohypoparathyroidism. Neuroradiology 27:32, 1985

54. Muenter MD, Whisnant JP: Basal ganglia calcification, hypoparathyroidism, and extrapyramidal motor manifestations. Neurology 18:1075, 1968

55. Connor TB, Rosen BL, Blaustein MP, et al: Hypocalcemia precipitating congestive heart failure. N Engl J Med 307:869, 1982

56. Horton WA, Wong V, Eldridge R: Von-Hippel Lindau disease: clinical and pathological manifestations in nine families with 50 affected members. Arch Intern Med 136:769, 1976

57. Thomas JE, Rooke ED, Kvale WF: The neurologist's experience with pheochromocytoma. JAMA 197:754, 1966

58. Bravo EL, Gifford RW: Pheochromocytoma: diagnosis, localization and management. N Engl J Med 311:1298, 1984

59. Gabrilove JL: Neurologic and psychiatric manifestations in the classic endocrine syndromes. Res Publ Assoc Res Nerv Ment Dis 43:419, 1966

60. Loli P, Berselli ME, Tagliaferri M: Use of ketoconazole in the treatment of Cushing's syndrome. J Clin Endocrinol Metab 63:1365, 1986

61. Melby JC: Diagnosis of hyperaldosteronism. Endocrinol Metab Clin North Am 20:247, 1991

62. Konomi H, Imai M, Nihei K, et al: Indomethacin causing pseudotumor in Bartter's syndrome. N Engl J Med 298:855, 1978

63. Dumas P, Archambeaud-Mouveroux F, Vallat JM, et al: Myasthenia gravis associated with adrenocortical insufficiency. J Neurol 232:354, 1985

64. Glaser GH: EEG activity and adrenocortical dysfunction. Electroencephalogr Clin Neurophysiol 10:366, 1958

65. Jefferson A: A clinical correlation between encephalopathy and papilloedema in Addison's disease. J Neurol Neurosurg Psychiatry 19:21, 1956

66. Gasc J-M, Renoir J-M, Radanyi C, et al: Progesterone receptor in the chick oviduct: an immunohistochemical study with antibodies to distinct receptor components. J Cell Biol 99:1193, 1984

67. McEwen BS: Gonadal and adrenal steroids and the brain: implications for depression. p. 239. In Halbreich U (ed): Hormones and Depression. Raven Press, New York, 1987

68. Nattero G: Menstrual headache. Adv Neurol 33:215, 1982

69. Welch KM, Darnley D, Simpkins RT: The role of estrogen in migraine: a review and hypothesis. Cephalalgia 4:227, 1984

70. Somerville B: The role of estradiol withdrawal in the etiology of menstrual migraine. Neurology 22:355, 1972

71. Somerville BW: Estrogen withdrawal migraine: I. Duration of exposure required and attempted prophylaxis by premenstrual estrogen administration. Neurology 25:239, 1975

72. Somerville BW: Estrogen-withdrawal migraine: II. Attempted prophylaxis by continuous estradiol administration. Neurology 25:245, 1975

73. Epstein MT, Hockaday JM, Hockaday TD: Migraine and reproductive hormones throughout the menstrual cycle. Lancet 1:543, 1975

74. Lance JW, Anthony M: Some clinical aspects of migraine. Arch Neurol 15:356, 1966

75. Saper J: Migraine: II. Treatment. JAMA 239:2480, 1978

76. Chancellor AM, Wroe SJ, Cull RE: Migraine occurring for the first time in pregnancy. Headache 30:224, 1990

77. Whitty CW, Hockaday JM, Whitty MM: The effect of oral contraceptives on migraine. Lancet 1:856, 1966

78. Bergeron RT, Wood EH: Oral contraceptives and cerebrovascular complications. Radiology 92:231, 1969

79. Bickerstaff E: Neurological Complications of Oral Contraceptives. Clarendon Press, Oxford, 1975

80. Silberstein SD: The role of sex hormones in headache. Neurology 42, suppl 2:37, 1992

81. Schipper HM: Neurology of sex steroids and oral contraceptives. Neurol Clin 4:721, 1986

82. Diamond S: Menstrual migraine and non-steroidal anti-inflammatory agents. Headache 24:52, 1984

83. Magos AL, Zilkha KJ, Studd JW: Treatment of menstrual migraine by oestradiol implants. J Neurol Neurosurg Psychiatry 46:1044, 1983

84. O'Dea JPK, Davis EH: Tamoxifen in the treatment of menstrual migraine. Neurology 40:1470, 1990

85. Carlton G, Burnett J: Danazol and migraine. N Engl J Med 310:721, 1984

86. Vincent FM: Migraine responsive to danazol. Neurology 35:618, 1985

87. Sartwell PE, Masi AT, Arthes FG, et al: Thromboembolism and oral contraceptives: an epidemiologic case-control study. Am J Epidemiol 90:365, 1969

88. Vessey MP, Doll R: Investigation of relation between use of oral contraceptives and thromboembolic disease: a further report. Br Med J 2:651, 1969

89. Collaborative Group for the Study of Stroke in Young Women: Oral contraception and increased risk of cerebral ischemia or thrombosis. N Engl J Med 288:871, 1973

90. Jick H, Porter J, Rothman KJ: Oral contraceptives and

nonfatal stroke in healthy young women. Ann Intern Med 89:58, 1978

91. Hedon B: The evolution of oral contraceptives: maximizing efficacy, minimizing risks. Acta Obstet Gynecol Scand Suppl 152:7, 1990

92. Mishell DR Jr: Oral contraception: past, present, and future perspectives. Int J Fertil 36, suppl 1:7, 1991

93. Lidegaard O: Oral contraception and risk of a cerebral thromboembolic attack: results of a case-control study. Br Med J 306:956, 1993

94. Meade TW, Berra A: Hormone replacement therapy and cardiovascular disease. Br Med Bull 48:276, 1992

95. Stubblefield PG: The effects on hemostasis of oral contraceptives containing desogestrel. Am J Obstet Gynecol 168:1047, 1993

96. Donaldson J: Neurology of Pregnancy. WB Saunders, Philadelphia, 1978

97. Schafer AI: The hypercoagulable states. Ann Intern Med 102:814, 1985

98. Elam MB, Viar MJ, Ratts TE, Chesney CM: Mitral valve prolapse in women with oral contraceptive-related cerebrovascular insufficiency. Arch Intern Med 146:73, 1986

99. Estanol B, Rodriquez A, Conte G, et al: Intracranial venous thrombosis in young women. Stroke 10:680, 1979

100. Kelly MA, Gorelick PB, Mirza D: The role of drugs in the etiology of stroke. Clin Neuropharmacol 15:249, 1992

101. Wren BG: The effect of oestrogen on the female cardiovascular system. Med J Aust 156:204, 1992

102. Green A, Bain C: Epidemiological overview of oestrogen replacement and cardiovascular disease. Baillieres Clin Endocrinol Metab 7:95, 1993

103. Beaumont V, Delplanque B, Lemort N, Beaumont JL: Blood changes in sex steroid hormone users: circulating immune complexes induced by estrogens and progestogens and their relation to vascular thrombosis. Atherosclerosis 44:343, 1982

104. Irey NS, Norris HJ: Intimal vascular lesions associated with female reproductive steroids. Arch Pathol 96:227, 1973

105. Royal College of General Practitioners' Oral Contraception Study: Further analysis of mortality in oral contraceptive users. Lancet 1:541, 1981

106. Ramcharan S, Pellegrin FA, Ray RM, Hsu JP: The Walnut Creek Contraceptive Drug Study: a prospective study of the side effects of oral contraceptives. J Reprod Med 25, suppl:345, 1980

107. Lombardo L, Mateos JH, Barroeta FF: Subarachnoid hemorrhage due to endometriosis of the spinal canal. Neurology 18:423, 1968

108. Gastaut H, Colomb H: Etude du comportement sexual chez les epileptiques psychomoteurs. Ann Med Psychol 112:657, 1954

109. Pritchard P: Hyposexuality: a complication of partial complex epilepsy. Trans Am Neurol Assoc 105:193, 1980

110. Herzog AG, Seibel MM, Schomer DL, et al: Reproductive endocrine disorders in women with partial seizures of temporal lobe origin. Arch Neurol 43:341, 1986

111. Bjerkedal T, Bahna SL: The occurrence and outcome of pregnancy in women with epilepsy. Acta Obstet Gynecol Scand 52:245, 1973

112. Mattson RH, Cramer JA, Darney PD, Naftolin F: Use of oral contraceptives by women with epilepsy. JAMA 256:238, 1986

113. Browne TR: Epilepsy, sexual function, and pregnancy. p. 333. In Browne TR, Feldman RG (eds): Epilepsy: Diagnosis and Management. Little, Brown, Boston, 1983

114. Mattson RH, Cramer JA: Epilepsy, sex hormones, and antiepileptic drugs. Epilepsia 26, suppl 1:S40, 1985

115. Backstrom T, Landgren S, Zetterlund B, et al: Effects of ovarian steroid hormones on brain excitability and their relation to seizure variation during the menstrual cycle. In Porter R, Ward A Jr, Mattson R, et al (eds): Advances in Epileptology: XVth Epilepsy International Symposium, Raven Press, New York, 1984

116. Gevorkyan ES, Nazaryan KB, Kostanyan AA: Modifying effect of estradiol and progesterone on epileptic activity of the rat brain. Neurosci Behav Physiol 19:412, 1989

117. Tauboll E, Lindstrom S: The effect of progesterone and its metabolite 5α-pregnan-3α-ol-20-one on focal epileptic seizures in the cat's visual cortex in vivo. Epilepsy Res 14:17, 1993

118. Dana-Haeri J, Richens A: Effect of norethisterone on seizures associated with menstruation. Epilepsia 24:377, 1983

119. Espir M, Walker ME, Lawson JP: Epilepsy and oral contraception. Br Med J 1:294, 1969

120. Herzog AG: Intermittent progesterone therapy and frequency of complex partial seizures in women with menstrual disorders. Neurology 36:1607, 1986

121. Levy RH, Yerby MS: Effects of pregnancy on antiepileptic drug utilization. Epilepsia 26, suppl 1:S52, 1985

122. De Leacy EA, McLeay CD, Eadie MJ, Tyrer JH: Effects of subjects' sex and intake of tobacco, alcohol and oral contraceptives on plasma phenytoin levels. Br J Clin Pharmacol 8:33, 1979

123. Ghanem Q: Recurrent chorea gravidarum in four pregnancies. Can J Neurol Sci 12:136, 1985

124. Gamboa ET, Isaacs G, Harter DH: Chorea associated

with oral contraceptive therapy. Arch Neurol 25:112, 1971

125. Riddoch D, Jefferson M, Bickerstaff ER: Chorea and the oral contraceptives. Br Med J 4:217, 1971

126. Bedard P, Langelier P, Villeneuve A: Oestrogens and extrapyramidal system. Lancet 2:1367, 1977

127. Quinn NP, Marsden CD: Menstrual-related fluctuations in Parkinson's disease. Mov Disord 1:85, 1986

128. Gomez-Mancilla B, Bedard PJ: Effect of estrogen and progesterone on L-dopa induced dyskinesia in MPTP-treated monkeys. Neurosci Lett 135:129, 1992

129. McDermott JL: Effects of estrogen upon dopamine release from the corpus striatum of young and aged female rats. Brain Res 606:118, 1993

130. Fahn S: Posthypoxic action myoclonus: review of the literature and report of two new cases with response to valproate and estrogen. Adv Neurol 26:49, 1979

131. Daube JR, Peters HA: Hereditary essential myoclonus. Arch Neurol 15:587, 1966

132. Quinn NP, Marsden CD: Dominantly inherited myoclonic dystonia with dramatic response to alcohol. Neurology 34, suppl 1:236, 1984

133. Koller WC, Barr A, Biary N: Estrogen treatment of dyskinetic disorders. Neurology 32:547, 1982

134. Robinson RO, Stutchfield P, Hicks B, Marsden CD: Estrogens and dyskinesia. Neurology 34:404, 1984

135. Zasorin NL, Baloh RW, Myers LB: Acetazolamide-responsive episodic ataxia syndrome. Neurology 33:1212, 1983

136. Schwabe MJ, Konkol RJ: Menstrual cycle-related fluctuations of tics in Tourette syndrome. Pediatr Neurol 8:43, 1992

137. Mizuta E, Yamasaki S, Nakatake M, Kuno S: Neuroleptic malignant syndrome in a parkinsonian woman during the premenstrual period. Neurology 43:1048, 1993

138. Kepes J: Meningiomas: Biology, Pathology, and Differential Diagnosis. Masson, New York, 1982

139. Schoenberg BS: Nervous system. p. 968. In Schottenfeld D, Fraumeni JF (eds): Cancer Epidemiology and Prevention. WB Saunders, Philadelphia, 1982

140. Poisson M: Sex steroid receptors in human meningiomas. Clin Neuropharmacol 7:320, 1984

141. Haddad G, Haddad F, Worseley K, Villemure JG: Brain tumours and pregnancy. Can J Neurol Sci 18:231, 1991

142. Bickerstaff E, Small J, Guest I: The relapsing course of certain meningiomas in relation to pregnancy and menstruation. J Neurol Neurosurg Psychiatry 21:89, 1958

143. Markwalder T-M, Seiler RW, Zava DT: Endocrine manipulation of inoperable and recurrent meningiomas—a pilot study. In Spitzy K, Karrer K (eds): Proceedings of the 13th International Congress of Chemotherapy. Egermann, Vienna, 1983

144. Lamberts SWJ, Tanghe HLJ, Avezaat CJJ, et al: Mifepristone (RU 486) treatment of meningiomas. J Neurol Neurosurg Psychiatry 55:486, 1992

145. Blankenstein MA, van der Meulen-Dijk C, Thijssen JHH: Effect of steroids and antisteroids on human meningioma cells in primary culture. J Steroid Biochem 34:419, 1989

146. Maiuri F, Montagnani S, Gallicchio B, et al: Oestrogen and progesterone sensitivity in cultured meningioma cells. Neurol Res 11:9, 1989

147. Adams EF, Schrell UMH, Fahlbusch R, Thierauf P: Hormonal dependency of cerebral meningiomas. Part 2. In vitro effect of steroids, bromocriptine, and epidermal growth factor on growth of meningiomas. J Neurosurg 73:750, 1990

148. Lamberts SW, Koper JW, de Jong FH: The endocrine effects of long-term treatment with mifepristone (RU 486). J Clin Endocrinol Metab 73:187, 1991

149. Michelsen JJ, New PF: Brain tumour and pregnancy. J Neurol Neurosurg Psychiatry 32:305, 1969

150. von Schoultz E, Bixo M, Backstrom T, et al: Sex steroids in human brain tumors and breast cancer. Cancer 65:949, 1990

151. Langub MC Jr, Watson RE Jr: Estrogen receptor-immunoreactive glia, endothelia, and ependyma in guinea pig preoptic area and median eminence: electron microscopy. Endocrinology 130:364, 1992

152. Glick RP, Molteni A, Fors EM: Hormone binding in brain tumors. Neurosurgery 13:513, 1983

153. Baltuch G, Shenouda G, Langleben A, Villemure JG: High dose tamoxifen in the treatment of recurrent high grade glioma: a report of clinical stabilization and tumour regression. Can J Neurol Sci 20:168, 1993

154. Verzat C, Courriere P, Hollande E: Heterotransplantation of a human oligoastrocytoma into nude mice: difference in tumour growth between males and females. Neuropathol Appl Neurobiol 18:37, 1992

155. Aronson NI, Kaplow S, Goldstein PJ: Brain tumors during pregnancy. p. 41. In Goldstein P (ed): Neurological Disorders of Pregnancy. Futura, Mt Kisco, NY, 1986

156. Shewchuk AB, Adamson GD, Lessard P, Ezrin C: The effect of pregnancy on suspected pituitary adenomas after conservative management of ovulation defects associated with galactorrhea. Am J Obstet Gynecol 136:659, 1980

157. Hansen SB, Galsgard H, von Eyben FE, et al: Tamoxifen for brain metastases from breast cancer. Ann Neurol 20:544, 1986

158. Pors H, von Eyben FE, Sorensen OS, Larsen M: Longterm remission of multiple brain metastases with tamoxifen. J Neurooncol 10:173, 1991

159. Lee L-S, Chi C-W, Chang T-J, et al: Steroid hormone receptors in meningiomas of Chinese patients. Neurosurgery 25:541, 1989

160. Kappas A, Sassa S, Granick S, Bradlow HL: Endocrine-gene interaction in the pathogenesis of acute intermittent porphyria. Res Publ Assoc Res Nerv Ment Dis 53:225, 1974

161. Welland F, Hellman E, Collins A, et al: Factors affecting the excretion of porphyrin precursors by patients with acute intermittent porphyria: II. The effect of ethinyl estradiol. Metabolism 13:251, 1964

162. Editorial: The Pill and porphyria. Br Med J 3:603, 1972

163. Tschudy DP, Valsamis M, Magnussen CR: Acute intermittent porphyria: clinical and selected research aspects. Ann Intern Med 83:851, 1975

164. Anderson KE, Spitz IM, Sassa S, et al: Prevention of cyclical attacks of acute intermittent porphyria with a long-acting agonist of luteinizing hormone-releasing hormone. N Engl J Med 311:643, 1984

165. Usuki F, Nakazato O, Osame M, Igata A: Hyperestrogenemia in neuromuscular diseases. J Neurol Sci 89:189, 1989

166. Reid RL, Yen SS: Premenstrual syndrome. Am J Obstet Gynecol 139:85, 1981

167. Muse KN, Cetel NS, Futterman LA, Yen SSC: The premenstrual syndrome: effects of "medical ovariectomy." N Engl J Med 311:1345, 1984

168. Glick ID, Quitkin FM, Bennett SE: The influence of estrogens, progestins, and oral contraceptives on depression. p. 339. In Halbreich U (ed): Hormones and Depression. Raven Press, New York, 1987

169. Young JK: Estrogen and the etiology of anorexia nervosa. Neurosci Behav Rev 15:327, 1991

170. Vinogradov S, Csernansky JG: Postpartum psychosis with abnormal movements: dopamine supersensitivity unmasked by withdrawal of endogenous estrogen? J Clin Psychiatry 51:365, 1990

171. Felthous AR, Robinson DB, Conroy RW: Prevention of recurrent menstrual psychosis by an oral contraceptive. Am J Psychiatry 137:245, 1980

172. Berlin FS, Bergey GK, Money J: Periodic psychosis of puberty: a case report. Am J Psychiatry 139:119, 1982

173. Dennerstein L, Judd F, Davies B: Psychosis and the menstrual cycle. Med J Aust 1:524, 1983

174. Schiff I, Regenstein Q, Tulchinsky D, Ryan KJ: Effects of estrogens on sleep and psychological state of hypogonadal women. JAMA 242:2405, 1979

175. Shaver J, Giblin E, Lentz M, Lee K: Sleep patterns and stability in perimenopausal women. Sleep 11:556, 1988

176. Pickett CK, Regensteiner JG, Woodard WD, et al: Progestin and estrogen reduce sleep-disordered breathing in postmenopausal women. J Appl Physiol 66:1656, 1989

177. Milerad J, Lagercrantz H, Lofgren O: Alveolar hypoventilation treated with medroxyprogesterone. Arch Dis Child 60:150, 1985

178. Lindvall-Axelsson M, Owman C: Actions of sex steroids and corticosteroids on rabbit choroid plexus as shown by changes in transport capacity and rate of cerebrospinal fluid formation. Neurol Res 12:181, 1990

179. Roof RL, Duvdevani R, Stein DG: Progesterone treatment attenuates brain edema following contusion injury in male and female rats. Restorative Neurol Neurosci 4:425, 1992

180. Roof RL, Duvdevani R, Stein DG: Gender influences outcome of brain injury: progesterone plays a protective role. Brain Res 607:333, 1993

181. Ziylan YZ, Lefauconnier JM, Bernard G, Bourre JM: Blood-brain barrier permeability: regional alterations after acute and chronic administration of ethinyl estradiol. Neurosci Lett 118:181, 1990

182. Emerson CS, Headrick JP, Vink R: Estrogen improves biochemical and neurologic outcome following traumatic brain injury in male rats, but not in females. Brain Res 608:95, 1993

21

Paraneoplastic Syndromes Involving the Nervous System

Jerome B. Posner

The term *paraneoplastic syndrome*[1,2] refers to a group of disorders that are caused by or associated with cancer but are not a direct effect of the primary tumor mass or of a metastasis to the involved organ. Paraneoplastic syndromes can affect many organs (Table 21-1). Using the broad definition above, any nervous system dysfunction caused by a nonmetastatic effect of cancer can be called a paraneoplastic syndrome (Table 21-2). Thus, metabolic disorders associated with cancer (e.g., hypercalcemia, inappropriate antidiuretic hormone secretion, and hypoglycemia), cerebral vascular disorders associated with hyper- or hypocoagulability, and opportunistic infections may all be considered paraneoplastic syndromes. The neurologist, however, usually uses the term *paraneoplastic syndrome* to refer to a group of neurological disorders that occur with increased frequency in patients with cancer and are not caused by infection, systemic metabolic disorders, vascular disease, or side effects of cancer therapy (Table 21-2). These disorders, also termed *remote effects* of cancer on the nervous system,[3–5] encompass a much less common and a clinically and pathologically more restricted group of disorders than other nonmetastatic effects of cancer. It is these remote effects of cancer on the nervous system that are addressed in this chapter. In common with the general usage of neurologists, the terms *remote effects* and *paraneoplastic syndrome* are used interchangeably.

Paraneoplastic syndromes can be classified according to the predominant clinical finding, as seen in Table 21-2, or according to pathological characteristics, the system used by Henson and Urich.[3] Often these two systems coincide, although at times clinical abnormalities are found that do not appear to have a pathological correlate (e.g., dementia in cerebellar degeneration); or pathological abnormalities, especially widespread perivascular inflammatory infiltrates, may not be associated with clinical findings. The major difference between the two classifications concerns the term *encephalomyelitis*, which Henson and Urich used to describe any paraneoplastic syndrome with inflammatory changes scattered throughout the nervous system, regardless of the clinical findings. In this chapter the term *encephalomyelitis* refers to those patients with clinical evidence of widespread central nervous system (CNS) dysfunction without predominant findings in one particular area.

GENERAL CONSIDERATIONS

Several studies have addressed the frequency of paraneoplastic syndromes. Data from these studies depend on (1) the definition of paraneoplastic syn-

Table 21-1 Some Nonneurological Paraneoplastic Syndromes

General physiological (host-reactive) syndromes
  Fever
  Anorexia and cachexia
  Fatigue and "weakness"
  Abnormalities of taste

Hematological and vascular syndromes
  Anemia
  Leukemoid reaction
  Thrombocytoses
  Hypercoagulability
  Hyperviscosity

Skin and connective tissue syndromes
  Acanthosis nigricans
  Erythemas
  Pruritus
  Vasculitis
  Flushing
  Poikiloderma
  Ichthyosis
  Hypertrichosis
  Pachydermoperiostosis

Endocrine-metabolic syndromes
  Cushing's syndrome
  Hypo- and hyperglycemia
  Antidiuretic hormone syndrome
  Carcinoid syndrome
  Hyper- and hypocalcemia
  Systemic nodular panniculitis
  Acromegaly

Gastrointestinal syndromes
  Malabsorption
  Exudative enteropathy
  Zollinger-Ellison syndrome

Collagen-vascular syndromes
  Arthritides
  Scleroderma
  Lupus erythematosus
  Amyloidosis
  Hypertrophic osteoarthropathy
  Palmar fasciitis

Renal syndromes
  Nephrotic syndrome
  Renal failure
  Hypokalemia

Bone syndrome
  Hypophosphatemic osteomalacia

See also Bunn and Ridgway.[2]
(Modified from Shnider BI, Manalo A: Paraneoplastic syndromes: unusual manifestations of malignant disease. DM 25:1, 1979, with permission.)

Table 21-2 Nonmetastatic Effects of Cancer on the Nervous System

Metabolic disorder
  Organ failure
  Endocrinopathies
  Nutritional problems
  Tumor secretions of ectopic substances

Vascular disorder
  Hypocoagulability (hemorrhage)
  Hypercoagulability (infarction)

Infection

Side effects of therapy
  Surgery
  Irradiation
  Chemotherapy

"Remote effects"
  Brain and cranial nerves
  Spinal cord and dorsal root ganglia
  Peripheral nerves
  Neuromuscular junction
  Muscle

dromes, (2) the rigor used to exclude other causes of neurological dysfunction, and (3) the care with which the neurological evaluation was performed. For example, the Lambert-Eaton myasthenic syndrome (LEMS) occurs in 3 percent or fewer of patients with small cell lung cancer[6] but when the symptom of paraneoplastic neuromuscular dysfunction is expanded to include any subjective or objective muscle weakness, the frequency rises to 44 percent. Croft and Wilkinson found that 7 percent of 1,476 patients with any type of cancer had a neuromyopathy as assessed by physical examination,[7] but Lipton and co-workers found abnormalities of peripheral nerve function by quantitative sensory testing in 44 percent,[8,9] and Gomm and colleagues found myopathic changes on muscle biopsy in 33 of 100 patients with lung cancer.[10] Such conflicting figures make it difficult to estimate the incidence of true neurological paraneoplastic syndromes, but clinically significant paraneoplastic syndromes probably occur in fewer than 1 percent of cancer patients.[11]

Pathogenesis

Although the etiology of most neurological paraneoplastic syndromes is unknown (Table 21-3), several potential mechanisms have been proposed, some

Table 21-3 Possible Pathogenesis of
Paraneoplastic Syndromes

Hypothesis	Example
"Toxin" secreted by tumor	ACTH → Cushing's syndrome Parathormone → hypercalcemia
Competition for essential substrate	Utilization of glucose by large intraabdominal sarcomas → hypoglycemia Carcinoid tumors compete with brain for tryptophan → pellagra-like syndrome
Opportunistic infection	Papovavirus → progressive multifocal leukoencephalopathy ?Subacute motor neuronopathy
Autoimmune process	Lambert-Eaton myasthenic syndrome ?Paraneoplastic cerebellar degeneration ?Subacute sensory neuronopathy ?Retinal degeneration

(Modified from Anderson NE, Cunningham JM, Posner JB: Autoimmune pathogenesis of paraneoplastic neurological syndromes. Crit Rev Neurobiol 3:245, 1987, with permission.)

of which cause neurological symptoms that are not now classified as paraneoplastic syndromes.

Oppenheim in 1888 proposed that some neurological disorders associated with cancer resulted from release by the tumor of a toxic substance.[12] That tumors can secrete substances that interfere with CNS function is now well established.[13]

In 1948, Denny-Brown, in describing what were probably the first cases of anti-Hu positive (see below) subacute sensory neuronopathy, noted a similarity between the dorsal root ganglionitis in his patients and that seen in swine deprived of pantothenic acid.[14] He suggested that the malignancy and the nervous system were competing for a vital nutrient. Metastatic carcinoid tumors[15] and large retroperitoneal sarcomas[16] appear to cause neurological symptoms by such a mechanism. However, no evidence indicates that small and occult cancers, such as those usually encountered with paraneoplastic syndromes, are capable of depriving the nervous system of any essential substrate.

Opportunistic viral infections involving the CNS complicate the clinical course of many patients whose immune systems are suppressed by cancer or its therapy. Progressive multifocal leukoencephalopathy, originally classified as a remote effect,[17] is one such infection. Subacute motor neuronopathy (see below) may be another. However, most paraneoplastic syndromes affect patients who are not immunosuppressed, making opportunistic infection unlikely unless these patients suffer isolated, currently unknown disorders of immunity. The absence of other opportunistic infections such as progressive multifocal leukoencephalopathy or herpes zoster also indicates a lack of significant immunosuppression in most patients with paraneoplastic syndromes.

Although individual paraneoplastic syndromes may have different etiologies and a given paraneoplastic syndrome such as paraneoplastic cerebellar degeneration may have more than one etiology, an immune mechanism is now the most attractive hypothesis as the cause of most, or perhaps all, remote effects of cancer on the nervous system. The hypothesis posits that antigenic molecules or epitopes known as onconeural antigens are shared between certain tumors and cells of the central or peripheral nervous system.[18] The immune system, recognizing the antigen in the tumor as foreign, directs a response at the tumor; the immune response is misdirected against the shared antigens or epitopes in the nervous system, causing neurological dysfunction. This immune response may be sufficient to retard tumor growth, thus also explaining why so many tumors associated with paraneoplastic syndromes are small and often hard to detect.

The evidence for the autoimmune hypothesis is best for the LEMS.[19] The presence of autoantibodies in the serum of many patients with CNS paraneoplastic syndromes suggests that immune mechanisms may participate in these disorders as well: in paraneoplastic cerebellar degeneration, for example, the antibodies react selectively with cerebellar Purkinje cells, the pathological target of the syndrome. The antibodies are found in both serum and cerebrospinal fluid (CSF) but at higher titer in CSF, suggesting CNS synthesis of the antibody. Inflammatory infiltrates found in the CNS also suggest that immune mechanisms play a role in pathogenesis,[20,21] and similar infiltrates found in the tumor of patients with paraneoplastic syndromes[22,23] suggest that the immune response is directed against the tumor as well as the nervous system. The immune response may also explain why patients with paraneoplastic syndromes usually have more limited and indolent cancers.[24,25] If paraneoplastic syndromes of the CNS are autoimmune, they would represent the end result of a multifactorial process including (1) expression of "immunologically privileged" neuronal antigen(s) by tumor cells; (2) a genetically determined propensity to generate self-reactive T-lymphocyte clones; (3) the presence of specific alleles in the major histocompatibility complex that allow binding and presentation of the autoantigen(s) to T cells; and (4) inherited or acquired abnormalities (or both) in immunoregulation that lead to activation of self-reactive T cells, deficient suppression of self-reactive T and B cells, and neuronal injury by immune effector elements.[26] The relative roles of cellular and humoral immune systems and the actual mechanism of neuronal destruction in these disorders is unknown and may differ from disorder to disorder.

Either an autoimmune process or an opportunistic infection, or both, seems to be the most likely etiology for most paraneoplastic syndromes. These two mechanisms could potentially coexist, for example, "molecular mimicry" between viral and CNS antigens could result in an immune response to an opportunistic virus, damaging the nervous system.[26]

Diagnosis

Paraneoplastic syndromes are encountered in patients not known to have cancer, in patients with active cancer, or in patients in remission after cancer treatment. The first is the most common situation. When they present in pure form, the classic syndromes are not easily confused with other causes of neurological disability. Frequently, however, patients present with one or more atypical or nonstereotypical features that obscure the diagnosis. In patients with known cancer, other cancer-associated processes need to be excluded before a diagnosis is made. Depending on the part of the nervous system affected, the workup should include computed tomography (CT) or magnetic resonance imaging (MRI) to exclude parenchymal or epidural metastasis, CSF examination to exclude leptomeningeal metastasis, measurement of metabolic and endocrine substances, coagulation studies, and electrophysiological testing. In patients without known cancer, if other causes of nervous system dysfunction have been excluded, a careful evaluation for systemic cancer must be performed. As will be detailed later, certain syndromes are associated with particular types of cancer; recognizing these associations helps to focus the search for an underlying neoplasm to a particular organ or organs.

Although the clinical presentation varies, several clinical features make diagnosing a paraneoplastic syndrome easier:

1. Most paraneoplastic syndromes are subacute in onset, progress over weeks to months, and then stabilize. Syndromes that begin acutely or are characterized by exacerbations and remissions are less likely to be paraneoplastic.

2. Most paraneoplastic syndromes are severe.

3. Paraneoplastic syndromes are often associated with an inflammatory CSF, including a pleocytosis, elevated levels of protein and myelin basic protein, or the presence of oligoclonal bands. Leptomeningeal metastases are excluded by cytological examination of the CSF.

4. Although patients with paraneoplastic encephalomyelitis have clinical evidence of widespread nervous system dysfunction and some patients with other paraneoplastic syndromes have pathological evidence of diffuse involvement of the neuraxis, most patients present with a clinical syndrome that predominantly affects one specific portion of the nervous system.

5. Several of the syndromes (e.g., LEMS) are so stereotypic that the correct diagnosis can be strongly suspected even before additional diagnostic testing has excluded alternative diagnoses.

In recent years, the diagnosis of at least some of the paraneoplastic syndromes has been aided by the detection of characteristic autoantibodies (see below). With the exception of the antibody found in the LEMS, the etiological significance of most of these autoantibodies is unknown. However, their presence helps confirm the clinical diagnosis of a paraneoplastic syndrome and further focuses the search for an underlying malignancy.

Treatment

Therapy for the individual paraneoplastic syndromes is discussed in the following sections. In general, treatment has been unrewarding; most patients with paraneoplastic syndromes are left with severe neurological disability. Most of the therapies tried have been forms of immunosuppression, particularly for those syndromes that are associated with autoantibodies.[27,28] However, with the exception of the LEMS, in which plasmapheresis is clearly effective, most patients do not benefit. It is possible that the rapid onset of these syndromes does not allow sufficient time for accurate early diagnosis and for treatment to begin before irreversible neuronal damage has occurred. With earlier diagnosis, as by specific laboratory tests for antibodies, therapy may be more successful.[29]

SPECIFIC SYNDROMES

Paraneoplastic syndromes that affect the nervous system are classified in Table 21-4. All these disorders are rare and some are the subject of only a few case reports. Only a few of the more common syndromes are considered in this chapter. More extensive reviews are available elsewhere.[3,11]

Paraneoplastic Cerebellar Degeneration

Although it is among the most common and best characterized of the paraneoplastic syndromes, paraneoplastic cerebellar degeneration is a rare disorder, with only about 300 cases reported in the literature.[30] It has become increasingly apparent that it comprises a group of related disorders that differ somewhat in their clinical features, prognosis, and types of associated malignancies. Some of the disorders can be separated on the basis of characteristic antibodies that react to particular tumor-associated antigens.

CLINICAL FINDINGS

Paraneoplastic cerebellar degeneration was first described in 1919, but the association between it and cancer was not recognized until 1938. Its clinical and pathological features were fully described in 1951; by 1982, 50 pathologically verified cases had been reported.[3] It can be associated with any cancer, but the most common culprits are lung cancer,[27,31] particularly small cell lung cancer; ovarian or uterine cancer[28]; and lymphomas, particularly Hodgkin's dis-

Table 21-4 Paraneoplastic Syndromes Affecting the Nervous System

Brain and cranial nerves
Subacute cerebellar degeneration[a]
Opsoclonus-myoclonus[a]
Limbic encephalitis[a] and other dementias
Brainstem encephalitis
Optic neuritis
Photoreceptor degeneration

Spinal cord and dorsal root ganglia
Necrotizing myelopathy
Subacute motor neuronopathy[a]
Motor neuron disease
Myelitis
Sensory neuronopathy[a]

Subacute peripheral nerve
Subacute or chronic sensorimotor peripheral neuropathy
Acute polyradiculoneuropathy (Guillain-Barré syndrome)
Mononeuritis multiplex and microvasculitis of peripheral nerve
Brachial neuritis
Autonomic neuropathy
Peripheral neuropathy with islet cell tumors
Peripheral neuropathy associated with paraproteinemia

Neuromuscular junction and muscle
Lambert-Eaton myasthenic syndrome[a]
Myasthenia gravis
Dermatomyositis, polymyositis
Acute necrotizing myopathy
Carcinoid myopathies
Myotonia
Cachectic myopathy
Stiff-man syndrome

Multiple levels of central and peripheral nervous system or unknown site
Encephalomyelitis[a]
Neuromyopathy

[a] Classic paraneoplastic syndrome.

ease.[32] It is the neurological symptoms that prompt most patients to seek medical care before the cancer itself causes symptoms. The cancer is usually found within months to a year after the neurological symptoms begin, but occasionally the cancer may elude detection for 2 to 4 or even more years and, in some instances, has been found only at autopsy. Typically, the disorder begins with slight incoordination in walking, evolving rapidly over weeks to a few months with progressive gait ataxia; incoordination in arms, legs, and trunk; dysarthria; and often nystagmus associated with oscillopsia.

Within a few months the illness reaches its peak and then stabilizes. By this time, most patients cannot walk without support, many cannot sit unsupported, handwriting is impossible, independent eating is difficult, and speech may be understood only with great effort. Oscillopsia may prevent reading or even watching television. The neurological signs are always bilateral and usually symmetrical, although at times one side may be more affected than the other. In occasional patients, the asymmetry is quite prominent. Diplopia is an early symptom in many patients, although abnormalities of ocular muscles are often not detected by the examiner.[28,33] Vertigo is also a common early symptom.[28]

The signs and symptoms are frequently limited to those of cerebellar or cerebellar pathway dysfunction but, in as many as 50 percent of the patients, other neurological abnormalities, usually mild, may be found on careful examination,[28,34] including sensorineural hearing loss, dysphagia, hyperreflexia with or without extensor plantar responses, extrapyramidal signs, peripheral neuropathy, dementia, and other mental status abnormalities. A recent study,[35] however, using formal cognitive testing found that dementia was not typical when testing was controlled for impaired motor and speech production, suggesting that perceived clinical changes in intellectual function may be more apparent than real. Despite this finding, positron emission tomography (PET) scanning, performed in a few patients, has revealed hypometabolism in all areas of the neuraxis including the cerebral cortex, cerebellum, and brainstem.[35]

Exceptions to the above statements do occur. The onset may occasionally be abrupt or more gradual, and the disorder itself may be relatively mild so that the patient can walk, write, and be understood, albeit with some difficulty.

LABORATORY EVALUATION

Early in the course of this disease, CT scans and MRI do not reveal an abnormality. If patients are followed for months to a few years, diffuse cerebellar atrophy appears.[36] Occasional patients have been reported in whom hyperintensity is found in cerebral and cerebellar white matter on T_2-weighted MR images.

In most patients who are studied early, the CSF contains an increased number of lymphocytes and slightly elevated protein and IgG concentrations. Oligoclonal bands may be present as well. The pleocytosis usually resolves with time.

Some patients with paraneoplastic cerebellar degeneration have autoantibodies in serum and CSF that react with Purkinje cells of the cerebellum and the causal tumor.[28] Some of these antibodies have been well characterized and appear to be specific for certain clinical syndromes and underlying cancers.[28] Some antibodies react predominantly or exclusively with Purkinje cells,[28] whereas others have neural reactivity well beyond the Purkinje cells of the cerebellum.[27] The presence or absence of specific antibodies allows the physician to subclassify the disorder.[33]

PATHOLOGY

The CNS may appear grossly normal when examined at autopsy, but usually the cerebellum is atrophic, with abnormally widened sulci and small gyri.

Microscopically, the hallmark of paraneoplastic cerebellar degeneration is severe and often complete loss of the Purkinje cells of the cerebellar cortex (Fig. 21-1).[3] Degenerating Purkinje cells may have swellings, called torpedoes, along the course of their axons. Other pathological features may include thinning of the molecular and granular layers of the cerebellar cortex, often without marked cell loss, and proliferation of Bergmann astrocytes. The deep cerebellar nuclei are usually well preserved, although rarefied white matter may surround the nuclei, caused by the loss of Purkinje cell axons. Basket cells and tangential fibers are usually intact. Lymphocytic infiltrates, if present in the cerebellum, are usually found in the leptomeninges and in the dentate nucleus and surrounding white matter, but not in the Purkinje cell layer.[3]

In many patients, the disorder is noninflammatory, with all pathological changes restricted to the Purkinje cell layer of the cerebellum. However, pathological changes outside the cerebellum do occur, differing from patient to patient.[3] Such abnormalities may include dorsal column and pyramidal tract degeneration in the spinal cord; degeneration of the basal ganglia, specifically the palladium; loss of pe-

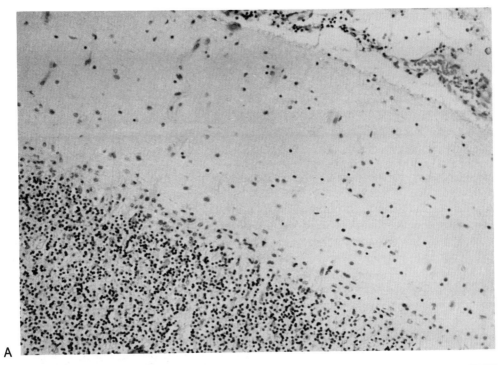

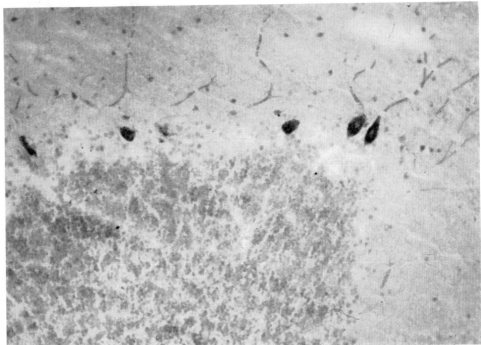

Fig. 21-1 Paraneoplastic cerebellar degeneration. **(A)** Section of cerebellum from a patient with autoantibody-positive paraneoplastic cerebellar degeneration. The molecular and granular cell layers are relatively normal, but Purkinje cells are absent and there is a slight increase in Bergmann's astroglia. There are some inflammatory cells in the leptomeninges. **(B)** Serum from the same patient reacted against human cerebellum by an indirect immunoperoxidase method (anti-Yo antibody). Note the staining of the cytoplasm of Purkinje cells in a granular pattern with sparing of the nucleus. There is also some peroxidase staining of Purkinje cell dendrites. Granule cells and molecular layer cells did not react but are counterstained with hematoxylin.

ripheral nerve fibers; and inflammatory infiltrates in brainstem, spinal cord, and cerebral cortex.

The tumors associated with paraneoplastic cerebellar degeneration do not differ histologically from similar tumors unassociated with paraneoplastic symptoms. However, in many patients the tumor, when identified, is still localized rather than widely metastatic. Hetzel and colleagues have reported that tumors in antibody-positive paraneoplastic cerebellar degeneration are more likely to be associated with lymphocytic infiltrates than similar histological tumors not associated with cerebellar degeneration.[22]

The diagnosis depends on recognizing the characteristic clinical syndrome and on excluding other cancer-associated causes of late-onset cerebellar dysfunction, such as parenchymal or leptomeningeal metastases, infections, and toxicity of therapy such as cytarabine. Etiologies unrelated to cancer, such as viral brainstem encephalitis or cerebellitis, demyelinating disease, Creutzfeldt-Jakob disease, infarction, hypothyroidism, and alcoholic and hereditary cerebellar degenerations must also be excluded.

A disorder clinically identical to paraneoplastic cerebellar degeneration may occur without a cancer being identified. How often "subacute cerebellar degeneration" is nonparaneoplastic is uncertain. Henson and Urich estimate 50 percent[3]; others believe the figure is higher.[37] In patients with paraneoplastic cerebellar degeneration the tumors are often very small.[38] Results of autopsy studies of "nonparaneoplastic" subacute cerebellar degeneration are few.

The clinical picture is sufficiently typical to allow the physician to predict, with or without confirmatory antibody studies, a 50 percent likelihood that the patient has paraneoplastic cerebellar degeneration, although the presence of a specific autoantibody in these studies confirms the diagnosis and identifies a specific neoplasm.

Once the disease has reached its peak, it usually does not change, and the patient remains neurologically stable despite treatment and even cure of the underlying cancer. Treatment directed at the cerebellar disorder, including immune suppression with corticosteroids and other drugs and plasmapheresis, usually does not help. Symptomatic improvement in the ataxia occurs in a few patients with clonazepam in doses varying from 0.5 to 1.5 mg/24 h. On occasion, the disorder may remit spontaneously or coincidentally with treatment of the tumor or administration

of thiamine, plasmapheresis, immunoglobulin, or corticosteroids.[29]

Subacute Sensory Neuronopathy/ Encephalomyelitis

Henson and co-workers introduced the term *encephalomyelitis with carcinoma* to describe patients with cancer associated with clinical signs of damage to several areas of the nervous system and with postmortem signs of inflammation within the brain, brainstem, spinal cord, dorsal root ganglia, and nerve roots.[21] Most of these patients had small cell lung cancer, although clinically and pathologically similar disorders have been described with a number of other tumors. At times the disorder is clinically and pathologically restricted to the dorsal root ganglion,[39] but in many patients both clinical and pathological signs of CNS damage may be present either with or without evidence of a sensory neuronopathy. The signs include dementia, cerebellar degeneration, brainstem dysfunction, myelopathy, and autonomic neuropathy. Some patients who suffer from this syndrome, particularly when associated with small cell cancer of the lung, harbor an antibody in their serum called anti-Hu (Fig. 21-2). The clinical features of the anti-Hu syndrome in 71 patients have recently been described by Dalmau and colleagues.[27] The same clinical and pathological picture can occur in patients without the anti-Hu antibody. At times the syndrome occurs in patients without clinically identifiable cancer even on autopsy examination.[27]

SUBACUTE SENSORY NEURONOPATHY

Sensory neuronopathy is a rare syndrome that can occur in previously healthy individuals and those with a variety of underlying autoimmune conditions including Sjogren's syndrome[40]; probably in fewer than one-third of patients is it a paraneoplastic syndrome. At least two-thirds of the patients with paraneoplastic sensory neuronopathy have small cell cancer of the lung.[3,27] Symptoms typically begin in middle age; men and women seem to be equally affected, although most patients who harbor the anti-Hu antibody are female.[27] In the majority the neurological syndrome precedes the diagnosis of cancer, and when the cancer is diagnosed it is small and limited in extent. Initial symptoms are dysesthetic pain and numbness that usually begin in the distal extremities but can begin in the arm(s) or face. The symptoms progress over days to several weeks to involve the limbs, trunk, and sometimes the face, causing a severe sensory ataxia resembling cerebellar degeneration. All sensory modalities are affected, distinguishing this disorder from cisplatin neuropathy, in which pin and temperature sensation are spared. Deep tendon reflexes are lost, but motor function is preserved. The CSF is typically inflammatory. Sensory nerve action potentials are low in amplitude or absent, whereas motor nerve action potentials are normal and electromyographic (EMG) evidence of denervation is absent.[41]

Early pathological changes are limited mostly to the dorsal root ganglia, in which both a loss of neurons and the presence of lymphocytic inflammatory infiltrates are noted (Fig. 21-2). As the disease progresses, the inflammatory process may advance to the dorsal root, posterior columns, and peripheral nerve. Paraneoplastic sensory neuronopathy can occur as a pure syndrome or as part of a more diffuse encephalomyelitis. About 50 percent of patients with paraneoplastic sensory neuronopathy have pathological changes that may be clinically inapparent in other regions of the nervous system. In most patients, treating the underlying tumor or removal of the autoantibody by plasmapheresis or immunosuppressive therapy does not alter the course of the neurological disease.

LIMBIC ENCEPHALITIS

Paraneoplastic limbic encephalitis is a rare complication of small cell cancer of the lung[27,42] or other cancers.[43] A similar clinical syndrome can occur without a neoplasm. The incidence of limbic encephalitis is approximately equal in men and women. Typically, subacute personality and mood changes are evident, with severe impairment of recent memory and occasional agitation, confusion, hallucinations, and complex partial seizures. Limbic encephalitis may occur in isolation or in association with encephalomyelitis or sensory neuronopathy. The diagnosis depends on recognizing the clinical syndrome and excluding other causes of encephalopathy. The CSF is typically inflammatory, at least early in the disease. CT scans

and MRI usually appear normal, although abnormalities in the medial temporal lobe(s) including hyperintensity on T_2-weighted MR images and, more rarely, contrast enhancement have been reported.[27]

The pathological changes of paraneoplastic limbic encephalitis are usually restricted to limbic and insular cortex, though other deep gray and sometimes white matter structures may be involved. Extensive loss of neurons with reactive gliosis, perivascular lymphocytic cuffing, and microglial proliferation also typify this syndrome.[3,20] No treatment has been consistently beneficial, although reports relate spontaneous remissions or improvement to treatment of the underlying tumor.

CEREBELLAR DEGENERATION

Prominent cerebellar signs occur in approximately 15 percent of patients with the anti-Hu syndrome.[27] The typical clinical findings of paraneoplastic cerebellar degeneration may occur as the first or only manifestation of encephalomyelitis.[27] The only differences between isolated paraneoplastic cerebellar degeneration as described above and cerebellar dysfunction associated with encephalomyelitis are that the patient with encephalomyelitis is more likely to have clinical evidence of widespread central and peripheral nervous system involvement, especially of sensory neuronopathy, and the pathological changes are more likely to be inflammatory.[3] In one patient with cerebellar signs associated with small cell cancer of the lung, infiltrates with T cells were found in the Purkinje cell layer of the cerebellum despite absent Purkinje cells.

BRAINSTEM ENCEPHALITIS

Paraneoplastic brainstem encephalitis characterized by the subacute development of bulbar, midbrain, or basal ganglia signs usually occurs as part of the more diffuse syndrome of encephalomyelitis, although it sometimes presents as the dominant or an isolated clinical finding.[27,44] Any cranial nerve can be affected. The syndrome usually affects the lower brainstem, causing diplopia, vertigo, oscillopsia, dysarthria, dysphagia, hypoventilation, hearing loss, and facial numbness. Movement disorders include chorea, dystonia, bradykinesia, and myoclonus. One of our patients with testicular cancer developed a typical parkinsonian syndrome; the only clinical differences

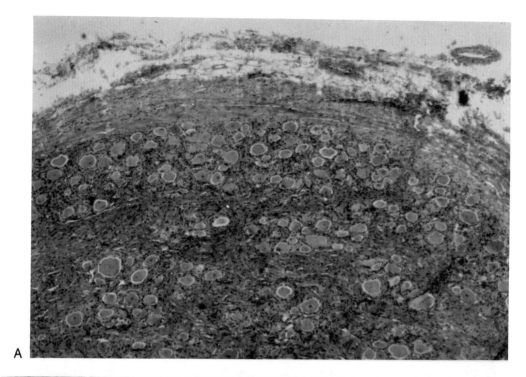

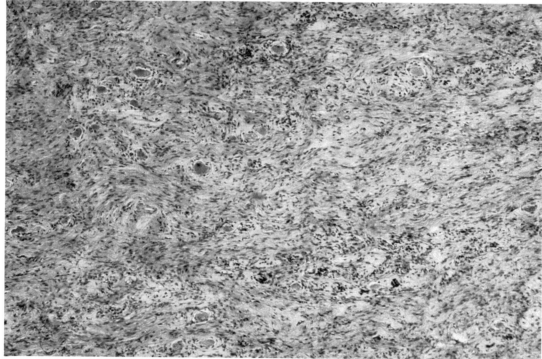

Fig. 21-2 Paraneoplastic sensory neuronopathy. **(A)** Dorsal root ganglion obtained at autopsy from a patient without neurological disease. **(B)** Dorsal root ganglion obtained from a patient with paraneoplastic sensory neuronopathy and an anti-Hu antibody. Note that there are virtually no normal dorsal root ganglion neurons in the entire section. There are a few scattered inflammatory infiltrates.

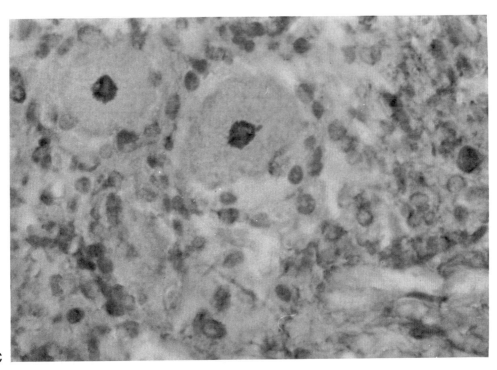

C

Fig. 21-2 (C) Frozen section of a trigeminal ganglion from a patient who died without neurological disease. The ganglion is reacted to serum of the patient whose dorsal root ganglion is shown in Fig. B and who died with paraneoplastic sensory neuronopathy and small cell lung cancer. The reaction is an indirect immunoperoxidase method and reveals reaction product in the nuclei of trigeminal ganglion neurons with sparing of the nucleolus and cytoplasm.

from idiopathic Parkinson's disease were his young age (28 years) and the rapid clinical evolution of his syndrome over a 3- to 4-week period with subsequent stabilization.

MYELITIS

Paraneoplastic nonnecrotizing myelitis occurs rarely as an isolated syndrome and more commonly as a part of diffuse encephalomyelitis. Patients present with progressive weakness, sometimes with lower motor neuron signs including fasciculations, in association with sensory loss and autonomic dysfunction (e.g., incontinence and postural hypotension). In at least one instance the disorder was episodic and primarily involved posterior column function. Early in its evolution, the disorder may resemble motor neuron disease clinically. The neurological disorder may precede or follow the diagnosis of cancer. Often

upper extremity findings predominate due to cervical cord involvement, and respiratory failure and death may occur. The differential diagnosis includes compressive or intrinsic spinal cord masses, other inflammatory or infectious myelopathies, and radiation injury in previously treated patients. The CSF is typically inflammatory. Neuroimaging usually shows a normal spinal cord but, occasionally, enlargement or hyperintensity of the spinal cord can be identified on T_2-weighted MR images and, rarely, contrast enhancement is present. No treatment is effective.

Pathologically, an intense inflammatory reaction and loss of neurons in the anterior and posterior horns is seen, with secondary nerve root degeneration and neurogenic muscle atrophy. Inflammation and degeneration of white matter tracts also occur.

Paraneoplastic myelitis with small cell cancer of the lung is associated with the anti-Hu antibody.[27] Babikian and colleagues described a patient with a different serum antibody that reacted with a 52-kd spinal cord antigen and a tumor-associated protein of the same molecular weight.[45]

AUTONOMIC NEUROPATHY

Paraneoplastic autonomic neuropathy is a rare syndrome that occurs alone or with a sensory neuronopathy.[27,46] Usually associated with small cell lung cancer, it may occur with other cancers and may present prior to or after the cancer is diagnosed. Patients present with the subacute onset of postural hypotension, intestinal immotility,[47] pupillary abnormalities, or a neurogenic bladder. The syndrome is generally progressive but may stabilize or improve with treatment of the underlying tumor. When autonomic neuropathy occurs with lung cancer, it is usually part of the anti-Hu syndrome. Among patients with the anti-Hu antibody, 28 percent had some autonomic dysfunction in one series.[27]

ANTI-Hu SYNDROME

The term *anti-Hu* was first applied by Graus and colleagues to describe an autoantibody in two patients with a subacute sensory neuronopathy associated with small cell cancer of the lung.[48] The antibody may have been the same one reported by Wilkinson and Zeromski in four of their patients with sensory neuropathy associated with cancer.[49] The antibody is a polyclonal, complement-fixing IgG that reacts predominantly with the nuclei of virtually all neurons in the central and peripheral nervous systems, sparing the nucleoli (Fig. 21-2). It shows a lesser reaction with the cytoplasm of neurons; glial cells and other nonneuronal components of the nervous system do not react. With Western blot analysis of extracts of cortical neurons and small cell lung cancer, the anti-Hu sera identify several bands between 35 and 40 kd.

Paraneoplastic Opsoclonus-Myoclonus

Opsoclonus, a disorder of saccadic stability, consists of involuntary, arrhythmic, multidirectional, high-amplitude conjugate saccades. Opsoclonus is often associated with diffuse or focal myoclonus and truncal titubation, with or without other cerebellar signs. It occurs primarily in children as a self-limited illness and is probably the result of a viral infection in the brainstem. This disorder also occurs as a paraneoplastic syndrome said to affect as many as 2 percent of children suffering from neuroblastoma. First recognized by Solomon and Chutorian[50] in 1968, subsequent reports indicate that nearly 50 percent of children with this syndrome harbor a neuroblastoma. Given the known tendency of neuroblastoma to differentiate and resolve spontaneously, one can question whether many cases of opsoclonus–myoclonus without tumor were truly paraneoplastic. The age of peak incidence is 18 months, with more girls than boys affected. Neurological signs precede identification of the tumor at least 50 percent of the time, making recognition of the neurological syndrome an important clue to the presence of neuroblastoma. Ataxia, irritability, vomiting, and dementia may accompany opsoclonus–myoclonus. Furthermore, when a neuroblastoma is associated with opsoclonus–myoclonus, there is a higher than expected incidence of intrathoracic tumors and of tumors with a benign histology. The prognosis of the neuroblastoma is better if opsoclonus–myoclonus is present than when the neurological complication is absent, an observation not explained by disease stage or earlier diagnosis as a consequence of neurological symptoms.[24] The neurological disorder responds to corticosteroid treatment, usually ACTH, and to treatment of the tumor, although 50 percent of patients suffer residual neurological damage.

The disorder is less commonly found in adults than children. A review of the literature identified 58 adults with opsoclonus–myoclonus, in 11 of whom it was believed to be paraneoplastic.[51] The most common tumor is lung cancer, but other cancers also cause the syndrome. Neurological symptoms usually precede the diagnosis of tumor and progress over several weeks, although more rapid or slower progression is observed in some instances. Opsoclonus is often associated with truncal ataxia, dysarthria, myoclonus, vertigo, and encephalopathy; some patients appear to have paraneoplastic cerebellar degeneration. The CSF has a mild pleocytosis in some patients and a mildly elevated protein level. The results of CT scans and MRI are usually normal; in a few reports, an abnormality in the brainstem or cerebellum is detected by MRI.[52] Paraneoplastic opsoclonus–myoclonus differs from most other paraneoplastic syndromes of adults in that remissions occur,[53] either spontaneously, following treatment of the tumor, or with clonazepam or thiamine treatment.

Neuropathological reports are conflicting.[53] In some patients, identifiable neuropathological abnormalities even of the omnipause neurons, the putative site of the physiological lesion, are not found. In other cases, pathological changes resemble those of paraneoplastic cerebellar degeneration, with a loss of Purkinje cells, gliosis of the Bergmann astrocytic layer, and loss of cells in the granular layer of the cerebellum and the inferior olive.

ANTI-RI SYNDROME

The anti-Ri antibody has been found in a small number of patients with eye movement disorders, usually opsoclonus, associated with truncal ataxia and sometimes other cerebellar signs.[54] It is histochemically identical to the anti-Hu antibody but identifies protein bands at 55 and 80 kd when cortical neurons are analyzed with the Western blot method, unlike the 35- to 40-kd band identified by anti-Hu sera.

Retinal Degeneration

The anti-Ri syndrome is primarily seen in women with gynecological malignancies, usually breast cancer. Paraneoplastic retinal degeneration, also called cancer-associated retinopathy, is a rare syndrome that usually occurs in association with small cell cancer of the lung,[55] melanoma,[56] and gynecological tumors. Typically, the visual symptoms—which include episodic visual obscurations, night blindness, light-induced glare, photosensitivity, and impaired color vision[57]—precede the diagnosis of cancer. The symptoms progress to painless visual loss. They may begin unilaterally but usually become bilateral. Visual testing demonstrates peripheral and ring scotomas and loss of acuity. Funduscopic examination may reveal arteriolar narrowing and abnormal mottling of the retinal pigment epithelium. The electroretinogram is abnormal. CSF is typically normal, although elevated immunoglobulin levels have been reported. Inflammatory cells are sometimes seen in the vitreous by slit-lamp examination. Pathologically, a loss of photoreceptors and ganglion cells with inflammatory infiltrates and macrophages is usually noted. The other parts of the optic pathway are preserved, although a loss of myelin and lymphocytic infiltration of the optic nerve may occur.

Serum antibodies that react immunohistochemically with antigens in retinal photoreceptor and ganglion cells have been found in some but not all patients with this disorder, although the antigens identified differ from patient to patient.[55] Retinal deposits of immunoglobulin suggest an immune-mediated mechanism. Some patients produce antibodies that react with a 23-kd calcium-binding protein called Recoverin that regulates guanylate cyclase resynthesis of cyclic guanosine monophosphate (GMP) in photoreceptors to allow recovery after light activation. Prednisone treatment reduces antibody titers and stabilizes vision.

Necrotizing Myelopathy

This rare syndrome occurs with lymphoma, leukemia, and lung or other cancers[58,59] (Fig. 21-3). A similar disorder also occurs in previously healthy patients without an underlying cancer. The onset of the paraneoplastic disorder may precede or follow the diagnosis of cancer. Patients typically present with rapidly ascending flaccid paraplegia; back pain or radicular pain may precede the onset of neurological dysfunction. The disease may ascend the spinal cord, leading to respiratory failure and death. Inflammatory cells are usually present in the CSF; malignant cells are absent. MRI is usually normal, although it may show spinal cord swelling or even contrast enhancement. The absence of an epidural mass or discrete intramedullary enhancement rules out metastatic myelopathy, which is much more common. Treatment is usually unsuccessful, although one patient is reported to have responded to intrathecal dexamethasone.[60] Pathologically, there is widespread spinal cord necrosis involving all components of the cord, but with some white matter predominance. Inflammatory lesions are not typical. The cause of this syndrome is unknown.

Subacute Motor Neuronopathy

Paraneoplastic subacute motor neuronopathy, or spinal muscular atrophy, occurs as a rare complication of Hodgkin's disease and other lymphomas[61] and occasionally of other cancers. Patients develop sub-

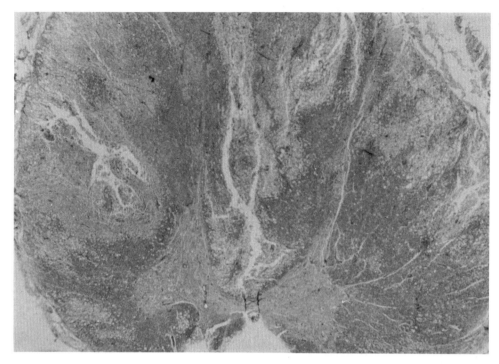

Fig. 21-3 Subacute necrotic myelopathy in a patient with carcinoma of the lung. Neurological symptoms of transverse myelopathy had evolved over several days and preceded the diagnosis of the cancer. Note the widespread necrotic changes of both gray and white matter in the cord. As in most instances, vascular changes and inflammatory infiltrates are absent.

acute, progressive, painless, and often patchy lower motor neuron weakness that usually affects the legs more than the arms. Atrophy is present, but fasciculations are not prominent; the bulbar musculature is spared. Although patients sometimes complain of paresthesias, sensory loss is mild despite often profound weakness. Motor and sensory nerve conduction velocities are normal or only mildly decreased; needle EMG shows denervation of affected muscles. The CSF is acellular with a mildly elevated protein concentration. MRI of the spinal cord is normal. The course is usually benign and independent of the activity of the underlying neoplasm. Unlike motor neuron disease, the neurological deficit usually does not incapacitate the patient; it often stabilizes or improves spontaneously after months or years. Treatment does not hasten recovery.

The main pathological characteristics are degeneration of neurons in the anterior horns of the spinal cord. Patchy mild demyelination of the white matter in the spinal cord sometimes occurs, particularly in the dorsal columns. In this condition—in contrast to motor neuron disease—the lateral columns of the spinal cord are typically spared. Indirect evidence suggests that the disorder may be caused by an opportunistic viral infection of neurons in the anterior horns. The disorder is typically associated with lymphoma, a tumor causing immunosuppression that permits opportunistic viral infections. Among our patients with the disorder, one died of progressive multifocal leukoencephalopathy and another of *Nocardia* infection. Furthermore, the pathological abnormalities resemble those of burnt-out poliomyelitis. A similar neurological disorder affecting spinal anterior horn cells in a strain of mice is caused by the murine leukemia virus.[62]

The relationship between this disorder and the lower motor neuron disorder associated with radiation therapy is unclear. Some of the patients reported to have subacute motor neuronopathy had received prior radiation therapy, raising the possibility that the radiation activated a latent virus.

Subacute Sensorimotor Neuropathy

Subacute sensorimotor neuropathy can be induced by many etiological mechanisms: diabetes mellitus, nutritional deficiency, alcoholism, chronic illness, vitamin B_{12} deficiency, toxin exposure, and chemotherapeutic agents, particularly vincristine and cisplatin. Because these disorders are more likely than a paraneoplastic syndrome to cause a peripheral neuropathy even in the cancer patient, the diagnosis of paraneoplastic neuropathy should be made with great caution and then only after carefully excluding all other causes. As a true paraneoplastic syndrome, the disorder is most frequently associated with lung cancer,[63] sometimes preceding the diagnosis of cancer by up to 5 years. The course is variable, with a few patients stabilizing or remitting after treatment of the underlying tumor.

This disorder is predominantly a distal symmetrical polyneuropathy, more marked in the lower extremities, with weakness, glove-and-stocking sensory impairment to all modalities, and a loss of tendon reflexes. Although the disorder may pursue the very slow course of idiopathic sensorimotor polyneuropathy, it is likely to progress rapidly and lead to more disability in patients with cancer than those with, for example, diabetes. Accordingly, a rapidly progressive or severe sensorimotor neuropathy should be given greater consideration as a possible paraneoplastic syndrome. Bulbar involvement is exceptional. A few patients with paraneoplastic sensorimotor neuropathy follow the remitting and relapsing course typical of chronic inflammatory demyelinating polyneuropathy. These patients may respond to corticosteroid therapy. The CSF is typically acellular, with normal or slightly elevated protein concentration. Nerve conduction studies are consistent with an axonal neuropathy, with low-amplitude or absent sensory nerve action potentials and normal or decreased motor nerve conduction velocities.[64] A few patients have marked slowing of motor conduction velocities consistent with a demyelinating process.[63]

Pathologically, there is usually axonal degeneration; in a few patients demyelination is prominent.[63]

Spinal root demyelination and lymphocytic infiltrates of peripheral nerves have also been reported.

A particular sensorimotor neuropathy is associated with breast cancer. Peterson and colleagues have described nine patients with a slowly progressive sensorimotor, predominantly sensory, neuropathy, some of whom had additional features suggesting a myopathy (e.g., proximal weakness) or CNS dysfunction (e.g., hyperreflexia and extensor plantar responses).[65] The disorder progressed very slowly over many years, was not disabling, and was frequently heralded by itching or muscle cramps. In one patient, itching, initially over the left breast and later diffusely, preceded identification of the cancer by 18 months. Most patients remained fully functional as neither the neuropathy nor the breast cancer was disabling.[65]

Bruera and colleagues, examining 61 consecutive patients with advanced breast cancer by electrophysiological tests, found abnormalities including fatigability, that they could not relate to nutritional status when compared with control subjects.[66]

Lambert-Eaton Myasthenic Syndrome

About 60 percent of patients with LEMS have small cell cancer of the lung. A few have other cancers. Some of the 40 percent who do not have cancer may have evidence of other autoimmune disease.[67] Patients present with progressive proximal weakness and fatigability, but, unlike myasthenia gravis, these symptoms do not significantly affect the bulbar musculature. Respiratory weakness may occur. Power initially increases with effort, so that reported weakness may seem out of proportion to the examiner's findings; however, with continued effort, weakness returns. Deep tendon reflexes, especially those in the legs, are diminished or absent but may reappear after exercise. Cholinergic dysautonomia occurs in more than 50 percent of patients, causing dry mouth and impotence. Characteristic abnormalities are found on electrophysiological testing, including very small compound muscle action potentials (CMAP) that may increase to normal after brief exercise. Repetitive stimulation causes a decrement of the CMAP at low rates of stimulation and an increment at high rates of stimulation.[68]

LEMS results from a reduced release of acetylcholine at presynaptic nerve terminals. In almost half of the patients, detectable antibodies react with the voltage-gated calcium channels at the nerve terminal.[19] Evidence that LEMS is actually an autoimmune disease includes its association with other autoimmune diseases, the clinical response to immunosuppression, and, most compellingly, the results of passive transfer experiments in which the disorder has been induced in animals by injection into them of IgG from patients with LEMS. Patients with small cell cancer produce IgG antibodies against calcium channel proteins that are expressed both by the cancer and the neuromuscular junction. The antibodies so produced bind specifically to calcium channels of the presynaptic neuromuscular junction, causing disarray that is visible by electron microscopy. Failure of calcium entry leads to diminished acetylcholine release. A gene coding for a protein similar in structure to the β subunit of the calcium channel has been cloned and characterized. Antibodies in the sera of about 50 percent of the LEMS patients react with this protein.[69]

Distinct from most paraneoplastic syndromes, LEMS usually responds to plasmapheresis or immunosuppressive therapy. Other treatments that increase transmitter release include guanidine hydrochloride, which mobilizes calcium, and 4-aminopyridine, which acts on potassium channels, but both have significant side effects. 3,4-Diaminopyridine also facilitates the release of transmitter, but with fewer side effects.[70] Cholinesterase inhibitors show minimal benefit in most patients. Treatment of the underlying malignancy in some instances improves the neurological syndrome. In some patients, LEMS develops in association with other paraneoplastic syndromes, including cerebellar degeneration and encephalomyelitis/sensory neuronopathy.

Dermatomyositis/Polymyositis

Polymyositis and dermatomyositis are common inflammatory, probably autoimmune muscle diseases.[71] Only a minority of patients suffering from these disorders have underlying malignancy as their cause.[71] Some investigators have concluded that the incidence of polymyositis or dermatomyositis is not increased in patients with cancer, but most believe that the incidence of cancer is substantially higher in patients with these disorders, particularly those in the older age group. Dermatomyositis with typical cutaneous changes is more likely than polymyositis to

be paraneoplastic. Females and males are affected in approximately equal numbers. Symptoms of the muscle weakness generally precede identification of the cancer. The tumor may be at any site, but breast, lung, ovarian, and gastric malignancies are the most common. Hodgkin's disease and prostate and colon cancer are also reported offenders.

The clinical and laboratory findings in dermatomyositis/polymyositis associated with malignancy resemble those in the idiopathic disease, although cancer patients often have more striking abnormalities on muscle biopsy. Patients characteristically present with proximal muscle weakness, elevated levels of serum creatine kinase (CK), and EMG evidence suggesting a myopathic process rather than nerve disease. A muscle biopsy specimen showing inflammatory myopathy confirms the diagnosis. Although laboratory findings do not distinguish paraneoplastic from nonparaneoplastic varieties, the presence of autoantibodies, particularly common in the disorder associated with lung disease,[72] is less common in patients with the paraneoplastic disorder. No laboratory test is absolutely diagnostic. Normal CK levels are occasionally found even in patients with profound muscle weakness, with or without malignancy; abnormal CK levels indicate a poor prognosis for the muscle disease. Toxoplasmosis may be a precipitating factor for the syndrome in some patients. As *Toxoplasma* infection is common in patients with malignancy, that diagnosis should be considered, because the muscle disease has sometimes responded to treatment of toxoplasmosis. The disorder has also been reported following bone marrow transplantation for Hodgkin's disease. Weakness of respiratory and pharyngeal muscles may contribute to death. The prognosis is less good for the paraneoplastic disorder than the nonparaneoplastic disorder.

The relationship between the course of the dermatomyositis/polymyositis and the underlying tumor is inconsistent. In some patients, muscle and dermatological symptoms improve coincident with treatment of the tumor; in others, improvement does not occur. Both paraneoplastic and nonparaneoplastic varieties are treated with immunosuppression. Corticosteroids, cyclosporine, and other immunosuppressants have been used successfully. Other reports suggest that high-dose intravenous γ-globulin is useful in patients unresponsive to other forms of immunosuppression.

Neuromyotonia

Muscle cramps are a common complication of cancer, sometimes related to electrolyte imbalance or induced by chemotherapy. A much rarer but clinically significant paraneoplastic disorder is acquired neuromyotonia, which is characterized by progressive aching and stiffness of muscles associated with spasms or severe rigidity that prevent muscle use.[73] EMG studies indicate continuous muscle fiber activity.[74] The muscle spasm and rigidity are sometimes precipitated by activity, forcing patients to become sedentary. The disorder can arise from peripheral nerves or the CNS and is sometimes a part of the encephalomyelitis syndrome.

Autoantibodies that react with cerebellum are found in both the paraneoplastic stiff-man syndrome usually associated with Hodgkin's disease[75] or breast cancer[76] and the nonparaneoplastic entity. The stiff-man syndrome has also been associated with lung cancer and thymoma; it can be distinguished by EMG from myoedema, an electrical contracture of muscle produced by percussion, and from myotonia, a rare manifestation of dermatomyositis/polymyositis.[77] The disorder can be treated successfully in many instances by phenytoin or diazepam. Plasmapheresis has also been reported to be successful.

Cachectic Myopathy

Chronic debilitating diseases, including cancer and anorexia nervosa, that are complicated by cachexia and malnutrition may be associated with diffuse muscle wasting with weakness as a late feature. Myoedema is also a frequent finding. Pathological changes include a loss or atrophy of large muscle fibers leading to a predominance of smaller fibers and grouping of atrophic fibers; noninflammatory fiber degeneration and vacuolization of muscles may also be present. Changes may be reversible when treatment of the underlying illness is possible.

Carcinomatous Neuromyopathy

Carcinomatous neuromyopathy is a syndrome characterized by the subacute onset of weakness, usually of proximal muscles, in patients who are well-nourished prior to the diagnosis of their cancer; it is associated with a decrease or absence of one or more reflexes.[7] During its course, some patients have spontaneous improvement in strength. Pathological changes in nerve and muscle are noninflammatory, nonspecific, and minor compared to the degree of clinical weakness. A neurogenic etiology has been suggested by the pathological finding of a distal intramuscular axonal neuropathy. The disorder is not well understood, and the etiology is not known. Some investigators believe that, in most patients, symptoms of neuromyopathy are related to weight loss that either precedes or follows diagnosis of the cancer.

REFERENCES

1. Shnider BI, Manalo A: Paraneoplastic syndromes: unusual manifestations of malignant disease. DM 25:1, 1979
2. Bunn PA Jr, Ridgway EC: Paraneoplastic syndromes. p. 2006. In DeVita VT Jr, Hellman S, Rosenberg SA (eds): Cancer: Principles and Practice of Oncology. 4th Ed. JB Lippincott, Philadelphia, 1993
3. Henson RA, Urich H: Cancer and the Nervous System. Blackwell Scientific Publications, London, 1982
4. Brain WR, Norris FH Jr (eds): The Remote Effects of Cancer on the Nervous System. Grune & Stratton, Orlando, FL, 1965
5. Posner JB, Furneaux HM: Paraneoplastic syndromes. p. 187. In Waksman BH (ed): Immunologic Mechanisms in Neurologic and Psychiatric Disease. Raven Press, New York, 1990
6. Elrington GM, Murray NMF, Spiro SG, Newsom-Davis J: Neurological paraneoplastic syndromes in patients with small cell lung cancer: a prospective survey of 150 patients. J Neurol Neurosurg Psychiatry 54:764, 1991
7. Croft PB, Wilkinson M: The incidence of carcinomatous neuromyopathy in patients with various types of carcinomas. Brain 88:427, 1965
8. Lipton RB, Galer BS, Dutcher JP, et al: Quantitative sensory testing demonstrates that subclinical sensory neuropathy is prevalent in patients with cancer. Arch Neurol 44:944, 1987
9. Lipton RB, Galer BS, Dutcher JP, et al: Large and small fibre type sensory dysfunction in patients with cancer. J Neurol Neurosurg Psychiatry 54:706, 1991
10. Gomm SA, Thatcher N, Barber PV, Cumming WJ: A clinicopathological study of the paraneoplastic neuromuscular syndromes associated with lung cancer. Q J Med 75:577, 1990

11. Anderson NE, Cunningham JM, Posner JB: Autoimmune pathogenesis of paraneoplastic neurological syndromes. Crit Rev Neurobiol 3:245, 1987

12. Oppenheim H: Uber Hirnsymptome bei carcinomatose ohne nachweisbare Veranderungen im Gehirn. Carite-Ann 13:335, 1888

13. Gelin J, Lundholm K: Cancer cachexia, what are the mediators? Top Support Care Oncol 3:4, 1991

14. Denny-Brown D: Primary sensory neuropathy with muscular changes associated with carcinoma. J Neurol Neurosurg Psychiatry 11:73, 1948

15. Castiello RJ, Lynch PJ: Pellagra and the carcinoid syndrome. Arch Dermatol 105:574, 1972

16. Chandalia HB, Boshell BR: Hypoglycemia associated with extrapancreatic tumors: report of two cases with studies on its pathogenesis. Arch Intern Med 129:447, 1972

17. Brain WR, Adams RD: Epilogue: a guide to the classification and investigation of neurological disorders associated with neoplasms. p. 216. In Brain WR, Norris FH Jr (eds): The Remote Effects of Cancer on the Nervous System. Grune & Stratton, Orlando, FL, 1965

18. Furneaux HM, Rosenblum MK, Dalmau J, et al: Selective expression of Purkinje-cell antigens in tumor tissue from patients with paraneoplastic cerebellar degeneration. N Engl J Med 322:1844, 1990

19. Leys K, Lang B, Johnston I, Newsom-Davis J: Calcium channel autoantibodies in the Lambert-Eaton myasthenic syndrome. Ann Neurol 29:307, 1991

20. Dalmau J, Furneaux HM, Rosenblum MK, et al: Detection of the anti-Hu antibody in specific regions of the nervous system and tumor from patients with paraneoplastic encephalomyelitis/sensory neuronopathy. Neurology 41:1757, 1991

21. Henson RA, Hoffman HL, Urich H: Encephalomyelitis with carcinoma. Brain 88:449, 1965

22. Hetzel DJ, Stanhope CR, O'Neill BP, Lennon VA: Gynecologic cancer in patients with subacute cerebellar degeneration predicted by anti-Purkinje cell antibodies and limited in metastatic volume. Mayo Clin Proc 65:1558, 1990

23. Szabo A, Dalmau J, Manley G, et al: HuD, a paraneoplastic encephalomyelitis antigen, contains RNA-binding domains and is homologous to Elav and Sex-lethal. Cell 67:325, 1991

24. Altman AJ, Baehner RL: Favorable prognosis for survival in children with coincident opso-myoclonus and neuroblastoma. Cancer 37:846, 1976

25. Dalmau J, Furneaux HM, Gralla RJ, et al: Detection of the anti-Hu antibody in the serum of patients with small cell lung cancer—a quantitative Western blot analysis. Ann Neurol 27:544, 1990

26. Sinha AA, Lopez MT, McDevitt HO: Autoimmune diseases: the failure of self tolerance. Science 248:1380, 1990

27. Dalmau J, Graus F, Rosenblum MK, Posner JB: Anti-Hu-associated paraneoplastic encephalomyelitis/sensory neuronopathy: a clinical study of 71 patients. Medicine (Baltimore) 71:59, 1992

28. Peterson K, Rosenblum MK, Kotanides H, Posner JB: Paraneoplastic cerebellar degeneration: I. A clinical analysis of 55 anti-Yo antibody-positive patients. Neurology 42:1931, 1992

29. Moll JWB, Henzen-Logmans SC, Van der Meche FGA, Vecht CH: Early diagnosis and intravenous immune globulin therapy in paraneoplastic cerebellar degeneration. J Neurol Neurosurg Psychiatry 56:112, 1993

30. Hammack JE, Posner JB: Paraneoplastic cerebellar degeneration. p. 475. In Platakis A (ed): Cerebellar Degenerations—Clinical Neurobiology. Kluwer, Boston, 1992

31. Clouston PD, Saper CB, Arbizu T, et al: Paraneoplastic cerebellar degeneration: III. Cerebellar degeneration, cancer, and the Lambert-Eaton myasthenic syndrome. Neurology 42:1944, 1992

32. Hammack J, Kotanides H, Rosenblum MK, Posner JB: Paraneoplastic cerebellar degeneration: II. Clinical and immunologic findings in 21 patients with Hodgkin's disease. Neurology 42:1938, 1992

33. Posner JB: Paraneoplastic cerebellar degeneration. In DeVita V (ed). PPO Updates. 5, (11):1, 1991

34. Hammack JE, Kimmel DW, O'Neill BP, Lennon VA: Paraneoplastic cerebellar degeneration: a clinical comparison of patients with and without Purkinje cell cytoplasmic antigens. Mayo Clin Proc 65:1423, 1990

35. Anderson NE, Posner JB, Sidtis JJ, et al: The metabolic anatomy of paraneoplastic cerebellar degeneration. Ann Neurol 23:533, 1988

36. Greenberg HS: Paraneoplastic cerebellar degeneration: a clinical and CT study. J Neurooncol 2:377, 1984

37. Ropper AH: Seronegative, non-neoplastic acute cerebellar degeneration. Neurology 43:1602, 1993

38. Anderson NE, Budde-Steffen C, Wiley RG, et al: A variant of the anti-Purkinje cell antibody in a patient with paraneoplastic cerebellar degeneration. Neurology 38:1018, 1988

39. Horwich MS, Cho L, Porro RS, Posner JB: Subacute sensory neuropathy: a remote effect of carcinoma. Ann Neurol 2:7, 1977

40. Font J, Valls J, Cervera R, et al: Pure sensory neuropathy in patients with primary Sjogren's syndrome: clinical, immunological, and electromyographic findings. Ann Rheum Dis 49:775, 1990

41. Donofrio PD, Alessi AG, Albers JW, et al: Electrodiagnostic evolution of carcinomatous sensory neuronopathy. Muscle Nerve 12:508, 1989

42. Corsellis JAN, Goldberg GJ, Norton AR: "Limbic encephalitis" and its association with carcinoma. Brain 91:481, 1968

43. Bakheit AM, Kennedy PG, Behan PO: Paraneoplastic limbic encephalitis: clinico-pathological correlations. J Neurol Neurosurg Psychiatry 53:1084, 1990

44. Reddy RV, Vakili ST: Midbrain encephalitis as a remote effect of a malignant neoplasm. Arch Neurol 38:781, 1981

45. Babikian VL, Stefansson K, Dieperink ME, et al: Paraneoplastic myelopathy: antibodies against protein in normal spinal cord and underlying neoplasm. Lancet 2:49, 1985

46. Siemsen JK, Meister L: Bronchogenic carcinoma with severe orthostatic hypotension. Ann Intern Med 58:669, 1963

47. Lennon VA, Sas DF, Busk MF, et al: Enteric neuronal autoantibodies in pseudoobstruction with small-cell lung carcinoma. Gastroenterology 100:137, 1991

48. Graus F, Cordon-Cardo C, Posner JB: Neuronal antinuclear antibody in sensory neuronopathy from lung cancer. Neurology 35:538, 1985

49. Wilkinson PC, Zeromski J: Immunofluorescent detection of antibodies against neurons in sensory carcinomatous neuropathy. Brain 88:529, 1965

50. Solomon GE, Chutorian AM: Opsoclonus and occult neuroblastoma. N Engl J Med 279:475, 1968

51. Digre KB: Opsoclonus in adults: report of three cases and review of the literature. Arch Neurol 43:1165, 1986

52. Hattori T, Hirayama K, Imai T, et al: Pontine lesion in opsoclonus-myoclonus syndrome shown by MRI. J Neurol Neurosurg Psychiatry 51:1572, 1988

53. Anderson NE, Budde-Steffen C, Rosenblum MK, et al: Opsoclonus, myoclonus, ataxia, and encephalopathy in adults with cancer: a distinct paraneoplastic syndrome. Medicine (Baltimore) 67:100, 1988

54. Luque FA, Furneaux HM, Ferziger R, et al: Anti-Ri: an antibody associated with paraneoplastic opsoclonus and breast cancer. Ann Neurol 29:241, 1991

55. Thirkill CE, Fitzgerald P, Sergott RC, et al: Cancer-associated retinopathy (CAR syndrome) with antibodies reacting with retinal, optic-nerve, and cancer cells. N Engl J Med 321:1589, 1989

56. Alexander KR, Fishman GA, Peachey NS, et al: "On" response defect in paraneoplastic night blindness with cutaneous malignant melanoma. Invest Ophthalmol Vis Sci 33:477, 1992

57. Jacobson DM, Thirkill CE, Tipping SJ: A clinical triad to diagnose paraneoplastic retinopathy. Ann Neurol 28:162, 1990

58. Hughes M, Ahern V, Kefford R, Boyages J: Paraneoplastic myelopathy at diagnosis in a patient with pathologic stage 1A Hodgkin disease. Cancer 70:1598, 1992

59. Mancall EL, Rosales RK: Necrotizing myelopathy associated with visceral carcinoma. Brain 87:639, 1964

60. Handforth A, Nag S, Sharp D, Robertson DM: Paraneoplastic subacute necrotic myelopathy. Can J Neurol Sci 10:204, 1983

61. Schold SC, Cho ES, Somasundaram M, Posner JB: Subacute motor neuronopathy: a remote effect of lymphoma. Ann Neurol 5:271, 1979

62. Gardner MB: Retroviral leukemia and lower motor neuron disease in wild mice: natural history, pathogenesis and genetic resistance. Adv Neurol 56:473, 1991

63. Croft PB, Urich H, Wilkinson M: Peripheral neuropathy of sensorimotor type associated with malignant disease. Brain 90:31, 1967

64. Campbell MJ, Paty DW: Carcinomatous neuromyopathy: 1. Electrophysiological studies. An electrophysiological and immunological study of patients with carcinoma of the lung. J Neurol Neurosurg Psychiatry 37:131, 1974

65. Peterson K, Forsyth PA, Posner JB: Paraneoplastic sensorimotor neuropathy associated with breast cancer. J Neurooncol, 1994 (in press)

66. Bruera E, Brenneis C, Michaud M, et al: Muscle electrophysiology in patients with advanced breast cancer. J Natl Cancer Inst 80:282, 1988

67. O'Neill JH, Murray NMF, Newsom-Davis J: The Lambert-Eaton myasthenic syndrome: a review of 50 cases. Brain 111:577, 1988

68. Lambert EH, Rooke ED: Myasthenic state of lung cancer. p. 67. In Brain WR, Norris FH Jr (eds): The Remote Effects of Cancer on the Nervous System. Grune & Stratton, Orlando, FL, 1965

69. Rosenfeld MR, Wong E, Dalmau J, et al: Cloning and characterization of a Lambert-Eaton myasthenic syndrome antigen. Ann Neurol 33:113, 1993

70. McEvoy KM, Windebank AJ, Daube JR, Low PA: 3,4-Diaminopyridine in the treatment of the Lambert-Eaton myasthenic syndrome. N Engl J Med 321:1567, 1989

71. Dalakas MC (ed): Polymyositis and Dermatomyositis. Butterworths, Boston, 1988

72. Hochberg MC, Feldman D, Stevens MB, et al: Antibody to Jo-1 polymyositis/dermatomyositis: association with interstitial pulmonary disease. J Rheumatol 11:663, 1984

73. Halbach M, Homberg V, Freund HJ: Neuromuscular, autonomic and central cholinergic hyperactivity associated with thymoma and acetylcholine receptor-binding antibody. J Neurol 234:433, 1987

74. Garcia-Merino A, Cabello A, Mora JS, Liano H: Continuous muscle fiber activity, peripheral neuropathy, and thymoma. Ann Neurol 29:215, 1991

75. Ferrari P, Federico M, Grimaldi LME, Silingardi V: Stiff-man syndrome in a patient with Hodgkin's disease: an unusual paraneoplastic syndrome. Haematologica 75:570, 1990

76. Folli F, Solimena M, Cofiell R, et al: Autoantibodies to a 128-kd synaptic protein in three women with the stiff-man syndrome and breast cancer. N Engl J Med 328:546, 1993

77. Partanen VSJ, Soininen H, Saksa M, Riekkinen P: Electromyographic and nerve conduction findings in a patient with neuromyotonia, normocalcemic tetany and small-cell lung cancer. Acta Neurol Scand 61:216, 1980

22

Neurological Complications of Chemotherapy and Radiation Therapy

Jean-Yves Delattre
Jerome B. Posner

Chemotherapy and radiation therapy are two of the major modalities used to treat cancer (Table 22-1). Their goal is kill or inactivate enough cancer cells that the body's own defenses can control the disease; this goal should be accomplished without unacceptable damage to normal tissue. Unfortunately, in most instances the goal is not fully achieved. The reason is that both radiation therapy and chemotherapy are relatively nonspecific and depend for their effect on their ability to do more damage to cancer cells than to normal cells. The therapeutic/toxic ratio is often low; even in highly sensitive tumors—such as acute lymphoblastic leukemia, Hodgkin's disease, testicular tumors, and choriocarcinoma, where the cure rate is high—many patients suffer serious side effects of therapy, either immediately or after months or years.

One might expect the nervous system to be relatively insensitive to side effects of cancer therapy. The nervous system is protected from exposure to many chemotherapeutic agents by the blood-brain, blood–cerebrospinal fluid (CSF), and blood-nerve barriers. Furthermore, most neurons do not repro-duce and glia reproduce only slowly, thus affording protection against agents that are directed at the DNA of reproducing cells. Nevertheless, nervous system toxicity is common and often dose-limiting for both radiation therapy and chemotherapy. The purpose of this chapter is to describe the side effects of these therapeutic modalities on the central and peripheral nervous system. The emphasis is on those chemotherapeutic agents and radiotherapeutic approaches that are widely used in clinical practice.

CHEMOTHERAPY

Table 22-2 classifies the major chemotherapeutic agents that have been reported to cause either central or peripheral nervous system toxicity as well as other commonly used agents that are not neurotoxic. The neurological complications caused by neurotoxic agents are detailed in the paragraphs below. More extensive reviews can be found elsewhere.[1-4]

Table 22-1 Modalities for Treating Cancer

Surgery

Radiation Therapy
    External beam radiation therapy
        Photons
        Neutron, protons, and other heavy particles
        Radiosurgery
    Interstitial radiation therapy
        High-intensity removable seeds
        Low-intensity permanent implants

Chemotherapy
    Hormones
    Nonhormonal agents

Biological therapy
    Monoclonal antibodies
    Immune potentiators
    Immune cells
    Vaccines
    Immune enhancers
    Differentiation agents
    Cytokines
    Immunosuppressants

Miscellaneous approaches
    Hyperthermia

Combinations of above approaches

Hormonal Agents

ADRENOCORTICOSTEROIDS (GLUCOCORTICOIDS)

The chemotherapeutic agents with which neurologists are most familiar are the glucocorticoids (corticosteroids). A 1-day prevalence study in 1986 indicated that 13 of 40 (33 percent) patients on the neurology in-patient service at The New York Hospital and 22 of 32 patients (69 percent) on the neuro-oncology service at Memorial Hospital (New York City) were receiving corticosteroids. These drugs are especially effective in treating clinical symptoms caused by brain tumors and epidural spinal cord compression. Because of their lympholytic activity, corticosteroids are also used to treat tumors of the lymphoid system, including acute lymphoblastic leukemia, Hodgkin's disease, and non-Hodgkin's lymphoma. Common effects of corticosteroids include increased appetite and improved sense of well-being, which, in patients being treated for cancer, are considered salutary.[5,6] Other less desirable effects are le-

gion[7–9] (Table 22-3). Only a few of neurological interest are discussed here.

Myopathy

The incidence of corticosteroid myopathy is unknown. The literature suggests that it occurs only after prolonged use of high-dose corticosteroids, particularly the fluorinated compounds such as dexamethasone.[10] Our experience has been that most patients on conventional doses (e.g., 16 mg of dexamethasone daily) for more than 2 or 3 weeks develop at least mildly myopathy. The syndrome is usually characterized by weakness of proximal muscles of the hip girdle with wasting of thigh muscles.[10] Patients complain of difficulty in arising from the toilet seat or from low chairs without using their hands. If the disorder is more severe, it may affect ability to climb stairs or to lift heavy objects above the head.[11] At its most florid, there is severe weakness of neck muscles, particularly the flexors, and of proximal muscles of the shoulder and pelvic girdle. The onset of weakness is usually gradual but, occasionally, it is acute and painful (myalgia). Distal weakness occurs rarely. In some instances, respiratory function is compromised.[11] Sensation is normal, as are deep tendon reflexes.

The differential diagnosis of proximal muscle weakness in a cancer patient being treated with corticosteroids must include metabolic and nutritional myopathies associated with the cancer, leptomeningeal tumor that may occasionally cause predominantly proximal weakness, and polymyositis as a remote effect of cancer. It is particularly important to rule out polymyositis because that disorder may be effectively treated by corticosteroids. The typical electromyographic (EMG) changes of increased insertional activity, elevated muscle enzyme concentrations in serum, and histological findings of muscle necrosis or inflammation indicate a paraneoplastic disorder. These findings are almost always absent in patients with corticosteroid myopathy. The treatment of corticosteroid myopathy is to discontinue the corticosteroids, if possible, after which the myopathy usually resolves over time.

Corticosteroid Psychosis

Psychotic changes associated with corticosteroids were common when adrenocorticotropic hormone (ACTH) and naturally occurring glucocorticoids

Table 22-2 Neurotoxicity of Chemotherapeutic Agents in Humans

Agents	Drug	Neurotoxicity[a]		
		PNS	CNS[b]	Muscle
Hormonal agents				
Adrenocorticosteroids	Prednisone	−	+ +	+
	Prednisolone	−	+ +	+
	Methylprednisolone	−	+ +	+
	Dexamethasone	−	+ +	+ +
Sex hormones	Diethylstilbestrol	−	−	−
	Ethinylestradiol	−	−	−
	Stilbestrol	−	−	−
Antiestrogens (receptor-binding agents)	Tamoxifen	−	+	−
	Megestrol	−	−	−
Progestins	Hydroxyprogesterone caproate	−	−	−
	Medroxyprogesterone acetate	−	−	−
	Norethindrone acetate	−	−	−
	Estramustine phosphate	−	−	−
Nonhormonal agents				
Plant alkaloids (mitotic inhibitors)				
Periwinkle derivatives	Vincristine	+ +	+	? +
	Vinblastine	+	−	−
	Desacetyl vinblastine amide (semisynthetic)	+	−	−
Podophyllotoxins	Epipodophyllotoxin VM-26	? +	? +	−
	Epipodophyllotoxin VP-16	? +	? +	−
Antibiotics	Bleomycin	−	−	−
	Actinomycin D	−	−	−
	Adriamycin	−	−	−
	Daunomycin	−	−	−
	Mithramycin	−	−	−
	Mitomycin C	−	−	−
Antimetabolites	Methotrexate	−	+ +	−
	5-Fluorouracil	−	+ +	−
	6-Mercaptopurine	−	−	−
	6-Thioguanine	−	−	−
	Cytarabine	+	+	−
	5-Azacytidine	+	+	? +
	Hydroxyurea	−	−	−
Alkylating agents	Cyclophosphamide	−	? +	−
	Melphalan	−	−	−
	Busulfan	−	−	−
	CCNU	−	+	−
	BCNU	−	+	−
	Thiotepa	−	+	−
	Chlorambucil	−	? +	−
	Cisplatin	+ +	+ +	−
	Aziridinylbenzoquinone	−	−	−
Miscellaneous	DTIC (dacarbazine)	−	? +	−
	mAMSA	? +	? +	−
	L-Asparaginase	−	+	−
	Procarbazine	+	+	−
	Hexamethylmelamine	+	+	−

[a] ? + = questionable; + = rare; + + common.
[b] CNS and cranial nerves.

Table 22-3 Some Side Effects of Corticosteroids

Neurological

Common
  Myopathy
  Behavioral
    alterations
  Hallucinations
    (with high
    dose)
  Withdrawal
    syndrome
    (Table 22-4)
  Hiccups
  Tremor
  Reduced taste and
    olfaction

Uncommon or Rare
  Psychosis
  Dementia
  Seizures
  Cerebral atrophy
  Dependence
  Paraparesis
    (epidural
    lipomatosis)
  Neuropathy

Cardiovascular
  Arrhythmia (with IV
    push)
  Hypertension
  Accelerated
    atherosclerosis

Rheumatological
  Avascular bone
    necrosis
  Osteoporosis
    (vertebral collapse)
  Growth retardation
  Tendinous ruptures

Ophthalmological
  Cataract
  Glaucoma
  Exophthalmos
  Uveitis
  Visual blurring

Endocrine/metabolic
  Adrenocortical
    insufficiency
  Diabetes
  Dyslipidemia
  Redistribution of
    body fat
  Hypernatremia,
    hypokalemia

Digestive
  Increased appetite
  Sensation of
    abdominal bloating
  Pancreatitis
  Liver hypertrophy
  Gastrointestinal
    perforation
  Gastrointestinal
    bleeding

Dermatological
  Striae, easy bruising
  Dermal atrophy
  Inhibition of wound
    healing
  Acne
  Hirsutism
  Kaposi's sarcoma;
    ?acanthosis
    nigricans
  Allergic contact
    dermatitis

Urogenital
  Genital burning (with
    IV push)
  Polyuria

Miscellaneous
  Hypersensitivity
    reactions
    (anaphylaxis)
  Neutrophilia,
    lymphopenia
  Opportunistic
    infections
  Night sweats

were widely used. With synthetic corticosteroids, the disorders are less common; with dexamethasone, florid psychosis is rare. The Boston Collaborative Group reported that the incidence of acute dose-related psychotic reaction was 3 percent in patients treated with prednisone.[12] A double-blind prospective trial of prednisone 80 mg/d for 5 days given to normal volunteers revealed, however, that 11 of 12 patients developed at least a mild psychiatric reaction during treatment or withdrawal.[13] Symptoms included irritability, anxiety, insomnia, difficulty concentrating, euphoria, and depression. More severe psychiatric reactions are of three general types: affective, schizophrenic-like, and delirious.[14] A reversible dementia unassociated with psychotic symptoms has also been reported.[15]

Affective disorders, either mania or, less commonly, depression (depression is more common in Cushing's syndrome than with exogenous corticosteroids), cannot be distinguished from psychiatric illness unassociated with corticosteroids. Affective disorders usually begin early in the course of therapy, are more likely to affect women, and are dose-related. They resolve when the corticosteroids are withdrawn. Neuroleptic drugs are effective in treating these disorders, but tricyclic agents may worsen symptoms. The affective disorder may begin during tapering of corticosteroids but almost always resolves once the corticosteroids are entirely discontinued. A persistent bipolar disorder after withdrawal of steroids has been described in one patient.[16] Three patients on alternate-day corticosteroids have been reported to cycle, with mood elevation on the "on days" and depression on the "off days".[17] One report suggests that use of lithium given prophylactically may prevent affective corticosteroid psychosis.[18] A history of corticosteroid psychosis does not predict recurrent psychosis with another course of corticosteroids.[14]

The second form of corticosteroid psychosis resembles *acute schizophrenia.* The patient may become withdrawn or paranoid and may experience auditory or visual hallucinations. The disorder cannot be distinguished from noniatrogenic psychiatric illness and responds to withdrawal of corticosteroids or to treatment with major tranquilizers.

The third form is *acute delirium.* The patient becomes distractible and unable to attend appropriately to environmental stimuli; confusion and visual hallucinations may also occur. Mild delirium is often not reported to the physician because the patient is neither surprised nor concerned about the hallucinations, correctly attributing them to the drug.

Aseptic Necrosis

Osteoporosis is a common side effect of prolonged corticosteroid use.[19] Although not a neurological disorder, aseptic necrosis of the hips[20] (occasionally shoulders, wrist, clavicle) may be confused with spinal cord compression or peripheral neuropathy. Patients have usually been on corticosteroids for a long time, although there are occasional reports of patients developing aseptic necrosis after only a few weeks of treatment.[21] The disorder is characterized by pain in the hip, often radiating down the anterior aspect of the thigh to the knee and resembling, in some respects, a femoral neuropathy or a lumbar radiculopathy. The pain causes difficulty in walking. The diagnosis can be made by reproducing the pain on rotation of the hip. Early during the course of the disorder, radiographs, radionuclide bone scans, and computed tomographic (CT) scan may be normal, but all will eventually reveal the necrosis. Magnetic resonance imaging (MRI) is the most sensitive diagnostic test.[22]

Lipomatosis

Corticosteroids cause redistribution of fat, and this sometimes leads to neurological symptoms and signs. Increased fat in the orbits causes proptosis and increased fat in the epidural space can cause spinal cord dysfunction[23]; mediastinal widening suggesting a mediastinal tumor has also been reported after treatment with corticosteroids. In all of these circumstances, fat can be distinguished from tumor on CT scan or MRI by its density. In a few instances, surgical decompression of the spinal cord has been necessary to relieve neurological symptoms.

Visual Changes

Corticosteroids can induce cataracts, increase intraocular pressure leading to glaucoma, and—occasionally—cause exophthalmos.[24] They are also often responsible for changes in visual acuity, leading patients to complain of visual blurring; patients may return to their ophthalmologist several times for a new prescription for glasses, particularly during the course of

a prolonged corticosteroid taper. The disorder appears to arise from changes in water content of the lens, leading to a difference in refraction depending on the dose of the corticosteroids.

Gastrointestinal Symptoms

Gastrointestinal bleeding and bowel perforation are well-recognized complications of corticosteroid usage.[25,26] The most serious complication in neurological patients receiving corticosteroids is bowel perforation[27]; the risk is particularly high in patients treated for spinal cord compression because they are prone to develop constipation, a predisposing factor for corticosteroid-induced perforation. Prevention of constipation might avert this serious complication.

Many patients on corticosteroids are given a histamine-blocking agent such as cimetidine or ranitidine in the questionable belief that it decreases the incidence of corticosteroid-induced peptic ulceration. The physician should be aware that these drugs occasionally cause encephalopathy and rarely coma.

Corticosteroid Withdrawal Syndrome

Withdrawal of patients from corticosteroids also causes neurological disability (Table 22-4). The most striking symptom of withdrawal is "pseudorheumatism," characterized by acute myalgia and arthralgia that may be so severe as to incapacitate the patient.[28] One of our patients was admitted to the hospital with a presumptive diagnosis of spinal cord compression because of severe pain in his legs and inability to walk. In other patients, the disorder is milder and can be ameliorated by increasing the dose of corticosteroids and tapering more slowly. Another withdrawal syn-

Table 22-4 Corticosteroid Withdrawal Syndrome

Headache
Lethargy
Nausea, vomiting, anorexia
Abdominal pain
Fever
Myalgia and arthralgia
Postural hypotension
Pseudotumor cerebri
Panniculitis

(Data from Amatruda and colleagues.[29])

drome, first described by Amatruda and associates in patients who had no neurological disability, is characterized by headache, lethargy, and sometimes low-grade fever.[29] It also occurs in patients with central nervous system (CNS) disease and may lead the physician to believe the symptoms are due to recurrent tumor rather than corticosteroid withdrawal. Withdrawal from prolonged corticosteroid treatment in children has been reported to cause the syndrome of pseudotumor cerebri.[30] Corticosteroid withdrawal in animals leads to decreased CSF absorption,[30] which may be the mechanism responsible for symptoms of increased intracranial pressure in this context.

SEX HORMONE AGONISTS AND ANTAGONISTS

Androgens and estrogens and their antagonists are not generally associated with neurological side effects. Tamoxifen, however, has been reported to cause visual disturbances[31] and, more rarely, encephalopathy.[32] Both are reversible.

Nonhormonal Chemotherapeutic Agents

Table 22-2 lists some nonhormonal chemotherapeutic agents. Most do not cause significant neurotoxicity. One reason is that when experimental drugs are discovered to cause major neurotoxicity, they rarely reach the market. However, several chemotherapeutic agents can produce substantial dysfunction of the central or peripheral nervous system and a few—such as the vinca alkaloids, methotrexate, and cisplatin—are major offenders. The specific neurotoxicity of these and other commonly used drugs is reviewed in the following paragraphs. Others are noted in Table 22-5. Specific details can be found either in the cited references or in recent reviews.[1–4]

METHOTREXATE

Methotrexate causes both acute and delayed neurotoxicity. The acute reactions are aseptic meningitis and transverse myelopathy, both of which are associated with intrathecal administration of the drugs[33] (more frequent after administration by lumbar puncture than via ventricular cannula), and a stroke-like

syndrome after intravenous high-dose methotrexate.[34]

Acute Toxicity

Aseptic meningitis (Table 22-6) begins 2 to 4 hours after the drug is injected and generally lasts for 12 to 72 hours. The symptoms are headaches, stiff neck, nausea, vomiting, fever, and lethargy. A CSF pleocytosis is often present and can mimic acute bacterial meningitis, except that it occurs too soon after injection to be caused by bacterial growth. The syndrome is common; in some series, more than 50 percent of patients treated with intrathecal methotrexate are affected. Curiously, a patient can have a florid reaction after one injection but may suffer no reaction after subsequent injections. The symptoms are self-limited and there is no specific treatment, although some inject hydrocortisone to prevent it.[35] Rarely, pulmonary edema (possibly neurogenic) has followed an intrathecal injection of methotrexate[36]; sudden death has also very rarely followed intrathecal instillation.[37]

Transverse myelopathy is a rare complication. Pain in the legs is followed by rapidly developing sensory changes, paraplegia, and neurogenic bladder dysfunction. The symptoms usually begin 30 minutes to 48 hours[38,39] after intrathecal treatment but may be delayed as long as 2 weeks. The pathological changes consist of a necrotic myelopathy without striking inflammation or vascular changes. The pathogenesis is believed to be an idiosyncratic reaction to the drug. A similar complication has been reported following intrathecal cytosine arabinoside or thiotepa.[40]

Delayed Toxicity

A *stroke-like syndrome* affecting adults or children occasionally follows systemic high-dose methotrexate infusion.[34] The disorder usually follows the second or third treatment by 5 or 6 days and is characterized by alternating hemiparesis associated with aphasia and sometimes encephalopathy or coma. Unequivocal seizure activity is rare. The electroencephalogram (EEG) is slow. Patients generally recover spontaneously in 48 to 72 hours. Surprisingly, in subsequent treatments the syndrome usually does not recur, although rare recurrences have been described. The pathogenesis of the disorder is unknown, but Phillips and his associates have shown marked changes in

Table 22-5 Neurotoxic Signs Caused by Agents Commonly Used in Cancer Patients

Acute encephalopathy (delirium)	Visual loss	Headaches without meningitis	Myelopathy (intrathecal drugs)
Glucocorticoids	Tamoxifen	Retinoic acid	Methotrexate
Methotrexate (high-dose IV, IT)	Gallium nitrate	Trimethoprim-sulfamethoxazole	Cytarabine
Cisplatin	Nitrosoureas (intra-arterial)	Cimetidine	Thiotepa
Vincristine	Cisplatin	Corticosteroids	**Peripheral neuropathy**
Asparaginase	**Cerebellar dysfunction—Ataxia**	Tamoxifen	Vinca alkaloids
Procarbazine	5-Fluorouracil (± levamisole)	**Seizures**	Cisplatin
5-Fluorouracil (±levamisole)	Cytarabine	Methotrexate	Hexamethylmelamine
Cytarabine (Ara-C)	Phenytoin	Etoposide (high-dose)	Procarbazine
Nitrosoureas (high-dose or arterial)	Procarbazine	Cisplatin	5-Azacytidine
Cyclosporin A	Hexamethylmelamine	Vincristine	Etoposide
Interleukin-2	Vincristine	Asparaginase	Tenoposide (VM-26)
Ifosfamide	Cyclosporin A	Nitrogen mustard	Misonidazole
Interferons	**Aseptic meningitis**	Carmustine	Methyl-G
Tamoxifen	Trimethoprim-sulfamethazole	Dacarbazine	Cytarabine
Etoposide (VP-16) (high-dose)	IVIG	m-AMSA	Taxol
PALA	NSAID	Busulphan (high-dose)	Suramin
Chronic encephalopathy (dementia)	Levamisole	Cyclosporin A	Mitotane
Methotrexate	Monoclonal antibodies	Mitro(miso)nidazole	
Carmustine (BCNU)	Metrizamide	Beta-lactam antibiotics	
Cytarabine	OKT-3	Iodinated contrast material (IV or IT)	
Carmofur	Cytarabine		
Fludarabine	Carbamazepine		
	Levamisole		
	Methotrexate (IT)		

Abbreviations: Ara-C, cytosine arabinoside or cytarabine; BCNU, carmustine; IV, intravenous; IVIG, intravenous γ-globulin; IT, intrathecal; m-AMSA, acridinylaniside or AMSA; NSAID, nonsteroidal anti-inflammatory drugs; OKT-3, orthoclone; PALA, phosphonacetyl-L-aspartate; VM-26, tenoposide; VP-16, etoposide.

Table 22-6 Methotrexate Toxicity[a]

Route of Administration	Dose	Toxic Effect
Oral or intravenous	Standard	Leukoencephalopathy (if prior brain irradiation)
Intravenous	High	Acute transient encephalopathy
		Chronic leukoencephalopathy
Intra-arterial	Standard	Hemorrhagic cerebral infarction
Intrathecal	Standard	Acute aseptic meningitis, paraplegia, seizures
		Chronic leukoencephalopathy, cerebral atrophy and calcification

[a] Toxicity may be enhanced by cranial irradiation and/or other systemic chemotherapeutic agents.

brain glucose metabolism following intravenous infusion of high-dose methotrexate to rats.[41]

Leukoencephalopathy is the major and most devastating delayed complication of methotrexate treatment. The disorder generally follows repeated doses of intravenous high-dose methotrexate injections or intrathecal methotrexate, but it may occur after standard-dose intravenous injection as well.[42,43] Although the syndrome can be caused by methotrexate alone, it is exacerbated by brain irradiation. Leukoencephalopathy may appear months to years following therapy, beginning insidiously or abruptly with personality changes and learning disability.[44] Children cured of leukemia who have received only intrathecal or high-dose intravenous methotrexate with cranial irradiation show a decreased IQ after therapy.[44] Seizures can occur, but usually do so late in the course. The clinical course varies. Patients may recover slowly over weeks or months, their symptoms may stabilize with a mild to moderate dementia, or there may be relentless progression with spastic hemi- or quadriparesis, severe dementia, and coma, ending in death.

The myelin basic protein concentration may be elevated in CSF, presumably due to myelin breakdown.[45] The CT scan reveals cerebral atrophy, bilateral and diffuse white matter hypodensities, ventricular dilatation, and, sometimes, cortical calcifications; similar findings may occasionally be seen in asymptomatic patients who have received methotrexate. Focal enhancement may be present in the early stages. These abnormalities are even more apparent on MRI.[46] While scans may be normal even in patients with diminished intellect, neurological signs are usually preceded by changes in white matter on the MRI.[47] These abnormal images should be a warning to the physician that the patient is at risk for clinical leukoencephalopathy. White matter changes on the MRI may be seen in patients years after prophylactic treatment with intrathecal or intravenous methotrexate, even in the absence of radiation therapy.

Several different pathological abnormalities have been reported.[48] The most common is disseminated foci of white matter degeneration characterized by demyelination, axonal swelling, and dystrophic mineralization of axonal debris. These necrotizing changes may occasionally be accompanied by fibrinoid necrosis of small blood vessels. Histologically, leukoencephalopathy from irradiation or methotrexate cannot easily be distinguished, although the presence of axonal swelling is much more characteristic of methotrexate-induced leukoencephalopathy. An unusual but now rarely encountered pathological and, sometimes, radiological change, virtually restricted to children, is mineralizing microangiopathy characterized by noninflammatory fibrosis and calcification of arterial capillaries and venules, particularly in the basal ganglia.

The pathophysiology of methotrexate neurotoxicity is poorly understood. Depletion of reduced folates in the brain, inhibition of cerebral protein or glucose metabolism, injury to cerebral vascular endothelium resulting in increased blood-brain barrier permeability, and inhibition of catecholamine neurotransmitter synthesis have all been implicated but not proved to be involved. No effective treatment exists.

CISPLATIN

Cisplatin is a drug with a heavy-metal base; thus, it is not surprising that, like other heavy metals, it causes a peripheral neuropathy[49] (Table 22-7). The disorder follows doses of cisplatin usually greater than 400 mg/m² and is characterized by numbness and tingling in the extremities, occasionally painful.[49] The first symptoms may not appear until cisplatin treatment is completed and then may progress for several months before stabilizing. The disorder affects predominantly the large sensory fibers; the deep tendon reflexes disappear and proprioception is lost, often to the point that patients cannot feed themselves or walk. Pin and

Table 22-7 Neurotoxicity of Cisplatin

Common
  Peripheral neuropathy (large fiber, sensory)
  Lhermitte's sign
  Hearing loss (high-frequency)
  Tinnitus

Uncommon
  Encephalopathy
  Visual loss (retinal-optic nerve, cortical)
  Seizures
  Herniation (hydration-related)
  Electrolyte imbalance (Ca^{++}, Mg^{++}, Na^+, SIADH)[a]
  Vestibular toxicity
  Autonomic neuropathy

Abbreviation: SIADH, syndrome of inappropriate antidiuretic hormone secretion.

temperature sensation are spared, however, and power may be entirely normal. Nerve conduction studies reveal decreased amplitude of sensory nerve action potentials and prolonged sensory latencies, compatible with a sensory axonopathy. If the patient survives the cancer, the neuropathy may improve and the patient's condition may even return to normal after many months. The disorder is often confused with paraneoplastic sensory neuronopathy but differs from that disorder in that paraneoplastic sensory neuronopathy usually affects all sensory modalities equally. There is no known treatment, nor is there an effective way of preventing the disorder. *Focal neuropathies* may follow arterial infusions in the extremities or neck.

Pathological examination of nerve roots reveals axonal loss with secondary demyelination.[50] Axonal loss is also found in posterior but not anterior roots, with secondary degeneration of posterior columns. Dorsal root ganglion cells are probably the primary site of pathology, and the predominant pathological abnormality is nuclear. A correlation exists between the degree of histological change and the levels of platinum found in dorsal roots and peripheral nerve.

Lhermitte's sign appearing during or shortly after treatment with cisplatin[51] suggests a transient demyelinating lesion in the posterior columns of the spinal cord. In some instances, patients may experience paresthesias down the arms when the upper limbs are abducted, suggesting that the brachial plexus may be demyelinated as well.

Muscle cramps not related to electrolyte imbalance (see below) are also common but, like Lhermitte's sign, they usually resolve spontaneously.[52]

Ototoxicity and *vestibulopathy* are also caused by cisplatin.[53] Hearing loss results from hair cell damage.[54] The hearing loss is often subclinical and affects primarily the high-frequency range—that is, frequencies greater than 4,000 Hz. Tinnitus may precede hearing loss; rarely, high-dose cisplatin causes acute deafness.

Vestibular toxicity is much less common than hearing loss. It is characterized by vertigo, oscillopsia, and ataxia. It may occur either with or without other symptoms of ototoxicity and may be exacerbated by prior usage of aminoglycoside antibiotics.

Ocular toxicity—which includes retinopathy (usually after intracarotid infusion),[55] papilledema, and retrobulbar neuritis—is rare. Color perception may be disturbed, probably as a result of retinal cone dysfunction. Cortical visual loss (homonymous hemianopia, cortical blindness) may be part of the encephalopathy sometimes caused by cisplatin.

Encephalopathy is rare following intravenous infusion[56] but more common following intra-arterial infusion. It is characterized by seizures and focal brain dysfunction, particularly cortical blindness, but the symptoms are usually reversible. Encephalopathy due to the drug must be differentiated from that caused by the hydration preceding cisplatin use—that is, water intoxication leading to cerebral herniation[57]—or by the nephropathy that often follows it. Hypocalcemia and hypomagnesemia are common after cisplatin and may rarely cause tetany, encephalopathy, or seizures. Hypozincemia has also been reported. Inappropriate antidiuretic hormone secretion (SIADH) with hyponatremia and seizures can also occur.

Cisplatin has been implicated in the late *vascular toxicity*—that is, Raynaud's phenomenon, cardiac infarction, and cerebral infarction—that sometimes follows multiagent chemotherapy. Some believe that the toxicity is caused by the cisplatin and probably related to hypomagnesemia; others believe that bleomycin is the major culprit. Other rare complications of cisplatin include irreversible *myelopathy, taste disturbances,* and a *myasthenic syndrome.*

VINCRISTINE

Vincristine affects primarily the peripheral nerves but can also be toxic to the CNS, cranial nerves, and autonomic nervous system (Table 22-8). (Vindesine and vinblastine are much less neurotoxic.) A dose-limiting *sensorimotor neuropathy* appears in virtually all patients.[58] The earliest complaint is tingling and paresthesias of the fingertips and later of the toes. Fine movements of the fingers and toes are often impaired.[59] Loss of ankle jerks is the earliest sign. With continued drug administration, other reflexes disappear as well. Muscle cramps, usually diurnal, affect arms and legs and may be the first symptom of neurotoxicity.[60] Objective sensory loss is uncommon, but weakness, especially of the extensors of the feet and wrist, is frequent. Foot drop is either unilateral or bilateral. Unilateral foot drop is especially common in patients who have lost weight and habitually sit with crossed legs, thereby causing compression of the peroneal nerve at the head of the fibula. The weakness

Table 22-8 The Spectrum of Vincristine Neurotoxicity

Toxic Effect	Subacute (1 day–2 weeks)	Intermediate (1–4 weeks)	Chronic (> 3 weeks)
Peripheral neuropathy	Depressed Achilles reflex (universal)	Other tendon reflexes depressed, paresthesias	Sensory loss, weakness, "foot drop" gait
?Myopathy	Muscle pain, tenderness, (especially quadriceps); jaw pain	—	—
Autonomic neuropathy	Ileus with cramping abdominal pain	Constipation, urinary hesitancy, impotence, orthostatic hypotension	—
Cranial neuropathy (uncommon)	—	—	Optic atrophy; ptosis; sixth, seventh, and eighth cranial nerve dysfunction; hoarseness; dysphagia
"Central" toxicity	—	Seizures, inappropriate ADH secretion	—

(Modified from Young DF, Posner JB: Nervous system toxicity of the chemotherapeutic agents. p. 91. In Vinken PJ, Bruyn GW (eds): Handbook of Clinical Neurology. Vol. 39. Elsevier, Amsterdam, 1980, with permission.)

is usually tolerable, but rare patients may become bedbound or quadriparetic, particularly if there is a preexisting neuropathy. The sensory symptoms, weakness, and lost reflexes are reversible, although they may require several months after the medication is stopped to improve. Agents used to relieve vincristine neurotoxicity, including gangliosides and glutamic acid, are not very effective.

Vincristine occasionally causes *focal neuropathies* of peripheral or cranial nerves.[61] The most common is mild oculomotor nerve involvement with ptosis. Less frequent is ophthalmoplegia with diplopia. The recurrent laryngeal nerve, facial nerve, acoustic nerve, and optic nerve are also occasionally affected. These various neuropathies may be bilateral or unilateral. Night blindness due to retinal damage has also been reported.

Autonomic neuropathy, characterized by colicky abdominal pain and constipation, occurs in as many as one-third of patients. Rarely, paralytic ileus develops in children and may be fatal. Amelioration of vincristine-induced ileus with metoclopramide has been reported[62] but prevention of constipation is essential; all patients receiving vincristine should receive a prophylactic bowel regimen of stool softeners and laxatives. Other manifestations of autonomic dysfunction which have been reported include bladder atony, impotence, and postural hypotension.

CNS toxicity may result from hyponatremia due to SIADH.[63] Encephalopathy[64] and focal or generalized seizures not due to SIADH have also been reported. Cortical blindness and other focal cerebral signs including athetosis, ataxia,[65] and parkinsonian-like symptoms usually reverse after treatment is discontinued.

The diagnosis of vincristine neurotoxicity is usually not difficult even when, as is common, the weakness develops a few weeks following therapy and progresses for several additional weeks. Neurophysiological studies are usually unnecessary but, when done, show the typical features of an axonal neuropathy. These findings have been confirmed by nerve biopsy.[66]

NITROSOUREAS

The nitrosoureas rarely cause neurological toxicity when given in conventional doses. However, in patients with brain tumors who have received radiation and are treated with intracarotid or high-dose intravenous bischloroethyl nitrosourea (BCNU), both *ocular toxicity* and *encephalopathy* have been reported.[67] After intracarotid treatment, the disorder is sometimes heralded by seizures and followed by slowly progressive neurological dysfunction, the exact signs depending

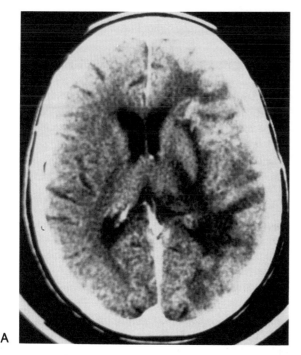 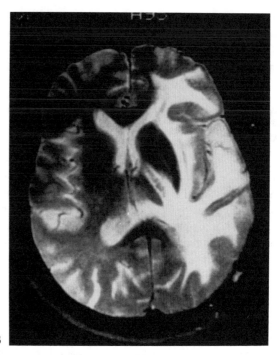

Fig. 22-1. Necrotizing encephalopathy following treatment with intracarotid BCNU. **(A)** CT scan and **(B)** T$_2$-weighted MRI of the brain. Note white matter hypodensity of the left hemisphere and irregular areas of contrast enhancement on CT. MRI shows diffuse hyperintensity of the left hemisphere, affecting primarily the white matter. The lesions are confined to the distribution of the treated carotid artery. No residual tumor was found at autopsy.

on the region infused. White matter abnormalities are often apparent on the CT scan or MRI, sometimes at a site distant from the tumor (Fig. 22-1); with time, the area of white matter hypodensity may develop calcification. The pathology is that of a necrotizing encephalopathy, giving an appearance similar to that of radiation damage[60] but strictly confined to the vascular territories perfused by the drug.

5-FLUOROURACIL

Neurotoxicity is rarely seen with conventional doses of the drug. The primary neurotoxicity with high doses is a *cerebellar syndrome,* clinically indistinguishable from paraneoplastic or cytarabine-induced cerebellar disorders, consisting of truncal and limb ataxia, dysmetria, nystagmus, and slurred speech.[68] The mechanism of this disorder or other neurotoxicity is unknown. The signs usually reverse within a week after the drug is discontinued but may recur with its reintroduction. In animals, the agent damages Purkinje cells, granule cells, and neurons of the inferior olive and vestibular nuclei.

Extraocular muscle abnormalities (particularly vergence disturbances), optic neuropathy, and extrapyramidal syndromes have been reported rarely with the administration of 5-fluorouracil. Encephalopathy, with diffuse slowing of the EEG but without cerebellar symptoms, has also been reported. Ocular toxicity includes blepharitis, conjunctivitis, lacrimal duct stenosis, and excessive lacrimation. Cerebral infarcts have been reported to complicate continuous infusion of the drug. Palmar-plantar erythrodysesthesia, a rare complication, may be confused with a peripheral neuropathy because of painful hands and feet. Acute neurological symptomatology—including somnolence, cerebellar ataxia, and upper motor neuron signs—has been reported following intracarotid arterial infusions. A diffuse encephalopathy occasionally follows conventional intravenous doses.

When levamisole is combined with 5-fluorouracil, a few patients develop an inflammatory multifocal leukoencephalopathy.[65] The disorder usually presents with confusion and focal signs, including ataxia or hemiparesis associated with multiple contrast-enhancing lesions on MRI that may be confused with metastases. Levamisole itself is rarely neurotoxic.[69]

CYTARABINE (CYTOSINE ARABINOSIDE OR ARA-C)

Aseptic meningitis and rarely *myelopathy*, both clinically similar to those induced by methotrexate, sometimes follow intrathecal ara-C.[70] Meningeal irritation causing headache, stiff neck, and pleocytosis has been encountered in approximately 30 percent of patients given the drug, but no direct relationship between this syndrome and the individual or cumulative dose has been established. The myelopathy begins with back pain or radicular leg pain. Weakness, sensory alterations, and bowel or bladder dysfunction occur at any time from a few days to months following treatment. The clinical picture usually evolves rapidly and sometimes renders the patient paraplegic. Signs typically persist, but some patients recover. Examination of the CSF usually reveals an elevated protein concentration and a modest pleocytosis; an elevated myelin basic protein has also been reported. Pathologically, portions of the spinal cord reveal demyelination with associated white matter vacuolization, histologically indistinguishable from methotrexate-induced myelopathy. One patient developed a "locked-in syndrome" (preserved consciousness but inability to move or communicate except by eye movement) 48 hours after a single dose of 100 mg intrathecal ara-C in conjunction with intravenous ara-C, cisplatin, and doxorubicin. At autopsy, there was extensive brainstem necrosis. Rarely, intrathecal administration of ara-C has been associated with seizures or an acute or subacute *encephalopathy*.[71]

Intravenous high-dose ara-C (3 g/m^2/12 h for 8 to 12 doses) may cause several neurological disorders.[72] *Cerebellar dysfunction* occurs most frequently in older patients and in those with preexisting renal dysfunction and usually at a cumulative dose of at least 36 g/m^2. However, it has been reported after a single dose of 3 g/m^2. Patients present with dysarthria, nystagmus, and appendicular and gait ataxia. They may also develop confusion, lethargy, and somnolence. With cessation of the drug, complete resolution of signs and symptoms generally occurs within 2 weeks. Neuro-

pathological changes in those patients who succumb to their underlying illness include widespread Purkinje cell loss, most pronounced in the deeper portion of the primary and secondary cerebellar sulci. The rest of the CNS appears to be largely unaffected, although white matter demyelination and filamentous degeneration of neurons in brainstem and spinal cord have been reported.

Peripheral neuropathy—either axonal, demyelinating, or both[73]—is a rare complication of ara-C; in most patients, high-dose ara-C was given along with other potentially neurotoxic agents, including fludarabine. Also reported occasionally are seizures; reversible ocular toxicity including blurred vision, photophobia, burning eye pain, and blindness; bulbar and pseudobulbar palsy; Horner's syndrome; the "painful legs, moving toes syndrome"; brachial plexopathy; reversible bilateral lateral rectus palsies; and acute aseptic meningitis (after intravenous injection). One patient who received a cumulative dose of 72 g developed a parkinsonian syndrome that resolved within 12 weeks.

The mechanism of ara-C toxicity is unknown. Some investigators believe that ara-C kills neurons by interfering with cytidine-dependent neurotrophic signal transduction.[74] There is no treatment for any of the neurotoxic effects of ara-C but, as indicated above, many patients recover spontaneously.

SURAMIN

Suramin causes a peripheral neuropathy in 40 percent of patients whose blood levels exceed 350 μg/L. This condition presents as a disorder like the Guillain-Barré syndrome, with rapid onset of a predominantly motor neuropathy leading to weakness or paralysis of the extremities,[75] and sometimes of bulbar and respiratory muscles. Paresthesias in the face and limbs are common prior to the weakness. The weakness often begins proximally. The disorder probably results from demyelination causing conduction block in peripheral nerves. It reverses after the drug is discontinued and can be prevented by monitoring blood levels carefully.

TAXOL AND TAXOTERE

Approximately 60 percent of patients receiving taxol at doses of 250 mg/m^2 or less develop paresthesias of the hands and feet that, in most patients, do not progress and may even resolve despite continued therapy.[76] A few patients also develop proximal muscle weakness that resolves. Acute arthralgia and myalgia of the legs that curtails activity (and is sometimes mistaken for peripheral neuropathy) may occur at 2 to 3 days after a course of taxol and last for 2 to 4 days. The neuropathy is predominantly sensory and, unlike cisplatin neuropathy, affects all sensory modalities. Taxol causes axonal damage with secondary demyelination, probably reflecting damage to the cell body. Taxotere appears to cause the same sensory neuropathy as does taxol. Nerve growth factor prevents taxol neuropathy in mice and is now in clinical trials.

BIOLOGICAL AGENTS

Several biological approaches may be used either to manipulate the immune system to destroy neoplastic cells (e.g., antibodies, cytokines, vaccines, and lymphocytes) or to combat the myelotoxic effects of chemotherapy (e.g., colony stimulating factors, bone marrow transplant). A few of these agents cause notable nervous system toxicity[77,78] (Table 22-9). Useful updates on the biological therapy of cancer are published frequently.[79]

Interleukin-2 causes capillaries, including those in the brain, to leak,[80] leading to increases in brain water content on MRI and to a severe encephalopathy.[81]

Interferons can also cause encephalopathy which at times is irreversible.[82] Nightmares, headache, myalgias, bilateral brachial plexopathy,[83] and oculomotor palsies are also side effects of interferons.

RADIATION THERAPY

Therapeutic ionizing irradiation may affect the nervous system in one of two settings: (1) Damage to neural structures may occur when those structures

Table 22-9 Neurological Complications of Immunotherapy

Agent	Acute (<1 week)	Intermediate (1–4 weeks)	Delayed (>1 month)
Levamisole	Encephalopathy	—	Leukoencephalopathy "MS-like" with 5-fluorouracil
Cyclosporin	Seizure[a] Burning feet and hands[c]	Tremor[b] "Cerebrocerebellar syndrome" Leukoencephalopathy Myelopathy	Myopathy Sensorimotor polyneuropathy
α-Interferon	Acute paresthesias Loss of taste/smell Encephalopathy[a] Leukoencephalopathy (IT)[d]	Brachial plexopathy	Chronic encephalopathy/dementia Parkinsonism Sensory and sensorimotor polyneuropathy 3rd-nerve palsy
Interleukin-2	Cerebral edema (ITU)[e] Encephalopathy (frequent) Leukoencephalopathy (rare) Nerve compression (during late vascular syndrome) Brachial plexopathy	Transient focal deficit	
CD3 Monoclonal	Aseptic meningitis Seizures Encephalitis (rare)		

[a] May also occur in the intermediate period.
[b] May also occur in the delayed period.
[c] Occurs during intravenous infusion.
[d] IT = with intrathecal administration.
[e] ITU = with intratumoral and systemic administration in patients with brain tumors.

are included in the radiation portal. This damage can occur whether the cancer undergoing radiation therapy is within or outside the nervous system. (2) Nervous system dysfunction can also occur secondarily when therapeutic irradiation damages blood vessels supplying the brain or endocrine organs necessary for appropriate nervous system function (usually the thyroid gland) or when the irradiation causes tumors that compress or destroy nervous system structures. Nervous system dysfunction caused by radiation therapy can occur acutely or be delayed by weeks, months, or even years following the successful completion of treatment. The likelihood that radiation therapy will damage the nervous system depends on many factors including the total dose delivered to the nervous system, the dose delivered with each treatment (higher doses with each treatment cause more damage to normal structures), the total volume of nervous system irradiated, the time after completion of radiation therapy, the presence of other systemic diseases which enhance the side effects of irradiation (e.g., diabetes, hypertension), and other unidentifiable host factors. The side effects of radiation therapy are detailed below. More extensive reviews can be found elsewhere.[4,84]

Primary Damage to the Nervous System

BRAIN

Encephalopathy caused by radiation therapy occurs in three forms: acute, early delayed (2 weeks to 4 months), and late delayed (4 months to 24 years) (Table 22-10).

Acute Encephalopathy

Acute encephalopathy usually follows large radiation therapy fractions given to patients with increased intracranial pressure from primary or metastatic brain tumor, particularly in the absence of corticosteroid coverage.[85] Immediately following treatment, susceptible patients develop headache, nausea, vomiting, somnolence, fever, and worsening of neurological symptoms rarely severe enough to culminate in cerebral herniation and death. Acute encephalopathy usually follows the first radiation fraction and becomes progressively less severe with each ensuing fraction. Usually the disorder is mild, with the patient only

reporting on the following morning the occurrence of headache and nausea on the evening following irradiation. The pathogenesis of the disorder is not certain. Some observers believe it is secondary to a rise in intracranial pressure, with cerebral edema following breakdown of the blood-brain barrier by ionizing radiation. Experimental evidence indicates that a single dose of 300 cGy delivered experimentally to an animal causes substantial breakdown of the blood-brain barrier if measured 2 hours after radiation; after 24 hours, the barrier has reconstituted itself. Corticosteroids will substantially prevent the breakdown of the blood-brain barrier.[86] A few observers have noted an increase in intracranial pressure following a single dose of radiation therapy,[85] but others have failed to document such an increase either in humans or animals even if clinical symptoms develop.[87] For the clinician there are two implications. First, patients harboring large brain tumors, particularly with signs of increased intracranial pressure, should probably not be treated with large doses per fraction. Doses of 200 cGy per fraction or less appear to be acceptable in such patients. Second, all patients undergoing brain irradiation should be protected with corticosteroids (8 to 16 mg dexamethasone daily or more if increased intracranial pressure is symptomatic), preferably for at least 24 hours before the start of radiation therapy. Both clinical and experimental evidence indicates that corticosteroids ameliorate the acute complications of irradiation.

Early Delayed Encephalopathy

Early delayed encephalopathy usually begins in the second or third month after irradiation but can begin anywhere from 2 weeks to 4 months after treatment. If the patient has a brain tumor, the symptoms of early delayed encephalopathy often simulate tumor progression.[88] For example, the patient may develop recurrence of headache, lethargy, and worsening of lateralizing signs. Changes on CT scan or MRI may include an increase in size of the lesion and sometimes the occurrence of contrast enhancement not previously present. These changes resolve spontaneously if the disorder is due to radiation encephalopathy rather than tumor recurrence, and this resolution can be hastened by the use of corticosteroids. The patient and the scan remain improved after corticosteroids are discontinued, indicating that the disorder was early

Table 22-10 Radiation-Induced Injury: Direct Damage to the CNS

Time After Radiation	Clinical Findings	Possible Mechanisms
Brain		
Acute (minutes to days)	Increased intracranial pressure	Acute vasogenic edema
Early delayed (weeks)	Diffuse: somnolence syndrome	Demyelination
	Focal: simulates recurrent tumor	
Delayed (months to years)		
Necrosis	Diffuse: dementia (rare)	Glial and vascular destruction
	Focal: simulates recurrent tumor	
?Hydrocephalus	Asymptomatic or dementia	Unknown
	Ataxia, dementia (rare)	Normal-pressure hydrocephalus
Spinal cord		
Early delayed (weeks)	Lhermitte's sign	Demyelination
Delayed (months to years)		
Spinal cord necrosis	Transverse myelopathy	Glial and vascular destruction
Epidural necrosis	Myelopathy (rare)	
Motor neuron disease	Flaccid paraparesis, amyotrophy	Unknown
Arachnoiditis	Often asymptomatic	Radiation-induced damage to the leptomeninges
?Hemorrhage	Acute myelopathy	Vascular lesions

delayed encephalopathy rather than tumor recurrence.

Early delayed encephalopathy also occurs in patients without brain tumors. Early delayed encephalopathy after prophylactic irradiation of the brain of children with leukemia has been called the "radiation somnolence syndrome."[89] This disorder is characterized by somnolence often associated with headache, nausea, vomiting and, sometimes, fever. The EEG may be slow, but there are no focal neurological signs. The syndrome is ameliorated by corticosteroids but will also resolve spontaneously. The disorder is sometimes seen in adults following prophylactic radiation therapy for small cell lung cancer.

A rare and serious neurological syndrome is brainstem encephalopathy following irradiation of posterior fossa tumors (or when the brainstem has been included in the irradiated field for head and neck cancer).[90] The most frequent symptoms are ataxia, diplopia, dysarthria, and nystagmus. Most patients recover spontaneously within 6 to 8 weeks. Rarely the symptoms progress to stupor, coma, and death.

The pathogenesis of early delayed encephalopathy is believed to be demyelination resulting from damage to oligodendroglia and subsequent breakdown of myelin sheaths. The best evidence supporting that hypothesis consists of pathological studies in patients with early delayed brainstem encephalopathy in which confluent areas of demyelination with varying degrees of axonal loss are found in areas receiving the radiation.[90] There is an associated loss of oligodendrocytes and abnormal and often multinucleated giant astrocytes.

Late Delayed Radiation Necrosis

Late delayed radiation necrosis usually begins a year or two after the completion of radiation therapy. The symptoms depend on the nature of the primary disease. In patients who were treated for primary or metastatic brain tumors, symptoms generally recapitulate those of the brain tumor, leading the physician to suspect tumor recurrence. In addition, the MRI or CT scan may suggest recurrence or enlargement of the original tumor[91,92] (Fig. 22-2). Occasionally, a lesion suggesting a tumor appears at a distant site. Positron emission tomography with glucose can help distinguish radiation necrosis from recurrent tumor, the former showing decreased glucose uptake (cold area), the latter an increased glucose uptake (hot area).[93,94]

Histologically, the typical lesion is an area of coagulative necrosis in the white matter, with relative sparing of the overlying cortex. Microscopically, the most striking abnormalities are found in blood vessels, with hyalinized thickening and fibrinoid necrosis of the walls often associated with vascular thrombosis, vascular hemorrhages, and accumulation of perivascular fibrinoid material.

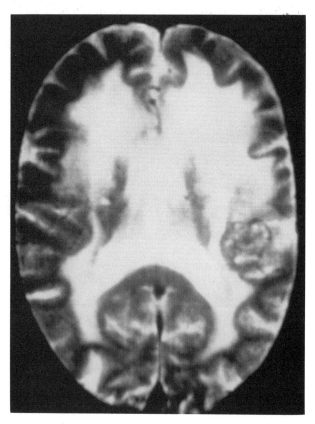

Fig. 22-2 Bilateral cerebral radiation necrosis 24 months after whole-brain irradiation (30 Gy delivered in six fractions). T$_2$-weighted MRI of the brain. Note diffuse hyperintensity of the white matter and anterior corpus callosum.

A second clinical picture has occurred when the patient's brain was included in the radiation portal but there was no underlying brain tumor. Examples include radiation of head and neck tumors, including pituitary tumors, and prophylactic irradiation of the brain.[93,95] Because only a portion of the brain has usually been irradiated and there was no previous brain damage, new focal neurological signs are the rule. For example, bilateral medial temporal destruction sometimes follows radiation for nasopharyngeal or pituitary tumors, and frontal or temporal lobe destruction follows treatment for ocular or maxillary sinus tumors. The clinical features are similar to those of a brain tumor, with signs of increased intracranial pressure and focal signs depending on the site of brain damage. The MRI usually reveals a mass, occasionally with contrast enhancement. An arteriogram may show vascular beading that suggests a vasculopa-

thy.[95] A definitive diagnosis can only be made pathologically. These patients do best when the area of radiation necrosis is resected.[93] Most patients respond transiently to corticosteroids, and there are reports of prolonged responses after corticosteroid therapy without surgery.[96] Other suggested treatments, such as aspirin and anticoagulation, that are based on the rationale that the disorder is primarily vascular, have not proved useful.

There are three hyeptheses concerning the pathogenesis of this disorder. The first is that the vascular changes lead to infarction and necrosis. The second is that radiation therapy directly damages glial cells, both astrocytes and oligodendrocytes, leading to destruction of tissue. The third is that the radiation causes release of brain antigens with subsequent antibody formation and immune destruction of the brain.

Cerebral Atrophy

Cerebral atrophy often follows whole-brain irradiation. The atrophy may occur in patients who are radiated prophylactically or in patients harboring brain tumors in whom irradiation has eradicated the tumor. It usually begins 6 to 12 months after radiation therapy. The patient may be asymptomatic but, more commonly, suffers memory loss and, in some instances, severe cognitive dysfunction.[97] Some patients have gait abnormalities and urgency incontinence, suggesting normal-pressure hydrocephalus.[97] MRI of virtually all patients receiving whole-brain irradiation in excess of 3,000 cGy shows cerebral atrophy with enlarged sulci and ventricles; there may also be symmetrical periventricular white matter hyperintense signals on T$_2$-weighted images. Symptomatic patients appear to have greater degrees of cerebral atrophy and ventricular dilatation. In some instances, the ventricular dilatation is out of proportion to sulcal atrophy; when such patients are symptomatic with dementia, gait apraxia, and incontinence they may respond to shunting of the ventricular system. Cerebral atrophy also occurs in children receiving prophylactic brain irradiation for acute leukemia. The atrophy is associated with learning disability.[98,99]

The pathogenesis of the cerebral atrophy is not clear. In some instances, true communicating hydrocephalus, perhaps from radiation-induced arachnoiditis or obliteration of pacchionian granulations, appears to be causal. In other instances, there is simply loss of cerebral substance. Except in those patients who respond to shunting, there is no treatment for the cerebral atrophy.

SPINAL CORD

There are no acute effects of radiation on the spinal cord. In the past, it was believed that, as with the brain, high doses of radiation delivered to the spinal cord for the treatment of epidural spinal cord compression might worsen neurological symptoms. Both clinical and experimental evidence have refuted this belief.[100,101]

Early Delayed Radiation Myelopathy

Early delayed radiation myelopathy is common after irradiation of the neck (Table 22-10). Several weeks after irradiation, the patient develops a Lhermitte's sign that persists for weeks or months and then spontaneously disappears.[102] Some investigators have reported prolonged sensory evoked potentials[103] but others have not.[104] Symptoms are believed to result from demyelination of the posterior columns of the spinal cord. Their presence does not predict the development of late delayed radiation spinal cord injury.

Late Delayed Radiation Myelopathy

Late delayed radiation myelopathy appears in two forms. The first and most common is characterized by progressive myelopathy, often beginning as a Brown-Séquard syndrome and progressing over weeks or months to cause paraparesis or quadriparesis.[105,106] Usually the symptoms progress subacutely but, in some instances, they progress over several years and, at times, may stabilize, leaving the patient with only mild or moderate paraparesis. The disorder probably never resolves spontaneously. Myelogram and MRI are usually normal, though rarely, in the acute stages, spinal cord swelling may be identified and the area of damage may enhance with contrast.[107] Spinal cord atrophy may occur at a later stage (Fig. 22-3). Pathologically, the lesions are characterized by confluent areas of necrosis with a predilection for the white matter, particularly the deeper parts of the posterior columns and superficial areas of the posterior lateral tracts. Vascular changes are similar to those in the brain but are usually less striking.[108] There is no effective treatment, although corticosteroids sometimes delay progression of the lesion.

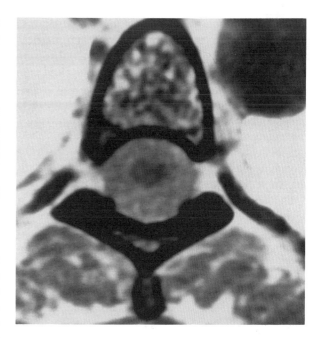

Fig. 22-3 Chronic radiation myelopathy. CT scan at the level of T5. Note atrophy of the spinal cord.

A few patients have been described with hemorrhage in the spinal cord developing many years after irradiation.[109] Characteristically, 8 to 30 years after radiation therapy to the spinal cord, a patient without prior neurological symptoms suddenly develops back pain and leg weakness. MRI suggests acute or subacute hemorrhage in the spinal cord. The cord may be slightly atrophic but no other lesions are found. After several days, the patient typically begins to improve, and the neurological symptoms may resolve entirely. A few patients have had recurrent episodes of spinal cord hemorrhage. The pathogenesis is probably related to vascular changes caused by the radiation therapy. A biopsy sample of the spinal cord from one patient was said to show an arteriovenous malformation.[109]

A second form of late delayed radiation myelopathy is a motor neuron syndrome that characteristically follows pelvic irradiation for testicular tumors[110,111] but has occurred after lumbosacral irradiation for other tumors[112,113] or after craniospinal irradiation for medulloblastoma.[114] This disorder occurs 3 months to 23 years following radiation and is characterized by the subacute onset of a flaccid weakness of the legs affecting both distal and proximal muscles, accompanied by atrophy, fasciculations, and areflexia. It is usually bilateral and symmetrical but may either begin in or remain restricted to one leg.[113] Sensory changes are absent. Sphincter and sexual functions are normal. The CSF may contain an increased protein concentration. The myelogram is normal. Although EMG reveals varying degrees of denervation, sensory and motor nerve conduction velocities are normal. The deficit usually stabilizes after several months to a few years; often patients are still able to walk, but some may become paraplegic.

The disorder is impossible to differentiate from a pure motor polyneuropathy or isolated motor neuron loss. It also resembles the paraneoplastic syndrome of subacute motor neuronopathy. A single report describes a motor neuron syndrome confined to the arms that developed 3 years following cervical irradiation and was associated with a cystic hypodense cavity affecting the spinal cord from C4 to C6.[115]

A single pathological report of a patient with a motor neuron syndrome in the lower extremities describes randomly distributed demyelination and axon loss in both sensory and motor roots, with areas of complete demyelination. The roots involved were primarily those of the cauda equina, with some anterior horn cells (motor neurons) in the lumbar cord exhibiting chromatolysis suggestive of secondary damage.[116]

CRANIAL NERVES

The clinical features of radiation injury to the cranial and peripheral nerves and the special senses are shown in Table 22-11. *Anosmia* may follow irradiation.[117] *Visual loss* may follow irradiation of the eye or brain. It may be caused by radiation-induced "dry eye syndrome," glaucoma, or cataract; more commonly, it may result from retinopathy or optic neuropathy.[118,119] The optic neuropathy following irradiation begins 7 to 26 months after the radiation and is characterized by painless monocular or bilateral blindness. Papilledema and retinal hemorrhages may be present. The likelihood of visual loss is probably increased by the use of concomitant chemotherapy, and visual loss can generally be prevented by shielding the eyes at the time of irradiation. *Hearing loss* also follows radiation therapy to the brain or ear.[120] Radiation-induced otitis media causes a conductive hearing loss that may require myringotomy for relief.[121,122] This disorder

Table 22-11 Radiation-Induced Injury: Damage to the Cranial and Peripheral Nerves and Organs of Special Sense

Cranial nerves
  Visual system
    Retinopathy
    Optic neuropathy
    Central retinal artery occlusion
  Taste and smell
    Acute, transient loss of taste and smell during radiation therapy
    Chronic loss of smell (rare)
  Hearing and vestibular system
    Radiation otitis
    Cochlear endarteritis
    8th-nerve neuropathy (rare)
  Involvement of the lower cranial nerves
    12th nerve most frequently affected (fibrosis)

Brachial plexus neuropathies
  ?Acute
  Early delayed (rare)
  Delayed brachial plexopathy (fibrosis)

Delayed lumbosacral plexopathy

Delayed sciatic neuropathy (after intraoperative irradiation)

usually appears during or shortly following radiation therapy. It is different from the sensorineural hearing loss that is a late delayed effect of radiation therapy and has been attributed to an endarteritis producing vascular damage of the cochlear or acoustic nerve. The *lower cranial nerves,* particularly the *hypoglossal* nerve, are often involved as a late delayed effect of radiation therapy delivered to the neck.[123] The pathogenesis appears to be radiation fibrosis. Recurrent laryngeal, vagal, and sympathetic fibers (Horner's syndrome) may be involved as well.

PERIPHERAL NERVES

There are no acute changes in peripheral nerve function following radiation therapy, although Haymaker and Lindgren mentioned that paresthesias may occur when patients are "under the beam."[124] *Early delayed brachial plexus dysfunction* is characterized by paresthesias in the hand and forearm, sometimes associated with pain and accompanied by weakness and atrophy in a C6 to T1 distribution.[125–127] Nerve conduction studies reveal segmental slowing, and the course is characterized by recovery over a few weeks or months. This disorder is particularly common when carcinoma of the breast is being treated. *Late delayed radiation plexopathy* has been reported after radiation of either the brachial[128,129] or lumbosacral plexus,[130,131] although the former is much more common. The disorder usually occurs a year or more after radiation therapy with doses of 6,000 cGy or greater. Brachial plexopathy is characterized by paresthesias and weakness of the hand or arm. There may be sensory loss in the thumb and index finger. This disorder is frequently accompanied by lymphedema and by palpable induration in the supraclavicular fossa. Myokymia in the territory of related nerves helps to differentiate radiation damage from tumor infiltration of the plexus.[132,133] The radiation-induced disorder is usually less painful than tumor recurrence but often progresses to a panplexopathy, rendering the entire arm useless. A CT scan or MRI may show a tumor mass but often simply reveals a diffuse loss of tissue planes that is nonspecific and can be seen with either plexopathy or tumor infiltration.[134] Diagnostic certainty requires surgical exploration of the plexus. Even this procedure may not exclude tumor if the nerves themselves are infiltrated and there is no perineural tumor. There is no treatment, although painful paresthesias may be relieved by amitriptyline.

Lumbosacral plexopathy causes weakness of one or both legs. As with radiation brachial plexopathy, pain is usually absent and, when present, is generally mild.[131,135] The disorder often affects the foot, and sensory disturbances as well as weakness are present in most cases. EMG frequently reveals myokymic discharges, which helps to differentiate the process from tumor recurrence. Radiation-induced lumbosacral plexopathy is often slowly progressive over many years. At times exploration is necessary to make the diagnosis. The pathogenesis of radiation plexopathy and peripheral nerve disease is believed to be related to fibrosis causing damage to Schwann cells rather than stemming from direct damage to the nerves themselves.

Secondary Involvement of the Nervous System

RADIOGENIC TUMORS

The manner in which the nervous system may be affected secondarily after radiation therapy is summarized in Table 22-12.

Table 22-12 Secondary Involvement of the Nervous System Following Radiation Therapy

Radiogenic tumors
    Meningiomas
    Sarcomas
    Gliomas
    Schwannomas

Vascular lesions
    Stenosis/occlusion of the supraclinoid internal carotid
    Moyamoya disease
    Extracranial stenosis/occlusion
    Carotid rupture (rare)

Endocrinopathy
    Primary hypothyroidism
    Hyperparathyroidism
    Hypothalamic pituitary dysfunction
        Growth hormone deficiency (most frequent)
        Hyperprolactinemia
        Cortisol deficiency (rare)
        Gonadotropin deficiency (rare)

Radiation-induced tumors—including meningiomas,[136] sarcomas, and, less frequently, gliomas[137] and malignant schwannomas[138]—may appear years to decades after irradiation of nervous system tissue; secondary tumors may develop after even low doses of radiation therapy. An epidemiological study following a group of children who received low-dose scalp radiation for tinea capitis demonstrated a 9.5-fold increase in the incidence of meningiomas as compared with a control group.[139] Malignant or atypical nerve sheath tumors may follow radiation of the brachial, cervical, or lumbar plexuses. Signs and symptoms of radiogenic tumors are no different from those tumors that arise without prior radiation therapy, and their surgical treatment is similar. Some patients may be able to tolerate additional radiation therapy or chemotherapy if the tumor is malignant and cannot be totally excised surgically.

VASCULAR ABNORMALITIES

Lesions of large intra- or extracranial blood vessels may follow radiation therapy by months to years.[140] Patients may develop transient ischemic attacks or cerebral infarcts. Arteriography reveals stenosis or occlusion of the artery within the radiation portal. A particularly vulnerable area is the supraclinoid portion of the internal carotid artery in children who have received brain irradiation. This occlusion is sometimes associated with moyamoya disease. The pathology of radiation-induced vascular occlusion is similar to that of severe atherosclerosis, although there may be marked periarterial fibrosis, so that at surgery it is difficult to separate the intima from the media.[141] This condition can be distinguished from other forms of atherosclerosis by its restriction to the segment of vessel within the radiation field without evidence of widespread atherosclerosis elsewhere, by the younger age of the patients affected, and by the atypical location of the stenotic carotid segments, which are often situated distal or proximal to the bifurcation.[141,142] If appropriate, endarterectomy can be successfully performed on these patients.

ENDOCRINOPATHIES

Primary *hypothyroidism* may appear many years after irradiation for Hodgkin's disease or head and neck tumors or, less frequently, after craniospinal irradiation.[143,144] The patient may not have typical stigmata of hypothyroidism but instead presents either with central or peripheral nervous system dysfunction, including encephalopathy, ataxia, and peripheral neuropathy. If the CSF protein concentration is elevated, as it often is in hypothyroidism, the patient may undergo an extensive workup prior to recognition that the neurological disorder is caused by hypothyroidism. Thyroid function should be studied in any patient with neurological symptoms who has undergone prior irradiation to the neck or head.

Hypercalcemic *hyperparathyroidism* has been reported to follow radiation therapy.[145] *Hypothalamic-pituitary dysfunction* is a frequent delayed complication of irradiation for head and neck or brain tumors, especially in children. In children, the most frequent endocrinopathy is growth hormone deficiency, which is more often symptomatic in patients irradiated for primary brain tumor than after prophylactic irradiation for acute leukemia because of the higher doses used to treat most brain tumors.[146] Growth should be carefully monitored in children irradiated for brain tumor and treatment given if symptomatic deficiency is detected. Growth hormone deficiency should be differentiated from growth failure resulting from spinal irradiation. Gonadotropin deficiency and secondary or tertiary hypothyroidism are less frequent endocrinopathies.

In adults, hypothalamic pituitary dysfunction is a common sequela of irradiation for head and neck tumors.[146] In a large study, it was found that 5 to 9 years after irradiation, 48 percent of patients had decreased growth hormone, 13 percent had decreased cortisol (two-thirds of them requiring cortisol replacement), 40 percent had increased prolactin, and 8 percent had decreased follicle-stimulating hormone and luteinizing hormone. Most studies suggest that the hypothalamus is preferentially damaged by radiation compared to the pituitary gland itself.

In adults, radiation-induced hypothalamic pituitary dysfunction also occurs in about one-third of long-term survivors of primary brain tumors. The most frequent abnormalities are hypothalamic hypogonadism associated with hyperprolactinemia and hypothyroidism.

REFERENCES

1. Rottenberg DA: Neurological Complications of Cancer Treatment. Butterworth-Heinemann, Boston, 1991
2. Hildebrand J (ed): Neurological Adverse Reactions to Anticancer Drugs. Springer-Verlag, Berlin, 1990
3. Chabner BA, Collins JM: Cancer Chemotherapy: Principles and Practice. JB Lippincott, Philadelphia, 1990
4. Posner JB: Neurologic Complications of Cancer. FA Davis, Philadelphia, in press
5. Bruera E: Current pharmacological management of anorexia in cancer patients. Oncology 6:125, 1992
6. Bruera E, Roca E, Cedaro L, et al: Action of oral methylprednisolone in terminal cancer patients: a prospective randomized double-blind study. Cancer Treat Rep 69:751, 1985
7. Bond WS: Toxic reactions and side effects of glucocorticoids in man. Am J Hosp Pharm 34:479, 1977
8. Baxter JD, Forsham PH: Tissue effects of glucocorticoids. Am J Med 53:573, 1972
9. Axelrod L: Glucocorticoid therapy. Medicine (Baltimore) 55:39, 1976
10. Bowyer SL, LaMothe MP, Hollister JR: Steroid myopathy: incidence and detection in a population with asthma. J Allergy Clin Immunol 76:234, 1985
11. Taylor LP, Posner JB: Phenobarbital rheumatism in patients with brain tumor. Ann Neurol 25:92, 1989
12. Boston Collaborative Drug Surveillance Program:

Acute adverse reactions to prednisone in relation to dosage. Clin Pharmacol Ther 13:694, 1972

13. Wolkowitz OM, Reus VI, Weingartner H, et al: Cognitive effects of corticosteroids. Am J Psychiatry 147:1297, 1990

14. Lewis DA, Smith RE: Steroid-induced psychiatric syndromes: a report of 14 cases and a review of the literature. J Affective Disord 5:319, 1983

15. Varney NR, Alexander B, MacIndoe JH: Reversible steroid dementia in patients without steroid psychosis. Am J Psychiatry 141:369, 1984

16. Pies R: Persistent bipolar illness after steroid administration. Arch Intern Med 141:1087, 1981

17. Sharfstein SS, Sack DS, Fauci AS: Relationship between alternate-day corticosteroid therapy and behavioral abnormalities. JAMA 248:2987, 1982

18. Falk WE, Mahnke MW, Poskanzer DC: Lithium prophylaxis of corticotropin-induced psychosis. JAMA 241:1011, 1979

19. Lukert BP, Raisz LG: Glucocorticoid-induced osteoporosis: pathogenesis and management. Ann Intern Med 112:352, 1990

20. Engel IA, Straus DJ, Lacher M, et al: Osteonecrosis in patients with malignant lymphoma: a review of twenty-five cases. Cancer 48:1245, 1981

21. O'Brien TJ, Mack GR: Multifocal osteonecrosis after short-term high-dose corticosteroid therapy. Clin Orthop 279:176, 1992

22. Robinson HJ Jr, Hartleben PD, Lund G, Schreiman J: Evaluation of magnetic resonance imaging in the diagnosis of osteonecrosis of the femoral head. J Bone Joint Surg [Am] 71:650, 1989

23. Haddad SF, Hitchon PW, Godersky JC: Idiopathic and glucocorticoid-induced spinal epidural lipomatosis. J Neurosurg 74:38, 1991

24. Slansky HH, Kolbert G, Gartner S: Exophthalmos induced by steroids. Arch Ophthalmol 77:578, 1967

25. Messer J, Reitman D, Sacks HS, et al: Association of adrenocorticosteroid therapy and peptic-ulcer disease. N Engl J Med 309:21, 1983

26. Carson JL, Strom BL, Schinnar R, et al: The low risk of upper gastrointestinal bleeding in patients dispensed corticosteroids. Am J Med 91:223, 1991

27. Fadul CE, Lemann W, Thaler HT, Posner JB: Perforation of the gastrointestinal tract in patients receiving steroids for neurological disease. Neurology 38:348, 1988

28. Dixon RA, Christy NP: On the various forms of corticosteroid withdrawal syndrome. Am J Med 68:224, 1980

29. Amatruda TT, Hurst MH, D'Esopo ND: Certain endocrine and metabolic facets of the steroid withdrawal syndrome. J Clin Endocrinol Metab 25:1207, 1965

30. Johnston I, Gilday DL, Hendrick EB: Experimental effects of steroids and steroid withdrawal on cerebrospinal fluid absorption. J Neurosurg 42:690, 1975

31. Pavlidis NA, Petris C, Briassoulis E, et al: Clear evidence that long-term, low-dose tamoxifen treatment can induce ocular toxicity. Cancer 69:2961, 1992

32. Ron IG, Inbar MJ, Barak Y, et al: Organic delusional syndrome associated with tamoxifen treatment. Cancer 69:1415, 1992

33. Boogerd W, vd Sande JJ, Moffie D: Acute fever and delayed leukoencephalopathy following low dose intraventricular methotrexate. J Neurol Neurosurg Psychiatry 51:1277, 1988

34. Walker RW, Allen JC, Rosen G, Caparros B: Transient cerebral dysfunction secondary to high-dose methotrexate. J Clin Oncol 4:1845, 1986

35. Pullen J, Boyett J, Shuster J, et al: Extended triple intrathecal chemotherapy trial for prevention of CNS relapse in good-risk and poor-risk patients with B-progenitor acute lymphoblastic leukemia: a Pediatric Oncology Group study. J Clin Oncol 11:839, 1993

36. Hamous JE, Guffy MM, Aschenbrener CA: Fatal acute respiratory failure following intrathecal methotrexate administration. Cancer Treat Rep 67:1025, 1983

37. Ten Hoeve RFA, Twijnstra A: A lethal neurotoxic reaction after intraventricular methotrexate administration. Cancer 62:2111, 1988

38. Skullerud K, Halvorsen K: Encephalomyelopathy following intrathecal methotrexate treatment in a child with acute leukemia. Cancer 42:1211, 1978

39. Sullivan MP, Windmiller J: Side effects of Amethopterin (methotrexate) administered intrathecally in the treatment of meningeal leukemia. Med Rec Ann 50:92, 1966

40. Hahn AF, Feasby TE, Gilbert JJ: Paraparesis following intrathecal chemotherapy. Neurology 33:1032, 1983

41. Phillips PC, Dhawan V, Strother SC, et al: Reduced cerebral glucose metabolism and increased brain capillary permeability following high-dose methotrexate chemotherapy: a positron emission tomographic study. Ann Neurol 21:59, 1987

42. Rubinstein LJ, Herman MM, Long TF, Wilbur JR: Disseminated necrotizing leukoencephalopathy: a complication of treated central nervous system leukemia and lymphoma. Cancer 35:291, 1975

43. Price RA, Jamieson PA: The central nervous system in childhood leukemia: II. Subacute leukoencephalopathy. Cancer 35:306, 1975

44. Ochs J, Mulhern R, Fairclough D, et al: Comparison of neuropsychologic functioning and clinical indicators of neurotoxicity in long-term survivors of child-

hood leukemia given cranial radiation or parenteral methotrexate: a prospective study. J Clin Oncol 9: 145, 1991

45. Gangji D, Reaman GH, Cohen SR, et al: Leukoencephalopathy and elevated levels of myelin basic protein in the cerebrospinal fluid of patients with acute lymphoblastic leukemia. N Engl J Med 303:19, 1980

46. Asato R, Akiyama Y, Ito M, et al: Nuclear magnetic resonance abnormalities of the cerebral white matter in children with acute lymphoblastic leukemia and malignant lymphoma during and after central nervous system prophylactic treatment with intrathecal methotrexate. Cancer 70:1997, 1992

47. Lien HH, Blomlie V, Saeter G, et al: Osteogenic sarcoma: MR signal abnormalities of the brain in asymptomatic patients treated with high-dose methotrexate. Radiology 179:547, 1991

48. Cruz-Sanchez FF, Artigas J, Cervos-Navarro J, et al: Brain lesions following combined treatment with methotrexate and craniospinal irradiation. J Neurooncol 10:165, 1991

49. Boogerd W, ten Bokkel Huinink WW, Dalesio O, et al: Cisplatin induced neuropathy: central, peripheral and autonomic nerve involvement. J Neurooncol 9: 255, 1990

50. Ongerboer de Visser BW, Tiessens G: Polyneuropathy induced by cisplatin. Prog Exp Tumor Res 29: 190, 1985

51. Walther PJ, Rossitch E, Bullard DE: The development of Lhermitte's sign during cisplatin chemotherapy. Cancer 60:2170, 1987

52. Siegal T, Haim N: Cisplatin-induced peripheral neuropathy. Cancer 66:1117, 1990

53. Moroso MJ, Blair RL: A review of cis-platinum ototoxicity. J Otolaryngol 12:365, 1983

54. Wright CG, Schaefer SD: Inner ear histopathology in patients treated with cis-platinum. Laryngoscope 92: 1408, 1982

55. Kupersmith MJ, Frohman LP, Choi IS, et al: Visual system toxicity following intra-arterial chemotherapy. Neurology 38:284, 1988

56. Highley M, Meller ST, Pinkerton CR: Seizures and cortical dysfunction following high-dose cisplatin administration in children. Med Pediatr Oncol 20:143, 1992

57. Walker RW, Cairncross JG, Posner JB: Cerebral herniation in patients receiving cisplatin. J Neurooncol 6:61, 1988

58. Holland JF, Scharlau G, Gailani S, et al: Vincristine treatment of advanced cancer: a cooperative study of 392 cases. Cancer Res 33:1258, 1973

59. DeAngelis LM, Gnecco C, Taylor L, Warrell RP Jr:

Evolution of neuropathy and myopathy during intensive vincristine/corticosteroid chemotherapy for non-Hodgkin's lymphoma. Cancer 67:2241, 1991

60. Haim N, Barron SA, Robinson E: Muscle cramps associated with vincristine therapy. Acta Oncol 30:707, 1991

61. Levitt LP, Prager D: Mononeuropathy due to vincristine toxicity. Neurology 25:894, 1975

62. Garewal HS, Dalton WS: Metoclopramide in vincristine-induced ileus. Cancer Treat Rep 69:1309, 1985

63. Robertson GL, Bhoopalam N, Zelkowitz LJ: Vincristine neurotoxicity and abnormal secretion of antidiuretic hormone. Arch Intern Med 132:717, 1973

64. Whittaker JA, Parry DH, Bunch C, Weatherall DJ: Coma associated with vincristine therapy. Br Med J 4:335, 1973

65. Hook CC, Kimmel DW, Kvols LK, et al: Multifocal inflammatory leukoencephalopathy with 5-fluorouracil and levamisole. Ann Neurol 31:262, 1992

66. McLeod JG, Penny R: Vincristine neuropathy: an electrophysiological and histological study. J Neurol Neurosurg Psychiatry 32:297, 1969

67. Burger PC, Kamenar E, Schold SC, et al: Encephalomyelopathy following high-dose BCNU therapy. Cancer 48:1318, 1981

68. Riehl J, Brown WJ: Acute cerebellar syndrome secondary to 5-fluouracil therapy. Neurology 14:961, 1964

69. Parkinson DR, Cano PO, Jerry LM, et al: Complications of cancer immunotherapy with levamisole. Lancet 1:1129, 1977

70. Dunton SF, Nitschke R, Spruce WE, et al: Progressive ascending paralysis following administration of intrathecal and intravenous cytosine arabinoside: a Pediatric Oncology Group study. Cancer 57:1083, 1986

71. Eden OB, Goldie W, Wood T, Etcubanas E: Seizures following intrathecal cytosine arabinoside in young children with acute lymphoblastic leukemia. Cancer 42:53, 1978

72. Barnett MJ, Richards MA, Ganesan TS, et al: Central nervous system toxicity of high-dose cytosine arabinoside. Semin Oncol 12:227, 1985

73. Borgeat A, De Muralt B, Stalder M: Peripheral neuropathy associated with high-dose ara-C therapy. Cancer 58:852, 1986

74. Damon LE, Plunkett W, Linker CA: Plasma and cerebrospinal fluid pharmacokinetics of 1-beta-D-arabinofuranosylcytosine and 1-beta-D-arabinofuranosyluracil following the repeated intravenous administration of high- and intermediate-dose 1-beta-D-arabinofuranosylcytosine. Cancer Res 51:4141, 1991

75. LaRocca RV, Meer J, Gilliatt RW, et al: Suramin-induced polyneuropathy. Neurology 40:954, 1990

76. Forsyth PA, Balmaceda C, Peterson K, et al: Prospective study of taxol-induced peripheral neuropathy (PN) with quantitative sensory testing (QST). Neurology 43, suppl 2:A397, 1993

77. Triozzi PL, Kinney P, Rinehart JJ: Central nervous system toxicity of biological response modifiers. Ann NY Acad Sci 594:347, 1990

78. DeVita VT Jr, Hellman S, Rosenberg SA (eds): Biologic Therapy of Cancer. JB Lippincott, Philadelphia, 1991

79. Schiller JH, Witt PL: Levamisole: clinical and biological effects. p. 1. In DeVita VT Jr, Hellman S, Rosenberg SA (eds): Biologic Therapy of Cancer Updates. Vol 2. JB Lippincott, Philadelphia, 1992

80. Saris SC, Patronas NJ, Rosenberg SA, et al: The effect of intravenous interleukin-2 on brain water content. J Neurosurg 71:169, 1989

81. Merrill JE: Interleukin-2 effects in the central nervous system. Ann NY Acad Sci 594:188, 1990

82. Merimsky O, Reider-Groswasser IR, Inbar M, Chaitchik S: Interferon-related mental deterioration and behavioral changes in patients with renal cell carcinoma. Eur J Cancer 26:596, 1990

83. Bernsen PL, Wong Chung RE, Vingerhoets HM, Janssen JT: Bilateral neuralgic amyotrophy induced by interferon treatment. Arch Neurol 45:449, 1988

84. Gutin PH, Leibel SA, Sheline GE (eds): Radiation Injury to the Nervous System. Raven Press, New York, 1991

85. Young DF, Posner JB, Chu F, Nisce L: Rapid-course radiation therapy of cerebral metastases: results and complications. Cancer 34:1069, 1974

86. Phillips PC, Delattre J-Y, Berger CA, Rottenberg DA: Early and progressive increases in regional brain capillary permeability following single- and fractionated-dose cranial radiation in the rat. Neurology 37, suppl 1:301, 1987

87. Hakansson CH: Effect of irradiation of brain tumours on ventricular fluid pressure. Acta Radiol Ther Phys Biol 6:22, 1967

88. Hoffman WF, Levin VA, Wilson CB: Evaluation of malignant glioma patients during the post-irradiation period. J Neurosurg 50:624, 1979

89. Mandell LR, Walker RW, Steinherz P, Fuks Z: Reduced incidence of the somnolence syndrome in leukemic children with steroid coverage during prophylactic cranial radiation therapy. Cancer 63:1975, 1989

90. Rider WD: Radiation damage to the brain—a new syndrome. J Can Assoc Radiol 14:67, 1963

91. Ashdown BC, Boyko OB, Uglietta JP, et al: Postradiation cerebellar necrosis mimicking tumor: MR appearance. J Comput Assist Tomogr 17:124, 1993

92. Constine LS, Konski A, Elkholm S, et al: Adverse effects of brain irradiation correlated with MR and CT imaging. Int J Radiat Oncol Biol Phys 15:319, 1988

93. Delattre J-Y, Fuks Z, Krol G, et al: Cerebral necrosis following neutron radiation of an extracranial tumor. J Neurooncol 6:113, 1988

94. DiChiro G, Oldfield E, Wright DC, et al: Cerebral necrosis after radiotherapy and/or intraarterial chemotherapy for brain tumors: PET and neuropathologic studies. AJR 150:189, 1988

95. Rottenberg DA, Chernik NL, Deck MD, et al: Cerebral necrosis following radiotherapy of extracranial neoplasms. Ann Neurol 1:339, 1977

96. Shaw PJ, Bates D: Conservative treatment of delayed cerebral radiation necrosis. J Neurol Neurosurg Psychiatry 47:1338, 1984

97. DeAngelis LM, Delattre J-Y, Posner JB: Radiation-induced dementia in patients cured of brain metastases. Neurology 39:789, 1989

98. Laukkanen E, Klonoff H, Allan B, et al: The role of prophylactic brain irradiation in limited stage small cell lung cancer: clinical, neuropsychologic, and CT sequelae. Int J Radiat Oncol Biol Phys 14:1109, 1988

99. Pavlovsky S, Fisman N, Arizaga R, et al: Neuropsychological study in patients with ALL. Am J Pediatr Hematol Oncol 5:79, 1983

100. Tefft M, Mitus A, Schulz MD: Initial high dose irradiation for metastases causing spinal cord compression in children. Am J Roentgenol Radium Ther Nucl Med 106:285, 1969

101. Ushio Y, Posner R, Kim J-H, et al: Treatment of experimental spinal cord compression by extradural neoplasm. J Neurosurg 47:380, 1977

102. Word JA, Kalokhe UP, Aron BS, Elson HR: Transient radiation myelopathy (Lhermitte's sign) in patients with Hodgkin's disease treated by mantle irradiation. Int J Radiat Oncol Biol Phys 6:1731, 1980

103. Dorfman LJ, Donaldson SS, Gupta PR, Bosley TM: Electrophysiologic evidence of subclinical injury to the posterior columns of the human spinal cord after therapeutic radiation. Cancer 50:2815, 1982

104. Lecky BR, Murray NM, Berry RJ: Transient radiation myelopathy: spinal somatosensory evoked responses following incidental cord exposure during radiotherapy. J Neurol Neurosurg Psychiatry 43:747, 1980

105. Dische S, Martin WMC, Anderson P: Radiation myelopathy in patients treated for carcinoma of bronchus

using a six fraction regime of radiotherapy. Br J Radiol 54:29, 1981

106. Sanyal B, Pant GC, Subrahmaniyam K, et al: Radiation myelopathy. J Neurol Neurosurg Psychiatry 42: 413, 1979

107. Michikawa M, Wada Y, Sano M, et al: Radiation myelopathy: significance of gadolinium-DTPA enhancement in the diagnosis. Neuroradiology 33:286, 1991

108. Schultheiss TE, Stephens LC, Maor MH: Analysis of the histopathology of radiation myelopathy. Int J Radiat Oncol Biol Phys 14:27, 1988

109. Allen JC, Miller DC, Budzilovich GN, Epstein FJ: Brain and spinal cord hemorrhage in long-term survivors of malignant pediatric brain tumors: a possible late effect of therapy. Neurology 41:148, 1991

110. Fossa SD, Aass N, Kaahlus O: Long-term morbidity after infradiaphragmatic radiotherapy in young men with testicular cancer. Cancer 64:404, 1989

111. Grunewald RA, Chroni E, Panayiotopoulos CP, Enevoldson TP: Late onset radiation-induced motor neuron syndrome. J Neurol Neurosurg Psychiatry 55: 741, 1992

112. Kristensen O, Melgard B, Schiodt AV: Radiation myelopathy of the lumbo-sacral spinal cord. Acta Neurol Scand 56:217, 1977

113. Lamy C, Mas JL, Varet B, et al: Postradiation lower motor neuron syndrome presenting as monomelic amyotrophy. J Neurol Neurosurg Psychiatry 54:648, 1991

114. Sadowsky CH, Sachs E, Ochoa J: Postradiation motor neuron syndrome. Arch Neurol 33:786, 1976

115. Malapert D, Brugieres P, Degos JD: Motor neuron syndrome in the arms after radiation treatment. J Neurol Neurosurg Psychiatry 54:1123, 1991

116. Berlit P, Schwechheimer K: Neuropathological findings in radiation myelopathy of the lumbosacral cord. Eur Neurol 27:29, 1987

117. Carmichael KA, Jennings AS, Doty RL: Reversible anosmia after pituitary irradiation. Ann Intern Med 100:532, 1984

118. Kinyoun JL, Kalina RE, Brower SA, et al: Radiation retinopathy after orbital irradiation for Graves' ophthalmopathy. Arch Ophthalmol 102:1473, 1984

119. Guy J, Mancuso A, Beck R, et al: Radiation-induced optic neuropathy: a magnetic resonance imaging study. J Neurosurg 74:426, 1991

120. Borsanyi SJ, Blanchard CL: Ionizing radiation in the ear. JAMA 181:958, 1962

121. Moretti JA: Sensorineural hearing loss following radiotherapy to the nasopharynx. Laryngoscope 86:598, 1976

122. Leach W: Irradiation of the ear. J Laryngol Otol 79: 870, 1965

123. Berger PS, Bataini JP: Radiation-induced cranial nerve palsy. Cancer 40:152, 1977

124. Haymaker W, Lindgren M: Nerve disturbances following exposure to ionizing radiation. p. 388. In Vinken PJ, Bruyn GW (eds): Handbook of Clinical Neurology. Vol 7. Elsevier, Amsterdam, 1980

125. Fulton DS: Brachial plexopathy in patients with breast cancer. Dev Oncol 51:249, 1987

126. Lachance DH, O'Neill BP, Harper CM, et al: Paraneoplastic brachial plexopathy in a patient with Hodgkin's disease. Mayo Clin Proc 66:97, 1991

127. Pezzimenti JF, Bruckner HW, DeConti RC: Paralytic brachial neuritis in Hodgkin's disease. Cancer 31:626, 1973

128. Bagley FH, Walsh JW, Cady B, et al: Carcinomatous versus radiation-induced brachial plexus neuropathy in breast cancer. Cancer 41:2154, 1978

129. Kori SH, Foley KM, Posner JB: Brachial plexus lesions in patients with cancer: 100 cases. Neurology 31:45, 1981

130. Glass JP, Pettigrew LC, Maor M: Plexopathy induced by radiation therapy. Neurology 35:1261, 1985

131. Jaeckle KA, Young DF, Foley KM: The natural history of lumbosacral plexopathy in cancer. Neurology 35:8, 1985

132. Albers JW, Allen AA, Bastron JA, Daube JR: Limb myokymia. Muscle Nerve 4:494, 1981

133. Lederman RJ, Wilbourn AJ: Brachial plexopathy: recurrent cancer or radiation? Neurology 34:1331, 1984

134. Cascino TL, Kori SH, Krol G, Foley KM: CT scans of the brachial plexus in patients with cancer. Neurology 33:1553, 1983

135. Thomas JE, Cascino TL, Earle JD: Differential diagnosis between radiation and tumor plexopathy of the pelvis. Neurology 35:1, 1985

136. Soffer D, Pittaluga S, Feiner M, Beller AJ: Intracranial meningiomas following low-dose irradiation to the head. J Neurosurg 59:1048, 1983

137. Liwnicz BH, Berger TS, Liwnicz RG, Aron BS: Radiation-associated gliomas: a report of four cases and analysis of postradiation tumors of the central nervous system. Neurosurgery 17:436, 1985

138. Devinsky O: Radiation-induced tumors of the central and peripheral nervous system. p. 79. In Rottenberg D (ed): Neurological Complications of Cancer Treatment. Butterworth-Heinemann, Boston, 1991

139. Ron E, Modan B, Boice JD, et al: Tumors of the brain and nervous system after radiotherapy in childhood. N Engl J Med 319:1033, 1988

140. McGuirt WF, Feehs RS, Bond G, et al: Irradiation-induced atherosclerosis: a factor in therapeutic planning. Ann Otol Rhinol Laryngol 101:222, 1992

141. Beyer RA, Paden P, Sobel DF, Flynn FG: Moyamoya pattern of vascular occlusion after radiotherapy for glioma of the optic chiasm. Neurology 36:1173, 1986

142. Atkinson JLD, Sundt TM Jr, Dale AJD, et al: Radiation-associated atheromatous disease of the cervical carotid artery: report of seven cases and review of the literature. Neurosurgery 24:171, 1989

143. Hancock SL, Cox RS, McDougall IR: Thyroid diseases after treatment of Hodgkin's disease. N Engl J Med 325:599, 1991

144. Maxon HR: Radiation-induced thyroid disease. Med Clin North Am 69:1049, 1985

145. Nader S, Schultz PN, Fuller LM, Samaan NA: Calcium status following neck radiation therapy in Hodgkin's disease. Arch Intern Med 144:1577, 1984

146. Lam K, Tse VK, Wang C, et al: Effects of cranial irradiation on hypothalamic-pituitary function—a 5-year longitudinal study in patients with nasopharyngeal carcinoma. Q J Med 286:165, 1991

23

Connective Tissue Diseases and the Nervous System

Kathleen M. Shannon
Christopher G. Goetz

Connective tissue diseases are usually characterized by striking changes in systemic organs, but nervous system dysfunction may be an early or presenting feature. Indeed, in some cases, nervous system dysfunction may be the sole manifestation of the autoimmune reactions that occur in these disorders. This chapter reviews the clinical, laboratory, and pathological features of some of the vasculitic and connective tissue diseases that may have peripheral and central nervous system (CNS) involvement.

There is no universally agreed classification for the connective tissue diseases and vasculitides. For the purposes of this chapter, the classification as outlined in Table 23-1 will be used. This is based on that of Fauci and co-workers[1] as modified by Scott.[2] Hypersensitivity vasculitis will not be discussed except in the context of the connective tissue diseases.

MECHANISMS OF AUTOIMMUNE DISEASES

The underlying basis of autoimmune connective tissue diseases is believed to be loss of immune system tolerance of self-antigens. The immune system then recognizes an endogenous antigen as foreign and pro-duces autoantibodies and autoreactive T cells. Autoimmune disorders represent a continuum with organ-specific autoimmunity (such as Hashimoto's thyroiditis) at one end and non-organ-specific autoimmunity (such as vasculitis and connective tissue diseases) at the other.[3] Most non-organ-specific autoimmune conditions have a predilection for kidney, muscle, and joint involvement.

The mechanisms of tissue injury in autoimmune vasculitis and connective tissue diseases include antigen-antibody immune complex formation and deposition, cell-mediated immunity, granuloma formation, and scarring. All mechanisms may be applicable to nervous system disorders. Antigen-antibody immune complex formation occurs under conditions of antigen excess. These soluble antigen-antibody complexes may be deposited in tissue or in blood vessel walls, where they activate complement, inducing inflammation and lysosomal enzyme–mediated tissue or blood vessel wall destruction. Circulating immune complexes have been implicated in the pathogenesis of systemic lupus erythematosus and systemic necrotizing vasculitis. In cell-mediated immunity, antigen reacts with sensitized lymphocytes, which release lymphokines. Mononuclear cells are attracted to the site and release damaging lysosomal enzymes or participate in granuloma formation. This mechanism

Table 23-1 Vasculitis and Connective Tissue Diseases

Vasculitis
    Systemic necrotizing vasculitis
        Polyarteritis
        Allergic angiitis and granulomatosis (Churg-Strauss syndrome)
        Overlap syndrome
        Wegener's granulomatosis
    Giant cell arteritis
        Temporal arteritis
        Takayasu's arteritis
    Nervous system vasculitis
        Primary CNS angiitis
        Primary PNS angiitis
    Hypersensitivity vasculitis
        Cutaneous vasculitis
        Henoch-Schönlein purpura
        Serum sickness
        Drug induced vasculitis
        Vasculitis associated with infection
        Vasculitis associated with malignancy
        Vasculitis associated with connective tissue disease
Connective tissue diseases
    Rheumatoid arthritis
    Systemic lupus erythematosus
    Progressive systemic sclerosis (scleroderma)
    Mixed connective tissue disease
    Dermatomyositis/polymyositis/inclusion body myositis
    Sjögren's syndrome
    Behçet's disease

may be responsible for granulomatous vasculitis. The reasons for the loss of immune tolerance of self-antigens in autoimmune disease are unknown, but they may involve a defect in the generation of T suppressor cells, a change in the ability of various cells to present antigen to T helper cells, exposure to foreign antigens that are closely analogous to endogenous antigens, or bypass of the normal T helper cell mechanism for stimulation of effector T and B cells.[3]

VASCULITIS

Vasculitic conditions are those in which autoimmune mechanisms are directed against blood vessel walls. They are differentiated by their propensity to affect blood vessels of a certain size, type, or location;

involvement of particular organ systems such as the skin or lung; granuloma formation; and association with other systemic diseases.[1,4] Vasculitis may occur as a primary disorder, as in systemic necrotizing vasculitis, giant cell arteritis, and isolated nervous system vasculitis[5]; as a hypersensitivity reaction to foreign proteins, drugs, infectious agents, or malignant processes; or as an inflammatory response to self-antigens in the context of other connective tissue diseases.

Systemic Necrotizing Vasculitis

POLYARTERITIS NODOSA, CHURG-STRAUSS SYNDROME, AND OVERLAP SYNDROME

General Medical Features

Polyarteritis nodosa (PAN) is a necrotizing vasculitis of small and medium-sized muscular arteries that preferentially involves branching points and vessel bifurcations. Estimates of incidence range between 1.8 to 6.3 per 100,000 in most populations, but they are as high as 7.7 per 100,000 in certain populations in which hepatitis B is endemic.[6,7] Men are affected twice as often as women. Onset is most commonly between the ages of 40 and 60 years.[6] Arteries are affected segmentally, with aneurysm formation. Unless secondarily involved by neighboring arteries, veins are spared. Renal and visceral arteries are usually involved. The kidney shows vasculitis, hypertensive changes, or glomerulonephritis in 70 percent of patients. There is cardiac involvement in 36 percent of patients. The pulmonary arteries are spared.[8]

Fever, weight loss, and malaise are seen in more than one-half of patients. Hypertension, musculoskeletal symptoms, gastrointestinal complaints, and skin rash occur in about 50 percent. Manifestations of heart disease include congestive heart failure, myocardial infarct, or pericarditis.[8]

Allergic angiitis and granulomatosis *(Churg-Strauss syndrome)* is similar to classic PAN with the following exceptions: (1) pulmonary vessels are frequently involved; (2) vasculitis affects veins, arteries, and venules in addition to small and medium-sized muscular arteries; (3) there are intra- and extravascular granulomas; (4) there may be eosinophilic tissue infiltrates; and (5) severe asthma and peripheral eosinophilia usually occur. The incidence is unknown but is considerably less than PAN.[7] Clinical manifestations are similar to those of PAN except that asthma and transient pulmonary infiltrates are common and often precede other clinical signs by up to 30 years. Skin rash, gastrointestinal involvement, and cardiac disease occur in a proportion similar to that in PAN patients, but renal disease is less common.[8]

A third type of systemic necrotizing vasculitis is the *overlap syndrome*. These patients have features characteristic of both conditions but fit neither PAN nor Churg-Strauss syndrome precisely.[8]

Although the clinical features of systemic involvement separate these syndromes, the neurological features are related to similar types of vasculitic involvement and are therefore discussed as a whole. Nervous system disease is common in these forms of systemic necrotizing vasculitis. The CNS is affected in 8 to 53 percent of patients,[9–12] usually later in the course of disease.[10,13–15] Eighty percent have signs or symptoms of central or peripheral nervous system dysfunction.

CNS Manifestations

In a 12-year retrospective and prospective study of 25 patients with systemic necrotizing vasculitis, 10 developed CNS disease, usually during the second to third year of the vasculitis. Two patterns of CNS disease emerged: 5 patients each had global and focal cerebral dysfunction.[13]

Of the *global symptoms,* headache is the major complaint in more than 50 percent of patients and may relate to sinusitis, uncontrolled hypertension, or, more commonly, inflammation of meningeal blood vessels.[10] Nearly 20 percent of patients have clinical and laboratory evidence of aseptic meningitis at some time during the course of the disease. Mental derangements, seen in nearly one-half of patients, tend to present in one of three way: dementia, psychosis, or generalized encephalopathy. Commonly, there is a global decline in cognitive function, with memory loss and personality change, but it is rare for the family to volunteer these mild complaints spontaneously. More marked psychiatric symptoms include depression or mania, hallucinatory states, and frank paranoid psychoses. Generalized encephalopathy may also present dramatically, with fluctuating level of consciousness, confusion, disorientation, and focal or generalized convulsions.[15] Localizing neurological

signs may be seen but are typically overshadowed by signs of global dysfunction.[10,13]

The electroencephalogram (EEG) shows generalized slow wave activity during periods of active encephalopathy or toxic delirium. Neuroimaging studies in patients with uncomplicated global CNS dysfunction are normal or show generalized atrophy. Cerebrospinal fluid (CSF) is often normal, but in patients with clinical evidence of aseptic meningitis it may be under increased pressure, with an elevated protein concentration and lymphocytic pleocytosis.

Focal CNS manifestations of systemic necrotizing vasculitis typically consist of an acute stroke syndrome, often in the setting of systemic hypertension. Any part of the brain may be affected. Common signs include aphasia, hemiparesis, visual field abnormalities, and sensory disturbances. Extrapyramidal signs, reported rarely, include chorea[10] and parkinsonism.[16] Brainstem and cerebellar syndromes may be seen.

Neuroimaging studies often show focal or multifocal areas of infarction or, less commonly, intraparenchymal hemorrhage. In some cases no obvious underlying lesion can be found.[13] Because of the size of vessels involved, angiography generally does not show evidence of vasculitis.

Areas of focal infarction of various ages are seen at necropsy, and there is evidence of widespread inflammation of small arteries and arterioles. Acute lesions characterized by polymorphonuclear leukocytes, lymphocytes, and plasma cells coexist with transitional and chronic lesions characterized by intimal thickening and occlusion of the vascular lumen.[17] Intracerebral, subarachnoid, or widespread petechial hemorrhage may be seen.[18]

There is clinical evidence of spinal cord involvement in about 2 percent of patients with systemic necrotizing vasculitis.[17] Transverse myelopathy can occur at any cord level and is usually acute or subacute in onset. Necropsy findings include severe myelomalacia, degeneration of anterior and lateral columns, and arteritis with thrombosis of spinal cord arteries. Severe involvement of spinal arteries may result in massive necrosis over large segments of the spinal cord.[19,20] Patchy necrosis and milder vasculitis may be present at autopsy in patients without history of myelopathic symptoms during life. Myelopathy has also been shown to result from cord compression by extramedullary hematoma secondary to ruptured arteritic spinal aneurysm.[21]

Peripheral Neurological Manifestations

Peripheral nerve disease is so common in systemic necrotizing vasculitis that it is thought by many authors to be a major criterion for diagnosis. Vasculitic neuropathy is seen in up to 60 percent of patients and usually is present at onset or develops within the first year of illness.[14,22] Vasculitic neuropathy presents as one of four clinical syndromes: (1) mononeuritis multiplex, (2) confluent or extensive mononeuritis multiplex, (3) distal polyneuropathy, or (4) cutaneous neuropathy.[13]

Mononeuritis multiplex has long been considered the hallmark of peripheral nerve involvement in systemic necrotizing vasculitis. Its onset is often accompanied by severe neuritic pain or dysesthesia and may be acute (developing over hours) or indolent. Involvement of several nerves simultaneously or the sequential development of multiple mononeuropathies leads to the clinical picture of patchy, asymmetrical neuropathy in which involvement of individual nerves is discernible.[23] Dysfunction of cranial nerves, especially the trigeminal, facial, and vestibuloacoustic, in the absence of signs of intramedullary brainstem disease suggests cranial mononeuritis multiplex.[10,13]

When mononeuritis becomes widespread, the clinical picture is that of asymmetrical neuropathy, sometimes affecting all extremities, without clear localization to major nerves. This pattern has been called confluent mononeuritis multiplex. Typically, there is distal weakness, with preferential involvement of the lower limbs. There may be a sensory level at the midportion of the extremities, reflecting a selective vulnerability to nerve infarction at this level.[13,23,24]

The clinical picture of a distal symmetrical polyneuropathy may emerge with evolution of a confluent mononeuritis multiplex. However, its appearance de novo in some patients early in the course of the disease suggests that it may be a separate syndrome. Cutaneous neuropathy is less common than the other forms of neuropathy. Generally, this presents as patchy areas of disrupted sensation that appear in the distribution of small cutaneous nerves. Most commonly, hyperesthetic patches appear on the digits or the soles of the feet.[13,24]

Other rarer syndromes of peripheral nerve involvement in systemic necrotizing vasculitis include brachial plexopathy,[25] radiculopathy,[11] cauda equina syndrome,[26] and ascending polyradiculoneuropathy.[27] Neuropathies may be transient, lasting only minutes, but more commonly they persist for weeks to months. Partial improvement may occur spontaneously or in response to treatment. A fluctuating course with sensory or motor residua, especially in the lower extremities, is common.

Electrophysiological studies are always abnormal in patients with symptomatic neuropathy and nearly always reveal subclinical neuropathy in the remaining patients with systemic necrotizing vasculitis.[28] Wees and associates evaluated 11 patients with this form of vasculitis. Although 59 percent had neuropathic signs and symptoms, all had abnormal electrophysiological studies suggestive of sensorimotor axonal neuropathy.[28]

Biopsy of the sural nerve in patients with abnormal sural nerve conduction studies usually discloses vasculitis of small epineural blood vessels.[28] Lesions in all stages of development from acute to chronic coexist in the same pathological specimen. Nerve bundle infarction is another common pathological sign. The arterial supply to nerves is so distributed that there is a watershed zone in the midextremity area. Infarction in this vulnerable area results in the characteristic midextremity sensory level.[23]

Etiology

Among patients with PAN, 30 percent are found to be positive for hepatitis B surface antigen. In hepatitis B–endemic populations, such as Alaskan eskimos, the incidence of polyarteritis approaches 7.7 per 100,000.[6,7] These data—combined with the demonstration of hepatitis B antigen and circulating hepatitis B antigen-antibody aggregates in the serum and antigen-antibody-complement deposits in vascular lesions—suggest that PAN results from complexes of antibodies and exogenous antigen, which at least in some patients with PAN is hepatitis B antigen. Other microbiological agents rarely associated with PAN include cytomegalovirus, hepatitis A, human T-cell leukemia-lymphoma virus, parvovirus, and human immunodeficiency virus.[6,7]

Treatment and Prognosis

Systemic necrotizing vasculitis is a chronic disease, the neurological features of which are multifocal and fluctuating. When it is untreated, the 5-year survival rate is 13 percent; nearly one-half of patients die within the first 3 months of onset.[14] Renal failure is the most common cause of death, with CNS disease the second most common cause. Corticosteroid treatment improves the 5-year survival rate to 50 to 60 percent.[6] It has been suggested that combined treatment with immunosuppressants and corticosteroids may increase 5-year survival to over 80 percent,[29] but this has not been conclusively proven, and some authors do not recommend the routine use of immunosuppressants.[23]

WEGENER'S GRANULOMATOSIS

General Medical Features

Wegener's granulomatosis is characterized by granulomatous vasculitis of the upper and lower respiratory tract together with glomerulonephritis. The incidence is unknown, but has been estimated at 0.4 cases per 100,000.[30] Men are affected 1.5 times as frequently as women. Onset can occur at any age but is usually between 30 and 40 years of age.

The commonest presentation is with sinus pain, bloody or purulent rhinorrhea, ear pain, otorrhea, otitis media, or hearing loss. Nasopharyngeal disease is progressive, leading to destruction of nasal cartilage, nasal septal perforation, and saddle-nose deformity. Bony destruction of the sinuses is apparent on radiological studies. Pulmonary symptoms, somewhat less common, include productive cough and hemoptysis. At presentation, there is usually evidence of renal disease, though symptoms are uncommon. Fever and malaise often accompany other early symptoms. Skin ulcers, rashes, and subcutaneous nodules are typical dermatological manifestations. Ocular signs include proptosis, nasolacrimal duct obstruction, ocular muscle dysfunction from adjacent granulomatous disease, keratoconjunctivitis, episcleritis, scleritis, corneal ulcers, uveitis, and retinitis. Transient arthralgias are common, but true arthritis is rare. Cardiac disease includes coronary vasculitis and pancarditis.[31]

Published data in several series of patients reveal neurological involvement in 20 to 56 percent of cases.[32–34] In a recent series of 324 patients with Wegener's granulomatosis, neurological signs or symptoms occurred in 33.6 percent and were multiple in 10.8 percent.[35] Three major mechanisms of neurological involvement have been identified: (1) vasculitis,

(2) extension of respiratory tract granulomas to contiguous nervous system structures, and (3) granuloma development remote from the respiratory tract granulomas.[33]

CNS Manifestations

The most common cause of CNS dysfunction is vasculitis of small to medium-size arteries. Cerebral arteritis usually presents late in the course of disease and may cause arterial thrombosis, intraparenchymal and subarachnoid hemorrhage,[33] or, rarely, global cognitive dysfunction.[36] One or more ischemic infarctions were seen in 4 percent of patients in the Mayo Clinic series.[35] Basilar meningitis and dural venous thrombosis result from extension of granulomas. Granulomas may also erode from the nasopharynx into the orbit, affecting the optic nerve in up to 12 percent of cases,[31,37] or from the temporal bone into the temporal lobe. Remote granulomas have been implicated in a case of multiple intracerebral mass lesions.[38]

Global CNS dysfunction with encephalopathy and seizures may result from metabolic derangements secondary to multiple organ system failure, especially in the terminal phase of the illness.[35]

Acute myelopathy with paraparesis has also been seen.[36]

Peripheral Neurological Manifestations

Peripheral neuropathy has been reported in 16 to 28 percent of patients[35,39] and commonly takes the form of a mononeuritis multiplex or of a pure motor, sensory, or mixed sensorimotor polyneuropathy.[35,36] Pathological studies reveal vasculitic changes in the vasa nervorum or axonal degeneration.[35,39]

Impairment of extraocular movements may occur due to extension of granulomas into the orbit, orbital cellulitis, pseudotumor, or cranial neuropathy. External ophthalmoplegia secondary to orbital pseudotumor is unique to Wegener's granulomatosis among the vasculitic syndromes.[35] Cranial neuropathies have been reported most frequently in the second, sixth and seventh nerves,[35,36] but there may be involvement of any of the cranial nerves, which may be affected by vasculitis or granulomas.[40]

Etiology

The demonstration of antineutrophil cytoplasmic antibody, elevated IgE and IgA levels, antigen-antibody complex deposition, and complement activation suggests that Wegener's granulomatosis may be a hypersensitivity reaction to an exogenous antigen.[41,42] Although no antigen has been identified, the clinical disorder frequently begins following a respiratory illness, suggesting that the initial antigen exposure is through the respiratory tract.

Prognosis and Treatment

The 2-year survival rate among untreated patients is 7 percent. The most common causes of death are renal and respiratory failure. Treatment with cyclophosphamide induces a remission in 90 percent of cases, with subsequent relapse in one-third.[7] Corticosteroids are used as adjunctive therapy early in the course of therapy. Treatment with immunosuppressants should be continued for at least 1 year after remission.

Giant Cell Arteritis

POLYMYALGIA RHEUMATICA AND TEMPORAL ARTERITIS

General Medical Features

Polymyalgia rheumatica is a common syndrome characterized by gradual onset of morning aching and stiffness in the muscles of the neck, shoulder, or pelvic girdle. Women are affected twice as often as men, usually during the sixth decade of life. Most patients have mild systemic symptoms including fever and malaise. Physical findings are scant, although tenderness to palpation of characteristic "trigger points" is common. Laboratory studies are remarkable for an elevated erythrocyte sedimentation rate (ESR).[43] Although the etiology is not known, histological evidence supports the concept that there may be a proximal synovitis.[44] An association between polymyalgia rheumatica and temporal arteritis has been recognized for more than 25 years. One-half of patients with temporal arteritis have polymyalgia,[45] and up to 15 percent of patients with polymyalgia rheumatica develop overt temporal arteritis.

Temporal arteritis is an inflammation of medium-sized and large arteries, characteristically involving but not limited to one or more branches of the carotid artery, especially the temporal artery. Reported incidence rates vary between 0.5 and 23.3 per 100,000.[7] This rare disease occurs mostly in patients over the age of 55 years,[46] though it has been reported in younger patients.[47] It is more common in women

and in family members of affected patients. In most patients there is insidious onset of malaise, fatigue, anorexia, weight loss, and myalgia. Low-grade fever occurs in 92 percent of patients. Prodromal symptoms may last for months.[45,48] Headache is the predominant symptom in 60 to 90 percent[45,47,49,50] and is described as a boring or throbbing pain predominantly temporal in location. Tongue, facial, and neck pain and jaw claudication are common. About one-half of patients have physical evidence of arteritis, with temporal artery tenderness, nodularity, or pulselessness. A few patients present only with constitutional symptoms or changes in affect.[50] Rarely, blindness is the presenting symptom.[51] Giant cell or temporal arteritis may also present as a systemic vasculitis. Aortitis, leg claudication, Raynaud's phenomenon, carotid[45] or coronary arteritis, and intestinal infarction have been reported.[52] The ESR is elevated in nearly all cases of temporal arteritis and is generally a reliable indicator of disease activity. However, 2 to 9 percent of patients do not have ESR elevation,[53] and some (particularly elderly) patients may have clinical and pathological improvement despite persistent ESR elevation.

Neurological manifestations are usually restricted to the CNS and to nerves within the orbit, but peripheral nervous system abnormalities may also occur.

CNS Manifestations

The most frequent and significant CNS complication of giant cell or temporal arteritis is blindness due to ischemic optic neuropathy, retinopathy, or retrobulbar neuritis.[54] In the past, blindness occurred in up to 60 percent of cases.[24,47,50] Because of increased recognition and appropriate treatment of this syndrome, more recent data suggest that the risk of blindness is much lower. In a recent series of 166 biopsy-proven cases, 8 percent developed permanent visual loss.[55] Amaurosis fugax, scintillating scotoma, and diplopia were also seen, but these symptoms did not presage the development of blindness.[55] Gradual onset of blindness over a period of months has also been reported.[56] Untreated, blindness in one eye is followed by blindness in the other in 25 percent of patients.

Involvement of large intracranial arteries produces transient or permanent brain ischemia in 7 percent of cases.[55] There is some evidence that temporal arteritis has a predilection to affect the posterior circulation.[57] Multi-infarct dementia has been reported.[58] Other less common manifestations of CNS dysfunction include encephalopathy, seizures,[52] tremor, and affective disorder.[55] Myelopathy is rare.[55]

Histologically, inflammatory infiltrate with lymphocytes, plasma cells, and histiocytes begins in the media and then extends into the intima and adventitia of affected vessels. The internal elastic lamina becomes segmented and necrotic. Multinucleated giant cells appear at the media–intima junction; fibrosis occurs in the media of the vessel wall, and the vascular lumen narrows.

Peripheral Neurological Manifestations

The most common signs and symptoms of peripheral nerve involvement reflect dysfunction of the innervation of the extraocular muscles. Ischemia of these cranial nerves probably results from arteritis of the meningohypophyseal trunk or recurrent collaterals of the ophthalmic artery.[52] Alternatively, ischemia of the extraocular muscles themselves may occur.[59] Peripheral neuropathy has been seen in 14 percent of cases in some series[55] and usually presents as a mononeuropathy or distal symmetrical polyneuropathy.[55] Cervical radiculopathy has also been described.[52]

Etiology

The etiology of temporal arteritis is unknown. It has been postulated that the disease results from circulating immune complex–mediated vasculitis or an immune reaction to elastin in arterial walls.[52]

Prognosis and Treatment

Temporal arteritis is a self-limited disease, usually running its course over 1 to 2 years. Death is rare but may occur from myocardial infarction or stroke in inadequately treated patients.[60] Corticosteroids should be instituted as soon as the diagnosis is suspected, because visual loss rarely reverses once it has occurred.[61] The ESR can be used as a marker of disease activity in some patients, but symptoms should be followed closely. Corticosteroids may be slowly tapered as tolerated. An alternate-day regime helps to reduce adverse effects.

Some authors have recommended that only clinically atypical cases and patients with known contraindications to corticosteroid therapy should be biop-sied.[62] A low threshold for consideration of temporal artery biopsy seems reasonable, however, because patients are generally elderly and prone to complications of corticosteroid therapy. Biopsy should be performed as soon as possible after initiation of corticosteroid therapy. Because the arteritis is patchy and segmental, a long biopsy sample should be obtained, and bilateral biopsy may be required.

TAKAYASU'S ARTERITIS

General Medical Features

Takayasu's arteritis, a rare disease of young women, is characterized by inflammation, scarring, and occlusion of the aorta and proximal portions of its major branches. The estimated annual incidence in Olmstead County, Minnesota, is 0.3 per 100,000,[63] but the condition is more common in Asian countries. Most patients present between the ages of 11 and 30 years with systemic symptoms including fever, malaise, night sweats, arthralgias, and weight loss. These symptoms may resolve for a period of time, during which the patient appears minimally affected. The patient then begins to manifest evidence of aortitis and branch occlusion including hypertension, valvular insufficiency, extremity claudication, angina, and visceral infarction. Postural dizziness and visual disturbance (blurring, diplopia, or amaurosis) are common. Clinical signs during this phase include diminished or absent pulse or blood pressure, a blood pressure discrepancy of more than 30 mmHg between the left and right arms, cardiac murmurs, diffuse bruits, and signs of congestive heart failure.[64–68] Funduscopic examination may reveal hypertensive retinopathy, microaneurysms, venous dilatation and beading, and retinal hemorrhages. Late ocular signs include optic atrophy, retinal detachment, and vitreous hemorrhage. Arthritis, skin lesions, coronary artery disease, pulmonary hypertension, and renal involvement may occur.[64] Mild anemia, leukocytosis, hypergammaglobulinemia, and an elevated ESR may accompany the systemic signs.

Takayasu's arteritis is a panarteritis that preferentially affects the aorta and aortic arch, subclavian and carotid arteries, and renal arteries. Other branches of the aorta are affected to a lesser degree. Diagnosis requires angiography with visualization of the entire aorta and the renal and visceral arteries.[64] Histologically, it is characterized by focal and segmental medial necrosis accompanied by infiltration of lymphocytes, plasma cells, and sometimes multinucleated giant cells. There is destruction of the internal elastic membrane as well as intimal thickening and fibrosis. The end result is obliteration of the vascular lumen.[69,70]

Neurological Features

Minor neurological complaints, including headache and orthostatic dizziness or syncope, are fairly common.[71,72] Significant neurological complications are restricted to the CNS. Up to 10 percent of patients have symptoms of transient ischemia in a carotid distribution or completed stroke with hemiplegia. Seizures have occurred in a few patients,[71,72] as has myelopathy.

Etiology

The discovery of circulating antiaorta antibodies and immunoglobulin deposition in arteritic lesions have added little to understanding the etiology of this unusual condition.[67] There have been some suggestions of an association with prior streptococcal infections or tuberculin skin test positivity. Rarely, circulating immune complexes have been reported.[64] However, the etiology of the disorder remains obscure.

Treatment and Prognosis

Takayasu's arteritis has a good prognosis. The 5-year survival rate is 83 percent.[73,74] The prognosis is worse in patients with severe complications or a progressive course.[64] Death usually results from major complications of the disease, including congestive heart failure, myocardial infarction, ruptured aortic aneurysm, and renal failure, often in patients in whom diagnosis or treatment was delayed.[74]

Treatment is with corticosteroids, which are instituted at a moderate daily dose and slowly tapered as tolerated. The ESR may be used to assess disease activity. Most patients require therapy for at least 2 years. There are currently no guidelines for treatment of established occlusive disease.[52]

Primary Angiitis of the Nervous System

PRIMARY ANGIITIS OF THE CNS

General Medical Features

Primary angiitis of the CNS is a rare vasculitis of unknown etiology, which, for the most part, is restricted to the small and medium-sized arteries of the CNS. Lie recently reported 15 pathologically proven cases and reviewed 108 cases from the literature.[75] These data suggest that the average age of onset is 45 years, with a slight male predominance of cases. Clinical onset is subacute, with headache, weakness, and changes in cognition and level of consciousness. Fewer than 25 percent of patients have fever or other systemic signs or symptoms. There have been occasional reports of an associated systemic vasculitis, but this is unusual. In contrast to earlier suggestions that the ESR is elevated in 70 percent of cases,[76] more recent data suggest that this test is rarely helpful.[5,75] Diagnosis rests on the demonstration of vasculitic changes by cerebral arteriogram and meningeal biopsy and on exclusion of systemic illness as a cause of vasculitis.[75]

Neurological Features

The disorder is rapidly progressive, even fulminant. Global deficits—such as, confusion, loss of memory, and delirium—are common.[75-78] Among untreated patients, 90 percent eventually develop focal CNS signs, which are multiple in 80 percent.[77] Focal weakness of at least one limb is present in more than 50 percent of patients.[52,76] Focal or generalized seizures occur in 25 percent.[52,76] Aphasia and hemiparesis are common. Cranial nerve dysfunction is either supranuclear in origin or secondary to increased intracranial pressure and brain herniation.[52,76] Progression to stupor or coma follows often. Extrapyramidal and cerebellar or brainstem signs develop in a few cases.[76] Myelopathy, which may have a relapsing and remitting course, is seen in up to 15 percent of patients and may lead to the erroneous diagnosis of multiple sclerosis.[78,79]

The EEG is abnormal in more than 80 percent of patients, showing generalized slowing, at times with focal predominance.[76] The CSF demonstrates lymphocytic pleocytosis in 90 percent of patients, and an elevated protein concentration is nearly as common. Computed tomography (CT) scans frequently show patchy areas of ischemia and edema, though these changes are nonspecific. Cerebral angiography may show arterial "beading," aneurysms, or arterial branch occlusions, but it may also be normal. Biopsy of the meninges and gray and white matter in an area thought clinically to be involved gives the definitive diagnosis.[75]

The small arteries and arterioles of the parenchyma and leptomeninges are affected predominantly, and the larger intracranial or extracranial arteries are rarely involved.[75] Segmental intimal proliferation and narrowing, with a dense inflammatory infiltrate consisting of lymphocytes, plasma cells, and multinucleated giant cells, are seen. Fibrinoid necrosis is present, with disruption of the internal elastic lamina. The media is relatively spared. Healing lesions appear in the same biopsy specimen as active arterial lesions.[75] The clinical manifestations can be explained on the basis of ischemia, with extensive small infarctions.[52] Although this condition is often referred to as a granulomatous angiitis, only 50 percent of biopsied cases demonstrate granulomatous changes; others show lymphomatous or necrotizing angiitis.[75]

Etiology

The etiology of the disorder is unknown. Associations have been reported with herpes zoster and Hodgkin's lymphoma.[75] Less commonly, the disorder has been linked to cytomegalovirus, human T-lymphotropic virus, and mycoplasma.[75,80,81]

Prognosis and Treatment

The prognosis is generally regarded as dismal, with inexorable progression to death within an average of 45 days.[52,76] However, corticosteroid therapy in combination with immunosuppressive agents has produced remissions of significant duration.[75,77,82] In one recent series of 48 cases, 95 percent of untreated patients, 46 percent of patients receiving corticosteroids, and 8 percent of patients treated with corticosteroids and immunosuppression died.[83] It is recommended that prednisone and cyclophosphamide be started, with the prednisone gradually changed to an alternate-day regimen after several weeks and then tapered after the disease has clinically remitted (usually in 6 to 12 months). The cyclophosphamide should be continued for 12 months after remission of the illness.[5]

PRIMARY ANGIITIS OF THE PERIPHERAL NERVOUS SYSTEM

General Medical Features

Primary angiitis of the peripheral nervous system is a rare disorder of unknown etiology. It is defined as the occurrence of vasculitic neuropathy in the absence of systemic arteritis. Clinical similarities to polyarteritis nodosa as well as the demonstration in some patients of vasculitis within muscle have led some authors to conclude that this entity represents a localized form of polyarteritis nodosa. However, others have noted differences in prognosis and pathology and have therefore suggested that this diagnostic entity be retained.[5,84]

Dyck and associates reviewed 20 cases with symptoms of persistent neuropathy in the absence of systemic signs and symptoms and with histopathological evidence of indolent necrotizing vasculitis of small epineural arterioles.[84] The disorder presented at about 50 years of age, affected women more commonly than men, and led to subacute symptoms of peripheral neuropathy.[84]

The ESR is commonly normal but may be elevated. Rheumatoid factor and other antibody studies are usually normal.

Neurological Manifestations

Neurological manifestations are limited to the peripheral nervous system. Paresthesias and pain are followed by pain and sensory deficits that progress over hours to days and then remain static or resolve. Onset is commonly in the lower extremity, usually in a sciatic nerve distribution. Progression leads to a multiple mononeuropathy. Symmetrical or asymmetrical distal sensory or sensorimotor neuropathy may be seen. Cranial nerves are occasionally affected.[5,84] Electrophysiological studies demonstrate multifocal axonal neuropathy.[84]

Prognosis and Treatment

In the series of Dyck and colleagues, the prognosis was good, with deterioration in 8 of 20 patients and improvement or no change in 9. Three patients died of unrelated illnesses.[84]

There has been no systematic study of therapy for this condition. Because the prognosis is often benign, therapy should be chosen based on the severity of individual symptoms and the nature and tempo of progression. Patients are best treated with corticosteroids; adjunctive immunosuppressant therapy is reserved for patients whose disorder progresses despite this initial approach.[84]

CONNECTIVE TISSUE DISEASES

Rheumatoid Arthritis

General Medical Features

Rheumatoid arthritis is a chronic multisystem disease of unknown etiology that affects 1 to 2 percent of the population. Women account for 75 percent of cases. Disease onset is between 35 and 50 years of age in 80 percent of cases. There is a genetic predisposition to developing the disorder: first-degree relatives of seropositive patients are four times more likely to acquire the disease than controls. Criteria for diagnosis are listed in Table 23-2.[86] The onset is typically insidious, with a variable duration of prodromal malaise, fatigue, and generalized weakness. Characteristic symmetrical polyarthritis develops within weeks to months. Articular signs and symptoms preferentially affect certain joints—metacarpophalangeal, proximal interphalangeal, wrist, elbow, knee, ankle, forefoot, and subtalar joints—and the cervical spine. Progression of joint disease leads to bony erosion and joint deformity. Extra-articular manifestations tend to occur in patients with high levels of circulating rheumatoid factor. Rheumatoid nodules may be found in the subcutaneous tissues, connective tissues of any organ, or serous membranes. Pleuropulmonary manifestations, typically occurring in men, include pleuritis, interstitial fibrosis, pneumonitis, and pulmonary nodules. Myocardial nodules and small pericardial effusions are frequent but usually asymptomatic. Felty's syndrome (rheumatoid arthritis, splenomegaly, neutropenia, anemia, and thrombocy-topenia) is seen in some patients with long-standing disease.

A few patients develop systemic vasculitis. Systemic rheumatoid vasculitis is diagnosed when a person who meets the criteria for rheumatoid arthritis develops ischemic skin lesions, mononeuritis multiplex, or documented visceral vasculitis.[87] While usually seen in men who have had rheumatoid arthritis for more than 10 years, it may occur in women or at disease presentation.[87] The course of vasculitis may be indolent or explosive.

Neurological manifestations occur in patients with moderate to severe rheumatoid arthritis. In addition to nervous system dysfunction directly caused by the disease (rheumatoid nodules, rheumatoid vasculitis), neurological dysfunction can be a secondary effect of joint or bone disease (synovitis, changes in bony architecture).

CNS Manifestations

Rheumatoid nodules frequently form in the dura mater, where they tend to be asymptomatic except in cases of extensive involvement with pachymeningitis.[88,89] Although most intracranial rheumatoid nodules are limited to the meninges, there have been reports of extensive intraparenchymal granulomas presenting with seizures[90] and obtundation.[88] The histological appearance of a rheumatoid nodule is a center of palisading histiocytes which is further enveloped in lymphocytes, plasma cells, and multinucleated giant cells.[88]

The occurrence of symptomatic CNS vasculitis is actually rare, even in the setting of active systemic vasculitis.[91,92] Twelve cases of CNS vasculitis have appeared in the literature.[93–95] CNS disease follows onset of the rheumatoid arthritis by 1 to 30 years. The CNS manifestations includes seizures, dementia, hemiparesis, cranial nerve palsy, blindness, hemispheric dysfunction, cerebellar ataxia, and dysphasia. Pathological examination reveals chronic perivasculitis, transmural chronic inflammatory cell infiltration, intimal collagen proliferation with luminal narrowing, and fibrinoid necrosis of the media of small arteries.[93] The coexistence of vasculitis and amyloid in the same CNS blood vessels has been noted,[93] but the significance of this finding is not known.

Changes in the articular architecture of the cervical spine may produce CNS dysfunction at the hemi-

Table 23-2 Criteria of the American Rheumatological Association for the Diagnosis of Rheumatoid Arthritis[a]

Morning stiffness
Arthritis of three or more joint areas
Arthritis of hand joints
Symmetrical arthritis
Rheumatoid nodules
Positive serum rheumatoid factor
Radiological changes

[a] The first four criteria must be present for at least 6 weeks. For diagnosis, patients must satisfy at least four criteria.

spheric, brainstem, or spinal cord level. Significant disease of the cervical spine is present in up to 70 percent of patients with advanced disease. The major changes in the cervical spine include vertebral body erosion and collapse,[96] rheumatoid discitis,[97] dural thickening and fibrosis with spinal cord compression,[98] and—most commonly—atlantoaxial subluxation.[99] Atlantoaxial subluxation occurs when rheumatoid changes affect the synovial joints between the dens and the atlas anteriorly and the dens and the transverse ligament posteriorly. Progressive changes include joint destruction, erosion of the dens, and lysis of the bony attachment of the transverse ligament. These changes, in concert with destruction of cervical facet joint capsules, result in four patterns of cervical subluxation: (1) anterior displacement of C1 on C2, (2) posterior movement of C1 on C2, (3) vertical subluxation resulting in protrusion of the odontoid process into the foramen magnum, and (4) subluxation of one vertebra on another at multiple levels (staircase subluxation).[100]

Cervical subluxation is often asymptomatic. In patients who are symptomatic, the most striking features are myelopathic. However, other symptoms have been reported, including occipital headache[101] and obstructive hydrocephalus.[102] Brainstem syndromes have been reported to result from pseudoaneurysm of the vertebral artery, attributed to cervical arthritis,[103] and from direct compression of the medulla by eroded, displaced odontoid fragments and rheumatoid granuloma.[104] Neurological manifestations more commonly result from intermittent or sustained anterior cord compression, sometimes complicated by ischemia in the distribution of branches of the anterior spinal artery, which may be compressed. Neck pain is common. Hyperreflexia, sometimes accompanied by extensor plantar responses, is seen in up to two-thirds of patients with radiological evidence of subluxation,[105] many of whom are asymptomatic. Weakness (affecting the arms before the legs), flexor spasms, sphincter disturbances, paresthesias, pain, and sensory changes are seen somewhat less frequently. More severe symptoms, including death, may result from extreme compression of the cord, snapping of the weakened odontoid process, or severe displacement of C1 due to marked hyperextension, as with endotracheal intubation. Patients with cervical subluxation tend to have more severe rheumatoid arthritis, but subluxa-

tion per se does not decrease life expectancy. Thus except in cases of extreme vertebral displacement, surgical fixation is probably not necessary. Among patients treated conservatively, 75 percent show no progression or actually improve over time.[106]

Peripheral Neurological Manifestations

Peripheral nerve disease is almost universal in rheumatoid arthritis. Its causes include nerve entrapment or compression, segmental demyelination, and vasculitic involvement of the vasa nervorum.

Entrapment or compression of peripheral nerves by inflamed synovial sacs occurs in 45 percent of patients.[107] Most commonly trapped is the median nerve, at the level of the carpal tunnel. Ulnar compression may occur at the cubital canal or canal of Guyon at the wrist. Radial nerve involvement usually presents as posterior interosseous syndrome. The tibial or common peroneal nerve may be compressed by a Baker's cyst, or there may be a common peroneal pressure palsy. In the distribution of the posterior tibial nerve, there may be tarsal tunnel syndrome or medial or lateral plantar syndrome.[100,107]

A mild distal sensorimotor polyneuropathy is common, occurring in more than 30 percent of patients, often as the sole extra-articular manifestation. Vibration may be impaired out of proportion to other sensory modalities, reflecting the primary underlying pathology, which is segmental demyelination, with lesser degrees of axonal damage. A more severe neuropathy may occur in the setting of systemic arteritis and is characterized histologically by wallerian degeneration. Vasculitic changes underlie both types of neuropathy, implying that both segmental demyelination and wallerian degeneration can result from lesions of the vasa nervorum.

A mononeuritis multiplex may develop in the setting of rheumatoid systemic vasculitis. Sudden onset of neuritic pain or dysesthesias is followed by marked weakness and sensory changes in the distribution of one or more named nerves. A patchy, asymmetrical neuropathy results and may progress to the pattern of a confluent mononeuritis.[108] Electrophysiological studies suggest predominantly axonal, sensorimotor involvement.

Myositis may be seen but is not usually a prominent feature of the disorder.

Etiology

Rheumatoid arthritis is an immune complex disease. Immune complexes are composed of IgG combined with IgM or IgG anti-IgG antibodies. Immune complex–mediated complement activation is localized to the synovial membrane. The original antigen responsible for inducing formation of anti-IgG antibody is unknown.

Prognosis and Treatment

Rheumatoid vasculitis with central or peripheral nervous system manifestations should be treated as any other systemic vasculitis. Immunosuppressant therapy is introduced along with corticosteroids; the corticosteroids are tapered after several weeks, the primary goal being monotherapy with immunosuppressants. The role of plasmapheresis is not known.[52] The prognosis is similar to that of systemic necrotizing vasculitis.

Cervical subluxation should be treated conservatively with analgesics, muscle relaxants, and neck immobilization. Protection from inadvertent and iatrogenic trauma is essential. So treated, 50 percent of patients stabilize, and 25 percent improve over time; 25 percent have progressive myelopathy.[106] Patients whose vertebral displacement is severe and associated with marked or progressive myelopathy are best treated with surgical fixation.

Patients with mild symmetrical polyneuropathy or mononeuritis multiplex should be treated conservatively, with attention to optimal treatment of the underlying disease and symptomatic treatment of neuritic complaints. Patients in whom neuropathy is severe and disabling should be treated as for systemic vasculitis.

Systemic Lupus Erythematosus

General Medical Features

Systemic lupus erythematosus (SLE) is an autoimmune multisystem inflammatory disease that predominantly affects women during the childbearing years.[109] Epidemiological studies in the United States suggest that SLE is more common in blacks than whites and that it occurs with increased frequency in family members of affected patients.[110] Articular and cutaneous signs and symptoms occur in more than 80 percent of patients. There is symmetrical arthritis of large and small joints, with deformity but without

Table 23-3 Criteria of the American Rheumatological Association for the Diagnosis of Systemic Lupus Erythematosus[a]

Malar rash
Discoid rash
Photosensitivity
Oral ulcers
Arthralgia/arthritis
Pleuritis/pericarditis
Persistent proteinuria/cellular casts
Seizures/psychosis
Hemolytic anemia/leukopenia/lymphopenia/thrombocytopenia
Positive LE cell preparation/anti-DNA/anti-Sm/false positive syphilis serology
Antinuclear antibody

[a] The presence of any four during any period of observation has an estimated specificity of 96 percent and sensitivity of 96 percent.

radiographic evidence of erosion. Although the malar "butterfly" rash is the hallmark of SLE, maculopapular rash, livedo reticularis, plaque-like (discoid) lesions, and oral and nasal ulcerations may occur as well. Renal and cardiopulmonary diseases occur in 50 to 60 percent of cases. Glomerulonephritis is the major determinant of morbidity and mortality. Cardiopulmonary involvement includes myocarditis, pericarditis, endocarditis, pneumonitis, pleuritis, and hemoptysis. Hematological abnormalities—including anemia, leukopenia, thrombocytopenia, and circulating anticoagulant—are common. Fever, malaise, or fatigue occurs in 80 percent of patients.[110] Diagnostic criteria are listed in Table 23-3.

Nervous system involvement can be documented at some point in the disease course in 25 to 75 percent of patients with SLE[111] and is second only to renal disease as a cause of death.[112] Neurological disorders appear within the first year of the disease in up to 63 percent of patients and are the initial manifestation in as many as 3 percent.[113] In most cases, there is evidence of increased systemic activity of the disease at the time that neurological signs develop.

CNS Manifestations

SLE affects the CNS at every level. The most common symptoms of cerebral pathology are *behavioral*. Occurring in up to 59 percent of patients with SLE, they include visual and auditory hallucinations, paranoid delusions, schizophreniform psychoses, and affective disorders.[114] Catatonia and conversion[115] symptoms have also been reported. Typically, psychiatric symptoms present early in the course of disease and are often accompanied by delirium, seizures, or evidence of focal neurological dysfunction.[114,115] Individual episodes last for weeks to months and may be recurrent.

Routine laboratory studies are consistent with active systemic disease. The EEG may be normal[116] or show nonspecific generalized slow wave activity.[117] CSF may be normal or show mild pleocytosis and elevated protein concentration.[116] CT scans and magnetic resonance imaging (MRI) may show generalized atrophy, evidence of cerebral infarction or intracranial hemorrhage, or no abnormality.[118]

At autopsy the major CNS findings relate to microvascular injury. More than one-half have vascular hyalinization, perivascular lymphocytosis, endothelial proliferation, and microvascular thrombosis. Large vessel involvement is not usually seen.[119]

Dementia has not been regarded as a prominent manifestation of cerebral lupus, but formal neuropsychiatric testing suggests that 66 percent of patients have cognitive impairment, which may be independent of other signs of CNS involvement.[120]

Signs of *increased intracranial pressure* may accompany focal pathology in the CNS or may occur in the setting of dural sinus thrombosis or CNS infection.[113] Pseudotumor cerebri, with papilledema and normal CSF, is seen in a small number of patients with SLE.

Although signs of meningeal inflammation are present in 18 percent of autopsied patients with SLE,[119] the clinical diagnosis of *aseptic meningitis* is made infrequently.[113,117] Often, although the CSF is abnormal, the clinical picture is overwhelmed by psychiatric or other neurological signs, and an alternative diagnosis is suggested. Aseptic meningitis is more likely to be diagnosed when it occurs early in the course of SLE and when headache, neck pain, and nuchal rigidity are the major presenting features. CSF analysis reveals a lymphocytic or, less commonly, neutrophilic pleocytosis and an elevated CSF protein concentration.[117]

Seizures may occur early or late in the course of SLE. The frequency increases with duration of disease, so that by the time of death, 30 to 54 percent of patients have had one or more seizures.[111,115,116]

Seizures may be partial or generalized and may occur in the setting of azotemia or systemic infection. They almost invariably occur during an active phase of the disease and frequently are accompanied by other neuropsychiatric symptoms and signs. Frequently, there is CSF pleocytosis, with increased protein concentration. The EEG is almost always abnormal, but often in a nonspecific way. When the clinical examination shows evidence of focal CNS involvement, neuroimaging studies may show focal pathology. Small vessel vasculopathy—with small infarctions in the cerebral cortex and subcortical white matter and intracranial and subarachnoid hemorrhage—is seen at autopsy.[116,119]

In a recent series of 91 patients with SLE, *stroke* occurred in 15 percent; it was multiple in 64 percent of these patients.[111] Stroke most often occurs at an intermediate stage of the illness, but in rare cases it may precede overt SLE. Its occurrence is significantly associated with cardiac valvular abnormalities, coagulopathy, and the lupus anticoagulant.[111] In some cases, stroke may be caused by true CNS vasculitis, though this is rare.[121] In 11 cases culled from the literature, vasculitis involved the branches of the anterior or posterior cerebral arteries, vessels in the circle of Willis, or spinal arteries. In nearly 50 percent of cases, presentation was with intracerebral or subarachnoid hemorrhage. Death occurred in 67 percent of cases.[121]

CSF may be normal or show increased protein concentration, a pleocytosis, or hemorrhage. CT and MRI scans are frequently abnormal, with evidence of focal infarction or hemorrhage. Strokes in SLE are usually small bland infarcts reflecting the underlying pathology, which is a vasculopathy of small vessels. However, when associated with vasculitis, they are larger and more likely to involve the territories of large named cerebral vessels.

Chorea, athetosis, or *ballism* complicate SLE in fewer than 2 percent of patients in large series.[116,122] Lusins and Szilagyi reported three cases of SLE-associated chorea and reviewed 25 well-documented cases from the literature. Chorea was a major presenting features of SLE in 14 cases and the sole presenting sign in another 7, preceding other signs of the disease by weeks to years.[122] Chorea in SLE often begins abruptly and may be self-limited. It may be unilateral or generalized and may affect the extremities or face. Neuropathological studies of seven patients showed the expected small vessel vasculopathy, but changes in the basal ganglia were surprisingly absent.[116] *Parkinsonian rest tremor* with or without cogwheel rigidity has also been reported in a few patients.[116]

Myelopathy is a rare manifestation of CNS lupus, found in only 1 of 57 autopsied cases in one series.[119] Provenzale and Bouldin reported 2 and reviewed 31 cases from the literature.[123] Myelopathy usually develops in the first several years of the illness. It may precede the diagnosis of SLE, but multiple organ system involvement is usually seen at presentation. Most patients develop pain and paresthesias which progress over a few days to paraplegia or, less commonly, quadriplegia. In an earlier series of patients, 50 percent died, most from such complications as infections or pulmonary embolism; among survivors, two-thirds remained disabled and one-third made significant recoveries.[124] CSF studies are usually abnormal. Elevated protein and depressed glucose levels and a lymphocytic pleocytosis are common, but there are no specific changes. Three types of pathological changes usually underlie the myelopathy of SLE. First, there may be segmental softening, accompanied by perivasculitis, fibrinoid arteritis, or thrombosis. Second, subdural hematoma may occur, with cord compression. Finally, there may be subpial white matter degeneration at multiple cord levels.[123] Spinal subarachnoid hemorrhage secondary to rupture of an arteritic posterior spinal artery has also been described.[125]

Peripheral Neurological Manifestations

Peripheral neuropathy affects 2 to 18 percent of patients with SLE.[126] Three major patterns have been reported. Most often there is an acute or subacute symmetrical demyelinating polyneuropathy. There may be a predominance of sensory or motor symptoms, or the picture may be that of a mixed sensorimotor neuropathy. Diminution of sensation in a "stocking-glove" distribution is accompanied by distal weakness. Autonomic insufficiency may also be present. The course is variable.[127]

A second pattern of involvement is reminiscent of acute Guillain-Barré syndrome with ascending motor radiculoneuropathy and autonomic dysfunction, sometimes following a rapidly progressive course.[128] With both modes of presentation, there is moderate to marked elevation in CSF protein concentration, without pleocytosis. Nerve conduction velocities are nearly always abnormal.

In some patients with SLE, peripheral nerve involvement presents as a mononeuropathy. The ulnar, radial, sciatic, or peroneal nerve may be involved. Multiple mononeuropathies may occur simultaneously, or single or multiple mononeuropathies may be superimposed on a symmetrical distal polyneuropathy.[116] Unilateral or bilateral optic neuropathy may also occur.

Pathological studies in SLE-associated neuropathy show two major types of lesions. In some cases there is clear evidence of vasculopathy. Mononuclear infiltrates surround perineural blood vessels, and rarely there is intimal thickening with vascular occlusion. In most there is loss of myelin in peripheral nerves, anterior and posterior roots, and posterior columns. The second type, however, shows little evidence of vasculopathy. Rather, there is axonal degeneration with infiltration and spreading of nerve fibers by amorphous material.[129]

Etiology

That no single pathophysiological mechanism accounts for all the nervous system manifestations of SLE is evidenced by the diversity of clinical presentations and pathological findings. Autoantibodies to ribosomal P proteins,[130] nucleic acids,[114] and neuronal antigens[131] have been found in the CSF and serum. Reduced levels of IgG and C4[114] and evidence of complement activation[132] have been demonstrated in the CSF. Antibodies to measles virus have also been found in the CSF.[114] The relationship of these abnormalities to the occurrence and clinical pattern of nervous system involvement is unknown.

Stoke in SLE may be associated with the lupus anticoagulant or anticardiolipin antibody. The lupus anticoagulant antibody is an IgG or IgM immunoglobulin that inhibits the generation of prothrombinase by disrupting calcium-dependent binding of prothrombin (factor II) and factor Xa to phospholipids. It is detected by a prolongation in the activated partial thromboplastin time in the presence of a normal or slightly prolonged prothrombin time.[133] Confirmatory tests include the kaolin clotting time, the dilute Russel viper venom time, and others.[133] Another type of antiphospholipid antibody is the anticardiolipin antibody, which can be detected by enzyme-linked immunosorbent assay (ELISA) in up to 61 percent of patients with SLE.[133] Although there is a correlation between these antibodies in some series, not all patients with anticardiolipin antibody have lupus anticoagulant antibody. Patients with SLE and either antibody have a propensity to develop venous and arterial thromboses. They are also prone to fetal loss and thrombocytopenia.[133]

Treatment and Prognosis
The 5-year survival rate in SLE ranges from 77 to 98 percent but is lower for those with nervous system involvement.[52,112] Corticosteroids in moderate doses are the mainstay of treatment. Although corticosteroids have been thought by some to contribute to the occurrence of psychosis,[134] this has largely been discounted.[115,116] Immunosuppressants and plasma exchange have been used in particularly severe or fulminant cases, but the value of the latter treatment is not known.[52] Because of the risk of recurrence in patients with SLE who have had a stroke, anticoagulation is recommended for such patients, especially those who are found to have lupus anticoagulant or anticardiolipin antibody.[111,113]

Progressive Systemic Sclerosis

General Medical Features
Progressive systemic sclerosis (scleroderma) is a disorder of excessive collagen deposition in the skin, blood vessels, and other organs.[135] The incidence ranges from 0.6 to 2.3 per 1,000,000.[136] Women, usually between the ages of 40 and 60 years, are affected three times as often as men. There may be several subtypes of the disorder. Some patients appear to have a form that is limited to cutaneous changes in the distal extremities; it carries a more benign prognosis. In the generalized form of the illness, cutaneous abnormalities may predominate, but systemic symptoms, including generalized malaise, are common. Vascular changes in the hands progress from Raynaud's phenomenon to frank necrosis and induration and fibrosis of the skin (sclerodactyly), with atrophy of the underlying muscle. Rigidity of ligamentous tissue in the inner ear leads to conductive hearing loss. There may be fibrotic changes in the myocardium, pericardium, pleura, or lung. Glomerulonephritis is

a frequent cause of morbidity and mortality. Mucosal gastrointestinal lesions occur, especially in the distal esophagus. Keratoconjunctivitis, lens subluxation, and cataracts make up the typical ocular signs. Musculoskeletal changes, including atrophy and osteolytic lesions, joint symptoms, and myopathy occur in 50 percent of patients.[135]

Nervous system disease is uncommon, occurring in only 6 of 727 patients in one large series.[135] In another study, neurological signs or symptoms occurred in 24 of 130 patients but in most cases could be attributed to other metabolic derangements or to iatrogenic causes.

CNS Manifestations
Although rare, CNS disease has been reported. It may present as global cognitive decline or as a focal lesion. Focal hemispheric or brainstem deficits may include pyramidal, sensory, extrapyramidal, and bulbar signs.[137,138] Three cases with presumed cerebral arteritis have been reported, one having a reversible encephalopathy with angiographic evidence of vasculitis[139]; the second with hemiplegia, aphasia and angiographic evidence of vasculitis; and the third with right thalamic hemorrhage at autopsy.[140]

Peripheral Neurological Manifestations
Trigeminal neuropathy is a frequent presenting feature of and the most common cranial neuropathy in progressive systemic sclerosis. It develops insidiously or acutely and affects primarily the central part of the face. Pain is common and may resemble that of tic douloureux.[141,142]

Evidence of direct involvement of scleroderma in producing clinically significant peripheral neuropathy is sparse. Symptomatic carpal tunnel syndrome and ulnar entrapment neuropathies at the wrist may relate to fibrosis and soft tissue edema.[143] Most peripheral neuropathies can otherwise be ascribed to metabolic and nutritional factors. However, some cases of sensorimotor neuropathy occurring before the onset of other symptoms or very early in the disease suggest that progressive systemic sclerosis may be responsible more directly.[144] In addition, prospective evaluation of 29 patients with limited or widespread systemic sclerosis demonstrated raised tactile thresholds in 28, suggesting that subclinical peripheral nerve dysfunction is common in this disorder.[145] Autonomic neuropathy may also occur. In a recent series, significant abnormalities were seen in cardiovascular reflexes, suggesting sympathetic and parasympathetic dysfunction in 25 patients with systemic sclerosis.[146]

Electrophysiological evaluation in most cases of sensorimotor neuropathy reveals an axonopathy. Histological features include collagenous infiltration of the peripheral nerves and the adventitia of vasa nervorum.

Etiology

The demonstration of antibodies to smooth muscle and cytotoxicity to cultured endothelial cells suggests that autoimmunity plays a role in pathogenesis. Cell-mediated cytotoxicity may play a role, but immune complex deposition has not been implicated.[52]

Prognosis and Treatment

The 5-year survival rate ranges between 50 and 94 percent. In some cases the disease is rapidly progressive and death occurs within 1 year. The most common causes of death are renal failure and cardiac complications. Symptomatic treatments include nonsteroidal anti-inflammatory drugs for arthritis and vasoactive drugs for Raynaud's phenomenon. Neuropathic pain, especially that associated with trigeminal neuropathy, can be treated with carbamazepine or tricyclic antidepressants. Penicillamine, colchicine, prednisone, and immunosuppressants have been used for more severe disease manifestations, but their relative effectiveness has not been determined.[52]

Mixed Connective Tissue Disease

General Medical Features

Mixed connective tissue disease is a syndrome that has overlapping features with other connective tissue diseases, including SLE, progressive systemic sclerosis, and rheumatoid arthritis. It is associated with a persistently high titer of antibody to RNAase-sensitive saline-extractable nuclear antigen, known as ribonucleoprotein (RNP) antibody. Most (80 percent) patients are women, and the mean age of onset is 37 years. Cutaneous manifestations include alopecia, lupus-like or heliotrope rashes, telangiectasias, and mild sclerodactyly. Nondeforming or deforming ar-

thritis occurs in most patients. Abnormal esophageal motility occurs in 80 percent of patients and pulmonary disease in 85 percent. Cardiac disease is somewhat less common. Renal disease is seen in fewer than one-third and uncommonly progresses to renal failure. Lymphadenopathy, hepatosplenomegaly, intestinal disorders, and fever occur in a small number of patients.[147] Most patients have high titers of antinuclear antibody with speckled pattern and anti-RNP antibodies. Rheumatoid factor is elevated in more than 50 percent. Anti–native DNA and anti-Sm antibodies are uncommon.

Neurological disease was not well recognized until Bennett and associates reported neuropsychiatric abnormalities in 11 of 20 patients with mixed connective tissue disease who were followed for 5 years.[148] It has now become apparent that patients may have nervous system involvement akin to that seen in SLE, with the exception that trigeminal neuropathy is common. In this last respect, nervous system involvement resembles that of progressive systemic sclerosis.

CNS Manifestations

The most common neurological abnormality is aseptic meningitis, the clinical features of which—fever, headaches, and nuchal rigidity—occur in nearly one-third of patients. The clinical episodes are associated with evidence of worsening of systemic disease, including fever, lymphadenopathy, alopecia, and nephropathy. Most patients have a CSF pleocytosis or increased protein concentration.[148]

In the series of Bennett and co-workers, paranoid psychosis occurred in three patients and convulsions in two patients; systemic disease flares accompanied two of the three psychoses and both convulsive disorders. Cerebellar ataxia and an altered level of consciousness each occurred in one patient.[148] Generalized choreoathetosis has been reported in a single case.[149] Rarely, transverse myelitis with loss of axons and myelin sheaths, gliosis, and dystrophic calcification has been seen.[150]

Peripheral Neurological Manifestations

Bennett and colleagues reported distal, symmetrical sensory polyneuropathy in two patients and trigeminal neuropathy in another two patients.[148] In neither of these disorders was there any relation to activity of the systemic disease. Trigeminal neuropathy has been noted to be an early[151] and persistent[152] feature of mixed connective tissue disease.

Prognosis and Treatment

The disorder has a relatively benign prognosis. Of 25 patients followed for 5 years after initial diagnosis, 8 died, but in only 2 was death clearly related to the mixed connective tissue disease. Morbidity among the survivors varied from no disability to persistent, severe disability.[152] In its early stages the disease follows a course like that of SLE, but subsequently systemic features become more quiescent and features of progressive systemic sclerosis become more prominent, with cutaneous sclerosis and esophageal dysmotility.

Treatment is dictated by the course of the individual patient. Severe SLE-like manifestations may require treatment with corticosteroids alone or in combination with immunosuppressants. Features like progressive systemic sclerosis are treated with the same drugs used to treat that disorder.

Inflammatory Myopathies

General Medical Features

The primary inflammatory myopathies comprise several clinically heterogeneous syndromes that have in common muscle weakness and pathological evidence of inflammation.[153] Inflammatory myopathy may occur in the setting of other connective tissue diseases or as a primary disorder. The incidence of primary inflammatory myopathy has been estimated at 0.2 per 100,000.[154]

Dermatomyositis may affect children or adults. Women are affected more commonly than men. Presentation is with progressive muscle weakness after or concurrent with a skin rash.[155,156] Characteristic skin rashes include an edematous, heliotrope facial rash, a macular red rash over the face or trunk, and a raised, erythematous, scaly rash over the knuckles.

Polymyositis differs from dermatomyositis in that there is no rash or other unique clinical sign. It represents a diagnosis of exclusion and is likely when progressive myopathy presents without extraocular muscle involvement, family history, endocrinopathy, toxic exposure, or biopsy changes suggestive of an alternative diagnosis.[153,156]

Inclusion body myositis is similar to polymyositis, except that distal muscle involvement is seen, especially with atrophy of the deep finger flexors.[153]

Systemic abnormalities are common in the primary inflammatory myopathies. Myocarditis or cardiomyopathy (with conduction defects, tachyarrhythmias, or congestive heart failure) reflects microscopic inflammation of cardiac muscle and may affect 40 percent of patients.[155] Dysphagia is common, especially in inclusion body myositis.[153] Respiratory symptoms result from weakness of accessory muscles of respiration or from the rare occurrence of interstitial lung disease.[153,157] Although it has long been believed that malignancies occur with increased frequency in patients with primary inflammatory myopathies, supportive evidence is scant except in cases of dermatomyositis.[153]

Neurological manifestations are limited to the peripheral nervous system in the primary inflammatory myopathies.

Peripheral Neurological Manifestations

The primary inflammatory myopathies present as subacute or chronic progressive, often symmetrical, proximal weakness. Distal weakness occurs late in the course of these disorders with the exception of inclusion body myositis, in which it may be an early feature. Facial and extraocular muscles are spared, but neck flexor weakness is seen. Myalgia is variable, and more likely to occur in dermatomyositis than other conditions. Wasting of involved muscles is common.

Electromyography demonstrates short-duration, low-amplitude, polyphasic motor unit action potentials, with an increase in spontaneous activity. At times, neuropathic changes accompany myopathic changes. Blood levels of muscle enzymes may be elevated, sometimes to very high values, but can be normal.[153] Muscle biopsy demonstrates inflammatory changes. In dermatomyositis, muscle fiber necrosis is accompanied by an inflammation of the perivascular regions and interfascicular septa. Perifascicular atrophy is the common pathological appearance.[153] The inflammatory infiltrates in polymyositis are mostly within fascicles. Vascular structures are normal, and there may be an increase in connective tissue.[153] Inclusion body myositis resembles polymyositis, but evidence of inflammation may be sparse. Basophilic granular inclusions surround slit-like vacuoles containing granular material. There are eosinophilic cytoplasmic inclusions.[153]

Etiology

The underlying abnormality in dermatomyositis appears to be a humorally mediated process against microvascular structures within muscle. Tissue destruction appears to be complement-mediated.[153] Autoantibodies to nuclear and cytoplasmic antigens have been demonstrated in the inflammatory myopathies but do not appear to be specific for these conditions.[153] The abnormal expression of major histocompatibility antigens on muscle fibers in regions of muscle inflammation suggest that T-cell–mediated cytotoxicity is directed against these antigens.[153]

It has been hypothesized that viruses, especially picornaviruses and retroviruses, trigger immune mechanisms in dermatomyositis and polymyositis. Picornaviruses share homologous regions with an antigen known as Jo-1, against which antibodies are demonstrated in some of these patients. Thus it is possible that cross reactivity between the viral and Jo-1 antigen has etiological importance.[153]

Treatment and Prognosis

The goal of therapy is to increase independence and comfort. High-dose corticosteroid treatment may control inflammation and clinical symptoms, but response to this treatment is not universal. Corticosteroids are the first line of therapy. Initially, high daily doses are employed, but these are tapered first to an alternate-day regimen, then to the lowest tolerated dose. Immunosuppressants are employed for steroid-unresponsive patients, for patients with steroid-induced adverse effects, and for rapidly progressive or resistant disease.[153]

Sjögren's Syndrome

General Medical Features

Sjögren's syndrome is defined by the clinical triad of xerophthalmia, xerostomia, and nondeforming arthritis. It is seen in 0.5 to 2.0 percent of the population. Among the connective tissue diseases, it is second in prevalence only to rheumatoid arthritis.[158]

Most (90 percent) patients are women. Onset usually occurs during middle age.[158] Sjögren's syndrome occurs in isolation in 50 percent of cases and in the context of rheumatoid arthritis, systemic lupus erythematosus, scleroderma, or another connective tissue disease in the remaining patients.[158]

Primary Sjögren's syndrome predominantly affects exocrine glands, with lymphocytic infiltration and fibrosis of lacrimal and salivary glands. Ocular, oral, and dental complications occur as a result of decreased tear and saliva production.[158]

Xerophthalmia can be demonstrated by Schirmer's test, staining of the corneal and conjunctival epithelium by Rose Bengal dye, or demonstration of epithelial strands by slit-lamp examination. Xerostomia can be assessed by nuclear scanning of the salivary glands, radiological sialography, or calculation of salivary flow rate. Biopsy of minor salivary glands, found on the inner aspect of the lower lip, is well tolerated and diagnostic when lymphocytic aggregation is demonstrated.

Extraglandular manifestations occur in at least 25 percent of patients. Lymphadenopathy and hepatosplenomegaly are common. Cutaneous vasculitis may present with a picture of nonthrombocytopenic purpura or urticaria. Arthritis of the small joints occurs in more than 80 percent of patients. Generally, there is symmetrical involvement, with mild synovitis and no deformity. Renal disease, usually interstitial nephritis, is seen in up to 40 percent of cases. Less commonly the lungs may be involved, with interstitial pneumonitis and restrictive or obstructive abnormalities of pulmonary function.[159] Vasculitis—usually localized to the skin, peripheral nervous system, and muscle—occurs in up to 20 percent of patients.[159] Lymphoproliferative disorders occur, and there is an increased risk of lymphoma in these patients.

Neurological disorders are usually associated with systemic vasculitis. Although thought to be a rare manifestation of Sjögren's syndrome, in some series they occur in as many as 25 percent of patients.[160]

CNS Manifestations

CNS complications are less frequent than peripheral neurological manifestations. Global neuropsychiatric changes are common and include affective and personality disorders. Nearly all patients have evidence of active extraglandular Sjögren's syndrome at the time of diagnosis of the psychiatric disorder.[160,161] Mild cognitive dysfunction is common, as is aseptic meningitis, which may be recurrent.[160,161] Focal cerebral deficits include hemiparesis, hemianopia, aphasia, and simple and complex partial seizures.[160] Nystagmus, ataxia, internuclear ophthalmoplegia, and movement disorders have occasionally been reported. Spinal cord involvement may take one of three forms: progressive myelopathy, acute transverse myelitis, or intraspinal hemorrhage.[160]

The EEG is abnormal in nearly one-half of patients with CNS dysfunction, but the findings are nonspecific. CT scans and MRI usually show focal regions of abnormality in patients with clinical evidence of localized pathology.[160] The CSF is characterized by elevation of protein concentration and evidence of intrathecal immunoglobulin synthesis, with increased IgG and oligoclonal bands.[160] Pathological studies are limited, but perivascular inflammation and diffuse vasculitis involving the cerebral blood vessels, as well as acute necrotizing arteritis of the spinal cord, have been described.[162]

Peripheral Neurological Manifestations

Signs and symptoms of peripheral nerve involvement occur in 10 to 32 percent of cases.[162] Most commonly, there is sensory or mixed sensorimotor polyneuropathy. Numbness and paresthesias are frequent; pain is a rarer complaint. Distal weakness in the lower extremities is generally mild.[163] Mononeuritis multiplex occurs somewhat less commonly. Entrapment neuropathy, particularly carpal tunnel syndrome, is well described. Cranial nerve involvement includes the trigeminal, oculomotor, and abducens nerves.[163]

Electrophysiological studies are consistent with demyelination, denervation, or both. The CSF may be normal or show a pleocytosis and an elevated protein concentration.

Peripheral nerve tissue shows demyelination and acute or chronic vasculitis or perivasculitis.[163] Dorsal root ganglionitis, with lymphocytic infiltration and degeneration of ganglion cells, has also been reported to accompany subacute sensory neuronopathy, which is a rare complication of Sjögren's syndrome.[164]

Etiology

The etiology of Sjögren's syndrome is unknown, but glandular inflammatory processes appear to be related to cell-mediated immunity or antibody-mediated cy-

totoxicity rather than immune complex deposition. The association with certain HLA class II antigens suggests a hereditary predisposition. Immune complex disease does appear to be responsible for rare cases of associated vasculitis.

Prognosis and Treatment

The prognosis of Sjögren's syndrome, when uncomplicated by systemic vasculitis, is good. Therapy is directed at sicca symptoms. Patients with vasculitis are best treated with corticosteroid and immunosuppressant medication.

Behçet's Disease

General Medical Features

Although originally believed to be a triad of relapsing ocular lesions and oral and genital ulcers, it has become apparent that Behçet's disease also affects other organ systems in more than 70 percent of patients.[165] The disorder affects 1 in 10,000 to 30,000 persons, men nearly twice as frequently as women. In most patients the first manifestation, usually oral or genital ulceration, appears between the ages of 20 and 35 years.[166] Ocular symptoms affect nearly 75 percent and include iridocyclitis, hypopyon, choroiditis, retinal phlebitis and arteritis, papillitis, cataracts, and glaucoma. Blindness occurs 4 to 8 years after the first ocular manifestation in one-third of cases. Skin lesions and recurrent deep venous thrombosis are common.[166] Many patients have nondeforming large-joint arthritis. The kidneys, lungs, heart, and gastrointestinal tract are affected less commonly.[166] Arterial involvement, with aneurysm of the aorta, femoral arteries, or pulmonary arteries, has also been seen.[166]

Neurological signs and symptoms occur in 4 to 29 percent of patients; in 5 percent they occur at presentation, but onset may be delayed for up to 20 years.

CNS Manifestations

CNS dysfunction occurs in 10 to 49 percent of patients with Behçet's disease.[167,168] CNS involvement is frequently heralded by headache, fever, and signs of aseptic meningitis. Pyramidal signs, pseudobulbar palsy, and cerebellar ataxia frequently accompany the meningitis.[167] Brainstem symptoms, seizures, delirium, aphasia, hemiparesis, extrapyramidal signs, and myelopathy also occur.[169] Rare manifestations include papilledema, subarachnoid hemorrhage, benign intracranial hypertension, tremor, and palatal myoclonus.[166,168–170] The onset of symptoms is commonly sudden but may be gradual. Fluctuation of CNS signs over days is common and may lead to the mistaken diagnosis of multiple sclerosis.[167]

The most consistent laboratory abnormality is a mild CSF pleocytosis, which occurs in more than 80 percent of patients. Increased protein concentration is seen in 65 percent of CSF samples. The EEG is frequently abnormal but in a nonspecific way. CT scan and MRI may demonstrate focal lesions, but are usually normal in the absence of focal clinical signs.[167,168] Pathologically, there are widely scattered foci of necrosis, demyelination, and scarring throughout the CNS, often in close proximity to small arterioles or venules that are infiltrated with inflammatory cells.[167]

Peripheral Neurological Manifestations

There have been only rare reports of peripheral neuropathy or mononeuritis multiplex occurring in association with Behçet's disease.[171]

Etiology

The etiology of Behçet's disease is unknown. Most likely, a hereditary susceptibility to the disorder coupled with lymphocyte sensitization to a viral antigen underlies the condition.[167]

Prognosis and Treatment

Progressive ocular involvement leads to blindness in many cases. Arteritis of the aorta or aortic aneurysm may be a cause of sudden death. The definitive treatment is unknown. Corticosteroids and immunosuppressants are used in concert in most patients with significant clinical disease activity. There is no agreement on the use of aspirin or anticoagulants in the treatment or prevention of thrombosis.[167]

REFERENCES

1. Fauci AS, Haynes B, Katz P: The spectrum of vasculitis: clinical, pathologic, immunologic and therapeutic considerations. Ann Intern Med 89:660, 1978
2. Scott DGI: Classification and treatment of systemic vasculitis. Br J Rheumatol 27:251, 1988
3. Brostoff J, Scadding GK, Male DK, Roitt IM: Clinical Immunology. Gower, London, 1991
4. Cohen SB, Hurd ER: Neurological complications of connective tissue and other "collagen-vascular" diseases. Semin Arthritis Rheum 11:190, 1981
5. Kissel JT, Rammohan KW: Pathogenesis and therapy of nervous system vasculitis. Clin Neuropharmacol 14:28, 1991
6. Conn DL: Polyarteritis. Rheum Dis Clin North Am 16:341, 1990
7. Michet CJ: Epidemiology of vasculitis. Rheum Dis Clin North Am 16:261, 1990
8. Cupps TR, Fauci AS: The Vasculitides. WB Saunders, Philadelphia, 1981
9. Arkin A: Clinical and pathological study of periarteritis nodosa: report of five cases, one histologically healed. Am J Pathol 6:401, 1930
10. Ford RG, Siekert RH: Central nervous system manifestations of periarteritis nodosa. Neurology 15:114, 1965
11. Sheehan B, Harriman DGF, Bardsaw JPB: Polyarteritis nodosa with ophthalamic and neurological complications. Arch Ophthalmol 60:537, 1958
12. Travers RL, Allison DJ, Brettle RP, Hughes GRV: Polyarteritis nodosa: a clinical and angiographic analysis of 17 cases. Semin Arthritis Rheum 8:184, 1979
13. Moore PM, Fauci AS: Neurologic manifestations of systemic vasculitis: a retrospective and prospective study of the clinicopathologic features and responses to therapy in 25 patients. Am J Med 71:517, 1981
14. Frohnert PP, Sheps SG: Long-term follow-up study of periarteritis nodosa. Am J Med 43:8, 1967
15. Prescott JE, Johnson JE, Dice WH: Polyarteritis nodosa presenting as seizures. Ann Emerg Med 12:642, 1983
16. Mayo J, Arias M, Leno C, Berciano J: Vascular parkinsonism and periarteritis nodosa. Neurology 36:874, 1986
17. Malamud N, Foster DB: Periarteritis nodosa: a clinicopathologic report, with special reference to the central nervous system. Arch Neurol Psychiatry 47:828, 1942
18. Tobias E: Periarteritis nodosa with special reference to the neurological complications. Excelsior, The Hague, 1956
19. Boyd LJ: Periarteritis nodosa: neuromyositic manifestations. Bull NY Med Coll 3:272, 1940
20. Ojeda VJ: Polyarteritis nodosa affecting the spinal cord arteries. Aust NZ J Med 13:287, 1983
21. Haft H, Finneson BE, Cramer H, Fiol R: Periarteritis nodosa as a source of subarachnoid hemorrhage and

spinal cord compression: report of a case and review of the literature. J Neurosurg 14:608, 1957

22. Chang RW, Bell CL, Hallett M: Clinical characteristics and prognosis of vasculitic mononeuropathy multiplex. Arch Neurol 41:618, 1984

23. Olney RK: Neuropathies in connective tissue disease. Muscle Nerve 15:531, 1992

24. Moore PM, Cupps TR: Neurological complications of vasculitis. Ann Neurol 14:155, 1983

25. Cohen RD, Conn DL, Ilstrup DM: Clinical features, prognosis, and response to treatment in polyarteritis. Mayo Clin Proc 55:146, 1980

26. Miller HG, Nelson MG: Polyarteritis nodosa developing during antisyphilitic treatment. Lancet 2:200, 1945

27. Patzold U, Haller P: Motorishe Polyneuropathie vom Landry-Typ und Querschnittssyndrom mit schlaffer Paraplegie: Seltene neurologische Syndrome bei der Panarteriitis nodosa. Dtsch Med Wochenschr 100:477, 1975

28. Wees SJ, Sunwoo IN, Oh SJ: Sural nerve biopsy in systemic necrotizing vasculitis. Am J Med 71:525, 1981

29. Guillevin L, Jarrousse B, Lok C, et al: Longterm followup after treatment of polyarteritis nodosa and Churg-Strauss angiitis with comparison of steroids, plasma exchange and cyclophosphamide to steroids and plasma exchange: a prospective randomized trial of 71 patients. The Cooperative Study Group for Polyarteritis Nodosa. J Rheumatol 18:567, 1991

30. Kurland LT, Chuang TY, Hunder GH: The epidemiology of systemic arteritis. p. 196. In Lawrence RC, Shulman LE (eds): Epidemiology of the Rheumatic Diseases. Gower, New York, 1984

31. Fauci As, Wolff SM: Wegener's granulomatosis: studies in eighteen patients and a review of the literature. Medicine (Baltimore) 52:535, 1973

32. Anderson JM, Jamieson DG, Jefferson JM: Non-healing granuloma and the nervous system. Q J Med 44: 309, 1975

33. Drachman DA: Neurological complications of Wegener's granulomatosis. Arch Neurol 8:145, 1963

34. Fauci AS, Haynes BF, Katz P, Wolff SM: Wegener's granulomatosis: prospective clinical and therapeutic experience with 85 patients for 21 years. Ann Intern Med 98:76, 1983

35. Nishino H, Rubino FA, DeRemee RA, et al: Neurological involvement in Wegener's granulomatosis: an analysis of 324 consecutive patients at the Mayo Clinic. Ann Neurol 33:4, 1993

36. Nishino H, Rubino FA, Parisi JE: The spectrum of neurologic involvement in Wegener's granulomatosis. Neurology 43:1334, 1993

37. Haynes BF, Fishman ML, Fauci AS, Wolff SM: The ocular manifestations of Wegener's granulomatosis. Am J Med 63:131, 1977

38. Case records of the Massachusetts General Hospital: Case 37511, Wegener's granulomatosis. N Engl J Med 245:978, 1951

39. Walton EW, Leggat PO: Wegener's granulomatosis. J Clin Pathol 9:31, 1956

40. Case records of the Massachusetts General Hospital: Case 87-1961, Wegener's granulomatosis. N Engl J Med 265:1156, 1961

41. Nolle B, Specks U, Ludemann J, et al: Anticytoplasmic autoantibodies: their immunodiagnostic value in Wegener granulomatosis. Ann Intern Med 111:28, 1989

42. van der Woude FJ, Rasmussen N, Lobatto S, et al: Autoantibodies against neutrophils and monocytes: tool for diagnosis and marker of disease activity in Wegener's granulomatosis. Lancet 1:425, 1985

43. Chuang T-Y, Hunder GG, Ilstrup DM, Kurland LT: Polymyalgia rheumatica: a 10-year epidemiologic and clinical study. Ann Intern Med 97:672, 1982

44. Henderson DRG, Tribe CR, Dixon AS: Synovitis in polymyalgia rheumatica. Rheumatol Rehabil 14:244, 1975

45. Huston KA, Hunder GG, Lie JT, et al: Temporal arteritis: a 25-year epidemiologic, clinical and pathologic study. Ann Intern Med 88:162, 1978

46. Fauci AS: The vasculitis syndromes. p. 1456. In Wilson JD, Braunwald E, Isselbacher KJ, et al (eds): Harrison's Principles of Internal Medicine. 12th Ed. McGraw-Hill, New York, 1991

47. Hollenhorst RW, Brown JR, Wagener HP, Shick RM: Neurologic aspects of temporal arteritis. Neurology 10:490, 1960

48. Eshaghian J: Controversies regarding giant cell (temporal, cranial) arteritis. Doc Ophthalmol 47:43, 1979

49. Andrews JM: Giant-cell ("temporal") arteritis: a disease with variable clinical manifestations. Neurology 16:963, 1966

50. Goodman BW: Temporal arteritis. Am J Med 67:839, 1979

51. Hamilton CR, Shelley WM, Tumulty PA: Giant cell arteritis: including temporal arteritis and polymyalgia rheumatica. Medicine (Baltimore) 50:1, 1971

52. Nadeau SE, Watson RT: Neurologic manifestations of vasculitis and collagen vascular syndromes. Ch. 59. In: Baker AB, Joynt RJ (eds): Clinical Neurology. Harper & Row, Philadelphia, 1985

53. Healey LA, Wilske KR: The Systemic Manifestations of Temporal Arteritis. Grune & Stratton, New York, 1978

54. Cohen DN, Damaske MM: Temporal arteritis: a

spectrum of ophthalmic complications. Ann Ophthalmol 7:1045, 1975

55. Caselli RJ, Hunder GG, Whisnant JP: Neurologic disease in biopsy-proven giant cell (temporal) arteritis. Neurology 38:352, 1988

56. Lipton RB, Solomon S, Wertenbaker C: Gradual loss and recovery of vision in temporal arteritis. Arch Intern Med 145:2252, 1985

57. Wilkinson IMS, Russell RWR: Arteries of the head and neck in giant cell arteritis: a pathological study to show the pattern of arterial involvement. Arch Neurol 27:378, 1972

58. Caselli RJ: Giant cell (temporal) arteritis: a treatable cause of multi-infarct dementia. Neurology 40:753, 1990

59. Barricks ME, Traviesa DB, Glaser JS, Levy IS: Ophthalmoplegia in cranial arteritis. Brain 100:209, 1977

60. Save-Soderbergh J, Malmvall BE, Andersson R, Bengtsson BA: Giant cell arteritis as a cause of death: report of nine cases. JAMA 255:493, 1986

61. Schneider HA, Weber AA, Ballen PH: The visual prognosis in temporal arteritis. Ann Ophthalmol 3: 1215, 1971

62. McDonnell PJ, Moore GW, Miller NR, et al: Temporal arteritis: a clinicopathologic study. Ophthalmology 93:518, 1986

63. Hall S, Barr W, Lie JT, et al: Takayasu arteritis. Medicine (Baltimore) 64:89, 1985

64. Hall S, Buchbinder R: Takayasu's arteritis. Rheum Dis Clin North Am 16:411, 1990

65. Lupi-Herrera E, Sanchez-Torres G, Marcushamer J, et al: Takayasu's arteritis: clinical study of 107 cases. Am Heart J 93:94, 1977

66. Marquis Y, Richardson J, Ritchie AC, Wigle ED: Idiopathic medical aortopathy and arteriopathy. Am J Med 44:939, 1968

67. Nakao K, Ikeda M, Kimata S-I, et al: Takayasu's arteritis: clinical report of eighty-four cases and immunological studies of seven cases. Circulation 35:1141, 1967

68. Judge RD, Currier RD, Gracie WA, Figley MM: Takayasu's arteritis and the aortic arch syndrome. Am J Med 32:379, 1962

69. Nasu T: Pathology of pulseless disease: a systematic study and critical review of twenty-one autopsy cases reported in Japan. Angiology 14:225, 1963

70. Rose AG, Sinclair-Smith CC: Takayasu's arteritis: a study of 16 autopsy cases. Arch Pathol Lab Med 104: 231, 1980

71. Currier RD, DeJong RN, Bole GG: Pulseless disease: central nervous system manifestations. Neurology 4: 818, 1954

72. Ross RS, McKusick VA: Aortic arch syndromes: diminished or absent pulses in arteries arising from arch of aorta. Arch Intern Med 92:701, 1953

73. Strachan RW: The natural history of Takayasu's arteriopathy. Q J Med 33:57,1964

74. Ishikawa K: Suvival and morbidity after diagnosis of occlusive thromboaortopathy (Takayasu's disease). Am J Cardiol 47:1026, 1981

75. Lie JT: Primary (granulomatous) angiitis of the central nervous system: a clinicopathologic analysis of 15 new cases and a review of the literature. Hum Pathol 23: 164, 1992

76. Sigal LH: The neurologic presentation of vasculitic and rheumatologic syndromes: a review. Medicine (Baltimore) 66:157, 1987

77. Cupps TR, Moore PM, Fauci AS: Isolated angiitis of the central nervous system: prospective diagnostic and therapeutic experience. Am J Med 74:97, 1983

78. Kolodny EH, Rebeiz JJ, Caviness VS, Richardson EP: Granulomatous angiitis of the central nervous system. Arch Neurol 19:510, 1968

79. Rawlinson DG, Braun CW: Granulomatous angiitis of the nervous system first seen as relapsing myelopathy. Arch Neurol 38:129, 1981

80. Sipe JC, Rosenberg JH: Granulomatous giant cell angiitis of the central nervous system. West J Med 127: 215, 1977

81. Thomas L, Davidson M, McCluskey RT: Studies of PPLO infection: I. The production of cerebral polyarteritis by Mycoplasma gallisepticum in turkeys: the neurotoxic property of the Mycoplasma. J Exp Med 123:897, 1966

82. Craven RS, French JK: Isolated angiitis of the central nervous system. Ann Neurol 18:263, 1985

83. Calabrese LH, Mallek JA: Primary angiitis of the central nervous system. Medicine (Baltimore) 67:20, 1988

84. Dyck PJ, Benstead TJ, Conn DL, et al: Nonsystemic vasculitic neuropathy. Brain 110:843, 1987

85. Kissel JT, Mendell JR: Vasculitic neuropathy. Neurol Clin 10:761, 1992

86. Lipsky PE: Rheumatoid arthritis. p. 1437. In Wilson JD, Braunwald E, Isselbacher KJ, et al (eds): Harrison's Principles of Internal Medicine. 12th Ed. McGraw-Hill, New York, 1991

87. Vollertsen RS, Conn DL: Vasculitis associated with rheumatoid arthritis. Rheum Dis Clin North Am 16: 445, 1990

88. Steiner JW, Gelbloom AJ: Intracranial manifestations in two cases of systemic rheumatoid disease. Arthritis Rheum 2:537, 1959

89. Bathon JM, Moreland LW, DiBartolomeo AG: Inflammatory central nervous system involvement in rheumatoid arthritis. Semin Arthritis Rheum 18:258, 1989

90. Ouyang R, Mitchell DM, Rozdilsky B: Central nervous system involvement in rheumatoid disease: report of a case. Neurology 17:1099, 1967

91. Bywaters EGL, Scott JT: The natural history of vascular lesions in rheumatoid arthritis. J Chronic Dis 16:905, 1963

92. Scott DGI, Bacon PA, Tribe CR: Systemic rheumtaoid vasculitis: a clinical and laboratory study of 50 cases. Medicine (Baltimore) 60:288, 1981

93. Ramos M, Mandybur TI: Cerebral vasculitis in rheumatoid arthritis. Arch Neurol 32:271, 1975

94. Watson P, Fekete J, Deck J: Central nervous system vasculitis in rheumatoid arthritis. Can J Neurol Sci 4:269, 1977

95. Beck DO, Corbett JJ: Seizures due to central nervous system rheumatoid meningovasculitis. Neurology 33:1058, 1983

96. Lorber A, Pearson CM, Rene RM: Osteolytic vertebral lesions as a manifestation of rheumatoid arthritis and related disorders. Arthritis Rheum 4:514, 1961

97. Bland JH: Rheumatoid arthritis of the cervical spine. Bull Rheum Dis 18:471, 1967

98. Hopkins JS: Lower cervical rheumatoid subluxation with tetraplegia. J Bone Joint Surg [Br] 49:46, 1967

99. Meikle JAK, Wilkinson M: Rheumatoid involvement of the cervical spine: radiological assessment. Ann Rheum Dis 30:154, 1971

100. Nakano KK: Neurologic complications of rheumatoid arthritis. Orthop Clin North Am 6:861, 1975

101. Santavirta S, Konttinen YT, Lindqvist C, Sandelin J: Occipital headache in rheumatoid cervical facet joint arthritis. Lancet 2:695, 1986

102. Collee G, Breedveld FC, Algra PR, Padberg GW: Rheumatoid arthritis with vertical atlanto-axial subluxation complicated by hydrocephalus. Br J Rheumatol 26:56, 1987

103. Fedele FA, Ho G, Dorman BA: Pseudoaneurysm of the vertebral artery: a complication of rheumatoid cervical spine disease. Arthritis Rheum 29:136, 1986

104. Kaiser MC, Veiga-Pires J, Capesius P: Atlanto-axial impaction and compression of the medulla oblongata and proximal spinal cord in rheumatoid arthritis evaluated by CT scanning. Br J Radiol 56:764, 1983

105. Stevens JC, Cartlidge NE, Saunders M, et al: Atlantoaxial subluxation and cervical myelopathy in rheumatoid arthritis. Q J Med 40:391, 1971

106. Smith PH, Benn RT, Sharp J: Natural history of rheumatoid cervical luxations. Ann Rheum Dis 31:431, 1972

107. Nakano KK: The entrapment neuropathies of rheumatoid arthritis. Orthop Clin North Am 6:837, 1975

108. Peyronnard JM, Charron L, Beaudet F, Couture F: Vasculitic neuropathy in rheumatoid disease and Sjogren syndrome. Neurology 32:839, 1982

109. Hahn BH: Systemic lupus erythematosus. p. 583. In Parker CW (ed): Clinical Immunology. WB Saunders, Philadelphia, 1980

110. Pisetsky DS: Systemic lupus erythematosus. Med Clin North Am 70:337, 1986

111. Futrell N, Schultz LR, Millikan C: Central nervous system disease in patients with systemic lupus erythematosus. Neurology 42:1649, 1992

112. Estes D, Christian CL: The natural history of systemic lupus erythematosus by prospective analysis. Medicine (Baltimore) 50:85, 1971

113. Feinglass EJ, Arnett FC, Dorsch CA, et al: Neuropsychiatric manifestations of systemic lupus erythematosus: diagnosis, clinical spectrum, and relationship to other features of the disease. Medicine (Baltimore) 55:323, 1976

114. Bennahum DA, Messner RP: Recent observations on central nervous system lupus erythematosus. Semin Arthritis Rheum 4:253, 1975

115. O'Connor JF, Musher DM: Central nervous system involvement in systemic lupus erythematosus: a study of 150 cases. Arch Neurol 14:157, 1966

116. Johnson RT, Richardson EP: The neurological manifestations of systemic lupus erythematosus: a clinical-pathological study of 24 cases and review of the literature. Medicine (Baltimore) 47:337, 1968

117. Gibson T, Myers AR: Nervous system involvement in systemic lupus erythematosus. Ann Rheum Dis 35:398, 1975

118. Kaell AT, Shetty M, Lee BCP, Lockshin MD: The diversity of neurologic events in systemic lupus erythematosus: prospective clinical and computed tomographic classification of 82 events in 71 patients. Arch Neurol 43:273, 1986

119. Ellis SG, Verity MA: Central nervous system involvement in systemic lupus erythematosus: a review of neuropathologic findings in 57 cases, 1955–1977. Semin Arthritis Rheum 8:212, 1979

120. Denburg JA, Carbotte RM, Denburg SD: Neuronal antibodies and cognitive function in systemic lupus erythematosus. Neurology 37:464, 1987

121. Weiner DK, Allen NB: Large vessel vasculitis of the central nervous system in systemic lupus erythematosus: report and review of the literature. J Rheumatol 18:748, 1991

122. Lusins JO, Szilagyi PA: Clinical features of chorea associated with systemic lupus erythematosus. Am J Med 58:857, 1975

123. Provenzale J, Bouldin TW: Lupus-related myelopathy: report of three cases and review of the literature. J Neurol Neurosurg Psychiatry 55:830, 1992

124. Andrianakos AA, Duffy J, Suzuki M, Sharp JT: Transverse myelopathy in systemic lupus erythema-

tosus: report of three cases and review of the literature. Ann Intern Med 83:616, 1975

125. Fody EP, Netsky MG, Mrak RE: Subarachnoid spinal hemorrhage in a case of systemic lupus erythematosus. Arch Neurol 37:173, 1980

126. Dubois EL, Tuffanelli DL: Clinical manifestations of systemic lupus erythematosus: computer analysis of 520 cases. JAMA 190:104, 1964

127. McCombe PA, McLeod JG, Pollard JD, et al: Peripheral sensorimotor and autonomic neuropathy associated with systemic lupus erythematosus: clinical, pathological, and immunological features. Brain 110: 533, 1987

128. Morgan SH, Kennett RP, Dudley C, et al: Acute polyradiculoneuropathy complicating systemic lupus erythematosus. Postgrad Med J 62:291, 1986

129. Scheinberg L: Polyneuritis in systemic lupus erythematosus: review of the literature and report of a case. N Engl J Med 255:416, 1956

130. Bonfa E, Golombeck SJ, Kaufman LD, et al: Association between lupus psychosis and anti-ribosomal P protein antibodies. N Engl J Med 317:265, 1987

131. Bluestein HG, Woods VL: Antineuronal antibodies in systemic lupus erythematosus. Arthritis Rheum 25: 773, 1982

132. Sanders ME, Alexander EL, Koski CL, et al: Detection of activated terminal complement (C5b-9) in cerebrospinal fluid from patients with central nervous system involvement of primary Sjogren's syndrome or systemic lupus erythematosus. J Immunol 138: 2095, 1987

133. Bowles CA: Vasculopathy associated with the antiphospholipid antibody syndrome. Rheum Dis Clin North Am 16:471, 1990

134. Sergent JS, Lockshin MD, Klempner MS, Lipsky BA: Central nervous system disease in systemic lupus erythematosus: therapy and prognosis. Am J Med 58: 644, 1975

135. Tuffanelli DL, Winkelmann RK: Systemic scleroderma: a clinical study of 727 cases. Arch Dermatol 84:359, 1961

136. Steen VD, Medsger TA: Epidemiology and natural history of systemic sclerosis. Rheum Dis Clin North Am 16:1, 1990

137. Benos J, Rettleback R, Suchenwirth R: Psychosen als zerebrale Manifestationen von Kollagenosen und verwandten Prozessen. Fortschr Med 88:279, 1970

138. Gordon RM, Silverstein A: Neurologic manifestations in progressive systemic sclerosis. Arch Neurol 22:126, 1970

139. Estey E, Lieberman A, Pinto R, et al: Cerebral arteritis in scleroderma. Stroke 10:595, 1979

140. Wise TN, Ginzler ME: Scleroderma cerebritis, an unusual manifestation of progressive systemic sclerosis. Dis Nerv Syst 36:60, 1975

141. Farrell DA, Medsger TA: Trigeminal neuropathy in progressive systemic sclerosis. Am J Med 73:57, 1982

142. Teasdall RD, Frayha RA, Shulman LE: Cranial nerve involvement in systemic sclerosis (scleroderma): a report of 10 cases. Medicine (Baltimore) 59:149, 1980

143. Machet L, Vaillant L, Machet MC, et al: Carpal tunnel syndrome and systemic sclerosis. Dermatology 185: 101, 1992

144. Richter RB: Peripheral neuropathy and connective tissue disease. J Neuropathol Exp Neurol 13:168, 1954

145. Schady W, Sheard A, Hassell A, et al: Peripheral nerve dysfunction in scleroderma. Q J Med 80:661, 1991

146. Klimiuk PS, Taylor L, Baker RD, Jayson MI: Autonomic neuropathy in systemic sclerosis. Ann Rheum Dis 47:542, 1988

147. Sharp GC: Mixed connective tissue disease. p. 1448. In Wilson JD, Braunwald E, Isselbacher KJ, et al (eds): Harrison's Principles of Internal Medicine. 12th Ed. McGraw-Hill, New York, 1991

148. Bennett RM, Bong DM, Spargo BH: Neuropsychiatric problems in mixed connective tissue disease. Am J Med 65:955, 1978

149. McKenna F, Eccles J, Neuman VC: Neuropsychiatric disorders in mixed connective tissue disease. Br J Rheumatol 25:225, 1986

150. Weiss TD, Nelson JS, Woolsey RM, et al: Transverse myelitis in mixed connective tissue disease. Arthritis Rheum 21:982, 1978

151. Searles RP, Mladinich EK, Messner RP: Isolated trigeminal sensory neuropathy: early manifestation of mixed connective tissue disease. Neurology 28:1286, 1978

152. Nimelstein SH, Brody S, McShane D, Holman HR: Mixed connective tissue disease: a subsequent evaluation of the original 25 patients. Medicine (Baltimore) 59:239, 1980

153. Dalakas MC: Clinical, immunopathologic, and therapeutic considerations of inflammatory myopathies. Clin Neuropharmacol 15:327, 1992

154. Benbassat J, Geffel D, Zlotnick A: Epidmiology of polymyositis-dermatomyositis in Israel, 1960–1976. Isr J Med Sci 16:197, 1980

155. Singsen B, Goldreyer B, Stanton R, Hanson V: Childhood polymyositis with cardiac conduction defects. Am J Dis Child 130:72, 1976

156. Pearson CM, Bohan A: The spectrum of polymyositis and dermatomyositis. Med Clin North Am 61:439, 1977

157. Salmeron G, Greenberg SD, Lidsky MD: Polymyositis and diffuse interstitial lung disease: a review of the pulmonary histopathologic findings. Arch Intern Med 141:1005, 1981

158. Talal N: Sjögren's syndrome: historical overview and clinical spectrum of disease. Rheum Dis Clin North Am 18:507, 1992

159. Stoltze CA, Hanlon DG, Pease GL, Henderson JW: Keratoconjunctivitis sicca and Sjögren's syndrome: systemic manifestations and hematologic and protein abnormalities. Arch Intern Med 106:513, 1960

160. Alexander E: Central nervous system disease in Sjögren's syndrome. Rheum Dis Clin North Am 18:637, 1992

161. Malinow KL, Molina R, Gordon B, et al: Neuropsychiatric dysfunction in primary Sjögren's syndrome. Arch Intern Med 103:344, 1985

162. Alexander GE, Provost TT, Stevens MB, Alexander EL: Sjögren syndrome: central nervous system manifestations. Neurology 31:1391, 1981

163. Kaltreider HB, Talal N: The neuropathy of Sjögren's syndrome: trigeminal nerve involvement. Ann Intern Med 70:751, 1969

164. Malinow K, Yannakakis GD, Glusman SM, et al: Subacute sensory neuronopathy secondary to dorsal root ganglionitis in primary Sjögren's syndrome. Ann Neurol 20:535, 1986

165. Kozin F, Haughton V, Bernhard GC: Neuro-Behçet disease: two cases and neuroradiologic findings. Neurology 27:1148, 1977

166. Wechsler B, Vidailhet M, Piette JC, et al: Cerebral venous thrombosis in Behçet's disease: clinical study and long-term follow-up of 25 cases. Neurology 42: 614, 1992

167. O'Duffy JD: Vasculitis in Behçet's disease. Rheum Dis Clin North Am 16:423, 1990

168. Serdaroglu P, Yazici H, Ozdemir C, et al; Neurologic involvement in Behçet's syndrome: a prospective study. Arch Neurol 46:265, 1989

169. Schotland DL, Wolf SM, White HH, Dubin HV: Neurologic aspects of Behçet's disease: case report and review of the literature. Am J Med 34:544, 1963

170. Wilkins MR, Gove RI, Roberts SD, Kendall MJ: Behçet's disease presenting as benign intracranial hypertension. Postgrad Med J 62:39, 1986

171. Takeuchi A, Kodama M, Takatsu M, et al: Mononeuritis multiplex in incomplete Behçet's disease: a case report and the review of the literature. Clin Rheumatol 8:375, 1989

24
Psychiatry and Neurology

Michael R. Trimble

As would be expected, there are many close links between neurology and psychiatry. Historically, neurology grew out of psychiatry (or, rather, neuropsychiatry), which was a well-established discipline by the nineteenth century. The divergence of the two disciplines, which in part related to the success of localization theories in predicting central nervous system (CNS) lesions, took place mainly during the twentieth century and was accelerated by the rapid acceptance of psychoanalytical theories into the main body of psychiatric thinking. Although this was predominantly an early-century phenomenon, its legacy has lingered, with the relative failure of many to appreciate that psychiatry, in contrast to psychology, has rediscovered its biological and neurological underpinnings during the last three decades, and the associations with neurology have become once again more obvious.

The cornerstone of pathogenesis for psychiatry and neurology in recent years has been the discovery of neurotransmitters, which has led to our acceptance of an entirely different kind of brain to that conceptualized by the neuroanatomical principles of earlier generations. Furthermore, the discovery of the limbic system, a series of interconnected neurons and pathways whose role it is, among others, to modulate emotional function, has provided a secure cornerstone for the neuroanatomical and neurochemical underpinnings of psychiatric disorders. It also has formed the basis for the extension of localizationalist neuropsychology into the discipline of behavioral

neurology. Thus, whereas biological psychiatry seeks an understanding of disturbances of the limbic system and related structures in association with primary psychiatric illness, behavioral neurology has become concerned not only with the consequences of cortical damage as reflected in the aphasias and other problems but also with the consequences of localized dysfunction of, for example, the temporal and frontal lobes of the brain and their behavioral correlates.

In this chapter we examine some of the relations between neurology and psychiatry, identifying two main areas. First, some psychiatric aspects of neurological disorders are presented, followed by neurological presentations of psychiatric disorders. Finally, the question "are psychiatry and neurology two sides of the same coin?" is discussed from a contemporary and historical point of view.

PSYCHIATRIC CONSEQUENCES OF NEUROLOGICAL DISEASE

Although the term *psychiatry* strictly refers to "the medical treatment of diseases of the mind," in its broader sense psychiatrists and neurologists deal with behavior problems. As a generalization it may be said that neurologists tend to be interested in the abnormal behavior of single elements of a person's repertoire and, on the whole, deal with negative symptoms (i.e., loss of function in the sense given to it by Hughlings

Jackson[1]), whereas the psychiatrists' concern lies in alterations of function of the whole person, with a particular interest in positive symptoms: those that "answer to activities of healthy nervous arrangements . . . [which] attend activities of all which is left intact in a nervous system maimed by dissolution. . . ."[1] The consequences of neurological disease for behavior may thus be broken down into two broad categories: general effects and those that are provoked by a focal lesion. Most interest has focused on focal lesions of the frontal and temporal lobes and the basal ganglia, and it is on these areas that attention is concentrated in this chapter.

Generalized Disturbances of Cerebral Function

In contrast to the focal symptoms described below, patients with neurological insults often display symptoms that appear to coalesce into a recognizable but variegated pattern. However, no specific symptom or group of symptoms is pathognomonic, and unless they are inquired about such symptoms are often not noticed or recorded; in many cases they are trivialized. These generalized disturbances were of particular interest to such authors as Goldstein.[2] He outlined several expressions of CNS disintegration, which he essentially saw as exhibiting the same features, regardless of the involved region of the brain (Table 24-1). Similarly, Mayer-Gross and Guttmann[3] and Lishman[4] discussed the cardinal features of the abnor-

mal mental state that follows cerebral disorders and which may be referred to as a generalized disturbance of cerebral function (Table 24-1). The pattern of symptoms depends on the premorbid personality of the patient, which tends to be exacerbated by any central neurological lesion, but also on the extent of the injury. However, Goldstein[2] and many others[5] have made the point that, although patients with severe brain damage may show such symptoms, mental symptoms are also seen in association with much less severe trauma. Some symptoms overlap with those of posttraumatic depression or posttraumatic stress disorder, particularly those observed in the postconcussional syndrome and later posttraumatic syndromes that follow minor head injury.

Typically, patients complain of "not being the same." They note that their memory is poor, although often underlying this problem is a disturbance of attention or concentration. They find prolonged attention to, for example, a book or a television program fatiguing and complain that they do not remember everyday events. Their emotional reactions appear labile, and, particularly with more severe damage, they may also appear "flattened." Outbursts of anxiety, recurrent depressive episodes, and irritability in interpersonal relationships are noted. Patients may become withdrawn from their usual company, preferring to spend more time alone in familiar surroundings, not looking forward to such everyday events as traveling or engaging in social activities. They complain that their mind is "empty," and they do not know what to say to people.

Table 24-1 Generalized Disturbances of the Mental State

Goldstein[2]	Mayer-Gross & Guttman[3]	Lishman[4]
Rise of threshold and retardation of excitation	Amnesia	Impairment of memory
Abnormal spread of excitation	Distrubed attention	Diminished social awareness
Performance influenced to greater extent by external stimuli	Disturbed spontaneity	Aggravation of premobid personality traits
Blurring of boundaries between "figure and ground"	Poverty of ideas	Loss of interest and initiative
Impaired abstracting attitude and "concretization"	Forced responsiveness to stimuli	Episodes of bizarre behavior
	Disturbed consciousness	Incapacity for decisive action
	Organic orderliness	Personal neglect
	Organic slovenliness	Labored thinking with loss of intellectual flexibility
	Disturbed affect	Stimulus binding
	"Catastrophe reaction"	Reduced vocabulary
	Perseveration	Emotional changes
	Fatigability	
	Iteration in speech	
	Haste in speech	
	Slowing down	

Disturbances of attention are common after cerebral injury. The term *stimulus binding* is sometimes used with reference to distractability, in which an environmental stimulus may lead to an altered sphere of attention for the patient. An impairment of mental agility leads to concretization, in which thoughts are bound to immediate experiences and mental flexibility is lost. For Goldstein, the patient is "unable to grasp the essential of a given whole," and abstracting common properties, with planning ahead ideationally, becomes difficult. He referred to the blurring of sharp boundaries and the difficulty of extracting the details from situations as a disturbance of figure/ground relations: The patient's judgment has become impaired, so that he cannot "see the wood for the trees." The patient's general behavior may be characterized by a lack of spontaneity, organic orderliness, personal neglect, diminished social awareness, and inappropriate behavior.

Following lesser head injury, where the posttraumatic amnesia is limited, patients may report symptoms that reflect a posttraumatic stress disorder and its interaction with the premorbid personality. Such patients also often report an increase in emotionality, disturbed affect with depressive symptoms, a tendency to withdraw from company, poor memory and concentration, increased distractability, irritability, and poor tolerance for ordinary environmental stimuli. For example, they may complain that everyday noise has become intolerable. In patients with subtle brain damage, such symptoms tend to blend with the mental symptoms of generalized organic damage described above, such that unraveling the organicity of the symptomatology becomes not only a fruitless enterprise but one that many authors have pointed out is fallacious. As Goldstein commented, "we must realise that the important question is whether a man is really suffering or not, really disturbed in his life and work or not, regardless of whether his symptoms have an organic cause or are psychogenic."[2]

Symptoms of Regional Dysfunction

FRONTAL LOBE SYMPTOMS

Although there are extensive accounts of frontal lobe syndromes,[6] it is surprising how often frontal lobe pathology goes unnoticed and frontal lobe symptoms are dismissed as unimportant. It was the primate observations of Jacobsen,[7] the reports of the consequences of head injuries, particularly during World War II, and information from patients examined after frontal leukotomy that led to delineation of the various syndromes associated with frontal lobe pathology. The clinical characteristics of three principal frontal lobe syndromes, as described by Cummings,[8] are shown in Table 24-2, although it should be noted that many patients show an admixture of symptoms, and such discrete syndromes are rarely observed.

One of the specific deficits of frontal lobe damage is poor attention; these patients also show increased distractibility. They often present with poor memory, the latter sometimes being referred to as "forget-

Table 24-2 Clinical Characteristics of the Three Principal Frontal Lobe Syndromes

Orbitofrontal syndrome (disinhibited)
Disinhibited, impulsive behavior ("pseudopsychopathic")
Inappropriate jocular affect, euphoria
Emotional lability
Poor judgment and insight
Distractibility

Frontal convexity syndrome (apathetic)
Apathetic (occasional brief angry or aggressive outbursts common)
Indifference
Psychomotor retardation
Motor perservation and impersistence
Loss of set
Stimulus boundedness
Discrepant motor and verbal behavior
Motor programming deficits
    Three-step hand sequence
    Alternating programs
    Reciprocal programs
    Rhythm tapping
    Multiple loops
Poor word-list generation
Poor abstraction and categorization
Segmented approach to visuospatial analysis

Medial frontal syndrome (akinetic)
Paucity of spontaneous movement and gesture
Sparse verbal output (repetition may be preserved)
Lower extremity weakness and loss of sensation
Incontinence

(From Cummings JL: Clinical Neuropsychiatry. Grune & Stratton, Orlando, FL, 1985, with permission.)

ting to remember." The thinking of patients with frontal lobe lesions tends to be concrete, and they may show perseveration and stereotypy of their responses. Perseveration, with inability to switch lines of thought, leads to difficulties with arithmetical calculations such as serial sevens or carryover subtractions.

Patients have no anomia, and repetition is intact, although they may have difficulty with spontaneous and conversational speech. This syndrome is similar to that referred to as transcortical motor aphasia and has been designated *dynamic aphasia* by Luria.[9]

Other features of frontal lobe syndromes include reduced activity, lack of drive, and inability to plan ahead. Patients show lack of concern and often display aimless uncoordinated behavior. Their affect is disturbed, with apathy, emotional blunting, and indifference. Clinically, this picture sometimes resembles that of a major affective disorder with psychomotor retardation.

In contrast, other patients may show euphoria and disinhibition, but the euphoria is not that of a mania, having an empty quality to it. The disinhibition can lead to markedly abnormal and sometimes antisocial behavior. Some authors have distinguished between lesions of the lateral frontal and orbital cortex. The lateral frontal cortex is closely linked to the motor structures of the brain, and lesions in that area therefore lead to disturbances of movement and action, with perseveration and inertia. Lesions of the orbital areas, which are linked with the limbic and reticular systems, lead to disinhibition and changes of affective life. The features of these two syndromes and that of the medial frontal syndrome are shown in Table 24-2.

Other clinical signs associated with frontal lobe damage include sensory inattention in the contralateral sensory field, abnormalities of visual searching, echophenomena, confabulation, hyperphagia, imitation behavior, and so-called utilization behavior, an exaggerated tendency to grope for objects and overuse them.

In clinical practice a variety of tests are used to detect frontal lobe damage. If only traditional neurological and neuropsychological testing is performed, frontal lobe pathology may go unnoticed. This point cannot be overemphasized—that the traditional neurological examination essentially seeks an alteration of function in the parietal and occipital cortices and

Table 24-3 Some Useful Tests on Frontal Lobe Function

Word fluency
Abstract thinking (If I have 18 books and 2 book-shelves, and I want twice as many books on one shelf as the other, how many books go on each shelf?)
Proverb and metaphor interpretation
Tests of cognitive estimates
Wisconsin card sorting task
Other sorting tasks
Block design
Maze test
Hand position test
Copying tasks (e.g., repetitive designs)
Rhythm tapping tasks

(Adapted from Cummings JL: Clinical Neuropsychiatry. Grune & Stratton, Orlando, FL, 1985, with permission.)

generally does not reflect frontal and temporal lobe function. When the latter areas of the brain are damaged, the patient's motor and psychic activities are influenced, and the resulting behavior disturbances reflect the pathology. Some useful tests of frontal lobe function are given in Table 24-3, fuller descriptions being given elsewhere.[6,8,10] A number of syndromes of abnormal awareness have been related to frontal pathology,[6] exemplified by Capgras' syndrome, in which patients acknowledge a person as looking like a relative or friend but maintain they are someone else in disguise. Another such disorder is reduplicative paramnesia, in which patients relocate their environment.

Various pathologies lead to frontal lobe damage, including trauma, tumors, cerebrovascular accidents, infections, and some degenerative diseases. Of the dementias, Pick's disease and normal-pressure hydrocephalus specifically affect this area. The frontal lobe dementias are more common than previously appreciated, although agreement has yet to be reached on terminology. Among various tumors, frontal meningiomas, especially if slowly growing, are likely to be missed and may lead to florid psychopathology. Anterior cerebral artery rupture is more likely to lead to frontal lobe damage than other cerebrovascular disorders, although the middle cerebral artery does supply the lateral parts of the orbital gyri and the inferior and middle frontal gyri. Intoxicants such as alcohol may preferentially damage frontal areas, and demyelinating conditions such as multiple sclerosis may also lead to frontal lobe problems.

The evidence for frontal lobe involvement in depressive illness, obsessive compulsive disorder, and schizophrenia is increasing.[10] Suffice it to say here that a number of the "negative" symptoms of schizophrenia (e.g., affective changes, impaired motivation, poor insight, and other "defect" syndromes) probably relate to abnormalities on the dorsolateral frontal cortex. Abnormalities of the frontal lobes in schizophrenic patients have been noted not only from neuropathological studies but also from clinical signs of frontal lobe deficits, neurophysiological studies, neuropsychological studies, and imaging studies that examined cerebral blood flow or evaluated metabolism [positron emission tomography (PET) scanning].

The frontal lobes are particularly likely to be damaged during head injury. The relative lack of movement in the frontal and temporal lobes, held rigid by the bony anterior fossae of the calvarium, leads to strains in cerebral tissue, with lacerations and damage at these sites on impact. Patients often complain of a number of symptoms reminiscent of frontal lobe damage, but traditional neuropsychological investigation as well as routine neurological examination and computed tomography (CT) scanning may be normal. It is in such patients that there should be a high level of alertness to the possibility of frontal lobe/limbic system damage, and symptoms should not be dismissed lightly. Tissue damage may be revealed by magnetic resonance imaging (MRI), which is now the most relevant imaging technique for investigating patients in these circumstances.

TEMPORAL LOBE SYNDROMES

Although a variety of pathologies affecting the temporal lobes lead to psychopathology, most interesting and perhaps most controversial are the changes of behavior that are secondary to epilepsy and that derive from the temporal lobes. This subject is reviewed in more detail elsewhere.[10,11]

Of the various psychopathologies related to epilepsy, it is the personality disorders and psychoses that have been the subject of most discussion. A considerable amount of confusion in the literature has been created by the failure of various authors to use precise terminology. Thus, with regard to personality disorder, there has been a confusion of two concepts. The first, a hangover from the earlier part of this century and the era of psychosomatic medicine, relates to the idea of disease-susceptible personalities. This concept was that patients with certain personality types and constitutions were susceptible to various diseases—hence the epileptic personality. There are few adherents to such concepts today, but the second belief is very much alive, in keeping with the ideas originally put forward by Gibbs and Stamps.[12] Essentially these authors proposed that patients with chronic brain lesions, especially in their temporal lobes, may develop personality changes as a direct manifestation of an organic brain syndrome. The precedent for this theory was set by the clear delineation of frontal lobe personality changes and the discovery of behavioral changes in animals following bilateral temporal lobectomy, as seen in the Kluver-Bucy syndrome.

Many of the investigations that have examined personality traits of patients with epilepsy have used standardized rating scales, but a number have failed to detect consistently abnormal profiles in comparison with normal subjects or other medically ill patients. Furthermore, attempts to show differences between patients with what used to be called temporal lobe epilepsy and generalized forms of seizure disorder using such methodologies have also produced inconsistent conclusions. Bear and Fedio developed their own scale of 18 behavioral traits drawn from the literature and supposedly associated with temporal lobe epilepsy.[13] Use of the latter scale has likewise produced inconsistent results.

The idea that there is a specific interictal syndrome or personality profile of patients with temporal lobe epilepsy has been most strongly argued from the clinical point of view by Geschwind.[14] He included hyposexuality, hyperreligiosity, and hypergraphia (the tendency toward extensive and compulsive writing) as its main features. Several studies have been carried out on hypergraphia, as reviewed by Trimble,[15] and these suggest that it occurs in a small number of patients and is probably more common in temporal lobe epilepsy. The writing tends to have an obsessional stereotypic quality to it and often has religious, moral, and philosophical content. Variations on hypergraphia include the hiring of a stenographer to take

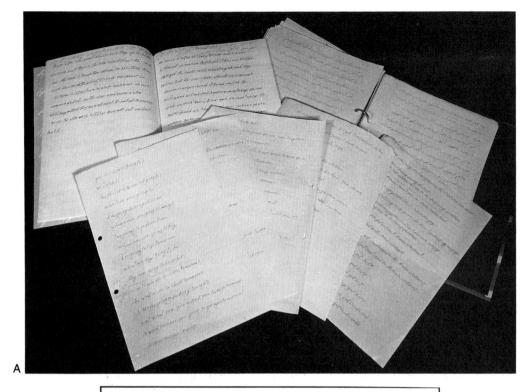

Fig. 24–1. (A) The kind of excessive output that patients with hypergraphia may bring to hospital with them. **(B)** The religious and repetitive nature of some of this writing is shown. This patient was Iranian, suggesting that such phenomenology is not confined to western cultures.

down extensive notes or compulsive repetitive painting or drawing (Fig. 24-1).

Hyposexuality is the predominant theme of any change of sexual behavior related to epilepsy, although there are few controlled studies. In those that have been carried out, significantly more patients with temporal lobe epilepsy reported hyposexuality compared to those with generalized forms of epilepsy, patients often reporting a global loss of sexual interest and showing little concern about it. Male epileptic patients reportedly have low levels of free testosterone in the presence of increased total testosterone levels, associated with higher sex hormone–binding globulin levels.[16] Thus the link between low libido and temporal lobe dysfunction requires further evaluation, taking into account these hormonal changes, which may themselves be consequent to a temporal lobe focus.

The relation between aggression and epilepsy is one that has caused considerable disagreement and has been well reviewed by Fenwick.[17] There is no doubt that aggressive behavior is a common cause of referral of epileptic patients to psychiatrists, and several authors have tried to correlate aggressive behavior with abnormal limbic system (especially amygdala) activity. As Fenwick pointed out, one of the difficulties has been in distinguishing the effects of diffuse brain damage from the effects of more discrete limbic system pathology. Fenwick concluded "that there is an association between poor impulse control and brain damage," taking the argument away from the more emotive area of aggression per se and placing it more firmly in relation to the control of a number of behaviors that may be impaired by epilepsy, its pathogenesis, or its treatment.

Another area of controversy has been that of the interictal psychoses. All neurologists have encountered acute psychotic disturbances in patients during the peri-ictal period; on occasion, and especially in complex partial status epilepticus, the phenomenology can resemble a schizophrenia-like illness in its entirety. However, the concept that patients with temporal lobe epilepsy may be more prone to the development of interictal psychotic disorders is less well recognized. The most extensive series so far published has been that of Slater and Beard.[18] They noted the absence of abnormal premorbid personality traits or a family history of psychiatric disturbance in their patients and an overrepresentation of temporal lobe

abnormalities. Their suggestion was that temporal lobe disturbance was somehow related to the development of the psychosis, but they did note certain phenomenological differences between patients with schizophrenia and the schizophrenia-like illness of epilepsy. In particular, they highlighted the preservation of warm affect and the lack of personality deterioration. Some 25 percent of patients in their series developed a psychosis as the frequency of generalized seizures was declining.

In recent years there have been several investigations of these psychoses.[11,19–23] In summary, it is suggested that psychoses of epilepsy are by no means rare, occurring in around 8 to 10 percent of patients with complicated temporal lobe epilepsy. The psychosis is not necessarily continuous but may be intermittent, and it may be provoked by a flurry of seizures. In other patients the development of the psychosis is insidious and chronic, and in a small percentage of patients it is related to a decline of seizure frequency.

Manic psychoses generally are rare. In 50 percent of patients with a psychosis related to epilepsy, the disorder resembles schizophrenia in nonepileptic patients, with the exceptions noted above. These schizophreniform presentations nearly always occur in patients with temporal lobe epilepsy who have complex partial seizures, often with secondary generalization. Further attempts to analyze the anatomical site of lesions in such patients suggest that it relates to a medial temporal[24] and often a dominant hemisphere focus. A dominant hemisphere link to a schizophreniform psychopathology has been demonstrated in clinical and electroencephalographic (EEG) studies,[21,22] in studies using PET,[25] and more recently those using MRI.[26]

Most authors agree that the psychosis develops a number of years after the onset of seizures, and there are few patients in whom seizures first occur following the onset of the psychosis. Of course, there are patients with schizophrenia who develop seizures secondary to the administration of neuroleptic drugs or electroconvulsive therapy. However, seizures otherwise are relatively uncommon in patients with schizophrenia with the exception of those who have a catatonic schizophrenia.

There has been a growing interest in temporal lobectomy as a treatment for intractable temporal lobe epilepsy. In many centers patients are now evaluated psychiatrically prior to surgery, and there is increasing recognition that a proportion of patients develop psychopathology after surgery. In many this is a transient affective disorder occurring in the first 3 months. However, severe depressive illness, manic states, suicidal ideation or acts, and occasional schizophrenia-like states that arise de novo are reported.[11] The necessity for psychiatric follow-up of these patients is clear.

Confusion in the literature regarding the relation between psychosis and epilepsy has been generated by the concept of forced normalization and the historical suggestion that electroconvulsive therapy (ECT) was introduced by von Meduna into psychiatric practice on the grounds that epilepsy and schizophrenia were antithetical conditions. This subject has recently been reviewed,[27] and the work of Landolt has been seen as being particularly important. He noted changes in the EEG during limited periods of overt psychoses lasting days or weeks. In particular, he reported improvement in previously abnormal EEGs during these episodes and referred to this phenomenon as "forced normalization." At the end of the psychotic episodes, the EEG again appeared abnormal. Although he was initially concerned with partial seizures, in his later writings he accepted the idea that forced normalization occurred with generalized seizures and could be provoked by the prescription of anticonvulsant drugs.

The term *alternative psychosis* has been used to emphasize the absence of seizures rather than normalization of the EEG. It implied that in some cases the control of seizures did not mean the cure of the clinical problems or inactivity of any underlying disease process of epilepsy, and that psychosis may occur as a result. These antagonisms occur in only a few patients but clinically are extremely important. Not only is the behavior disturbance in such patients often misunderstood and not interpreted in the light of seizure control, but it is now recognized that this phenomenon relates not only to psychoses but also to many other behavior disturbances that may be provoked by control of seizures. Common examples are behavior disturbances in children and depressive illnesses or the sudden presentation of pseudoseizures in adults who are taking a variety of anticonvulsant drugs to bring their epileptic seizures under control. The drugs most commonly involved are phenobarbital, benzodiazepines, and vigabatrin.

DISORDERS OF THE BASAL GANGLIA

It has been long been recognized that the basal ganglia have an important role in the development of psychiatric symptoms, and that patients with basal ganglia disorders often present with psychopathology. In recent years neuroanatomical techniques have unraveled some of the neurobiological underpinnings of this relationship. In particular, recognition of multiple parallel circuitry involving cortical structures and the basal ganglia has permitted distinction of the dorsal striatum (with its interconnections with the neocortex) from the ventral striatum (with its largely limbic, orbitofrontal, and cingulate connections). Further, it is recognized that there is considerable cross-talk between the limbic system and the basal ganglia, allowing an understanding of the relationship between emotional and motor disorders. The concept that the basal ganglia are purely motor in function has long ceased to be part of neurological dogma.

Huntington's disease exemplifies a neurological disorder that frequently presents with a psychiatric disturbance. Up to 50 percent of patients with Huntington's disease present with psychopathology before they develop motor disorders.[28] This ranges from behavioral disturbances, with psychopathic behavior and alcoholism, to more obvious manic-depressive psychoses and paranoid and schizophrenia-like states. Eventually these cease to be the predominant clinical features, as the dementia progresses. *Parkinson's disease* is known to be associated with a depressive illness in up to 60 percent of patients. This is often an atypical affective disorder with considerable associated anxiety, but it may also take the form of a classic unipolar depression. Psychotic states are increasingly recognized, particularly in patients with Parkinson's disease who have been on dopamine agonists for several years.[28] The extent to which medication and the underlying disease processes are interlinked with these phenomena is unclear. The psychiatric disorder may be extremely difficult to treat, as drugs that control the psychoses are likely to exacerbate the movement disorder. A new range of antipsychotics, exemplified by clozapine, are proving useful in these conditions.

The *Gilles de la Tourette syndrome,* a condition of multiple motor and vocal tics that starts in childhood and waxes and wanes over time, is associated with obsessive compulsive disorder. It is now suggested that underlying these states may be an autosomal dominant gene that has varying phenotypes which include Gilles de la Tourette syndrome, multiple motor tics, and obsessive compulsive disorder.[29]

There is a growing literature in psychiatry showing disturbed frontal-striatal function in obsessive compulsive disorder. A number of other disorders of the basal ganglia are associated with obsessive compulsive behaviors, including Parkinson's disease, Fahr's syndrome, neuroacanthocytosis, Wilson's disease, and Sydenham's chorea. Other psychopathologies are also sometimes seen with these states.[30]

It is important to note that the drugs used to treat psychoses, particularly the neuroleptics, are associated with the development of movement disorders, notably tardive dystonia and tardive dyskinesia. Biological associations can therefore be postulated between such neurotransmitters as dopamine and both motor dysfunction and severe psychopathology.

SUMMARY

Certain regional CNS disorders have been reviewed to emphasize one important aspect of the relation between psychiatry and neurology—that is, the way that neurological illness can precipitate or predispose to behavior disturbances. These areas need assessment by physicians who are familiar with the vagaries of behavior disorders and their prognosis and differing modes of presentation. The fact that a number of neurological conditions present with behavior disorders that phenomenologically resemble psychiatric conditions (e.g., the schizophrenia-like psychoses of epilepsy) makes them important models for understanding the neurological underpinning of psychiatric illnesses and emphasizes the close links between psychiatry and neurology.

The counterpart to this idea is the increasing evidence that many patients with psychiatric disorders have impaired neurological function or structural changes in the brain, as detected by the newer investigative techniques. In essence, this argument is merely continuing the progress made from previous centuries, so that behavior disorders have increasingly come to be associated with recognized neuropathology. Obvious examples from the last century include Parkinson's disease, multiple sclerosis, and general paralysis of the insane (earlier "neuroses"), while in this century the neurological underpinnings of de-

mentia are becoming clearer. Furthermore the evidence is now overwhelming that schizophrenia represents the outcome of neuropathological processes as yet to be clearly defined.[10] Most investigators view it as a neurodevelopmental disorder, with subtle neuropathological changes in the hippocampus leading to the later onset of the psychotic state. An interesting analogy is with temporal lobe epilepsy. In that condition, specific pathology (mesial temporal sclerosis) may be the seed for the later onset of seizures (and in some patients with temporal lobe epilepsy, a psychosis). It is important to emphasize that it is disturbances of the limbic system in particular that are most likely to present with behavior disorders. Nevertheless, there are other neurological states that have obvious behavioral counterparts, such as nondominant hemisphere parietal lesions.[10] Unfortunately, space limitations preclude further discussion of these disorders here.

NEUROLOGICAL PRESENTATIONS OF PSYCHIATRIC ILLNESS

The last half-century has seen an expansion of psychiatric units in general hospitals and the recognition that a large number of psychiatric problems can be found in patients with general medical disorders. In general, some 30 to 60 percent of inpatients and 50 to 80 percent of outpatients may be suffering from some form of psychic distress or overt psychiatric problem. Using rating scales, Knights and Folstein showed that 33 percent of patients admitted to general medical wards showed cognitive impairments, and 46 percent had psychiatric disorders.[31] In many cases the physician in charge of the patient had not identified these abnormalities.

De Paulo and Folstein studied 126 patients admitted to hospital for neurological disorders, using rating scale assessments to detect psychopathology. They noted that 30 percent had cognitive deficits and 50 percent emotional disorders.[32] Rates of referral to psychiatrists were minimal, around 15 percent in the studies of De Paulo and Folstein.[32] Bridges and Goldberg examined 100 neurological admissions, both clinically and with rating scales, and noted that 43 scored high on the General Health Questionnaire, the estimated prevalence of psychiatric disability being 39 percent from the psychiatrist and 11 percent from the admitting neurologist.[33] Of the psychiatric morbidity, 72 percent went undetected by the admitting neurologist. Schiffer applied DSM III criteria to 241 inpatients and outpatients on a neurology service and noted 42 percent to have sufficient symptomatology to justify a DSM III diagnosis.[34] Ten of 57 inpatients and 32 of 184 outpatients were evaluated with a chief complaint that could be classified as primarily psychiatric. In this group the most common diagnoses were conversion disorders, anxiety disorders, and somatoform disorders. In general, as determined in various series, organic brain syndromes and depression are the commonest causes for psychiatric referral in a liaison unit, followed by personality disorders and psychoneuroses. Schizophrenia and paranoid psychoses are reported with much less frequency. Depression is the most common diagnosis; it often presents with somatic symptoms but may also coexist with neurological disease (see below).

Pain, especially headache, is a frequently reported psychiatric symptom and, unrelated to overt somatic pathology, may be found as a presenting symptom in 45 to 60 percent of psychiatric patients. Psychiatric illness itself is a major factor in determining the onset of pain. In one survey, 46 percent of patients who presented with the cardinal symptom of headache were found to be suffering from an endogenous depression.[35] In addition, pain presenting as a symptom in medical clinics is often associated with psychiatric illness and thus may be equally indicative of psychiatric or somatic illness. Contrary to the commonly held view, patients with chronic pain often have some form of hypochondriacal illness with somatic preoccupation or some underlying personality disorder rather than a depressive illness.

The concept that some patients are particularly susceptible to pain was advocated by Engel.[36] He assumed that from birth an individual builds up a library of pain experiences that are of importance not only for development but also because they later influence pain interpretation. Pain has a number of meanings for the individual. It serves as a warning of damage to the body, a means of communication especially leading to comfort by a loved person, a means of punishment, a means for expressing aggression and power, an expression of sexual feeling, and a signal for badness and guilt and sometimes for the expiation of guilt. In other words, pain is seen as a

mechanism to achieve certain gratifications and to attain psychic equilibrium. According to Engel, the "pain-prone" patient shows some or all of the following features: (1) a prominence of guilt, with pain serving as the means of atonement; (2) a background of predisposition to the use of pain for such purposes; (3) a history of defeat and suffering and an inability to tolerate success; (4) unfulfilled aggression; (5) development of pain as a replacement for loss; (6) sadomasochistic sexual development; (7) the location of pain often determined by identification with another; and (8) a variety of psychiatric illnesses.

Patient Response to Illness

Such explanations and ways of looking at medical problems, particularly neurological problems, border on the concepts of psychosomatic medicine and an era of medical psychiatry that did a great deal of injustice to the subject. In clinical terms, there are many patients who develop symptoms of somatic disease without any obvious somatic underpinnings. Furthermore, a patient's psychological reaction to a known illness may itself lead to alteration of the symptoms of that illness and bring with it secondary symptoms that need evaluation in their own right. The patient's premorbid personality is an important variable that influences the response to disease.[37] Hence assessment of a patient's personality and individual coping style has relevance for understanding symptoms as they present. For the patient, any disease represents injury or threat of injury and often a threat of loss of some ideal—either body function, body image, psychosocial role, or occupation. In this respect, neurological illness is particularly stressful and may lead to psychiatric symptoms, the latter manifesting as depression or an anxiety state, and to lesser degrees of behavior change as shown by frustration, anger, withdrawal, denial, regression, or dependence.

A patient's response to disease may be related to the meaning and importance for the patient of the affected part of the body or of the actual lesion and its relation to the body image. In neurological patients the idea of damage to the highest integrative function of the self (i.e., the brain) is particularly threatening. Additional variables include beliefs about the cause of the disease, which depend in part on cultural and educational factors, the state of the patient's current interpersonal relationships and social support systems, the extent of any mutilation and loss of ability and consequent socioeconomic disability, previous experience of disease, the patient's state of awareness and cognitive functioning, and the degree of acceptance by the patient of his or her "sick role." The fact that in some instances illness paradoxically provides gain or relief for the patient must not be overlooked, and this assumption is implicit to understanding the presentation of certain varieties of hysteria.

Hysteria

Although it is one of the oldest words in medicine, *hysteria* is difficult to define. A number of contemporary definitions—for example, that in the International Classification of Diseases[38]—refer to psychological mechanisms and imply that the symptoms have either some form of symbolic value or represent the outcome of some Freudian mechanism based on psychological conflict. Generally it is assumed that a diagnosis of hysteria implies a medically unexplainable condition[39] manufactured from the metaphysical context of the patient's interpersonal relationships. In reality, it is a diagnosis most frequently made by non-psychiatrists, often being the outcome of either a failure of the doctor-patient relationship or a frustration of the regular diagnostic process because clinical and laboratory evaluations reveal no abnormality. Hence the diagnosis is made on purely negative grounds. A number of advances have been made in understanding hysteria and are briefly reviewed here. A fuller account is given elsewhere.[40]

An important step forward was made by Chodoff and Lyons.[41] They highlighted the problem that historically two independent aspects had been confused—that is, a personality style (referred to as hysterical) and certain symptoms (referred to as conversion or dissociative). In other words, simply because a patient displayed a flamboyant personality style referred to as hysterical did not mean that the symptoms were necessarily those of hysteria.

The hysterical personality includes a dramatic and emotional style of presentation, with excessive gestures and exaggerated, imprecise verbal responses. It is precisely these latter qualities that make history–taking difficult, and patients with elusive neurological symptoms provide the unwary doctor with a poorly defined account of their problems. Their affect appears shallow and labile but without the emptiness associated with a pseudobulbar palsy, and patients can be seductive and demanding in their interpersonal relationships.

Terms such as *conversion* or *dissociative,* when applied to symptoms, are best used in a metaphorical sense without any underlying concept in regard to pathogenesis either from a physiological or a psychological point of view. In other words, the term *conversion* is applied to the symptom pattern with no underlying need to explain what precisely is "converted" to what.

There is some relation between the hysterical personality and conversion symptoms, but it is not strong. Results from several studies have suggested that around 19 percent of patients presenting with conversion phenomena show the hysterical personality style.[40] Thus conversion symptoms may occur in patients of different personalities, including obsessional personalities.

An important association of conversion symptoms is with organic, especially neurological, disease, although this is not as strong as is often supposed. Several investigators have commented on this phenomenon, including Gowers,[42] who said, "there is hardly a single disease of the nervous system by which such symptoms (hysteria) may not be evoked in predisposed subjects." The high frequency of later development of organic disease found in the follow-up study of Slater was the reason for his suggestion that hysteria was "a myth."[43] Of his original 85 patients, nearly 60 percent had an associated recognizable organic disease at the time of diagnosis of hysteria or developed one during the follow-up interval. Slater was led to conclude that "the diagnosis of hysteria is a disguise for ignorance and a fertile source of clinical error."

Thus, a diagnosis of hysteria can be made in the presence of associated neurological disease. Such a diagnosis should not automatically lead to instant discharge from the clinic and failure of follow-up. Over time, patients may develop recognizable neuropathology, and an alternative diagnosis may become more appropriate.

One of the arguments for assuming some underlying neurophysiological abnormality in patients with hysteria relates to the persistent reporting of an over-representation of symptoms on the left side of the body. These observations have been noted with regard to anesthetic patches[44] and other symptoms such as pain.[45] The sensory loss may affect several modalities, is overrrepresented on the left side, and may be associated with diminished taste, smell, and hearing on that side. Further examination may reveal restricted visual fields with tubular vision, and the tendon reflexes may also be diminished on the affected side. Although there are several potential explanations for this unequal distribution of the anesthesia, including the special properties of the nondominant hemisphere for processing unconscious information, it is certainly of interest that disorders of the body image that occur after lesions to the nondominant parietal cortex—for example, anosognosia—are unilateral. Those seen after lesions of the dominant parietal cortex—such as autotopagnosia and finger agnosia—tend to be bilateral. Furthermore, anosognosia and its milder variant anosodiaphoria (denial of illness and hemiplegia) have some resemblance to the intense denial so often reported in association with hysteria, referred to as "la belle indifference." Clinically the important point is that the anesthetic areas, which do not correspond to normal neuroanatomical boundaries, have diagnostic significance and should not be merely discarded by an innocent intern as the result of "suggestion." They have been observed in patients who receive a diagnosis of hysteria for well over 100 years and may reflect some underlying neurophysiological change in patients who tend to somatize.

HYSTERICAL SEIZURES

Patients with hysterical seizures (usually called *pseudoseizures* but more properly designated as *nonepileptic seizures*) are being referred increasingly for evaluation.[46] This has resulted from technical advances permitting the long-term EEG monitoring of patients with intractable seizures. Such monitoring has revealed that many patients, some of whom have carried a diagnosis of epilepsy for many years and been treated with multiple anticonvulsants drugs, do not have epilepsy at all. Among such patients, many have only pseudoseizures, but a few also have epilepsy. Evaluation of these patients can only be undertaken with the full knowledge of the psychiatric conditions that may present as seizures, including particularly panic disorder with agoraphobia, depersonalization, other anxiety states, depression, and seizures as a manifestation of dissociation.[47] The importance of

early recognition of these patients is clear, since treatment is with psychotropic medications, psychotherapy, or behavior therapy; anticonvulsant drugs should be avoided.

BRIQUET'S SYNDROME

Briquet's syndrome is a polysymptomatic disorder that begins during early life. It usually affects female subjects and is characterized by recurrent multiple somatic complaints that are inexplicable in terms of current knowledge of pathological processes. Patients make repeated visits to physicians, are prescribed a large number of medications, and undergo frequent hospitalizations and operative procedures. In the current diagnostic and statistical manual of the American Psychiatric Association (DSM IIIR),[39] it is referred to as somatization disorder, the diagnostic features of which are shown in Table 24-4. In practice such patients are not difficult to discern, and Briquet's syndrome is reported in 1 to 2 percent of consecutive female patients attending hospitals for investigations. It is rare in men. First-degree female relatives have a 10-fold increase in the same syndrome, whereas male relatives show a preponderance of antisocial personalities and alcoholism. Monozygotic twins have a greater concordance rate than dizygous pairs.[48]

Briquet's syndrome assumes importance among patients presenting with neurological symptoms, as seizures, fainting, reports of loss of consciousness, visual symptoms, weakness, headaches, anesthesia, and paralysis are commonly reported by patients with the disorder. The importance of recognizing the diagnosis is that it has prognostic validity, and individual symptoms must be assessed in the full knowledge of the overall medical and psychiatric history of such patients. Management includes avoidance of any form of invasive procedure that could lead to secondary iatrogenic damage, resistance to further surgical exploration of any symptoms, and avoidance of any addictive medications.

ABNORMAL ILLNESS BEHAVIOR

The term "abnormal illness behavior" is popular, particularly in the setting of liaison psychiatry, and it is briefly discussed here. It was Pilowsky who introduced the concept based on ideas that derived from social psychology.[49] Abnormal illness behavior is de-

Table 24-4 Diagnostic Criteria for Somatization Disorder (Briquet's Syndrome)

A history of many physical complaints or a belief that one is sickly, beginning before the age of 30 and persisting for several years.

At least 13 symptoms from the list below. To count a symptom as significant, the following criteria must be met:

1. No organic pathology or pathophysiologic mechanism (e.g., a physical disorder or the effects of injury, medication, drugs, or alcohol) to account for the symptom or, when there is related organic pathology, the complaint or resulting social or occupational impairment is grossly in excess of what would be expected from the physical findings
2. Has not occurred only during a panic attack
3. Has caused the person to take medicine (other than over-the-counter pain medication), see a doctor, or alter life-style

Symptom list

Gastrointestinal symptoms
1. Vomiting (other than during pregnancy)
2. Abdominal pain (other than when menstruating)
3. Nausea (other than motion sickness)
4. Bloating (gassy)
5. Diarrhea
6. Intolerance of (gets sick from) several different foods

Pain symptoms
7. Pain in extremities
8. Back pain
9. Joint pain
10. Pain during urination
11. Other pain (excluding headaches)

Cardiopulmonary symptoms
12. Shortness of breath when not exerting oneself
13. Palpitations
14. Chest pain
15. Dizziness

Conversion or pseudoneurologic symptoms
16. Amnesia
17. Difficulty swallowing
18. Loss of voice
19. Deafness
20. Double vision
21. Blurred vision
22. Blindness
23. Fainting or loss of consciousness
24. Seizure or convulsion
25. Trouble walking
26. Paralysis or muscle weakness
27. Urinary retention or difficulty urinating

Sexual symptoms for the major part of the person's life after opportunities for sexual activity
28. Burning sensation in sexual organs or rectum (other than during intercourse)
29. Sexual indifference
30. Pain during intercourse
31. Impotence

Female reproductive symptoms judged by the person to occur more frequently or severely than in most women
32. Painful menstruation
33. Irregular menstrual periods
34. Excessive menstrual bleeding
35. Vomiting throughout pregnancy

(From American Psychiatric Association: Diagnostic and Statistical Manual of Mental Disorders, Third Edition, Revised. APA, Washington, DC, 1987, with permission.)

fined as "the persistence of an inappropriate mode of perceiving, evaluating, acting in relation to one's state of health, despite the fact that a doctor has offered a reasonably lucid explanation of the nature of the illness, and the appropriate course of management to be followed, based on a thorough medical examination."[49] This broad definition covers a number of medical conditions such as hysteria, hypochondriasis, malingering, and the Munchausen syndrome, in which an abnormality in the way patients evaluate and act in relation to their symptoms (illness behavior) is central. Pilowsky pointed out that these diagnoses are usually made by nonpsychiatrists on the basis of a discrepancy between detectable somatic pa-

thology and the patient's reaction; in other words "the doctor does not believe that the sick role that the patient assumes is appropriate to the objective pathology detected."[50] Use of the term *abnormal illness behavior* makes it unnecessary to question the nature or existence of hysteria and places understanding of these conditions in a wider context.

SOMATOFORM DISORDER

In any neurological setting there are several kinds of patient who present under the rubric of somatoform disorder (DSM IIIR). There are those with obvious psychiatric disorders, the main one being a major affective disorder with somatization, in whom there is little evidence of underlying neurological illness. Anxiety states frequently present with neurological symptoms, and hyperventilation itself provokes somatic symptoms. By contrast, psychotic conditions, in particular schizophrenia, rarely present to the neurologist with conversion phenomena. There are also patients with Briquet's syndrome, the chronic long-standing stable form of hysteria, who are best viewed as having a severe form of a personality disorder with a poor prognosis.

Patients with neurological illness who present with conversion symptoms are generally of three sorts. First, there are those whose neuroticism threshold has been lowered in a nonspecific way by cerebral lesions and who are thus more likely to present with a neurotic illness, of which hysteria is one, in a setting of stress. This explanation may reflect one reason for the high association between a diagnosis of hysteria and underlying neurological disease in some series and may be particularly important with such illnesses as multiple sclerosis, epilepsy (especially with anticonvulsant intoxication), head injury, and early dementia. Second, there are those patients whose conversion symptoms replicate their existing neurological illness, such as the occurrence of nonepileptic seizures in a patient with epilepsy or motor weakness in a patient with mild multiple sclerosis. The onset of the conversion symptoms may relate to the development of an underlying anxiety state or affective disorder or an alternative psychiatric problem. Finally, as Slater noted, there are patients who have undiagnosed neurological disease and in whom the diagnosis of hysteria is made.[43] It is particularly because of these patients that the diagnosis of hysteria should be made on positive grounds. This requires clearly demonstrating discrepancies between neurological signs and symptoms as expected and as displayed and establishing firmly, by careful dissection of the past history and current mental state, some clear evidence of psychopathology and predisposition. Anesthetic patches should always be noted and not dismissed. Earlier episodes of abnormal illness behavior should be sought, and an extensive surgical history should be viewed skeptically. The finding of secondary gain, although interesting and important, is itself insufficient to make a diagnosis of hysteria and in many settings is purely in the eye of the beholder. Where there is no positive evidence to make the diagnosis, it is perhaps better to wait before committing the patient to a diagnosis of hysteria that may have unfortunate consequences.

Affective Disorders

Disorders of affect, in particular depression, are frequently encountered in neurological practice, and two aspects merit consideration here: (1) the quality of the depressive symptoms reported by patients and (2) the relation of any change of affect to underlying CNS disease. In clinical practice a common and important error is to confuse depression as an illness with depressive symptoms occurring as a reaction. The essential criterion for a *depressive illness* is disturbance of mood, which, moreover, must be prolonged and continuous. Episodes of more transient mood change or chronic mild changes of mood are best referred to as *dysthymic disorder*. For the assessment of depressive symptoms, personality factors are often poorly taken into account, in particular premorbid neuroticism. Thus, many patients suffering from dysphoric symptoms and complaining of depression in reality have long-standing personality disorders and tolerate life's stresses poorly. These patients are best not diagnosed as having depressive illness and are not helped by the prescription of psychotropic medications.

With depressive illness the change of mood is associated with loss of vitality, the patient ceasing to enjoy life and admitting to a loss of emotional well-being. Concentration difficulty with complaints of poor memory, increased apathy with diminution of movements, and change of appetite, food intake, and sleep pattern are found. Sleep may be disturbed in a variety of ways, the commonest being nocturnal restlessness with periodic waking, or the more typical early morning waking with morbid ruminations and inability to get to sleep again. Patients lose interest in their food, complain that it is tasteless, and often lose weight. Feelings of anxiety and tension are invariably present; and sometimes, in contrast to the typical psychomotor retardation, agitation with indecision and excessive motor activity is seen. In an extreme form, intense aimless pacing is noted. Patients complain of loss of energy, fatigability, and tiredness; often there is a diurnal variation, the symptoms improving as the day passes.

Suicidal thoughts and preoccupations are frequent and should always be inquired about. Thoughts of worthlessness, guilt, and letting people down are typical, but crying is often not reported and should be asked about, especially in men. Increased irritability, hostility, and aggressive episodes, especially within the family setting, become troublesome. Libido is diminished. A low-dose dexamethasone test may reveal a failure of cortisol suppression.

When strictly defined, the diagnosis of depressive illness among patients in neurological units is less common than is suggested by the number who are actually given that diagnosis but who in reality are suffering from more long-standing personality disturbances or understandable reactions to neurological disability. However, there are patients with a more direct association between neurological illness and depression, and this association touches on the fundamental biochemical and neurological underpinnings of affective expressions. With regard to tumors, meningiomas (especially frontal meningiomas) are notoriously liable to induce a picture typical of major depressive disorder, and diencephalic tumors have been reported to lead to an affective disorder with hypomanic swings. The association between disorders of the basal ganglia and depression is of particular interest.

Cerebrovascular accidents have also been reported as leading to a depressive illness. In a controlled study in which comparison was made with similarly disabled orthopedic patients, patients with stroke had a significantly higher incidence of depression than controls (45 versus 10 percent), suggesting that the mood change is not simply a reaction to disability.[51] In a series of studies, Robinson and colleagues found that with lesions in the dominant hemisphere, the nearer the lesion was to the frontal pole, the more severe was the depression.[52] In the nondominant hemisphere, the farther away the lesion was from the frontal pole, the higher was the frequency of depression. There was no association with aphasia, although depression has been reported to be more frequent in association with Broca's aphasia.[53] These findings were largely related to depression of early onset; longer-term follow-up studies suggest the depression associated with stroke is linked to psychosocial factors and difficulty with rehabilitation.

It should be noted that patients with an affective disorder can present with a marked cognitive disturbance with complaints of poor memory, impaired concentration, difficulty with planning and decision making, and poor abstracting abilities. The term *pseu-*

dodementia has been used to specify this disorder, although it can be argued that it is better referred to as a reversible dementia and categorized as subcortical. The presentation can so resemble the dementia of Alzheimer's disease that it may be misdiagnosed and left untreated. Important clues that help distinguish this disorder from Alzheimer's disease include a history of affective disorder, a relatively acute onset with little evidence of decline prior to the development of affective symptoms, the patient's distress and complaints about cognitive function (in contrast to the lack of insight often seen in dementia), the response to questions in the mental state examination (patients often using "don't know" as an answer, whereas in dementia the answers are more evasive), and the performance on more structured psychological tests (which do not reveal the focal deficits of early Alzheimer's disease and suggest patchy and inconsistent impairments). Although no clear pattern of cognitive change emerges, the subjective complaints of patients are often worse than is warranted by their performance on objective tests, and they in particular show difficulty with attention, speed of mental processing, attention to detail, abstraction, and memory, especially on tasks that require effort, motivation, and active processing.[54]

The EEG findings can be deceptive in patients with an affective disorder. Certain waveforms that some authors have associated with affective symptoms are occasionally misinterpreted as being related to epilepsy, whereas other authors regard them as normal variants. Rhythmic midtemporal discharges are said to be associated with a generalized increased risk for psychopathology, including hypochondriasis and depression.[55] Small sharp waves that are sometimes exclusively temporal in location and that occur during drowsy states or light sleep have also been associated with affective symptoms and a tendency to suicide. Furthermore, 43 percent of patients with bipolar affective disorder have been reported as showing small sharp waves, which may be significantly related to a family history of affective disorder.[56] Finally, Struve and colleagues reported a highly significant positive relation between paroxysmal EEG abnormalities and suicidal ideation and acts, as well as associated destructive acts, unrelated to medications.[57] Thus, patients with an affective disorder who present with paroxysmal episodes of poor concentration and coordination may be thought to have complex partial seizures, and their EEGs may be "abnormal." Close attention to the total clinical picture, the family history, and past history of the patient reveals the appropriate diagnosis.

Posttraumatic Stress Disorder

Patients who are involved in life-threatening accidents sometimes go on to develop one of a number of posttraumatic syndromes. Posttraumatic stress disorder is one of the most important; its diagnostic criteria are delineated elsewhere.[39] A number of patients with symptoms of this disorder have also had head injuries, and distinguishing between symptoms secondary to organic brain damage and those of posttraumatic stress disorder may then be difficult.

The cardinal features of posttraumatic stress disorder relate to re-experiencing the traumatic event, increased autonomic arousal (particularly on exposure to environmental triggering stimuli or reminders of the event) and the development of avoidance phenomena, social withdrawal, and difficulty in making affective contact with relatives and friends. The disorder often comes on several weeks after the trauma and frequently is intertwined with depressive symptoms. In neurological practice it may also be interlinked with a somatoform disorder. In such cases the underlying constellation of symptoms of the posttraumatic stress disorder may be missed unless sought specifically.

PSYCHIATRY AND NEUROLOGY: TWO SIDES OF THE SAME COIN

Psychiatry and neurology have always been closely intertwined, the discipline of neurology evolving from the work of the neuropsychiatrists of the seventeenth, eighteenth, and nineteenth centuries. It was the middle to late nineteenth century that saw the beginnings of a division between the two disciplines. The continuing pursuit of localization and the anatomical/pathological correlations based on these ideas led to the evolution of neurology as a separate discipline. The failure of strict localization principles to provide a satisfactory explanation for mental disorders and the reaction to the pessimism of the earlier degeneracy theories that had permeated neuropsy-

chiatric thinking for a half-century led to renewed hopes of understanding and treating neuropsychiatric illnesses through the discipline of psychoanalysis, founded by the neurologist Sigmund Freud. Psychoanalytical theory, modified and diluted, came to dominate psychiatry, particularly in the United States, through the early part of this century, when the divisions between neurology and psychiatry considerably magnified. North America was crucial to this development, first on account of the "optimistic" social climate that has always characterized that region of the world. In contrast to the European emphasis on hereditary factors and biological determinism, America was seen as the great egalitarian society where background made no difference to one's achievements or failures. Mental illness could thus be seen only in terms of epigenetic principles and sociological developments. Second, there was the financial aspect, in the sense that psychoanalytical treatment was expensive, and it was only the economic climate of North America that was fertile enough for its growth. The United States also provided fertile ground for the growth of neurology, not only with the development of lucrative private practices but during the 1940s with the development of EEG for clinical use (and financial reward).

Although a number of physicians have trod an intermediate ground between neurology and psychiatry, they have been few and far between. Putnam was interested in psychoanalysis and in part responsible for inviting Freud to deliver lectures at Clarke University in Worcester in 1909. Jelliffe too was deeply interested in psychoanalysis; and both Cobb and Schilder, in their own ways, sought integration between the two disciplines. Gradually, however, mind and body, the Cartesian dualism that has always undermined this area, became separated, and the idea arose, particularly in lay minds, that the psychiatrist dealt only with the metaphysical ("it's all in my mind") and the neurologist with "real diseases." It is only during the last three decades that there has been a dramatic change in this relation, accelerated by several important discoveries.

First and foremost was the discovery of neurotransmitters and the way in which they influence behavior, followed by the introduction of psychotropic drugs. These have dramatically altered and improved the prognosis for many patients with both neurological and psychiatric disability. Second, there was the discovery of the limbic system (see above), which provided a cerebral representation for emotional disorders, a concept similar to the cerebral representation for speech disorders. When a patient is referred with a speech disorder, the cerebral underpinnings are now at least partially understood. However, with an "emotional disorder," the logic of attributing it to some cerebral disruption still evades many practitioners. Third, neurology and psychiatry have come to share technological developments, not only in terms of the neurochemical advances of recent years but also in terms of investigative techniques such as EEG, CT, MRI, magnetic resonance spectroscopy, single photon emission computed tomography (SPECT), and PET scanning.

The division between neurology and psychiatry left many patients dissatisfied, particularly those whose diagnoses fell on the borderline of the two disciplines. A number of physicians similarly found the split unsatisfactory or misguided. To fill the needs of patients, there has been a growth of interest in the borderline problems and of practitioners who deal with them. New disciplines have sprung up—variously termed *neuropsychiatry, organic psychiatry, biological psychiatry,* and *behavioral neurology*—each with a slightly different emphasis. Behavioral neurology, in particular, has been dominant in North America, deriving principally from the school of Geschwind and colleagues, who view behavior from a strictly neurological standpoint and whose interest is largely represented by the section above on behavioral consequences of neurological illness. In contrast, neuropsychiatry has a tradition firmly rooted in brain function and pathology, but it also embraces an interest in changes of function as well as structure. It has a tendency to embrace holism with regard to understanding the way the brain behaves, as opposed to following a strictly localizationalist approach.

If psychiatry and neurology represent two sides of the same coin, an appropriate apophthegm may be that psychiatry represents heads and neurology tails. However, it is probably more appropriate to suggest that, like a trick coin on which half of a symbol is printed on one side and half on the other side, a fuller appreciation of the role of the brain and its diseases in the human condition will come about only when the coin is spun and the ensuing gestalt becomes visible.

REFERENCES

1. Jackson JH: In Taylor J (ed): Selected Writings of John Hughlings Jackson. p. 382. Hodder & Stoughton, London, 1931
2. Goldstein K: After Effects of Brain Injuries in War. Grune & Stratton, New York, 1942
3. Mayer-Gross W, Guttmann E: The problem of general as against focal symptoms in cerebral lesions: a contribution to general symptomatology. J Ment Sci 82:222, 1936
4. Lishman WA: Organic Psychiatry. Blackwell Scientific Publications, Oxford, 1978
5. Trimble MR: Post-Traumatic Neurosis. John Wiley & Sons, Chichester, 1981
6. Stuss DT, Benson DF: Frontal Lobes. Raven Press, New York, 1986
7. Jacobsen CF: Functions of the frontal association cortex. Arch Neurol Psychiatry 33:558, 1935
8. Cummings J: p. 57. In: Clinical Neuropsychiatry. Grune & Stratton, Orlando, FL, 1985
9. Luria AR: The Working Brain. Basic Books, New York, 1973
10. Trimble MR: Biological Psychiatry. John Wiley & Sons, Chichester, 1988
11. Trimble MR: The Psychoses of Epilepsy. Raven Press, New York, 1991
12. Gibbs FA, Stamps FW: Epilepsy Handbook. Charles C Thomas, Springfield, IL, 1958
13. Bear DM, Fedio P: Quantitative analysis of interictal behavior in temporal lobe epilepsy. Arch Neurol 34:454, 1977
14. Geschwind N: Behavioral changes in temporal lobe epilepsy. Psychol Med 9:217, 1979
15. Trimble MR: Hypergraphia. p. 75. In Trimble MR, Bolwig T (eds): Aspects of Epilepsy and Psychiatry. John Wiley & Sons, Chichester, 1986
16. Toone BK, Edeh J, Fenwick P, et al: Hormonal and behavioral changes in epileptics. p. 283. In Porter RJ, Mattson RH, Ward AA, Dam M (eds): Advances in Epileptology, 15th International Epilepsy Symposium. Raven Press, New York, 1984
17. Fenwick P: Aggression and epilepsy. p. 31. In Trimble MR, Bolwig T (eds): Aspects of Epilepsy and Psychiatry. John Wiley & Sons, Chichester, 1986
18. Slater E, Beard AW: The schizophrenia-like psychoses of epilepsy. Br J Psychiatry 109:95, 1963
19. Trimble MR: Psychiatric aspects of epilepsy. Psychiatr Dev 4:285, 1987
20. Toone BK, Garralda ME, Ron MA: The psychoses of epilepsy and the functional psychoses: a clinical and phenomenological comparison. Br J Psychiatry 141:256, 1982

21. Flor-Henry P: Psychosis of temporal lobe epilepsy. Epilepsia 10:361, 1969
22. Perez MM, Trimble MR: Epileptic psychosis—diagnostic comparison with process schizophrenia. Br J Psychiatry 137:245, 1980
23. Perez MM, Trimble MR, Murray NMF, Reider I: Epileptic psychosis: an evaluation of PSE profiles. Br J Psychiatry 146:155, 1985
24. Hermann BP, Dikman S, Schwartz MS, Karnes WE: Interictal psychopathology in patients with ictal fear: a quantitative investigation. Neurology 32:7, 1982
25. Gallhofer B, Trimble MR, Frackowiak R, et al: A study of cerebral blood flow and metabolism in epileptic psychosis using positron emission tomography and oxygen. J Neurol Neurosurg Psychiatry 48:201, 1985
26. Conlon P, Trimble MR: A study of epileptic psychosis using MRI. Br J Psychiatry 156:231, 1990
27. Wolf P, Trimble MR: Biological antagonism and epileptic psychosis. Br J Psychiatry 146:272, 1985
28. Trimble MR: Neuropsychiatry. John Wiley & Sons, Chichester, 1981
29. George MS, Trimble MR, Ring HA, Sallee FR, Robertson MM: Obsessions in obsessive-compulsive disorder with and without Gilles de la Tourette's syndrome. Am J Psychiatry 150:93, 1993
30. Cummings JL. Clinical Neuropsychiatry. Grune & Stratton, Orlando, FL, 1985
31. Knights EB, Folstein MF: Unsuspected emotional and cognitive disturbance in medical patients. Ann Intern Med 87:723, 1977
32. De Paulo JR, Folstein MF: Psychiatric disturbances in neurological patients: detection, recognition and hospital course. Ann Neurol 4:225, 1978
33. Bridges THW, Goldberg DP: Psychiatric illness in inpatients with neurological disorders. Br Med J 289:656, 1984
34. Schiffer RB: Psychiatric aspects of clinical neurology. Am J Psychiatry 140:205, 1983
35. Haack HP, Kick H: How frequently are headaches expression of an endogenous depression? JAMA 256:765, 1986
36. Engel GL: "Psychogenic" pain and the pain-prone patients. Am J Med 26:899, 1959
37. Lipowski ZJ: Review of consultation psychiatry and psychosomatic medicine: 2. Clinical aspects. Psychosom Med 29:201, 1967
38. World Health Organization: Mental disorders: glossary and guide to their classification. In: International Classification of Diseases. 9th Ed. WHO, Geneva, 1980
39. American Psychiatric Association: Diagnostic and Statistical Manual of Mental Disorders, 3rd Ed. Revised. APA, Washington, DC, 1987
40. Trimble MR: Hysteria. p. 159. In Reynolds EH, Trimble MR (eds): The Bridge between Neurology and Psychiatry. Churchill Livingstone, Edinburgh, 1989
41. Chodoff P, Lyons H: Hysteria, the hysterical personality and "hysterical" conversion. Am J Psychiatry 114:734, 1958
42. Gowers WR: A Manual of Diseases of the Nervous System. 2nd Ed. Churchill, London, 1893
43. Slater E: Diagnosis of hysteria. Br Med J 1:1395, 1965
44. Purves-Stewart J: The Diagnosis of Nervous Diseases. Butler & Tanner, London, 1920
45. Merskey H, Boyd DB: Emotional adjustment of chronic pain. Pain 5:173, 1978
46. Trimble MR: Pseudoseizures. Neurol Clin 4:531, 1986
47. Trimble MR: Hysteria. p. 159. In Reynolds EH, Trimble MR (eds): The Bridge between Neurology and Psychiatry. Churchill Livingstone, Edinburgh, 1989
48. Torgersen S: Genetics of somatoform disorders. Arch Gen Psychiatry 43:502, 1986
49. Pilowsky I: The diagnosis of abnormal illness behavior. Aust NZ J Psychiatry 9:135, 1975
50. Pilowsky I: Dimensions of abnormal illness behavior. Aust NZ J Psychiatry 9:141, 1975
51. Folstein MF, Maiberger R, McHugh PR: Mood disorder as a specific complication of stroke. J Neurol Neurosurg Psychiatry 40:1018, 1977
52. Robinson RG, Kubos KL, Starr LB, et al: Mood disorders in stroke patients: importance of location of lesion. Brain 107:81, 1984
53. Benson DR: Aphasia, Alexia and Agraphia. Churchill Livingstone, Edinburgh, 1979
54. Caine E: Pseudodementia: current concepts and future directions. Arch Gen Psychiatry 38:1359, 1981
55. Hughes JR, Hermann BP: Evidence for psychopathology in patients with rhythmic mid-temporal discharges. Biol Psychiatry 19:1623, 1984
56. Small JG, Small IF, Milstein V, et al: Familial associations with EEG variants in manic depressive disease. Arch Gen Psychiatry 32:43, 1975
57. Struve FA, Saraf KR, Arko RS, et al: Relationships between paroxysmal electroencephalographic dysrhythmia and suicide ideation and attempts in psychiatric patients. p. 199. In Shagass C, Gershon S, Friedhoff AJ (eds): Psychopathology and Brain Dysfunction. Raven Press, New York, 1977

25

Neurological Aspects of Sleep

Bruce J. Fisch

Within a relatively short period of time, the centuries-old concept of sleep as a passive, monolithic, restorative process has been replaced by a view of sleep as a dynamic process in which cerebral activity at times exceeds that of waking levels and at other times decreases to levels only encountered in coma. This conceptual awakening has been led by remarkable advances in knowledge about the functional anatomy of sleep, such as the discovery of the role of the suprachiasmatic hypothalamic nucleus in regulating the sleep-wake cycle. These advances now provide a scientific basis for the neurological practice of sleep disorders medicine.

Although sleep disorders medicine is an emerging field, it is already an important part of the practice of neurology. This is due partly to the striking prevalence of sleep disorders. Approximately 60 million Americans experience serious insomnia, as many as 10 million suffer from sleep apnea, 20 million have sleep schedule disorders, and over 250,000 have narcolepsy. Thousands of others suffer from a variety of sleep disorders, many of which complicate common neurological disorders. The International Classification of Sleep Disorders[1] currently lists 88 separate disorders of sleep, most of which are primarily disorders of the nervous system.

SLEEP PHYSIOLOGY

As in other areas of medicine, a knowledge of sleep physiology forms the basis for effective diagnostic and therapeutic decision making. This information, when summarized for the patient, can also alleviate anxiety, provide reassurance, and enhance compliance.

The current era of sleep physiology began in the mid-1930s with the discovery by Loomis and colleagues that sleep is separated into different electroencephalographic states now referred to as stages I, II, III, and IV of non-rapid eye movement (NREM) sleep.[2] Following their discovery, efforts to understand sleep continued to focus on dividing it into more elemental components. Initially, this was accomplished by recording over extended periods of time using additional physiological monitors. The recording of eye movements led to the first description of rapid eye movement (REM) sleep by Aserinsky and Kleitman in 1953.[3] Electromyographic (EMG) monitoring resulted in the discovery of muscle atonia in REM sleep.[4,5] The subsequent addition of respiratory, blood pressure, thermal, and cardiac monitoring further revealed the dramatic autonomic variability of REM sleep. Monitoring sleep over extended periods led to the discovery that the stages of sleep recur in cycles throughout the night.

Currently, sleep is divided into five stages: I, II, III, and IV, and REM sleep. This division is based on variations in three physiological functions: (1) electroencephalogram (EEG), (2) chin EMG, and (3) eye movements. According to currently accepted guidelines, the polysomnogram is scored by assigning a particular stage of sleep to each 20- or 30-second epoch or recording according to set criteria provided in the guidelines.[6] This allows for the quantitation of sleep states and for the graphical displays of sleep stages, sometimes referred to as hypnograms, as shown in Figure 25-1.[7] The physiological characteristics of the various stages of sleep are summarized below.

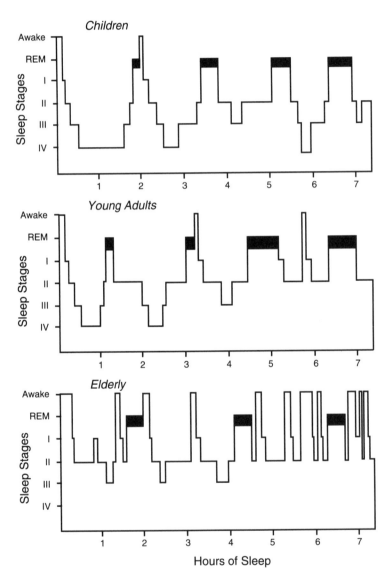

Fig. 25-1 Hypnograms representing normal sleep at different ages. As age increases, nocturnal arousals and awakenings increase and stages III and IV sleep decrease. REM sleep continues to occur in approximately 90-minute cycles. (From Kales A, Kales JD: Recent findings in the diagnosis and treatment of disturbed sleep. N Engl J Med 209:487, 1974 with permission.)

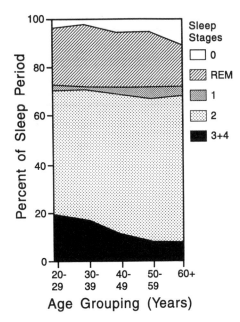

Fig. 25-2 Sleep stages obtained from the second consecutive night of PSG (the second night reduces problems related to adaptation to the laboratory environment). Sleep stages are shown as a percentage of the sleep period—defined as the time between sleep onset and final awakening. (From Hirshkowitz M, Moore CA, Hamilton CR, et al: Polysomnography of adults and elderly: sleep architecture, respiration, and leg movement. J Clin Neurophysiol 9:56, 1992, with permission.)

STAGE I SLEEP

Stage I sleep is referred to as light sleep or drowsiness. Stage I sleep is defined as a dropout of the alpha rhythm often associated with slow wandering lateral eye movements and a diminution of EMG activity.[8] Not all individuals perceive themselves to be asleep during these changes and some maintain awareness of the environment. Increases in nocturnal stage I sleep occur in a variety of sleep disorders, particularly sleep apnea. The percentage of total sleep occupied by stage I sleep increases with age, as illustrated by Figure 25-2.[9]

STAGE II SLEEP

Stage II sleep is defined by the appearance of K complexes (prominent biphasic waveforms that are at least 0.5 second in duration, with an initial negative phase followed by a positive phase appearing maximally over the central head regions) or sleep spindles (complexes of 12- to 14-Hz waveforms in runs exceeding 0.5 seconds in duration, appearing maximally

over the central head regions). Occasionally slow lateral eye movements from stage I sleep persist into stage II sleep. Sleep spindles first appear at 1 to 3 months after birth and peak at 7 to 8 months of age, when they may be present for more than 50 percent of the time during stage II sleep. In adult sleep they typically occur 2 to 8 times each minute, whereas K complexes occur 2 to 3 times per minute. EMG activity in stage II sleep is present but reduced from waking and stage I levels. The percentage of total sleep occupied by stage II sleep increases with age.

STAGES III AND IV SLEEP

Stages III and IV sleep, also referred to as *slow-wave sleep* or *delta sleep,* are defined by the appearance of 2-Hz or slower EEG waveforms that are at least 75 μV in amplitude when recorded from electrode derivations A1 to C4 or A2 to C3. To distinguish stage III from stage II, the delta waves must occupy at least 20 percent of the recording. When they occupy more than 50 percent of each epoch, sleep is scored as stage

IV. The EMG is often active but less so than in stage I sleep. Sleep spindles and K complexes may be present but occur less frequently as sleep deepens. Eye movements are absent.

Slow-wave sleep is most prominent in childhood and declines with age (Fig. 25-2). Indeed, it may be absent in normal individuals over 60 years of age. This decline in slow-wave sleep roughly parallels the normal decline in amplitude of the waking EEG and may be due in part to reduced synaptic connectivity. The largest decline in slow-wave sleep occurs during the second decade of life. The arousal threshold to various stimuli is higher in slow-wave sleep than in stage I or II sleep. Children in slow-wave sleep are normally difficult to arouse and may remain confused for prolonged periods following arousal (see below, under Confusional Arousals). Benzodiazepines reduce slow-wave sleep and abrupt withdrawal may produce excessive slow-wave sleep.

Growth hormone has its greatest 24-hour peak at the beginning of the night, during the initial period of slow-wave sleep. This may explain why individuals who are allowed to sleep after a period of sleep deprivation recover slow-wave sleep first. If slow-wave sleep is consistently interrupted, symptoms of fibrositis may arise. Thus, slow-wave sleep has been referred to as restorative sleep.

REM SLEEP

REM sleep is distinct from the other stages of sleep. Only three stages of sleep can be consistently distinguished in the neonatal period: active sleep, quiet sleep, and indeterminate or transitional sleep. Active sleep is the forerunner of REM sleep. As in adults, it is characterized by abrupt, rapid eye movements, irregular respiration and heart rate, penile tumescence, muscular atonia (absent EMG activity), and a low-amplitude, irregular EEG pattern. Thermal regulation is markedly suppressed, so that neither shivering nor sweating is typically seen. In the neonate, sleep onset is usually in active sleep, whereas in the child or adult, REM sleep rarely occurs during the first 60 minutes of sleep. Sleep onset with REM sleep beyond early childhood is therefore abnormal. Active sleep first appears at approximately 20 weeks conceptual age. At 30 weeks gestational age, 80 percent of sleep time is in active sleep. At term, REM (active) sleep occupies 50 percent of sleep time. After the first

year of life, the majority of REM sleep occurs during the second half of the night, and REM sleep occupies 20 to 25 percent of total sleep time (Figs. 25-2). During REM sleep, brain metabolism increases dramatically to near waking levels. The combination of atonia, active cerebral metabolism, and an EEG pattern that at times resembles alert wakefulness has led to the characterization of REM sleep as a metabolically awake brain in a paralyzed body.

REM sleep is suppressed by tricyclic antidepressant medications and monoamine oxidase inhibitors. Alcohol ingestion immediately before sleep suppresses REM sleep during the first half of the night but then results in excessive REM activity later in the night. Prolonged REM suppression (produced by repeatedly awakening individuals from REM sleep or by pharmacological means) is followed by a period of excessive REM sleep, often referred to as REM rebound. These observations have important implications for sleep testing. For example, the sudden withdrawal of tricyclic antidepressant medication before testing may lead to the erroneous impression of narcolepsy because of early onset and excessive REM sleep.

Sleep Stage Distributions

The stages of sleep are distributed across the night in approximately four to five cycles (Fig. 25-1). Each cycle begins with NREM sleep and ends with REM sleep. After infancy, sleep begins with stage I sleep and then usually progresses from stage II to stage IV sleep, with a return to stage II sleep before the occurrence of REM sleep. As sleep continues through the night, the contribution of slow-wave sleep to each cycle decreases and REM sleep increases. REM sleep during the first cycle lasts only several minutes, whereas slow-wave sleep often lasts over 30 minutes. The duration of the first cycle is typically 70 to 110 minutes, whereas subsequent cycles last closer to 90 to 120 minutes.

When viewed across the entire night, the total percentages of the stages of sleep are distributed approximately as follows: stage I, 5 percent; stage II, 45 to 55 percent; stage III, 3 to 8 percent; stage IV, 10 to 15 percent; and REM, 20 to 25 percent.[10] Sleep epochs with EEG awakenings or excessive artifact caused by patient movement are scored as arousals or movement time, respectively. Increases in either stage I sleep, arousals, movement time, or wakefulness after sleep onset are all common nonspecific indicators of abnormally disrupted sleep.

As illustrated in Figure 25-2, the ability to consolidate all of one's sleep time into a single continuous major sleep period declines with age. Even though elderly individuals often appear to be excessively sleepy because of daytime napping, their total 24-hour sleep time is approximately the same as during middle age. Various strategies have been used to enhance sleep consolidation in the elderly, with limited success.

Circadian Rhythms and the Sleep-Wake Cycle

Circadian rhythms (*circa*: "around," *dia*: "day") are biological time cycles which have a period of approximately 24 hours, such as the sleep-wake cycle.[11] Biological cycles that repeat more than once every 24 hours, such as the cycling of sleep stages throughout the night, are referred to as *ultradian* rhythms. The study of biological rhythms is referred to as *chronobiology*.

One of the major advances in chronobiology has been the discovery of the biological clock, which regulates the sleep-wake cycle: the suprachiasmatic nucleus of the hypothalamus. In animals, bilateral ablation of this nucleus causes an immediate and total loss of the circadian sleep-wake cycle.[12,13] Equally remarkable, replacement of the suprachiasmatic nucleus using fetal transplant tissue restores circadian rhythmicity.[14,15] The nucleus, like all circadian clocks, is synchronized by an external cue or *zeitgeber* ("time giver"). The zeitgeber of the suprachiasmatic nucleus is light. Thus, the nucleus is set according to the day-night light cycle of the earth. Light reaches the suprachiasmatic nucleus by a projection from the retina that is separate from the primary visual pathway.[16]

Core body temperature appears to have a strong synchronizing effect on the sleep-wake cycle. Core body temperature fluctuates over an approximately 24-hour period, with the lowest temperature occurring prior to awakening, between 4 and 5 AM, and the highest in the late afternoon, near 5 PM. The ability of most individuals to fall asleep is greatest at the nadir or as core body temperature declines. REM sleep, more so than the other stages of sleep, is strongly regulated by core body temperature. REM sleep is most likely to occur during the upward swing in temperature between 4 to 6 AM. This relationship is easily demonstrated by delaying sleep onset until the end of the night, at which time REM sleep tends to predominate and may even initiate sleep onset.

When individuals are placed in time isolation without zeitgebers (external time cues), the sleep-wake cycle continues to parallel the temperature cycle for weeks to months. Thereafter an abrupt dissociation occurs in which the sleep-wake cycle increases to greater than 24 hours even though the temperature rhythm remains stable. Thus, it appears that although circadian temperature rhythms can be entrained by the suprachiasmatic nucleus, the circadian rhythm for temperature is modulated by more than one biological clock.

The clinical relevance of circadian rhythmicity to sleep becomes apparent when one tries to change a sleep-wake schedule abruptly. Difficulties arise not only because the "sleep debt" is altered but also because biological rhythms that ordinarily influence the sleep-wake cycle continue to cycle for varying periods of time on their own established schedules. This makes adaptations to new situations—such as time-zone changes (jet lag) or shift work—highly problematic. Elderly individuals who have difficulty consolidating sleep and individuals with neurological disorders that disrupt the normal cycling of sleep (see below, under Alzheimer's Disease) exemplify circadian rhythm disorders. One promising approach to regulating the sleep-wake cycle externally is the use of strategically timed exposure to bright light. Although still experimental, it has been demonstrated that light exposure can lead to dramatic shifts in the circadian rhythms for body temperature and cortisol secretion[17] and can thereby speed the resetting of the sleep-wake cycle. Future treatment strategies will probably include pharmacological agents and perhaps surgical interventions (e.g., transplantation of the suprachiasmatic nucleus).

Functional Anatomy of Sleep

The nervous system structures most important for initiating and maintaining NREM sleep are the basal forebrain, anterior hypothalamus-preoptic region, midline brainstem, and dorsolateral medullary reticular formation. Severe insomnia can be induced in animals by destruction of the midbrain, pontine, and medullary tegmental serotonergic raphe nuclei or by pharmacologically depleting brain serotonin.[18] The putative role of serotonin in sleep generation in humans is also supported by reports of insomnia associated with lesions in the midline mesencephalic and pontine tegmentum.[19] In one such report, natural sleep was temporarily restored by the administration of the serotonin precursor 5-hydroxytryptophan.[20] In animals, spontaneous recovery from such lesions further suggests that serotonin is only one of several important factors in sleep generation.

The presence of sleep-inducing substances in cerebrospinal fluid (CSF) has been established by experiments in which intraventricular injection of CSF taken from a sleep-deprived animal induced sleep in an alert animal. Several substances produced within the nervous system—including melanocyte stimulating hormone, prostaglandin D_2, and uridine—have been shown to have sleep-inducing effects. However, no single endogenous substance has been identified that is necessary or sufficient for the generation or maintenance of sleep.[21]

Structures essential for the generation of REM sleep are located primarily within the dorsolateral pons. Animal studies and anecdotal reports of pontine lesions in humans indicate that REM initiation and maintenance (i.e., rapid eye movements and muscle atonia) can be eliminated by lesions of the dorsolateral pons ventral to the locus ceruleus. Smaller pontine lesions than those required to block REM sleep can produce REM sleep without atonia in animals.[22] Such animals may thus exhibit complex aggressive behaviors during REM sleep which appear to be the enactment of dream content and are analogous to those which occur in humans with REM behavior disorder. Conversely, injections of cholinesterase inhibitors into the same location within the pons may induce atonia in the absence of sleep.[23] Using intracellular recording, such experiments have established that the atonia occurring in REM sleep is produced by the pontine activation of medullary inhibitory centers, which in turn induce postsynaptic hyperpolarization of brainstem and spinal motor neurons.

Several disorders of REM sleep function in humans have been delineated that were, in part, predicted by animal experimentation. Spinal motor neuron inhibition, absent H reflexes, and suppressed or absent tendon reflexes of REM atonia occur as discrete attacks of cataplexy or sleep paralysis in narcolepsy and rarely in other neurological disorders. In narcolepsy, these

attacks, together with the sudden onset of dream-like hallucinations (hypnagogic hallucinations), represent the sudden intrusion of REM sleep phenomena (atonia and dream mentation) during wakefulness. Thus, narcolepsy is actually a REM sleep disorder in which dissociated states occur. In REM behavior disorder, in which sometimes violent physical activity occurs during REM sleep, the atonia of REM sleep fails and the patient becomes physically active while dreaming. The discovery of dissociated sleep states in which certain features that should be present are absent (such as the lack of atonia in REM behavior disorder) or in which one state appears to intrude upon another (as in the atonia of REM sleep during wakefulness in cataplexy) underscores our current understanding of wakefulness, NREM sleep, and REM sleep as variable associations of physiological processes rather than "all or none" states.

DIAGNOSIS AND CLASSIFICATION OF SLEEP DISORDERS

A sleep disorder is generally defined as a disturbance of sleep that is deleterious to the individual's health or psychosocial well-being. Although some sleep disorders are life-threatening due to cardiovascular complications (e.g., sleep apnea) or the effects of sleepiness (e.g., industrial and automobile accidents), others may involve only temporary discomfort (e.g., jet lag). Currently, a patient who either complains of or is observed to have disturbed nocturnal sleep, excessive daytime sleepiness, or some other problem related to sleep is considered to have a sleep disorder. This broad definition even includes those who actually have no difficulty sleeping but believe they do (referred to as sleep misperception disorder, pseudo-insomnia, or sleep hypochondriasis).

The International Classification of Sleep Disorders groups disorders into the following four categories: dyssomnias, parasomnias, medical or psychiatric sleep disorders, and proposed sleep disorders.[1] Table 25-1 provides an outline of the classification as well as selected examples within each category. Dyssomnias are disorders that cause either excessive sleepiness or an inability to initiate or maintain sleep. Parasomnias are disorders intruding into the sleep process that

Table 25-1 The International Classification of Sleep Disorders

Classification	Selected Disorders
I. Dyssomnias	
A. Intrinsic sleep disorders	Narcolepsy, obstructive sleep apnea, restless legs syndrome, psycho-physiological insomnia
B. Extrinsic sleep disorders	Insufficient sleep syndrome, hypnotic-dependent sleep disorder
C. Circadian rhythm sleep disorders	Shift-work sleep disorder, delayed sleep-phase syndrome
II. Parasomnia	
A. Arousal disorders	Sleepwalking, sleep terrors
B. Sleep-wake transition disorders	Rhythmic movement disorder ("head banging")
C. Parasomnias usually associated with REM sleep	REM sleep behavior disorder, sleep paralysis
D. Other parasomnias	Nocturnal paroxysmal dystonia
III. Medical/psychiatric sleep disorders	
A. Associated with mental disorders	Depression, anxiety disorder, schizophrenia
B. Associated with neurological disorders	Sleep-related epilepsy, parkinsonism, electrical status epilepticus of sleep
C. Associated with other medical disorders	Sleep-related asthma, fibrositis syndrome, sleep-related gasteroesophageal reflux
IV. Proposed sleep disorders	Sleep-related laryngospasm, short sleeper, long sleeper

(Modified from Diagnostic Classification Steering Committee of the American Sleep Disorders Association: International Classification of Sleep Disorders: Diagnostic and Coding Manual. American Sleep Disorders Association, Rochester, MN, 1990, with permission.)

appear to be related to difficulties with partial arousal. Sleepwalking is an example of a parasomnia.

A more practical approach to classifying sleep disorders from the clinician's point of view is according to major symptomatology. A differential listing based on clinical distinctions is provided in Tables 25-2 and 25-3. It is beyond the scope of this review to discuss all the disorders listed, but summary descriptions can be found in the international classification.[1] The clinical manifestations of disorders of primary concern to the neurologist are presented below under specific headings.

The diagnosis of sleep disorders begins and often ends with the patient's history. Patients with sleep disorders will present with one or more of three complaints: (1) "I cannot get enough sleep"; (2) "I'm sleepy during the day;" or "I fall asleep all the time"; or (3) there is some unusual sleep behavior, often best described by a bed partner. Certain disorders may be associated with all three complaints. For example, patients with obstructive sleep apnea may complain of daytime sleepiness as well as an inability to sleep because of frequent awakenings gasping for air. As in the evaluation of a patient with epilepsy, an observer (i.e., the bed partner) should be encouraged to attend the initial interview. If possible, prior to the initial clinic visit, the patient should be sent a structured sleep questionnaire and a sleep diary to fill out. The former should contain questions concerning the patient's sleep habits, usual hours of sleep, sleep problem, current medications, other medical problems, weight gain in the last 30 years, alcohol intake, conditions under which sleep occurs, dietary stimulants (coffee, caffeinated beverages, etc.), activities other than those pertaining to sleep or sex that take place while in bed (e.g., eating and writing), occurrence or history of various abnormal sleep behaviors (e.g., enuresis and sleepwalking), and occurrence of other relevant symptoms (e.g., sleep paralysis, cataplexy, hypnagogic hallucinations, early morning headache, loud snoring, and difficulty in breathing at night). The sleep diary, which lists times of getting in and out of bed and of sleep onset and cessation, should be maintained for 1 week prior to the visit.

Observing patients after they have been allowed to sit for a few minutes in a quiet waiting room often provides a rough measure of sleepiness. Patients with moderate to severe sleepiness will be asleep, and those with sleep apnea will probably be snoring loudly.

Table 25-2 The Differential Diagnosis of Insomnia

Associated with psychological disorders
    Adjustment sleep disorder
    Psychophysiological insomnia
    Inadequate sleep hygiene
    Limit-setting sleep disorder
    Sleep-onset association disorder
    Nocturnal eating syndrome
	Associated with disorders of timing of the
	  sleep-wake pattern
	    Short sleeper
	    Time-zone change
	    Shift-work sleep disorder
	    Delayed sleep-phase syndrome
	    Non-24-hour sleep-wake syndrome
	    Irregular sleep-wake pattern

Associated with psychiatric disorders
    Psychoses
    Mood disorders
    Anxiety disorders
    Panic disorders
    Alcoholism
	Associated with parasomnias
	    Confusional arousals
	    Sleep terrors
	    Nightmares
	    Sleep hyperhidrosis

Associated with environmental factors
    Environmental sleep disorder
    Food allergy insomnia
    Toxin-induced sleep disorder
	Associated with disorders of the central
	  nervous system
	    Parkinsonism
	    Dementia
	    Cerebral degenerative disorders
	    Sleep-related epilepsy
	    Fatal familial insomnia

Associated with drug dependency
    Hypnotic-dependent sleep disorder
    Stimulant-dependent sleep disorder
    Alcohol-dependent sleep disorder	

Associated with sleep-induced respiratory impairment
    Obstructive sleep apnea syndrome
    Central sleep apnea syndrome
    Central alveolar hypoventilation syndrome
    Chronic obstructive pulmonary disease
    Sleep-related asthma
    Altitude insomnia
	Associated with no objective sleep
	  disturbance
	    Sleep state misperception
	    Sleep choking syndrome

Associated with movement disorders
    Sleep starts
    Restless legs syndrome
    Periodic limb movement disorder
    Nocturnal leg cramps
    Rhythmic movement disorder
    REM sleep behavior disorder
    Nocturnal paroxysmal dystonia
	Idiopathic insomnia, other causes
	    Sleep-related gasteroesophageal reflux
	    Fibrositis syndrome
	    Menstrual-associated sleep disorder
	    Pregnancy-associated sleep disorder
	    Terrifying hypnagogic hallucinations
	    Sleep-related abnormal swallowing
	    Sleep-related laryngospasm

(Modifed from Diagnostic Classification Steering Committee of the American Sleep Disorders Association: International Classification of Sleep Disorders: Diagnostic and Coding Manual. American Sleep Disorders Association, Rochester, MN, 1990, with permission.)

Prior to performing the physical examination, the sleep questionnaire, sleep diary, psychosocial situation (occupation, current and recent life stresses, presence of drug or alcohol abuse), and medical and psychiatric history should be reviewed. As in other areas of neurology, if the diagnosis has not been limited to two or three possibilities before the physical examination is performed, it is unlikely that a correct diagnosis will be reached.

The physical examination should include the patient's weight, vital signs, neurological examination, auscultation of the heart, and inspection of the nasal and oral airways. The presence of redundant tissue, tonsillar hypertrophy, micrognathia, malocclusion, and erythema of the soft palate and posterior pharynx (due to snoring) should be noted as risk factors for sleep apnea. In most cases, routine laboratory studies should include determination of plasma electrolytes,

Table 25-3 The Differential Diagnosis of Sleepiness

Associated with
  psychological disorders
  Inadequate sleep
    hygiene
  Insufficient sleep
    syndrome
  Limit-setting sleep
    disorder
Associated with psychiatric
  disorders
  Psychoses
  Mood disorders
  Alcoholism
Associated with
  environmental factors
  Environmental sleep
    disorder
  Toxin-induced sleep
    disorder
Associated with drug
  dependency
  Hypnotic-dependent
    sleep disorder
  Stimulant-dependent
    sleep disorder
Associated with sleep-
  induced respiratory
  impairment
  Obstructive sleep
    apnea
  Central sleep apnea
    syndrome
  Central alveolar
    hypoventilation
    syndrome
  Sleep-related
    neurogenic
    tachypnea
Associated with movement
  disorders
  Periodic limb
    movement disorder

Associated with disorders
  of the central nervous
  system
  Narcolepsy
  Idiopathic
    hypersomnia
  Posttraumatic
    hypersomnia
  Recurrent
    hypersomnia
  Subwakefulness
    syndrome
  Fragmentary
    myoclonus
  Parkinsonism
  Dementia
  Sleeping sickness
Associated with disorders
  of the timing of the
  sleep-wake pattern
  Long sleeper
  Time-zine change
  Shift-work sleep
    disorder
  Delayed sleep-phase
    syndrome
  Advanced sleep-
    phase syndrome
  Non-24-hour sleep-
    wake syndrome
  Irregular sleep-wake
    pattern

(Modified from Diagnostic Classification Steering Committee of the American Sleep Disorders Association: International Classification of Sleep Disorders: Diagnostic and Coding Manual. American Sleep Disorders Association, Rochester, MN, 1990, with permission.)

renal and hepatic function, and a complete blood count. In some cases additional tests for endocrine function, rheumatological disease, or infectious disease will be suggested by the patient's medical history and physical examination. Thyroid function tests should be obtained in all patients with sleep apnea.

SLEEP LABORATORY TESTING

The most useful tests for diagnosing sleep disorders are the overnight polysomnogram (PSG), multiple sleep latency test (MSLT), and actigraphy. PSG is used to determine whether nocturnal sleep is disturbed and to identify any specific causes for the sleep disturbance. The MSLT is used to determine whether the patient has excessive daytime sleepiness or the likelihood that the patient has narcolepsy. Actigraphy is used to establish objectively the patient's sleep-wake schedule over a period of 1 or more weeks.

Polysomnography

The PSG evaluation includes staging of sleep; assessment of respiratory, cardiac, and cerebral activity; and detection of movement disorders or other abnormal behaviors associated with sleep or arousal. In the past, due to technological limitations, the range of routinely monitored functions has been limited. Although this is no longer the case, some patients have difficulties in sleeping in the laboratory environment, and this will be made worse with the placement of additional monitoring devices. The likelihood of a "first-night effect" can be reduced before testing by taking time to explain to the patient what will happen in the sleep laboratory before testing. Patients who are anxious should be encouraged to visit the sleep laboratory and talk to the technologists about testing. They should also be encouraged to bring their own sleeping clothes, pillow, or whatever else they feel might make them comfortable. There should be some provision for another adult to accompany the patient to the laboratory. In some cases patients actually sleep far better in the laboratory than at home. This phenomenon is referred to as a "reverse first-night effect" and is most often associated with psychophysiological insomnia, an environmental sleep disorder (e.g., noise and allergies), sleep state misperception, or a psychiatric disorder.

Sleep is staged using at least one channel of EEG,

eye movement monitors (electrodes placed around the eyes), and submental EMG (electrodes placed under the chin). Because one channel is insufficient for assessing other cerebral activity and because the EEG changes of sleep are facilitated by additional channels of recording, PSGs typically use three or four channels of EEG recording. Respiratory functions are monitored by placing a small device between the nose and mouth that has separate channels for detecting nasal and oral air flow. This device registers the presence of airflow by detecting temperature changes. Respiratory effort is monitored by placing mercury strain gauge or piezoelectric belts around the chest and abdomen to detect changes in circumference. Intercostal EMG electrodes may be added as a backup monitor for the belts, which may become displaced during the night. Intercostal EMG may also be helpful in assessing actual effort. Oxygen saturation is monitored with a clip-on pulse oximeter, which is usually worn on the finger. Leg movements are monitored with a pair of disk electrodes placed over the pretibial surface of each leg. Finally, a video camera with low-light recording capability is used to record continuously for any behavioral changes that might occur. Video monitoring is also used by the technologist in the control room to monitor the patient's activities.

In selected situations additional physiological monitors may be used. In patients with gastroesophageal reflux, a pH probe inserted nasogastrically will register sudden increases in acidity of the lower esophagus. In certain patients with subtle obstructive apnea (i.e., upper airway resistance syndrome), frequent arousals may occur with little evidence of upper airway obstruction in airflow or chest-wall or abdominal monitors. In such cases it is helpful to place an esophageal balloon transducer that can detect slight changes in intrathoracic pressure and thereby confirm the presence of airway obstruction.

Although there are normative values for the distribution of sleep stages[24] and abnormalities of breathing in sleep,[25-27] the interpretation and clinical significance of the PSG usually depends on the patient's presenting complaint, current medications, medical and neurological evaluation, and adaptation to the laboratory environment. Thus, the PSG in isolation infrequently provides a diagnosis. The interpretation of specific PSG findings is discussed below, in the sections on specific disorders.

Multiple Sleep Latency Testing

The MSLT is performed using PSG monitoring during four or five daytime nap opportunities at 2-hour intervals beginning 1.5 to 3 hours after the patient arises from nocturnal sleep. For accurate interpretation, the MSLT is performed following overnight PSG. As with the PSG, the recording montage includes EEG (C3-A2 or C4-A1), submental EMG, and eye movement monitors for staging sleep. Additional channels of EEG recording—such as T3-Cz, Cz-T4, and O1-A2 or O2-A1—are used to facilitate the recognition of sleep onset. For clinical testing, the nap is concluded if sleep does not occur after 20 minutes or 15 minutes after the first 30-second epoch of sleep. An average latency to sleep onset for each of the four or five naps (five are performed if REM sleep occurs during one of the preceding four naps) is then calculated. An average latency of less than 5 minutes is clearly abnormal, whereas an average latency of more than 10 minutes is clearly normal. Patients with excessive daytime somnolence typically have an average latency of less than 8 minutes. The occurrence of REM sleep during any nap is abnormal. Two or more naps containing REM sleep is virtually diagnostic of narcolepsy unless the patient suffers from another severe sleep disorder associated with either REM deprivation, such as sleep apnea, or a circadian rhythm disturbance.[28]

Actigraphy

Actigraphy is a simple and relatively inexpensive test that allows the physician to make an objective assessment of the patient's sleep-wake activity outside the laboratory. The actigraphic device is a small motion detector that is usually worn like a wristwatch. An on-board memory chip is used to store motion information. After being worn for 1 to 2 weeks it is inserted into a computer, which generates a graphic display of motility—the actigram. Persistent quiescent periods indicate sleep, and high levels of activity correlate with wakefulness. In normal individuals the actual correlation between wrist actigraphy and polysomnography may exceed 90 percent.[29] This correlation is less perfect in individuals with abnormal sleep and during times other than active wakefulness or slow-wave sleep.[30] Nevertheless, accuracy is sufficient to allow for a reliable objective assessment of sleep-wake patterns over long periods of time. Actigraphy is most useful in the evaluation of insomnia and sleep schedule disorders.

INSOMNIA

Insomnia is a symptom often associated with complaints of daytime sleepiness, headache, irritability, difficulty with concentration and memory, frequent nocturnal awakenings, early morning awakening, and nonrefreshing sleep. Because insomnia is a manifestation of so many disorders, an organized approach to diagnosis is essential. The first step is to understand clearly what the patient means by insomnia and to determine the significance of the complaint. The initial history should focus on nocturnal experiences and daytime sequelae. The pattern of insomnia may be important. Early morning awakening is typical of depression, whereas delayed sleep onset suggests psychophysiological insomnia (see below). Disorder-specific symptoms such as snoring, gastrointestinal discomfort, polyuria, breathing difficulties, paresthesias, itching, and involuntary movements should be sought. Because the largest proportion of patients with serious insomnia suffer from psychiatric disorders, it is important to obtain a psychiatric history. As with most disorders, duration is an important consideration in diagnosis and therapy. Transient insomnia has a duration of days and is usually related to changes in the environment, emotional stress, or changes in the timing of sleep (e.g., time-zone changes). Short-term insomnia has a duration of several weeks and is usually related to stress associated with acute illness, family life, or work. Chronic insomnia has a duration of more than 1 month and is often related to a primary psychiatric, neurological, or medical disorder.

Most individuals who seek help at a sleep disorders center suffer from chronic insomnia. Common causes of serious insomnia (Table 25-4) are psychiatric disorders, psychophysiological factors, drug and alcohol abuse, restless legs syndrome, and sleep apnea.[31] The diagnosis of drug and alcohol abuse may only become apparent when the patient enters the sleep laboratory or may require blood and urine toxicology screening. Table 25-5 provides a list of common medications that may interfere with sleep.

Table 25-4 Disorders of Initiating and Maintaining Sleep

Diagnosis	Percent Diagnosed
Psychiatric disorders	34.9
Psychophysiological insomnia	15.3
Drug or alcohol dependency	12.4
Periodic movements of sleep with or without restless legs syndrome	12.2
No insomnia	9.2
Sleep apnea	6.2
Medical, toxic, or environmental causes	3.8
Other	5.9

(From Coleman RM, Roffwarg HP, Kennedy SJ, et al: Sleep-wake disorders based on a polysomnographic diagnosis: a national cooperative study. JAMA 247:997, 1982, with permission.)

Psychophysiological Insomnia

Psychophysiological insomnia is a behaviorally conditioned sleep disorder in which sleep-preventing associations have become internalized and persist even though the initial cause of insomnia has been removed. Sleep-incompatible behavior that maintains the insomnia may be manifested by obvious poor sleep hygiene or by a subtle conditioned response to the bedroom environment. In the latter situation, patients find that they sleep better in unfamiliar environments. Psychophysiological insomnia usually develops out of periods of stress in which anxious thoughts keep the patient awake. After several nights, increased concern over an inability to sleep develops. Thereafter, a vicious cycle develops in which worry over the inability to sleep keeps the patient awake. As the insomnia develops, simple activities performed routinely before going to bed (setting the clock,

Table 25-5 Drugs That May Cause Insomnia

Stimulants	Tricyclic antidepressants
Caffeine	MAO inhibitors
Amphetamines	Meprobamate
Methylphenidate	Hypnotics
Sympathomimetics	Anxiolytics
Anticholinergics	Chemotherapeutic agents
Diphenhydramine	Opiates
Cimetidine	Methyldopa
Theophylline	Reserpine
Alcohol	β-Adrenergic blockers

brushing the teeth, etc.) become associated with an inability to sleep and eventually evoke a conditioned response. A focused absorption on the inability to sleep that overshadows other medical or social problems is a distinguishing feature of this disorder.

Patients with psychophysiological insomnia rarely have significant daytime sleepiness but do experience other common findings in insomnia: depression and irritability, fatigue, decreased motivation, memory impairment, and poor concentration. They may also have neurasthenic symptoms such as tension headache or cold hands and feet. Sleep occurs at times when no effort to sleep is put forth, as while reading or watching television. The PSG is characterized by an increased sleep latency (exceeding 30 minutes), increased wakefulness after sleep onset, a sleep efficiency of less than 85 percent (the ratio of total sleep time to time in bed), and increased stage I sleep.[1,32] If a reverse first-night effect occurs, the patient will be aware of it; by contrast, a patient with sleep state misperception will report poor sleep.

The treatment of psychophysiological insomnia includes sleep hygiene, behavioral therapy, and occasional hypnotics. Common rules of sleep hygiene for facilitating sleep are listed in Table 25-6.[33] These rules actually apply to most patients with insomnia. Behavioral intervention consists of relaxation therapy

(e.g., meditation, muscle relaxation, and breathing techniques), sleep restriction (allowing only several hours of sleep per night to improve sleep efficiency), and stimulus control therapy (patients are asked to get out of bed whenever they cannot sleep). Hypnotics may be helpful in breaking the cycle of insomnia but should be used only on one or two occasions per week. If the patient intends to attempt sleep before taking the hypnotic, then one with a rapid onset should be considered. If the patient knows that he or she will need a hypnotic ahead of time because of a potentially stressful event the next day, then the hypnotic is selected by its duration of effect.

Special care must always be taken when using hypnotics to treat patients with chronic insomnia. If the diagnosis is not clear, they should be avoided so as to lessen the risk of exacerbating sleep apnea or a substance abuse disorder. Sedation in either instance may be dangerous. Many patients with chronic insomnia develop paradoxical worsening of insomnia several weeks after the introduction of benzodiazepines or barbiturates. This occurs either because tolerance has developed and the initial dosage is now too low or because the patient tries to stop the medication only to encounter withdrawal symptoms. In either case the best approach is to withdraw medication slowly and treat the underlying cause of insomnia.

Table 25-6 Rules of Sleep Hygiene for Patients

1. Sleep only as long as needed to feel refreshed the next day. Avoid excessively long times in bed.
2. Maintain a regular arousal time in the morning in order to establish a constant circadian sleep pattern.
3. Maintain a steady daily amount of exercise.
4. Eliminate noise in the bedroom environment.
5. Keep the bedroom temperature comfortable. Avoid a sleeping environment that is too warm.
6. Use the bedroom for sleep only. Do not perform other activities in bed such as writing letters or eating.
6. Do not go to bed hungry.
7. Avoid the frequent use of sleeping pills.
8. Avoid caffeine in the evening, even if you think it does not disturb sleep.
9. Do not use alcohol as a sedative. It facilitates the onset of sleep but later acts as a stimulant.
10. Avoid the frequent use of tobacco.
11. If you feel upset because you cannot sleep, get up, turn on the light, and do something else.

(Adapted from Hauri PJ: The Sleep Disorders. 2nd Ed. Upjohn, Kalamazoo, MI, 1982, with permission.)

Periodic Leg Movement Disorder and the Restless Legs Syndrome

Periodic leg movement disorder and restless legs syndrome are leading causes of insomnia. The former consists of repetitive, stereotyped movements that cause repeated arousals from sleep. Each periodic leg movement resembles a Babinski reflex response, with dorsiflexion of the great toe and foot often accompanied by flexion of the ankle, knee, and hip. The movement may occur as a sustained contraction or as a rapid series of clonic contractions. EMG monitoring of the tibialis anterior reveals activity lasting 0.5 to 5 seconds and recurring every 4 to 90 seconds (usually every 15 to 40 seconds), mainly during stage II sleep. The contractions may affect only one leg but more often occur asynchronously in both. Interestingly, Babinski responses can be elicited in normal individuals in NREM sleep.[34] The resemblance to the Babinski reflex response has led to the hypothesis that the periodic leg movements are caused by transient lapses in cortically mediated motor inhibition.[35]

It was originally thought that the occurrence of more than five periodic leg movements per hour was clinically significant. However, it soon became apparent that such movements occur more frequently with increasing age in otherwise normal individuals. In view of these findings, the significance of these movements now depends on whether they are associated with arousals and complaints of daytime sleepiness. Therapeutic intervention is generally warranted when 15 or more periodic leg movements associated with arousals occur per hour of sleep.[36]

Patients with restless legs syndrome present with complaints of unusual and severe leg sensations, such as creeping, crawling, crushing, or searing pains. Infrequently, the pain may extend to the arms or remain unilateral. Relief is gained temporarily by walking, rubbing the legs, or applying heat. As soon as these maneuvers stop, the discomfort returns. Thus, a hallmark of this disorder is the irresistible urge to move the legs to relieve discomfort. The discomfort increases throughout the day until patients find they are unable to tolerate being stationary. Thus, not only is sleep interrupted but normal activities such as business meetings or long car rides become impossible. Restless legs syndrome is a relatively common disorder, affecting over 5 percent of the population. Its onset may occur in childhood, but the peak onset is in middle age. The course is somewhat unpredictable, with long remissions lasting for months or years, during which symptoms are greatly diminished. A family history should be sought, as the disorder is frequently familial. Unfortunately, familial cases tend to be more resistant to therapy.[37] Almost all patients with restless legs syndrome have periodic leg movements during sleep.

The restless legs syndrome is usually idiopathic but has been associated with pregnancy, uremia, rheumatoid arthritis, iron deficiency anemia, fibromyositis, peripheral neuropathy, myelopathy, leukemia, and withdrawal from anticonvulsants, benzodiazepines, barbiturates, and other hypnotics. Stimulants such as caffeine, as well as physical and emotional stress, may exacerbate the underlying condition.

The restless legs syndrome and periodic leg movement disorder respond to three main classes of medication: antiparkinsonian medications,[38] benzodiazepines, and opiates. Levodopa/carbidopa, bromocriptine, and selegiline may all be effective, but treatment is usually initiated with levodopa/carbidopa, beginning in the evening 1 to 2 hours before bedtime. If symptoms recur later at night or during the day, then a longer-acting preparation should be tried and if necessary taken also in the morning. Benzodiazepines have been used frequently, particularly clonazepam, but in our experience have not proven as efficacious. Moreover, sedative medications may cause daytime sleepiness or, rarely, insomnia. Opiates were used successfully by Ekbom,[39] who first described the restless legs syndrome, and remain a viable therapeutic alternative. If opiates are necessary, those with long half-lives or low addictive potential should be tried first. In some instances it may be necessary to combine medications.

Parkinsonism

As summarized by Aldrich,[40] patients with parkinsonism are at risk for disrupted sleep due to one or more of the following: (1) degeneration of the neural systems that regulate sleep, resulting in sleep fragmentation and reduced REM and slow-wave sleep; (2) bradykinesia and rigidity, and a reduction in the normal number of body shifts during sleep, causing discomfort and frequent arousals; (3) periodic leg movements, tremors, or medication-induced movement disorders, causing frequent and prolonged arousals; (4) abnormal muscle tone, which facilitates breathing abnormalities that may awaken the patient; and (5) disorders of circadian rhythm and the sleep-wake schedule, which may arise from medications or the disease itself. Improved sleep is often achieved by treating the underlying disorder with levodopa in the evening. Any improvement in sleep that occurs is probably due in part to increased nocturnal mobility.[41] Some patients may also respond to other dopamine agonists (e.g., pergolide, bromocriptine) or selegiline. Insomnia due to involuntary movements may respond to benzodiazepines or reduced doses of dopamine agonists. For sleep-wake schedule disturbances, a brief course of a short-acting benzodiazepine hypnotic may be helpful. Breathing disturbances should be approached as in other individuals; continuous positive airway pressure or upper airway surgery may be necessary.

One of the more difficult aspects of sleep disorders in patients with parkinsonism is that each of the medications used can potentially disrupt sleep. Low-dose dopamine agonists facilitate sleep, but high doses lead to sleep disruption. Dopamine agonists may cause nightmares, night terrors, nocturnal hallucinations, or dyskinesias. Benzodiazepine hypnotics may exacerbate sleep apnea. Tricyclic antidepressants are often useful for insomnia in parkinsonism, particularly because of their cholinergic side effects, but occasionally lead to an increase in periodic leg movements with arousal. These problems can usually be detected by careful history taking, but testing in the sleep laboratory may ultimately be required.

Alzheimer's Disease

The cognitive decline in Alzheimer's disease is paralleled by a decline in slow-wave sleep and REM sleep and an increase in the number of nocturnal awakenings and amount of time spent awake during normal sleep time.[42] As the disease advances, there is a progressive disruption of the circadian sleep-wake cycle, with reduced nocturnal sleep and increased daytime sleep. In addition to the gradual breakdown of the normal sleep process, patients with Alzheimer's disease experience the phenomenon of "sundowning." Although there is no formal definition for sundowning, it generally consists of evening attacks of delirium in which the patient experiences emotional and perceptual disturbances with irrational thinking, disorganized speech, and agitation.

The physiological basis for the deterioration of sleep in Alzheimer's disease appears to be the degeneration of brainstem and basal forebrain pathways that are crucial for initiating and maintaining sleep. Autopsy studies demonstrate degeneration of the brainstem midline raphe nuclei, locus ceruleus, and reticular formation, all of which play a critical role in sleep control.[42] Although the physiological basis for sundowning remains unclear, histological evidence suggests that it may be caused by degeneration of the suprachiasmatic nucleus.[43] Destruction of this nucleus would also explain the circadian sleep-wake schedule disturbance.

The first step in the treatment of sundowning is to rule out treatable causes such as drug-induced, infectious, or metabolic disorders. Behavioral and environmental treatments should be used whenever possible. These include maintaining a constant and familiar environment, increasing daytime activity, restricting daytime sleep, and increasing exposure to bright light during the day. Nocturnal agitation is usually treated with neuroleptics such as haloperidol or phenothiazines. There appears to be little evidence that one neuroleptic is superior to another.[44] Because of the potential for undesirable side effects such as orthostatic hypotension and extrapyramidal disorders (e.g., tardive dyskinesia, parkinsonism, and akasthisia), neuroleptics should be used intermittently or occasionally withdrawn to determine whether they are still necessary.

DISORDERS OF EXCESSIVE SLEEPINESS

Sleep Apnea

The most commonly diagnosed organic disorder of excessive daytime sleepiness is the obstructive sleep apnea syndrome,[31] which has a prevalence estimated to be between 1 and 8.5 percent.[45] Sleepiness in this syndrome is due to sleep deprivation caused by repeated arousals from struggling against a closed airway. In the original description of the pickwickian syndrome (i.e., obesity, daytime sleepiness, and cardiorespiratory failure), sleepiness was erroneously attributed to the effects of hypercarbia.[46] Although hypercarbia is known to impair cerebral function, somnolence is not an outstanding feature.[47] The true cause of sleepiness in the obstructive sleep apnea syndrome was discovered in 1965 when Gastaut and colleagues[48] in France and Jung and Kuhlo[49] in Germany, studying a series of pickwickian patients, found frequent intermittent airway obstruction during sleep, associated with repeated EEG arousals.

Obstructive apnea occurs when the upper airway collapses during inspiration. Respiratory effort continues against the closed airway until inspiratory pressures trigger an arousal. The arousal restores tone in the upper airway dilators, the genioglossus and geniohyoideus muscles, and airflow resumes. The site of airway collapse varies among patients; in approximately half it is at the level of the palate (velopharynx), and in the other half it is below the palate.[50,51] Airway collapse is often most severe during REM sleep, when muscle atonia of the upper airway occurs,[52] and is coupled with a reduced ventilatory drive to hypercarbia and hypoxia.[53] In approximately 60 percent of patients, the apneas are more frequent and more prolonged in the supine position during NREM sleep. During REM sleep, the occurrence of apnea is less dependent on position.[54] Obstructive apnea appears in the PSG as a cessation of airflow in the nasal and oral thermistor channels, with a continuation and buildup of respiratory effort in the channels monitoring chest and abdominal motion and intercostal EMG (Fig. 25-3). As the patient struggles to overcome the obstruction, paradoxical breathing occurs and the chest and abdominal circumferences enlarge and contract out of phase with each other. If the apnea is

prolonged, there is a fall in oxygen saturation as measured by pulse oximetry. An apnea is defined on the PSG as a cessation of airflow for at least 10 seconds. Other significant respiratory events include mixed apneas and hypopneas.

Mixed apneas consist of an initial cessation of both airflow and effort (i.e., a central apnea), followed several seconds later by the appearance of effort without airflow (i.e., an obstructive apnea). Mixed apneas have the same significance as obstructive apneas in patients with obstructive sleep apnea syndrome. Patients with this syndrome also experience episodic

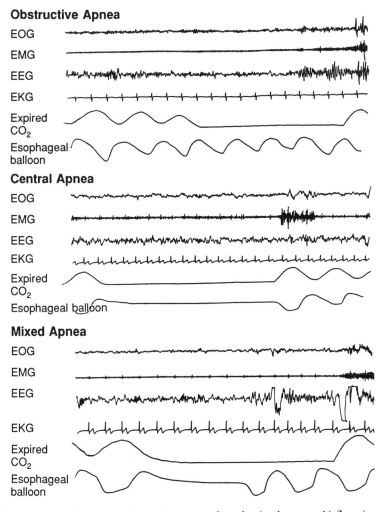

Fig. 25-3 Differences between obstructive, central, and mixed apnea. Airflow is monitored by CO_2 analysis and respiratory effort by an esophageal balloon transducer. (From Orr WC: Disorders of excessive somnolence (DOES). p. 52. In Hauri PJ (ed): The Sleep Disorders. Upjohn, Kalamazoo, MI, 1982, with permission.)

partial airway obstructions referred to as hypopneas. Hypopneas are variously defined on the PSG as (1) a decline of more than 50 percent in airflow; (2) a decline in airflow accompanied by a decline in oxygen saturation (SaO_2) exceeding 3 percent; or (3) a decline in airflow terminated by an EEG arousal. Occasional patients with the clinical presentation of obstructive sleep apnea syndrome appear to have central apneas on the PSG. In many instances this is because routine respiratory monitoring techniques fail to detect low-amplitude respiratory effort. Indeed, the only definitive technique for ruling out the presence of airway obstruction is esophageal pressure monitoring (Fig. 25-3). This is accomplished by inserting an esophageal balloon transducer attached to the end of a nasogastric tube. Esophageal pressure monitoring equipment has only recently become commercially available.

Interestingly, patients can present with the clinical findings of obstructive sleep apnea syndrome in the absence of polygraphically defined sleep apnea. This has been termed the upper airway resistance syndrome by Guilleminault and colleagues.[55,56] Esophageal pressure monitoring in such patients reveals frequent episodes of decreased pressure during inspiration that end with an EEG arousal. Recurrent arousals cause sleep deprivation. The upper airway resistance syndrome may be difficult to detect on a routine PSG because the polysomnographer has to look for subtle signs of airway resistance, such as recurrent EEG arousals, that may be associated with a buildup of snoring or increased intercostal EMG activity. Patients with upper airway resistance syndrome respond to the same therapeutic interventions used for obstructive sleep apnea.

In contrast to adults, complete airway obstruction with apnea is a rare event in children with clinically significant airway resistance during sleep. In a group of 20 children with obstructive sleep apnea syndrome, a mean apnea index (apneas per hour of sleep) of 2 was found by Rosen and colleagues.[57] In contrast, oxygen desaturations occurred frequently and the mean minimum SaO_2 was 66 percent (normal range in children is 92 to 100 percent). Clinical manifestations during sleep included loud snoring and labored breathing. Thus, the diagnosis in children depends more on changes in oxygen saturation and EEG arousals than the presence of apneas. Snoring in any child should always raise the suspicion of obstructive sleep apnea.

A useful summary measure of the severity of sleep-disordered breathing is the respiratory disturbance index (RDI), also referred to as the apnea-hypopnea index (AHI). The RDI is the number of apneas plus hypopneas that occur per hour of sleep. Although it was originally thought that obstructive sleep apnea could be diagnosed by an RDI of 5, it has become apparent that this would include almost 40 percent of normal individuals over 60 years of age[25,27,58] and would exclude the majority of children with obstructive sleep apnea. The number of apneas per hour of sleep (the apnea index) normally increases with age; it should be less than 1 in children,[59] less than 5 in adults aged between 20 and 60 years, and less than 10 in adults over 60 years. The presence of daytime sleepiness correlates most closely with the degree of sleep fragmentation rather than with the number of apneas or frequency or degree of oxygen desaturation. Thus, as in the upper airway resistance syndrome, the diagnosis can be made in the appropriate clinical setting even with an RDI of less than 5 as long as there are frequent awakenings or arousals associated with other respiratory findings (e.g., crescendo snoring, bradytachycardia, oxygen desaturation).

A number of symptoms arise as a direct consequence of sleep deprivation. These include impaired cognitive abilities, memory difficulties, delayed reaction times, irritability, aggressiveness, confusional awakenings, fatigue, and sexual dysfunction (reduced drive or impotence). If sleep deprivation is severe enough, there may be hypnagogic hallucinations or episodes of automatic behavior in which the patient performs complex activities with no subsequent recollection of them. Restless sleep occurs as a consequence of struggling to overcome a closed airway. During the apneic episode, body movements may be slight or massive. In the latter instance the patient may assume an upright sitting position and make loud choking sounds as the apnea terminates. Occasionally the patient awakens in a panic-stricken state and may run breathless to a window. Bed partners often report being kicked during the night and that bedcovers are torn off the bed. Excessive body movements during sleep cause excessive sweating in most patients. Nocturia occurs in approximately one-fourth of patients[60] and is rarely associated with episodes of urinary incontinence. Urinary incontinence is probably caused by increases in intra-abdominal pressure that occur during apneic episodes. Headache upon awakening is a frequent complaint and may be a consequence of recurrent elevations of intracranial pressure that occur with each instance of obstructive apnea (see below). The headaches are usually bifrontal and last for 1 to 3 hours after awakening.

Patients with clinically significant obstructive sleep apnea syndrome usually present with the complaint of daytime sleepiness. Less often there is a complaint of difficulty in initiating and maintaining sleep due to the arousing effects of airway obstruction. Rarely, there is a denial of difficulties with daytime sleepiness, even though family members and friends are well aware of the problem. With growing awareness among the lay public, patients are increasingly being brought to the physician by concerned bed partners who notice lapses in breathing or episodes of choking. More unusual presentations encountered in the hospital or emergency room include postanesthetic respiratory failure and anoxic nocturnal seizures. Patients with acute stroke may develop obstructive or central apneas with severe oxygen desaturations. The incidence of apnea in stroke is unknown, but the disorder is probably underdiagnosed. Because of the physiological consequences of obstructive apnea in stroke, treatment should be instituted without delay. Patients with severe, long-standing obstructive sleep apnea may also present with right-sided heart failure from pulmonary hypertension either caused or exacerbated by the apneic episodes. Approximately 50 percent of patients with obstructive sleep apnea have hypertension, and up to 7 percent have polycythemia.[60]

Nearly all patients with obstructive sleep apnea snore, and in many cases the snoring is loud enough to drive the bed partner from the bedroom. Over two-thirds of patients are also overweight or obese.[60] Thus, in many instances a presumptive diagnosis can be made upon finding an overweight patient sitting in a chair, asleep and snoring loudly in the waiting room. It should be emphasized, however, that patients need not be obese or have a history of snoring. Indeed, one of the more common surgical interventions regularly cures snoring but infrequently rids the patient of sleep apnea (see below).

The immediate danger of sleep deprivation from this syndrome is accidental injury or death. The automobile accident rate for individuals with severe obstructive sleep apnea is approximately three times that of the normal population,[61] and a history of falling asleep while driving or at traffic lights is frequently obtained. Serious aviation and industrial accidents

may also occur. He and colleagues found a 37 percent cumulative 8-year mortality in patients with obstructive sleep apnea syndrome and more than 20 apneas per hour, compared with a 4 percent mortality with less than 20 apneas per hour.[62] Partinen and colleagues found an 11 percent mortality at 5 years in patients with obstructive sleep apnea treated conservatively with weight reduction, compared with 0 percent mortality among those treated with tracheostomy.[63]

During obstructive apneas, a number of events occur that are thought to contribute to mortality and morbidity. Systolic and diastolic blood pressures increase by an average of 25 percent during an obstructive apnea.[64] As has been shown by direct recordings from sympathetic nerves in patients with obstructive sleep apnea, elevations in blood pressure are mediated by the sympathetic nervous system.[65] The role of hypoxemia in blood pressure elevation appears to be limited, because elevations in blood pressure continue even when SaO_2 is maintained at levels greater than 90 percent with supplemental oxygen.[66] That obstructive sleep apnea causes chronic hypertension is not as well established; however, its treatment consistently reverses daytime hypertension in children as well as in many adults.[67] Various cardiac arrhythmias have been reported in patients with obstructive apneas, including sinus pauses of up to 13 seconds, second-degree atrioventricular block, and ventricular ectopy, although all of these may occur in similar-aged control subjects. The most common arrhythmia is a bradytachycardia that results from increased vagal output during the apnea[68] and increased sympathetic output upon resumption of breathing. Of all the effects on heart rhythm, the most serious is an increase in ventricular ectopy, which occurs when SaO_2 levels decline below 60 to 65 percent.[69,70]

Individuals with obstructive sleep apnea syndrome have a greater risk of stroke compared to unaffected individuals. Impaired cerebral blood flow and cerebrovascular autoregulation have also been reported in patients with this syndrome.[71] Several epidemiological studies indicate that snoring alone appears to be a risk factor for stroke.[72–74] Established risk factors for stroke, hypertension, and cardiac arrhythmias are commonly associated with obstructive sleep apnea. A somewhat more tenuous link between this syndrome and stroke is the observation that approximately one-third of strokes are present upon awakening and that peak occurrences of myocardial infarction and stroke are between 3 AM and 9 AM.[75] Possible mechanisms for stroke in this context include reduced blood flow and impaired autoregulation, cyclical increases in intracranial pressure,[76] and anoxia during apneic episodes in combination with either atherosclerotic occlusive disease, polycythemia, or cardiac arrhythmias.

Permanent cognitive impairment may also be a consequence of the obstructive sleep apnea syndrome. Montplaisir and colleagues have found that deficits in cognitive tasks requiring planning abilities, verbal fluency, and manual dexterity persist despite correction of daytime sleepiness with continuous positive airway pressure.[77] They believe that persistent cognitive dysfunction is probably due to irreversible anoxic cerebral damage.

In most cases obstructive sleep apnea appears to be idiopathic, with the main contributing factor being obesity. Fatty infiltration in the neck decreases the size of the pharyngeal lumen, which then predisposes the airway to collapse during sleep. There is often a history of weight gain that parallels the onset and severity of the disorder. Weight loss usually results in a substantial improvement in symptoms.[78,79] Unfortunately, most patients achieve only limited success in weight loss by dieting alone. Gastric surgery may be beneficial for certain patients, particularly those with extreme obesity.[80] In approximately two-thirds of patients the apneas are more frequent or severe in the supine position. It may be helpful to outfit such patients with a shirt that has tennis balls sewn into a pocket in the back to keep them from assuming the supine position.

In some cases specific causes of obstructive sleep apnea can be identified. Neurological disorders associated with both obstructive and central sleep apnea syndromes are listed in Table 25-7.[81] Anatomical abnormalities and medical disorders associated with these syndromes are listed in Table 25-8. Most surgical disorders are diagnosed during the clinical examination, which should include inspection of the nasal passages, oropharynx, and larynx.

The current treatment of choice for the obstructive sleep apnea syndrome is continuous positive airway pressure (CPAP). Nasal CPAP forces air through the nose into the pharynx and acts as a pneumatic splint to keep the airway open. To use CPAP, the patient must wear either a mask that covers the nose or "nasal pillows" that rest against the nares. CPAP therapy is

Table 25-7 Sleep Apnea Syndromes and Neurological Diseases

Disorder	Obstructive	Central
Hemispheric lesions	+	+
Diencephalic lesions		+
Olivopontocerebellar atrophy	+	+
Brainstem lesions		+
Parkinson's dysautonomia	+	
Postencephalitic parkinsonism		+
Shy-Drager syndrome	+	+
Multiple sclerosis	+	
Familial dysautonomia	+	+
Diabetic autonomic neuropathy	+	+
Bulbar poliomyelitis	+	+
Syringobulbia	+	+
Syringomyelia	+	+
Arnold-Chiari malformation	+	+
Motor neuron disease	+	+
Myotonic dystrophy	+	+
Muscular dystrophy	+	+

(Adapted from Langevin B, Sukkar F, Leger P, et al: Sleep apnea syndromes (SAS) of specific etiology: review and incidence from a sleep laboratory. Sleep 15, suppl:S25, 1992, with permission.)

initiated in the sleep laboratory, where pressures are gradually adjusted throughout the night until apneas are suppressed. CPAP pressures are usually effective within a range of 7.5 to 14 cmH$_2$O. Approximately 85 percent of patients are able to tolerate CPAP.[82] Of those who do not, some will be able to tolerate bimodal positive airway pressure (BiPAP). The BiPAP device detects exhalation and immediately reduces the positive air pressure to a preset level that is lower than the pressure during inhalation, so that breathing does not occur against a resistance. The main reasons that patients are unable to tolerate CPAP or BiPAP are (1) a sensation of claustrophobia; (2) irritation from dry throat and nasal passages; (3) nasal congestion (self-limited in the majority of cases); or (4) esthetic concerns. Newer CPAP and BiPAP devices are readily portable and are relatively quiet. Irritation from dryness can be addressed by warming and humidifying the air from the CPAP device. Nasal congestion usually responds to corticosteroid or vasoconstrictor nasal sprays. A return to normal daytime vigilance as measured by the MSLT usually takes approximately 1 to 2 weeks after beginning CPAP. Although tracheostomy is no longer the therapy of choice, it is still

Table 25-8 Medical Conditions Associated with Sleep Apnea

Specific disorder	Obstructive	Central
Upper airway obstruction		
Nasopharyngeal carcinoma	+	
Adenoidal hypertrophy	+	+
Nasal obstruction	+	+
Tonsillar hypertrophy	+	
Neoplasms	+	
Lymphomas of tonsils	+	
Lingual cysts	+	
Macroglossia	+	
Lipoma of neck	+	
Storage diseases	+	
Laryngeal edema	+	
Vocal cord paralysis	+	
Craniofacial abnormalities		
Basicranium angulation	+	
Micrognathia	+	
Retrognathia	+	+
Macroglossia	+	
Pierre Robin syndrome	+	+
Franceschetti syndrome	+	
Treacher Collins syndrome	+	
Klippel-Feil syndrome	+	
Achondroplasia	+	
Prader-Willi syndrome	+	+
Other medical disorders		
Hypothyroidism	+	+
Acromegaly	+	+
Hurler's syndrome	+	
Amyloidosis	+	
Scheie's syndrome	+	
Obesity	+	+
End-stage renal failure	+	+
Acid-maltase deficiency	+	+

(Adapted from Langevin B, Sukkar F, Leger P, et al: Sleep apnea syndromes (SAS) of specific etiology: review and incidence from a sleep laboratory. Sleep 15, suppl:S25, 1992, with permission.)

commonly used in severe cases when CPAP is ineffective or not tolerated.

The most commonly performed surgery for obstructive sleep apnea is uvulopalatopharyngoplasty (UPPP). The goal of UPPP is to increase the size of the airway via a resection of the uvula, soft palate, tonsils, and redundant soft tissue within the posterior pharynx. Unfortunately, success in terms of a greater than 90 percent suppression of apneas occurs in less than 30 percent of patients. However, in approximately 50 percent of patients the number of apneas is reduced by more than 50 percent.[83,84] For some patients, particularly young adults facing a lifelong disorder, it may be considered as a useful adjunctive measure to other treatments including weight loss and CPAP. The UPPP is also extremely effective for eliminating snoring. The most commonly encountered untoward effect is nasal regurgitation. In children, enlargement of the adenoids and tonsils is an important cause of obstructive sleep apnea that responds readily to surgical resection.

Other surgical procedures that address specific anatomical defects, such as retrognathia or micrognathia, have been found to be useful adjunctive measures. Pharmacological therapy has been aimed primarily toward suppressing REM sleep with tricyclic antidepressants or stimulating respiratory drive in patients with hypoventilation at rest with medroxyprogesterone acetate.[85] At present the role for pharmacological intervention is quite limited.

Patients with sleep apnea should be warned that sedatives and alcoholic beverages will exacerbate their condition. The danger of an accident while driving is increased if the patient has a history of recent accidents or near misses or clearly has excessive daytime sleepiness. Under such conditions the physician is obligated to warn the patient and discourage driving until daytime vigilance can be restored. This often takes 1 to 2 weeks after the initiation of CPAP. For medicolegal reasons, instructions to the patient should be clearly documented in the physician's notes. In some locales it may also be appropriate to report the patient's condition to the driver licensing agency or state health department, but it is advisable in such cases to discuss the legal ramifications with a local attorney.

As with obstructive sleep apnea, the approach to central sleep apnea is initially directed toward treating potential underlying causes such as nasal obstruction, congestive heart failure, or metabolic disturbances (Tables 25-7 and 25-8). If a treatable cause cannot be found and there are no contraindications, treatment for adults should be initiated with acetazolamide 250 mg four times daily and the PSG repeated to determine the efficacy of the response.[86] Nasal CPAP should also be tried and may be effective in some cases.[87] If neither of these approaches is successful, supplemental oxygen is prescribed and may abolish or greatly diminish central apneas.[88] Tracheostomy with mechanical ventilation may be necessary in severe cases. The usefulness of ventilatory stimulant medications has not been established.

Narcolepsy

The term *narcolepsy* was first used by Gelineau in 1880 to describe a condition of recurrent attacks of irresistible sleep.[89,90] Until the mid-20th century, narcolepsy was widely considered to be a psychiatric disorder. It is now understood to be a central disorder of sleep-wake regulation and REM sleep. The International Classification of Sleep Disorders[1] defines narcolepsy as essentially "a disorder of unknown etiology, characterized by excessive sleepiness typically associated with cataplexy and other REM sleep phenomena such as sleep paralysis and hypnagogic hallucinations." The first symptoms usually occur in the second decade, with the peak age of onset between 15 and 25 years of age. However, onset may occur as early as 5 years or after 50 years of age. Excessive sleepiness is usually the presenting symptom. Cataplexy may follow the onset of sleepiness by more than 20 years or, less often, appear in advance of sleepiness.

The salient feature of narcolepsy is excessive daytime somnolence. The narcoleptic patient typically takes short naps lasting for 10 to 20 minutes (rarely longer than 1 hour) that restore vigilance for up to 2 to 3 hours. Sleep occurs most readily in monotonous environments, especially when physical activity is not required. Remarkably, many patients with narcolepsy can remain awake if engaged in a stimulating task. Sometimes the onset of sleep is precipitous. Such "sleep attacks" occur without warning in situations in which sleep rarely occurs normally (e.g., while eating, talking, or driving).

The symptom that is most specific for narcolepsy is cataplexy. Cataplexy occurs in approximately 70 percent of patients with narcolepsy[91] and may precede or follow the onset of daytime sleepiness by months or years. Cataplexy is characterized by a sudden loss of muscle tone, which may last from seconds to several minutes. The distribution and severity of atonia vary from mild localized weakness (e.g., arm or leg weakness, dysarthria, buckling of the knees) to complete postural collapse. The most common cataplectic attacks are subtle and often go unnoticed by nearby individuals. As in sleep paralysis (see below), extraoc-

ular movements and respiration are largely unaffected during the attack, but there may be blurring of vision, ptosis, or rarely diplopia. If the weakness is limited to the muscles of speech, the patient may present with stuttering attacks. If attacks are limited mainly to the arms, the patient may complain of intermittent clumsiness. Although consciousness and memory are usually preserved, prolonged attacks may be accompanied by dream-like hallucinations (visual, auditory, or tactile) or lead directly into an episode of REM sleep. Cataplectic attacks are always associated with an emotional precipitant such as excitement, surprise, fear, anger, elation, or pride; the most common is laughter. Persistent strong emotions may even trigger a series of cataplectic attacks lasting for hours to days (status cataplecticus). The interindividual frequency of cataplexy varies widely from several attacks per year to numerous attacks each day. Attacks are more likely to occur during periods of exhaustion or sleepiness. As with epileptic attacks, the sudden loss of motor control may lead to serious injury. Depending on the severity and frequency of attacks, certain precautions may therefore be necessary.

Sleep paralysis and hypnagogic hallucinations occur in approximately 25 and 30 percent, respectively, of all patients with the narcoleptic syndrome.[91] Together with excessive sleepiness and cataplexy, they complete the so-called tetrad of the narcoleptic syndrome (which actually occurs in less than 20 percent of patients). Sleep paralysis is a frightening experience in which the patient is unable to open the eyes, move, speak, or take a deep breath. Fright is commonly intensified by a sensation of being unable to breathe and by simultaneous hypnagogic hallucinations. The attacks occur during the transition between wakefulness and sleep and may last from several seconds to several minutes (rarely longer than 10 minutes). With repeated attacks the patient becomes less concerned, and the attacks are ultimately viewed simply as an inconvenience. As in cataplexy, the H reflex and tendon reflexes are suppressed or absent during the attack. The EEG is remarkable only for the apparent preservation of consciousness during patterns of drowsiness. Sleep paralysis also occurs in the absence of narcolepsy in approximately 5 percent of normal individuals,[92] as a rare X-linked genetic syndrome (familial sleep paralysis), and rarely in association with the obstructive sleep apnea syndrome.

Hypnagogic hallucinations occur during the transition between wakefulness and sleep and are primarily visual. The visual content may range from simple forms to fantastic scenes. Other components of the experience may include simple or complex auditory hallucinations, feelings of being touched, changes in the location of body parts, and a sensation of levitation or being outside of one's body. Awareness that these experiences represent hallucinations is usually preserved, but they may be so unpleasant that the patient begins to dread going to bed at night.

Automatic behavior, memory problems, and disturbed nocturnal sleep complete the clinical picture of narcolepsy. Automatic behavior consists of semipurposeful activity associated with amnesia that occurs in up to 80 percent of patients.[28] It occurs in monotonous environments conducive to sleep and may last from seconds to more than 30 minutes. During attacks there may be irrelevant gestures and remarks, lapses in speech, and illogical activity (e.g., placing a magazine in the refrigerator). More complex activities such as driving may also occur. Memory problems occur in over 50 percent of patients due to drowsiness and brief episodes of sleep. Indeed, both automatic behavior and memory problems are encountered in other sleep disorders as a consequence of sleep deprivation. Disturbed nocturnal sleep parallels the severity of narcolepsy and is manifested by frequent awakenings and increased body movements.

Daytime sleepiness is almost always lifelong, but its severity stabilizes within several years of onset. Worsening sleepiness after a period of stability should therefore prompt reevaluation for a new sleep problem such as sleep apnea. Cataplexy, hypnagogic hallucinations, and sleep paralysis improve with age in about one-third of patients. The progressive disruption of sleep that naturally occurs with aging is accelerated in some cases of narcolepsy.

The prevalence of narcolepsy varies from 1 in 600 persons in Japan, to 1 in 3,000 in North America and Europe, to 1 in 500,000 in Israel.[93–96] Although complaints of excessive sleepiness are eight times more likely to be elicited in relatives of patients with narcolepsy compared with the general population, earlier reports of a high rate of familial narcolepsy appear to have been inaccurate. More recently, Guilleminault and colleagues conducted the first large-scale study in which sleep recordings were used to confirm the diagnosis.[97] They found that only 3 percent of patients had one first-degree relative with narcolepsy-cataplexy, and only 1 percent had more than one affected first-degree relative.

Despite the finding of a relatively low familial incidence of narcolepsy, there is ample evidence for a genetic predisposition. The HLA-DR2 and HLA-DQw1 histocompatibility antigens on chromosome 6 are present in 100 percent of Japanese patients with narcolepsy[98] and over 90 percent of white patients.[99] The DQw1 antigen is also present in over 90 percent of blacks and DR2 is present in approximately 65 percent.[100] DR2 is present in 10 to 35 percent of general populations studied thus far. Although the association of specific histocompatibility antigens with narcolepsy raises the question of an immune-mediated process, evidence for immune system involvement is currently lacking.

Rarely, narcolepsy is caused by a structural lesion of the rostral brainstem, often in association with invasion of the third ventricle.[101,102] Lesions reported to cause sleep attacks and cataplexy have included pituitary adenoma, midbrain glioma, sarcoidosis, colloid cyst of the third ventricle, craniopharygioma of the floor of the third ventricle, and glioma of the third ventricle.[101] Rarely, symptoms may occur in a protracted manner, as in the "limp man syndrome" of continuous cataplexy reported by Stahl and colleagues.[102] Tumors, in general, may cause sleep-wake disturbances by the direct invasion of sleep modulating structures or as a remote effect of intracranial hypertension.[103] Peduncular hallucinosis, characterized by vivid visual and auditory hallucinations, may resemble hypnagogic hallucinations. It usually results from a vascular lesion of the rostral brainstem, most commonly "top of the basilar" artery occlusion. Hallucinations similar to those encountered in the syndrome of peduncular hallucinosis also occur as a side effect of levodopa medication. Prolonged episodes of repeated hypnagogic hallucinations have been misdiagnosed as schizophrenia.[104]

The diagnosis of narcolepsy is relatively straightforward when cataplexy and excessive sleepiness are present. This diagnostic opportunity is sometimes missed because the manifestations of cataplexy are often subtle and are therefore ignored or not understood by the physician. In approximately 10 to 15 percent of cases, cataplexy does not develop until 10 or more years after the onset of sleepiness.[28] Cataplectic attacks accompanied by vivid hallucinations (with or without progression directly into REM sleep) and episodes of automatic behavior have been misdiagnosed as epileptic. Cataplectic attacks have also been misinterpreted as drop attacks associated with vertebrobasilar insufficiency or periodic paralysis. More subtle cataplectic episodes may be mistaken for myasthenia gravis. The duration of attacks, preservation of consciousness, and precipitating emotional factors help to distinguish cataplexy from other disorders.

A secure diagnosis of narcolepsy in the absence of cataplexy can be made when the following are present: (1) a complaint of excessive sleepiness; (2) recurrent daytime sleep almost daily for at least 3 months; (3) sleep paralysis, hypnagogic hallucinations, automatic behavior, and disrupted sleep; (4) an absence of any medical or psychiatric disorder that could explain the aforementioned symptoms; and (5) a sleep latency of less than 10 minutes, REM sleep latency less than 20 minutes, or an MSLT that demonstrates either a mean sleep latency of less than 5 minutes or two or more naps with REM sleep. For reliable PSG and MSLT findings, the patient should be free of any sleep-altering drugs (particularly those that interfere with REM sleep such as amphetamines or tricyclic antidepressants) for 15 days, the sleep-wake schedule should be standardized for at least 7 days prior to testing, and the MSLT should be performed on the day following the PSG. Interpretation of the sleep studies is complicated by the observation that sleep apnea and periodic limb movements occur in up to one-half of individuals with narcolepsy.[28] However, if narcolepsy is present, the treatment of these disorders will not restore daytime vigilance.

Because the DR2 and DQw1 histocompatibility agents occur frequently in the general population and may be absent in some affected individuals (except perhaps in those of Japanese descent), their role in the diagnostic evaluation is limited. Currently the main indication for testing is in high-risk individuals in families of narcoleptic patients who are DR2- or DQw1-positive. A family member without the antigens is extremely unlikely to develop the disorder.

The treatment of narcolepsy includes patient education. Self-help groups should be encouraged. Advice regarding safety precautions should be carefully considered and based on the severity of the disorder. It is not necessary to curtail essential activities such as driving if sleepiness is mild or can be anticipated and cataplectic attacks are controlled. In most cases the initial treatment of daytime sleepiness does not include pharmaceutical agents. Strategically timed short naps lasting 15 to 20 minutes one to three times a day will usually provide adequate relief for up to 2 hours.[105] Indeed, it has never been demonstrated that stimulant medications are more effective in achieving short-term relief from sleepiness. Exercise, even in the form of a brief walk, also has a useful alerting effect. If driving or attendance at a conference is anticipated, heavy meals should be avoided, as they tend to be sedating. Finally, caffeinated beverages in combination with the aforementioned strategies alone may provide sufficient relief that medications are unnecessary.

Stimulant medications are indicated if the aforementioned strategies fail. The only way to determine the efficacy of stimulant medication is the patient's perceived response (MSLT testing remains largely unchanged despite reports of clinical improvement). Unfortunately, complete relief from daytime sleepiness is rarely achieved. Treatment is often initiated with pemoline (Cylert) because side effects are less likely with it than with other, stronger agents. A beginning dose of 18.75 mg is given in the morning and then increased by 18.75 mg increments as needed every 1 to 2 weeks. If a dosage of 75 mg in the morning and 37.5 mg in the early afternoon is reached without substantial improvement, treatment with this agent should be discontinued and a trial of methylphenidate begun. Methylphenidate has a more rapid onset of action and is associated with fewer side effects than amphetamine. A typical starting dose in adults is 5 mg taken three times daily. If this is unsuccessful after a dosage of 60 to 90 mg/d is reached, dextroamphetamine (beginning at 5 mg twice daily) is initiated and increased as necessary to a maximum total dose of 60 mg/d. Chronic stimulant use may result in addiction, habituation, irritability, psychosis, or hypertension. Habituation can often be avoided with a drug holiday for 1 day each week. Remarkably, most patients with narcolepsy are able to take stimulants for decades without encountering serious side effects.[28]

Tricyclic antidepressants are effective in the treatment of both sleep paralysis and cataplexy in over 80 percent of patients.[28] Protriptyline (5 to 30 mg/d) is often used because its stimulant side effect helps in the treatment of daytime sleepiness. Otherwise, imipramine, nortriptyline, and desipramine are probably equally effective. Newer, more selective antidepressants such as viloxazine (which inhibits serotonin uptake) and fluoxetine (which inhibits norepinephrine uptake) are associated with fewer anticholinergic side effects and may be preferable in some cases. Rarely, tolerance develops, necessitating a 1- to 2-week drug holiday. Caution should be exercised when withdrawing tricyclic antidepressants because abrupt withdrawal may precipitate cataplectic attacks or even status cataplecticus.

Disrupted sleep contributes to both daytime sleepiness and associated symptoms such as cataplexy. Short-term sedatives are frequently used to facilitate sleep, but their effect on daytime symptoms has not been established. Benzodiazepines such as temazepam (Restoril) and triazolam (Halcion) or the newer nonbenzodiazepine zolpidem (Ambien) are currently the preferred agents. Sedatives may actually worsen morning sleepiness, and those with relatively long half-lives should be avoided.

PARASOMNIAS

Disorders associated with prominent physical phenomena during sleep but not with the primary complaints of insomnia or daytime somnolence are referred to as parasomnias (Table 25-1). There are 24 separate parasomnias; the most common that present with neurological manifestations are discussed below.

Confusional Arousals, Sleepwalking, and Sleep Terrors

Confusional arousals, sleepwalking, and sleep terrors are considered arousal disorders because the patient manifests certain aspects of waking behavior yet fails to awaken fully. A common feature of the arousal disorders is that they occur during NREM sleep, particularly stages III and IV. Confusional arousals, sometimes referred to as sleep drunkenness, are characterized by inappropriate behaviors, disorientation, slowed speech, and amnesia following partial arousal

from slow-wave sleep that may last from minutes to several hours. They are most likely to occur following sleep deprivation, with sedative medications, in metabolic/toxic encephalopathies, or in association with narcolepsy or sleep apnea. They are normally present in children under 5 years of age and can be precipitated by arousal from sleep during the first one-third of the night. Rarely, frequent confusional arousals occur in association with brain lesions in areas subserving sleep control, including the periventricular gray matter, the midbrain reticular area, and posterior hypothalamus.[1] Personal injuries have occasionally occurred and, as in any confusional state, individuals may become aggressive if restrained.

Sleepwalking (somnambulism) consists of walking and other complex behaviors occurring in stage III or IV sleep. Episodes may be relatively benign or the patient may appear frantic, attempting to escape from an imagined threat. Patients are difficult to arouse and remain in a confusional state after arousal. The prevalence of sleepwalking is between 1 and 15 percent and, as with the other arousal disorders, it is most common in children and adolescents.[1] Rarely, the onset of sleepwalking occurs in adulthood. A genetic predisposition for sleepwalking is suggested by the observation that the incidence approaches 60 percent when both parents are affected.[1] Serious injuries may result in a number of ways including walking into the street, off a balcony, or through a window. Aggressive behavior toward others is rare in the absence of physical restraint. Rarely, homicide has been reported. The main consideration in differential diagnosis is epilepsy with ambulatory automatisms; these automatisms can be distinguished clinically by their relatively short duration and by the presence of epileptiform EEG activity during attacks.[106]

Sleep terrors, also referred to as night terrors or pavor nocturnus, are characterized by a sudden partial arousal from slow-wave sleep and a subsequent attack heralded by a piercing scream or cry with behavioral and autonomic manifestations of intense fear. Unlike nightmares, sleep terrors tend to occur during the first one-third of the night, when slow-wave sleep predominates; there is little or no recollection of dream content, and the patient is difficult to arouse. Indeed, attempts to arouse the patient usually intensify the attack. The entire episode usually lasts no more than 3 to 5 minutes. Following arousal there is confusion and amnesia for the event. Sleep terrors occur most often in children between the ages of 2 and 12. The occurrence of sleep terrors in childhood, unlike adulthood, does not suggest the presence of psychopathology.

Confusional arousals, sleep terrors, and sleepwalking may all occur in varying combinations in a given individual. Their treatment depends upon the frequency and severity of their occurrence. In children the events may be prevented by the use of a benzodiazepine at bedtime. The response to psychotherapy is often favorable. Unfortunately, in adults, medications and psychotherapy often meet with mixed results. Isolated reports of success in adults with various agents, such as tricyclic antidepressants or anticonvulsants, raise the question of an undetected underlying condition (e.g., depression or epilepsy). Precipitating factors such as sleep deprivation, loud noises during sleep, or bladder fullness should be avoided, as should certain medications known to exacerbate or cause sleepwalking, including thioridazine, prolixin, perphenazine, desipramine, chloral hydrate, and lithium.

REM Sleep Behavior Disorder

REM sleep behavior disorder is characterized by the loss of atonia during REM sleep, with elaborate motor activity and dream mentation. The behavioral activities that occur are consistent with dream enactment and may at times be quite violent. Frequent manifestations include leaping, running, kicking, and punching. The disorder occurs far more often in men than in women. Usually medical attention is sought at the urging of a bed partner because of disturbed sleep or physical injury. The attacks usually occur after the first 90 minutes of sleep, at which time REM sleep normally begins. Just as there are usually four REM cycles during a normal night, attacks often occur four or more times a night. Consistent with REM sleep, patients are difficult to arouse fully during an attack, awakening is not associated with a prolonged confusional state, and there is detailed dream recall. Most patients have a typical repetitive dream, which usually consists of being attacked. Because the episodes are often violent, this may result in the ironic situation in which the patient dreams of defending a bed partner only to find, upon awakening, that they have inflicted injuries instead.[107]

REM behavior disorder may present as an acute transient form, usually associated with drug intoxication or withdrawal, or as a chronic form. The acute form has been associated with withdrawal of alcohol, meprobamate, pentazocine, and nitrazepam or intoxication from biperiden, tricyclic antidepressants, and monoamine oxidase inhibitors.[107] The chronic form usually first appears in the sixth or seventh decade of life and is a progressive disorder in terms of the complexity, intensity, and frequency of expressed behaviors.[107,108] One-third of affected individuals have had a history of neurological disorder including dementia, subarachnoid hemorrhage, ischemic cerebrovascular disease, olivopontocerebellar degeneration, brainstem astrocytoma, multiple sclerosis, and Guillain-Barré syndrome. Although bilateral lesions in the vicinity of the locus ceruleus might be anticipated from animal experiments, these are rarely found in affected humans. Instead, involvement of suprapontine structures seems to play a more important role.[109]

The diagnosis can be made in the presence of limb or body movements associated with dream mentation and either harmful or potentially harmful sleep behaviors, dreams that appear to be "acted out," or sleep behaviors that disrupt sleep continuity. The PSG during REM sleep typically demonstrates excessive augmentation of tonic submental EMG activity and excessive phasic EMG activity (Fig. 25-4).[107] Simultaneous video monitoring reveals excessive limb or body jerking or more complex, vigorous, violent behaviors.

Treatment with clonazepam has been uniformly effective, emphasizing the utility of proper diagnosis. The initial starting dosage is 0.5 mg and the maximal effective dosage is 2.0 mg administered at bedtime. Administration up to 2 hours before before bedtime is helpful for patients complaining of excessive morning sedation, limb jerking at sleep onset, or difficulty in initiating sleep. The efficacy of clonazepam is probably due to its serotonergic effects. Disinhibition of REM phasic activity in cats has been induced by serotonin-depleting drugs and by lesions of serotonergic neurons of the brainstem raphe nuclei.[107] In one reported instance, the effective dosage of clonazepam was successfully reduced using the serotonin precursor L-tryptophan.[107] Habituation does not appear to be a significant problem even after years of treatment, whereas withdrawal leads to immediate relapse.

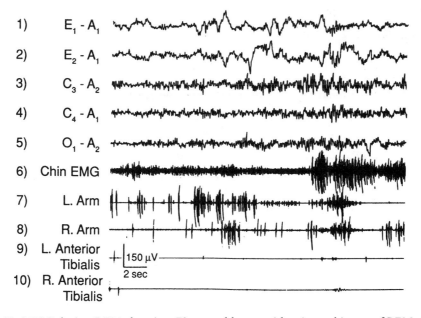

Fig. 25-4 PSG during REM sleep in a 70-year-old man with a 6-year history of REM sleep behavior disorder following a subarachnoid hemorrhage. Chin atonia is absent and there are abundant left and right arm movements. Rapid eye movements consistent with REM sleep are seen, but there is excessive alpha activity. (From Mahowald MW, Schenck CH: REM sleep behavior disorder. p. 389. In Kryger MH, Roth T, Dement WC (eds): Principles and Practice of Sleep Medicine. WB Saunders, Philadelphia, 1989, with permission.)

Nocturnal Paroxysmal Dystonia

Nocturnal paroxysmal dystonia is a heterogeneous and somewhat controversial syndrome of nocturnal attacks that all share the distinction of being marked by stereotyped dystonic, ballistic, or choreoathetoid movements that arise out of stage II sleep (or, less frequently, slow-wave sleep or the transition from slow-wave sleep to REM sleep) and often occur nightly, frequently several times per night. At least two varieties exist: in one the attacks are brief, lasting 40 to 50 seconds, whereas in the other the attacks are prolonged and last for up to 60 minutes.[109]

The short-lasting attacks begin with an EEG arousal from sleep, often preceded by a K complex. Initially there is eye opening and neck flexion. Shortly thereafter the patient begins to flail the limbs and trunk wildly with ballistic movements, dystonic posturing, and accompanying vocalizations.[110] The attacks may be preceded by tachycardia or bradycardia or a central apnea. Following the attack, the patient usually goes back to sleep. If the patient is awakened

immediately afterwards, he or she may have partial recall of the ictal events and show little evidence of postictal confusion. In some patients, similar attacks occur during wakefulness. The attacks are differentiated from epileptic seizures by the absence of ictal electrographic activity. Although the prevalence is unknown, the disorder is rare. The attacks do not subside spontaneously and have been known to occur over periods of 20 years or more. When frequent, the attacks may result in severe sleep disruption. The movements may disturb or injure the bed partner as well as the patient.

Although it was originally thought that short-lasting attacks might represent a new nonepileptic syndrome, it now seems more likely that they represent frontal lobe seizures.[110] This conclusion is based on the following observations: (1) the attacks respond to carbamazepine (albeit sometimes in relatively low dosage and not to other anticonvulsants); (2) frontal lobe seizures may also involve bizarre behavior with torsion, flailing, and side-to-side movements, vocalizations, and movements involving both hands and feet, sometimes with dystonic posturing (particularly when arising from supplementary motor cortex)[111,112]; (3) frontal lobe seizures are typically nocturnal, brief, and repetitive; and (4) the EEG frequently fails to show epileptiform changes during frontal lobe seizures that produce behaviors resembling those seen during nocturnal paroxysmal dystonic attacks.[113] Finally, in a series of 12 patients with nocturnal paroxysmal dystonia studied with polygraphic and video monitoring, two-thirds experienced focal sensorimotor daytime seizures and one-third had generalized tonic-clonic seizures during sleep.[114]

Attacks lasting for 2 to 60 minutes are extremely rare and differ further from shorter attacks in their poor response to carbamazepine. Prolonged motor attacks with dystonic features arising out of sleep are currently considered to be a sleep-induced movement disorder.

REFERENCES

1. Diagnostic Classification Steering Committee of the American Sleep Disorders Association: International Classification of Sleep Disorders: Diagnostic and Coding Manual. American Sleep Disorders Association, Rochester, MN, 1990
2. Loomis AL, Harvey EN, Hobart GA: Electrical potentials of the human brain. J Exp Psychol 19:249,1936
3. Aserinsky E, Kleitman N: Regularly occurring periods of eye motility, and concomitant phenomena, during sleep. Science 118:273, 1953
4. Berger RJ: Tonus of extrinsic laryngeal muscles during sleep and dreaming. Science 134:840, 1961
5. Jouvet M, Michel M: Correlations electromyographiques du sommeil chez le chat decortique et mesencephalique chronique. C R Soc Biol 153:422, 1959
6. Rechtschaffen A, Kales A (eds): A Manual of Standardized Terminology, Techniques and Scoring System for Sleep Stages of Human Subjects. UCLA Brain Information Service/Brain Research Institute, Los Angeles, 1968
7. Kales A, Kales JD: Recent findings in the diagnosis and treatment of disturbed sleep. N Engl J Med 290: 487, 1974
8. Hauri PJ: Basic facts on sleep. p. 6. In: The Sleep Disorders. 2nd Ed. Upjohn, Kalamazoo, MI, 1982
9. Hirshkowitz M, Moore CA, Hamilton CR, et al: Polysomnography of adults and elderly: sleep architecture, respiration, and leg movement. J Clin Neurophysiol 9:56, 1992
10. Carskadon MA, Dement WC: Normal human sleep: an overview. p. 3. In Kryger MH, Roth T, Dement WC (eds): Principles and Practice of Sleep Medicine. WB Saunders, Philadelphia, 1989
11. Monk T: Chronobiology. p. 139. In Kryger MH, Roth T, Dement WC (eds): Principles and Practice of Sleep Medicine. WB Saunders, Philadelphia, 1989
12. Moore RY, Eichler VB: Loss of a circadian adrenal corticosterone rhythm following suprachiasmatic lesions in the rat. Brain Res 42:201, 1972
13. Stephan FK, Zucker I: Circadian rhythms in drinking behavior and locomotor activity of rats are eliminated by hypothalamic lesions. Proc Natl Acad Sci USA 69: 1583, 1972
14. DeCoursey PJ, Buggy J: Restoration of locomotor rhythmicity in SCN-lesioned golden hamsters by transplantation of fetal SCN. Soc Neurosci Abstr 12: 210, 1986
15. Lehman MN, Silver R, Gladstone WR, et al: Circadian rhythmicity restored by neural transplant: immunocytochemical characterization of the graft and its integration with the host brain. Soc Neurosci Abstr 12:210, 1986
16. Moore RY: Retinohypothalamic projection in mammals: a comparative study. Brain Res 49:403, 1973
17. Czeisler CA, Allan JS, Strogatz SH, et al: Bright light resets the human circadian pacemaker independent of the timing of the sleep-wake cycle. Science 233:667, 1986
18. Jouvet M: The role of monoamines and acetylcholine-containing neurons in the regulation of the sleep-waking cycle. Ergeb Physiol 64:166, 1972
19. Markand ON, Dyken ML: Sleep abnormalities in patients with brain stem lesions. Neurology 26:769, 1976
20. Fischer-Perroudon C, Mouret J, Jouvet M: Sur un cas d'agrypnie (4 mois sans sommeil) au cours d'une maladie de Morvan: effet favorable du 5-hydroxy-tryptophane. Electroencephalogr Clin Neurophysiol 36:1, 1974
21. Jones B: Basic mechanisms of sleep-wake states. p. 121. In Kryger MH, Roth T, Dement WC (eds): Principles and Practice of Sleep Medicine. WB Saunders, Philadelphia, 1989
22. Henley K, Morrison AR: A re-evaluation of the effects of lesions of the pontine tegmentum and locus coeruleus on phenomena of paradoxical sleep in the cat. Acta Neurobiol Exp 34:215, 1974
23. Mitler MM, Dement WC: Cataplectic-like behavior

in cats after micro-injection of carbachol in pontine reticular formation. Brain Res 68:335, 1974

24. Williams RL, Karacan I, Hursch CJ: Electroencephalography (EEG) of Human Sleep: Clinical Applications. John Wiley & Sons, New York, 1974
25. Bery DT, Webb WB, Block AJ: Sleep apnea syndrome: a critical review of the apnea index as a diagnostic criterion. Chest 86:529, 1984
26. Knight H, Millman RP, Gur RC, et al: Clinical significance of sleep apnea in the elderly. Am Rev Respir Dis 136:845, 1987
27. Krieger J, Turlot JC, Mangin P, Kurtz D: Breathing during sleep in normal young and elderly subjects: hypopneas, apneas, and correlated factors. Sleep 6: 108, 1983
28. Aldrich MS: Narcolepsy. Neurology 42, suppl 6:34, 1992
29. Mullaney DJ, Kripke DF, Messin S: Wrist-actigraphic estimation of sleep time. Sleep 3:83, 1980
30. Hauri PJ: Actigraphy. p. 263. In Shepard JW (ed): Atlas of Sleep Medicine. Futura, Mount Kisco, NY, 1991
31. Coleman RM, Roffwarg HP, Kennedy SJ, et al: Sleep-wake disorders based on a polysomnographic diagnosis: a national cooperative study. JAMA 247:997, 1982
32. Hauri PJ: Primary insomnia. p. 442. In Kryger MH, Roth T, Dement WC (eds): Principles and Practice of Sleep Medicine. WB Saunders, Philadelphia, 1989
33. Hauri P, Fisher J: Persistent psychophysiologic (learned) insomnia. Sleep 9:38, 1986
34. Fujiki A, Shimizu A, Yamada Y, et al.: The Babinski reflex during sleep and wakefulness. Electroencephalogr Clin Neurophysiol 31:610, 1971
35. Smith RC: Relationship of periodic movements in sleep (nocturnal myoclonus) and the Babinski sign. Sleep 8:239, 1985
36. Radtke RA: Sleep disorders: laboratory evaluation. p. 561. In Daly D, Pedley TA (eds): Current Practice of Clinical Electoencephalography. 2nd Ed. Raven Press, New York, 1990
37. Montplaisir J, Godbout R: Restless legs syndrome and periodic movements during sleep. p. 400. In Kryger MH, Roth T, Dement WC (eds): Principles and Practice of Sleep Medicine. WB Saunders, Philadelphia, 1989
38. Brodeur C, Montplasisir J, Godbout R, Marinier R: Treatment of restless legs syndrome and periodic movements during sleep with L-dopa: a double-blind controlled study. Neurology 38:1845, 1988
39. Ekbom K: Restless legs syndrome after partial gastrectomy. Acta Neurol Scand 2:79, 1966
40. Aldrich MS: Parkinsonism. p. 351. In Kryger MH, Roth T, Dement WC (eds): Principles and Practice of Sleep Medicine. WB Saunders, Philadelphia, 1989
41. Askenasy JJM, Yahr MD: Reversal of sleep disturbance in Parkinsons's disease by antiparkinsonian therapy: a preliminary study. Neurology 35:527, 1985
42. Vitiello MV, Bliwise DL, Prinz PN: Sleep in Alzheimer's disease and the sundown syndrome. Neurology 42, suppl 6:83, 1992
43. Swaab DF, Fliers E, Partiman TS: The suprachiasmatic nucleus of the human brain in relation to sex, age and senile dementia. Brain Res 342:37, 1985
44. Devanard DP, Sackeim HA, Mayeux R: Psychosis, behavioral disturbance, and the use of neuroleptics in demential. Compr Psychiatry 29:387, 1988
45. Partinen M, Telakivi T: Epidemiology of obstructive sleep apnea syndrome. Sleep 15, suppl:S1, 1992
46. Burwell CS, Robin ED, Whaley RD, Bickelmann AG: Extreme obesity associated with alveolar hypventilation: a pickwickian syndrome. Am J Med 21: 811, 1956
47. Dement WC: A personal history of sleep disorders medicine. J Clin Neurophysiol 7:17, 1990
48. Gastaut H, Tassinari C, Duron B: Etude polygraphique des manifestations episodiques (hypniques et respiratoires) du syndrome de Pickwick. Rev Neurol (Paris) 112:568, 1965
49. Jung R, Kuhlo W: Neurophysiological studies of abnormal night sleep and the pickwickian syndrome. Prog Brain Res 18:140, 1965
50. Chaban R, Cole P, Hoffstein V: Site of upper airway obstruction in patients with idiopathic obstructive sleep apnea. Laryngoscope 98:641, 1988
51. Hudgel DW: Variable site of airway narrowing among obstructive sleep apnea patients. J Appl Physiol 61:1403, 1986
52. Orem J, Lydic K: Upper airway function during sleep and wakefulness: experimental studies on normal and anesthetized cats. Sleep 1:49, 1978
53. White DP: Occlusion pressure and ventilation during sleep in normal humans. J Appl Physiol 61:1279, 1986
54. Pevernagie DA, Shepard JW: Relations between sleep stage, posture and effective nasal CPAP levels in OSA. Sleep 15:162, 1992
55. Stoohs R, Guilleminault C: Obstructive sleep apnea syndrome or abnormal upper airway resistance during sleep? J Clin Neurophysiol 7:83, 1990
56. Guilleminault C, Stoohs R, Clerk A, et al: From obstructive sleep apnea syndrome to upper airway resistance syndrome: consistency of daytime sleepiness. Sleep 15, suppl:S13, 1992
57. Rosen CL, D'Andrea L, Haddad GG: Adult criteria for obstructive sleep apnea do not identify children with serious obstruction. Am Rev Respir Dis 146: 1231, 1992
58. Carskadon MA, Dement WC: Respiration during sleep in the aged human. J Gerontol 36:420, 1981

59. Marcus CL, Omlin KJ, Basinki DJ, et al: Normal polysomnographic values for children and adolescents. Am Rev Respir Dis 146:1235, 1992

60. Guilleminault C: Clinical features and evaluation of obstructive sleep apnea. p. 552. In Kryger M, Roth T, Dement WC (eds): Principles and Practice of Sleep Medicine. WB Saunders, Philadelphia, 1989

61. Findley LJ, Fabrizio M, Thommi G, Surratt PM: Severity of sleep apnea and automobile crashes. N Engl J Med 320:868, 1989

62. He J, Kryger MH, Zorick FJ, et al: Mortality and apnea index in obstructive sleep apnea: experience in 385 male patients. Chest 94:9, 1988

63. Partinen M, Jamieson A, Guilleminault C: Long-term outcome for obstructive sleep apnea syndrome patients. Mortality. Chest 94:1200, 1988

64. Shepard JW Jr: Gas exchange and hemodynamics during sleep. Med Clin North Am 69:1243, 1985

65. Hedner J, Ejnell H, Sellgren J, et al: Is high and fluctuating muscle nerve sympathetic activity in the sleep apnoea syndrome of pathogenetic importance for the development of hypertension? J Hypertens 6, suppl: S529, 1988

66. Ringler J, Basner RC, Shannon R, et al: Hypoxemia alone does not explain blood pressure elevations after obstructive apneas. J Appl Physiol 69:2143, 1990

67. Guilleminault C, Suzuki M: Sleep-related hemodynamics and hypertension with partial or complete upper airway obstruction during sleep. Sleep 15, suppl:S20, 1992

68. Schroeder JS, Motta J, Guilleminault C: Hemodynamic studies in sleep apnea. p. 177. In Guilleminault C, Dement WC (eds): Sleep Apnea Syndromes. Alan R Liss, New York, 1978

69. Shepard JW Jr, Garrison MW, Grither DA, Dolan GF: Relationship of ventricular ectopy to nocturnal O_2 desaturation in patients with obstructive sleep apnea. Chest 88:335, 1985

70. Guilleminault C, Connolly SJ, Winkle RA: Cardiac arrhythmia and conduction disturbances during sleep in 400 patients with sleep apnea syndrome. Am J Cardiol 52:490, 1983

71. Daly JA, Giombetti R, Miller B, et al: Impaired awake cerebral perfusion in sleep apnea. Am Rev Respir Dis 141:A376, 1990

72. Koskenvuo M, Kaprio J, Telakivi T, et al: Snoring as a risk factor for ischaemic heart disease and stroke in men. Br Med J 294:16, 1987

73. Partinen M, Palomaki H: Snoring and cerebral infarction. Lancet 2:1325, 1985

74. Palomaki H, Partinen M, Juvela S, Kaste M: Snoring as a risk factor for sleep-related brain infarction. Stroke 20:1311, 1989

75. Marler JR, Price TR, Clark GL, et al: Morning increase in onset of ischemic stroke. Stroke 20:473, 1989

76. Jennum P, Borgesen SE: Intracranial pressure and obstructive sleep apnea. Chest 95:279, 1989

77. Montplaisir J, Bedard MA, Richer F, Rouleau I: Neurobehavioral manifestations in obstructive sleep apnea syndrome before and after treatment with continuous positive airway pressure. Sleep 15, suppl:S17, 1992

78. Browman CP, Sampson MG, Yolles SF, et al: Obstructive sleep apnea and body weight. Chest 85:435, 1984

79. Harman E, Wynne JW, Block AJ: The effect of weight loss on sleep-disordered breathing and oxygen desaturation in morbidly obese men. Chest 82:291, 1982

80. Sugerman HJ, Fairman RP, Baron PL, Kwentus JA: Gastric surgery for respiratory insufficiency in obesity. Chest 90:81, 1986

81. Langevin B, Sukkar F, Leger P, et al: Sleep apnea syndromes (SAS) of specific etiology: review and incidence from a sleep laboratory. Sleep 15, suppl:S25, 1992

82. Krieger J: Long-term compliance with nasal continuous positive airway pressure (CPAP) in obstructive sleep apnea patients and nonapneic snorers. Sleep 15, suppl:S42, 1992

83. Fujita S, Conway W, Zorick F, Roth T: Surgical correction of anatomic abnormalities in obstructive sleep apnea syndrome: uvulopalatopharyngoplasty. Otolaryngol Head Neck Sug 89:923, 1981

84. Sher AE, Thorpy MJ, Shprintzen RJ, et al: Predictive value of Muller maneuver in selection of patients for uvulopalatopharyngoplasty. Laryngoscope 95:1483, 1985

85. Rajagopal KR, Abbrecht PH, Jabbari B: Effects of medroxyprogesterone acetate in obstructive sleep apnea. Chest 90:815, 1986

86. White DP, Zwillich CW, Pickett CK, et al: Central sleep apnea: improvement with acetazolamide therapy. Arch Intern Med 142:1816, 1982

87. Issa FG, Sullivan CE: Reversal of central sleep apnea using nasal CPAP. Chest 90:165, 1986

88. Martin RJ, Sanders MH, Gray BA, Pennock BE: Acute and long-term ventilatory effects of hyperoxia in the adult sleep apnea syndrome. Am Rev Respir Dis 125:175, 1982

89. Gelineau J: De la narcolepsie. Gaz Hop (Paris) 53:626 and 54:635, 1880

90. Guilleminault C: Narcolepsy syndrome. p. 338. In Kryger M, Roth T, Dement WC (eds): Principles and Practice of Sleep Medicine. WB Saunders, Philadelphia, 1989

91. Yoss RE, Daly DD: Criteria for the diagnosis of the narcoleptic syndome. Proc Mayo Clin 32:320, 1957
92. Goode GB: Sleep paralysis. Arch Neurol 6:228, 1962
93. Dement WC, Carskadon MA, Ley R: The prevalence of narcolepsy. Sleep Res 2:147, 1973
94. Dement WC, Zarcone V, Varner V, et al: The prevalence of narcolepsy. Sleep Res 1:148, 1972
95. Honda Y. Census of narcolepsy, cataplexy, and sleep life among teenagers in Fujisawa City. Sleep Res 8:191, 1979
96. Lavie P, Peled R: Narcolepsy is a rare disease in Israel. Sleep 10:608, 1987
97. Guilleminault C, Mignot E, Grumet FC: Familial patterns of narcolepsy. Lancet 2:1376, 1989
98. Juji T, Matsuki K, Tokunaga K, et al: Narcolepsy and HLA in the Japanese. Ann NY Acad Sci 540:106, 1988
99. Kramer RE, Dinner DS, Braun WE, et al: HLA-DR2 and narcolepsy. Arch Neurol 44:853, 1987
100. Neely S, Rosenberg R, Spire J-P, et al: HLA antigens in narcolepsy. Neurology 37:1858, 1987
101. Aldrich MS, Naylor MW: Narcolepsy associated with lesions of the diencephalon. Neurology 39:1505, 1989
102. Stahl MS, Layzer RB, Aminoff MJ, et al: Continuous cataplexy in a patient with a midbrain tumor: the limp man syndrome. Neurology 30:1115, 1980
103. Culebras A: Neuroanatomic and neurologic correlates of sleep disturbances. Neurology 42, suppl 6:19, 1992
104. Douglass AB, Hays P, Pazderka F, et al: A schizophrenic variant of narcolepsy. Sleep Res 18:173, 1989
105. Roehrs T, Zorick F, Wittig R, et al: Alerting effects of naps in patients with narcolepsy. Sleep 9:194, 1986
106. Pedley TA, Guilleminault C: Episodic nocturnal wanderings responsive to anticonvulsant drug therapy. Ann Neurol 2:30, 1977
107. Mahowald MW, Schenck CH: REM sleep behavior disorder. p. 389. In Kryger MH, Roth T, Dement WC (eds): Principles and Practice of Sleep Medicine. WB Saunders, Philadelphia, 1989
108. Culebras A, Moore JT: Magnetic resonance findings in REM sleep behavior disorder. Neurology 39:1519, 1989
109. Mahowald MW, Schenck CH: Dissociated states of wakefulness and sleep. Neurology 42, suppl 6:44, 1992
110. Montagna P: Nocturnal paroxysmal dystonia and nocturnal wandering. Neurology 42, suppl 6:61, 1992
111. Morris HH, Dinner DS, Luders H, et al: Supplementary motor seizures: clinical and electroencephalographic findings. Neurology 38:1075, 1988
112. Waterman K, Purves SJ, Koska B, et al: An epileptic syndrome caused by mesial frontal lobe seizure foci. Neurology 37:577, 1987
113. Williamson PD, Spencer DD, Spencer SS, et al: Complex partial seizures of frontal lobe origin. Ann Neurol 18:497, 1985
114. Lugaresi E, Cirignotta F, Montagna P: Nocturnal paroxysmal dystonia. J Neurol Neurosurg Psychiatry 49:375, 1986

26

Sphincter Disorders and the Nervous System

Michael Swash
Susan Mathers

Disorders of the urinary and anorectal sphincters are common, consisting of incontinence or difficulty expelling urine or feces (Table 26-1). Retention of urine is usually due to mechanical obstruction of the urethra but may also result from failure of sphincter relaxation or incoordination of the urinary detrusor and urinary sphincter mechanisms. A similar functional disorder of the anorectal sphincter musculature is a common cause of intractable constipation, termed *anismus*. In this disorder colonic transit is normal but, during attempted defecation, there is failure of relaxation of the striated anal sphincter musculature. Incontinence of urine or feces is a devastating disability. Individuals with incontinence are reluctant to go out, are fearful of making social contacts, and often become depressed and housebound. Incontinence is not a subject that patients find easy to discuss with friends or relatives, and the symptom thus often remains hidden for many months or even years before being brought to medical or nursing attention. It is particularly common in aged populations, but even in this group it cannot be regarded as an invariable consequence of the normal aging process.

In order to understand the pathogenesis of the various sphincter disorders, it is important to recognize the complexity of the normal control systems governing sphincter function.

SPHINCTER CONTROL SYSTEMS IN HUMANS

The urinary and anal sphincter systems consist of smooth and striated muscles innervated by autonomic and somatic efferent neurons. These muscular sphincters are modulated by spinal centers with central connections that reach conscious levels. There are extensive afferent connections from sensory receptors in the bladder and urethra and in the anal canal and bowel that relate to spinal and more rostral levels of this neuronal control system.[1] There is a close relation between the autonomic and somatic nervous systems in the control of continence and the orderly evacuation of the bladder and bowel. Earlier accounts of the normal mechanisms of micturition and defecation have tended to neglect the role of the somatic nervous system in these functions.

Functional Anatomy of Continence

ANAL CONTINENCE

The involuntary *smooth muscle sphincter* of the anal canal consists of a thickened ring of smooth muscle derived from the circular layer of smooth muscle of

521

Table 26-1 Sphincter Dysfunction and Related Disorders

Incontinence
    Sphincter incompetence
        Stress urinary incontinence
        Idiopathic anorectal incontinence
        Double incontinence
        Sphincter injuries, e.g., obstetrical tears
        Cauda equina lesions
    Disordered sphincter control
        Idiopathic detrusor hyperreflexia
        Central nervous system disorders (Table 26-2)

Retention
    Sphincter incoordination
        Detrusor-sphincter dyssynergia
        Anismus-type constipation
    Loss of propulsive force
        Idiopathic detrusor weakness
        Progressive autonomic failure
        Idiopathic visceral myopathies
        Idiopathic visceral neuropathies
        Hirschsprung's disease

the rectum and anal canal. Tonic contraction of this smooth muscle ring holds the inner layers of the anal canal in apposition.[2]

The smooth muscle of the anal canal is richly innervated by sensory nerves and nerve endings derived from the pudendal nerves.[3] These sensory receptors subserve discriminative sensation, so that the upper anal canal functions as a sampling organ to discern the arrival of fecal matter and its consistency[4]; thus liquid stool, solid stool, and gas can be readily discerned in the healthy individual. The smooth muscle of the anal canal and internal anal sphincter may be particularly important for modulating sensitivity of these sensory receptors by maintaining apposition of the anal squamous epithelium.

The *striated anal sphincter* consists of a complex ring of striated muscle fibers forming the external anal sphincter muscle. The superficial layers of this muscle ring insert into the skin of the perianal region, and the deeper layers interdigitate in the midline anteriorly and posteriorly. The external anal sphincter muscle is not the major voluntary muscle of continence. The puborectalis muscle sling is a larger muscle, arising from the posterior surface of the pubis on each side and passing posteriorly beside the urethra and vagina to fuse with the opposite homologous muscle

behind the anorectum at the anorectal junction. This muscle sling forms the innermost margin of the pelvic floor diaphragm, differing from the levator ani muscle diaphragm itself in that it does not insert into the sacrum.[2] The puborectalis muscle, separated from the external anal sphincter by a fascial layer, is innervated by direct somatic efferent nerves from the sacral plexus,[5,6] whereas the external anal sphincter muscle receives its innervation from the inferior rectal branches of the pudendal nerves. In addition, there are differences in the size and fiber-type distribution of muscle fibers in these three muscles.[7,8]

The external anal sphincter and puborectalis muscles are in a constant state of low-level tonic resting contraction, even during sleep.[9] Tonic contraction of the puborectalis muscle (puboanal sling) pulls the anal canal forward toward the pubis, thus maintaining a sharp rectoanal angulation. This angulation is such that the normal downward pressure of the abdominal contents results in apposition of the mucosa of the anterior and posterior walls of the anorectum, against the resistance of the tonic contraction of the puborectalis muscle, thus maintaining a flap-valve mechanism at this site. Parks suggested that this flap-valve mechanism at the level of the puborectalis muscle was the major mechanism of fecal continence in humans,[10] the tonic contraction of the external anal sphincter serving a minor role except in emergencies or in the presence of liquid stool, since the anal canal is usually empty.[11] There has been much subsequent controversy about this concept, mainly centered around whether there is a zone of high pressure at the level of the flap valve.[12] However, the flap valve does not require a zone of pressure to maintain the integrity of the valve because the forces playing on it vary considerably during changes in posture, with abdominal activity, and according to the pull of the puborectalis muscle. Thus increased contraction of the puborectalis and the external anal sphincter muscles occurs during a period of increased abdominal pressure, as with straining against a closed anal canal, coughing, and changes of posture.[9,13–15] Only in tabes dorsalis is the resting tonic activity of these muscles abolished.[9]

URINARY CONTINENCE

The mechanism of urinary continence is still imperfectly understood.[1,16] It is probably dependent on tonic contraction of the periurethral striated sphincter musculature, resulting in a sharply angled bladder neck.[16–19] However, tonic contraction of the intramural component of the striated urethral sphincter is also important.[18] These two muscles seem to be analogous to the external anal sphincter and puborectalis muscles, respectively, in function and innervation; the periurethral striated sphincter muscle is innervated by perineal branches of the pudendal nerves, and the intramural striated sphincter by direct motor branches of the somatic efferent pelvic nerves. Combined contraction of these two muscles may result in slight kinking of the proximal urethra, in addition to the closure and angulation of the bladder neck that results from contraction of the periurethral striated sphincter muscle. Kinking of the urethra itself would be an effective means of ensuring "no flow" in the urethra with a minimal externally applied force, whereas squeezing the urethra by contraction of a circular muscle would be an inefficient means of closing this relatively high-pressure system. Kinking the urethra is analogous to kinking a garden hose to stop the flow of water; a small applied force produces cessation of flow by a flap-valve mechanism. Conversely, relaxation of these muscles is necessary before micturition can commence.[1,16,20,21]

Like the voluntary anal sphincter musculature, the periurethral striated sphincter and intramural striated sphincter muscles are in a state of tonic basal activity; and, like these muscles, they consist largely of type 1 tonic muscle fibers.[18,22] The only other muscles in the human that show similar continuous basal activity are the cricopharyngeal sphincter muscles (which are responsible for closure of the upper esophagus during respiration), the muscles of the floor of the mouth (which maintain the upper airway), and the intrinsic abductor muscles of the vocal cords in the larynx.

The internal urethral sphincter muscle is clearly also important in the maintenance of urinary continence, but its precise role in the integration of muscular activity that takes place at the proximal urethra is unknown.[1] This smooth muscle sphincter was thought formerly to be the major factor in normal urinary continence. It is evident, however, that the role of the striated sphincter musculature has been neglected and that both internal and external sphincters are important. As in the case of the anal sphincter musculature, little is known of the reflex and other mechanisms that integrate the activity of the somatic and autonomic nervous systems in the control of urinary continence.

Neural Organization of Sphincter Control Systems

The conventional view of the neural organization for the control of the bladder and bowel sphincters is that there are neural systems overlaid on one another in the spinal cord, brainstem, basal ganglia, and cerebral cortex. Although control systems of this type exist, it is likely that control of the sphincter musculature is organized in a network of distributive systems such that each component can be related in functional motor programs that are connected in parallel rather than in series.[23] This arrangement encourages flexibility of response and the capacity for learning and behavioral responsiveness because it allows input for decision making at several functional and anatomical levels.[24]

ONUF'S SACRAL NUCLEUS

The peripheral components of the innervations of the anal and urinary sphincters, including both autonomic and somatic components, are organized in Onuf's sacral nuclei.[25] These consist of bilateral symmetrical groups of anterior horn cells making up a distinct nucleus in the S2 and S3 spinal segments. The Onuf nucleus is situated medially in the anterior horn on each side. The specialized groups of somatic efferent motor neurons in the ventromedial parts of the nucleus innervate the striated components of the vesical and anorectal sphincter musculature[26,27] and the perineal muscles (e.g., the ischiocavernosus and bulbocavernosus muscles).[28] The dorsal component of this nucleus contains motor neurons that innervate the periurethral striated sphincter muscle. The site of the neurons that innervate the puborectalis muscle is unknown but, since it has the same root origin, it is probably adjacent to the Onuf nucleus.

The neurons of Onuf's nucleus are smaller than other somatic neurons and have dense dendritic bundles that project rostrocaudally while remaining within the confines of the column of the nucleus.[29] These prominent and unusual dendritic arrays provide direct pathways for interconnection of the neurons of the nucleus. These profuse connections may provide the anatomical basis for the synchronization of neuronal activity in the nucleus for the maintenance of rhythmic and repetitive output and perhaps for metabolic and developmental functions.[28,29] Other dendrites extend radially from the main body of the nucleus and make contact with fibers descending rostrocaudally from brainstem and cerebral centers, especially from the ipsilateral paraventricular hypothalamic nucleus, ipsilateral caudal pontine lateral reticular formation, and caudal nucleus retroambiguus. Afferents from the pudendal nerve (e.g., muscle spindle and other muscular afferents) and input from the pudendal sensory innervation of the anal canal also synapse in this nucleus.[30,31] Muscle spindles are present, but only in small numbers, in the external anal sphincter muscle,[32,33] so that primary and secondary afferent input to this nucleus is probably relatively sparse. The neurotransmitters in these terminals are not characterized. Histological studies in humans have suggested that the Onuf nucleus contains both autonomic and somatic efferent neurons (see below), although Holstege and Tan found that in the cat this nucleus consists only of autonomic neurons.[30]

Terminals containing leucine-enkephalin, somatostatin, and vasopressin intestinal peptide are found in relation to these neurons but not in the somatic motor neurons just adjacent to the Onuf nucleus.[34] Similar peptidergic terminals are found in relation to the parasympathetic neurons themselves. It has been suggested that the leucine-enkephalin terminals are derived from collaterals of parasympathetic neurons that innervate the bladder detrusor[35] and perhaps the smooth muscle of the colon through connections with the enteric nervous system established from the parasympathetic innervation of the myenteric plexus (Auerbach's plexus). The parasympathetic neurons innervating colonic smooth muscle probably contain both leucine-enkephalin and somatostatin. These peptides may be important in mediating reciprocal inhibition of urethral and anorectal sphincter neurons during defecation and micturition. The origin of the terminals containing vasopressin intestinal peptide is uncertain, but they may represent interneuronal connections.[28]

SUPRASEGMENTAL ORGANIZATION OF SPHINCTER CONTROL SYSTEMS

The sacral nuclei subserving urinary smooth and striated sphincter and detrusor (smooth muscle) activity are modulated by descending pathways that traverse the spinal cord from the brain.[1,36] In the human, most of these fibers belong to the corticospinal tract and are situated in the most mesial portion of this tract.[37,38] The enteric nervous system[39] is separated from the somatic and visceral nervous systems at an early stage of ontogenesis, but is modulated by vagal and sacral parasympathetic efferents and by sympathetic efferents derived from the thoracic outflow.[40,41] Afferent fibers that subserve sensation in the bladder and urethra and presumably also in the anorectum probably travel in the superficial ventral part of the lateral funiculus.[37,38] The different paths followed by parasympathetic and sympathetic afferents, and by somatic afferents, from the bladder and anorectum are not yet fully understood.[1]

Many attempts to locate centers for the control of micturition and defecation in the central nervous system (CNS) have been made during the last century, and several supposed centers for these functions have been described in the cortex, basal ganglia, and region of the third ventricle. In addition, several complex systems of neuronal circuits have been suggested as being important to micturition, involving brainstem relays with so-called spinal centers. Loops of excitation and inhibition have been proposed, with relays extending through the length of the CNS from cortex to pons and to the sacral nuclei.[1] However, there is little anatomical evidence to support these concepts, which depend on an underlying notion of nuclei and interconnecting telephone-like systems of relays, with fixed responses resulting from activity in any part of the system.

Excitatory effects in the basal ganglia may produce detrusor hyperreflexia,[42] but the urinary hesitancy and incontinence with constipation that often occurs in idiopathic Parkinson's disease is probably the result of associated degeneration in dopaminergic autonomic pathways, rather than from the lesion in the substantia nigra that characterizes the disease.[43] Connections probably exist from the anorectum and bladder to nuclei in the limbic system, hypothalamus, and cerebellum.[1]

More is known about the brainstem systems concerned with micturition,[1,31,36,44–46] and it is presumed that these pathways are closely integrated with those concerned with defecation.[37,38] A lateral-dorsal tegmental nucleus in the pons, rostral to the nucleus of the locus ceruleus, is probably the site of origin of the neuronal system that descends in the intermediolateral tract of the spinal cord to supply parasympathetic innervation to the sacral outflow[38] and thus to the detrusor muscle of the bladder (the voiding pathway). This autonomic outflow connects with the neurons of Auerbach's myenteric plexus that modulate the enteric innervation of the colonic and anorectal smooth muscle.[39] It has also been suggested that this autonomic innervation to the bladder detrusor muscle travels in the reticulospinal tract.[1]

Hald and Bradley tried to integrate current information on these neuronal systems in the control of bladder function and suggested that there are four loop control systems: two for the detrusor muscle and two for the periurethral striated sphincter muscle.[1] They all involve connections through the pudendal nuclei and the pontine brainstem. Loop 1 connects the brainstem to the frontal lobe, loop 2 connects detrusor muscle afferents to the brainstem, loop 3 consists of detrusor afferents connecting with the pudendal nucleus in the sacral cord, and loop 4 consists of afferents and efferents connecting the periurethral striated muscles with the pudendal and pontine nuclei. Clearly, this suggestion is not entirely supported by the known neurophysiology and neuroanatomy and does not explain the complex coordinated mechanisms required for successful urinary and fecal continence and for micturition and defecation.

Barrington described brainstem reflexes induced by bladder distension and by running water through or distending the urethra.[45,46] In addition, he recognized that thoracic spinal cord section would temporarily abolish micturition and that low thoracic section would permanently abolish it. These features are observed in the spinal patient, and the pathways suggested by Barrington for these reflexes have been largely confirmed by physiological, evoked potential, and morphological studies.[47–49]

The cortical localization of the functions of micturition and defecation was placed by Foerster, following the work of Kleist on head injuries sustained by German soldiers during World War I,[50] on the medial surface of the cerebral hemisphere in the paracentral lobule, just anterior to the central sulcus. This localization is consistent with that of the motor representation of the sacral muscles on the cortical surface and has been confirmed in normal human subjects by transcutaneous electrical stimulation of the motor cortex.[51] The cortical localization of the sensory input from these organs is less certain but is probably in the adjacent sensory cortex, also on the medial surface

of the hemisphere. Penfield and Rasmussen reported that patients had sensations of bladder and rectal fullness when the sensory cortex on the upper part of the medial surface of the cerebral hemisphere was stimulated.[52] The localization of the sensory input from the pelvic area can be investigated in the intact human by cerebral evoked potential studies involving stimulation of the pudendal nerve (dorsal nerve of the penis or clitoris) or the pelvic detrusor nerve.[49] Stimulation of the latter nerve results in a response in the frontal lobe,[1] but the cortical localization of the parasympathetic detrusor innervation of the bladder and bowel is not known.[53]

Lesions of the superior parts of the medial surface of the hemispheres in the rolandic areas are uncommon, but frontal lobe lesions produce characteristic effects on bladder and bowel continence,[54,55] particularly loss of social inhibition, so that micturition and defecation occur at inappropriate times and places. These clinical syndromes overshadow the effects of lesions in other parts of the brain because they are so common, occurring especially frequently as a result of stroke, subarachnoid hemorrhage from anterior communicating aneurysms, frontal lobe tumors, and trauma.[54,55] Kuroiwa and associates reported that lesions of the right hemisphere were more likely to cause urgency and frequency of micturition than lesions of the left hemisphere.[56] Lesions in other parts of the brain are less likely to cause major problems with continence. Only lesions in the spinal cord, conus medullaris, or cauda equina are likely neurological causes of urinary or fecal retention.[1]

CLINICAL ASSESSMENT AND INVESTIGATION OF SPHINCTER DISORDERS

Clinical examination is important in terms of providing evidence of CNS disease and in suggesting the possibility of urinary infection or colonic disorders, including fecal retention with overflow, in which the anus is often patulous and the anorectum laden with feces. In patients who have urinary retention with overflow, the bladder may be palpable, regardless of the underlying etiology. Inspection of the perineum may reveal local causes, such as traumatic damage to the sphincter musculature, perhaps associated with injury during childbirth, local infection, or surgical damage. In addition, the response of the perineum to coughing and straining downward (as though defecating) is a useful clinical test for weakness of the perineal musculature. When there is weakness of these muscles, the perineal plane bulges downward toward the examiner during a cough, a feature termed "perineal descent."[57]

Anorectal Function

Clinical examination is supplemented by measurement of function and other neurophysiological variables.

ANAL MANOMETRY

Anorectal pressures can be measured with closed or open-tipped catheter probes connected to a pressure transducer. Resting anal pressure in the anal sphincter region is largely a measure of internal anal sphincter tone. The voluntary squeeze pressure corresponds to recruitment of activity in the external anal sphincter muscle. It can be sustained for only a few seconds at a time. Distension of an air-filled balloon within the rectum causes relaxation of the internal anal sphincter; this rectoanal relaxation reflex is mediated through intramural nerves in the myenteric plexus of the anorectum.[40] It is absent in Hirschsprung's disease, in which there is focal absence of the myenteric plexus in the anorectum, leading to obstruction of the lower bowel. Inflation of the rectal balloon also causes an initial burst of activity in the external anal sphincter muscle due to stretch-induced activation of its muscle spindles. This inflation reflex is absent in tabes dorsalis and in some patients with diabetic neuropathy.[53]

PERINEAL DESCENT

The plane of the perineum at rest and during a straining effort can be measured with respect to the plane of the ischial tuberosities using a perineometer.[58]

ELECTROMYOGRAPHY

Concentric needle electromyography (EMG) with motor unit potential analysis can be used to examine the external anal sphincter and puborectalis muscles

in studies of the anal sphincter system and the striated urethral sphincter muscle in vesicourethral investigations.[59] We have preferred to use single-fiber EMG because fiber density is a relatively robust measure that has good concordance between examiners and between serial investigations.[60-62] Furthermore, it is a good index of reinnervation in a muscle (Fig. 26-1).[60,61]

Vesicourethral Function

Assessment of vesicourethral function has received a great deal of attention since the pioneering studies of Denny-Brown and Robertson.[47] Urodynamic methods are commonly applied to the investigation of voiding disorders. A number of techniques are used, especially cystometry, urine flow-rate measurement, urethral pressure profile, and integrated pelvic floor muscle EMG. These methods provide complementary information on parts of the filling, storage, and voiding cycle that comprise normal vesicourethral function.

URODYNAMICS

Cystometry, using gas or more commonly liquid (e.g., water or radiological contrast),[1] may be utilized to study the relation between intravesical pressure and bladder filling volume, which represents the detrusor activity in response to change in bladder volume. Cystometric abnormalities are not diagnostic of any underlying lesion but describe the functional disturbance itself. There are five main categories of information derived from urodynamic studies.

1. *Residual urine volume.* This is a measure of the completeness of bladder emptying.
2. *Bladder sensation.* Normal subjects can first sense bladder filling at volumes of 100 to 200 ml. As filling continues, the desire to void increases and becomes urgent at maximum bladder capacity. Loss of these bladder sensations occurs with lesions in the peripheral or central nervous system and with a chronically distended, obstructed bladder.
3. *Maximum bladder capacity.* This varies greatly, ranging from 300 to 600 ml. Impairment of this storage capacity leads to frequency.

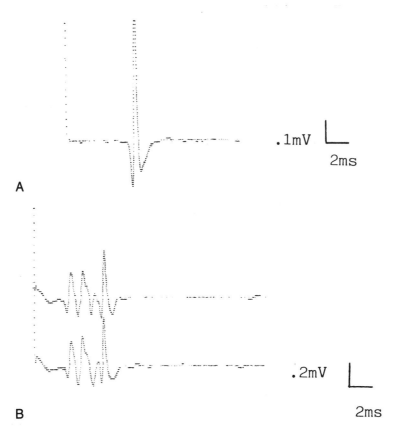

Fig. 26-1 Single-fiber EMG recording of the external anal sphincter muscle. **(A)** Normal subject. **(B)** Idiopathic anorectal incontinence—the motor unit potentials are abnormally complex, and the fiber density is increased.

4. *Bladder compliance.* The term *compliance* describes the change in pressure with any given change in volume during bladder filling, corresponding to the slope of the cystometrogram. It reflects the stretch characteristics of the bladder wall. In the normal bladder, pressure should not increase by more than 10 cmH$_2$O until full capacity is reached. Stiffening of the bladder wall after infection or radiotherapy reduces compliance, so that intravesical pressure rises more sharply than normal. This action results in urgency.

5. *Detrusor contractility.* Intravesical pressure results from the sum of intra-abdominal pressure and bladder detrusor pressure. The former can be measured with an anorectal pressure probe, allowing derivation of detrusor pressure by subtraction. Detrusor pressure is high when there is bladder outlet obstruction; intra-abdominal pressure is high when there is a weak detrusor muscle, so that micturition is accomplished by abdominal straining rather than detrusor contraction. Abdominal straining is also a feature of bladder outlet obstruction. Normal micturition is under voluntary control. The normal individual is able to sense bladder filling and to initiate or inhibit detrusor contractions.

URINARY FLOW RATE

Measurement of urinary flow rate is an inexpensive, noninvasive method for assessing detrusor function and outflow obstruction. The rate of flow and the total volume of urine voided can be measured.

URETHRAL PRESSURE PROFILE

Open-tipped catheters can be used to measure pressure in the urethra during micturition. This method resembles that used for anorectal manometry and gives information about the length of the functional sphincter zone in the urethra (normally 2.5 to 3.0 cm in women and 4 to 6 cm in men). Abnormalities in the pressure gradient in the urethra can be directly correlated with fluoroscopic imaging of the urethra during micturition. However, there is no direct correlation between abnormalities in the urethral pressure profile and urinary incontinence.

PELVIC FLOOR MUSCLE EMG: STUDIES OF VESICOURETHRAL FUNCTION

Surface or needle EMG recordings from pelvic floor muscles can be used to monitor the function of striated muscle during cystometry and micturition. The external anal sphincter or urethral striated sphincter muscles are commonly studied. Basal EMG activity in the external anal sphincter muscle normally increases during micturition. Conversely, at the start of micturition, basal activity in the urethral striated sphincter muscle is inhibited at the commencement of detrusor contraction and reestablished at the end of micturition. The normal patient can interrupt the flow of urine during micturition. Such interruption is accompanied by a burst of EMG activity in the urethral striated sphincter muscle. EMG activity in this muscle also increases during bladder filling and responds briskly to changes in body posture and intra-abdominal pressure, as during that induced by coughing.[21] This reflex modulation of activity in the urethral striated sphincter muscle is similar to that found in the external anal sphincter and puborectalis muscles and is important to the maintenance of continence during the normal stresses of daily life.

Abnormalities in the relation between modulation of EMG activity in these muscles and changes in filling pressure in the anorectum and bladder are found with functional disorders of voiding and defecation, for example, detrusor-sphincter dyssynergia and anismus (see below). Study of the configuration of motor unit potentials in the urethral striated sphincter muscle has been used to detect abnormalities in the innervation of this muscle in patients with stress urinary incontinence and certain types of functional obstruction to micturition.[63]

Other Neurophysiological Investigations

When there are abnormalities in motor unit configuration in the external anal sphincter, puborectalis, or urethral striated sphincter muscles, it is appropriate to investigate the innervation of these muscles directly. Such investigation can be achieved with techniques that utilize standard EMG equipment.

PUDENDAL AND PERINEAL NERVE TERMINAL MOTOR LATENCIES

The terminal motor latency in the pudendal and perineal nerves is a measure of function in the distal parts of the nerve supply of the external anal sphincter and periurethral striated sphincter muscles (Fig. 26-2). The evoked compound action potentials in these muscles are recorded after stimulation of the pudendal nerves in the pelvis.[64–67] This measurement is accomplished using a finger-mounted array of recording and stimulating electrodes with fixed interelectrode distances (3.5 cm). The two stimulating electrodes are mounted at the tip of the finger, with the cathode arranged distally; the recording electrodes are mounted side by side at the base of the finger so as to be in a suitable position to pick up the response in the external anal sphincter muscle. Stimulation of the pudendal nerves is achieved on either side of the pelvis by directing the exploring finger in the rectum toward the lateral rim of the pelvis (i.e., toward the ischial spine). The onset of the stimulus is used to trigger the oscilloscope. Stimuli of square wave pulses, 0.1 ms in duration and about 50 V (but always supramaximal), are used to find the shortest latency of the response in the external anal sphincter muscle. The perineal nerve terminal motor latency (Fig. 26-2) can be measured using a similar technique, recording the response with a pair of catheter-mounted recording electrodes placed in the urethra. Normal values for terminal motor latencies in these nerves are published elsewhere.[65,68]

TRANSCUTANEOUS SPINAL STIMULATION

The innervation of the puborectalis, which is derived from pelvic branches of the sacral plexus, is not accessible to intrarectal electrical stimulation techniques.

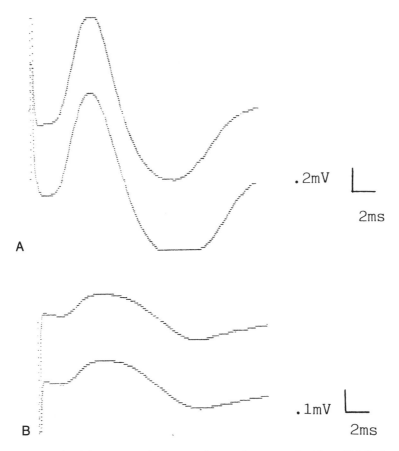

Fig. 26-2 (A) Pudendal nerve terminal motor latency in a normal subject. **(B)** Perineal nerve terminal motor latency in a normal subject. The terminal latency in this nerve is slightly longer than that in the pudendal nerve, reflecting its greater length from the point of stimulation in the perirectal space.

The nerves innervating this and other muscles of the perineum or legs can be excited transcutaneously by applying stimulation over the cauda equina, thereby allowing the motor latency to these muscles to be measured.[69,70]

With our method, direct electrical stimulation of the cauda equina is achieved by transcutaneous spinal stimulation (Fig. 26-3).[69,70] The patient is placed in the left lateral position, and single shocks are delivered through two saline-soaked gauze electrode pads, 1 cm in diameter, arranged 5 cm apart and placed with the cathode at the level of the first and fourth lumbar vertebrae, respectively. The anode is directed cranially. An initial 500-V stimulus is applied and increased by 200-V increments (up to 1,500 V) until the response amplitude and latency of the pelvic sphincter muscles do not change with further stimulus increments. Three consecutive responses elicited by a stimulus that is 20 percent greater in voltage than required to produce a maximal response are used for latency measurements. The muscle responses in the external anal sphincter muscle (Fig. 26-3) are recorded with the electrode array used for measuring terminal motor latency of the pudendal nerve or with an anal plug electrode. The puborectalis response (Fig. 26-3) is recorded with a glove-mounted electrode array similar to that used for studying the pudendal nerve. The finger bearing this device is inserted into the rectum so that the electrode array is in contact with the puborectalis muscle (i.e., the recording surfaces face

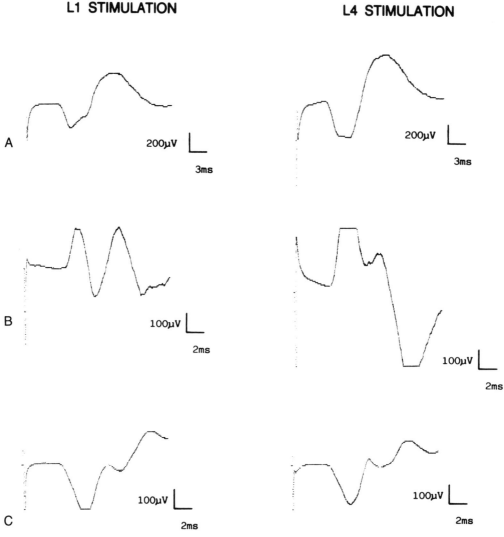

L1 STIMULATION

L4 STIMULATION

Fig. 26-3 Transcutaneous spinal (cauda equina) stimulation at the L1 and L4 levels, with responses recorded from **(A)** external anal sphincter muscle, **(B)** puborectalis muscle, and **(C)** periurethral striated sphincter muscle. Note the different latencies to these muscles from the L1 and L4 sites of stimulation, reflecting the different lengths of these lower motor neuron pathways.

posteriorly).[71] A catheter-mounted electrode can be used to assess responses in the periurethral striated sphincter muscle (Fig. 26-3).

The L1 and L4 vertebral levels of stimulation represent the conus medullaris and the lumbosacral nerve roots of the cauda equina, respectively. With currently available electrical or magnetic stimulators, it is not possible to reliably stimulate these nerve roots at a more caudal vertebral level, presumably because of attenuation of current by the bony mass of the sacrum. It is particularly appropriate to record from the external anal sphincter and puborectalis muscles because these muscles are innervated by the most caudal segments of the spinal cord and thus represent the nerve fibers with the longest course through the cauda equina. Furthermore, studies of these nerve roots have obvious application in patients presenting with sphincter dysfunction and with other pelvic floor problems that might be associated with cauda equina disease.[70]

The stimulating electrodes, situated on the skin overlying the cauda equina, are several centimeters distant from the underlying excitable nervous tissue,[70,72] so that the precise site of stimulation of the nerve roots is not necessarily represented by the surface marking of the cathode. Moreover, measurement of the length of the cauda equina between the two stimulation points is likely to be inaccurate.[69,70] We have therefore used latency measurements rather than calculated conduction velocities to study the findings in various clinical contexts.

SPINAL LATENCY RATIO

The difference in motor latency of the responses in the external anal sphincter, puborectalis, and urethral striated sphincter muscles from stimulation at the L1 and L4 levels represents the conduction time in the S2, S3, and S4 cauda equina nerve roots between these vertebral levels (Fig. 26-3). We have found it useful to express this as a ratio of the two latencies because the absolute values of the latencies from L1 and L4 stimulation are modified not only by damage to these nerve roots but by variations in height, pelvic size, and other morphometric features of the subject under investigation. The spinal latency ratio (SLR) obviates these difficulties without introducing error from measurements of the interelectrode distance.

$$SLR = \frac{\text{latency to puborectalis after L1 stimulation}}{\text{latency to puborectalis after L4 stimulation}}$$

In the presence of a distal conduction delay, both L1 and L4 motor latencies increase similarly, and the SLR therefore becomes slightly smaller. However, with a proximal conduction delay due to a lesion of the cauda equina between the L1 and L4 vertebral levels, the L1 motor latency is increased compared to the L4 motor latency, and consequently the SLR is increased. Stimulation at these two vertebral sites can thus be used to determine if there is a conduction delay within or distal to the L1 to L4 portion of the cauda equina. The SLR is also increased in patients with slowed motor conduction both proximally and distally (Fig. 26-4), as the increased proximal (terminal) motor latency is then contained only in the measurement from the L1 stimulus.[70]

The variance of the SLR between normal subjects is relatively small, and the motor conduction velocity in the motor nerve roots of the cauda equina derived from these latency measurements is 58 m/s (SD 10 m/s). The SLR to the external anal sphincter or urethral striated sphincter muscles from stimulation at the same vertebral sites is comparable to the SLR to the puborectalis muscle.[70,73]

CORTICAL STIMULATION

The sphincter musculature can be excited by electrical[74–77] or magnetic stimulation[78] of the motor cortex. The cortical motor representation of the striated sphincter and pelvic floor musculature is close to the median sagittal plane of the skull. Surface electrodes, preferably of disposable type, placed within the anal canal can be used to record the response of the external anal sphincter muscle. The shortest latency of the response is at about 20 ms in normal subjects.[74,76] The response is therefore probably monosynaptic, since it occurs at a latency consistent with that of other striated muscles known to have corticospinal innervation, allowing for differences in length of the intervening pathways. Ertekin and colleagues reported a longer latency,[75] but this is probably attributable to the lower-powered electrical stimulator that they used in their experiments. In patients with multiple sclerosis associated with incontinence or with other spinal disorders (see below), the motor latency to the external anal sphincter muscle from cortical stimulation is usually increased.

SENSORY EVOKED POTENTIALS

The sensory pathway to the cerebral cortex can be investigated using evoked response techniques with computer averaging. This technique can be applied to stimulation in the anorectum, at the bladder neck, at the dorsal nerve of the penis or clitoris (pudendal nerve), or at the trigone of the bladder. All these methods are uncomfortable for the patient, and they have not therefore been generally applied to investigation of voiding or defecatory disorders except in patients with spinal injuries in whom sensation is impaired.[79] Anorectal sensory evoked potentials have proved inconsistent in form and latency in clinical studies.[80]

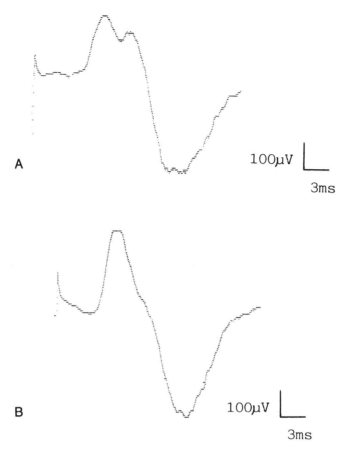

Fig. 26-4 Transcutaneous spinal stimulation. The latencies to the puborectalis muscle are increased from the L1 level **(A),** but normal from the L4 level **(B),** suggesting a lesion in the spinal canal between these two levels.

SPINAL MOTOR CONDUCTION VELOCITY IN SPHINCTER PATHWAYS

The corticospinal fibers of the spinal cord can be excited by transcutaneous electrical stimulation using the method introduced by Merton and Morton.[81] Stimulation can be achieved at the lumbar (T12/L1 and L4), midthoracic, and cervical (C6) levels, thereby allowing calculation of the motor conduction velocity between these levels. Using these methods and recording from the puborectalis or external anal sphincter muscles, we found that mean corticospinal motor conduction velocity between the C6 and L1 vertebral levels in 21 normal adults with a mean age of 55 years was 67.4 m/s (SD 9.1 m/s).[82] Although there was a trend for the spinal motor conduction velocity to decrease with increasing age, the change was not statistically significant.

CLINICAL DISORDERS OF SPHINCTER FUNCTION

Sphincter disorders are frequent although often unvoiced. The two basic symptoms of sphincter dysfunction are sphincter incompetence, leading to incontinence, and incoordination between sphincter relaxation and detrusor activity, leading to retention of urine or feces (Table 26-1). A discussion of disorders of other sphincters (e.g., cricopharyngeal sphincter) and other muscles concerned with the process of swallowing; the coordination of laryngeal activity with breathing, swallowing, and talking; and the control of the diaphragmatic sphincter at the lower end of the esophagus is not within the scope of this chapter. Similarly, management is not considered here, but in general it consists of treatment of the underlying disorder and the symptomatic measures discussed in most standard medical textbooks.

Incontinence

Surveys of the prevalence of urinary and fecal incontinence in the general population suggest that incontinence is much more common than has generally been supposed, especially among women.[83] As many as 10 percent of women older than 50 years experience two or more episodes of incontinence of urine each month; in elderly populations in nursing homes, a prevalence figure for incontinence of more than 50 percent is common. Fecal incontinence is less common, but the observation of Leigh and Turnberg[84] that 51 percent of patients presenting to a gastroenterology clinic with the complaint of diarrhea were, in reality, incontinent suggests that the incidence of fecal incontinence has been greatly underestimated. Surveys have confirmed the commonly held view that incontinence is much more common in women than in men.[83–85]

Incontinence itself is relatively commonly found in association with disorders of the CNS (e.g., multiple sclerosis). Incontinence occurs in these patients in response to cutaneous or other stimuli, often as part of a generalized reflex activity (e.g., in association with flexor or extensor spasms). In patients with neurological disorders such as multiple sclerosis, the possibility that incontinence may develop is sometimes a greater threat to self-esteem than the potential loss of mobility. Incontinence may also develop when there is damage to the motor or sensory pathways in the cauda equina. However, most patients with incontinence have no evident neurological disorder, and they experience incontinence particularly when the sphincter system is stressed, as during a cough or other sudden increase in intra-abdominal pressure. This idiopathic form of incontinence is usually called *idiopathic stress urinary incontinence* or *idiopathic anorectal incontinence,* terms that suggest ignorance of both the underlying causative factors and the functional disturbances leading to the sphincter disorder. A classification of fecal incontinence is given in Table 26-2, and a similar approach can be used to classify urinary incontinence.

Classifications of clinical symptoms[86] are generally not useful in the diagnostic process. Unfortunately, it is not yet possible to construct classifications of urinary and fecal incontinence that are relevant to

Table 26-2 Fecal Incontinence

Local sphincter dysfunction
Congenital anorectal anomalies
Sphincter trauma
Obstetrical
Surgical
Accidental
Perianal suppuration
Rectal or anal cancer

Enteric disorder
Overwhelming diarrhea

Neurological disorders
Upper motor neuron lesions
Cerebral lesions
Dementia
Cerebrovascular disease
Hydrocephalus
Multiple sclerosis
Tumors (especially frontal)
Traumatic encephalopathy
Cerebral infections
Spinal cord lesions
Trauma
Spinal cord compression
Multiple sclerosis
Ischemia
Lower motor neuron lesions
Onuf's nucleus/conus medullaris lesions
Multiple sclerosis
Ischemia
Spinal dysraphism
Degenerative disease: primary autonomic failure and multisystem atrophy
Cauda equina disease
Lumbosacral trauma
Lumbosacral disc prolapse
Lumbar canal stenosis and spondylosis
Ankylosing spondylitis
Peripheral lesions
Pudendal/perineal nerve stretch injury
Childbirth injury to pudendal/perineal nerves
Intrapelvic tumor, sepsis, and endometriosis
Proximal diabetic neuropathy
Autonomic neuropathy ?

Multifactorial causes
Incontinence in the elderly
Incontinence in confusional states
Fecal impaction
Immobility

functional and anatomical concepts and yet can be used in clinical practice. The four-loop theory of sphincter control[1] can be loosely related to older concepts of the uninhibited, or reflex, bladder, corresponding to lesions in the connections between the frontal region and the brainstem or sacral detrusor nucleus (loops 1 and 2) and to the motor or sensory "paralytic" bladder defects that characterize more distal (lower motor or sensory neuron) lesions. In addition, it is helpful to recognize that more rostral lesions are generally associated with failure of storing urine or feces, and more distal lesions with failure of voiding urine or feces. Thus, frontal lesions result in micturition in inappropriate circumstances, whereas conus or cauda equina lesions initially cause retention of urine, with overflow. Central lesions in brain, brainstem, or spinal cord may cause detrusor hyperreflexia (Fig. 26-5), which is characterized by detrusor contractions that occur during the filling phase of the cystometrogram. These contractions are only partially inhibited and may lead to involuntary micturition, especially if there is incompetence of the sphincter mechanism. This feature is often referred to as "bladder instability" by urologists. It is also found in patients in whom the normal pressure–flow relations are disturbed by the presence of partial outflow obstruction due to prostatic enlargement or urethral stricture: a similar functional disorder occurs when the bladder wall is irritable (e.g., with infection).

With some disorders (e.g., multiple sclerosis), lesions may be present in both the frontal lobe white matter and the conus medullaris, accounting for any difficulty in understanding the basis of sphincter disturbances. Mathers and co-workers found electrophysiological evidence for damage to both upper and lower motor neuron pathways subserving sphincter control in multiple sclerosis.[76] Furthermore, incontinence is more likely to develop in women with multiple sclerosis who have borne children,[87] probably because of damage to the pudendal nerves.

FRONTAL LOBE LESIONS

Frontal lobe tumors[55] arising from the falx cerebri or olfactory groove that impinge on the medial or inferior surface of the frontal lobe are well known causes of incontinence. Indeed, the tumor may present with incontinence, sometimes consisting in voiding at inappropriate times or inappropriate places, rather than frank urge incontinence. Incontinence also occurs in patients with intrinsic disease of the cerebral hemispheres (e.g., intrinsic tumors, multiple strokes, multiple sclerosis, or uncompensated hydrocephalus). With the latter there is ventricular enlargement, and the corticospinal and other fibers running from the cortex to the brainstem are stretched around the enlarged ventricles. The fibers to the sacral spinal cord are particularly vulnerable to this lesion, and treatment is followed by recovery of sphincter function. Incontinence in uncompensated hydrocephalus is

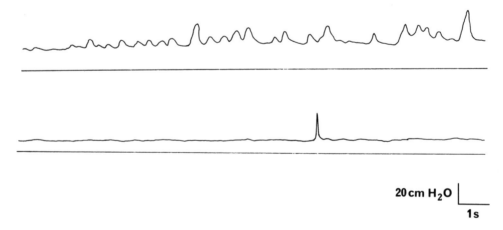

20 cm H₂O

1s

Fig. 26-5 Urodynamics. In this cystometrogram *(upper trace)* the detrusor muscle contracts during small increments of fluid during the filling phase. In the normal bladder *(lower trace)* the detrusor muscle is relaxed during this early phase of filling; a single sharp spike of increased pressure represents a cough during the procedure.

commonly accompanied by gait apraxia, probably reflecting damage to frontal lobe motor connections, and by extensor plantar responses and other signs of mild corticospinal dysfunction in the legs.[88] There may be a mild dementia. With degenerative brain diseases, especially Alzheimer's dementia, the location of the lesions responsible for incontinence is undefinable.

BRAINSTEM LESIONS

Lesions in the brainstem (e.g., infarcts) are not likely to cause incontinence unless there is pseudobulbar palsy with the associated abnormality of affect; the latter often implies the presence of lesions rostral to the brainstem. However, pontine lesions may present with incontinence as one of their clinical manifestations. This may reflect involvement of neurons in the pontomedullary centers concerned with suprasegmental control of the Onuf sacral nucleus and interruption of descending pathways from frontal and hypothalamic regions to this nucleus. These brainstem neurons are located in the locus ceruleus and the medullary medial reticular formation.[30] These neurons and pathways are also important in the control of the enteric nervous system by the CNS, especially in relation to gut motility.[39,89]

SPINAL CORD LESIONS

With spinal cord lesions, there is loss of supranuclear control of the sacral centers for micturition and defecation so that, in the absence of obstruction or infection, an automatic pattern of micturition and defecation is established. However, micturition and defecation are both abnormal in the presence of partial or complete spinal cord lesions. The absence of the normal sensation of filling of the bladder and anorectum, because afferent pathways are interrupted through the damaged cord, often results in overdistension and injury to these organs, with consequent secondary functional effects. Loss of viscoelasticity of the wall of the bladder and anorectum and loss of the normal smooth muscle responses to filling and inflation lead to abnormal compliance and incontinence (e.g., as with fecal impaction). There is thus not only reflex incontinence from an absence of supraspinal control mechanisms but loss of storage function from local effects on the bladder and anorec-

tum. In addition, spinal lesions produce abnormalities in the reflex interrelations of the detrusor and sphincter systems, causing detrusor-sphincter dyssynergia (see below).

LOWER MOTOR NEURON LESIONS

Incontinence results from damage to the somatic afferent and efferent pathways to the striated sphincter musculature of the anorectum in the pelvic floor and the external anal sphincter muscles, and to the striated muscles at the bladder neck and periurethral striated sphincter muscles. This damage may occur with congenital anomalies (e.g., myelomeningocele), spondylosis, narrow spinal canal syndromes, primary or secondary sacral tumors, sacral bony anomalies, or trauma. Similarly, incontinence may occur as part of the clinical syndrome of involvement of the sacral plexus and nerve roots in proximal neuropathies (e.g., diabetic neuropathy), in association with malignant infiltration of these nerves, or with pelvic trauma. Other features (e.g., pain, weakness, and sensory loss) are major features of these syndromes.

In progressive autonomic failure (Shy-Drager syndrome), there is selective damage to the innervation of the striated urinary sphincter musculature similar to that found in the abductor muscles of the larynx. The external anal sphincter seems to be spared, at least in the early stages of the disease. This observation implies selective vulnerability within the somatic efferent component of the neurons of the Onuf nucleus in this disease.[90] In motor neuron disease (amyotrophic lateral sclerosis) and the spinal muscular atrophies, the converse occurs in that the striated pelvic floor sphincter muscles are relatively spared, as are the external ocular muscles, the cricopharyngeal sphincter, and the diaphragmatic sphincter muscles. These features have implications for selective vulnerability in degenerative disorders of anterior horn cells.[91,92]

When incontinence results from lesions in the S2 to S4 nerve roots, whether in the spinal canal or the pelvis, it is important to recognize that conventional neurological examination is normal. Sensory disturbance is evident only on testing in the gluteal cleft. The anal reflex, although much relied on, is often absent even in normal subjects, with the relatively crude technique generally used clinically. Tone is reduced in the external anal sphincter muscle during a maximal squeeze and during a cough, and there may be palpable atrophy of the puborectalis muscle. Atrophy of the posterior thigh muscles is difficult to appreciate, and tendon reflexes cannot be reliably elicited from these muscles even in normal subjects. It is in these syndromes that the electrophysiological tests, described above, are useful when deciding how far to pursue investigation. EMG features of denervation in the external anal sphincter and puborectalis muscles, and the slowing of nerve conduction in the motor innervation of the perianal sphincter muscles comprise useful confirmatory evidence of the site of the causative disease and may indicate the need for myelography, computed tomography (CT) scanning, or magnetic resonance imaging (MRI) of the sacral canal and pelvis.[70]

IDIOPATHIC STRESS INCONTINENCE

In patients with stress urinary or fecal incontinence (idiopathic anorectal incontinence), there is denervation of the striated pelvic floor sphincter muscles (Fig. 26-1). It is usually due to damage to the innervation of these muscles during childbirth.[73] The nerves involved are the inferior rectal and perineal branches of the pudendal nerves and the somatic, direct pelvic branches of the sacral nerves. Injury is caused by direct force applied to these nerves during passage of the fetal head through the birth canal and by stretching during elongation of the birth canal and descent of the perineum as part of the normal process of childbirth.[73] Difficulty during childbirth (e.g., prolonged labor, a large baby, and especially the application of forceps to the head and sphincter tears) is particularly associated with damage to the perineal and pudendal nerves.[68,73] Anal endosonography has brought to attention the frequency of associated tears in the external anal sphincter in these patients.[93]

Weakness of the pelvic floor muscles from denervation causes loss of tone in these muscles, descent of the pelvic floor during simulated defecation straining and during coughing, and other symptoms such as genital, urinary, or anorectal prolapse, nagging pain, and difficulty with defecation because of mucosal prolapse. A pattern of straining during defecation is thus initiated that leads to frequent, pronounced perineal descent and to further recurrent stretch-induced injury to the pelvic floor muscles, and eventually to the development of incontinence of feces or urine or to double incontinence.[69] The clinical deficit depends on the relative amount of damage to the innervations of the urethral and anal striated sphincter muscles. Because the pelvic floor sphincters are weak, the anorectal and vesicourethral angles are increased (flattened), and urine and feces are voided during sudden straining, coughing, twisting, laughing, or other movements that increase intra-abdominal pressure.

Not all patients with stress incontinence have given birth; indeed the syndrome occurs in men, though rarely. In these patients there is often a history of straining during defecation or of intractable constipation (see below). This form of the disorder is associated with the same features of denervation due to nerve injury as in most women in whom the association with childbirth has been established. Pelvic floor descent during straining or coughing is also a feature in these patients.[58] Thus, constipation or an abnormal bowel habit with a straining pattern of defecation also leads to stretch injury to the pelvic floor muscles (Fig. 26-6).

In about 10 percent of our patients referred for investigation of stress incontinence, there is electrophysiological evidence of damage not only to the distal parts of the innervation of the pelvic floor striated sphincter muscles but also to the cauda equina nerve roots in the sacral spinal canal.[69] This is probably due to lumbosacral spondylosis, but its relevance to the clinical syndrome is as yet uncertain. It is important to recognize that the cystometric and anal manometric findings of stress incontinence do not differentiate between these patient groups, as they give information concerning only the functional state of the bladder-sphincter relations and the compliance of the bladder and anorectal walls.

SENSORY ABNORMALITIES

Damage to the somatic sensory innervation of the anorectum and bladder would be expected when there is denervation of the pelvic floor muscles due to a neuropathy.[94] However, the somatic sensory innervation of these organs is restricted to the anal canal itself and to the trigone of the bladder and urethra. Sensory abnormalities in these areas are well recognized in some patients with proximal diabetic neuropathy. The rectum and bladder receive sensory innervation from the autonomic and enteric nervous systems,[1,4] which is probably the main source of the

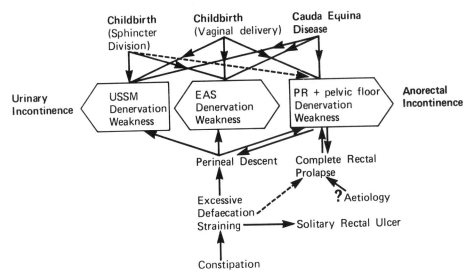

Fig. 26-6 Algorithm of stress incontinence. Fecal and urinary incontinence are shown associated with denervation and weakness of the pelvic floor muscles and especially of the striated sphincter muscles. This condition results from damage to the innervation of these muscles sustained during childbirth, during excessive straining at defecation, and from disease in the pelvis and cauda equina. The relative involvement of the different innervations of the sphincter muscles accounts for the occurrence of predominantly urinary and fecal incontinence. *USSM,* urethral striated sphincter muscle; *EAS,* external anal sphincter; *PR,* puborectalis muscle.

sensations of filling and urgency and of visceral pain. The role of sensory deficit in urinary and anorectal stress incontinence is controversial[95]; but because continence may be partially restored by biofeedback conditioning in idiopathic anorectal incontinence, enough sensory input must be present to allow access to central control mechanisms.[96] Lack of awareness of bladder or anorectal filling could be important in some patients with autonomic neuropathies, as in those with an idiopathic visceral neuropathy and patients with progressive autonomic failure.

Retention

Inability to void may be a feature of both bladder and anorectal dysfunction (Table 26-1). It may be due to sphincter incoordination in relation to the detrusor mechanism or to detrusor weakness causing loss of propulsive force.

DETRUSOR-SPHINCTER DYSSYNERGIA

Successful micturition depends on adequate detrusor contraction, with synchronous relaxation of the smooth and striated urinary sphincter muscles. De-

trusor-sphincter dyssynergia results from an involuntary increase in urinary sphincter tone during attempted voiding, so that the detrusor muscle contracts against a tightly closed sphincter and urine flow is poor or absent.[36] Contraction of the periurethral striated sphincter musculature can be recognized by the presence of bursts of EMG activity in this muscle during attempted micturition, at a time when intravesical pressure is high from detrusor muscle contraction.[97,98] Simultaneous pressure recordings and EMG recordings are therefore required for accurate recognition of this functional disturbance.

The most commonly recognized cause of detrusor-sphincter dyssynergia is spinal cord disease, the lesion being above the level of the conus medullaris.[1] The syndrome has been explained as due to separation of the sacral micturition center from the brainstem and its central connections, preventing the normal integration of detrusor and sphincter muscle functions.[99] From the theoretical standpoint, detrusor-sphincter dyssynergia is of special interest because it represents the dissociation of the central control of the functional interrelation of the visceral detrusor muscle control system from the somatic sensorimotor system that controls the striated external sphincter system.[31] Little is known about the anatomy and physiology of the interactions of these two nervous systems in health or disease. The syndrome also occurs in patients with other CNS lesions, in particular stroke, dementia, multiple sclerosis, and Parkinson's disease. However, these patients, more commonly have detrusor hyper-reflexia with urge incontinence.[100]

Despite the assumption that detrusor-sphincter dyssynergia is due to neurological disease, most cases appear idiopathic in that there is no demonstrable neurological lesion. They appear in children presenting with hesitancy of micturition, straining, and encopresis, and in otherwise healthy adults who develop voiding dysfunction after a previously normal pattern of micturition. The cause of the functional disturbance of micturition in these patients is not known. Detrusor-sphincter dyssynergia is important because it leads to an increase in intravesical pressure, with persistent residual urine. In some patients intermittent catheterization may be required to achieve bladder emptying and so reduce the risk of recurrent urinary tract infection. Nonetheless, there is a substantial risk of the development of hydronephrosis from the back-pressure effect on the upper urinary and renal tracts, a problem that may cause chronic renal failure if untreated (e.g., by α-blocking agents or sphincterotomy).

Detrusor-sphincter dyssynergia must be differentiated from other disordered patterns of micturition.[1] For example, some patients show an abnormal straining pattern of micturition in which other pelvic floor muscles are recruited into the act of micturition[20]; external sphincter spasm also occurs in some patients with detrusor hyporeflexia in whom there is no evidence of any organic lesion in the detrusor innervation and no dyscoordination between the detrusor and the external urinary sphincter. Spasm of the external urinary sphincter muscle also occurs when there is urethritis or cystitis.[1,20]

ANISMUS-TYPE CONSTIPATION

There are various causes of constipation (Table 26-3). Constipation is difficult to define, but a useful working definition states that a person is constipated if he or she strains at stool more than 25 percent of defecating time or passes fewer than two stools per week.[101] In one study, patients with constipation were given radiopaque markers in the diet. Eighty

Table 26-3 Classification of Severe, Chronic Constipation

Slow-transit constipation (diet, pregnancy, aging, irritable bowel syndrome, systemic sclerosis, idiopathic)

Local disease of anorectum and colon (anal stenosis, aganglionosis, and megacolon syndromes)

Functional pelvic outlet obstruction (anismus, Parkinson's disease, rectocele, and rectal prolapse)

Other (CNS disorders, psychiatric disorders, drug effects)

percent of the markers were visible on plain abdominal radiographs 10 days later; in normal subjects these markers are voided within 4 days. The location of the markers in the colon gives information concerning the cause of the functional disorder.[102]

Constipation may be of the slow-transit type, in which there is a delay in passage of fecal matter through the colon as a whole, or of the normal-transit type, in which colonic motility is normal but there is a functional obstruction to defecation at the pelvic outlet.[102,103] This syndrome of pelvic outlet obstruction, termed *anismus,* is a common cause of constipation, especially in women.[103,104] Defecating proctography in patients with anismus has shown that the anorectal angle retains its acuteness during attempted defecation rather than opening to allow passage of the fecal bolus.[103] This is due to paradoxical recruitment of the puborectalis muscle during defecation, a phenomenon that is not found exclusively in pelvic outlet obstruction but that also occurs in some patients with intractable pelvic and perineal pain and in those with solitary rectal ulcer syndrome.[105]

A similar functional disturbance of defecation occurs in Parkinson's disease.[106] With both anismus and Parkinson's disease, paradoxical recruitment of the puborectalis muscle is accompanied by recruitment of other pelvic floor muscles and of the glutei and anterior abdominal wall muscles. This form of constipation thus resembles a focal dystonia in the widespread muscle recruitment that occurs during the attempted motor task and in the inappropriate contraction of the puborectalis muscle.[106] Attempts to weaken the puborectalis muscle by surgical division[107] and by local injection of botulinum toxin have had some success in relieving the disordered defecation.

A long history of straining at stool in patients with the anismus syndrome is associated with the later development of fecal incontinence, probably because of the perineal descent that occurs during straining. The latter can lead to progressive denervation of the pelvic floor sphincter muscles and so to weakness.[108]

LACK OF PROPULSIVE FORCE

Disease of the enteric innervation of the gut (e.g., of the colon) results in reduced motor activity and slowing of intestinal transit.[39,109] Similarly, abnormalities in the bladder wall can cause weakness of the bladder detrusor muscle. Autonomic neuropathies involving the parasympathetic nervous system may also cause these symptoms. Thus, detrusor weakness and lack of intestinal motility are common features of autonomic involvement in Guillain-Barré syndrome and occur in diabetic autonomic neuropathy, in the hereditary autonomic and sensory neuropathies, and in patients with progressive autonomic failure. Weakness of the bladder detrusor muscle may occur without other clinical deficits (detrusor areflexia); although investigation usually fails to reveal any systemic or local cause, it is often assumed that it results from degeneration in the parasympathetic innervation of the bladder detrusor muscle.

In Chagas' disease, due to infestation with *Trypanosoma cruzi,* there is widespread destruction of ganglia in the myenteric plexus and of neurons in the peripheral autonomic ganglia, leading to megacolon and impaired colonic transit as one of the manifestations of the gastrointestinal disorder.[110] Megacolon is also a feature of patients with idiopathic visceral neuropathy, a syndrome in which constipation and slowed intestinal transit results from inflammatory or noninflammatory degeneration of the intrinsic neurons of the whole gut, especially of the myenteric plexus.[111–114] Some cases, with inflammatory change in the plexus, are associated with neoplasia, representing a paraneoplastic syndrome.[113] Slow-transit constipation has been associated with degeneration of the myenteric neurons in the colon, a degenerative, noninflammatory disorder that affects young women and that may even require colectomy to achieve relief.[115] Its cause is unknown. A few families have been reported in which visceral neuropathy was the predominant clinical feature of an unclassified type of hereditary autonomic neuropathy.

Hirschsprung's disease presents with colonic obstruction during the first few days or weeks of life.

It is due to congenital absence of ganglion cells from a segment of the terminal portion of the bowel. This anomaly leads to massive dilatation proximal to the region of aganglionosis because peristalsis is interrupted in this region. The disorder is probably due to an abnormality in the migration of neurons into the gut from the neural crest during development. It is not associated with other abnormalities of neural development and may be due to abnormalities in the basal laminae of smooth muscle cells in this region of the gut.[116] Congenital pyloric stenosis may have a similar origin.

In another group of poorly understood disorders, megacolon, with extensive involvement of other parts of the gastrointestinal tract, seems to be due to degeneration of the smooth muscle of the gut wall.[114] The innervation of the smooth muscle by the autonomic and enteric nervous systems in these disorders appears to be normal, but there is involvement of the smooth muscle of the wall of the bladder, leading to detrusor areflexia and weakness, with megacystis and megaureter. Peristalsis is abnormal and intestinal pseudo-obstruction develops, sometimes requiring surgical excision of redundant loops of gut.[115]

REFERENCES

1. Hald T, Bradley WE: The Urinary Bladder: Neurology and Dynamics. Williams & Wilkins, London, 1982
2. Wood BA: Anatomy of the pelvic floor. p. 3. In Henry MM, Swash M (eds): Coloproctology and the Pelvic Floor. Butterworths, London, 1985
3. Duthie HL, Gairns FW: Sensory nerve endings and sensation in the anal region of man. Br J Surg 47:585, 1960
4. Miller R, Bartolo DCC, Cervero F, Mortensen NJMcC: Anorectal sampling: comparison of normal and incontinent patients. Br J Surg 75:44, 1988
5. Percy J, Neill ME, Swash M, Parks AG: Electrophysiological study of motor nerve supply of pelvic floor. Lancet 1:16, 1981
6. Snooks SJ, Swash M: The innervation of the muscles of continence. Ann R Coll Surg Engl 68:45, 1986
7. Parks AG, Swash M, Urich H: Sphincter denervation in anorectal incontinence and rectal prolapse. Gut 18:656, 1977
8. Beersiek F, Parks AG, Swash M: Pathogenesis of idiopathic anorectal incontinence: a histometric study of

the anal sphincter musculature. J Neurol Sci 42:111, 1979

9. Floyd WF, Walls EW: Electromyography of the sphincter ani externus in man. J Physiol (Lond) 122:599, 1953

10. Parks AG: Anorectal incontinence. Proc R Soc Med 68:681, 1975

11. Kerremans R: Morphological and Physiological Aspects of Anal Continence and Defaecation. Editions Arscia, Brussels, 1969

12. Bannister JJ, Read NW: Is there a role for a flap valve in maintaining normal continence? Gut 28:1242, 1987

13. Taverner D, Smiddy FG: An electromyographic study of the normal function of the external anal sphincter and pelvic diaphragm. Dis Colon Rectum 2:153, 1959

14. Beck A: Elektromyographische Untersuchungen am Sphinkter Ani. Arch Physiol 224:278, 1930

15. Parks AG, Porter NH, Melzack J: Experimental study of the reflex mechanism controlling the muscles of the pelvic floor. Dis Colon Rectum 5:407, 1962

16. McGuire E: Electromyographic evaluation of sphincter function and dysfunction. Urol Clin North Am 6:121, 1979

17. Vereecken RL, Verduyn H: The electrical activity of the para-urethral and perineal muscles in normal and pathological conditions. Br J Urol 42:457, 1970

18. Gosling J: The structure of the bladder and urethra in relation to function. Urol Clin North Am 6:31, 1979

19. Kuru M: Nervous control of micturition. Physiol Rev 45:425, 1965

20. Abrams P, Feneley R, Torrens M: Urodynamics. Springer-Verlag, Berlin, 1983

21. Hutch JA, Elliott HW: Electromyographic study of the electrical activity in the para-urethral and perineal muscles prior to and during voiding. J Urol 99:759, 1968

22. Schroder HD, Reske-Nielsen EC: Fiber types in the striated urethral and anal sphincters. Acta Neuropathol (Berl) 60:278, 1984

23. Ito M: Neural systems controlling movement. Trends Neurosci 9:515, 1986

24. Kennard C, Swash M (eds): Jacksonian Hierarchies in Neurology. Springer-Verlag, London, 1989

25. Onuf (Onufrowicz) B: Notes on the arrangement and function of the cell groups in the sacral region of the spinal cord. J Nerv Ment Dis 26:498, 1899

26. Schroder HD: Organisation of the motoneurons innervating the pelvic muscles of the male rat. J Comp Neurol 192:567, 1980

27. De Groat WC, Kawatani M, Hisamitsu T, et al: The role of neuropeptides in the sacral autonomic reflex pathways of the cat. J Auton Nerv Syst 7:339, 1983

28. Roppolo JR, Nadelhaft I, de Groat WC: The organisation of pudendal motoneurons and primary afferent projections in the spinal cord of the rhesus monkey revealed by horseradish peroxidase. J Comp Neurol 234:475, 1985

29. Kuzuhara S, Kanazawa I, Nakanishi T: Topographical localization of the Onuf's nuclear neurons innervating the rectal and vesical striated sphincter muscles: a retrograde fluorescent double labeling in cat and dog. Neurosci Lett 16:125, 1980

30. Holstege G, Tan J: Supraspinal control of motoneurons innervating the striated muscles of the pelvic floor including urethral and anal sphincters in the cat. Brain 110:1323, 1987

31. Holstege G, Kuypers HGJM: The anatomy of brain stem pathways to the spinal cord in the cat: a labelled amino acid tracing study. Prog Brain Res 57:145, 1982

32. Winckler G: Remarques sur la morphologie et l'innervation du muscle releveur de l'anus. Arch Anat Histol Embryol 41:77, 1958

33. Swash M: Histopathology of the pelvic floor muscles. p. 129. In Henry MM, Swash M (eds): Coloproctology and the Pelvic Floor. Butterworths, London, 1985

34. Schroder HD: Somatostatin in the caudal spinal cord: an immunohistochemical study of the spinal centers involved in the innervation of pelvic organs. J Comp Neurol 223:400, 1984

35. Erdman SL, Kawatani M, Thor KB, et al: Identification of neuropeptides in Onuf's nucleus in cat: an autoradiographic study. J Neurosci 5:1993, 1984

36. Blaivas JG: The neurophysiology of micturition: a clinical study of 550 patients. J Urol 127:958, 1982

37. Nathan PW, Smith MC: The centripetal pathway from the bladder and urethra within the spinal cord. J Neurol Neurosurg Psychiatry 14:262, 1951

38. Nathan PW, Smith MC: The centrifugal pathway for micturition within the spinal cord. J Neurol Neurosurg Psychiatry 21:177, 1958

39. Furness JB, Costa M: The Enteric Nervous System. Churchill Livingstone, Edinburgh, 1987

40. Lubowski DZ, Nicholls RJ, Swash M, Jordan MJ: Neural control of internal anal sphincter function. Br J Surg 74:668, 1987

41. Lubowski DZ, Swash M, Henry MM: Neural mechanisms in disorders of defaecation. Baillieres Clin Gastroenterol 2:183, 1988

42. Bradley WE, Teague CT: Cerebellar regulation of the micturition reflex. Exp Neurol 23:399, 1969

43. Andersen JT, Bradley WE: Cystometric, sphincter and electromyographic abnormalities in Parkinson's disease. J Urol 116:75, 1976

44. Barrington FJF: The effect of lesions of the hind and midbrain on micturition in the cat. Q J Exp Physiol 15:181, 1925
45. Barrington FJF: The relation of the hind brain to micturition. Brain 44:23, 1921
46. Barrington FJF: The component reflexes of micturition. Brain 54:177, 1931
47. Denny-Brown D, Robertson EG: The physiology of micturition. Brain 56:149, 1933
48. Denny-Brown D, Robertson EG: An investigation of the nervous control of defaecation. Brain 58:256, 1935
49. Haldeman S, Bradley WE, Bhatia NN, Johnson BK: Pudendal evoked responses. Arch Neurol 39:280, 1982
50. Kleist K: Kriegsverletzungen des Gehirns. p. 1343. In Bonhoeffer K (ed): Handbuch der ärztlichen Erfahrungen im Weltkriege 1914/1918, Vol IV: Geistes- und Nervenkrankheiten. Barth, Leipzig, 1922/1934.
51. Merton PA: Electrical stimulation through the scalp of pyramidal fibres supplying pelvic floor muscles. p. 125. In Henry MM, Swash M (eds): Coloproctology and the Pelvic Floor. Butterworths, London, 1985
52. Penfield W, Rasmussen T: The Cerebral Cortex of Man. Macmillan, New York, 1950
53. Bradley WE, Teague CT: Electrophysiology of the pelvic and pudendal nerves in the cat. Exp Neurol 56:237, 1972
54. Andrew J, Nathan PW: Lesions of the anterior frontal lobes and disturbances of micturition and defaecation. Brain 87:233, 1964
55. Maurice-Williams RS: Micturition symptoms in frontal tumours. J Neurol Neurosurg Psychiatry 37:431, 1974
56. Kuroiwa Y, Toghi H, Ono S, Itoh M: Frequency and urgency of micturition in hemiplegic subjects: relationship to hemisphere laterality of lesions. J Neurol 234:100, 1987
57. Henry MM, Swash M: Coloproctology and the Pelvic Floor. Butterworths, London, 1985
58. Henry MM, Parks AG, Swash M: The pelvic floor in the descending perineum syndrome. Br J Surg 69:470, 1982
59. Bartolo DCC, Jarratt JA, Read NW: The use of conventional EMG to assess external sphincter neuropathy in man. J Neurol Neurosurg Psychiatry 46:1115, 1983
60. Stalberg E, Trontelj V: Single Fibre Electromyography. Mirvalle Press, Old Woking, England, 1979
61. Swash M, Schwartz MS: Neuromuscular Disorders: A Practical Approach to Diagnosis and Management. 2nd Ed. Springer-Verlag, London, 1988
62. Neill ME, Swash M: Increased motor unit fibre density in external anal sphincter muscle in anorectal in-

continence: a single fibre EMG study. J Neurol Neurosurg Psychiatry 43:343, 1980
63. Fowler CJ, Kirby RS: Decelerating bursts and complex repetitive discharges in the striated muscle of the urethral sphincter, associated with retention of urine in women. J Neurol Neurosurg Psychiatry 48:1004, 1985
64. Kiff ES, Swash M: Normal proximal and delayed distal conduction in the pudendal nerves of patients with idiopathic (anorectal) incontinence. J Neurol Neurosurg Psychiatry 47:820, 1984
65. Snooks SJ, Swash M: Abnormalities in the innervation of the urethral striated sphincter musculature in incontinence. Br J Urol 56:401, 1984
66. Snooks SJ, Barnes PRH, Swash M: Damage to the innervation of the voluntary anal and periurethral striated sphincter musculature in incontinence: an electrophysiological study. J Neurol Neurosurg Psychiatry 47:1269, 1984
67. Snooks SJ, Badenoch D, Tiptaft R, Swash M: Perineal nerve damage in genuine stress urinary incontinence. Br J Urol 57:422, 1985
68. Snooks SJ, Swash M, Setchell M, Henry MM: Injury to innervation of pelvic floor sphincter musculature in incontinence. Lancet 2:546, 1984
69. Snooks SJ, Swash M, Henry MM: Abnormalities in peripheral and central nerve conduction in anorectal incontinence. J R Soc Med 78:294, 1985
70. Swash M, Snooks SJ: Slowed motor conduction in lumbosacral nerve roots in cauda equina lesions: a new diagnostic technique. J Neurol Neurosurg Psychiatry 49:808, 1986
71. Henry MM, Snooks SJ, Barnes PRH, Swash M: Investigation of disorders of the anorectum and colon. Ann R Coll Surg Engl 67:355, 1985
72. Maertens de Noordhout A, Rothwell JC, Thompson PD, et al: Percutaneous electrical stimulation of lumbosacral roots in man. J Neurol Neurosurg Psychiatry 51:174, 1988
73. Snooks SJ, Swash M: Perineal and transcutaneous nerve stimulation: new methods for the investigation of the striated urethral sphincter musculature. Br J Urol 56:406, 1984
74. Merton PA: Electrical stimulation through the scalp of pyramidal tract fibres supplying pelvic floor muscles. p. 125. In Henry MM, Swash M (eds): Coloproctology and the Pelvic Floor. Buttersworths, London, 1985
75. Ertekin C, Hansen MV, Larsson LE, Sjodahl R: Examination of the descending pathway to the external anal sphincter and pelvic floor muscles by transcranial cortical stimulation. Electroencephalogr Clin Neurophysiol 75:500, 1990

76. Mathers SE, Ingram DA, Swash M: Electrophysiology of motor pathways for sphincter control in multiple sclerosis. J Neurol Neurosurg Psychiatry 53:955, 1990

77. Ingram DA: Neurophysiological investigation of central motor pathways controlling pelvic floor sphincter muscles. p. 244. In Henry MM, Swash M (eds): Coloproctology and the Pelvic Floor. 2nd Ed. Butterworth-Heinemann, London, 1992

78. Herdmann J, Bielefeldt K, Enck P: Quantification of motor pathways to the pelvic floor in humans. Am J Physiol 260:G720, 1991

79. Light JK: Restorative procedures for neuropathic bladder dysfunction: an overview. p. 128. In Eccles J, Dimitrijevic MR (eds): Recent Achievements in Restorative Neurology, Vol 1: Upper Motor Neuron Functions and Dysfunctions. Karger, Basel, 1985

80. Speakman CTM, Kamm MA, Swash M: Rectal sensory evoked potentials: an assessment of their clinical value. Int J Colorect Dis 8:23, 1993

81. Merton PA, Morton HB: Stimulation of the cerebral cortex in the intact human subject. Nature 285:227, 1980

82. Snooks SJ, Swash M: Motor conduction velocity in the human spinal cord: slowed conduction in multiple sclerosis and radiation myelopathy. J Neurol Neurosurg Psychiatry 48:1135, 1985

83. Thomas M, Egan M, Walgrove A, Meade TW: The prevalence of faecal and double incontinence. Community Med 6:216, 1984

84. Leigh PJ, Turnberg LA: Faecal incontinence: the unvoiced symptom. Lancet 1:349, 1982

85. Brocklehurst JC: Management of anal incontinence. Clin Gastroenterol 4:479, 1975

86. ICS Standardisation Committee: The standardisation of human investigations related to lower urinary tract function: first report. Scand J Urol Nephrol 11:193, 1977

87. Swash M, Snooks SJ, Chalmers DHK: Parity as a factor in incontinence in multiple sclerosis. Arch Neurol 44:504, 1987

88. Hakim S, Adams RD: The special clinical problem of symptomatic hydrocephalus with normal cerebrospinal fluid pressure. J Neurol Sci 2:307, 1965

89. Gershon MD, Erde SM: The nervous system of the gut. Gastroenterology 80:1571, 1981

90. Chalmers DHK, Swash M: Selective vulnerability of urinary Onuf motoneurons in Shy-Drager syndrome. J Neurol 234:259, 1987

91. Mannen T, Iwata M, Toyokura Y, Nagashima K: Preservation of a certain motoneurone group of the sacral cord in amyotrophic lateral sclerosis: its clinical significance. J Neurol Neurosurg Psychiatry 40:464, 1977

92. Swash M, Leader M, Brown A, Swettenham KW: Focal loss of anterior horn cells in the cervical cord in motor neuron disease. Brain 109:939, 1986

93. Law PJ, Kamm MA, Bartram CI: Anal endosonography in the investigation of faecal incontinence. Br J Surg 78:312, 1991

94. Read MG, Read NW: Role of anorectal sensation in preserving continence. Gut 23:345, 1982

95. Rogers J, Henry MM, Misiewicz JJ: Combined sensory and motor deficit in primary neuropathic faecal incontinence. Gut 29:5, 1988

96. Schuster MM: Biofeedback for fecal incontinence. JAMA 238:2595, 1977

97. Andersen JT, Bradley WE: The syndrome of detrusor-sphincter dyssynergia. J Urol 116:493, 1976

98. Blaivas JG, Sinha HP, Zayed AAH, et al: External sphincter dyssynergia: detailed EMG study. J Urol 125:545, 1980

99. Yalla SV, Rossier AB, Fam B: Dyssynergic vesicourethral responses during bladder rehabilitation in spinal cord injury patients: effect of suprapubic percussion, Credé method and bethanechol chloride. J Urol 115:575, 1976

100. Bors E: Neurogenic bladder. Urol Surv 7:177, 1957

101. Drossman DA, Sandler RS, McKee DC, Lovitz AJ: Bowel patterns among subjects not seeking health care. Gastroenterology 83:529, 1982

102. Lennard-Jones JE: Constipation: pathophysiology, clinical features and treatment. p. 350. In Henry MM, Swash M (eds): Coloproctology and the Pelvic Floor. Butterworths, London, 1985

103. Preston DM, Lennard-Jones JE: Anismus in chronic constipation. Dig Dis Sci 30:413, 1985

104. Kuijpers JH, Bleijenberg G: The spastic pelvic floor syndrome. Dis Colon Rectum 28:669, 1985

105. Jones PN, Lubowski DZ, Swash M, Henry MM: Is paradoxical contraction of puborectalis muscle of functional importance? Dis Colon Rectum 30:667, 1987

106. Mathers S, Kempster P, Swash M, Lees A: Constipation in anismus and Parkinson's disease: a focal dystonia. J Neurol Neurosurg Psychiatry (in press)

107. Barnes PRH, Hawley PR, Preston DM, Lennard-Jones JE: Experience of posterior division of the puborectalis muscle in the management of chronic constipation. Br J Surg 72:475, 1985

108. Snooks SJ, Barnes PRH, Swash M, Henry MM: Damage to the innervation of the pelvic floor musculature in chronic constipation. Gastroenterology 89:971, 1985

109. Wood JD: Physiology of the enteric nervous system. p. 67. In Johnson LR, Christensen J, Jackson M (eds):

Physiology of the Gastrointestinal Tract. Raven Press, New York, 1987

110. Earlam RJ: Gastrointestinal aspects of Chagas' disease. Am J Dig Dis 17:559, 1972

111. Mayer EA, Schuffler MD, Rotter JI, et al: Familial visceral neuropathy with autosomal dominant transmission. Gastroenterology 91:1528, 1986

112. Smith B: The neuropathology of pseudo-obstruction of the intestine. Scand J Gastroenterol 17, Suppl 71: 103, 1982

113. Schuffler MD, Baird HW, Fleming CR, et al: Intestinal pseudo-obstruction as the presenting manifestation of small cell carcinoma of the lung: a paraneoplastic neuropathy of the gastrointestinal tract. Ann Intern Med 98:129, 1983

114. Stanghellini V, Corinaldesi R, Barbara L: Pseudo-obstruction syndromes. Baillieres Clin Gastroenterol 2: 225, 1988

115. Preston DM, Hawley PR, Lennard-Jones JE, Todd IP: Results of colectomy for severe idiopathic constipation in women (Arbuthnot Lane's disease). Br J Surg 71:547, 1984

116. Gershon MD: The pathogenesis of Hirschsprung's disease and hypertrophic pyloric stenosis. Presented at Symposium on Gastrointestinal Motility, Annenberg Medical Center, Palm Springs, CA, February 1988

27

Sexual Dysfunction and the Nervous System

P. C. Gautier-Smith
Clare J. Fowler

Human sexual behavior has preoccupied theologians, philosophers, physicians, anthropologists, writers, and indeed the general population throughout the ages, and its every facet has been subjected to the closest scrutiny. Why then is so little known about it even today? There are many reasons, not the least of which is that it is complex and has therefore proved difficult to measure.

It is an activity that is in large part biological, being under the influence of genetic and hormonal factors, with considerable differences between the sexes. Males are much more sexually aggressive than females, and they are more interested in the so-called perversions; although the explanations put forward have been many and various, androgens probably play the most important role. In addition, sexual activity is subject to environmental influences, and its expression, both quantitative and qualitative, varies widely from individual to individual. As it usually occurs with another person in a social setting, social influences play a particularly important part in relation to education, acceptable practices, and prohibitions, and all of these factors may vary from one generation to another. For example, in England during the eighteenth century, women were expected to reach orgasm, conception being thought to be difficult without it. During the nineteenth century, how-

ever, many considered that orgasm was not a proper response in wives and mothers, and it was relegated to the demimonde. Finally, during the last three decades, it has become an obsession in some quarters, women being expected to achieve multiple orgasms regularly.

Organized religions have also had a great deal to say about human sexuality, all of them exercising strict taboos on their followers. Interestingly, though, several surveys have shown that the sexual behavior of people in a particular culture appears to be much the same whether or not they practice religion.[1] In referring to the powerful effect of orgasm, which clearly affected the whole man, St. Augustine considered that any follower of wisdom and holy joy would prefer to beget children without lust of that kind.[2] With the advent of effective contraception, sexual activity as an expression of love and of physical play has become separated from its role in procreation, although several of the major religions still do not view it in this light at all, condemning sexual relations outside marriage—even though such sexual activity may be fully accepted in secular circles within the same culture. Attitudes to male homosexuality have also fluctuated in various cultures and religious groups over the centuries, from being extolled as the purest form of love to being considered disgusting and against natural law. Some religions have taken a more liberal view than others, but the acquired immunodeficiency syndrome (AIDS) epidemic intensified the debate. Greater acceptance and understanding in some quarters has been balanced by the hardening of attitudes, both social and religious, in others. The recent suggestion that a gene carried by females and expressed in some of their male offspring is an important factor in the genesis of male homosexuality is certain to fuel debate about the place of homosexuals in society.

Governments and their lawmakers have also sought to regulate sexual behavior. In the United Kingdom, the important Wolfenden committee on homosexual offenses and prostitution stated that, "It is not in our view the function of the law to interfere in the private lives of citizens, or to seek to enforce any particular patterns of behavior."[3] Despite this, however, heterosexual anal intercourse is still illegal, even between married couples, whereas it is not illegal between consenting male homosexuals over the age of 21 years. Recently, several men have received prison sentences for having carried out mutually acceptable sadomasochistic acts on each other. In some parts of the United States, heterosexual orogenital contact is also illegal under statute, although this activity is practiced regularly by many couples.[1] This situation is an example of the clear contrast between what is prescribed by the lawmakers and what people are, in fact, doing and what little effect such prohibitions have. Certainly, laws designed to limit sexual behavior are constantly flouted. The age of consent for heterosexual intercourse in the United Kingdom is 16 years, but pregnancies below that age are common, and evidence from questionnaires and family planning clinics makes it clear that sexual activity in this group is widespread.

Doctors and, more recently, social workers have not been without influence either. The supposedly fearful consequences of masturbation—including blindness, epilepsy, and feeble-mindedness—were a popular theme in the nineteenth century; birth control was fiercely attacked in the early twentieth century; and in the 1990s, some have jumped on the bandwagon of the sexual abuse of children. In their zeal in the pursuance of what is undoubtedly an appalling problem, they have themselves abused children psychologically by removing them from their parents and then forcing them to make incriminating statements. They have also carried out degrading and questionable physical examinations with neither explanation nor consent. Satanic pedophilia is currently in the news, but despite all the reports and media interest, not a single case has been upheld in a court of law in the United Kingdom.

Because sexual behavior is to a considerable extent learned, education must have an important part to play in its expression. The accent in schools is usually on the biology of reproduction and the mechanisms of intercourse rather than its psychological and emotional aspects. Much inaccurate information is culled from peers and as the result of clumsy experimentation. Many parents are reluctant to discuss the topic at all, finding it embarrassing; and in any case, they are worried that their children might become sexually active too soon if they are told too much about sexuality. The question of whether comprehensive sex education at an early age, as provided in Scandinavia, leads to better sexual adjustment during adult life has yet to be answered.

The earliest attempts at sex research were detailed case studies of neurotic patients, in whom fact and fantasy were inextricably intertwined. Knowledge of normal variations and function was limited, and some of the theories—such as that of Freud that foreplay and the pleasure women gained from it was infantile and that only vaginal orgasm was mature—were based on both anatomical and physiological ignorance. Nevertheless, such studies paved the way for later work, and it was Kinsey and associates who provided the first reliable evidence of the sexual behavior of a group of people at a particular time in a particular culture.[4,5] They used self-reporting questionnaires, and although this approach has been criticized in that samples may be biased in various ways—those responding may be only a small percentage of those who have been sent the questionnaire and their very interest in the research may make them unrepresentative—their work was an important milestone. Comparison with studies two decades later permitted assessment of the effect that changes of attitude and public opinion had on sexual behavior.[6,7] This and other work on people who were not psychiatrically ill but who had unusual sexual interests made it clear that not only was the range of "normal" much wider than had been generally realized[1,8] but that there was no absolute standard of normality. In other words, "normality" varied according to cultural, social, and economic pressures. Many "normal" couples who have never sought advice also have major sexual difficulties.[9]

The most recent approach to research into sexual function has been by means of physiological measurements. As with other methods, it has also been fraught with difficulty. Although such work had been carried out long before, it was Masters and Johnson who were largely responsible for publicizing it and making it respectable. Despite this fact, many criticisms of it have been voiced, including the difficulty of assessing the normality of the responses of volunteers or prostitutes under laboratory conditions, the concern that the behavior of some couples in the bedroom is so idiosyncratic that it is impossible to extrapolate to people in general, and the belief that sexual responses, particularly arousal in women, are too personal to be assessed objectively by such means. Ethics committees have also refused to sanction such investigations on normal volunteers. However, using these techniques, important insights have been gained into the physiology and pathology in both sexes.

Despite this general interest, relatively little has been written about sexual dysfunction and neurological illness[10]; in contrast to psychiatric aspects, it has received scant attention in many standard textbooks. Neurologists frequently work in large cities, and with the ever-increasing mobility of population, their patients are already a fascinating mix of ethnic, religious, and cultural groups and will become more so. All these factors have an important effect on people's perceptions of sexual function and the extent to which physical illness impinges on it and them. In many cultures nowadays, people have a more open attitude to sexual matters, are more knowledgeable, and have greater expectations; it follows, then, that neurologists will be consulted more frequently about these matters. The support and counseling of patients with chronic, disabling, and often progressive illness have always been important parts of the work of any neurologist, but unfortunately this has not often been extended to the effects of these illnesses on sexual function. Some neurological and rehabilitation units have established clinics for sexual dysfunction, and this trend should be extended; physicians, clinical physiologists, urologists, and counselors of both sexes should work in them together.

PHYSIOLOGICAL AND ANATOMICAL CONSIDERATIONS

For conception to occur, viable spermatozoa must come into contact with an ovum; for this contact to be accomplished naturally by sexual intercourse, the man must be able to achieve a strong enough erection to permit vaginal intromission and then ejaculate. On the female side, all that is required is the ability to relax sufficiently to allow vaginal penetration. Such an event on its own is a far cry from a rewarding and satisfactory sexual experience, which couples may achieve in a wide variety of ways, from the conventional to the unconventional, and which may change with the development of the relationship and with aging. Sexual expression varies according to the strength of the sex drive and the types of erotic stimuli required to produce arousal and orgasm; it is conditioned by social and cultural factors and the highly complex human emotions of love and affection. A satisfactory sexual relationship may even exist between two people without conventional intercourse at all, an important point to remember with reference to counseling those who are physically disabled. That part of the AIDS awareness campaign that promotes "safe sex" should prove helpful in making such behavior both more widely known and acceptable.

It is convenient to consider the physiology in terms of the ability of the two sexes to reach orgasm, which may be achieved by heterosexual, homosexual, or autosexual activity, given that there is adequate libido and arousal.

Libido

In the present context, *libido* is taken to mean the degree to which an individual has sexual appetite—how much or how easily he or she responds to or seeks out erotic stimuli. Libido is difficult to assess; not only does it vary in an individual from time to time and in response to circumstances but its measurement depends on self-ratings on such items as the frequency of spontaneous sexual thoughts and the excitement provoked by them and masturbation. The incidence of intercourse is a poor measure unless it is achieved with the mutual satisfaction of the two partners. Although the evidence is far from conclusive, there appears to be a genetic factor in relation to libido, and libido is enhanced by sexual activity itself, new sexual partners and exciting circumstances, hypomania, and by some focal brain lesions, particularly of the frontal and temporal lobes. It has often been stated that no true aphrodisiac exists, but depressed patients may develop more than their premorbid levels of libido in response to antidepressant medication,[11,12] and there are scattered reports of similar effects with levodopa in patients with Parkinson's disease.[13] Libido may be lowered by lack of opportunity, as in a prison population; by the effects of age and many of the sedative drugs and those of addiction; by malnutrition and any debilitating illness; by depression; and by epilepsy and some focal brain lesions. Libido also decreases in couples when their relationship has become unhappy or stale. There has been a good deal of publicity in the media recently concerning loss of libido in couples who both have demanding jobs and who have neither the time nor the energy for sexual activity. Although this may happen in some cases, only a few years ago the same people were stating that with women having been liberated from the shackles of generations of repression, couples were more active sexually, with greater reward than ever before. Sexual behavior in a given culture, though, is probably a good deal more stable than suggested by these opinions.

The extent to which hormones affect libido in both sexes has been discussed by Bancroft.[14] Their role in normal sexual function in the two sexes is complicated and still has not been worked out satisfactorily, particularly in women. Androgens are necessary for both the development and maintenance of sexual interest. Men with primary testicular failure do not develop libido, and it is diminished or lost if such changes are secondary, although androgens produced by the adrenal glands may be sufficient to allow some retention of sex drive. Sexual appetite in these patients is restored by testosterone.[15] There is evidence from studies on patients being treated by antiandrogens that even though sexual interest and appetite are reduced, erections in response to visual stimuli are maintained, whereas they are diminished in response to erotic fantasies, suggesting that androgens may facilitate erotic imagery.[16] Androgens are also probably responsible for libido in women. Removal of the ovaries does not consistently reduce sex drive, and the role of estrogens in its maintenance is not clear.

Even less is known about the effects of peptide hormones on sexual function, particularly in women. Elevated levels of prolactin certainly interfere with sexual function in men either by a direct effect on the Leydig cells or indirectly by their action on the pituitary.

Arousal

Sexual arousal may be defined as the psychological and physiological response to erotic stimuli. It consists of feelings of mounting excitement and physiological changes: tachycardia and hyperventilation in both sexes, with penile tumescence in men and clitoral and labial engorgement and vaginal lubrication in women. In order for arousal to occur, a person must have sufficient interest, sexual appetite, or libido to be able to respond to an appropriate stimulus, and the central and peripheral nervous pathways must be intact. "Erotically colored" sensations from the genital region are conveyed by the spinothalamic pathways, and patients with selective damage to these tracts may complain of anorgasmia and ejaculatory failure.[17,18]

MEN

Evidence from epileptic patients and those having suffered brain injuries,[19] as well as electrical stimulation experiments in primates[20] and humans,[21] suggest that sexual arousal and psychogenic erections depend on the limbic system, including the hypothalamus and temporal lobes. The efferent pathway follows the medial forebrain bundle to the substantia nigra and into the ventrolateral part of the pons. Studies of patients and those who have been treated by cordotomy[17,22] suggest that both the efferent and afferent pathways are in the lateral columns. Psychogenic erection is a highly complex phenomenon and may be triggered by visual, auditory, and olfactory stimuli as well as memories of previous experiences.

Reflex erection, which may provoke psychic reinforcement, is mediated on the afferent side by somatosensory impulses from the glans penis; these pass through the pudendal nerves to the second, third, and fourth sacral segments of the spinal cord. The main efferent pathway is by way of the parasympathetic pelvic nerves, also arising from S2 to S4. In a proportion of paraplegic men in whom a Brindley anterior root stimulator has been implanted, strong stimulation of the S2 and S3 ventral roots, at an intensity higher than that required for maximal contraction of skeletal muscle, causes erection.[23] The parasympathetic erectile pathway, unlike other parasympathetic innervation, does not release acetylcholine as the postganglionic transmitter. Indeed, the postganglionic transmitter has yet to be identified with certainty, although vasoactive intestinal polypeptide (VIP)[24] and nitric oxide have been suggested.[25]

Although sympathetic fibers from the thoracolumbar spinal cord also supply the penile vasculature, their exact role is not clear. Stimulation of the hypogastric plexus by a surgically implanted device induces erection or penile enlargement, indicating that there is a sympathetic erectile pathway. However, men who have had surgical dissection of the para-aortic lymph nodes or other surgery damaging the sympathetic outflow have failure of seminal emission, but erectile function and orgasmic sensation usually remain intact. This may be interpreted as indicating that parasympathetic activity alone can be sufficient for erectile function. Men with sacral cord lesions may be capable of psychogenic but not reflex erection, presumably mediated via the sympathetic erectile pathway.[26] There is also antierectile sympathetic activity, which is continuously active when the penis is flaccid and may be blocked by α-adrenergic blocking agents.[27]

WOMEN

Sexual arousal is less easy to measure in women than in men, but vaginal plethysmography appears to be a reliable technique and has produced some interesting data. It has been shown that women report greater levels of arousal to erotic films with increasing levels of blood alcohol despite physiological measurements showing the reverse,[28] and that sexual ictal manifestations are more common in women than in men.[29] These findings and the fact that in some women sufficient arousal can be achieved by fantasy and hypnosis[30] to induce orgasm without genital manipulation suggest that both arousal and orgasm may be more cerebrally determined in women than in men.

It seems reasonable to assume that the neurophysiological basis of the mechanisms that are responsible for the hemodynamic changes that occur during sexual arousal in women are the same as those in men, although they have not been studied to the same degree. It has been thought that vasocongestion of the clitoris and labia and vaginal lubrication are under the control of cholinergic pelvic nerves, but it has been shown that, as in men, sexual arousal in women is atropine-resistant,[31] suggesting that other pathways and neurotransmitters are also involved.

Orgasm

Orgasm in both sexes is difficult to describe in that it is a cortical sensory experience with input from the smooth muscles of the internal sex organs and the voluntary perineal muscles. This sensory experience is very variable from individual to individual and from one occasion to another. Its intensity may vary from a mild pulsation in the genital organs with ejaculation in men to extreme tension, opisthotonos, clonic spasms of the muscles, and complete loss of control. Anorgasmia is rare in physiologically normal men, but 13 percent of women between the ages of 18 to 26 years have never achieved orgasm, with the incidence declining to a minimum of 3 percent in women between the ages of 51 and 64 years.[1] The reasons for this are not clear. Certainly, masturbation is much more common in men than women; moreover, ejaculation is a prerequisite of fertilization, whereas female orgasm is not, and so the biological role of orgasm is much more clearly defined in men. Brain mechanisms are important for orgasm, which may occur in both sexes without genital stimulation as part of an epileptic seizure, and phantom orgasms have also been reported in paraplegics. Centrally acting drugs (e.g., monoamine oxidase inhibitors) may prevent orgasm without interfering with arousal in both sexes, probably as the result of α-adrenergic blockade.[32]

Ejaculation in men is a reflex and, although influenced by central mechanisms, can occur even if the spinal cord is transected in the midthoracic region. The spinal center for ejaculation is thought to be situated between the lower thoracic and upper lumbar segments of the spinal cord. Afferent impulses reach it by way of the pudendal nerves; when threshold is reached, efferent pathways through the sympathetic nerves produce contraction of the smooth muscles of the epididymis, vas deferens, seminal vesicles, and prostate. Semen is expelled into the posterior urethra, and there is partial closure of the bladder neck. Finally, ejaculation occurs because of contraction of the somatic pelvic musculature, which is supplied by the pudendal nerves arising in the sacral cord. Electromyographic recording of the pelvic floor muscles during orgasm in the normal woman shows intermittent activity associated with orgasmic contractions on a background of continuous activity occurring soon after the onset of vibratory clitoral stimulation.[33] Such measurements have not been carried out in paraplegic women, but it seems likely that a spinal reflex similar to that in men is present.

SEXUAL DISORDERS IN NEUROLOGICAL ILLNESS

Many forms of sexual dysfunction—including disinhibition, lowered or heightened libido, and disorders of arousal and orgasm—are common in neurological disease. The same is true of psychiatric illness, particularly in anxiety states and depression. From a therapeutic point of view, it is important to distinguish one from the other and to be aware that neurological and psychiatric disorders may coexist; it may be the anxiety and depression provoked by the neurological condition that is producing the dysfunction and not the neurological illness itself. There have been numerous surveys showing that sexual dysfunction is common in the general population.[1,9,34,35]; assessment must therefore take into account the premorbid pattern of patients' sexual behavior. Those with neurological disorders are frequently taking medication such as anticonvulsants, hypotensive agents, and psychotropic drugs, all of which may have an influence on sexual function.

Specific Neurological Conditions

FOCAL CEREBRAL LESIONS

Alterations of sexual behavior in patients with focal brain lesions have been reported in cases of trauma,[36] cerebral tumors,[36,37] vascular disorders,[19,38] encephalitis,[19] leukotomy,[39] and temporal lobectomy.[40] The fact that a focal brain lesion and an abnormality of sexual function may coexist does not necessarily imply a causal relation; but if the latter appears at the same time as the former and is relieved by its surgical treatment, such a relation seems likely. The sexual problem may be related to the lesion itself, epilepsy produced by it, or a combination of the two.

Frontal Lobe

Lesions of the frontal lobe often lead to euphoria and a lack of concern for the present or the future. Disinhibition and failure to foresee the consequence of actions reduce control and may lead to outspokenness and uncontrolled sexual activity. Exhibitionistic behavior has been reported, with public masturbation and inappropriate sexual overtures to members of the same and opposite sex.[19] Such symptoms occurring with frontal tumors and hemorrhage from anterior communicating artery aneurysms, and resolving after treatment, is strong evidence that the abnormal behavior is secondary to frontal lobe dysfunction. Lesions in the same site, often in elderly patients and secondary to degenerative disorders, hydrocephalus, and cerebral infarction, may also explain some of the sad instances of socially unacceptable behavior that bring these patients into conflict with the law.

Some patients, in whom the sexual response is inhibited by obsessional preoccupation with cleanliness and who are incapable of relaxing and "letting go," have found that they are able to achieve orgasm for the first time following frontal lesions.[36] Such improvement has been noted after head injury, hemorrhage, and leukotomy and has not been associated with undesirable behavioral changes.

A true increase in libido with a constant desire for and attempts at sexual intercourse has been reported in patients with frontal lobe lesions,[19] but more commonly libido is decreased or lost.

Temporal Lobe

In almost all the reports in the literature concerning sexual function and temporal lobe lesions, epilepsy has been present as well. As a result, it is difficult to differentiate the effects of the lesion itself from the epileptic discharges it produces. In these cases, interictal sexual behavioral abnormalities are common; these are considered in the section on epilepsy. Hypersexuality in patients with unilateral nonepileptic lesions has been described only on rare occasions.[36,37]

In 1937 Kluver and Bucy removed the temporal lobes, including most of the uncus and hippocampus, in the rhesus monkey and noted the development of strong oral tendencies, loss of fear and aggression, and an increase in sexual activity.[41] A similar syndrome has since been described in humans following bilateral surgical temporal lobectomy[40] and with a variety of encephalopathies of which herpes simplex encephalitis and Pick's disease are the most common.[42] In all the autopsied cases the temporal cortex and white matter have been involved bilaterally, as has the amygdala, lesions of which correlate best with the sexual disorders.

EPILEPSY

Epilepsy may be associated with sexual sensations and activity in a wide variety of ways (Table 27-1). Hyperventilation is routinely used to provoke latent electroencephalographic abnormalities in patients suspected of having epilepsy, and it is not surprising that overbreathing during sexual excitement should occasionally induce seizures in those susceptible.[36]

Tactile genital sensations may occur in either sex as a manifestation of a focal discharge provoked by lesions of the medial surface of the postcentral gyrus.[43] The sensations consist of emotionally neutral or unpleasant unilateral paresthesias in the genital region and are unassociated with erotic feeling or activity. Lesions in the same site may also produce paroxysmal scrotal pain,[44] which may be associated with contraction of the cremaster muscle, producing retraction of the testis on that side.[45]

Orgasm and other sexual sensations may occur as manifestations of an epileptic attack with or without spread to a generalized seizure. The attacks are spontaneous without preceding sexual stimulation, and during them genital warmth and swelling, penile erection, genital lubrication, breast engorgement, ejaculation, and anal muscular contraction have been described.[21,36,46] The experience may be intensely

Table 27-1 Epilepsy and Sexual Function

Hyperventilation-provoked seizures during sexual activity
Tactile genital sensations as part of the aura
Orgasm and sexual hallucinations as part of the aura
Reflex epilepsy provoked by orgasm and other sexual
  stimuli
Sexual automatisms during or after seizures
Postictal sexual activity
Abnormal interictal sexual behavior
Effects of anticonvulsant drugs

pleasurable or occasionally unpleasant.[46] Sexual imagery during an attack has also been reported.[36] When sexual arousal and orgasm are present with seizures, the provoking lesion is almost invariably in the right temporal lobe; such seizures do not occur before puberty, and it seems that hormonal priming of the brain is necessary for their production. The sensations described above are much more common in women than in men, and it has been suggested that the neural organization of psychosexual behavior is different in the two sexes.[21]

Epilepsy may be triggered by orgasm induced by masturbation,[36,37] coitus,[47] and hypnosis.[29] In these cases it is the orgasm itself that provokes the seizure, not hyperventilation or tactile genital manipulation. Seizures may occur under other circumstances, but in one case orgasm was the only trigger.[36] The sight or fantasy of a fetishistic object may also precipitate seizures.[48] Seizure activity induced by these stimuli also arises in the temporal lobe[29,48]; because the part of the brain functionally associated with orgasm is at the same site, it seems likely that the threshold of the lesion is lowered by these powerful afferent stimuli.

Sexual automatisms that occur during or immediately after seizures are usually poorly structured and consist of masturbatory movements and verbal sexual approaches to people of the same or opposite sex, accompanied by clumsy gestures.[49–51] The patient has no memory of the events. Undressing after a seizure, again without memory, is not uncommon following a psychomotor attack.[52,53]

Remembered and directional sexual activity also occurs after temporal lobe seizures.[54] The patient feels intensely aroused (more so than usual) immediately or a few minutes after the attack and seeks sexual relations. The quality of the behavior is no different from the subject's usual pattern and can be suppressed if circumstances are not propitious.

Abnormal interictal sexual behavior is common in patients with temporal lobe epilepsy, and it is difficult to be certain how closely it is related to the epilepsy on the one hand and the underlying lesions on the other. Sometimes the dysfunction clears with control of the seizures and sometimes with excision of the causative pathology. The most common disorder is hyposexuality or sexual apathy, with a decrease or absence of sexual curiosity, erotic fantasies, and desire for sexual activity.[55] Impotence with normal libido has also been reported,[56] as has hypersexuality,[37] homosexuality,[55] and transvestite[57] and exhibitionistic[58] behavior.

The influence of anticonvulsant drugs on sexual activity in epileptics has proved difficult to assess. Both hyposexuality and reproductive endocrine disorders are more common in patients with complex partial seizures than in those with other types of epilepsy. Increased androgen metabolism as a result of hepatic enzyme induction and reduced free testosterone due to an increase in sex hormone–binding globulin synthesis secondary to the medication have been suggested as possible causes.[59] However, hypogonadotropic hypogonadism has been found in temporal lobe epileptics not on medication, and it has been suggested that dysfunction of the medial temporal structures, particularly the amygdala, may modulate hypothalamopituitary secretion. Another possibility is that reproductive endocrine disorders favor the development of temporal lobe epilepsy.[60] There seems little evidence to support the view that hyperprolactinemia plays a significant role in the hyposexuality associated with temporal lobe epilepsy.[61]

The relation of epilepsy to sexual dysfunction is highly complex, but it seems reasonable to suggest that inhibitory and facilitatory mechanisms related to sexual activity reside in the temporal lobes and limbic system and that irritative lesions in these sites may alter behavior in different directions. The frontal lobes and hypothalamopituitary system also have modulating roles.

MULTIPLE SYSTEM ATROPHY

Multiple system atrophy is a progressive degenerative disorder of the central nervous system (CNS) with a varied clinical presentation that may include extrapyramidal, cerebellar, or pyramidal features together with autonomic failure and marked bladder involvement. Shy-Drager syndrome is one form of this disease.

In a retrospective study of the duration of symptoms in 46 men clinically diagnosed as suffering from multiple system atrophy, 44 (96 percent) were impotent by the time of diagnosis. Impotence alone was the first symptom in 37 percent but was part of the presenting symptom complex in 59 percent.[62] Figure 27-1 shows the duration of symptoms before diagnosis in this group of 46 men. It can be seen that the onset of impotence often predated the onset of other neurological symptoms by several years. The mean age of this study group at the time of diagnosis was 55 years, with a range of 38 to 68 years; many of these men had therefore developed impotence in their early fifties or late forties. Many spoke with mild resentment of the way they had been told at the time that their sexual problem was due to "stress." The reason that erectile failure should be such an early symptom in this disease is unknown. There are insufficient clinical grounds for attributing it to part of a general autonomic failure because symptomatic or laboratory-proven autonomic failure occurred much later in most instances. By the time of diagnosis, 30 percent of these men were unable to ejaculate.

Electromyographic examination of either the urethral or anal sphincter has been demonstrated to be a valuable diagnostic test.[63,64] This is because the pathology of multiple system atrophy involves Onuf's nucleus,[65] the sacral spinal nucleus innervating both the urethral and anal sphincters. The reason for the selective involvement of the anterior horn cells in this nucleus is unknown, but their degeneration reflects some interesting aspect of their neurobiology because these same cells are spared in motor neuron disease or amyotrophic lateral sclerosis.[66] The progressive loss of cells in Onuf's nucleus that occurs in multiple system atrophy results in denervation and reinnervation of the tonically firing motor units of the sphincters, and these changes can be readily demonstrated electromyographically in much the same way as the changes of reinnervation in somatic muscle can be demonstrated in amyotrophic lateral sclerosis. However, there is a notable electromyographic difference between the two conditions: in amyotrophic lateral sclerosis, motor unit action potentials are usually reduced in number but of high amplitude, whereas in multiple system atrophy the reinnervated motor units of the sphincter do not compact to the same extent, so that typically motor unit action potentials are of highly prolonged duration. Because the sphincter units fire tonically, analysis of individual motor unit action potentials using a trigger and delay line is convenient. We have found that the most discriminating analysis is to measure the mean duration of the action potentials of 10 motor units as well as to plot the number out of 10 that are excessively prolonged (i.e., more than 10 ms in duration).[64]

Whether this test is abnormal in men with early multiple system atrophy and no symptoms other than

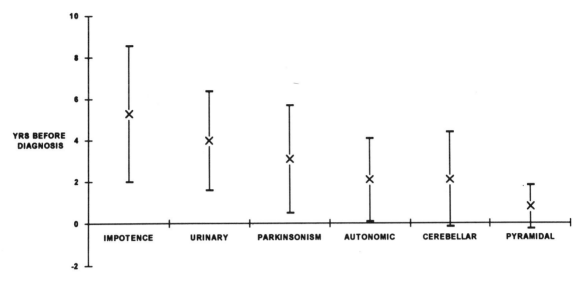

Fig. 27-1 The duration of symptoms (mean + 2 SD) in 46 men with multiple system atrophy. This information was obtained by inquiring retrospectively at the time of diagnosis. (From Beck RO, Betts CD, Fowler CJ: Genitourinary dysfunction in multiple system atrophy: clinical features and treatment in 62 cases. J Urol 151:1336, 1994, with permission.)

impotence is unknown. In the absence of specific treatment of the underlying neurological degeneration, however, nothing would be gained from making the diagnosis at this stage. The natural history of this disease should nevertheless be borne in mind when a man in middle life presents with impotence, especially if he himself doubts that his problem is due to "stress." Once bladder symptoms start and urological surgery (which is inadvisable in this disorder) is being contemplated, sphincter electromyography is a worthwhile test.

SPINAL CORD INJURIES

The subject of sexual function following spinal cord injury in men has been well studied over the years, presumably because this neurological catastrophe most commonly occurs in active young men. One of the earliest studies was by Talbot, who wrote in 1949 that "with no intent to exaggerate its importance, the value of a reasonable degree of sexual readjustment in connection with the rehabilitation of these men [200 paraplegics] is beyond question. They seem hitherto to have been more or less written off in this respect. This study . . . suggests that for many of them the door to reasonable gratification or even paternity need not be arbitrarily closed."[67]

In 1960 Bors and Comarr published an extensive review of the literature which amounted to reports of some 1,000 men and added to this their own observations on sexual function in 529 men with spinal cord injury.[26] It had been variously reported in the literature that erection was possible following spinal cord injury in 63 to 94 percent of men and that intercourse was possible in 23 to 33 percent. Ejaculation was possible in only 3 to 20 percent and orgasm in between 3 and 14 percent. Their own studies generally supported these figures and they were able to make further fundamental neurological observations. The level of the lesion was important with regard to erection—men with complete high spinal injuries had reflex erections with no descending psychogenic contribution, whereas men with a complete cord lesion below T12 to L2 could have psychogenic erections but not reflex erections. Ejaculation was thought to be more vulnerable to neural damage than erection but was best preserved in men with partial lower motor neuron lesions (i.e., lesions of the cauda equina or sacral cord). Orgasm or some form of it could occur as long as the autonomic innervation of the genitalia or the somatic innervation of the pelvic floor was intact.

Use of the Brindley root stimulator has shown that in 30 percent of paraplegic men with otherwise normal sacral root responses, no erectile response can be produced by appropriate electrical stimulation of S2 and S3 motor roots.[23] This has been interpreted as evidence that the sacral parasympathetic pathway is subject to considerable individual variation.

The problems of fertility following spinal cord injury are beyond the scope of this chapter, but these are well reviewed in an article by Bennett and colleagues, which also includes an updated review of sexual dysfunction in men with spinal cord injury.[68] The menstrual cycle usually continues after spinal cord trauma in women, with normal conception and full-term pregnancies reported.[68]

MULTIPLE SCLEROSIS

The prevailing view of the incidence of impotence in multiple sclerosis is very different now from that reported 70 years ago.[69] The striking increases in acknowledged prevalence of this problem over the years is clearly shown in Figure 27-2. This must surely reflect an increased willingness by patients to report their difficulty and a greater ease of clinicians in discussing the topic, rather than a change in the natural history of the disease.

The more recent studies referred to in Figure 27-2 have found that between 60 and 65 percent of men

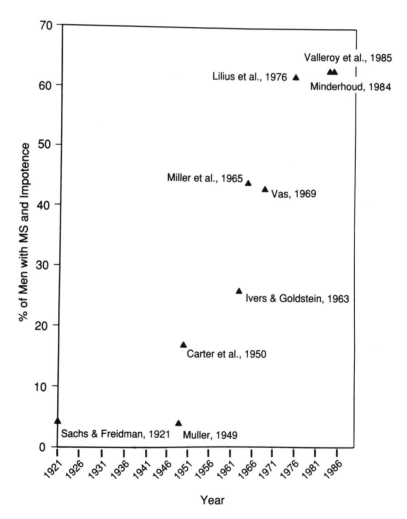

Fig. 27-2 The reported incidence of erectile difficulties in men with multiple sclerosis in papers published between 1921 and 1985.

with multiple sclerosis, unselected for their neurological disability, have erectile difficulties. In 1965 Miller and associates reviewed the urogenital symptoms of 297 patients with multiple sclerosis and found that 62 percent of men had erectile difficulties, but the report goes on to say, without any further explanation, that in 18 percent the problem was "psychological."[70] Three questionnaire surveys disclosed erectile problems in 62 percent[71] and 63 percent[72,73] of men with multiple sclerosis.

Only a few studies have looked at the neurological features associated with this common problem. Vas described an association between sensory disturbance and erectile dysfunction as well as between the distribution of anhidrosis and impotence.[74] Men with complete impotence did not sweat below the iliac crests, whereas those with partial impotence had a normal pattern of sweating except on the lower limbs. Of the questionnaire studies, two[71,72] found an association between lower limb dysfunction and a disturbance of sexual function, whereas one[73] did not.

We have recently completed a study of 48 men with clinically definite multiple sclerosis who presented for advice on the management of their impotence.[75] Among them, 46 (96 percent) had unequivocal, bilateral pyramidal signs in the legs; whereas there was a definite correlation between pyramidal dysfunction and the presence of impotence in this group, no other Kurtzke function score was so consistently abnormal. From these clinical data alone it was possible to conclude that spinal cord disease was the major underlying cause of erectile failure in these men, but confirmatory neurophysiological evidence of spinal cord disease was also obtained. Recordings of the tibial and pudendal somatosensory evoked potentials were made in 44 patients and some abnormality found in 73 percent. Of particular interest was the finding that the pudendal evoked potential was not abnormal more often than the tibial evoked responses, indicating that the responsible spinal cord disease was suprasacral. Furthermore, there were seven men with impotence who had normal neurophysiological investigations, four of whom had unequivocal clinical evidence of bilateral pyramidal tract dysfunction in the lower limbs. This finding should be borne in mind by urologists and andrologists who have perhaps overrated the usefulness of the pudendal evoked potential.

Miller and colleagues found that impotence was al-

ways associated with urinary symptoms.[70] In our study, 41 patients (85 percent) had urodynamically proven hyperreflexia, a problem that is also associated with spinal cord involvement in multiple sclerosis.[76]

Treatment of the erectile dysfunction in our group of men by means of intracorporeal papaverine injections revealed the extent of ejaculatory failure, and information about ejaculation was available from 40. Among these, 6 were unable to ejaculate and 20 reported variable difficulty. Preservation of ejaculatory function appeared to be associated with less severe spinal cord disease as measured both by the Kurtzke pyramidal function score and the extent of abnormality of the evoked potentials (Fig. 27-3). The ability to ejaculate was lost in those with severe spinal cord disease.[75] These results are consistent with the findings of the very few other studies that have looked at this problem: the three questionnaire surveys found that ejaculation was either difficult or impossible in 37 to 77 percent.[71-73]

A diagnosis of multiple sclerosis is unlikely in men presenting with impotence but no other symptoms and signs of spinal cord disease. In our series[75] and in the course of encountering many hundreds of patients with urogenital symptoms and established multiple sclerosis, no patient has presented with impotence as an isolated complaint.

Little is known about sexual dysfunction in women with multiple sclerosis; although the questionnaire studies[71-73] mentioned above included women, there is only a single publication to date researching exclusively the sexual problems of women with multiple sclerosis.[77] Loss of sacral sensation seems to be associated with loss of ability to achieve orgasm, and the questionnaire surveys showed that anxiety about incontinence and spasticity and adductor spasm of the lower limbs may all be contributory difficulties.

OTHER NONTRAUMATIC SPINAL CORD LESIONS

Many other nontraumatic causes of spinal cord disease produce genitourinary dysfunction similar to that occurring in multiple sclerosis. Bors and Commar were of the view that there is a hierarchy of vulnerability of these spinal cord functions, with sexual and then bladder functions being most vulnerable and bowel function least vulnerable.[78] Thus, following transverse myelitis, lower limb function may recover

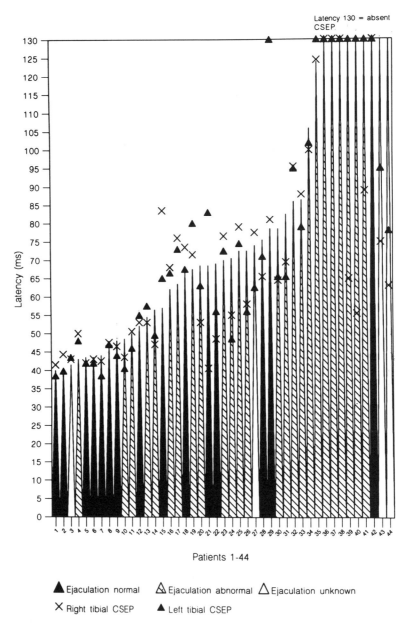

Fig. 27-3 The latencies of the pudendal and tibial cortical sensory evoked potentials (CSEPs) in 44 men with multiple sclerosis and erectile dysfunction. The upper limits of normal for the tibial and pudendal evoked potentials have been taken as 45 and 48 ms respectively. (From Betts CD, Jones SJ, Fowler CG, Fowler CJ: Erectile dysfunction in multiple sclerosis; associated neurological and neurophysiological deficits and treatment of the condition. Brain, in press, with permission.)

well but the patient may be left with urinary symptoms and, if male, erectile difficulties. Conversely, mild or evolving lesions such as an intrinsic or extrinsic spinal tumor or arteriovenous malformation[79] may present with erectile dysfunction as an early symptom. Patients with tethered cords, however, do not seem to follow this general rule. Men presenting in adult life may well have preservation of sexual function in the presence of quite severe neurogenic disorders of bladder function, due presumably to preservation of the thoracic sympathetic outflow.

CAUDA EQUINA AND PELVIC NERVE INJURY

A complete lesion of the cauda equina will damage the parasympathetic erectile pathways to the penis and cause sacral sensory loss. However, a number of men (approximately one-quarter) may still be able to achieve an erection psychogenically.[26] This is thought to be mediated by a sympathetic erectile pathway via the hypogastric plexus.

The pelvic plexus, which supplies the corpora cavernosa with both sympathetic and parasympathetic innervation, can be damaged by deep pelvic surgery such as an abdominoperineal resection, panproctocolectomy, or low anterior resection. The damage may be transient or permanent, resulting in erectile failure, which is often accompanied by impaired bladder function. The benefits and disadvantages of a "nerve-sparing" radical prostatectomy are currently the subject of debate among urologists. The close adherence to the prostatic capsule of the nerves to the corpora cavernosa means that radical prostatectomy for malignancy may lead to erectile failure, unless special precautions are taken to spare the nerves.[80]

DIABETES

All studies that have examined the incidence of impotence in diabetic men agree that the problem is very common, with estimates of between one-quarter to over one-half of diabetic men being affected[81-83] and the incidence increasing with age.[84] Erectile dysfunction may be a presenting symptom of diabetes, and in one study of men attending an impotence clinic, 11 percent were found to have an abnormal glucose tolerance test.

Typically the history is of a gradual deterioration in the strength of erections over the course of some months, followed by complete failure which is usually irreversible.[85] In contrast to men with partial spinal lesions who often have ejaculatory difficulties as well as erectile failure, ejaculation in diabetic men is usually well preserved, although retrograde ejaculation may be a problem.[86] The reason for the high incidence of erectile failure in diabetics is uncertain, but there are several possible pathogeneses and in some men the problem may be multifactorial.

Opinion about the basis of impotence in diabetes is a good example of how views have changed over the years. Although a psychogenic component may exacerbate difficulties for some men, there is little reason to believe that a primary psychogenic cause is any more common in diabetic than in nondiabetic men. Current investigative methods are relatively insensitive in identifying pathology (see below), and lack of abnormality in such studies should not be taken to imply that the problem is psychogenic.

At one time a hormonal factor was thought to be significant, but this has now been disproved,[87] and there is certainly no therapeutic effect to be gained from treatment with testosterone in diabetics with normal testosterone levels. The accelerated development of arteriosclerosis and hence of vascular insufficiency in diabetes has been proposed as a major factor, and internal pudendal artery stenosis has been shown to be more common in impotent than in potent diabetics. Small vessel disease is probably also a contributory factor, and an association has been shown between diabetic retinopathy and impotence.[84] Furthermore, andrologists who teach men to self-inject with intracorporeal vasoactive agents such as papaverine report that diabetic men are likely to need a considerably higher dose of papaverine than men with a pure neurogenic problem and that a significant proportion will not respond at all to intracorporeal papaverine. Despite the various techniques of investigating penile hemodynamics (such as dynamic cavernosography and cavernosometry, computerized Doppler waveform analysis, duplex color imaging ultrasonography, and radionuclide evaluation performed during pharmacologically induced erection),[88] no clear picture has emerged of the role of small vessel disease in causing impotence in diabetics. However, those studies that have looked at the relative incidence of hemodynamic and neurogenic disorders have concluded that neurogenic disorders are the more common and a peripheral nerve disorder seems to be a highly significant factor.[82,89]

In the simplest terms, the responsible neurological lesion is probably a defect of the autonomic innervation of the penis, which in health receives a rich nerve supply from the sympathetic and parasympathetic nervous system as well as somatic afferent innervation. Current research is directed at examining the nonadrenergic, noncholinergic (NANC) neurotransmitters in the penis, including VIP, calcitonin gene-related peptides, neuropeptide-Y,[90] and the role of endothelium-dependent responses.[25] It seems likely that the final theory of neurogenic impotence in diabetes will include the view that it results from disease of that class of fibers which is important in neuropeptide release as well as in the endothelial mechanisms controlling vascular tone.

Clinical studies to identify a neurogenic basis for impotence have involved testing of autonomic function and neurophysiological studies of conduction in the somatic innervation of the genitalia, and, more recently, in autonomic nerves. The early work of Ewing and colleagues who measured the response to the Valsalva maneuver and sustained hand grip, revealed no abnormality in those diabetic men with impotence alone.[91] Many groups since have investigated the integrity of various cardiovascular reflexes in diabetics and found such tests to be imperfectly sensitive but to provide information unavailable by other means. A recent study has shown that single breath beat-to-beat variation in heart rate is especially valuable in detecting autonomic abnormality in diabetics.[92]

Electrophysiological measurement of the bulbocavernosus reflex was one of the first tests to be used to identify neuropathy in men with impotence. In the early studies, abnormalities were found in a proportion of patients,[93–98] but the test lacks sufficient sensitivity to be of value in investigating an individual patient.[99,100] Its sensitivity is undoubtedly improved if visceral afferents at the bladder neck are stimulated rather than the dorsal nerve of the penis, but this involves passing a stimulator mounted on a catheter into the urethra.[89,101]

When first introduced, the pudendal somatosensory evoked potential[102] was hailed with enthusiasm as a valuable test in the investigation of impotence. It was claimed that by recording the pudendal somatosensory evoked potential and the bulbocaverno-sus reflex, all neural pathways important for physiological sexual function could be tested. However, these tests examine the wrong group of nerve fibers: both the bulbocavernosus reflex and somatosensory evoked potentials examine conduction in large myelinated afferents that are less important for sexual function than the unmyelinated or small unmyelinated fibers which convey the autonomic innervation. Studies have shown that there is no significant abnormality of central conduction in diabetes[103] and the pudendal evoked potential probably has little useful role in the investigation of impotence in diabetics.[104]

Various tests have been devised to examine the function of small and unmyelinated nerve fibers, and these are now being applied in diabetics to detect either generalized neuropathy or specific defects of innervation of the genital region. The value of thermal thresholds in this regard is now well accepted and testing thermal thresholds on the soles of the feet offers a sensitive means of detecting a length-dependent neuropathy, such as occurs in diabetes. In a series of men attending an impotence clinic, abnormal thermal thresholds on the feet were found in all patients with diabetes or small fiber neuropathy in whom the response to papaverine had excluded a significant vascular component.[98] Others have demonstrated alterations of thermal thresholds in the genital region.[105]

More recently the value of recording the sympathetic skin response in the genital region has been investigated.[106] Although it has limitations,[107] it is an easily performed test with some merits. Ertekin and his colleagues showed that a sympathetic skin response was present in all healthy controls but absent in a high proportion of impotent diabetics; in some men it was unrecordable from the genital region when it could be recorded from the feet. However there were also some diabetics with impotence who did have genital sympathetic skin responses.[108] It seems that this test is neither entirely specific nor sensitive, but it may well prove to be useful. Certainly it seems to be more sensitive than the bulbocavernosus reflex.[109]

Most recently claims have been made that the "cavernosal electromyogram" can be recorded and that this is of value in assessing neurogenic impotence. This electrical activity was recorded with an ordinary concentric needle electrode sited in the corpus cavernosum.[110] It was suppressed during the development of erection in response to visually erotic stimuli and the timing of its activity was abnormal in diabetics with erectile failure.[111] It was subsequently discovered that the same type of activity could be recorded with surface electrodes placed over the shaft of the penis.[112] A longer time base for recording was used and individual potentials of the trace were identified, so that the recording technique was given the acronym SPACE (single potential analysis of cavernous electrical activity). The full biological significance of this activity remains uncertain, but the activity recorded from the penis may represent the continuous ongoing changes in sympathetic skin activity because similar traces can be obtained from nongenital extremities.

Research is currently in progress to examine the potential usefulness of laser Doppler recorded changes in microcirculatory blood flow in the genital region following sympathetic stimulation. This is technically more demanding than recording the sympathetic skin responses, requiring more elaborate equipment and meticulous attention to minimize movement artifact. There is also a wide range for normal, making individual comparison difficult, although the mean values of reactive vasoconstriction in groups of patients with diabetes or central autonomic failure are less than controls. However, the results so far suggest that this test will not be any more sensitive than the sympathetic skin response in detecting genital neuropathy.[113]

In summary, therefore, the evidence that neuropathy is a major contributing factor in diabetic impotence seems convincing, but the role of small vessel disease remains uncertain. The most helpful studies in patients with diabetic impotence are probably the recording of parasympathetically mediated cardiovascular reflexes, and a genital recording of the sympathetic skin response, but until the latter becomes widely available thermal thresholds on the feet should also be measured to demonstrate small fiber neuropathy.

RECOMMENDED NEUROLOGICAL APPROACH TO PATIENTS PRESENTING WITH SYMPTOMS OF SEXUAL DYSFUNCTION

History

Loss of interest in sex in both men and women is most commonly related to depression or a breakdown in the interpersonal relationship. However, should it occur without mood change, sleep disturbance, or the start of medication, a medical cause should be considered. Heightened libido or disinhibition may appear in hypomania and patients with behavior disorders, but its appearance should alert the physician to the possibility of a cerebral lesion.

Erectile failure in men and lack of arousal in women are common in states of anxiety and sexual disharmony; pointers to a nonpsychogenic origin are (1) the presence of organic symptoms such as impairment of lower limb function, bladder dysfunction, or alteration in genital sensation; (2) normal libido; and (3) gradual onset. Loss of nocturnal and early morning erections suggests an organic basis, but men with partial spinal lesions may have erections at these times and yet be unable to obtain a willed erection or sustain it adequately for intercourse. Normal sexual function with a different partner and nonintercourse sexual activity strongly suggest a psychogenic explanation.

Clinical Examination

Sexual dysfunction has many different possible neurological causes. As with any complaint, a detailed history will often lead to a tentative diagnosis that assists in directing the examination to the site of suspected disease. In a patient with isolated sexual dysfunction in whom there are no clues from the history, it is necessary to perform a full neurological examination, looking for evidence of cerebral, spinal, or peripheral nerve disease. Because physiological sexual function is highly dependent on the integrity of the spinal cord, special attention should be given to examination of the lower limb reflexes and the plantar responses. Absence of the ankle reflexes and impaired vibration perception in the toes are valuable in suggesting a peripheral neuropathy. Acquired sacral anesthesia is likely to be accompanied by symptoms, but sensation in the saddle area should nevertheless be tested in all cases of cauda equina injury. Lack of anal tone on rectal examination should alert the clinician to the possibility of a cauda equina lesion. If there is any suggestion that impotence is due to autonomic dysfunction, the patient should be examined for postural hypotension. Impotence may occur as the first symptom of multiple system atrophy, and early signs of extrapyramidal or cerebellar dysfunction should therefore be carefully sought. The patient's leg pulses should always be checked to avoid embarking on inappropriate neurological investigation of a complaint due to peripheral vascular disease. Similarly, ophthalmoscopic examination may detect relevant small vessel disease in an undiagnosed diabetic.

Investigations

If no investigations have been carried out prior to referral to the neurologist, serum prolactin, testosterone, FSH, and LH should be measured to exclude testicular failure or hyperprolactinemia, and random blood sugar level determined.

The introduction of intracorporeal injection therapy for the treatment of erectile failure has led to changes in the investigation of impotence. Many andrologists or urologists now take a pragmatic approach to treatment: if the response to a small dose of papaverine is good, the problem is assumed to be nonvascular and therefore either psychogenic or neurological in origin and thus potentially responsive to therapy. It may then only be for research purposes or to satisfy the curiosity of patient or physician that investigations are carried out. Nocturnal penile tumescence studies should no longer be considered a "gold standard" for investigation because nocturnal erections do occur in impotent men with spinal cord disease.

Many different investigations, as described in the foregoing sections, have been used to identify a neurological cause. The bulbocavernosus reflex recorded electrophysiologically has been severely criticized—the mistaken rationale for performing this test and its demonstrated poor sensitivity mean there is little to be gained from it.[99] It is our impression that the presence or absence of the ankle reflex is as good a means of identifying relevant neuropathy as this neurophysiological investigation. The pudendal evoked potential is delayed or absent in the presence of spinal cord disease that is causing erectile failure. The response is readily produced using a repetitive stimulus at 2.5 times threshold to the dorsal nerve of the penis or clitoris and is technically no more difficult to record than the tibial evoked potentials. However it may be of no greater usefulness than the latter in detecting spinal cord disease causing sexual dysfunction and perhaps no better than a good clinical neurological examination.[75,114]

Whether newer tests such as measurement of thermal thresholds or sympathetic skin responses prove to be more sensitive in detecting relevant peripheral nerve disease remains to be established. Autonomic function tests may be abnormal in either peripheral nerve disease with small fiber involvement or central causes of autonomic failure. Because cortical lesions can produce abnormalities of sexual function, an electroencephalogram may occasionally be of some contributory value in demonstrating an interictal focal abnormality. If impotence is accompanied by any clinical features of extrapyramidal or cerebellar disease and multiple system atrophy is suspected, sphincter electromyography may show characteristic changes in motor unit action potentials.

MANAGEMENT AND TREATMENT OF SEXUAL DISORDERS

Even if no specific cause of sexual dysfunction can be found, it is usually apparent whether patients are best referred for some form of physical treatment or whether a psychiatric opinion or referral for psychosexual counseling is more appropriate.

If patients with sexual dysfunction are known to have neurological disease, it is often helpful to spend some time in explaining the mechanism by which the organic pathology has produced their disability; discussion alone may do much to help them adjust to their disability and may considerably ease tensions between partners who have begun to suspect alternative explanations. Sometimes discussion of the problem and an explanation of the management options is sufficient. Although there are several different ways in which men with erectile failure may be helped, there are other patients for whom no physical treatment is available, such as women with perineal sensory loss. It may be patients such as these who particularly benefit from counseling by a sex therapist and advice on maximizing sensory input from other erogenous regions.

Yohimbine

Yohimbine is obtained from the yohimbine tree (*Pausinystalia yohimbine* of the Rubaceae family), which grows in West Africa. It is an α_2-adrenergic blocker which, it is claimed, facilitates male sexual arousal. This is thought to be achieved by its effect on noradrenergic transmission, decreasing sympathetic activity and thereby resulting in increased penile blood inflow and reduced outflow. Pharmacologically, its action is similar to the peripheral action of reserpine, but it also has a pronounced central action and may have a mood stimulating effect. Brindley states that the drug makes orgasm easier to achieve.[115]

The recommended dosage is either 10 mg (increasing to 20 mg) taken approximately 2 hours before intercourse is attempted or 5 mg three times daily taken on a regular basis. Its side effects include a feeling of general excitation, anxiety, nausea, and tremulousness. The case report of a young man who took 350 mg of yohimbine in a suicide attempt described how, after a delay of 17 hours, the patient had a self-limiting period of atrial fibrillation, drowsiness, confusion, and a reduction in body temperature. On recovery, he had a 24-hour period of retrograde amnesia which lasted for 4 days.[116]

A controlled trial of the effect of yohimbine in the treatment of organic erectile impotence showed a small effect when compared to placebo.[117] This is probably sufficient to justify a trial of treatment, particularly in men who still have some partial erectile function or in those with anorgasmia. Trial of an oral preparation is often helpful in men seeking treatment who are initially unwilling to perform intracorporeal self-injection.

Intracorporeal Vasoactive Injection Therapy

The introduction of treatment by injection of intracorporeal vasoactive agents has transformed the management of erectile failure. In the United Kingdom, papaverine is most commonly used, but prostaglandin E_1 is an alternative agent[118] that has some advantages as well as disadvantages.

Under hospital (outpatient) supervision, a trial dose of between 7 to 10 mg of papaverine is injected using a fine needle (a 1-ml insulin syringe is very suitable) and the effect observed. Usually several visits by the patient are required to establish a suitable dose (between 5 and 120 mg) and to teach him the technique of self-injection. The most serious ill effect is of inducing a prolonged erection lasting more than 4 to 6 hours and a risk of venous thrombosis and priapism. Abnormally prolonged erections may be reversed by

aspiration from the corpus cavernosum; if this fails, injection of an α-adrenergic agent such as metaraminol or phenylephrine is likely to be effective. It is uncommon for surgical intervention to be necessary in the management of priapism resulting from intracorporeal injection. More minor side effects of these injections are bruising of the penis, which may then lead to fibrosis and so cause curvature. Since papaverine is not licensed for intracorporeal injection, the patient should sign a consent form before embarking on this form of therapy and should also be given an information sheet with clear instructions on where to go if a prolonged erection occurs.

Vacuum Pump

Vacuum pump devices require a rigid cylinder to be placed over the penis; tumescence is induced by the creation of negative pressure by a hand pump. A band is then placed around the base of the penis and the cylinder removed. Several different devices are available. Published reports of the satisfaction achieved with vacuum pump devices are varied,[119–121] and their success probably reflects to some extent the enthusiasm of the supervising clinician for this method of treatment.

Prostheses

There are a variety of penile prostheses, ranging from a relatively simple semirigid device to a complex, and accordingly more expensive, inflatable device. Details of these devices and how they are implanted can be found in urological textbooks.[88] Some facts that should be known to the physician referring a man for consideration of such surgery is that implantation of the device requires replacing the corpora of the penis by the implant, so that the procedure is irreversible. Moreover, the erection that can be achieved by such a device lacks the warmth of the penis, which is a feature of a physiological erection. Nevertheless there are many men who have been well pleased by the performance of their implants.[122] Implantation of such a device is probably inadvisable in a man with a progressive neurological disease such as multiple sclerosis, who may become embarrassed by it if he later becomes more disabled and needs assistance with personal care.

NEUROLOGICAL PROBLEMS ASSOCIATED WITH SEXUAL ACTIVITY

Headache

The development of headache during sexual activity, particularly if it is of sudden onset and occurs at the time of orgasm, is an alarming symptom for patients; many are convinced that they have had a cerebral hemorrhage. In fact, although this may be the case, most headaches that occur under these circumstances are benign.

Vascular mechanisms are thought to be the cause of headache that occurs during sexual arousal in cases of unruptured aneurysms, cerebral tumors, and subdural hematomas. The combination of hyperventilation, the Valsalva maneuver, and exertion increases the cerebrospinal fluid (CSF) pressure, which may produce traction on pain-sensitive structures, giving rise to short-duration, well-localized pain.

Masters and Johnson found that in both sexes the heart rate increased at orgasm to 110 to 180 beats per minute and that the blood pressure rose by 40 to 100 mmHg systolic and 20 to 50 mmHg diastolic.[123] Arousal and with it these cardiovascular changes are increased if the circumstances are novel and unusual; subarachnoid hemorrhages in patients with aneurysms and angiomas are more common in those situations than they are in domestic circumstances and with familiar sexual activity. The reported incidence varies from 3.8 to 12 percent.[124,125] Primary intracranial hemorrhage should also be considered as a cause of sudden headache.

Benign coital cephalalgia is also considered to have a vascular cause. It consists of a severe, usually sudden occipital headache that occurs at or near orgasm and lasts from a few minutes to several hours. The pain is pulsatile and is thought to be due to sudden vasodilatation secondary to acute alterations between the sympathetic and parasympathetic systems, with circulating agents also playing a part.[126] It is often recurrent but usually self-limiting. There have been no controlled studies of treatment, but propranolol is worth a trial.

Postcoital migraine is well documented and may occur in patients with benign coital cephalalgia. Its character is identical with the patient's usual pattern of migraine, and the onset is postorgasmic, commencing minutes or hours after the event. On occasion, particularly in women, sexual arousal forms part of the aura of migraine.

Ampules of amyl nitrite, crushed and inhaled immediately before the event, are sometimes used in an attempt to enhance orgasm. A potent vasodilator, this drug may produce severe vascular headache.[127]

Low-pressure postcoital headache, analogous to that which may follow lumbar puncture, may also occur. Symptoms are relived by recumbency. Tearing of the arachnoid membrane and leakage of CSF has been postulated as the cause.[128]

Transient Global Amnesia

Fisher studied 85 episodes of transient global amnesia in 78 patients and found that 26 of the attacks were provoked by such events as emotional experiences, pain, and bathing in cold water.[129] In seven cases the trigger was sexual intercourse. It has been suggested that the amnesia is secondary to cerebral ischemia, but a more likely explanation is that it is due to a hippocampal seizure,[130] which is well recognized as occasionally being provoked by intense emotions.

Drugs

Many drugs interfere with normal sexual function, including some prescribed for the treatment of neurological disorders. Further comment on this aspect is provided in Chapter 29.

ACKNOWLEDGMENTS

Dr. Clare Fowler would like to thank Mr. C. D. Betts, F.R.C.S., and Mr. R. O. Beck, F.R.C.S., for their advice about the text and for kindly supplying Figures 27-1, 27-2, and 27-3.

REFERENCES

1. Janus SS, Janus CL: The Janus Report on Sexual Behavior. John Wiley & Sons, New York, 1993
2. McCall A: The Medieval Underworld. Hamish Hamilton, London, 1979
3. Report of the Committee on Homosexual Offences and Prostitution, HMSO, London, 1957

4. Kinsey AC, Pomeroy WB, Martin CE: Sexual Behaviour in the Human Male. WB Saunders, Philadelphia, 1948

5. Kinsey AC, Pomeroy WB, Martin CE: Sexual Behaviour in the Human Female. WB Saunders, Philadelphia, 1953

6. Schmidt G, Sigusch V: Changes in sexual behaviour among young males and females between 1960–1970. Arch Sex Behav 2:27, 1972

7. Schofield M: The Sexual Behaviour of Young Adults. Allen Lane, London, 1973

8. Gosselin C, Wilson G: Sexual Variations: Fetishism, Sado-masochism and Transvestism. Faber & Faber, London, 1980

9. Frank E, Anderson C, Rubinstein D: Frequency of sexual dysfunction in "normal" couples. N Engl J Med 299:111, 1978

10. Boller F, Frank E: Sexual Dysfunction in Neurological Disorders. Raven Press, New York, 1982

11. Freed E: Increased sexual function with nomifensine. Med J Aust 1:551, 1983

12. Gartrell N: Increased libido in women receiving trazodone. Am J Psychiatry 143:781, 1986

13. Brown E, Brown GM, Kofman O, Quarrington B: Sexual function and affect in parkinsonian men treated with L-dopa. Am J Psychiatry 135:1552, 1978

14. Bancroft J: Endocrinology of sexual function. Clin Obstet Gynaecol 7:253, 1980

15. Nieschlag E, Mauss J, Coert A, Kicovic P: Plasma androgen levels in men after oral administration of testosterone or testosterone undecanoate. Acta Endocrinol (Copenh) 79:366, 1975

16. Bancroft J, Tennent G, Loucas K, Cass J: Control of deviant sexual behaviour by drugs: behavioural changes following oestrogens and anti-androgens. Br J Psychiatry 125:310, 1974

17. Brindley GS: Pathophysiology of erection and ejaculation. p. 1083. In Whitfield HN, Hendry WF (eds): Textbook of Genito-urinary Surgery. Churchill Livingstone, Edinburgh, 1985

18. Beric A, Light JK: Anorgasmia in anterior spinal cord syndrome. J Neurol Neurosurg Psychiatry 56:548, 1993

19. Miller BL, Cummings JL, McIntyre H, et al: Hypersexuality or altered sexual preference following brain injury. J Neurol Neurosurg Psychiatry 49:867, 1986

20. Dua S, MacLean PD: Localization for penile erection in medial frontal lobe. Am J Physiol 207:1425, 1964

21. Remillard GM, Andermann F, Testa GF, et al: Sexual ictal manifestations predominate in women with temporal lobe epilepsy: a finding suggesting sexual dimorphism in the human brain. Neurology 33:323, 1983

22. Olivecrona H: The surgery of pain. Acta Psychiatr Neurol Suppl 46:268, 1947

23. Brindley GS, Polkey CE, Rushton DN, Cardozo L: Sacral anterior root stimulators for bladder control in paraplegia: the first 50 cases. J Neurol Neurosurg Psychiatry 49:1104, 1986

24. Polak JM, Gu J, Mina S, Bloom SR: VIPergic nerves in the penis. Lancet 2:217, 1981

25. Saenz de Tejada I, Goldstein I, Azadzoi K, et al: Impaired neurogenic and endothelium-mediated relaxation of penile smooth muscle from diabetic men with impotence. N Engl J Med 320:1025, 1989

26. Bors EH, Comarr AE: Neurological disturbances of sexual function with special references to 529 patients with spinal cord injury. Urol Survey 10:191, 1960

27. Brindley GS: Pilot experiments on the actions of drugs injected into the human corpus cavernosum penis. Br J Pharmacol 87:495, 1986

28. Wilson GT: Alcohol and sexual function. Br J Sex Med 11:56, 1984

29. Hoenig J, Hamilton C: Epilepsy and sexual orgasm. Acta Psychiatr Scand 35:448, 1960

30. Levin RJ: The physiology of sexual fucntion in women. Clin Obstet Gynaecol 7:213, 1980

31. Wagner G, Levin RJ: Effect of atropine and methylatropine on human vaginal blood flow, sexual arousal and climax. Acta Pharmacol Toxicol 46:321, 1980

32. Barnes TRE, Bamber RWK, Watson JP: Psychotropic drugs and sexual behaviour. Br J Hosp Med 21:594, 1979

33. Gillan P, Brindley GS: Vaginal and pelvic floor responses to sexual stimulation. Psychophysiology 16:471, 1979

34. Master WH, Johnson VE: Human Sexual Inadequacy. Little, Brown, Boston, 1970

35. Kaplan HS: The New Sex Therapy. Bailliere Tindall, London, 1974

36. Gautier-Smith PC: Atteinte des fonctions cérébrales et troubles du comportement sexuel. Rev Neurol (Paris) 136:311, 1980

37. Van Reeth P, Dierkens J, Luminet D: L'hypersexualite dans l'epilepsie et les tumeurs du lobe temporal. Acta Neurol Belg 58:194, 1958

38. Monga TN, Monga M, Raina MS, Hardjasudarma M: Hypersexuality in stroke. Arch Phys Med Rehabil 67:415, 1986

39. Levine J, Albert H: Sexual behaviour after lobotomy. J Nerv Ment Dis 113:332, 1951

40. Terzian H, Ore GD: Syndrome of Kluver and Bucy reproduced in man by bilateral removal of the temporal lobes. Neurology 5:373, 1955

41. Kluver H, Bucy PC: Psychic blindness and other symptoms following bilateral temporal lobectomy in rhesus monkeys. Am J Psychiatry 119:352, 1937

42. Lilly R, Cummings JL, Benson DF, Franklin M: The human Kluver-Bucy syndrome. Neurology 33:1141, 1983

43. Penfield W, Jasper HH: Epilepsy and the Functional Anatomy of the Human Brain. Little, Brown, Boston, 1954

44. York, GK, Gabor AJ, Dreyfus PM: Paroxysmal genital pain: an unusual manifestation of epilepsy. Neurology 29:516, 1979

45. Bhaskar PA: Scrotal pain with testicular jerking: an unusual manifestation of epilepsy. J Neurol Neurosurg Psychiatry 50:1233, 1987

46. Ruff RL: Orgasmic epilepsy. Neurology 30:1252, 1980

47. Bancaud J, Favel P, Bonis Aea: Manifestations sexuelles paroxystiques et epilepsie temporale. Rev Neurol (Paris) 123:217, 1970

48. Mitchell W, Falconer M, Hill D: Epilepsy with fetishism relieved by temporal lobectomy. Lancet 2:626, 1954

49. Freemon FR, Nevis AH: Temporal lobe sexual seizures. Neurology 19:87, 1969

50. Currier RD, Little SC, Suess JF, Andy OJ: Sexual seizures. Arch Neurol 25:260, 1971

51. Anson JA, Kuhlman DT: Post-ictal Kluver-Bucy syndrome after temporal lobectomy. J Neurol Neurosurg Psychiatry 56:311, 1993

52. Spencer SS, Spencer DD, Williamson PD, Mattson RH: Sexual automatisms in complex partial seizures. Neurology 33:527, 1983

53. Hooshmand H, Brawley BW: Temporal lobe seizures and exhibitionism. Neurology 19:1119, 1969

54. Blumer D: Hypersexual episodes in temporal lobe epilepsy. Am J Psychiatry 126:1099, 1970

55. Blumer D, Walker AE: Sexual behavior in temporal lobe epilepsy. Arch Neurol 16:37, 1967

56. Hierons R, Saunders M: Impotence in patients with temporal-lobe lesions. Lancet 2:761, 1966

57. Davies BM, Morgenstern FS: Case of acquired transvestism associated with cysticercosis and temporal lobe epilepsy. J Neurol Neurosurg Psychiatry 23:247, 1960

58. Gautier-Smith PC: Parasagittal and Falx Meningiomas. Butterworths, London, 1970

59. Toone BK, Wheeler M, Nanjee M, et al: Sex hormones, sexual activity and plasma anticonvulsant levels in male epileptics. J Neurol Neurosurg Psychiatry 46:824, 1983

60. Herzog AG, Seibel MM, Schomer DL, et al: Reproductive endocrine disorders in men with partial seizures of temporal lobe origin. Arch Neurol 43:347, 1986

61. Berkovic SF, Bladin PF, Vajda FJE: Temporal lobe epilepsy in hyposexual men. Lancet 1:622, 1984

62. Beck RO, Betts CD, Fowler CJ: Genitourinary dysfunction in multiple system atrophy: clinical features and treatment in 62 cases. J Urol 151:1336, 1994

63. Kirby R, Fowler C, Gosling J, Bannister R: Urethrovesical dysfunction in progressive autonomic failure with multiple system atrophy. J Neurol Neurosurg Psychiatry 49:554, 1986

64. Eardley I, Quinn NP, Fowler CJ, et al: The value of urethral sphincter electromyography in the differential diagnosis of parkinsonism. Br J Urol 64:360, 1989

65. Onufrowicz B: On the arrangement and function of the cell groups of the sacral region of the spinal cord in man. Arch Neurol Psychopathol 3:387, 1900

66. Sakuta M, Nakanishi T, Toyokura Y: Anal muscle electromyograms differ in amyotrophic lateral sclerosis and Shy-Drager syndrome. Neurology 28:1289, 1978

67. Talbot H: A report on sexual function in paraplegics. J Urol 61:265, 1949

68. Bennett CJ, Seager SW, Vasher EA, McGuire EJ: Sexual dysfunction and electroejaculation in men with spinal cord injury: review. J Urol 139:453, 1988

69. Sachs B, Friedman ED: The general symptoms of multiple sclerosis. Assoc Res Nerv Ment Dis 2:49, 1921

70. Miller H, Simpson CA, Yeates WK: Bladder dysfunction in multiple sclerosis. Br Med J 1:1265, 1965

71. Lilius HG, Valtonen EJ, Wikstrom J: Sexual problems in patients suffering from multiple sclerosis. J Chronic Dis 29:643, 1976

72. Valleroy ML, Kraft GH: Sexual dysfunction in multiple sclerosis. Arch Phys Med Rehabil 65:125, 1984

73. Minderhoud JM, Leemhuis JG, Kremer J, et al: Sexual disturbances arising from multiple sclerosis. Acta Neurol Scand 70:299, 1984

74. Vas CJ: Sexual impotence and some autonomic disturbances in men with multiple sclerosis. Acta Neurol Scand 45:166, 1969

75. Betts C, Jones S, Fowler C: Erectile dysfunction in multiple sclerosis; associated neurological and neurophysiological deficits and treatment of the condition. Brain, in press

76. Betts CD, D'Mellow MT, Fowler CJ: Urinary symptoms and the neurological features of bladder dysfunction in multiple sclerosis. J Neurol Neurosurg Psychiatry 56:245, 1993

77. Lundberg PO: Sexual dysfunction in female patients with multiple sclerosis. Int Rehabil Med 3:32, 1981

78. Bors E, Comarr AE: Neurological Urology. Karger, Basel, 1971

79. Aminoff MJ, Logue V: Clinical featues of spinal vascular malformations. Brain 97:197, 1974

80. Walsh PC, Donker PJ: Impotence following radical

prostatectomy: insight into etiology and prevention. J Urol 128:492, 1982

81. Rubin A, Babbott D: Impotence and diabetes mellitus. JAMA 168:498, 1958

82. Ellenberg M: Impotence in diabetes: the neurologic factor. Ann Intern Med 75:213, 1971

83. Faerman I, Glocer L, Fox D, et al: Impotence and diabetes. Histological studies of the autonomic nervous fibers of the corpora cavernosa in impotent diabetic males. Diabetes 23:971, 1974

84. McCulloch DK, Campbell IW, Wu FC, et al: The prevalence of diabetic impotence. Diabetologia 18: 279, 1980

85. McCulloch DK, Young RJ, Prescott RJ, et al: The natural history of impotence in diabetic men. Diabetologia 26:437, 1984

86. Greene LF, Kelalis PP: Retrograde ejaculation of semen due to diabetic neuropathy. J Urol 98:696, 1967

87. Maatman TJ, Montague DK, Martin LM: Erectile dysfunction in men with diabetes mellitus. Urology 29:589, 1987

88. Kirby RS, Carson CC, Webster GD (eds): Impotence: Diagnosis and Management of Male Erectile Dysfunction. Butterworth-Heinemann, Oxford, 1991

89. Bemelmans BL, Meuleman EJ, Anten BW, et al: Penile sensory disorders in erectile dysfunction: results of a comprehensive neuro-urophysiological diagnostic evaluation in 123 patients. J Urol 146:777, 1991

90. Lincoln J, Crowe R, Burnstock G: Neuropeptides and impotence. p. 3. In Kirby RS, Carson CC, Webster GD (eds): Impotence: Diagnosis and Management of Male Erectile Dysfunction. Butterworth-Heinemann, Oxford, 1991

91. Ewing DJ, Campbell IW, Bell AA, Clarke BF: Vascular reflexes in diabetic autonomic neuropathy. Lancet 2:1354, 1973

92. Nisen HO, Larsen A, Lindstrom BL, et al: Cardiovascular reflexes in the neurological evaluation of impotence. Br J Urol 71:199, 1993

93. Ertekin C, Reel F: Bulbocavernosus reflex in normal men and in patients with neurogenic bladder and/or impotence. J Neurol Sci 28:1, 1976

94. Kaneko S, Bradley WE: Penile electrodiagnosis: value of bulbocavernosus reflex latency versus nerve conduction velocity of the dorsal nerve of the penis in diagnosis of diabetic impotence. J Urol 137:933, 1987

95. Tackmann W, Porst H, Van Ahlen H: Bulbocavernosus reflex latencies and somatosensory evoked potentials after pudendal nerve stimulation in the diagnosis of impotence. J Neurol 235:219, 1988

96. Parys BT, Evans CM, Parsons KF: Bulbocavernosus reflex latency in the investigation of diabetic impotence. Br J Urol 61:59, 1988

97. Nogueira MC, Herbaut AG, Wespes E: Neurophysiological investigations of two hundred men with erectile dysfunction: interest of bulbocavernosus reflex and pudendal evoked responses. Eur Urol 18:37, 1990

98. Fowler CJ, Ali Z, Kirby RS, Pryor JP: The value of testing for unmyelinated fibre, sensory neuropathy in diabetic impotence. Br J Urol 61:63, 1988

99. Fowler CJ: Electrophysiologic evaluation of sexual dysfunction. p. 279. In Low PA (ed): Evaluation and Management of Clinical Autonomic Disorders. Little, Brown, Boston, 1993

100. Vardi Y, Yarnitsky D, Simri W, et al: Bulbocavernous reflex latency in evaluation of diabetic impotence. Int J Impot Res 4:97, 1992

101. Sarica Y, Karacan I: Bulbocavernosus reflex to somatic and visceral nerve stimulation in normal subjects and in diabetics with erectile impotence. J Urol 138:55, 1987

102. Haldeman S, Bradley WE, Bhatia N: Evoked responses from the pudendal nerve. J Urol 128:974, 1982

103. Ziegler D, Muhlen H, Dannehl K, Gruies FA: Tibial nerve somatosensory evoked potentials at various stages of peripheral neuropathy in insulin dependent diabetic patients. J Neurol Neurosurg Psychiatry 56: 58, 1993

104. Vodusek DB, Ravnik-Oblak K, Oblak C: Pudendal versus limb nerve electrophysiological abnormalities in diabetics with erectile dysfunction. Int J Impot Res 5:37, 1993

105. Robinson LQ, Woodcock JP, Stephenson TP: Results of investigation of impotence in patients with overt or probable neuropathy. Br J Urol 6:583, 1987

106. Ertekin C, Ertekin N, Mutlu S, et al: Skin potentials (SP) recorded from the extremities and genital regions in normal and impotent subjects. Acta Neurol Scand 76:28, 1987

107. Schondorf R: The role of the sympathetic skin response in the assessment of autonomic functions. p. 231. In Low PA (ed): Clinical Autonomic Disorders: Evaluation and Management. Little, Brown, Boston, 1993

108. Ertekin C, Ertekin N, Almis S: Autonomic sympathetic nerve involvement in diabetic impotence. Neurourol Urodynam 8:589, 1989

109. Ertekin C, Almis S, Ertekin N: Sympathetic skin potentials and bulbocavernosus reflex in patients with chronic alcoholism and impotence. Eur Neurol 30: 334, 1990

110. Wagner G, Gerstenberg T, Levin RJ: Electrical activity of corpus cavernosum during flaccidity and erection of the human penis: a new diagnostic method? J Urol 142:723, 1989

111. Gerstenberg TC, Nordling J, Hald T, Wagner G:

Standardized evaluation of erectile dysfunction in 95 consecutive patients. J Urol 141:857, 1989

112. Stief CG, Djamilian M, Anton P, et al: Single potential analysis of cavernous electrical activity in impotent patients: a possible diagnostic method for autonomic cavernous dysfunction and cavernous smooth muscle degeneration. J Urol 146:771, 1991

113. Beck R: Laser Doppler (in preparation)

114. Kunesch E, Reiners K, Muller-Mattheis V, et al: Neurological risk profile in organic erectile impotence. J Neurol Neurosurg Psychiatry 55:275, 1992

115. Brindley G: Personal communication, 1991

116. Varkey S: Overdose of yohimbine. Br Med J 304:548, 1992

117. Morales A, Condra M, Owen JA, et al: Is yohimbine effective in the treatment of organic impotence? Results of a controlled trial. J Urol 137:1168, 1987

118. Ishii N, Watanabe H, Irisawa C, et al: Intracavernous injection of prostaglandin E1 for the treatment of erectile impotence. J Urol 141:323, 1989

119. Nadig P: Vacuum erection devices. World J Urol 8:114, 1990

120. Price DE, Cooksey G, Jehu D, et al: The management of impotence in diabetic men by vacuum tumescence therapy. Diabet Med 8:964, 1991

121. Wiles PG: Successful non-invasive management of erectile impotence in diabetic men. Br Med J 296:161, 1988

122. Wilson SK, Wahman GE, Lange JL: Eleven years of experience with the inflatable penile prosthesis. J Urol 139:951, 1988

123. Master WH, Johnson VE: Human Sexual Response. Little, Brown, Boston, 1966

124. Locksley HB: Natural history of subarachnoid hemorrhage, intracranial aneurysms and arteriovenus malformations: based on 6368 cases in the Cooperative Study. J Neurosurg 25:219, 1966

125. Lundberg PO, Osterman PO: The benign and malignant forms of orgasmic cephalgia. Headache 14:164, 1974

126. Braun A, Klawans HL: Headaches associated with exercise and sexual activity. p. 373. In Vinken PJ, Bruyn GW, Klawans HL (eds): Handbook of Clinical Neurology. Vol 48. Elsevier, Amsterdam, 1986

127. Pearlman JT, Adams GL: Amyl nitrite inhalation fad. JAMA 212:160, 1970

128. Paulson GW, Klawans HL: Benign orgasmic cephalgia. Headache 13:181, 1974

129. Fisher CM: Transient global amnesia: precipitating activities and other observations. Arch Neurol 39:605, 1982

130. Fisher C, Adams R: Transient global amnesia. Acta Neurol Scand 40, suppl 9:1, 1964

28

Pregnancy and Disorders of the Nervous System

Michael J. Aminoff

Neurological disorders may first present during pregnancy, and their investigation and treatment may be complicated by concerns for the safety of the developing fetus. Furthermore, the natural history of certain preexisting diseases may be affected by pregnancy, and obstetrical management may be influenced by the neurological disturbance. These aspects are considered in this chapter.

EPILEPSY

Pregnancy may affect the natural history and management of patients with epilepsy in several ways. First, it may affect the frequency of seizures in known epileptics. Knight and Rhind studied 153 pregnancies in 59 epileptic patients and found that seizure frequency increased in 45 percent, decreased in 5 percent, and was unchanged in the remainder.[1] More recently, Schmidt and associates reported that during 136 pregnancies in 122 epileptic women, seizure frequency increased in 37 percent of pregnancies, often in association with poor compliance with anticonvulsant drug regimens.[2] In other recent series, an increase in seizures occurred during pregnancy in between 23 and 75 percent of cases.[3]

There is no way of predicting in advance whether or how seizure frequency will be altered during preg-

nancy, but certain general points can be made. Seizure frequency is more likely to increase in poorly controlled epileptics than in those with infrequent seizures, and any increase is most likely to occur during the first trimester. Any change in seizure frequency usually reverses after the birth of the baby, although occasional patients whose seizures increase during pregnancy remain more difficult to control thereafter. The influence of a particular pregnancy cannot be predicted by the outcome of previous pregnancies, any relation between seizures and the menstrual cycle, or maternal age. Seizures may occur for the first time during or immediately after pregnancy and in some instances occur only in relation to pregnancy. Even in patients with such true gestational epilepsy, however, it is not possible to predict the course of subsequent pregnancies from the occurrence of seizures during one pregnancy.

Status epilepticus may complicate pregnancy and sometimes occurs before there is any other evidence that seizures have become more difficult to control. As in the nonparous woman, it is important to obtain control of the seizures rapidly, but therapeutic termination of pregnancy is usually unnecessary. There is no evidence that anticonvulsant drugs administered intravenously to treat status epilepticus affect the fetus adversely.

The reason that seizure frequency sometimes in-

567

creases during pregnancy is not clear, but a change in drug requirements during the gestational period may be responsible in some patients. For example, the amount of phenytoin and phenobarbital required to maintain total plasma drug levels increases during the gestational period and decreases during the puerperium.[4] This is true for all first-line antiepileptic drugs.[5] However, free or unbound drug concentrations decline less often, and do so significantly only for phenobarbital.[5] Other possible reasons for the increased dose requirements of these drugs during pregnancy include poor compliance with the anticonvulsant drug regimen, changes in drug absorption and excretion, and the dilutional effects of increasing plasma volume and extracellular fluid volume. An increased metabolic capacity of maternal liver and metabolism of part of the anticonvulsant dose by the fetus, placenta, or both may also be important. Folic acid therapy, prescribed routinely by many obstetricians, sometimes lowers the plasma phenytoin level. Whether hormonal factors also contribute to an increase in seizure frequency is unclear, but estrogens are epileptogenic in experimental animals, and progesterone is said to have both convulsant and anticonvulsant properties. Finally, fatigue and sleep deprivation may influence seizure frequency during pregnancy.

The reason that seizure frequency decreases in some epileptic patients is also unclear, but improved compliance with the anticonvulsant drug regimen may be responsible.

A second major concern in the management of epileptic women during pregnancy is the possible effect of the seizure disorder and of anticonvulsant drugs on the developing fetus. It is difficult to determine the precise risk that the offspring of epileptic parents will also develop a seizure disorder. The risk depends in part on whether the parental epilepsy is idiopathic (constitutional) or acquired in nature; such risk appears to be increased among the offspring of epileptic mothers but not when only the father is epileptic. The reason for the increased risk is unclear, but genetic factors may be important, as may the consequences of maternal seizures or anticonvulsant drugs taken during pregnancy.

For many years there has been concern that anticonvulsant drugs are teratogenic. Epidemiological studies are difficult to interpret because epilepsy occurs for many reasons, varies markedly in severity,

may itself increase the risk of fetal malformation, and is treated by many drugs in different doses and combinations; environmental factors also bear on the development of fetal malformations and are difficult to control for. Nevertheless, numerous reports suggest that anticonvulsant drugs are indeed teratogenic in humans,[6–8] and the risk of malformation among the offspring of epileptic women is about double that for nonepileptic women. Trimethadione has been incriminated particularly clearly as being teratogenic and should be avoided during pregnancy; fortunately, it is now rarely used. Among the major anticonvulsant drugs in current use, phenytoin and phenobarbital may lead especially to congenital heart disease and to cleft lip and cleft palate; carbamazepine may be associated with craniofacial defects, fingernail hypoplasia, and developmental delay[9] and—when used in combination with other anticonvulsants—with spina bifida.[10] Valproic acid has been associated especially with neural tube defects.[11,12] It is probably best avoided in women of childbearing potential; if pregnancy occurs in a woman taking it, amniocentesis is advised so that therapeutic abortion can be considered if the α-fetoprotein level suggests a high risk of neural tube defect. The mechanisms involved in teratogenesis of anticonvulsant drugs are not known but may include folate deficiency (Fig. 28-1) or antagonism[13] and production of toxic intermediary metabolites during biotransformation of the parent compound.[14] Specific oxidative intermediates such as epoxide, for example, have been suggested as the ultimate teratogen in patients receiving phenytoin.[14]

A specific syndrome has been described among some of the offspring born to mothers taking phenytoin or phenobarbital during pregnancy and bears some resemblance to the fetal alcohol syndrome. It is characterized by prenatal and postnatal growth deficiency, microcephaly, dysmorphic facies, and mental deficiency.[15,16] A somewhat similar syndrome has been ascribed to carbamazepine.[9] A characteristic facial phenotype in children exposed to valproic acid or sodium valproate in utero has also been described.[17]

A clinical or subclinical bleeding disorder may occur in neonates exposed to anticonvulsant drugs in utero, without evidence of coagulopathy in the mothers. For example, Mountain and colleagues reported that 7 of 16 infants born to mothers taking anticonvulsant drugs had a severe coagulopathy, one had a mild defect, and the remainder were normal.[18] Factors II,

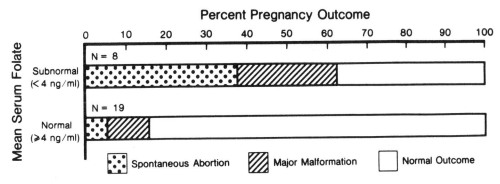

Fig. 28-1 Percent pregnancy outcome in relation to mean serum folate levels in the first trimester dichotomized as less than 4 (subnormal) or at least 4 ng/ml. N = number of pregnancies with subnormal or normal serum folate levels. A significantly higher number of pregnancies with subnormal levels resulted in an abnormal outcome than did pregnancies with normal levels. Using Fisher's exact test, $p = 0.05$ for spontaneous abortion and $p = 0.03$ for total abnormal outcomes. (From Dansky LV, Andermann E, Rosenblatt D, et al: Anticonvulsants, folate levels, and pregnancy outcome: a prospective study. Ann Neurol 21: 176, 1987, with permission.)

VII, IX, and X were decreased in affected infants, whereas factors V and VIII and fibrinogen were normal. Bleeding usually occurred within 24 hours of birth, sometimes in unusual sites (e.g., the pleural or abdominal cavities). Bleeding has also been reported to occur in utero, leading to stillbirth.[19] The bleeding disorder may be prevented by the maternal ingestion of vitamin K_1 during the last month of pregnancy.[20] Because of the risk of such hemorrhagic complications, vitamin K_1 (1 mg/kg intramuscularly) is sometimes given routinely to newborns of women receiving anticonvulsant drugs during pregnancy. Alternatively, the prothrombin time of cord blood should be measured at delivery of such children; if it is subnormal or there is clinical evidence of bleeding during the neonatal period, intravenous vitamin K_1 should be given. Treatment with infusion of fresh frozen plasma or concentrates of factors II, VII, IX, and X is sometimes necessary also.

Maternal use of barbiturates may be associated with barbiturate withdrawal symptoms in the neonate, with restlessness, irritability, tremulousness, difficulty sleeping, and vasomotor instability, usually beginning a week after birth.

Although anticonvulsant drugs taken by the mother may be present in breast milk, their concentrations are usually too low to have any clinically significant effect on neonates. The rate of transmission into breast milk varies with the drug.[21] Breast-feed-ing need not be discouraged on this basis; however, when obvious sedation develops in an infant and could relate to anticonvulsants in the maternal milk, breast-feeding should be discontinued and the baby observed for signs of drug withdrawal.

Management of Epilepsy During Pregnancy

Epilepsy must be managed during pregnancy, as at other times, by prophylactic anticonvulsant drugs. As indicated earlier, trimethadione and valproic acid are best avoided, but available data concerning relative safety and therapeutic utility of the various anticonvulsant drugs during pregnancy are insufficient to provide any more detailed guidelines at this time for the management of epileptics or of women wishing to become pregnant. Moreover, there is little point in substituting one anticonvulsant drug for another after the first 2 to 3 months of pregnancy because major fetal malformations will probably have occurred already if they are going to occur at all. Folate supplementation (4 mg daily) may help, however, to reduce the risk of teratogenicity.[13]

It is important to monitor anticonvulsant drug treatment during pregnancy by serial measurement of plasma drug levels. Patients should be seen monthly, and as the pregnancy continues, the dose of medication may need to be increased to maintain plasma concentrations at previously effective levels. If increases are made during pregnancy, dose reductions will be necessary at some point following delivery to prevent toxicity, but at a time that must be determined individually based on clinical evaluation and plasma drug levels.

If patients inquire, it is appropriate to indicate that there is a slightly increased risk of fetal malformation due either to the seizure disorder itself or to the drugs used in its treatment. Nevertheless, there is still a very good chance (90 to 95 percent) that offspring will be normal. It must also be emphasized that the risks to both mother and fetus of noncompliance with anticonvulsant drug regimen are considerable, in that an increased seizure frequency or even status epilepticus may occur, with its associated morbidity and mortality.

Obstetrical Management of Epileptic Women

Increased incidences of vaginal hemorrhage and toxemia were reported in epileptic women by Bjerkedal and Bahna,[22] but others have found the incidence of toxemia to be unchanged.[23] There is a significantly increased stillbirth rate in epileptic women, but the incidence of low-birthweight infants is not increased.[24-26] An increased incidence of neonatal death has also been reported,[19,22] perhaps owing to an increased incidence of congenital malformations, iatrogenic neonatal hemorrhage, the metabolic or toxic effects of seizures or anticonvulsant drugs, or socioeconomic factors.

Interactions Between Oral Contraceptives and Anticonvulsant Agents

Certain anticonvulsants (including phenytoin, carbamazepine, phenobarbital, and primidone) may alter the effectiveness of oral contraceptives, leading to unwanted pregnancy.[21] Oral contraceptives may also affect seizure frequency or blood levels of anticonvulsant medication, but this is less clear.

MIGRAINE

Migraine is often influenced by pregnancy. Most commonly, symptoms improve after the first trimester, but occasionally they worsen or occur for the first time during pregnancy. The influence of pregnancy on migraine does not depend on any relation of migraine to the menstrual cycle. Similarly, it does not relate to the sex of the fetus or to differences in plasma progesterone levels, although there may be some relation to changes in the pattern of circulating estrogens.[27] Treatment of migraine during pregnancy is similar to that at other times, with emphasis on the avoidance of precipitating factors together with the use of simple analgesics as necessary. However, acetaminophen should be used in preference to aspirin because there is some evidence that aspirin usage in large dosage in the later stages of pregnancy may prolong labor and increase the incidence of stillbirth.[28] Ergot-containing preparations should be avoided where possible because of the effect that this drug may have on the gravid uterus. There is no evidence that the frequency and nature of congenital abnormalities in the offspring of women taking ergotamine during the first trimester of pregnancy is increased.[29] Propranolol is also best avoided during pregnancy when possible because it may impair fetal growth,[30] and β-adrenergic blockade may inhibit the normal responsiveness of the fetus to asphyxia or other stresses.[31] Other reported complications in neonates include prematurity, respiratory depression, hypoglycemia, and hyperbilirubinemia.[32,33]

Many women, often with a past or family history of migraine,[34] experience mild bifrontal headaches in the week following delivery. These headaches generally respond to simple analgesics and settle spontaneously.

TUMORS

Although any type of intracranial tumor occasionally presents during pregnancy, pituitary adenomas, meningiomas, neurofibromas, hemangioblastomas, and certain vascular malformations sometimes lead to relapses during pregnancy, with partial or complete remission occurring after delivery. The basis of this relation is unclear, but it seems likely that pregnancy produces a slight increase in tumor size. The enlargement of certain pituitary adenomas during pregnancy may be due to the trophic effects of increased circulating estradiol.[34,35] Similarly, an increase in size of meningiomas may relate to a direct trophic effect of gonadal hormones on tumor cells; sex steroid–binding sites have been found in human meningiomas, but there are marked differences in their reported prevalence and concentration.[34] Tumors with symptoms that show a consistent temporal relation to pregnancy are usually so situated that significant neurological involvement, with the development of new symptoms or signs, occurs with only slight expansion of the underlying lesion. Thus, spinal meningiomas are more likely than convexity meningiomas to show a relation of symptoms to pregnancy.

Patients with suspected intracranial neoplasms should be managed during pregnancy as at other times. Magnetic resonance imaging (MRI) is generally the best noninvasive means of establishing the diagnosis and does not involve exposing the fetus to irradiation. Essential operative treatment should not be delayed. However, surgery for pituitary adenomas or other benign tumors diagnosed toward the end of pregnancy can often be delayed until after delivery provided that the patient is followed closely. Radiation therapy may be required during pregnancy and carries a teratogenic risk for the developing fetus, especially if administered during the first trimester. If such therapy cannot be delayed to the latter half of pregnancy or postponed until after delivery, consideration may have to be given to aborting the fetus.

The pregnancy itself can usually be managed normally in patients with intracranial tumors. Concerns that vaginal delivery may exacerbate any existing increase in intracranial pressure due to the tumor are usually misplaced, especially if adequate regional anesthesia is employed and low forceps are used, if necessary, to shorten the second stage of labor. The necessity and justification of therapeutic abortion should be considered on an individual basis in patients with malignant tumors.

The long survival associated with low-grade gliomas suggests that some women with such tumors may wish to become pregnant after the diagnosis has been established. Such decisions need to be made on an individual basis, but patients with these lesions may certainly go through pregnancy without further complications.

PSEUDOTUMOR CEREBRI

Benign intracranial hypertension has a clear association with pregnancy and is especially likely to occur during the first trimester or the postpartum period. Headache and visual disturbances due to papilledema may be accompanied by diplopia due to sixth nerve palsy. Investigations reveal no space-occupying lesion, but the cerebrospinal fluid (CSF) pressure is increased. The disorder is self-limiting, but it may not remit for weeks after delivery, and there may be recurrences during subsequent pregnancies. Treatment, as in the nonpregnant woman, consists of measures to lower the intracranial pressure in order to prevent secondary optic atrophy. It may require the use of acetazolamide, furosemide, corticosteroids, repeated lumbar punctures, or a surgical shunting procedure. Optic nerve decompression and early delivery of the fetus may have to be considered if the intracranial pressure remains high despite these measures. There are no specific obstetrical complications, and a normal birth can be expected.

Intracranial venous sinus thrombosis may simulate pseudotumor cerebri (discussed below).

CEREBROVASCULAR DISEASE

An increased incidence of stroke has been associated with pregnancy and the puerperium as well as with the use of oral contraceptive preparations. The extent to which this increase relates to hormonal changes is unclear. However, sex steroids can certainly affect several physiological and metabolic factors that predispose to cerebral thromboembolic or venous infarction. Estrogens and perhaps some progestogens increase blood coagulability and platelet aggregation, increase the blood pressure, affect serum lipid profiles, and may lead to pathological changes in blood vessels.[35] Sex hormones may also predispose to aneurysm formation or rupture, as suggested by the report of case clustering during the first 5 days of the menstrual cycle.[36] The underlying mechanism is unknown, but suggestions include the possibility that fluctuations in circulating levels of sex hormones have a direct effect on the integrity of cerebral arteries, causing them to become more susceptible to rupture.[35,37] Whether pregnancy influences intracranial arteriovenous malformations (AVMs) is unclear, but it may certainly aggravate spinal AVMs (discussed on p. 574). The microangiopathic syndromes of preeclampsia, thrombotic thrombocytopenic purpura, and hemolytic-uremic syndrome are considered briefly on p. 582.

Occlusive Arterial Disease

Most cases of nonhemorrhagic hemiplegia developing during pregnancy or the postpartum period are due to arterial occlusion.[38] As in nonpregnant patients, this may relate to thrombus formation on an atheromatous plaque; inflammatory disorders such as arteritis or meningovascular syphilis; hematological disorders such as polycythemia and sickle cell disease; and cardiac disorders such as a cardiomyopathy, rheumatic or ischemic heart disease, cardiac dysrhythmias, subacute bacterial endocarditis, and cardiac myxoma. During pregnancy, in addition, stroke may be predisposed to by anemia, hormonal factors, changes in blood coagulation factors, increased platelet aggregation, hypertension, and puerperal septicemia.

The blood is said to be in a hypercoagulable state during pregnancy; there is a rise in all procoagulant factors except XI and XIII, and increased thrombin activity. Circulating inhibitors of coagulation, such as protein C and protein S, are reduced during normal pregnancy, and antithrombin III is reduced under certain circumstances.[39] The activity of the fibrinolytic system is also reduced during pregnancy.[39] These various changes will predispose pregnant women to stroke. Other factors also become important risk factors for stroke during the gestational period. Hemoglobinopathies, for example, may lead to significant maternal morbidity during pregnancy. Thus, women with sickle cell disease are especially likely to experience crises, usually vaso-occlusive, during pregnancy.[40] Sickle cell disease is also associated with an increased incidence of obstetrical complication—including abortion, growth retardation, preterm birth, and stillbirth—although fetal wastage has been reduced considerably in recent years by improved prenatal care.[40] The presence of circulating antiphospholipid autoantibodies is similarly associated with a high rate of maternal arterial and venous thrombotic events and of transient ischemic attacks,[41] as well as with obstetrical complications such as a high rate of spontaneous abortion and of early-onset, atypical preeclampsia.[42] Pregnancy may represent an especially high risk for thromboembolic disease in patients with these antibodies.[42]

A peripartum cardiomyopathy may occur during the last trimester of pregnancy or the puerperium, especially in the presence of twinning, toxemia, or postpartum hypertension[43]; it sometimes presents with embolic phenomena necessitating anticoagulation.[44] Its precise cause is unclear, but nutritional, hormonal, viral, and immunological mechanisms have been suggested in the past.[43]

Rare cases have been described of segmental cerebral vasoconstriction ("vasospasm") of uncertain cause in young adults.[45] Such a syndrome may occur during pregnancy or the postpartum period and lead to a fatal outcome.[46] A reversible intimal hyperplasia of the cerebral vasculature during pregnancy has also been described as a rare cause of stroke or transient ischemic attack during the gestational period,[47] but such cases are poorly documented and hard to interpret. There are rare reports of arterial occlusion by paradoxical embolization from a pelvic vein via a patent foramen ovale. Fat, air, or amniotic fluid embolism may also occur during childbirth[48] but usually present with dyspnea, shock, and acute encephalopathy.

As in nonpregnant women, transient cerebral ischemic attacks may precede occlusion of one of the major intracranial arteries. Neurological investigation and management should not be influenced by the pregnancy, but special shielding during radiological studies may help to protect the developing fetus. Angiographic delineation of degenerative atherosclerotic disease in a localized arterial segment that is surgically accessible may permit disobliterative surgery. If surgery is decided against or there is more widespread atherosclerotic disease, treatment with aspirin may be commenced. A cardiac source of emboli usually necessitates treatment with warfarin. This drug is associated with risks of teratogenicity and fetal wastage when used during the first trimester, and it crosses the placenta, thereby increasing the risk of hemorrhagic complications. Accordingly, patients requiring anticoagulation during pregnancy are best maintained on subcutaneous heparin, which is discontinued with the onset of labor and restarted about 12 hours after vaginal delivery (or 24 hours after cesarean section).

The optimal mangement of labor and delivery in patients who have had a stroke during pregnancy is unclear. In most cases, vaginal delivery assisted by forceps is probably satisfactory. The blood pressure will need to be monitored closely, however, to avoid excessively high or low levels.

Occlusive Venous Disease

Aseptic intracranial venous thrombosis may occur during pregnancy for reasons that are unclear. It has been attributed to coagulation abnormalities, changes in the constituents of peripheral blood, and intimal damage to dural sinuses. The extent to which it relates to hormonal changes is unknown. In only 7 of 34 cases of autopsy-verified cerebral venous thrombosis was there any evidence that pelvic or leg veins were thrombosed.[49]

Intracranial venous thrombosis occurs most commonly during the third trimester of pregnancy or the postpartum period, sometimes in relation to preeclampsia.[49] Although it may, in fact, occur at any time during a normal pregnancy, when it develops during the first trimester it usually is in relation to some complication such as spontaneous or therapeutic abortion. It is characterized clinically by headache, seizures, obtundation, confusion, and sometimes focal neurological disturbances. Examination commonly reveals papilledema, and there may be signs of meningeal irritation from subarachnoid bleeding secondary to cortical infarction. CSF pressure is often increased, and its protein or cell content may be increased. Radiological imaging procedures [computed tomography (CT) scan, MRI, and arteriography] confirm the diagnosis and help to exclude arterial pathology.

Treatment of intracranial venous thrombosis is controversial. Anticonvulsant drugs and antiedema agents may be helpful. Anticoagulation with dose-adjusted intravenous heparin may also be helpful despite the risk of provoking hemorrhagic complications.[50] About one-third of patients do not survive, and survivors may experience recurrence of thrombosis later in the same pregnancy or in subsequent ones.[51,52]

Cesarean section may be necessary if venous thrombosis has occurred before or during labor. If it occurs early in the pregnancy, labor can generally be allowed to commence spontaneously, delivery being assisted with forceps if necessary.

Pituitary Infarction or Hemorrhage

Acute infarction or hemorrhage of the pituitary gland, especially around the time of delivery, is a well recognized complication that leads to hypopituitarism if the patient survives the acute event. The disorder may occur in patients with preexisting diabetes or in those who experience such obstetrical complica-

tions as postpartum hemorrhage with vascular collapse. It may also occur in patients with coagulopathies or with a pituitary adenoma. The extent of pituitary damage governs the severity of pituitary hypofunction. The initial symptom may be failure of lactation. Emergency treatment with corticosteroids and transsphenoidal decompression of the intrasellar content may need to be considered to preserve life and vision. Management otherwise is with hormone replacement therapy.

Disseminated Intravascular Coagulation

Disseminated intravascular coagulation may occur in patients with a variety of obstetrical complications. It is discussed in Chapter 12, and further consideration here is unnecessary.

Subarachnoid Hemorrhage From Intracranial Vascular Anomalies

Subarachnoid hemorrhage may occur during pregnancy from an aneurysm or cerebral AVM. The morbidity and mortality is greater with the former. Although Robinson and associates suggested that pregnancy had an adverse effect on intracranial AVMs, making them more likely to bleed,[53] this has not been substantiated by others.[54–56]

Symptoms and signs of subarachnoid hemorrhage are as in nonpregnant patients. The hemorrhage may be the first indication of the underlying lesion. An AVM is somewhat more likely than an aneurysm to be responsible if subarachnoid hemorrhage is accompanied by a major focal neurological deficit (suggesting an intracerebral hematoma). CT scan of the head is a reliable means of detecting recent subarachnoid or intracerebral bleeding and may permit the causal lesion to be identified and localized. Arteriography permits the identity of the lesion to be confirmed and provides information about its anatomical characteristics that is especially important in planning operative treatment. All of the major intracranial vessels should be opacified because feeders to AVMs sometimes arise from the contralateral side, and aneurysms may be multiple. Special shielding during radiological studies is necessary for pregnant women in order to protect the developing fetus.

The management of subarachnoid hemorrhage is as for nonpregnant women. Because of the high risk of rebleeding in survivors of a ruptured aneurysm, operative treatment should not be delayed because of pregnancy if the clinical and arteriographic findings indicate its feasibility. Although ruptured AVMs may also bleed again, this may not be for months or years after the initial hemorrhage, and neurosurgical treatment can often be postponed until the pregnancy is over.

The obstetrical management of survivors of a subarachnoid hemorrhage is controversial. In patients with aneurysms that have been successfully treated by surgery or in whom rupture occurred before the last trimester, pregnancy and delivery can generally be permitted to continue normally. In patients with unoperated or incompletely obliterated aneurysms that ruptured during the last trimester of pregnancy, cesarean section at 38 weeks' gestation is probably appropriate. Some have also suggested delivery by cesarean section at 38 weeks for women with AVMs, with subsequent sterilization to prevent further pregnancies,[53] but this measure seems unjustified.

Intracranial hemorrhage during pregnancy or the postpartum period may also occur in association with hypertension, vasculitis, various hematological disorders, mycotic aneurysms, cocaine abuse,[57,58] moyamoya disease,[59] or as a manifestation of choriocarcinoma.[60] Treatment is of the underlying cause.

Intracranial Dural AVMs

Dural AVMs may present during pregnancy, sometimes following abortion, or during the postpartum period.[61,62] The anomalous arteriovenous shunt may involve either the anterior-inferior group of dural sinuses (cavernous, intercavernous, sphenoparietal, superior and inferior petrosal, and basilar plexus) or the superior-posterior group (superior and inferior sagittal, straight, transverse, sigmoid, and occipital).[63] Anomalies involving the former group lead typically to unilateral orbital or head pain, diplopia, a proptosed or red eye, tinnitus, or some combination of these symptoms. Malformations involving the superior-posterior dural sinuses may lead to subarachnoid hemorrhage, increased intracranial pressure, tinnitus, seizures, or focal neurological deficits due to cerebral ischemia. In either case, there may be papilledema, and a bruit is often present either over the eye (with involvement of the anterior-inferior sinuses) or about the mastoid region or ear (superior-posterior sinuses involved).

Arteriography is necessary to localize the shunt with certainty and determine its anatomical features. With shunts to the anterior-inferior dural sinuses, embolization of feeding vessels may help to preserve vision or relieve intolerable symptoms. Ligation or embolization of feeding vessels is often helpful in relieving symptoms from shunts to the superior-posterior dural sinuses, and a direct surgical approach is also sometimes feasible.

Spinal AVMs

Spinal AVMs are usually either dural or intradural in location. They may lead to spinal subarachnoid hemorrhage or to a myeloradiculopathy that can either present acutely or develop insidiously. Symptoms are generally progressive. At least one-half of the survivors of subarachnoid hemorrhage from a spinal AVM have further episodes of bleeding, and one-half of the subsequent survivors bleed again unless the underlying lesion is treated.[64] Similarly, once there is any functional impairment in the legs due to the myeloradiculopathy, disability is likely to worsen, so that 50 percent of patients become unable to walk at all or require two sticks or crutches to do so, within 3 years.[64] Cord or root symptoms may show a characteristic relation to exercise or posture and occasionally to pregnancy or the menstrual cycle.[64]

Typically, examination reveals a mixed upper and lower motor neuron deficit in the legs, often with an associated sensory disturbance that occasionally has a radicular distribution. There may be a coexisting cutaneous malformation that sometimes relates segmentally to the spinal lesion. A spinal bruit may be present.

Unruptured spinal AVMs probably produce symptoms by causing venous hypertension. Although they are usually extramedullary, their draining veins connect with veins draining the spinal cord. The increased venous pressure leads to a reduction in the arteriovenous pressure gradient across the cord and thus to a reduction in spinal blood flow.[64] Pressure on pelvic or abdominal veins by the gravid uterus could aggravate symptoms of caudally situated AVMs by obstructing venous return to the heart, thereby reducing still more the arteriovenous pressure gradient across the cord.[64] Whether anemia and hemodilution are also partly responsible for exacerbations of symptoms during pregnancy is unclear, and it is not known if sex hormones exert direct trophic influences on AVMs.

Recent advances in imaging procedures have revealed that the nidus of many spinal AVMs is situated durally, and these lesions are thus readily accessible to embolization or surgical intervention. Treatment is indicated in patients with progressive symptoms, functional incapacity, or a history of hemorrhage. Treatment is clearly more difficult for AVMs located anteriorly or within the cord, but in some of these, also, the actual nidus of the lesion is dural and thus operable.

INFECTIONS

A variety of organisms may infect the nervous system, as discussed in Chapters 33 to 41. Pregnancy is reportedly associated with a depression of cell-mediated immunity[65] that may interfere with resistance to specific infectious agents (as well as permitting fetal retention), thereby endangering maternal health. Treatment of various infections may also be complicated during pregnancy because of the need to avoid certain antimicrobial agents if possible. When infection occurs during pregnancy, it may pose risks to the developing fetus from the infective organism and the drugs used in its treatment. Thus, obstetrical management may be complicated. The evidence that there are changes in the immune system during pregnancy and that resistance to certain infections is reduced has recently been reviewed by Weinberg,[65] but there is no general agreement concerning the subject.

Pregnancy increases the susceptibility of women to clinical *poliomyelitis,* but it is not clear whether this is because pregnant women are more susceptible to the initial viral infection or to invasion of the nervous system. Weakness tends to be more severe and widespread when poliomyelitis develops during the late stages of pregnancy. Poliomyelitis affects the course of pregnancy. During the first trimester, spontaneous abortion may occur with apparently mild nonparalytic attacks of the disease or in conjunction with a febrile reaction in its acute phase. Abortion or fetal loss may also occur during later stages of pregnancy,

but usually in conjunction with severe poliomyelitis. The uterine muscle is not paralyzed in women with poliomyelitis, and labor can usually be managed as in normal women unless there are specific obstetrical indications for cesarean section or induction of labor. Normal offspring can be anticipated, although neonatal poliomyelitis may occur.[66] Neonatal involvement within the first 5 days of life is generally assumed to follow transplacental transmission of the virus and is associated with a 50 percent or greater mortality rate.

Tetanus is an important complication of abortion or delivery, especially in the developing countries, and is associated with a high mortality rate. In addition to treating the tetanus, any retained products must be evacuated from the uterus, and hysterectomy is sometimes necessary. Neonatal tetanus results from contamination of the umbilical cord, and in some areas the mortality is so high that it approaches 10 percent of all births. Infants are usually diagnosed within 10 days; the history is typically that of increased irritability for up to 48 hours, followed by cessation of sucking and crying, accompanied by convulsions and often by fever.[67] Improved maternity facilities and the active immunization of pregnant women are important public health measures to counter this disorder.

Maternal infection with *Listeria monocytogenes* may lead to abortion or stillbirth and in neonates to either an early-onset, predominantly septicemic infection or a late-onset, predominantly meningitic or meningoencephalitic infection.[68] The bacteriological and serological findings suggest the diagnosis, and treatment is with appropriate antibiotics.

Maternal *rubella,* especially during the first trimester, may lead to congenital fetal malformations. Ocular abnormalities, seizures, mental retardation, deafness, focal neurological deficits, and other abnormalities including cardiac anomalies occur in a variety of combinations. Much more rarely, a panencephalitic illness has been reported during the second decade of life in patients with congenital rubella and leads to pyramidal and extrapyramidal signs, seizures, and dementia. High antibody titers to rubella virus occur in the blood and CSF, and the virus may be isolated from the brain.[69,70]

Congenital *toxoplasmosis* may lead to meningoencephalitis, chorioretinitis, obstructive hydrocephalus, and cerebral calcification. Pregnant women should therefore be advised to keep away from cat feces and to avoid ingestion of raw or undercooked meat or eggs.

Fetal infection with *cytomegalovirus* may lead to a variety of somatic manifestations. Neurological involvement may be manifest by cerebral malformation, microcephaly, mental retardation, seizures, obstructive hydrocephalus, cerebral calcification, deafness, chorioretinitis, or some combination of these disorders.

Neonatal infection with *herpes simplex virus* leads primarily to visceral involvement. When there is neurological involvement, manifestations may include seizures, irritability, increased intracranial pressure, depressed level of consciousness, and motor deficits.

Maternal *syphilis* is an important disorder to recognize and treat. It is associated with an increased rate of spontaneous abortion and increased perinatal mortality. Offspring of affected mothers may have symptomatic congenital syphilis. Infection may also occur at birth if infants come into contact with an infective lesion. The clinical features of congenital neurosyphilis are similar to those of neurosyphilis in adults. They may become apparent at any time after the first few weeks of life, or they can be delayed for several years. Treatment is of the underlying infection, penicillin being the drug of choice. Fetal infection usually occurs in the second half of pregnancy. Thus, treatment at an early stage of pregnancy generally prevents fetal involvement, emphasizing the importance of serological testing during antenatal care.

Tuberculous meningitis may occur during pregnancy and is then associated with a higher mortality and neurological morbidity than otherwise.[71] Its treatment is discussed further in Chapter 35.

Children born to women with *acquired immunodeficiency syndrome* (AIDS) are at risk of developing the disease after an interval that varies from several months to several years. Infection may occur during fetal development, at birth, or from breast milk.[72] Neurological manifestations of the disorder are particularly frequent in such children and are due to a progressive encephalopathy that leads to developmental delay or regression, with CT evidence of cortical atrophy. Calcification of the basal ganglia also occurs. Other manifestations of the disease include failure to thrive, interstitial pneumonitis, hepatosplenomegaly, and increased susceptibility to bacterial infections.[73]

Children of women infected with human T-cell leukemia virus, type I (HTLV-I) may acquire the infection through breast-feeding and develop a resulting myelopathy in adult life. This is considered further in Chapter 39.

METABOLIC DISORDERS

Clinical presentation of the neurological manifestations of *vitamin B$_{12}$ deficiency* (myelopathy, polyneuropathy, mental changes, optic neuropathy) do not differ during pregnancy, but any accompanying megaloblastic anemia may be obscured by folic acid supplements. As in the nonpregnant patient, treatment is with parenteral vitamin B$_{12}$ to arrest progression and correct reversible neurological deficits. Maternal vitamin B$_{12}$ deficiency during pregnancy may lead to similar deficiency in neonates, exacerbated in breast-fed infants by the reduced content of vitamin B$_{12}$ in maternal milk. Clinically, such infants exhibit apathy, developmental delay or regression, involuntary movements, cutaneous pigmentation, and megaloblastic anemia.[74] Treatment is with vitamin supplementation.

Phenylketonuria, with its autosomal recessive inheritance, is an important cause of mental retardation. Neonatal screening programs can identify affected infants so they can be treated before intellectual function deteriorates.[75] Affected women have a high rate of spontaneous abortion. Offspring of untreated women have a high incidence of mental retardation, microcephaly, and congenital heart disease, which correlates with maternal blood levels of phenylalanine.[76] Dietary treatment during pregnancy has not prevented these fetal effects, and it may be that treatment must be initiated before conception occurs. To ensure that the diagnosis is not missed, antenatal screening for maternal phenylketonuria, or testing at the first antenatal visit of women with a positive family history, low intelligence of uncertain cause, or a history of microcephalic offspring is probably justifiable.[77] The homozygous offspring of an affected mother requires a diet low in phenylalanine, but the most appropriate nutritional management of heterozygotes is less certain. In any event, the affected mother should avoid breast-feeding because of the high concentration of phenylalanine in her milk.[77]

MOVEMENT DISORDERS

Movement disorders of any type may occur during pregnancy, as at other times. Comment here is restricted to those related more specifically to pregnancy or posing obstetrical problems.

Chorea gravidarum occurs most often in primigravidas, frequently without evidence of preceding streptococcal infection, as a variant of Sydenham's chorea. About two-thirds of patients have a history of chorea or rheumatic fever, and most of the others have signs of rheumatic heart disease. Symptoms usually begin early in pregnancy; they remit after delivery but may recur during subsequent pregnancies. Altered patterns of circulating sex hormones during pregnancy may account for the chorea by their effects on previously damaged basal ganglia. Such a notion is supported by the observation that the chorea improves following delivery or abortion, as sex hormone levels return to prepregnancy values, and by the occurrence of chorea in women taking oral contraceptives.[35] The prognosis relates to cardiac complications. The neurological disorder generally benefits from bed rest and sedation. It is not an indication for termination of pregnancy and there are no specific obstetrical complications.

Chorea developing for the first time during pregnancy does not necessarily represent a variant of Sydenham's chorea. Huntington's chorea may occasionally present during pregnancy, and chorea may also develop at this time due to systemic lupus erythematosus, polycythemia vera rubra, thyrotoxicosis, hypocalcemia, encephalitis, cerebrovascular disease, or Wilson's disease, or as a drug-induced reaction.

Chorea may be induced by oral contraceptives, sometimes in women with preexisting abnormalities of the basal ganglia. It usually begins about 3 months after starting on the contraceptives, tends to evolve subacutely, may be asymmetrical or unilateral, and settles with discontinuation of the causal agent. Its pathophysiological basis is unknown, but vascular or immunological mechanisms or a hormone-dependent alteration in central dopaminergic activity have been proposed.[78]

A number of pregnant women develop the *restless legs syndrome,* usually during the latter part of pregnancy.[79] Unpleasant creeping sensations occur in the legs and occasionally the arms, usually at night or during relaxation, leading to a compelling need to move about. The cause is unknown. Neurological examination reveals no abnormalities. Treatment of coexisting anemia or iron deficiency may improve symptoms, and treatment with diazepam or clonazepam is sometimes worthwhile. Other drugs that may be helpful include carbidopa-levodopa (Sinemet), bromocriptine, carbamazepine, propranolol, and baclofen, but these drugs are usually best avoided during pregnancy.[79]

Untreated *Wilson's disease,* an autosomal recessive disorder, is associated with a high miscarriage rate, but pregnancy poses no special problems in patients receiving adequate chelation treatment. There have been some concerns that chelating agents may cause fetal abnormalities by inhibiting the synthesis and maturation of collagen,[80] but use during pregnancy does not lead to fetal connective tissue abnormalities.[81,82] Nevertheless, some have suggested that penicillamine dosage be reduced to 250 mg daily about 6 weeks before delivery if cesarean section is planned in order to avoid any impairment of wound healing.[81]

When acute *dystonia* develops during pregnancy, the most probable cause is use of a dopamine-antagonist antiemetic (or neuroleptic), such as metoclopramide. In patients with long-standing dystonia of either the idiopathic or secondary variety, there is no evidence that pregnancy will affect the neurological outcome adversely. Pregnant patients with dystonia should be offered genetic counseling if the disorder has a hereditary basis; the conduct of labor will depend on the severity and nature of the abnormal posturing.

Parkinson's disease may develop in women who are still young enough to bear children, and concerns are sometimes expressed about the possible effects of pregnancy on the neurological disorder. A recent study has shown no consistent effect on overall parkinsonian disability, although some patients did show a worsening of their neurological symptoms; among the series of patients that was studied, there was no increase in the incidence of obstetrical complications or fetal defects.[83]

MULTIPLE SCLEROSIS

The classic, unpredictable relapses and remissions that occur in multiple sclerosis make it difficult to determine if pregnancy influences the disorder. However, several epidemiological studies have suggested that there is an increased frequency of relapses during the 3 to 6 months immediately after childbirth.[84-88] Neither pregnancy itself nor the number of pregnancies affects the degree of subsequent neurological disability,[89,90] and multiple sclerosis does not influence the course of pregnancy or childbirth.[91-93]

Pregnant women with multiple sclerosis are often concerned about their offspring developing the disease. Although multiple sclerosis may indeed show a familial incidence, this association is uncommon and tends to involve siblings rather than different generations, so that firm reassurance can generally be given. Pregnancy and parenthood should not be discouraged unless the patient is incapable of coping with the demands involved. Neurological management during pregnancy is as at other times, but patients with sphincter disturbances or a paraparesis may pose particular problems. The method of delivery should be guided by obstetrical factors alone.

OPTIC NEURITIS

Optic neuritis of any type may occur fortuitously during pregnancy. Optic nerve involvement is a rare complication of hyperemesis gravidarum, and uncontrollable vomiting may necessitate termination of pregnancy.[94] Optic nerve involvement may occur during pregnancy or the postpartum period in patients with multiple sclerosis or tumors that enlarge slightly during the gestational period. Genetic counseling is important if there is a family history of hereditary optic atrophy.

TRAUMATIC PARAPLEGIA

When spinal injury occurs during pregnancy, the patient must be investigated and managed with her own best interests in mind. Despite concerns that radiological studies might affect the developing fetus, such studies should not be postponed if indicated neurologically.

Patients with established paraplegia should be educated about (1) the importance of avoiding urinary infection by ensuring a minimal amount of residual urine after micturition and (2) the best means of avoiding pressure sores. Care should be taken to prevent anemia during pregnancy. Unless a paraplegic woman has a gross impairment of renal function, however, she need not be discouraged from pregnancy if she wishes to have a family.

The conduct of labor is complicated in paraplegic women. With complete cord lesions above T10, onset of labor will be unrecognized and labor will be painless. For this reason, the cervix is usually examined at each antenatal visit after about the 26th week of pregnancy; patients are hospitalized if the cervix is dilated or routinely after about 32 weeks of pregnancy. With cord lesions below T10, uterine contractions are accompanied by normal pain sensations.

Complete cord lesions above T5 or T6 may be associated with autonomic hyperreflexia. Headache, sweating, nasal congestion, hypertension, reflex bradycardia, and cutaneous vasodilatation and piloerection above the level of the lesion are often conspicuous during the uterine contractions of labor, becoming especially marked just before delivery. If unrecognized, the disorder is sometimes mistaken for preeclampsia. Symptoms have been attributed to release of catecholamines. Treatment has included reserpine (to deplete catecholamines from sympathetic nerve terminals), atropine, clonidine, glyceryl trinitrate, or hexamethonium. Continuous lumbar epidural anesthesia has also been used to block autonomic hyperreflexia.

Cesarean section is not necessarily indicated by the paraplegia itself but may be required if there is bony deformity of the spine or pelvis. Forceps delivery may be necessary to compensate for paralysis of muscle involved in the expulsive efforts of the second stage or to shorten delivery time because of severe hypertension. Paraplegic or even quadriplegic patients have a normal milk ejection reflex during suckling and can breast-feed their babies.

ROOT AND PLEXUS LESIONS

Acute prolapse of a lumbar intervertebral disc is rare during pregnancy. Management of the acute prolapse is as in nonpregnant women, but it is important to distinguish the disorder from conditions simulating it. Compressive injuries of the lumbosacral plexus may occur during labor and can be difficult to distinguish from an acutely prolapsed lumbar intervertebral disc. However, the latter is associated with tenderness and rigidity of the lumbar spine, sciatica, and signs of root tension. Electrophysiological studies may also clarify the diagnosis, depending on whether there is evidence of involvement of the paraspinal muscles (which are supplied proximally from the nerve roots).

Lumbosacral plexus lesions result from compression by the fetal head or obstetrical forceps of the roots of the sciatic nerve. This injury is especially likely when there is minor disproportion or when midforceps are used during delivery because of malpresentation. Anatomical features of the pelvis that predispose to this complication include a straight sacrum, a flat, wide posterior pelvis, posterior displacement of the transverse diameter of the inlet, wide sacroiliac notches, and prominent ischial spines.[95] Symptoms are usually unilateral and develop immediately after delivery. There is often predominant involvement of peroneal fibers, as reflected by the distribution of motor and sensory findings. With mild injuries the prognosis for recovery is excellent, but recovery may be prolonged and incomplete if axonal degeneration has occurred. Electrophysiological studies therefore assist in determining prognosis. Treatment of severe cases with calipers and a night cast prevents contractures.

Despite an obstetrical lumbosacral plexus palsy, delivery in subsequent pregnancies need not be by cesarean section. However, cesarean section is appropriate if the infant is large or there are premonitory symptoms suggesting nerve compression with attempted engagement of the fetal head during the last 4 weeks of pregnancy.

Brachial plexopathy may occur on a familial basis, and in some of the reported cases there has been a clear association of attacks with pregnancy or the puerperium.[96]

PERIPHERAL NERVE DISORDERS

Entrapment Neuropathies

Two entrapment neuropathies are especially likely to occur during pregnancy. *Carpal tunnel syndrome* occurs often, possibly because of fluid retention. Nocturnal pain and paresthesias in the hand disturb sleep. Weakness of the thenar muscles occurs in more advanced cases. The clinical and electrophysiological features of the disorder do not require description here. When the syndrome develops during pregnancy, it often settles within about 3 months of delivery, and treatment should therefore be conservative. The use of a nocturnal wrist splint is often helpful for alleviating symptoms, the splint being placed on the dorsal surface with the aim of maintaining the wrist in a neutral or slightly flexed position. Local injection of corticosteroids into the carpal tunnel or treatment with diuretics sometimes helps. The patient should be reassured about the benign nature of her symptoms. Surgical division of the anterior carpal ligament is usually unnecessary unless symptoms become intolerable or continue to progress in the weeks following delivery.

Entrapment of the lateral femoral cutaneous nerve is also common during pregnancy, especially in its later stages, and leads to the syndrome of *meralgia paresthetica*. Pain, paresthesias, and numbness occur about the outer aspect of the thigh, usually unilaterally, and are sometimes relieved by sitting. Clinical examination reveals no abnormality except in advanced cases, when cutaneous sensation may be disturbed in the affected area. Symptoms generally settle spontaneously within a few weeks of delivery, and the patient can therefore be reassured. In rare instances, however, the pain has reportedly been so severe that labor has been induced early. Local injection of hydrocortisone about the region where the nerve lies medial to the anterior superior illiac spine may provide temporary benefit.

Traumatic Mononeuropathies

A number of isolated nerve lesions may occur as a complication of various obstetrical maneuvers. The *obturator nerve* may be injured when the patient is in the lithotomy position, because of angulation as the nerve leaves the obturator foramen. It may also be compressed between the fetal head and the bony pelvic wall. Similarly, an isolated *femoral neuropathy* may occur by angulation and pressure from the inguinal ligament when the thighs are markedly flexed and abducted, as when anesthetized patients are placed in the lithotomy position; stretch of the nerve by excessive hip abduction and external rotation may also be important.[97] The *saphenous nerve* may be injured by pressure from leg braces when the patient is improperly suspended in the lithotomy position. The most common cause of a *sciatic nerve* palsy is a misplaced deep intramuscular injection, but this nerve can also be injured by stretch when a patient is placed in stirrups on the obstetrical table. Burkhart and Daly have cautioned that, to avoid such injury, the knee and hip joints should be well flexed and extreme external rotation of the hip avoided.[98] The *common peroneal nerve* may be injured in the region of the head of the fibula by pressure from the leg braces of the obstetrical table, especially in anesthetized women. The clinical features of all these neuropathies are well known and are not recapitulated here.

Damage during labor and delivery to the innervation of the sphincter muscles in the pelvic floor may be responsible for stress incontinence of urine or feces, as discussed in Chapter 26.

Bell's Palsy

Idiopathic lower motor neuron facial palsy is common and shows a definite association with pregnancy. The incidence of Bell's palsy among nonpregnant women of childbearing age was reported by Hilsinger and associates as 17.4 per 100,000 per year, whereas during pregnancy the rate was 45.1 per 100,000 births.[99] Considered in terms of year of exposure, the risk to pregnant women was more than three times that to nonpregnant women of similar age. About 85 percent of cases occurred during the third trimester of pregnancy or the puerperium. Most patients with Bell's palsy recover completely without treatment. Despite questions concerning the validity of trials assessing its therapeutic efficacy, treatment with corticosteroids is generally prescribed for Bell's palsy, especially if a poor prognosis is anticipated because of severe pain or a clinically complete palsy and if patients are seen within the first week of the disorder. It is this author's policy to prescribe corticosteroids only to patients with a poor prognosis for recovery.

Polyneuropathies

There is no specific polyneuropathy of pregnancy, but any type may occur during the gestational period. *Nutritional deficiency* is probably the most likely cause in patients from one of the developing nations or in those with hyperemesis. There may be evidence of peripheral nerve involvement in patients with hyperemesis gravidarum complicated by Wernicke's en-

cephalopathy and sometimes by Korsakoff's syndrome. Diagnosis is confirmed by finding a marked reduction in blood transketolase activity and a marked thiamine pyrophosphate effect. As in nonpregnant women, treatment is with thiamine, 50 mg being given once intravenously and then intramuscularly for several days until a satisfactory diet is ensured. Vitamin B_{12} deficiency was discussed earlier (see p. 576).

Guillain-Barré syndrome may occur during pregnancy, but it does not do so more commonly than at other times, and its course is not influenced by pregnancy. About 3 percent of patients have one or more relapses, sometimes several years after the initial illness, and they occasionally occur in relation to pregnancy.[100,101] A recent study suggested that there is an increased risk of relapse of *chronic inflammatory demyelinating polyneuropathy* during pregnancy.[102]

Pregnancy may lead to acute exacerbations in the hepatic type of *porphyria*. The usual neurological manifestation is a polyneuropathy that is predominantly motor but sometimes has pronounced autonomic accompaniments. Cerebral manifestations may also occur. In many patients with hepatic porphyria, however, pregnancy is well tolerated. Relapses may occur at any time, but are most likely to do so during early pregnancy and may then lead to spontaneous abortion. Patients with this disorder who are contemplating pregnancy must therefore understand the implications and uncertain outcome, and they must be monitored closely during the gestational period. Caution must also be exercised in the medications used during and after labor, as they may provoke exacerbations.

MYASTHENIA GRAVIS

Exacerbations of myasthenia gravis may occur in relation to the menstrual period. The disorder may be influenced in an unpredictable manner by pregnancy, and the effect of pregnancy may vary in the same patient on different occasions. Osserman reported that definite remission occurred during pregnancy in about one-third of cases, relapse in another one-third, and there was no change in the remainder.[103] Somewhat similar findings were reported in a more recent study, but a significant additional number of relapses occurred in the postpartum period, when they tended to be particularly severe.[104] Severe relapse of the disorder may suggest the need for termination of pregnancy, but termination does not necessarily lead to clinical benefit.

Myasthenia gravis has little effect on pregnancy itself, but there is sometimes a marked contrast between the strength of uterine contractions during the second stage of labor and the severity of skeletal muscle weakness. Enemas should not be given, as they may precipitate a myasthenic crisis. Cesarean section should be reserved for patients in whom it is indicated for obstetrical reasons. Regional anesthesia rather than general anesthesia is desirable, and the use of muscle relaxant drugs should be avoided if possible. Magnesium sulfate should not be used in myasthenic patients with toxemia because of its effects on neuromuscular transmission.

Neonatal myasthenia, a transient disorder that may relate to placental transfer of maternal antibodies against acetylcholine receptors, occurs in about 10 to 15 percent of the newborn babies of myasthenic women, regardless of the duration or severity of the maternal illness.[105] Infants of myasthenic mothers should therefore be watched carefully for clinical signs of the disorder: a poor cry, respiratory difficulties, weakness in sucking, feeble limb movements, and a weak Moro reflex. Symptoms generally become apparent within the first 3 days of birth but are not usually apparent immediately after birth. The neonatal disorder can be treated with anticholinesterase drugs if necessary, and it usually subsides within 6 weeks of delivery. Its occurrence in one child does not imply that subsequent children born to the same mother will also have the disorder.

The transient neonatal form of myasthenia is distinct from congenital myasthenia, which is rare, occurs in children born to healthy mothers, and is a lifelong disorder that varies in type with age of onset, severity, and pathogenesis.

MYOTONIC DYSTROPHY

The weakness and myotonia of myotonic dystrophy may worsen during pregnancy, and the course of the disorder sometimes appears to accelerate during the gestational period. A number of obstetrical complications have been reported, including threatened, spontaneous, and habitual abortion. Hydramnios has been attributed to diminished fetal swallowing.[106] Premature onset of labor in patients with myotonic dystrophy has sometimes been attributed to abnormalities of uterine muscle.[107] The uterus may fail to contract normally during labor, so that the first stage is prolonged, and retention of the placenta and postpartum hemorrhage may occur. Skeletal muscle weakness may also lead to difficulties during the second stage of labor. If anesthesia is required for obstetrical reasons, depolarizing muscle relaxant drugs should be avoided because they may cause myotonic spasm,[108] and nondepolarizing drugs are given in reduced dosage to patients who are taking quinine for their myotonia. Electrocardiographic monitoring facilitates the early recognition of cardiac arrhythmias, to which patients with myotonic dystrophy are prone. General anesthetics may lead to marked respiratory depression,[106] and regional analgesia is the preferred method of management.

Myotonic dystrophy may occur congenitally among the offspring of mothers with the disease. There may be a history of hydramnios or reduced fetal activity during late pregnancy. Affected infants may die within hours or a few days of birth. Clinical features of the disorder in such infants include facial diplegia, hypotonia, respiratory distress, difficulty feeding, delayed motor development, and mental retardation.[106] Talipes is also common. Myotonia is absent clinically in neonates with the congenital form of myotonic dystrophy but is uniformly present in children aged 10 years or more.

In congenital myotonic dystrophy, transmission is generally via the mother. The data suggest that the disorder results from the combination of the gene responsible for the disorder in adults with some additional maternally transmitted factor.[106]

Genetic counseling is an important consideration for women with myotonic dystrophy who are contemplating pregnancy. Recent advances in molecular biology have permitted prenatal detection of the disorder,[109–111] thereby providing the opportunity for abortion of an affected fetus.

ECLAMPSIA AND PREECLAMPSIA

Reference has not been made in this chapter to eclampsia, which is usually treated by obstetricians rather than neurologists. The pathophysiological basis of the seizures or coma that occur in patients with eclampsia is unclear, but the cerebral dysfunction has been attributed to a number of factors including intensive vasoconstriction, cerebral edema, and disseminated intravascular coagulation in the cerebral microcirculation.[112] The relationship between hypertension, seizures, and cerebral dysfunction is unclear and unpredictable. Treatment generally consists in controlling hypertension, preventing convulsions, and reducing cerebral edema. In extreme cases, termination of pregnancy may be necessary. In general, seizures can be controlled with intravenous diazepam, with the addition of phenytoin if necessary. Many obstetricians prefer to use magnesium sulfate to control eclamptic seizures, although the justification for this method has been questioned.[112] Magnesium sulfate has not been shown in controlled studies in humans to be an effective anticonvulsant drug and, until adequately designed therapeutic trials have been performed, treatment of the patient with eclampsia should be based on the use of anticonvulsant drugs of established efficacy.

Preeclampsia may present with a variety of manifestations due to involvement of such different organs as the kidney, liver, heart, CNS, or blood clotting system. There is increasing evidence that preeclampsia is characterized by a subclinical, chronic consumptive coagulopathy associated with endothelial damage.[113] It may be clinically impossible to distinguish between preeclampsia and either thrombotic thrombocytopenic purpura or the hemolytic-uremic syndrome. Hematologically, however, preeclampsia is characterized by disseminated intravascular coagulation and reduction of plasma antithrombin III activity, in contrast to thrombotic thrombocytopenic purpura and hemolytic-uremic syndrome.[114]

Thrombotic thrombocytopenic purpura is characterized by fever, Coombs-negative hemolytic anemia, thrombocytopenic purpura, fluctuating neurological involvement, and renal disease, and it may simulate preeclampsia. Its neurological features are discussed in Chapter 12. Thrombotic thrombocytopenic purpura may develop during the antepartum period, often before about 24 weeks of gestation, and may result in infant death, although successful treatment may permit prolongation of the pregnancy. Treatment is by plasma infusion, plasma exchange, or plasmapheresis. Platelet transfusions should be avoided because they may trigger an exacerbation.[115] Anti-platelet agents (such as aspirin or dipyridamole) are generally not effective, but treatment with corticosteroids may be helpful. Postpartum *hemolytic-uremic syndrome* is very similar to thrombotic thrombocytopenic purpura, and many consider it within the same spectrum.[113]

Weiner has recommended that if the differential diagnosis is between thrombotic thrombocytopenic purpura and preeclampsia and the gestational age is 34 weeks or greater, the plasma antithrombin III activity level should be determined and the patient delivered.[113] The correct diagnosis will probably be preeclampsia, in which case the plasma antithrombin III activity level will be diminished, and the patient will begin to recover soon after delivery. If the antithrombin III level is normal and the patient does not recover quickly, it should be assumed that the correct diagnosis is thrombotic thrombocytopenic purpura, and plasma therapy should be initiated. If the patient is less than 28 weeks pregnant when she presents, the plasma antithrombin III activity level should be measured before delivery, and if the fetal condition is satisfactory, plasma therapy is tried; if the patient's response is rapid, a diagnosis of thrombotic thrombocytopenic purpura is supported. By contrast, if there is no response to therapy, the probable diagnosis is preeclampsia and the patient should be delivered.

REFERENCES

1. Knight AH, Rhind EG: Epilepsy and pregnancy: a study of 153 pregnancies in 59 patients. Epilepsia 16: 99, 1975
2. Schmidt D, Canger R, Avanzini G, et al: Change of seizure frequency in pregnant epileptic women. J Neurol Neurosurg Psychiatry 46:751, 1983
3. Yerby MS: Pregnancy and epilepsy. Epilepsia 32, suppl 6:S51, 1991
4. Lander CM, Edwards VE, Eadie MJ, Tyrer JH: Plasma anticonvulsant concentrations during pregnancy. Neurology 27:128, 1977
5. Yerby MS, Friel PN, McCormick K: Antiepileptic drug disposition during pregnancy. Neurology 42, suppl 5:12, 1992
6. Kaneko S, Otani K, Kondo T, et al: Malformation in infants of mothers with epilepsy receiving antiepileptic drugs. Neurology 42, suppl 5:68, 1992
7. Koch S, Lösche G, Jager-Román E, et al: Major and

minor birth malformations and antiepileptic drugs. Neurology 42, suppl 5:83, 1992

8. Janz D: On major malformations and minor anomalies in the offspring of parents with epilepsy: review of the literature. p. 211. In Janz D, Bossi L, Dam M, et al (eds): Epilepsy, Pregnancy and the Child. Raven Press, New York, 1982

9. Jones KL, Lacro RV, Johnson KA, Adams J: Pattern of malformation in the children of women treated with carbamazepine during pregnancy. N Engl J Med 320:1661, 1989

10. Rosa FW: Spina bifida in infants of women treated with carbamazepine during pregnancy. N Engl J Med 324:674, 1991

11. Lindhout D, Omtzigt JGC, Cornel MC: Spectrum of neural-tube defects in 34 infants prenatally exposed to antiepileptic drugs. Neurology 42, suppl 5:111, 1992

12. Omtzigt JGC, Los FJ, Grobbee DE, et al: The risk of spina bifida aperta after first-trimester exposure to valproate in a prenatal cohort. Neurology 42, suppl 5:119, 1992

13. Dansky LV, Rosenblatt DS, Andermann E: Mechanisms of teratogenesis: folic acid and antiepileptic therapy. Neurology 42, suppl 5:32, 1992

14. Finnell RH, Buehler BA, Kerr BM, et al: Clinical and experimental studies linking oxidative metabolism to phenytoin-induced teratogenesis. Neurology 42, suppl 5:25, 1992

15. Hanson JW, Myrianthopoulos NC, Harvey MAS, Smith DW: Risks to the offspring of women treated with hydantoin anticonvulsants, with emphasis on the fetal hydantoin syndrome. J Pediatr 89:662, 1976

16. Seip M: Growth retardation, dysmorphic facies and minor malformations following massive exposure to phenobarbitone in utero. Acta Paediatr Scand 65:617, 1976

17. DiLiberti JH, Farndon PA, Dennis NR, Curry CJR: The fetal valproate syndrome. Am J Med Genet 19:473, 1984

18. Mountain KR, Hirsh J, Gallus AS: Neonatal coagulation defect due to anticonvulsant drug treatment in pregnancy. Lancet 1:265, 1970

19. Speidel BD, Meadow SR: Maternal epilepsy and abnormalities of the fetus and newborn. Lancet 2:839, 1972

20. Deblay MF, Vert P, Andre M, Marchal F: Transplacental vitamin K prevents haemorrhagic disease of infant of epileptic mothers. Lancet 1:1247, 1982

21. Janz D, Beck-Mannagetta G, Andermann E, et al: Guidelines for the care of epileptic women of childbearing age. Epilepsia 30:409, 1989

22. Bjerkedal T, Bahna SL: The occurrence and outcome of pregnancy in women with epilepsy. Acta Obstet Gynecol Scand 52:245, 1973

23. Watson JD, Spellacy WN: Neonatal effects of maternal treatment with the anticonvulsant drug diphenylhydantoin. Obstet Gynecol 37:881, 1971

24. Niswander KR, Gordon M: The Collaborative Perinatal Study of the National Institute of Neurological Diseases and Stroke. The Women and Their Pregnancies. DHEW Publ. No. NIH 73-379. Department of Health, Education and Welfare, Washington, DC, 1972

25. Monson RR, Rosenberg L, Hartz SC, et al: Diphenylhydantoin and selected congenital malformations. N Engl J Med 289:1049, 1973

26. Shapiro S, Slone D, Hartz SC, et al: Anticonvulsant and parental epilepsy in the development of birth defects. Lancet 1:272, 1976

27. Somerville BW: A study of migraine in pregnancy. Neurology 22:824, 1972

28. Niederhoff H, Zahrodnik H-P: Analgesics during pregnancy. Am J Med 75, suppl (on antipyretic analgesic therapy):117, 1983

29. Wainscott G, Sullivan FM, Volans GN, Wilkinson M: The outcome of pregnancy in women suffering from migraine. Postgrad Med J 54:98, 1978

30. Schoenfeld N, Epstein O, Nemesh L, et al: Effects of propranolol during pregnancy and development of rats: I. Adverse effects during pregnancy. Pediatr Res 12:747, 1978

31. Rosen TS, Lin M, Spector S, Rosen MR: Maternal, fetal, and neonatal effects of chronic propranolol administration in the rat. J Pharmacol Exp Ther 208:118, 1979

32. Ueland K, McAnulty JH, Ueland FR, Metcalfe J: Special considerations in the use of cardiovascular drugs. Clin Obstet Gynecol 24:809, 1981

33. Jackson CD, Fishbein L: A toxicological review of beta-adrenergic blockers. Fundam Appl Toxicol 6:395, 1986

34. Stein GS: Headaches in the first post partum week and their relationship to migraine. Headache 21:201, 1981

35. Schipper HM: Neurology of sex steroids and oral contraceptives. Neurol Clin 4:721, 1986

36. Heyman A, Stadel B, Odom G, et al: The relation of subarachnoid hemorrhage in young women to phases of the natural menstrual cycle—a preliminary report. Neurology 26:358, 1976

37. Petitti DB, Wingerd J: Use of oral contraceptives, cigarette smoking, and risk of subarachnoid haemorrhage. Lancet 2:234, 1978

38. Jennett WB, Cross JN: Influence of pregnancy and oral contraception on the incidence of strokes in women of childbearing age. Lancet 1:1019, 1967

39. Finley BE: Acute coagulopathy in pregnancy. Med Clin North Am 73:723, 1989

40. Perry KG, Morrison JC: The diagnosis and management of hemoglobinopathies during pregnancy. Semin Perinatol 14:90, 1990

41. Levine SR, Welch KMA: Antiphospholipid antibodies. Ann Neurol 26:386, 1989

42. Branch DW: Antiphospholipid antibodies and pregnancy: maternal implications. Semin Perinatol 14:139, 1990

43. Homans DC: Current concepts: peripartum cardiomyopathy. N Engl J Med 312:1432, 1985

44. Hodgman MT, Pessin MS, Homand DC, et al: Cerebral embolism as the initial manifestation of peripartum cardiomyopathy. Neurology 32:668, 1982

45. Call GK, Fleming MC, Sealfon S, et al: Reversible cerebral segmental vasoconstriction. Stroke 19:1159, 1988

46. Geraghty JJ, Hoch DB, Robert ME, Vinters HV: Fatal puerperal cerebral vasospasm and stroke in a young woman. Neurology 41:1145, 1991

47. Brick JF: Vanishing cerebrovascular disease of pregnancy. Neurology 38:804, 1988

48. Wiebers DO: Ischemic cerebrovascular complications of pregnancy. Arch Neurol 42:1106, 1985

49. Carroll JD, Leak D, Lee HA: Cerebral thrombophlebitis in pregnancy and the puerperium. Q J Med 35:347, 1966

50. Einhaupl KM, Villringer A, Meister W, et al: Heparin treatment in sinus venous thrombosis. Lancet 338:597, 1991

51. Goldman JA, Eckerling B, Gans B: Intracranial venous sinus thrombosis in pregnancy and puerperium: report of fifteen cases. J Obstet Gynaecol Br Commonw 71:791, 1964

52. Garcin R, Pestel M: Thrombo-phlebites Cerebrales. Masson, Paris, 1949

53. Robinson JL, Hall CS, Sedzimir CB: Arteriovenous malformations, aneurysms, and pregnancy. J Neurosurg 41:63, 1974

54. Horton JC, Chambers WA, Lyons SL, et al: Pregnancy and the risk of hemorrhage from cerebral arteriovenous malformations. Neurosurgery 27:867, 1990

55. Parkinson D, Bachers G: Arteriovenous malformations: summary of 100 consecutive supratentorial cases. J Neurosurg 53:285, 1980

56. Kelly DL, Alexander E, Davis CH, Maynard DC: Intracranial arteriovenous malformations: clinical review and evaluation of brain scans. J Neurosurg 31:422, 1969

57. Henderson CE, Torbey M: Rupture of intracranial aneurysm associated with cocaine use during pregnancy. Am J Perinatol 5:142, 1988

58. Mercado A, Johnson G, Calver D, Sokol R: Cocaine, pregnancy, and postpartum intracerebral hemorrhage. Obstet Gynecol 73:467, 1989

59. Enomoto H, Goto H: Moyamoya disease presenting as intracerebral hemorrhage during pregnancy: case report and review of the literature. Neurosurgery 20:33, 1987

60. Seigle JM, Caputy AJ, Manz HJ, et al: Multiple oncotic intracranial aneurysms and cardiac metastases from choriocarcinoma: case report and review of the literature. Neurosurgery 20:39, 1987

61. Newton TH, Hoyt WF: Dural arteriovenous shunts in the region of the cavernous sinus. Neuroradiology 1:71, 1970

62. Taniguchi RM, Goree JA, Odom GL: Spontaneous carotid-cavernous shunts presenting diagnostic problems. J Neurosurg 35:384, 1971

63. Aminoff MJ: Angiomas and fistulae involving the nervous system. p. 296. In Ross Russell RW (ed): Vascular Disease of the Central Nervous System. 2nd Ed. Churchill Livingstone, Edinburgh, 1983

64. Aminoff MJ: Spinal Angiomas. Blackwell Scientific Publications, Oxford, 1976

65. Weinberg ED: Pregnancy-associated depression of cell-mediated immunity. Rev Infect Dis 6:814, 1984

66. Abramson H, Greenberg M, Magee MC: Poliomyelitis in the newborn infant. J Pediatr 43:167, 1953

67. Athavale VB, Pai PN: Tetanus neonatorum—clinical manifestations. J Pediatr 67:649, 1965

68. Linnan MJ, Mascola L, Lou XD, et al: Epidemic listeriosis associated with Mexican-style cheese. N Engl J Med 319:823, 1988

69. Townsend JJ, Baringer JR, Wolinsky JS, et al: Progressive rubella panencephalitis: late onset after congenital rubella. N Engl J Med 292:990, 1975

70. Weil ML, Itabashi HH, Cremer NE, et al: Chronic progressive panencephalitis due to rubella virus simulating subacute sclerosing panencephalitis. N Engl J Med 292:994, 1975

71. Kingdom JCP, Kennedy DH: Tuberculous meningitis in pregnancy. Br J Obstet Gynaecol 96:233, 1989

72. MacDonald MG, Ginzburg HM, Bolan JC: HIV infection in pregnancy: epidemiology and clinical management. J Acquir Immune Defic Syndr 4:100, 1991

73. Shannon KM, Amman AJ: Acquired immune deficiency syndrome in childhood. J Pediatr 106:332, 1985

74. Jadhav M, Webb JKG, Vaishnava S, Baker SJ: Vitamin B$_{12}$ deficiency in Indian infants: a clinical syndrome. Lancet 2:903, 1962

75. Scriver CR, Clow CL: Phenylketonuria: epitome of human biochemical genetics. N Engl J Med 303:1336, 1980

76. Lenke RR, Levy HL: Maternal phenylketonuria and hyperphenylalaninemia: an international survey of the outcome of untreated and treated pregnancies. N Engl J Med 303:1202, 1980

77. Editorial: The growing problems of phenylketonuria. Lancet 1:1381, 1979
78. Nausieda PA, Koller WC, Weiner WJ, Klawans HL: Chorea induced by oral contraceptives. Neurology 29:1605, 1979
79. Ekbom K: Restless legs. p. 543. In Vinken PJ, Bruyn GW, Klawans HL (eds): Handbook of Clinical Neurology. Vol. 51. Elsevier, Amsterdam, 1987
80. Marsh L, Fraser FC: Chelating agents and teratogenesis. Lancet 2:846, 1973
81. Scheinberg IH, Sternlieb I: Pregnancy in penicillamine-treated patients with Wilson's disease. N Engl J Med 298:1300, 1975
82. Walshe JM: Pregnancy in Wilson's disease. Q J Med 46:73, 1977
83. Golbe LI: Parkinson's disease and pregnancy. Neurology 37:1245, 1987
84. Schapira K, Poskanzer DC, Newell DJ, Miller H: Marriage, pregnancy and multiple sclerosis. Brain 89:419, 1966
85. Korn-Lubetzki I, Kahana E, Cooper G, Abramsky O: Activity of multiple sclerosis during pregnancy and puerperium. Ann Neurol 16:229, 1984
86. Birk K, Rudick R: Pregnancy and multiple sclerosis. Arch Neurol 43:719, 1986
87. Birk K, Ford C, Smeltzer S, et al: The clinical course of multiple sclerosis during pregnancy and the puerperium. Arch Neurol 47:738, 1990
88. Roullet E, Verdier-Taillefer M-H, Amarenco P, et al: Pregnancy and multiple sclerosis: a longitudinal study of 125 remittent patients. J Neurol Neurosurg Psychiatry 56:1062, 1993
89. Thompson DS, Nelson LM, Burns A, et al: The effects of pregnancy in multiple sclerosis: a retrospective study. Neurology 36:1097, 1986
90. Weinshenker BG, Hader W, Carriere W, et al: The influence of pregnancy on disability from multiple sclerosis: a population-based study in Middlesex County, Ontario. Neurology 39:1438, 1989
91. Sweeney WJ: Pregnancy and multiple sclerosis. Am J Obstet Gynecol 66:124, 1953
92. Kulig K, Schaltenbrand G: Statistische Untersuchungen zum Problem der Multiplen Sklerose. Dtsch Z Nervenheilk 174:460, 1956
93. Poser S, Poser W: Multiple sclerosis and gestation. Neurology 33:1422, 1983
94. Walsh FB, Hoyt WF: Clinical Neuro-Ophthalmology. 3rd Ed. Williams & Wilkins, Baltimore, 1969
95. Whittaker WG: Injuries to the sacral plexus in obstetrics. Can Med Assoc J 79:622, 1958
96. Taylor RA: Heredofamilial mononeuritis multiplex with brachial predilection. Brain 83:113, 1960
97. Al Hakim M, Katirji MB: Femoral mononeuropathy induced by the lithotomy position: a report of 5 cases with a review of literature. Muscle Nerve 16:891, 1993
98. Burkhart FL, Daly JW: Sciatic and peroneal nerve injury: a complication of vaginal operations. Obstet Gynecol 28:99, 1966
99. Hilsinger RL, Adour KK, Doty HE: Idiopathic facial paralysis, pregnancy and the menstrual cycle. Ann Otol Rhinol Laryngol 84:433, 1975
100. Calderon-Gonzalez R, Gonzalez-Cantu N, Rizzi-Hernandez H: Recurrent polyneuropathy with pregnancy and oral contraceptives. N Engl J Med 282:1307, 1970
101. Jones MW, Berry K: Chronic relapsing polyneuritis associated with pregnancy. Ann Neurol 9:413, 1981
102. McCombe PA, McManis PG, Frith JA, et al: Chronic inflammatory demyelinating polyradiculoneuropathy associated with pregnancy. Ann Neurol 21:102, 1987
103. Osserman KE: Pregnancy in myasthenia gravis and neonatal myasthenia gravis. Am J Med 19:720, 1955
104. Plauché WC: Myasthenia gravis in mothers and their newborns. Clin Obstet Gynecol 34:82, 1991
105. Namba T, Brown SB, Grob D: Neonatal myasthenia gravis: report of two cases and review of the literature. Pediatrics 45:488, 1970
106. Harper PS: Myotonic Dystrophy. 2nd Ed. WB Saunders, Philadelphia, 1989
107. Shore RN, MacLachlan TB: Pregnancy with myotonic dystrophy: course, complications and management. Obstet Gynecol 38:448, 1971
108. Hook R, Anderson EF, Noto P: Anesthetic management of a parturient with myotonia atrophica. Anesthesiology 43:689, 1975
109. Norman AM, Floyd JL, Meredith AL, Harper PS: Presymptomatic detection and prenatal diagnosis for myotonic dystrophy by means of linked DNA markers. J Med Genet 26:750, 1989
110. Caskey CT, Pizzuti A, Fu Y-H, et al: Triplet repeat mutations in human disease. Science 256:784, 1992
111. Shelbourne P, Davies J, Buxton J, et al: Direct diagnosis of myotonic dystrophy with a disease-specific DNA marker. N Engl J Med 328:471, 1993
112. Kaplan PW, Lesser RP, Fisher RS, et al: No, magnesium sulfate should not be used in treating eclamptic seizures. Arch Neurol 45:1361, 1988.
113. Weiner CP: Thrombotic microangiopathy in pregnancy and the postpartum period. Semin Hematol 24:119, 1987
114. Byrnes JJ, Moake JL: Thrombotic thrombocytopenic purpura and the haemolytic-uraemic syndrome: evolving concepts of pathogenesis and therapy. Clin Haematol 15:413, 1986
115. Harkness DR, Byrnes JJ, Lian EC-Y, et al: Hazard of platelet transfusion in thrombotic thrombocytopenic purpura. JAMA 246:1931, 1981

29

Iatrogenic (Drug-Induced) Disorders of the Nervous System

Frank L. Mastaglia

Adverse drug reactions are a frequent cause of morbidity and admission to hospital.[1] The introduction in many countries of spontaneous reporting schemes has led to increasing awareness of such reactions, and these schemes have played an important role in identifying new drug hazards and risk factors that predispose to them.[2]

Drug reactions commonly involve the nervous system, resulting in a variety of manifestations that may mimic many naturally occurring diseases of the nervous system. Unlike many of the latter, most drug-induced disorders are potentially reversible if the offending agent is withdrawn. It is therefore essential that the possibility of an iatrogenic condition should be considered in any patient presenting with neurological symptoms, and a full drug history should always be obtained with this possibility in mind. The spectrum of drug-induced neurological disorders is very wide, ranging from disturbances of neuromuscular or autonomic function to seizures, movement disorders, and syndromes of raised intracranial pressure, stroke, cognitive dysfunction, and encephalopathic states.

HEADACHE

Various drugs may cause headache by inducing vasodilatation, increased intracranial pressure, or rarely acute aseptic meningitis.[3]

Vascular Headaches

Drugs that cause headache through vasodilatation include antihistamines, sympathomimetic agents, amyl nitrate, nicotinic acid, hydralazine, bromides, histamine, nifedipine, perhexiline, theophylline, aminophylline, and terbutaline.[3] Similar headaches may occur following withdrawal of amphetamines, ergotamine, caffeine, methysergide, or benzodiazepines.

Headache may also occur during treatment with bromocriptine, dopamine, and the nonsteroidal anti-inflammatory drugs indomethacin, phenylbutazone, naproxen, ketoprofen, diclofenac, alclofenac, and ibuprofen, particularly when treatment is first commenced.[3] A severe persistent headache has been reported in some patients treated with H_2-receptor antagonists such as cimetidine and ranitidine.

Severe headaches associated with hypertension may occur when patients taking monoamine oxidase inhibitors are treated with amphetamines, imipramine, ephedrine, or other sympathomimetic agents, or when they consume food with a high tyramine content.

Oral contraceptives and female hormonal preparations may cause migrainous headaches or exacerbate a preexisting migrainous tendency, as may vasodilators and some of the other drugs already discussed. A paradoxical increase in frequency of headaches commonly occurs in migraine sufferers taking excessive ergotamine-containing preparations on a regular basis and is an indication for gradual ergotamine withdrawal.[4]

Benign Intracranial Hypertension (Pseudotumor Cerebri)

A number of drugs may be associated with the development of benign intracranial hypertension, which is characterized by headache, papilledema, and, at times, diplopia and impairment of vision.[3] These include oral contraceptives, estrogens and progestational agents,[5] tetracyclines,[6] nalidixic acid, nitrofurantoin, ketamine, nitrous oxide, excessive vitamin A, etretinate,[3] danazol,[7] amiodarone,[8] perhexiline,[5] ampicillin, thyroxine,[9] and corticosteroids, particularly in children.[3] In the case of corticosteroids, this complication may occur when the drug is withdrawn abruptly.[3]

Aseptic Meningitis

There have been a number of reports of an aseptic meningitic illness with headache, neck stiffness, photophobia, and pyrexia developing in patients with systemic connective tissue diseases treated with ibuprofen, sulindac, tolmetin, or cotrimoxazole,[3,10] and also with intravenous immunoglobulin therapy.[11]

STROKE

Women taking oral contraceptives have an increased risk of cerebral venous thrombosis and ischemic stroke, although the absolute risk is small.[3] It has been suggested that the risk of thrombotic stroke is greater with the higher-dose estrogen contraceptive preparations, although there is evidence that the progestogen component may also be involved.[3] Oral contraceptives may also predispose to stroke in some women by causing hypertension, and have been implicated in causing subarachnoid hemorrhage, particularly in women who smoke.[3] There also appears to be an increased risk of cerebral thromboembolism in perimenopausal women taking estrogen preparations and in men treated with stilbestrol for prostatic carcinoma.

The inappropriate use of antihypertensive drugs is an important cause of iatrogenic stroke, particularly in the elderly and in patients with cerebrovascular disease.[12,13] These drugs should be used with caution, particularly in individuals with previous symptoms of cerebral ischemia, and should only be administered when there is sustained and significant elevation of the systemic blood pressure. The mild to moderate elevation of blood pressure that occurs following a stroke is usually self-limiting and does not require antihypertensive therapy.

Patients taking anticoagulant drugs have an increased risk of intracerebral and other intracranial hemorrhages, particularly with poorly controlled or long-term therapy. Intracerebral or subarachnoid hemorrhage may also occur after intravenous or even oral or intranasal administration of amphetamines and related compounds that can cause transient hypertension.[14] Intracranial hemorrhage has also been reported in patients taking diet pills, decongestants, or stimulants containing the sympathomimetic drug pheylpropanolamine (which may cause acute hypertension and cerebral vasospasm[15]), and pseudoephedrine. Intracerebral hemorrhage or ischemic stroke has also been reported in patients abusing ephedrine-containing preparations[16] or addicted to cocaine[17,18] or "T's and Blues" (i.e., pentazocine and tripelennamine).[19]

Myocardial and cerebral ischemia may occur in patients given cisplatin-based combination chemotherapy.[20] Combination chemotherapy including L-asparaginase has been associated with the development of cerebral venous or arterial thrombosis and hemorrhage.[21] Cerebral ischemic lesions have been reported following prolonged intake of high doses of ergotamine[22] and after subcutaneous administration of sumatriptan.[23]

SEIZURES

Numerous drugs may induce seizures in otherwise healthy individuals and are more likely to do so in those with preexisting epilepsy or a low seizure threshold[3,24] (Table 29-1). The Boston Collaborative Drug Surveillance Program reported an incidence of drug-induced seizures of only 0.18 per thousand.[25] However, in a large hospital series, drug-induced seizures accounted for 1.7 percent of all seizure admissions.[26] In this series, single (45 percent) or multiple (40 percent) generalized seizures occurred, and 15 percent of patients had status epilepticus. Generalized seizures with focal features were common, but simple partial seizures occurred in only 4 percent of patients. Absence seizures and status have been reported in patients treated with the third-generation cephalosporin ceftazidime.[27]

Some drugs are more likely than others to precipitate seizures, particularly those administered in high doses by the intrathecal or intravenous routes and those that cross the blood-brain barrier. In the case of a number of the drugs listed in Table 29-1, seizures have been reported only rarely and the association remains circumstantial. A number of factors appear to predispose to the occurrence of drug-induced seizures. Patients who have such seizures often have a family history of epilepsy, suggesting that they may have a genetically determined low seizure threshold.

Individuals with preexisting cerebral or systemic disease may also have a lowered seizure threshold. Penicillin-induced seizures are more likely to develop with high-dose intravenous or intrathecal administration of the drug and in patients with renal failure who develop high blood levels due to reduced excretion. Other drugs that may accumulate as a result of renal failure and cause convulsions include imipenem, nalidixic acid, cimetidine, cephalosporins, lithium, and recombinant erythropoietin.[28]

Intravenous administration of lidocaine, mepivacaine, or theophylline may cause convulsions, especially in patients with liver disease or heart failure.[3] Water intoxication caused by oxytocin or carbamazepine, or overhydration due to the use of hyperosmolar parenteral solutions, may also induce seizures.[3] Withdrawal of certain drugs such as benzodiazepines, barbiturates, tricyclic antidepressants, alcohol, and baclofen is an important cause of seizures, particularly if these drugs are discontinued too abruptly.[3] Withdrawal of anticonvulsant drugs in epileptic patients is an important cause of seizures or status epilepticus and should always be carried out gradually. Conversely, excessively high doses and serum concentrations of phenytoin may exacerbate epilepsy or even precipitate status epilepticus.[29]

The convulsant effects of isoniazid, aminophylline, local anesthetics, phencyclidine, and meperidine are dose-related.[26] A number of other drugs may cause

Table 29-1 Drugs Reported to Cause Seizures

Antidepressants	Imipramine, amitriptyline, doxepin, nortryptyline, maprotiline, mianserin, nomifensine, bupropion
Antipsychotics	Chlorpromazine, thioridazine, perphenazine, trifluoperazine, prochlorperazine, haloperidol
Analgesics	Fentanyl, meperidine, pentazocine, propoxyphene, cocaine, mefenamic acid
Local anesthetics	Lidocaine, mepivacaine, procaine, bupivacaine, etidocaine
General anesthetics	Ketamine, halothane, althesin, enflurane, propanidid, methohexital, propofol
Antimicrobials	Penicillin, synthetic penicillins (oxacillin, carbenicillin, ticarcillin), ampicillin, cephalosporins, imipenem, metronidazole, nalidixic acid, isoniazid, cycloserine, pyrimethamine
Antineoplastics	Chlorambucil, vincristine, methotrexate, cytosine arabinoside, misonidazole, BCNU, PALA
Bronchodilators	Aminophylline, theophylline
Sympathomimetics	Ephedrine, terbutaline, phenylpropanolamine
Others	Insulin, antihistamines, anticholinergics, baclofen, cyclosporin A, lithium, atenolol, disopyramide, phencyclidine, amphetamines, domperidone, doxapram, ergonovine, folic acid, camphor, methylxanthenes, TRH, vitamin K oxide, aqueous iodinated contrast media, oxytocin, hyperosmolar parenteral solutions, hyperbaric oxygen, anticonvulsants, methylphenidate, erythropoietin

(Based on material presented elsewhere.[3,24,119,189])

seizures even with therapeutic doses and serum levels. These include theophylline[30]; tricyclic antidepressants, which cause seizures in about 1 percent of patients; and phenothiazines, which induce seizures in 1 to 2 percent of patients.[26] The aliphatic phenothiazines chlorpromazine, promazine, and prochlorperazine are more likely to induce seizures than those of the piperazine group, such as fluphenazine and trifluoperazine.[3] In addition to the tricyclic antidepressants, the tetracyclic drugs mianserin and maprotiline have also been implicated in causing seizures,[3,31] as has the aminoketoalkyl agent bupropion.[32] It has been suggested that doxepin or the monoamine oxidase inhibitors are the safest drugs for treating the depressed patient who is at risk of seizures.[33]

COMA

Drugs are a common and important cause of coma, which may result from accidental overdosage of drugs such as insulin or oral hypoglycemic agents in patients with diabetes mellitus or, more frequently, from self-administered overdosage with hypnotics, sedatives, antidepressants, analgesics, or drug combinations.[34] Whereas barbiturates were once the most common cause of drug-induced coma, the benzodiazepines and other nonbarbiturate hypnotics or sedatives and the antidepressant drugs are now more commonly taken in overdose. Other drugs that may produce depression of consciousness and coma include phenothiazines, salicylates, acetaminophen (which produces severe hepatic damage with resulting coma), paraldehyde, chlormethiazole,[35] acyclovir,[36] and intrathecal baclofen.[3,37]

Certain patterns of neurological findings are characteristic of drug-induced coma. The pupils are typically small and reactive, although they may be dilated and fixed in severe barbiturate or glutethimide intoxication or pinpoint in opiate poisoning. The corneal reflexes are preserved and symmetrical, though they may be lost in cases of profound drug-induced coma. Ocular movements, both spontaneous and reflex, are depressed at an early stage, particularly with barbiturate, tricyclic antidepressant, and phenytoin intoxication, the eyes being typically fixed and divergent without spontaneous roving eye movements and with impaired or absent oculocephalic (doll's head) or oculovestibular (caloric) reflexes.[34] Muscle tone is

usually reduced and the deep tendon reflexes depressed, with flexor plantar responses, although in some cases there may be hypertonia, hyperflexia, decerebrate posturing, and extensor plantar responses, particularly if there has been superadded hypoxia.[34] Muscle twitching, choreoathetosis, myoclonus, and seizures may occur in coma caused by tricyclic antidepressants.[34,38]

The electroencephalogram (EEG) may show diffuse slowing of cerebral rhythms or, in cases of barbiturate or benzodiazepine intoxication, prominent generalized beta activity. Alpha coma, with preservation of background alpha activity but with an altered distribution and reactivity, or a combination of alpha and beta activity, occurs in some cases of intoxication with benzodiazepines or chlormethiazole.[35]

DIFFUSE ENCEPHALOPATHY

Certain drugs such as lithium and acyclovir may cause a diffuse disturbance of cerebral function leading to tremor, asterixis, myoclonus, seizures, primitive reflexes, ataxia, mental confusion, and obtundation, at times progressing to coma. Such a syndrome may be caused by lithium toxicity and, at times, occurs even when blood levels are within the therapeutic range.[39,40] In some patients with lithium toxicity, the combination of cognitive impairment, myoclonus, mutism, primitive reflexes, and periodic sharp wave complexes in the EEG may resemble Creutzfeldt-Jakob disease.[41] Although the neurological abnormalities are usually reversible when treatment is discontinued, cerebellar dysfunction and other neurological deficits may persist and are irreversible in some cases.[40]

A reversible myoclonic encephalopathy has also been reported in patients with a prolonged exposure to bismuth-containing preparations. This was first reported from Australia in colostomy patients taking bismuth subgallate orally,[42] and there have been subsequent reports of a similar syndrome developing in patients using bismuth-containing cosmetic creams,[43] antidiarrheal mixtures containing bismuth subsalicylate,[44] and bismuth subnitrate for the treatment of constipation.[43]

Other drugs that may cause an encephalopathy include penicillin and cephaloridine[45] when administered in high doses, particularly in patients with renal failure, lidocaine and its oral analogue tocainide,[46] benzodiazepines in patients on hemodialysis,[47] vigabatrin,[48] as well as the antineoplastic agents L-asparaginase, thymidine, 5-fluorouracil, carmustine (BCNU), mechlorethamine, N-phosphacetyl aspartic acid (PALA), cytosine arabinoside,[49] fludarabine,[50] and doxorubicin.[51]

A severe progressive leukoencephalopathy characterized by dementia, dysarthria, ataxia, and paralysis, at times followed by seizures, coma and death, may occur in patients treated with high-dose intrathecal, intraventricular, or intravenous methotrexate, particularly if cranial or craniospinal radiotherapy has previously been administered.[49,52] A severe, progressive, and, at times, fatal spongiform leukoencephalopathy has been described from the Netherlands in individuals inhaling heroin pyrolysate.[53]

PSYCHIATRIC DISORDERS

For a detailed review and chart of psychiatric side effects of all commonly used drugs, the reader is referred to the account published recently in *The Medical Letter*.[54]

Behavioral Toxicity

The term *behavioral toxicity* has been used to cover a variety of nonspecific symptoms such as listlessness, drowsiness, insomnia, irritability, restlessness, anxiety, euphoria, mild depression, excitement, vivid dreams and nightmares, increased sensitivity to light and sound, mood changes, and impaired psychomotor performance, which may occur during treatment with a wide range of drugs.[55,56] Although such symptoms may be the prelude to a more florid delirious state, they usually subside gradually if the dose of the offending drug is reduced. The drugs most frequently implicated include tricyclic antidepressants, lithium, amphetamines, barbiturates and other hypnotics, oral contraceptives, cholinergic drugs, amantadine, levodopa, digitalis derivatives, anticonvulsants, antihistamines, reserpine, clonidine, methyldopa, propranolol, isoniazid, ethionamide, cycloserine, bromides, and acyclovir. Similar symptoms may be caused by withdrawal of a number of drugs such as benzodiazepines.

Delirious/Confusional States

Drugs are an important cause of delirium and confusional states, which are characterized by a fluctuating level of consciousness, diminished awareness, impairment of attention and memory, disorientation, and, at times, illusions, hallucinations, and paranoid delusions.[55] The elderly are particularly prone to develop such reactions, presumably being predisposed because of the presence of age-related degenerative cerebral changes. As shown in Table 29-2, a wide range of drugs may produce these reactions, the tranquilizers and hypnotics collectively being the most important groups.[55] Other important causes include the benzodiazepines and the antiparkinsonian drugs benzhexol, amantadine, and levodopa.

Table 29-2 Drugs That May Cause Delirious/Confusional States

Cardiovascular drugs	**Anticonvulsants**
Digitalis	Phenytoin
Diuretics	Sodium valproate
β-blockers	**Miscellaneous drugs**
Disopyramide	Disulfiram
Amiodarone	Piperazine
Anticholinergic drugs	Cimetidine
Atropine and	Ranitidine
homatropine eyedrops	Chloroquine
Scopolamine	Oral hypoglycemics
Benzhexol	Nitrous oxide
Benztropine	**Drug withdrawal**
Tricyclic antidepressants	Barbiturates
Dopamine agonists	Benzodiazepines
Levodopa	Chlormethiazole
Bromocriptine	
Amantadine	
Tranquilizers, hypnotics	
Barbiturates	
Benzodiazepines	
Bromides	
Phenothiazines	
Antimicrobial drugs	
Isoniazid	
Cycloserine	
Rifampicin	
Procaine penicillin	
Streptomycin	
Sulfonamides	

(Adapted from Davison K: Drug-induced psychiatric disorders. Medicine (UK) 35:1823, 1980, with permission.)

Affective Disorders

Depressive reactions are common during drug therapy. Reserpine and subsequently methyldopa were among the first drugs recognized to cause depression. Depression is less common in patients treated with some of the newer antihypertensive agents such as clonidine, propranolol, and the calcium channel blockers verapamil and nifedipine. Depression may also occur in patients on corticosteroids but is less common than euphoria. It is the commonest psychiatric symptom in patients on levodopa. Other drugs that may induce depression include oral contraceptives, digoxin, indomethacin, sulfonamides, disulfiram, antituberculous drugs (in particular cycloserine), and the phenothiazines and butyrophenones.[55] Benzodiazepine, amphetamine, and fenfluramine withdrawal may also cause depression.[55]

Although some degree of euphoria is common in patients on various drugs, actual manic or hypomanic reactions are uncommon.[55] Such reactions may, however, occur in patients treated with corticosteroids or corticotropin, levodopa and other dopaminergic agents, opiates, pentazocine, monoamine oxidase inhibitors, tricyclic antidepressants, iproniazid, sympathomimetic amines, trazolobenzodiazepines, procyclidine, and hallucinogens.[55,57]

Paranoid and Schizophreniform Psychoses

Various drugs have been reported to cause paranoid and schizophreniform psychotic reactions characterized by delusions, hallucinations, and emotional and thought disorder in the absence of impaired consciousness.[55] Although the drug-induced disorders closely resemble the naturally occurring psychoses, individuals who develop these conditions do not appear to be predisposed to develop idiopathic psychotic disorders subsequently.[55] The drugs that may precipitate such reactions are listed in Table 29-3.

Hallucinatory States

Certain drugs may cause hallucinations without other features of delirium or psychosis.[55] The hallucinations, which are usually visual, tend to be extremely vivid, are often colored, and are often of animals, sometimes having a microptic or lilliputian

Table 29-3 Drugs That May Induce Paranoid or Schizophrenia-like Psychoses

Hallucinogens	Antimicrobials
LSD	Isoniazid
Mescaline	Cycloserine
Phencyclidine	Ethionamide
Dimethoxymethyl-	Atabrine
amphetamine	Mepacrine
CNS stimulants	Chloroquine
Amphetamines	**Cardiovascular drugs**
Cocaine	Digitalis
Diethylpropion	Hydralazine
Phenmetrazine	Disopyramide
Ephedrine	Methyldopa
Pseudoephedrine	**Antiparkinsonian drugs**
Propylhexedrine	Benzhexol
CNS depressants	Benztropine
Ethyl alcohol	Levodopa
Barbiturates	Bromocriptine
Bromides	**Miscellaneous drugs**
Chloral hydrate	Corticosteroids[a]
Antihistamines	ACTH
Anticonvulsants	Indomethacin
(phenytoin,	Disulfiram
sulthiame,	Dextropropoxyphene
ethosuximide)	Tocainide

[a] Including corticosteroid withdrawal.
(Adapted from Davison K: Drug-induced psychiatric disorders. Medicine (UK) 35:1823, 1980, with permission.)

dimension.[55] The drugs most frequently involved include tricyclic antidepressants, benzodiazepines, bromides, atropine and other anticholinergic drugs after parenteral or even topical administration into the eye, amantadine, bromocriptine, levodopa, digoxin, β-blockers, disopyramide, pentazocine, buprenorphine, indomethacin, salicyclates, cimetidine, aminophylline, and cyproheptadine, as well as cannabis and lysergic acid diethylamide (LSD).[55,58] Hallucinations, usually auditory and less often visual, are also a feature of withdrawal from alcohol, barbiturates, benzodiazepines, and baclofen.

Pseudodementia

A number of drugs may cause transient memory impairment—for example, clioquinol, isoniazid, and drugs with a central anticholinergic action, such as benzhexol. More severe, but still reversible, cognitive impairment that may mimic dementia may develop in some patients with chronic intake of benzodiazepines, barbiturates, bromides, and major tranquilizers such as chlorpromazine, with anticonvulsant overdosage in epileptics, and with interleukin administration.[55,59] Some degree of cognitive impairment is common in treated epileptics, particularly those taking phenytoin or barbiturate derivatives, even when these drugs are administered in therapeutic doses and there are no other signs of toxicity. Carbamazepine and sodium valproate are less likely to produce cognitive deficits.[29] There are rare reports of irreversible cognitive impairment due to levodopa therapy in Parkinson's disease and to combined treatment with lithium and haloperidol.

EXTRAPYRAMIDAL SYNDROMES

Several groups of drugs may induce involuntary movements or abnormalities of posture or muscle tone that may resemble those associated with naturally occurring extrapyramidal disorders.[60–63] All of the major classes of psychotropic drugs (phenothiazines, reserpine, benzoquinolizines, thioxanthenes, and butyrophenones) as well as the dopaminergic antiparkinsonian agents and tricyclic antidepressants have the ability to induce such syndromes, which may take a number of different forms[64] (Table 29-4). The reported incidence of these disorders varies considerably according to the diagnostic criteria used and the patient groups studied.[64] It is well-recognized that there is a marked individual variability in the susceptibility to these extrapyramidal reactions; some

Table 29-4 Drug-Induced Extrapyramidal Disorders

Acute dystonic-dyskinetic reactions
Akathisia
Tardive dyskinesia
Tardive dystonia
Chorea and choreoathetosis
Drug-induced parkinsonism
Neuroleptic malignant syndrome
Tremor
Tics
Myoclonus

patients develop side effects even after small doses of a drug, whereas many others take much higher doses and are unaffected. The factors responsible for this variable susceptibility are not fully understood, but there is some evidence that age, gender, and genetic factors play a part. For example, acute dystonic-dyskinetic reactions are more likely to occur in patients under the age of 20 years and in females, whereas drug-induced parkinsonism is more frequent in patients over the age of 65 years.[2]

Acute Dystonic-Dyskinetic Reactions

An acute dystonic syndrome is a well-recognized complication of treatment with many neuroleptic drugs such as the phenothiazines and butyrophenones, as well as the tricyclic antidepressants, metoclopramide, and less frequently phenytoin, carbamazepine, propranolol, chlorzoxazone,[3,65,66] the calcium channel blockers flunarizine and cinnarizine,[67] and diazepam.[68] The onset is usually within the first few days of starting treatment and may be quite abrupt and alarming. The dystonia may be confined to the muscles of the head and neck, causing facial grimacing, trismus, abnormal movements and spasms of the tongue, oculogyric crises, orofacial dyskinesias, torticollis, and retrocollis; or it may be more generalized, with slow writhing movements of the limbs and more prolonged tonic contractions of the axial and limb muscles leading to opisthotonos, lordosis, tortipelvis, and a bizarre gait. The bizarre and protean nature of the manifestations may lead to a mistaken diagnosis of hysteria, tetanus, tetany, or epilepsy. The incidence of this type of extrapyramidal reaction has been estimated to be of the order of 2.5 percent in patients treated with neuroleptic drugs[69] and is considerably lower in patients treated with metoclopramide, prochlorperazine, and haloperidol.[65,70] Despite their dramatic and at times alarming nature, the acute dystonias are usually self-limited and remit once the drug is discontinued. Particularly severe reactions may be terminated by the intravenous administration of benztropine or diazepam.

Acute dyskinetic reactions involving the lips, face, and tongue, and at times the limbs and trunk, occur commonly in parkinsonian patients treated with levodopa and are dose-related. These dyskinesias may develop early during the course of treatment with levodopa (or with various dopamine agonists) and they respond to a reduction in dose. With prolonged treatment, dyskinesias become an increasing problem, tending to occur at times of maximal response to the levodopa and alternating with periods of akinesia and severe rigidity (the "on-off" phenomenon). The administration of small, frequent doses of levodopa or a reduction in the overall dose and the introduction of bromocriptine is sometimes helpful in alleviating this common complication of prolonged levodopa therapy.

Reversible forms of dyskinesia involving the face, mouth, and tongue and at times the limbs and trunk have also been reported in patients treated with phenytoin,[29] flunarizine, and the antimalarials chloroquine and amodiaquine.[71]

Akathisia

Akathisia is a state of motor restlessness, characterized by an inability to be still and an urge constantly to move about, pace, or even run incessantly.[72] The condition is seen particularly after the administration of phenothiazine derivatives such as fluphenazine, trifluoperazine, and prochlorperazine, and less frequently with the butyrophenones, reserpine, tricyclic antidepressants, levodopa, monoamine oxidase inhibitors, and vigabatrin. It may also occur with amoxapine and oxazepam withdrawal.[3] The reported incidence of akathisia in groups of patients treated with antipsychotic drugs has ranged from 12.5 to 45 percent.[72] Akathisia may be associated with other extrapyramidal manifestations such as parkinsonism, tremor, and dystonia. The pathophysiological basis for akathisia is uncertain. Experimental work in the rat has produced evidence linking the phenomenon with a disturbance of the mesocortical dopaminergic system.[72]

Akathisia usually remits within days or weeks of withdrawal of the neuroleptic drug, although in some cases it persists for several months or occasionally is permanent.[72] Anticholinergic drugs such as benztropine or diphenhydramine are usually effective in controlling akathisia when given by the intramuscular or intravenous route. Amantadine and propranolol have also been reported to be effective.[72]

Tardive Dyskinesia

The distinctive involuntary movement disorder called tardive dyskinesia occurs most frequently after prolonged treatment with dopamine antagonists, par-

Table 29-5 Drugs Associated with the Development of Tardive Dyskinesia

Phenothiazines
Chlorpromazine
Triflupromazine
Fluphenazine
Perphenazine
Trifluoperazine
Pericyazine
Promazine
Thiopropazate
Thioridazine
Mesoridazine

Thioxanthines
Thiothixene
Chlorprothixene

Butyrophenones
Droperidol
Haloperidol

Dibenzapines
Loxapine

Diphenylbutylpiperidines
Pimozide

Indolones
Molindone

Antiemetics
Metoclopramide
Phenothiazines
Prochlorperazine
Thiethylperazine
Promethazine

ticularly the antipsychotic drugs, but also with antiemetic drugs such as metoclopramide and prochlorperazine (Table 29-5).[73] Some studies have found tardive dyskinesia in up to 50 percent of patients treated with antipsychotic drugs.[73]

In contrast to the acute dystonic-dyskinetic syndrome, tardive dyskinesia usually develops after more than 12 months of continuous therapy, although it has been reported with periods as short as 3 months; it occasionally develops after cessation of therapy. The condition is more common and more severe in the elderly, in whom it is less likely to remit than in younger individuals.[73]

The condition typically takes the form of an orofaciolingual dyskinesia with lip smacking and pursing; sucking; jaw opening and closing; protruding, side-to-side, or writhing movements of the tongue; and facial grimacing. The movements tend to be rather stereotyped and, when severe, may interfere with speech or swallowing. In some cases more generalized choreoathetotic movements of the limbs and trunk and repetitive foot tapping are present, and the condition may resemble Huntington's chorea. Less frequently, dystonic posturing of the neck and myoclonic jerking of the distal extremities are also present, and concomitant akathisia or parkinsonism may also occur.[74] A related syndrome (the "withdrawal emergence" syndrome) characterized by choreoathetoid and myoclonic movements of the limbs, trunk, and mouth has been described after sudden withdrawal of antipsychotic drugs in children.

The pathophysiological basis for tardive dyskinesia has not been clearly established. The most widely held theory is that, as a result of prolonged dopamine receptor blockade in the corpus striatum, a state of hypersensitivity to endogenous dopamine develops due to changes in receptor properties or numbers.[73–75]

The severity of tardive dyskinesia is variable and the condition is not often disabling. It may remit in up to 40 percent of cases, even on continued therapy. In cases where it is possible to withdraw the offending drug, there is usually gradual resolution of the dyskinesia over a period of several weeks or months, but in some cases the condition persists. Occasionally a remission occurs even several years after withdrawal of antipsychotic drugs. Interruption of therapy when dyskinesia first develops may be beneficial, but there is some evidence that repeated interruption leads to an increased prevalence and persistence of dyskinesia.[73]

Although many pharmacological agents have been used to treat tardive dyskinesia, none has proved to be consistently beneficial. The drugs used include, on the one hand, agents with an effect on dopaminergic transmission, such as reserpine, tetrabenazine, bromocriptine, and levodopa, and, on the other hand, drugs with a cholinergic action, including deanol, choline, and lecithin. Other drugs reported to be beneficial in some cases include baclofen, propranolol, diazepam, α-tocopherol, sodium valproate, and the calcium channel blockers verapamil and diltiazem.[73,76]

Chorea and Choreoathetosis

A number of drugs may produce chorea, which is characterized by irregular, multifocal, nonstereotyped, semipurposive "fidgety" or jerky movements.[3] At times, chorea is associated with the slower, more sinuous movements of athetosis or with dystonia. These involuntary movements are thought to result from dopamine overactivity or cholinergic underactivity in the basal ganglia. Chorea or choreoathetosis has been reported with phenytoin intoxication and clonazepam withdrawal,[3,77] treatment with high doses of benzhexol,[3] and treatment with amphetamines, methadone, methylphenidate, amoxapine, pemoline, cimetidine, neuroleptics,

the androgenic steroid oxymetholone, and oral contraceptives.[3,78] Contraceptive-induced chorea is rare and may occur with high- or low-dose estrogen preparations.[79] Some patients who develop the condition have a past history of rheumatic chorea.[79] The occurrence of contraceptive-induced chorea may be followed by the development of chorea gravidarum in some women.

It is not uncommon for the dyskinesia occurring in parkinsonian patients treated with levodopa to have a choreic quality. Similarly, the orofacial and other involuntary movements of tardive dyskinesia may also resemble chorea, although in general they tend to be more repetitive and stereotyped.[74]

Parkinsonism

Parkinsonism can occur at all ages but is most frequent in the elderly and is probably the most common form of drug-induced movement disorder. The condition resembles naturally occurring Parkinson's disease very closely, bradykinesia usually being the most prominent feature, with a variable degree of rigidity, tremor, facial masking, and abnormal gait. Although tremor has been said to be less prominent than in idiopathic Parkinson's disease, in some series the incidence of tremor has been as high in cases of drug-induced parkinsonism as in the naturally occurring variety.[80] The drugs most frequently implicated are the neuroleptics including almost all of the phenothiazines (the most frequent being prochlorperazine), haloperidol, the tricyclic antidepressants, metoclopramide, methyldopa, lithium, and the calcium channel blockers cinnarizine and flurarizine.[81] The condition is usually reversible after drug withdrawal or dose reduction. In a group of 48 cases, Stephen and Williamson found that the condition resolved over a mean period of 7 weeks (1 to 36 weeks).[80] Five patients who initially improved subsequently developed idiopathic parkinsonism after an interval of 3 to 18 months, suggesting that the drug had unmasked a latent form of idiopathic parkinsonism.

The antidepressant drug fluoxetine has been reported to worsen drug-induced parkinsonism when used with neuroleptics.[82] Anticholinergic agents such as benzhexol or benztropine may reverse parkinsonian symptoms in patients who need to continue on neuroleptic therapy. In some cases spontaneous improvement occurs even if the causative agent is continued. Prophylactic treatment with anticholinergic agents may predispose to the development of an irreversible form of tardive dyskinesia and is not advocated, and treatment with levodopa may aggravate an underlying psychotic disorder.[3]

Neuroleptic Malignant Syndrome

The neuroleptic malignant syndrome, a serious and potentially lethal complication of treatment with antipsychotic drugs, is characterized by hyperpyrexia, severe rigidity, bradykinesis, tremor, and autonomic manifestations.[83–85] The serum creatine kinase (CK) activity is typically elevated, with levels of up to 15,000 IU/L being recorded. The drugs most frequently implicated are haloperidol, fluphenazine, chlorpromazine or other phenothiazines, and thioxanthenes, or combinations of these drugs with each other or with lithium and less frequently metoclopramide,[86] loxapine, or a tricyclic antidepressant.[87] The condition may occur with both high and low doses of either high- or low-potency neuroleptic drugs and may develop after commencing neuroleptic therapy, after an increase in dose, or following the introduction of a second, more potent drug. A similar syndrome has been reported after abrupt levodopa withdrawal in patients with Parkinson's disease.[84,88] The syndrome of "lethal catatonia" that has been described in patients on long-term antipsychotic therapy may be related to the neuroleptic malignant syndrome.[3]

Although in mild forms of the condition complete recovery may occur within days or weeks of stopping the causative drug, severe cases may develop various complications including metabolic acidosis, acute myoglobinuria with renal failure, coagulation defects, respiratory failure, shock, seizures, and coma. A mortality rate of up to 20 percent has been reported in some series[84] but has declined in the past decade.[85] Persisting neurological sequelae occur in up to 10 percent of survivors.[86]

The pathophysiological mechanism responsible for the neuroleptic malignant syndrome is uncertain. The current view is that the condition is due to profound dopamine receptor blockade in the corpus striatum as well as in thermoregulatory and vasomotor centers in the hypothalamus.[3,83,84] Treatment involves discontinuation of the causative drug or drugs together with vigorous cooling and correction of fluid and electrolyte balance and other complications. Specific measures that may be beneficial in reversing the rigidity and akinesia include the use of bromocriptine, levodopa, pancuronium, or dantrolene sodium, or a combination of these drugs (e.g., dantrolene with small doses of bromocriptine or levodopa).[84] The calcium channel blocker nifidepine has also been reported to be effective in some cases.

Tremor

A number of drugs may aggravate physiological or essential tremor. These include sympathomimetic agents, theophylline, doxapram, levodopa, corticosteroids, thyroxine, tricyclic antidepressants, caffeine, phenothiazines, butyrophenones, amphetamines, hypoglycemic agents, amiodarone, and Adriamycin, as well as benzodiazepine or alcohol withdrawal.[3,38,89,90] A postural or resting tremor resembling essential tremor and involving the hands, head, and trunk is not uncommon in patients treated with sodium valproate. The tremor usually develops over a period of several months and remits when the drug is stopped or the dose is reduced.[29] Treatment with propranolol or amantadine may alleviate the tremor.[91] Cimetidine and terfenadine may induce a severe postural and action tremor by aggravating physiological or essential tremor.[92] Postural or action tremor is an early manifestation of lithium intoxication and is also common in patients taking therapeutic doses of the drug.[93] Tremor with cerebellar ataxia may occur in patients on cyclosporin A.[94]

Asterixis may occasionally occur in patients treated with phenytoin, phenobarbital, carbamazepine, sodium valproate,[29] lithium, or tocainide.[46] Asterixis and head bobbing that failed to recover have been reported following metrizamide myelography.[95]

Tics

A syndrome resembling Gilles de la Tourette's syndrome has been reported following the administration of dextroamphetamine, methylphenidate, pemoline, or haloperidol in children.[3]

Myoclonus

Drug-induced myoclonus is rare but may occur in patients treated with antipsychotic and tricyclic antidepressant drugs or lithium carbonate. Myoclonus has been reported in patients treated with amitriptyline and in imipramine toxicity.[38] A clinical picture resembling that of Creutzfeldt-Jakob disease with myoclonus, coarse tremor, cerebellar and extrapyramidal manifestations, cognitive impairment, and periodic sharp wave complexes in the EEG has been reported in patients with lithium toxicity.[41] Complete resolution of the clinical and EEG changes occurred in these cases after withdrawal from the drug. Posturally induced myoclonic jerks in the upper limbs have been described in patients on long-term antipsychotic drug therapy and may be a component of tardive dyskinesia in some patients.[96] Myoclonus may also occur in some patients with Parkinson's disease who are treated with levodopa or bromocriptine.[97]

CEREBELLAR SYNDROMES

Various drugs may cause ataxia, incoordination, and other manifestations of cerebellar dysfunction. Sedatives (e.g., chloral hydrate, barbiturates, benzodiazepines, and paraldehyde) and anticonvulsants (e.g., phenytoin, carbamazepine, primidone, ethosuximide, and methosuximide) are most often responsible, their effects being dose-dependent. Individual tolerance to these drugs varies considerably, but in general symptoms are more likely to develop when high doses are administered too quickly. This is particularly important in the case of carbamazepine, which should be commenced in a low dose and then slowly increased over a period of at least a week. Ataxia and drowsiness may occur during administration of high doses of most tranquilizers, including diazepam, chlordiazepoxide, and meprobamate; signs of cerebellar dysfunction may be caused more rarely by phenothiazines, monoamine oxidase inhibitors, reserpine, thioxanthenes, and lithium salts. The latter may cause an isolated cerebellar ataxia or a more diffuse encephalopathy, even with blood levels within the therapeutic range.[98] These disorders are usually reversible when the causative agent is withdrawn or the dose adjusted, but there are occasional reports of permanent cerebellar atrophy or dysfunction in patients treated with phenytoin or lithium. Cerebellar ataxia has also been reported in bone marrow transplant recipients treated with cyclosporin A and has been associated with hypomagnesemia.[94]

A reversible cerebellar syndrome has been described in patients with leukemia or lymphoma treated with high doses of cytosine arabinoside; in some patients the drug causes an irreversible cerebellar degeneration.[99] Cerebellar dysfunction has also been reported in cancer patients treated with high- or low-dose fluorouracil[49,100] and in patients with impaired renal function receiving colistin; it may be associated with a peripheral neuropathy in certain patients taking nitrofurantoin or perhexiline.[101]

OTOTOXICITY

Drug-induced ototoxicity has been the subject of a number of recent reviews.[102,103] Many drugs may have ototoxic effects, causing damage to the cochlear or vestibular portions of the inner ear. Tinnitus is usually the earliest symptom of cochleotoxicity and, when persistent, is suggestive of impending hearing loss. Vestibulotoxicity may result in vertigo, oscillopsia, imbalance, and impairment of caloric responses. The most important group of ototoxic drugs are the aminoglycoside antibiotics, which may cause inner ear damage that is often irreversible after parenteral or oral administration or even after topical application, introduction into the peritoneal cavity or bronchial tree, or local application to burned areas or into the middle ear. All of the aminoglycosides can damage both the cochlear and vestibular portion of the inner ear; some (e.g., neomycin, kanamycin, and vancomycin) are more cochleotoxic, whereas others (e.g., streptomycin, gentamicin, and tobramycin) are preferentially more vestibulotoxic (Table 29-6). A vertical oscillation of the surroundings on movement ("bobbing oscillopsia") is highly characteristic of the vestibular disturbance produced by the aminoglycoside antibiotics. Hearing loss affects the high frequencies initially and is usually irreversible. It may develop within a few days of commencing treatment but is more often delayed and may even develop after administration of the drug has ceased. As a group, the aminoglycosides cause a degeneration of the sensory hair cells of the cochlea, the outer hair cells being most severely affected, accounting for the preferential loss of high frequencies. Experimental studies have shown that the primary site of action of these drugs is on the hair cell membrane, but they also interfere with the mechanical properties of the sensory hairs and the mechanoelectrical transduction process.[104]

Table 29-6 Major Ototoxic Drugs in Order of Decreasing Incidence of Toxicity[a]

Drug	Cochlear Toxicity	Vestibular Toxicity
Minocycline		4+
Kanamycin	3+	+
Amikacin	4+	
Neomycin	3+	+
Streptomycin	+	3+
Viomycin	2+	2+
Gentamicin	+	3+
Tobramycin	+	3+
Ethacrynic acid	3+	+
Furosemide	4+	
Vancomycin	4+	
Quinine	4+	
Salicylates	4+	
Polymyxin B[b]		4+
Colistin[b]		4+

[a] Ototoxicity is indicated on a scale of 0 to 4+.
[b] Applied topically.
(From Friedlander IR: Ototoxic drugs and the detection of ototoxicity. N Engl J Med 301:213, 1979, with permission.)

Other ototoxic antibiotics include minocycline (which is almost exclusively vestibulotoxic), erythromycin (which occasionally produces reversible deafness after oral or intravenous administration), metronidazole, and rarely, procaine penicillin, cephalexin, and chloramphenicol.

The loop diuretics furosemide and ethacrynic acid may cause hearing loss of rapid onset that is usually reversible and that may be due to electrolyte changes in the cochlear endolymph. Salicylates, in particular aspirin, may cause tinnitus, deafness, and vertigo when the serum concentration approaches 300 mg/L. Hearing loss is usually reversible, although recovery may be delayed or incomplete, and there are occasional reports of permanent hearing loss. There are also reports of deafness occurring following the use of salicylate-containing ointments. Quinine may cause tinnitus and reversible low-tone hearing loss in a small proportion of patients taking the drug; an idiosyncratic mechanism seems to be involved. Prolonged high-dose administration of chloroquine may cause tinnitus and perceptive deafness that is usually irreversible. A number of cytotoxic drugs including cisplatin, vincristine, misonidazole, bleomycin, and mustine hydrochloride may also cause hearing loss.

Cisplatin has been reported to cause a high incidence of tinnitus and high-tone hearing loss; brainstem auditory evoked potential recording is helpful in detecting early involvement of the auditory pathway, particularly in children.[105]

Other ototoxic drugs include quinidine, deferoxamine,[106] and the β-blocker practolol, which caused combined sensorineural deafness and conductive hearing loss due to serous otitis media when it was in general use. There are also rare reports of hearing loss or vestibular dysfunction in patients taking propoxyphene, naproxen, indomethacin, metoprolol, nortriptyline, propylthiouracil, flecainide acetate, or sulindac, and after vaccination.

VISUAL DISORDERS

Drug-induced visual disorders may result from effects on the pupil, refractive mechanisms, retina, optic nerve, or central visual pathways. Drug-induced disorders of the cornea and lens are discussed elsewhere.[58]

Pupillary Changes

Parasympathomimetic drugs such as carbachol and neostigmine produce miosis, as may morphine, chloral hydrate, and phenothiazines.[58] Mydriasis is more often drug-induced and potentially more serious, as it may precipitate an attack of acute angle-closure glaucoma in susceptible individuals.[58] Drugs that may cause mydriasis and cycloplegia with blurring of near vision include anticholinergics such as atropine, hyoscine hydrobromide, antihistamines, monoamine oxidase inhibitors, tricyclic antidepressants, chlorpropamide, indomethacin, hexamethonium, fenfluramine, oral contraceptives, amphetamines, and LSD derivatives.[58]

Refractive Changes

In addition to the drugs mentioned above that may cause cycloplegia and induced hypermetropia, certain drugs may cause a transient myopia as a result of fluid shifts between the lens and the aqueous humor. These include oral diuretics (chlorothiazide, hydrochlorothiazide, chlorthalidone, and acetazolamide), tetracyclines, sulfonamides, corticosteroids and corticotropin, stilbestrol, phenytoin, thiamine, bromocriptine, and arsenicals, as well as insulin and oral hypoglycemic agents in diabetics.[58]

Retinopathy

Chloroquine and related drugs such as hydroxychloroquine, mepacrine, and amodiaquine may produce a pigmentary maculopathy and retinopathy with central and peripheral field defects and impairment of central vision after prolonged administration in patients with rheumatoid arthritis or discoid lupus erythematosus. Patients treated with these drugs should have regular neuro-ophthalmic examinations as well as electroretinography and electrooculography to detect early signs of retinopathy. Phenothiazines in high doses may produce a progressive chorioretinopathy; cardiac glycosides, methylphenidate, and cephaloridine have also been reported to cause a pigmentary retinopathy. Macular edema may be caused by oral contraceptives and, rarely, by chlorothiazide and acetazolamide. Other drugs that may interfere with vision through effects on the retina include indomethacin, quinine, tamoxifen, ethambutol, diethylcarbamazine,[107] and, in experimental animals, hexachlorophene and perhexiline.

Optic Neuropathy

An optic neuropathy leading to optic atrophy occurred in the subacute myeloptic neuropathy (SMON) syndrome that was prevalent in Japan. A number of antibiotics may also cause optic neuropathy. These include chloramphenicol (which may produce slowly progressive optic atrophy with constriction of the visual fields after prolonged administration), isoniazid, paraminosalicylate, streptomycin, ethambutol, sulfonamides, griseofulvin, dapsone, and chlorpropamide.[58] In the case of chloramphenicol, prophylactic administration of vitamin B_{12} may prevent the onset of optic neuropathy.[58] Prolonged high-dose treatment with the iron-chelating agent deferoxamine has been reported to cause optic neuropathy with marked reduction in visual acuity, loss of color vision, and delayed visual evoked potentials in addition to hearing loss.[106] Bilateral ischemic optic neuropathy has been reported in a patient taking Cafergot (a combination of ergotamine and caffeine).[108]

Other drugs implicated in causing optic neuropathy include chlorambucil,[109] penicillamine, disulfiram, phenylbutazone, indomethacin, ibuprofen, benoxaprofen, morphine, monoamine oxidase inhibitors, organic arsenicals, cardiac glycosides, hexamethonium, and barbiturates,[58,110] as well as dideoxyinosine (ddI).[111]

Disorders of Color Vision

Disturbances of color vision may result from the effects of drugs on the retinal cone receptors or from optic nerve dysfunction. Xanthopsia (yellow vision) may be caused by a number of drugs including sulfonamides, streptomycin, methaqualone, barbiturates, digitalis derivatives, thiazide diuretics (in particular, chlorothiazide), and the antihelminthic agent santonin.[58] Other drugs that may cause disturbances of color vision include nalidixic acid, oral contraceptives, cannabis, LSD, and the anticonvulsants troxidone and paramethadione, which also cause an increased dazzle effect and impairment of color discrimination.[58]

Cortical Blindness

Cortical blindness may rarely occur following episodes of severe hypotension during anesthesia and has also been reported as a complication of chemotherapy during childhood or of excessive doses of salicylates or barbiturates.[58]

Diplopia

Certain drugs commonly cause diplopia by leading to breakdown of a latent squint. These include indomethacin, chlorpropamide, diazepam, quinine, methaqualone, fenfluramine, tricyclic antidepressants, and anticonvulsant drugs.[58] Rarely, diplopia may be due to an extraocular muscle palsy or gaze palsy.[58]

Nystagmus

Drug-induced nystagmus is common, particularly in hospital practice. Horizontal vestibular nystagmus is commonly found in patients on high doses of barbiturates, benzodiazepines, anticonvulsants, and other sedative and hypnotic drugs. It is a useful sign of toxicity in patients on anticonvulsant therapy but may occur even with therapeutic doses of some of the other drugs. Other drugs reported to cause nystagmus include monoamine oxidase inhibitors, salicylates, gold, neostigmine, chlordiazepoxide, fenfluramine, and amitryptyline, as well as the ototoxic antibiotics.[58] Lithium and a number of other drugs may cause downbeat nystagmus.[112]

DISORDERS OF TASTE AND SMELL

Drug-induced disorders of taste are common. Many drugs may cause metallic, bitter, or salty taste sensations (phantogeusias) or distortions of taste.[113–115] These include biguanides, ethambutol, vitamin D, gold, allopurinol, penicillin, metronidazole, timidazole, lincomycin, clindamycin, aspirin, and phenindione. A number of other drugs may cause a reduction or loss in taste, the perception of sweetness being most often affected. These include D-penicillamine (which causes marked hypogeusia in up to 30 percent of patients receiving it; this is corrected by the administration of copper), levodopa, captopril, enalapril, etidronate, oxyfedine, methimazole, carbimazole, thiouracil, phenylbutazone, amphotericin B, griseofulvin, terbinafine, azathioprine, salazosulfapyridine, chlormezanone, carbamazepine, and baclofen.

Distortion of the sense of smell or complete anosmia, which may be irreversible, has been associated with the administration of a number of drugs including augmentin, intranasal beclomethasone, captopril, doxycycline, and erythromycin.[116]

SPINAL DISORDERS

Intrathecal injections of certain drugs may be complicated by infective or aseptic meningitis, adhesive arachnoiditis, or toxic effects of the drug on the spinal cord or nerve roots. Intrathecal injection of corticosteroid preparations such as Depo-Medrol causes an acute meningial reaction that is thought to be due to the polyethylene glycol detergent in the preparation and is associated with back and leg pain and paresthesias, bladder dysfunction, and a polymorphonuclear pleocytosis and raised protein level in the cerebrospinal fluid (CSF).[117] Intrathecal Depo-Medrol has also been implicated in causing a chronic adhesive arachnoiditis.[117,118]

Epidural injections, which are now preferred in the treatment of patients with chronic lumbar radicular pain, are not associated with such reactions unless there is inadvertent penetration of the dura. Spinal anesthesia is associated with a low incidence of lower limb numbness, paresthesias, or weakness that has been attributed to toxic effects of the anesthetic agent on the lumbosacral roots.[119] Symptoms usually develop immediately after operation and persist for several months in some cases. The incidence of such complications is even lower following epidural anesthesia.[119]

Intrathecal chemotherapy with methotrexate or cytosine arabinoside may cause aseptic meningitis or transient or permanent paraplegia.[49,120] An acute transverse myelopathy may also occur in heroin addicts and has been attributed to ischemia of the cord due to vasculitis.[121]

A syndrome of myeloneuropathy with sensory dysesthesias, Lhermitte's sign, leg weakness and spasticity, ataxia, and sphincter disturbances has been described in dentists after prolonged exposure to nitrous oxide.[122] The condition is thought to be due to the inhibitory effects of nitrous oxide on vitamin B_{12} utilization and, in some cases, hematological changes of vitamin B_{12} deficiency are also found.[122] Recovery usually occurs after exposure to nitrous oxide is stopped. Lhermitte's sign has also been reported in association with peripheral neuropathy in patients treated with high doses of cisplatin.[123]

Spinal cord compression, attributed to increased extradural adipose tissue, has been reported rarely in patients on prolonged corticosteroid therapy.[124]

AUTONOMIC DISORDERS

Postural Hypotension

Many drugs may precipitate or aggravate postural hypotension, resulting in giddiness, falls, or syncope; focal cerebral ischemic events sometimes occur in patients with cerebrovascular disease. The drugs which most frequently produce this side effect are the antihypertensive agents, vasodilators, diuretics, antidepressants, and levodopa.[125]

Bladder Dysfunction

Drugs with an anticholinergic action may cause urinary retention by inhibiting parasympathetic postganglionic cholinergic neurons and decreasing bladder tone, particularly if there is already some degree of bladder outflow obstruction due to prostatic hypertrophy.[3] These include atropine, hyoscine, propantheline, benzhexol, benztropine, methixene, orphenadrine, dicyclomine, and other derivatives of belladonna alkaloids. In addition, tricyclic antidepressants and phenothiazines may cause difficulty with micturition and urinary retention because of their anticholinergic effects. Other drugs that may cause urinary retention include monoamine oxidase inhibitors, disopyramide, ephedrine, salbutamol, terbutaline, and theophylline.[3]

A number of other drugs may interfere with the control of micturition and cause urinary incontinence. These include prazosin, metoprolol, benoxaprofen, depot phenothiazines, clonazepam, and the combination of phenoxybenzamine and methyldopa.[3]

Disorders of Sexual Function

Many drugs interfere with normal sexual function, causing loss of or decreased libido, impotence, impaired ejaculation, or orgasmic dysfunction. The drugs implicated in causing these side effects have been reviewed elsewhere.[126,127] Those most commonly involved are antihypertensive agents, tricyclic antidepressants, monoamine oxidase inhibitors, major tranquilizers, antihistamines, and anticholinergics, as well as baclofen, cimetidine, clofibrate, disopyramide, bromocriptine, and levodopa.

NEUROMUSCULAR DISORDERS

Many drugs can affect the peripheral nerves, neuromuscular junctions, or muscles, resulting in sensory symptoms, weakness, or fatigability.[128–130] Patients with a preexisting neuromuscular disorder are more likely to develop such adverse effects.

Peripheral Neuropathies

Various drugs used in clinical practice may interfere with peripheral nerve function and cause a neuropathy.[131] Some have an effect principally on sensory nerve function, causing peripheral paraesthesias and in some cases other signs of a sensory neuropathy (Table 29-7). Conversely, other drugs such as dapsone and gold may produce a motor neuropathy with absent or inconspicuous sensory findings. Most drugs, however, produce a mixed sensory and motor polyneuropathy that manifests initially with sensory symptoms; signs of motor involvement develop at a later stage if the drug is not stopped. Muscle pain and cramps are prominent early symptoms in some cases. The tendon reflexes may be preserved in the early stages but are subsequently depressed or absent, even when motor involvement is absent or inconspicuous. In general, drugs that cause peripheral neuropathy do so either by interfering with axonal or Schwann cell metabolism or, less frequently, through a vascular effect.[132] Localized forms of neuropathy may occur as a complication of intramuscular, intravenous, or intra-arterial injections of certain drugs.[132]

ANTIMICROBIAL AGENTS

More than a dozen antimicrobial drugs may cause a peripheral neuropathy. The best-known example is the mixed sensorimotor neuropathy caused by isoniazid, which is due to the effect of the drug on pyridoxine metabolism and which can be prevented by giving vitamin B_6 supplements. Ethambutol may also cause a sensory or sensorimotor neuropathy or an optic neuropathy. Ethionamide and streptomycin may rarely also cause a peripheral neuropathy, although in the case of streptomycin this is less frequent than the ototoxic effects of the drug. Peripheral neuropathy is a well-documented complication of treatment with nitrofurantoin. The neuropathy is usually of mixed sensorimotor type but occasionally is predominantly motor; it is more likely to develop in patients with renal insufficiency. Although peripheral neuropathy was a well-recognized complication of treatment with sulfonamides in the past, none of the sulfonamides in current clinical use have this effect. There have been several reports of a reversible sensory neuropathy in patients treated with metronidazole. Peripheral neuropathy was also part of the SMON syndrome caused by clioquinol that was prevalent in Japan during the 1950s and 1960s and has been reported only rarely from other countries.[133]

Table 29-7 Drug-Induced Peripheral Neuropathies

Clinical Syndrome	Antimicrobial Drugs	Antineoplastic Drugs	Antirheumatic Drugs	Hypnotics and Psychotropics	Cardiovascular Drugs	Other Drugs
Sensory neuropathy	Ethionamide Chloramphenicol Thiamphenicol Diamines	Procarbazine Misonidazole Cisplatin Ormaplatinum Dideoxycytidine Taxotere	Sulindac	Thalidomide	Enalapril	Calcium carbimidine Sulfoxone Ergotamine Propylthiouracil Pyridoxine Almitrine Simvastatin Gemfibrozil
Paresthesias only	Colistin Streptomycin Nalidixic acid	Cytosine arabinoside		Phenelzine	Propranolol	Sulthiame Chlorpropamide Methysergide Acetazolamide Gemfibrozil
Sensorimotor neuropathy	Isoniazid Ethambutol Streptomycin Nitrofurantoin Clioquinol Metronidazole	Vincristine Vinblastine Podophyllin Chlorambucil Laetrile Cisplatin Hexamethylmelamine Taxotere Suramin	Gold Indomethacin Colchicine Chloroquine Phenylbutazone D-Penicillamine	Thalidomide Methaqualone Glutethimide Amitriptyline Lithium Phenelzine Perazine	Perhexiline Hydralazine Amiodarone Disopyramide	Phenytoin Disulfiram Carbutamide Tolbutamide Chlorpropamide Methimazole Methylthiouracil Cimetidine Clofibrate Tetanus toxoid
Predominantly motor neuropathy	Sulfonamides Amphotericin B Streptomycin Dapsone	Azathioprine	Gold Sulindac	Imipramine Amitriptyline		Cimetidine
Localized neuropathy	Penicillin Amphotericin B Mustine	Ethoglucid				Anticoagulants
Guillaine-Barré syndrome			D-Penicillamine	Zimeldine	Streptokinase	? Danazol ? Captopril ? Gangliosides ? Epidural anesthesia

(Adapted from Argov Z, Mastaglia FL: Drug-induced neuromuscular disorders in man. p. 981. In Walton JN (ed): Disorders of Voluntary Muscle. 5th Ed. Churchill Livingstone, Edinburgh, 1988, with permission.)

ANTINEOPLASTIC DRUGS

Vincristine and other vinca alkaloids are particularly neurotoxic, and most patients treated with these drugs for long enough will develop a sensorimotor polyneuropathy with early loss of tendon reflexes and in some cases postural hypotension and constipation due to autonomic nervous system involvement.[48,134,135] Muscle cramps may be a prominent symptom in the early stages and in some cases there is an associated painful proximal myopathy. Recovery may occur if the drug is stopped or the dose reduced, but areflexia and mild sensory symptoms usually persist.

Procarbazine, which is structurally related to isoniazid, and nitrofurazone, a congener of nitrofurantoin, can cause a sensory neuropathy, as may cisplatin,[135,136] ormaplatinum,[137] and Taxotere.[138] Misonidazole and related compounds, which are chemically related to metronidazole and are used as radiosensitizing agents in cancer therapy, may also induce a sensory neuropathy.[132] The experimental chemotherapeutic agent suramin produces a dose-related axonal sensorimotor neuropathy associated with lamellar inclusions in dorsal root ganglia and Schwann cells.[139] Podophyllin derivatives, which have been used to treat disseminated malignancy and are also constituents of certain laxative preparations and topical agents, may cause a peripheral neuropathy of variable severity, sometimes associated with signs of spinal cord involvement. Peripheral neuropathy and Lhermitte's sign may also occur in patients treated with high-dose cisplatin.[123]

ANTIRHEUMATIC DRUGS

Peripheral neuropathy is a well-recognized complication of gold treatment in patients with rheumatoid arthritis, occurring in 0.5 to 1 percent of patients. Motor involvement is prominent, with inconspicuous sensory symptoms. The onset may be abrupt and the progression rapid, so that in some cases the condition mimics the Guillain-Barré syndrome, particularly in patients who develop facial diplegia and have elevated CSF protein levels.[132]

Chloroquine may cause a mild sensorimotor neuropathy as well as a more severe proximal myopathy in some cases. A neuropathy may also occur rarely in patients treated with D-penicillamine, which is known to have an antipyridoxine action, but this is less common than the myasthenic syndrome that may occur in patients on long-term treatment with this drug. There has been a report of the Guillain-Barré syndrome developing in a patient on D-penicillamine.[132]

CARDIOVASCULAR DRUGS

A demyelinating sensorimotor polyneuropathy occurred in about 0.1 percent of patients treated with the coronary vasodilator perhexiline, which is no longer widely used.[81] Associated findings in some cases included papilledema, dysgeusia, deafness, cerebellar signs, autonomic dysfunction, and raised CSF protein levels. A demyelinating sensorimotor neuropathy is also well documented in patients treated with the antiarrhythmic agent amiodarone.[140,141] Peripheral neuropathy may rarely develop in patients treated with disopyramide, hydralazine, flecainide,[142] enalapril, and captopril.[143]

HYPNOTIC AND PSYCHOTROPIC DRUGS

There have been occasional reports of peripheral neuropathy developing in patients taking phenelzine,[144] methaqualone, glutethimide, imipramine, amitriptyline, lithium carbonate,[132] thalidomide,[145] and perazine.[146] Administration of the antidepressant drug zimeldine has been associated with the development of the Guillain-Barré syndrome in Sweden, the risk of developing this condition being increased 25-fold in patients taking the drug.[147]

OTHER DRUGS

Various other drugs have occasionally been implicated in causing a peripheral neuropathy (Table 29-7). A mild peripheral neuropathy with depression of the tendon reflexes and minor sensory changes may occur in patients on long-term treatment with phenytoin but is only rarely symptomatic. Disulfiram, used in the treatment of alcoholism, may cause a sensorimotor polyneuropathy of axonal type as well as optic neuropathy.[132] Dapsone, used in the treatment of leprosy and of certain dermatological conditions, may cause a predominantly motor peripheral neuropathy after prolonged high-dose therapy.

Chronic administration of high doses of pyridoxine has been reported to cause a severe sensory polyneuropathy of insidious onset and course, and paresthesias may develop even in some patients taking conventional doses of this vitamin.[148] A severe irreversible sensory neuropathy has also been reported in patients treated with massive doses of pyridoxine parenterally.[148] An inflammatory demyelinating polyneuropathy has also been found to occur in many patients with the *eosinophilia myalgia syndrome* caused by certain preparations of L-tryptophan.[135]

Almitrine bismesylate, a drug used in the treatment of patients with chronic respiratory insufficiency, has been reported to cause a sensory polyneuropathy.[149] Colchicine, a neurotubular toxin, may cause a neuromyopathy characterized by progressive proximal muscle weakness and suppression of deep tendon reflexes.[150] The condition is potentially reversible after withdrawal of the drug.

Captopril, danazol,[151] and epidural anesthesia[152] have been associated with the development of the Guillain-Barré syndrome, as have streptokinase[153] and gangliosides[154]; the causative role of gangliosides remains unproven.

Disorders of Neuromuscular Transmission

A variety of drugs used in clinical practice may interfere with neuromuscular transmission by causing a postsynaptic block or through an additional presynaptic effect[129,132] (Table 29-8). The most frequently encountered clinical syndrome is the postoperative respiratory depression that sometimes occurs in patients being treated with antibiotics, particularly those of the aminoglycoside group, or with various other drugs including some that potentiate the action of muscle relaxants used during anesthesia. Many of the drugs shown in Table 29-8 may also unmask or aggravate a preexisting myasthenic disorder by further reducing the safety factor for neuromuscular transmission and should therefore be avoided or used with caution in such patients. Patients with myasthenia are also excessively sensitive to the effects of muscle relaxants and in some patients the occurrence of prolonged postoperative respiratory depression is the first indication that the patient has myasthenia.

A syndrome which is clinically indistinguishable from myasthenia gravis may develop in some patients treated with D-penicillamine for prolonged periods. Most reported cases have been in patients with rheumatoid arthritis, who have usually recovered gradually over a period of several months after withdrawal of the drug. These patients develop acetylcholine receptor antibodies in the serum, similar to those found in naturally occurring myasthenia gravis, suggesting that the drug initiates an autoimmune response through an effect on immunoregulatory mechanisms or, possibly, by altering the antigenic properties of the acetylcholine receptor.[132]

Muscle Disorders

Certain drugs cause muscular symptoms through a direct toxic effect on muscle. Other drugs that are not intrinsically myotoxic may lead to muscle damage secondary to an immunological process, to severe hypokalemia or ischemia, to muscle compression ("crush syndrome") as a result of prolonged periods of immobility following drug overdose, or to excessive neural driving or accumulation of acetylcholine at the neuromuscular junction.[155]

MYALGIA AND CRAMPS

Various drugs have been reported to cause muscle pain, stiffness, and cramping that are reversible when the drug is withdrawn (Table 29-9). In some cases the serum CK activity is elevated transiently, indicating a direct effect of the drug on muscle. Similar symptoms may occur in patients with drug-induced myotonia and may also be the initial symptoms heralding the onset of a more severe necrotizing myopathy[132,155] (see below).

Muscle pain and fasciculation are commonly induced by suxamethonium during anesthesia. The incidence of these side effects may be reduced by the use of *d*-tubocurarine, diazepam, or calcium gluconate. Fasciculations and myokymia have also been reported in patients treated with gold[156] or D-penicillamine.[157]

ACUTE RHABDOMYOLYSIS

Acute rhabdomyolysis, the most acute and severe form of necrotizing myopathy, may occur following general anesthesia, ethanol intoxication, prolonged drug-induced coma, self-administration of heroin or other narcotic drugs, or treatment with various other

Table 29-8 Drugs Associated with Neuromuscular Transmission Disorders

Clinical Syndrome	Antibiotics	Antirheumatic Drugs	Cardiovascular Drugs	Anticonvulsants	Psychotropic Drugs	Anesthetics	Other Drugs
Drug-induced myasthenic syndrome	Neomycin Streptomycin Kanamycin Gentamicin Polymyxin B Colistin	D-Penicillamine	Oxyprenolol Practolol Trimethaphan	Trimethadione Phenytoin			? Busulfan ? Oral contraceptive D,L-Carnitine
Aggravation or unmasking of myasthenia gravis	Streptomycin Kanamycin Colistin Rolitetracycline Oxytetracycline Gentamicin Ampicillin Erythromycin Imipenem/cilistatin	Chloroquine	Quinidine Procainamide Propranolol	Phenytoin	Lithium Chlorpromazine		Methoxyflurane ACTH Corticosteroids Thyroid hormones Acetylcholinesterase inhibitors Timolol Magnesium salts Iodinated contrast media
Postoperative respiratory depression Antibiotic-induced respiratory arrest syndrome	Neomycin Streptomycin Kanamycin Colistin						
Potentiation of muscle relaxants	Lincomycin Clindamycin	Chloroquine	Quinidine Trimethaphan		Lithium Promazine Phenelzine	Diazepam Ketamine Propanidid Ether	Oxytocin Trasylol Cholinesterase inhibitors Procaine Lidocaine Timolol Magnesium salts

(Adapted from Argov Z, Mastaglia FL: Disorders of neuromuscular transmission caused by drugs. N Engl J Med 301:409, 1979; and Argov Z, Mastaglia FL: Drug-induced neuromuscular disorders in man. p. 981. In Walton JN (ed): Disorders of Voluntary Muscle. 5th Ed. Churchill Livingstone, Edinburgh, 1988, with permission.)

Table 29-9 Drugs Reported to Cause Myalgia or Muscle Cramps

Suxamethonium	Isoetherine
Danazol	Zimeldine
Clofibrate[a]	Labetalol
Salbutamol	Procainamide
Lithium	Clonidine
Captopril	Pindolol
Enalapril	Cimetidine
Bumetadine	D-penicillamine
Metolazone	Gold
Cytotoxics	Nifedipine
Colchicine	Merceptopropionyl glycine
Zidovudine	Ethchlorvynol
Rifampicin	L-tryptophan

[a] And other hypocholesterolemic agents.

Table 29-10 Drugs Implicated in Causing Acute Rhabdomyolysis and Myoglobinuria

Rhabdomyolysis associated with coma, seizures, dyskinesia	Hypokalemia and rhabdomyolysis
Barbiturates	Diuretics
Heroin	Carbenoxolone
Methadone	Amphotericin B
Glutethimide	Licorice
Chlorpromazine	**Other drugs**
Diazepam	Amphetamines
Rohypnol	Phenmetrazine
Lithium	Phencyclidine
Amoxapine	Phenylpropanolamine
Phenelzine	Morphine
Phenformin/	Dihydrocodeine
fenfluramine	LSD
Meprobamate	Salicylates
Antihistamines/	Clofibrate/bezafibrate/
acetaminophen	fenofibrate
Oxprenolol	Lovastatin
Ethanol	Gemfibrozil
Postanesthetic rhabdomyolysis	ε-Aminocaproic acid
Suxamethonium	Isoniazid
Malignant hyperpyrexia	Loxapine
Neuroleptic malignant syndrome	Theophylline
Haloperidol	Pentamidine
Stelazine	Vasopressin
Fluphenazine	
Other neuroleptics	

drugs[158–160] (Table 29-10). The condition is characterized by severe widespread muscle pain, weakness, and areflexia usually developing over a period of 24 to 48 hours. Swelling of limb muscles may occur and is sometimes so severe that it causes secondary ischemia and peripheral nerve entrapment ("compartment syndromes"), necessitating fasciotomy. Myoglobinuria is an early feature, leading to brownish discoloration of the urine and a blood-positive orthotolidine (Hematest) reaction in the absence of hematuria or hemoglobinuria; it can be confirmed by radioimmunoassay. Patients with severe myoglobinuria frequently develop acute oliguric renal failure and require dialysis. Hyperkalemia, hyperphosphatemia, and hypocalcemia are also common, and hypercalcemia may develop during the recovery phase.[158,161] The serum CK activity is markedly elevated, and muscle biopsy shows severe necrosis that may be associated with regenerative changes and mild inflammation. The prognosis for recovery is generally good, but some patients with severe renal failure die as a result of multiple organ failure and other complications.

SUBACUTE NECROTIZING MYOPATHY

A less acute syndrome characterized by symmetrical proximal or generalized weakness, myalgia, preserved tendon reflexes, elevated serum CK levels, and, in some severe cases, myoglobinuria has been reported in patients treated with a number of hypocholesterolemic agents, ε-aminocaproic acid, emetine, and cardiac glycosides, as well as in heroin or opiate addicts.

Hypocholesterolemic Drugs

A myopathy with severe muscle pain, cramps, weakness and markedly elevated serum CK activity may occur in hyperlipidemic patients treated with clofibrate or other fibric acid derivatives—such as fenofibrate, bezafibrate, and gemfibrozil (Lopid)[160,162]—and nicotinic acid (niacin).[163] Clofibrate myopathy is more likely to occur in patients with renal failure, nephrotic syndrome, or hypothyroidism, situations in which serum levels of the active metabolite chlorophenoxyisobutyric acid are increased. Symptoms usually develop abruptly within

3 weeks of commencing treatment; withdrawal of the drug or reduction in dose is followed by gradual recovery. A painful myopathy, at times with myonecrosis and myoglobinuria, has also been reported in patients and animals treated with the newer HMG-CoA reductase inhibitors lovastatin, simvastatin, and pravastatin and is potentiated by coadministration of cyclosporine.[164,165]

ε-Aminocaproic Acid

Myopathy is an uncommon complication of treatment with ε-aminocaproic acid, an antifibrinolytic agent, usually developing after 4 to 6 weeks of continuous treatment with doses over 18 g/d in patients with subarachnoid hemorrhage or hereditary angioneurotic edema.[132,160] The mechanism of the myopathy is uncertain but may be related to incorporation of the drug into cellular membranes in place of lysine, leading to altered membrane function. Muscle biopsy has shown capillary occlusions and fibrinogen deposition, suggesting an ischemic basis for the myopathy in some cases.[160]

Emetine

Muscle weakness is a common side effect of treatment with emetine, an ipecac alkaloid, in patients with amebiasis. A severe myopathy has also been reported in patients using ipecac syrup as an emetic agent[132,166] and may be associated with cardiomyopathy.[167] Experimental studies have shown that the drug interferes with protein synthesis and causes mitochondrial, cell membrane, and myofibrillar changes in muscle.[132,160]

Cardiac Glycosides

A proximal myopathy with myalgia or myasthenic features and marked elevation of the serum CK activity has been reported in drug addicts consuming large quantities of the cough suppressant codeine linctus, one of the components of which is squill, which contains the cardiac glycosides scillarin A and B.[168] The cardiac glycosides as a group inhibit the cell membrane Na^+-K^+ pump, and the myopathy in these cases may therefore be due to the effects of scillarin on muscle cell membranes.

MITOCHONDRIAL MYOPATHY

A myopathy characterized by myalgia, proximal or generalized weakness, and elevated serum CK levels may occur in patients with human immunodeficiency virus (HIV) infection who are on long-term treatment with zidovudine (AZT)[165,169,170]; it usually improves when the drug is withdrawn.[171] Muscle biopsy shows ragged red fibers and mitochondrial inclusions and allows differentiation from HIV-associated myopathy.[172] Zidovudine inhibits mDNA replication, leading to depletion of mDNA.[173]

POTASSIUM MYOPATHY

Hypotonic weakness with depression of tendon reflexes and marked elevation of serum CK activity may develop in patients who become hypokalemic as a result of treatment with diuretics or nasal sprays containing fluoroprednisolone, or as a result of purgative abuse or the consumption of large quantities of licorice or licorice extracts, which are ingredients of some traditional Chinese drugs and which contain the potent mineralocorticoid analogue glycyrrhizinic acid.[160,174,175] Profound muscle weakness due to hyperkalemia has also been reported in patients treated with potassium-retaining diuretics.

INFLAMMATORY MYOPATHIES

An inflammatory myopathy may develop in patients with rheumatoid arthritis, scleroderma, or Wilson's disease treated with D-penicillamine, the condition being indistinguishable clinically and pathologically from other forms of polymyositis and dermatomyositis.[160,176] An interstitial form of myositis characterized clinically by muscle pain, stiffness, and mild weakness has been reported rarely in patients treated with procainamide, hydralazine, phenytoin, or levodopa. There are also reports of the onset of dermatomyositis following treatment with penicillin.[176]

An interstitial form of eosinophilic myositis and fasciitis characterized by severe myalgia, edema and induration of the skin, and a peripheral blood eosinophilia has recently been recognized in patients taking certain preparations of L-tryptophan (the *eosinophilia-myalgia syndrome*).[160,177,178] The condition has been most prevalent in the United States, where more than 1,500 cases have been reported,[177] and has been attributed to a chemical contaminant.[179] Neuropathic symptoms occur in up to two-thirds of cases due to an associated inflammatory polyneuropathy.[135]

DRUG-INDUCED MYOTONIA

Certain drugs may induce myotonia in humans or animals. These include the hypocholesterolemic agents 20,25-diazacholesterol, clofibrate, triparanol, and zuclomiphene. In addition, a number of drugs may exacerbate or unmask previously undetected myotonia. These include depolarizing muscle relaxants such as suxamethonium, which may markedly exacerbate myotonia during general anesthesia, the β-adrenergic blockers propranolol and pindolol, and the β$_2$-agonists fenoterol and ritodrine. A number of diuretics including furosemide, ethacrynic acid, mersalyl, and acetazolamide induce myotonia in animals and should therefore be used with caution in patients with hereditary forms of myotonia.[180]

CORTICOSTEROID MYOPATHY

Corticosteroid myopathy is probably the commonest drug-induced myopathy encountered in clinical practice. A symptomatic myopathy is most likely to develop in patients treated with 9-α-fluorinated steroids such as triamcinolone, betamethasone, and dexamethasone, but may also occur when other corticosteroids are administered for prolonged periods. Patients treated for long periods with more than 10 mg of prednisolone per day, or its equivalent of another corticosteroid, may develop a myopathy. Those taking daily doses of 40 mg or more of prednisolone are at particular risk, while patients on an alternate-day regime are not usually affected.[181] The muscles of the pelvic girdle and thighs are most severely affected; pain is not usually a feature. Muscles innervated by the cranial nerves are spared, although involvement of the laryngeal muscles leading to dysphonia has been reported in patients using inhaled corticosteroids such as beclomethasone. Diaphragmatic weakness may develop in asthmatic patients on corticosteroids.[181] A severe generalized myopathy has been reported in asthmatics after prolonged courses of high-dose intravenous hydrocortisone, particularly in patients also receiving nondepolarizing neuromuscular blocking agents ("blocking agent–corticosteroid myopathy").[160,165,182]

Serum CK levels are usually normal in corticosteroid myopathy; elevated levels should suggest the possibility of some other type of myopathy. Creatine and 3-methylhistidine excretion in the urine is increased. Muscle biopsy shows selective atrophy of type IIB muscle fibers.

The myopathy is usually reversible if the drug can be withdrawn or the dose reduced, or to some extent if an alternate-day regime can be implemented. Recent studies have shown that disuse of muscles due to physical inactivity may render them more susceptible to the effects of corticosteroids and that steroid-induced muscle atrophy and weakness can be at least partially prevented or reversed by a regular program of physical training.[183,184] The mechanism of the myopathy is thought to be related to the basic cellular action of corticosteroids in inhibiting mRNA synthesis, as a result of which the translation and synthesis of muscle-specific proteins is impaired.[183]

AUTOPHAGIC MYOPATHY

A number of drugs with amphiphilic cationic properties lead to autophagic degeneration and accumulation of phospholipid in muscle and other tissues.[155,160] These include chloroquine, which can cause a painless proximal myopathy or neuromyopathy after prolonged periods of administration, and perhexiline and amiodarone, which lead to the development of a demyelinating sensorimotor peripheral neuropathy with an associated proximal myopathy in some patients. Vincristine and colchicine may also cause an autophagic myopathy or neuromyopathy.[160]

MALIGNANT HYPERPYREXIA

Malignant hyperpyrexia is a condition in which susceptible individuals may develop a potentially fatal state of severe generalized muscular rigidity, hyperpyrexia, metabolic acidosis, and myoglobinuria when exposed to certain anesthetic agents or other drugs.[185,186] Susceptibility is usually transmitted as an autosomal dominant trait and may be associated with either a clinically apparent or subclinical myopathy. The most reliable method of identifying individuals at risk in affected families is by the demonstration of abnormal sensitivity of muscle tissue to anesthetic agents in vitro. A similar susceptibility to anesthetic reactions may rarely also occur in patients with Duchenne muscular dystrophy, myotonia congenita, myotonic dystrophy, central core disease, Noonan syndrome, and osteogenesis imperfecta.[132,155]

The malignant hyperpyrexia crisis is thought to be due to an intrinsic abnormality of the excitation-contraction coupling mechanism in skeletal muscle, as a result of which exposure to anesthetic agents leads to the excessive release of calcium ions from the sarcoplasmic reticulum, causing sustained myofibrillar contraction. Various drugs which reduce myoplasmic calcium levels may be used to treat malignant hyperpyrexia. These include procaine, procainamide, hydrocortisone, dexamethasone, and dantrolene sodium, which is the drug of choice.[187]

FOCAL MYOPATHY

Localized areas of muscle damage occur after intramuscular injection of various drugs as a result of needle trauma ("needle myopathy") and local effects of the agent injected.[155] Severe muscle fibrosis and contracture may develop after repeated intramuscular injections in drug addicts or after prolonged courses of antibiotic injections in children.

OTHER DRUGS

Other drugs that have been reported to cause a myopathy include vincristine and colchicine (which may also cause a neuropathy or neuromyopathy), rifampicin, cimetidine, tetracycline, mercaptoproprionyl glycine, adenine arabinoside, and ethchlorvynol.[132,160] Cyclosporine has also been reported to cause a reversible dose-dependent myopathy characterized by myalgia and weakness or elevated serum CK and myoglobinuria when it is administered with lovastatin.[188]

ACKNOWLEDGMENTS

I am grateful to Mr. Roger Hall of the Sir Charles Gairdner Hospital Drug Information Office and Mrs. Beverley Laing for their help in reviewing the literature on drug-induced disorders.

REFERENCES

1. Ives TJ, Bentz EJ, Gwyther RE: Drug-related admissions to a family medicine inpatient service. Arch Intern Med 147:1117, 1987
2. Rawlins MD: Spontaneous reporting of adverse drug reactions. Q J Med 59:531, 1986
3. Blain PG, Stewart-Wynne E: Neurological disorders. p. 494. In Davies DM (ed): Textbook of Adverse Drug Reactions. 3rd Ed. Oxford University Press, Oxford, 1985
4. Saper JR: Ergotamine dependency—a review. Headache 27:435, 1987
5. Vespignani H, Lepori JCI, Gehin PH, et al: Benign intracranial hypertension: apropos of 4 drug-induced cases. Rev Oto Neuro-Ophthalmol 56:277, 1984
6. Walters BNJ, Gubbay SS: Tetracycline and benign intracranial hypertension: report of five cases. Br Med J 282:19, 1981
7. Shah A, Roberts T, McQueen INF, et al: Danazol and benign intracranial hypertension. Br Med J 294:1323, 1987
8. Fikkers BG, Bogousslavsky J, Regli F, Glasson S: Pseudotumour cerebri with amiodarone. J Neurol Neurosurg Psychiatry 49:606, 1986
9. Van Dop C, Conte FA, Koch TK, et al: Pseudotumor cerebri associated with initiation of levothyroxine therapy for juvenile hypothyroidism. N Engl J Med 308:1076, 1983
10. Gordon MF, Allon M, Coyle PK: Drug-induced meningitis. Neurology 40:163, 1990
11. Vera-Ramirez M, Charlet M, Parry GJ: Recurrent aseptic meningitis complicating intravenous immunoglobulin therapy for chronic inflammatory demyelinating polyradiculoneuropathy. Neurology 42:1636, 1992
12. Jansen PA, Schulte BP, Meyboom RH, Gribnau FW: Antihypertensive treatment as a possible cause of stroke in the elderly. Age Ageing 15:129, 1986
13. Hankey GJ, Gubbay SS: Focal cerebral ischaemia and infarction due to antihypertensive therapy. Med J Aust 146:412, 1987
14. Delaney P, Estes M: Intracranial hemorrhage with amphetamine abuse. Neurology 30:1125, 1985
15. Kase CS, Foster TE, Reed JE, et al: Intracerebral hemorrhage and phenylpropanolamine use. Neurology 37:399, 1987
16. Bruno A, Nolte KB, Chapin J: Stroke associated with ephedrine use. Neurology 43:1313, 1993
17. Wojak JC, Flamm ES: Intracranial hemorrhage and cocaine use. Stroke 18:712, 1987
18. Levine SR, Brust JCM, Futrell N, et al: A comparative study of the cerebrovascular complications of cocaine: alkaloidal versus hydrochloride—a review. Neurology 41:1173, 1991
19. Caplan LR, Thomas C, Banks G: Central nervous system complications of addiction to "T's and Blues." Neurology 32:623, 1982

20. Doll DC, List AF, Greco FA, et al: Acute vascular ischemic events after cisplatin-based combination chemotherapy for germ-cell tumors of the testis. Ann Intern Med 105:48, 1986

21. Feinberg WM, Swenson MR: Cerebrovascular complications of L-asparaginase therapy. Neurology 38:127, 1988

22. Fincham RW, Perdue Z, Dunn VD: Bilateral focal cortical atrophy and chronic ergotamine abuse. Neurology 35:720, 1985

23. Luman W, Gray RS: Adverse reactions associated with sumatriptan. Lancet 341:1091, 1993

24. Zaccara G, Muscas GC, Messori A: Clinical features, pathogenesis and management of drug-induced seizures. Drug Saf 5:109, 1990

25. Porter J, Jick H: Drug-induced anaphylaxis, convulsions, deafness, and extrapyramidal symptoms. Lancet 1:587, 1977

26. Messing RO, Closson RG, Simon RP: Drug-induced seizures: a 10-year experience. Neurology 34:1582, 1984

27. Jackson GD, Berkovic SL: Ceftazidime encephalopathy: absence status and toxic hallucinations. J Neurol Neurosurg Psychiatry 55:333, 1992

28. Eschbach JW, Abdulhadi MH, Browne JK, et al: Recombinant human erythropoietin in anemic patients with end-stage renal disease: results of a phase III multicenter clinical trial. Ann Intern Med 111:992, 1989

29. Reynolds EH, Trimble MR: Adverse neuropsychiatric effects of anticonvulsant drugs. Drugs 29:570, 1985

30. Bahls FH, Ma KK, Bird TD: Theophylline-associated seizures with "therapeutic" or low toxic serum concentrations: risk factors for serious outcome in adults. Neurology 41:1309, 1991

31. Richens A, Nawishy S, Trimble M: Antidepressant drugs, convulsions and epilepsy. Br J Clin Pharmacol 15, suppl 2:2958, 1983

32. Peck AW, Stern WC, Watkinson C: Incidence of seizures during treatment with tricyclic antidepressant drugs and bupropion. J Clin Psychiatry 44:197, 1983

33. Markowitz JC, Brown RP: Seizures with neuroleptics and antidepressants. Gen Hosp Psychiatry 9:135, 1987

34. Cartlidge NEF: Drug-induced coma. Adverse Drug React Bull 88:320, 1981

35. Carroll WM, Mastaglia FL: Alpha and beta coma in drug intoxication uncomplicated by cerebral hypoxia. Electroencephalogr Clin Neurophysiol 46:95, 1979

36. Haefeli WE, Schoenenberger RAZ, Weiss P, Ritz RF: Acyclovir-induced neurotoxicity: concentration–side effect relationship in acyclovir overdose. Am J Med 94:212, 1993

37. Romijn JA, van Lieshout JJ, Velis DN: Reversible coma due to intrathecal baclofen. Lancet 2:696, 1986

38. Koller WC, Musa MN: Amitriptyline-induced abnormal movements. Neurology 35:1086, 1985

39. Speirs J, Hirsch SR: Severe lithium toxicity with "normal" serum concentrations. Br Med J 1:815, 1978

40. Donaldson IMacG, Cunningham J: Persisting neurologic sequelae of lithium carbonate therapy. Arch Neurol 40:747, 1983

41. Fear CF: Drug-induced Creutzfeldt-Jakob like syndrome: a review. Hum Psychopharmacol 7:89, 1992

42. Burns R, Thomas DW, Barron VJ: Reversible encephalopathy possibly associated with bismuth subgallate ingestion. Br Med J 1:220, 1974

43. Kruger G, Thomas DJ, Weinhardt F, Hoyer S: Disturbed oxidative metabolism in organic brain syndrome caused by bismuth in skin creams. Lancet 2:485, 1976

44. Hasking GJ, Duggan JM: Encephalopathy from bismuth subsalicylate. Med J Aust 2:167, 1982

45. Taylor R, Arze R, Gokal R, Stoddart JC: Cephaloridine encephalopathy. Br Med J 283:409, 1981

46. Vincent FM, Vincent T: Tocainide encephalopathy. Neurology 35:1804, 1985

47. Taclob L, Needle M: Drug-induced encephalopathy in patients on maintenance haemodialysis. Lancet 2:704, 1976

48. Sälke-Kellermann A, Baier H, Rambeck B, et al: Acute encephalopathy with vigabatrin. Lancet 342:185, 1993

49. Shapiro WR, Young DF: Neurological complications of antineoplastic therapy. Acta Neurol Scand 70:125, 1984

50. Cohen RB, Abdallah JM, Gray JR, Foss F: Reversible neurologic toxicity in patients treated with standard-dose fludarabine phosphate for mycosis fungoides and chronic lymphocytic leukemia. Ann Intern Med 118:114, 1993

51. Barbui T, Rambaldi A, Parenzan L, et al: Neurological symptoms and coma associated with doxorubicin administration during chronic cyclosporin therapy. Lancet 339:1421, 1992

52. Boogerd W, vd Sande JJ, Moffie D: Acute fever and delayed leukoencephalopathy following low dose intraventricular methotrexate. J Neurol Neurosurg Psychiatry 51:1277, 1988

53. Wolters EC, van Wijngaarden GK, Stam FC, et al: Leucoencephalopathy after inhaling "heroin" pyrolysate. Lancet 2:1233, 1982

54. The Medical Letter on Drugs and Therapeutics: Drugs that cause psychiatric symptoms. Med Lett Drugs Therapeut 31:113, 1989

55. Davison K: Drug-induced psychiatric disorders. Medicine (UK) 35:1823, 1980

56. Johnson DAW: Drug-induced psychiatric disorders. Drugs 22:57, 1981

57. Sultzer DL, Cummings JL: Drug-induced mania —causative agents, clinical characteristics and management: a retrospective analysis of the literature. Med Toxicol Adverse Drug Exp 4:127, 1989

58. Crombie AL: Eye disorders. p. 516. In Davies DM (ed): Textbook of Adverse Drug Reactions. 3rd Ed. Oxford University Press, Oxford, 1985

59. Denicoff KD, Rubinow DR, Papa MZ, et al: The neuropsychiatric effects of treatment with interleukin-2 and lymphokine-activated killer cells. Ann Intern Med 107:293, 1987

60. Ross RT: Drug-induced parkinsonism and other movement disorders. Can J Neurol Sci 17:155, 1990

61. Miller LG, Jankovic J: Neurologic approach to drug-induced movement disorders: a study of 125 patients. South Med J 83:525, 1990

62. Gershanik OS: Drug-induced movement disorders. Curr Opin Neurol 6:369, 1993

63. Lang AE, Weiner WJ: Drug-Induced Movement Disorders: Futura, Mt Kisco, NY, 1991

64. Ganzini L, Casey DE, Hoffman WF, McCall AL: The prevalence of metoclopramide-induced tardive dyskinesia and acute extrapyramidal movement disorders. Arch Intern Med 153:1469, 1993

65. Bateman DN, Rawlins MD, Simpson JM: Extrapyramidal reactions with metoclopramide. Br Med J 291:930, 1985

66. Pratty JS, O'Brien JE, Ananth J: Drug-induced dystonic reactions. Adv Ther 6:242, 1989

67. Micheli F, Pardal MF, Gatto M, et al: Flunarizine- and cinnarizine-induced extrapyramidal reactions. Neurology 37:881, 1987

68. Hooker EA, Danzl DF: Acute dystonic reaction due to diazepam. J Emerg Med 6:491, 1988

69. Rupniak NM, Jenner P, Marsden CD: Acute dystonia induced by neuroleptic drugs. Psychopharmacology 88:403, 1986

70. Bateman DN, Rawlins MD, Simpson JM: Extrapyramidal reactions to prochlorperazine and haloperidol in the United Kingdom. Q J Med 59:549, 1986

71. Osifo NG: Drug-related transient dyskinesias. Clin Pharmacol Ther 25:767, 1979

72. Ball R: Drug-induced akathisia: a review. J R Soc Med 78:748, 1985

73. Barnes TRE: Tardive dyskinesia. Br Med J 296:150, 1988

74. Jankovic J: Drug-induced and other orofacial-cervical dyskinesias. Ann Intern Med 94:788, 1981

75. Casey DE, Gerlach J: Is tardive dyskinesia due to dopamine hypersensitivity? Clin Neuropharmacol 9:134, 1986

76. Ames D, Webber J: Sodium valproate and tardive dyskinesia. Med J Aust 140:350, 1984

77. O'Flaherty S, Evans M, Epps A, Buchanan N: Choreaoathetosis and clonazepam. Med J Aust 142:453, 1985

78. Tilzey A, Heptonstall J, Hamblin T: Toxic confusional state and choreiform movements after treatment with anabolic steroids. Br Med J 283:349, 1981

79. Nausieda PA, Koller WC, Weiner WJ, Klawans HL: Chorea induced by oral contraceptives. Neurology 29:1605, 1979

80. Stephen PJ, Williamson J: Drug-induced parkinsonism in the elderly. Lancet 2:1082, 1984

81. Negrotti A, Calzetti S, Sasso E: Calcium-entry blockers-induced parkinsonism: possible role of inherited susceptibility. Neurotoxicology 13:261, 1992

82. Choulnard G, Sultan S: A case of Parkinson's disease exacerbated by fluoxetine. Hum Psychopharmacol 7:63, 1992

83. Knezevic W, Mastaglia FL, Lefroy RB, Fisher A: Neuroleptic malignant syndrome. Med J Aust 140:28, 1984

84. Gibb WRG, Lees AJ: The neuroleptic malignant syndrome—a review. Q J Med 56:421, 1985

85. Schrader GD: The neuroleptic malignant syndrome. Med J Aust 154:301, 1991

86. Friedman LS, Weinrauch LA, D'Elia JA: Metoclopramide-induced neuroleptic malignant syndrome. Arch Intern Med 147:1495, 1987

87. Baca L, Martinelli L: Neuroleptic malignant syndrome: a unique association with a tricyclic antidepressant. Neurology 40:1797, 1990

88. Reutens DC, Harrison WB, Goldswain PRT: Neuroleptic malignant syndrome complicating levodopa withdrawal. Med J Aust 155:53, 1991

89. Jankovic J, Fahn S: Physiologic and pathologic tremors. Ann Intern Med 93:460, 1980

90. Koller W, Cone S, Herbster G: Caffeine and tremor. Neurology 37:169, 1987

91. Karas BJ, Wilder BJ, Hammond EJ, Bauman AW: Treatment of valproate tremors. Neurology 33:1380, 1983

92. Bateman DN, Bevan P, Longley BP, et al: Cimetidine induced postural and action tremor. J Neurol Neurosurg Psychiatry 44:94, 1981

93. Tyrer P, Lee I, Trotter C: Physiological characteristics of tremor after chronic lithium therapy. Br J Psychiatry 139:59, 1981

94. Thompson CB, June CH, Sullivan KM, Thomas ED: Association between cyclosporin neurotoxicity and hypomagnesaemia. Lancet 2:1116, 1984

95. Davis CE Jr, Smith C, Harris R: Persistent movement disorder following metrizamide myelography. Arch Neurol 39:128, 1982

96. Buchman AS, Bennett DA, Goetz CG: Bromocriptine-induced myoclonus. Neurology 37:885, 1987

97. Tominaga H, Fukuzako H, Izumi K, et al: Tardive myoclonus. Lancet 1:322, 1987

98. Jacome DE: Cerebellar syndrome in lithium poisoning. J Neurol Neurosurg Psychiatry 50:1722, 1987

99. Winkelman MD, Hines JD: Cerebellar degeneration caused by high-dose cytosine arabinoside: a clinicopathological study. Ann Neurol 14:520, 1983

100. Goldberg ID, Bloomer WD, Dawson DM: Nervous system toxic effects of cancer therapy. JAMA 247:1437, 1982

101. Graebner RW, Herskowitz A: Cerebellar toxic effects from nitrofurantoin. Arch Neurol 29:195, 1973

102. Friedlander IR: Ototoxic drugs and the detection of ototoxicity. N Engl J Med 301:213, 1979

103. Huang MY, Schacht J: Drug-induced oxotoxicity. Curr Ther 32(10):71, 1991

104. Kroese ABA, van den Bercken J: Dual action of ototoxic antibiotics on sensory hair cells. Nature 283:395, 1980

105. Kovnar EH, Horowitz ME, Tate J, McHaney VA: Brainstem auditory evoked responses (BAER), audiometry, and ototoxicity in children receiving cisplatin. Ann Neurol 20:399, 1986

106. Olivieri NF, Buncic JR, Chew E, et al: Visual and auditory neurotoxicity in patients receiving subcutaneous deferoxamine infusions. N Engl J Med 314:869, 1986

107. Bird AC, El-Sheikh H, Anderson J, Fuglsang H: Visual loss during oral diethylcarbamazine treatment for onchocerciasis. Lancet 2:46, 1979

108. Gupta DR, Strobos RJ: Bilateral papillitis associated with Cafergot therapy. Neurology 22:793, 1972

109. Yiannakis PH, Larner AJ: Visual failure and optic atrophy associated with chlorambucil therapy. Br Med J 306:109, 1993

110. Dodd MJ, Griffiths ID, Howe JW, Mitchell KW: Toxic optic neuropathy caused by benoxaprofen. Br Med J 283:193, 1981

111. Lafeuillade A, Aubert L, Chaffanjon P, Quilichini R: Optic neuritis associated with dideoxyinosine. Lancet 337:615, 1991

112. Halmagyi GM, Rudge P, Gresty MA, Sanders MD: Downbeating nystagmus—a review of 62 cases. Arch Neurol 40:777, 1983

113. Rollin H: Drug-related gustatory disorders. Ann Otol Rhinol Laryngol 87:37, 1978

114. Jones PBB, McCloskey EV, Kanis JA: Transient taste-loss during treatment with etidronate. Lancet 2:637, 1987

115. Ottervanger JP, Stricker BHC: Loss of taste and terbinafine. Lancet 340:728, 1992

116. Australian Adverse Drug Reactions Bulletin: Drugs that leave a bad taste in the mouth. 11:14, 1992

117. Bernat JL: Intraspinal steroid therapy. Neurology 31:168, 1981

118. Gronow DW, Mendelson G: Epidural injection of depot corticosteroids. Med J Aust 157:417, 1992

119. Steen PA, Michenfelder JD: Neurotoxicity of anesthetics. Anesthesiology 50:437, 1979

120. Hahn AF, Feasby TE, Gilbert JJ: Paraparesis following intrathecal chemotherapy. Neurology 33:1032, 1983

121. Ell JJ, Uttley D, Silver JR: Acute myelopathy in association with heroin addiction. J Neurol Neurosurg Psychiatry 44:448, 1981

122. Blanco G, Peters HA: Myeloneuropathy and macrocytosis associated with nitrous oxide abuse. Arch Neurol 40:416, 1983

123. Walther PJ, Rossitch E, Bullard DE: The development of Lhermitte's sign during cisplatin chemotherapy: possible drug-induced toxicity causing spinal cord demyelination. Cancer 60:2170, 1987

124. Guegan Y, Fardoun R, Launois B, Pecker J: Spinal cord compression by extradural fat after prolonged corticosteroid therapy. J Neurosurg 56:267, 1982

125. Davies DM: Drug-induced hypotension. p. 162. In Davies DM (ed): Textbook of Adverse Drug Reactions. 3rd Ed. Oxford University Press, Oxford, 1985

126. Buffum J: Pharmacosexology update: prescription drugs and sexual dysfunction. J Psychoactive Drugs 18:97, 1986

127. Smith PJ, Talbert PL: Sexual dysfunction with antihypertensive and antipsychotic agents. Clin Pharm 5:373, 1986

128. Lane RJM, Mastaglia FL: Drug-induced myopathies in man. Lancet 2:562, 1978

129. Argov Z, Mastaglia FL: Disorders of neuromuscular transmission caused by drugs. N Engl J Med 301:409, 1979

130. Argov Z, Mastaglia FL: Drug-induced peripheral neuropathies. Br Med J 1:663, 1979

131. Olesen LL, Jensen TS: Prevention and management of drug-induced peripheral neuropathy. Drug Saf 6:302, 1991

132. Argov Z, Mastaglia FL: Drug-induced neuromuscular disorders in man. p. 981. In Walton JN (ed): Disorders of Voluntary Muscle. 5th Ed. Churchill Livingstone, Edinburgh, 1988

133. Rose EC, Gawel M: Clioquinol neurotoxicity: an overview. Acta Neurol Scand 70:137, 1984

134. Postma TJ, Benard BA, Huijgens PC, et al: Long-term effects of vincristine on the peripheral nervous system. J Neurooncol 15:23, 1993

135. Kuncl RW, George EB: Toxic neuropathies and myopathies. Curr Opin Neurol 6:695, 1993

136. Daugaard GK, Petrera J, Trojaborg W: Electrophysi-

ological study of the peripheral and central neurotoxic effect of cis-platin. Acta Neurol Scand 76:86, 1987

137. Seharaseyan J, New P, Barohn R, et al: Sensory neuronopathy induced by ormaplatinum. Neurology 43, suppl 2:A174, 1993

138. New PZ, Barohn R. Neurotoxicity of Taxotere. Neurology 43, suppl 2:A191, 1993

139. Russell JW, Windebank AJ: Electrophysiological and pathological characteristics of suramin-induced neuropathy. Neurology 43, suppl 2:A174, 1993

140. Palakurthy PR, Iyer V, Meckler RJ: Unusual neurotoxicity associated with amiodarone therapy. Arch Intern Med 147:881, 1987

141. Pellissier JF, Pouget J, Cros D, et al: Peripheral neuropathy induced by amiodarone chlorhydrate: a clinicopathological study. J Neurol Sci 63:251, 1984

142. Palace J, Shah R, Clough C: Flecainide induced peripheral neuropathy. Br Med J 305:810, 1992

143. Hormigo A, Alves M: Peripheral neuropathy in a patient receiving enalapril. Br Med J 305:1332, 1992

144. Goodheart RS, Dunne JW, Edis RH: Phenelzine associated peripheral neuropathy—clinical and electrophysiologic findings. Aust NZ J Med 21:339, 1991

145. Hess CW, Hunziker T, Kupfer A, Ludin HP: Thalidomide-induced peripheral neuropathy: a prospective clinical, neurophysiological and pharmacogenetic evaluation. J Neurol 233:83, 1986

146. Roelcke U, Hornstein C, Hund E, et al: Acute neuropathy in perazine-treated patients after sun exposure. Lancet 340:729, 1992

147. Fagius J, Osterman PO, Siden A, Wiholm BE: Guillain-Barré syndrome following zimeldine treatment. J Neurol Neurosurg Psychiatry 48:65, 1985

148. Albin RL, Albers JW, Greenberg HS, et al: Acute sensory neuropathy-neuronopathy from pyridoxine overdose. Neurology 37:1729, 1987

149. Petit H, Leys D, Hurtevent JF, et al: Neuropathies et almitrine. Rev Neurol (Paris) 143:508, 1987

150. Kuncl RW, Duncan G, Watson D: Colchicine myoneuropathy. Lancet 2:668, 1987

151. Hory B, Blanc D, Boillot A, Panouse-Perrin J: Guillain-Barré syndrome following danazol and corticosteroid therapy for hereditary angioedema. Am J Med 79:111, 1985

152. Steiner I, Argov Z, Cahan C, Abramsky O: Guillain-Barré syndrome after epidural anesthesia: direct nerve root damage may trigger disease. Neurology 35:1473, 1985

153. Roquer J, Herraiz J, Arnau D, Serrat R: Guillain-Barré syndrome after streptokinase therapy. Acta Neurol Scand 82:153, 1990

154. Figueras A, Morales-Olivas FJ, Capella D, et al: Bovine gangliosides and acute motor polyneuropathy. Br Med J 305:1330, 1992

155. Mastaglia FL: Adverse effects of drugs on muscle. Drugs 24:304, 1982

156. Mitsumoto H, Wilbourn AJ, Subramony SH: Generalized myokymia and gold therapy. Arch Neurol 39: 449, 1982

157. Pinals RS: Diffuse fasciculations induced by D-penicillamine. J Rheumatol 10:809, 1983

158. Gabow PA, Kaehny WD, Kelleher SP: The spectrum of rhabdomyolysis. Medicine (Baltimore) 61:141, 1982

159. Koppel C: Clinical features, pathogenesis and management of drug-induced rhabdomyolysis. Med Toxicol Adverse Drug Exp 4:108, 1989

160. Mastaglia FL: Toxic myopathies. p. 595. In Rowland LP, DiMauro S (eds): Handbook of Clinical Neurology. Vol 62. Elsevier, Amsterdam, 1992

161. Knochel JP: Rhabdomyolysis and myoglobinuria. Annu Rev Med 33:435, 1982

162. Blane GF: Comparative toxicity and safety profile of fenofibrate and other fibric acid derivatives. Am J Med 83, suppl 5B:26, 1987

163. Litin SC, Anderson CF: Nicotinic acid-associated myopathy. Am J Med 86:481, 1989

164. Marais GE, Larson KK: Rhabdomyolysis and acute renal failure induced by combination lovastatin and gemfibrozil therapy. Ann Intern Med 112:228, 1990

165. Dalakas MC: Inflammatory and toxic myopathies. Curr Opin Neurol Neurosurg 5:645, 1992

166. Palmer EP, Guay AT: Reversible myopathy secondary to abuse of ipecac in patients with major eating disorders. N Engl J Med 313:1457, 1985

167. Dresser LP, Massey EW, Johnson EE, Bossen E: Ipecac myopathy and cardiomyopathy. J Neurol Neurosurg Psychiatry 56:560, 1993

168. Kilpatrick C, Braund W, Burns R: Myopathy with myasthenic features possibly induced by codeine linctus. Med J Aust 2:410, 1982

169. Dalakas MC, Illa I, Pezeshkpour GH, et al: Mitochondrial myopathy caused by long-term zidovudine therapy. N Engl J Med 322:1098, 1990

170. Panegyres PK, Papadimitriou JM, Hollingsworth PN, et al: Vesicular changes in the myopathies of AIDS. Ultrastructural observations and their relationship to zidovudine treatment. J Neurol Neurosurg Psychiatry 53:649, 1990

171. Chalmers AC, Greco CM, Miller RG: Prognosis in AZT myopathy. Neurology 41:1181, 1991

172. Simpson DN, Citak KA, Godfrey E, et al: Myopathies associated with human immunodeficiency virus and zidovudine: can their effects be distinguished? Neurology 43:971, 1993

173. Arnaudo E, Dalakas M, Shanske S, et al: Depletion of muscle mitochondrial DNA in AIDS patients with zidovudine-induced myopathy. Lancet 337:508, 1991

174. Valeriano J, Tucker P, Kattah J: An unusual cause of hypokalemic muscle weakness. Neurology 33:1242, 1983

175. Vita G, Bartolone S, Santoro M, et al: Hypokalemic myopathy in pseudohyperaldosteronism induced by fluoroprednisolone-containing nasal spray. Clin Neuropathol 6:80, 1987

176. Mastaglia FL, Argov Z: Immunologically mediated drug-induced neuromuscular disorders. p. 62. In Dukor P, Kallos P, Schlumberger HD, West GB (eds): Pseudo-allergic Reactions. Involvement of Drugs and Chemicals. Vol 3. Karger, Basel, 1982

177. Kaufman LD: Neuromuscular manifestations of the L-tryptophan-associated eosinophilia-myalgia syndrome. Curr Opin Rheumatol 2:896, 1990

178. Hertzman PA, Blevins WL, Mayer J, et al: Association of the eosinophilia-myalgia syndrome with the ingestion of tryptophan. N Engl J Med 322:869, 1990

179. Belongia EA, Hedberg CW, Gleich GJ, et al: An investigation of the cause of the eosinophilia-myalgia syndrome associated with tryptophan use. N Engl J Med 323:357, 1990

180. Bretag AH, Dawe SR, Moskwa AG: Chemically induced myotonia in amphibia. Nature 286:625, 1980

181. Bowyer SL, LaMonthe MP, Hollister JR: Steroid myopathy: incidence and detection in a population with asthma. J Allergy Clin Immunol 76:234, 1985

182. Panegyres PK, Squier M, Mills KR, Newsom-Davis J: Acute myopathy associated with large parenteral dose of corticosteroid in myasthenia gravis. J Neurol Neurosurg Psychiatry 56:702, 1993

183. Karpati G: Denervation and disuse atrophy of skeletal muscles—involvement of endogenous glucocorticoid hormones? Trends Neurosci 7:61, 1984

184. Horber FF, Scheidegger JR, Grunig BE, Frey FJ: Thigh muscle mass and function in patients treated with glucocorticoids. Eur J Clin Invest 15:302, 1985

185. Nelson TE, Flewellen EH: The malignant hyperthermia syndrome. N Engl J Med 309:417, 1983

186. Britt BA (ed): Malignant Hyperthermia. Martinus Nijhoff Publishing, Boston, 1987

187. Kolb ME, Horne ML, Martz R: Dantrolene in human malignant hyperthermia. Anesthesiology 56:254, 1982

188. Arellano F, Krupp P: Muscular disorders associated with cyclosporin. Lancet 337:915, 1991

189. Chadwick DW: Convulsions associated with drug therapy. Adverse Drug React Bull 87:316, 1981

30

Alcohol and the Nervous System

Robert O. Messing
David A. Greenberg

Who could have foretold, from the structure of the brain, that wine could derange its functions?

Seneca

The ability of alcohol to interfere with neuronal function is no longer a surprise, but the wide variety of alcohol-related neurological disorders and their underlying mechanisms remain puzzling. As illustrated in Figure 30-1, alcohol abuse has been implicated in neurological diseases affecting every level of the neuraxis, including brain, peripheral nerve, and muscle. Despite its protean nature, alcoholic neurological disease often involves discrete anatomical structures or cell populations, suggesting that multiple, discrete pathophysiological processes are at work.[1,2]

Intoxication results from acute, pharmacological effects of alcohol, and enhancement of neurotransmission in γ-aminobutyric acid (GABA) systems may be especially important in this respect.[3] Adaptation at the cellular level to alcohol's acute effects leads to clinical withdrawal syndromes when alcohol intake is reduced or terminated; these syndromes may result from chronic upregulation of calcium channels or glutamate receptors.[4,5] A direct, cytotoxic action of alcohol has been proposed as a pathogenetic mechanism in alcoholic myopathy and fetal alcohol syndrome, whereas other neurological complications appear unrelated to the amount of alcohol consumed.[6] Several neurological disorders are related to systemic effects of alcohol (such as hepatic cirrhosis, nutritional deficiency, or electrolyte disturbances); these include dementia due to pellagra or acquired hepatocerebral degeneration, Wernicke's encephalopathy, Korsakoff's amnestic syndrome, cerebellar degeneration, central pontine myelinolysis, and polyneuropathy.

Genetic factors may also operate in the pathogenesis of alcohol-related neurological disease. First, evidence exists for an inherited predisposition to alcoholism in certain individuals.[7] In addition, genetically determined predilections could explain why individual alcoholics develop a particular neurological disorder or escape neurological complications altogether. While genetic factors may therefore influence the occurrence of these disorders, the role of alcohol itself is primary: not all at-risk individuals develop either alcoholism or neurological complications, and cessation of alcohol abuse can arrest or reverse neurological deficits in many instances.

This chapter summarizes the clinical features of the major alcohol-related neurological disorders.

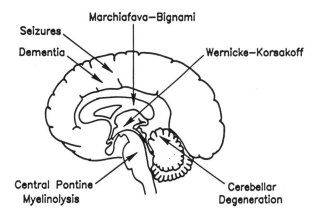

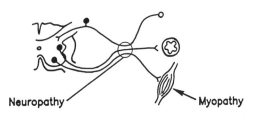

Fig. 30-1 Alcohol-related disorders affecting different levels of the neuraxis.

ALCOHOL INTOXICATION AND WITHDRAWAL

Intoxication

Early signs of alcohol intoxication include euphoria, mood swings, loss of social inhibition, mild ataxia, nystagmus, dysarthria, flushing, tachycardia, and mydriasis.[8] In nonalcoholics, measurable impairment of coordination and cognition occurs with blood concentrations of 31 to 65 mg/dl.[9] With increasing blood alcohol levels, findings of central nervous system (CNS) depression predominate, leading to coma, hyporeflexia, respiratory compromise, and hypotension.[8]

Although the behavioral effects of alcohol generally correlate with blood concentrations, tolerance may occur rapidly and greatly modify the clinical response. Acute tolerance may develop during a single bout of drinking, causing the drinker to become sober at blood alcohol concentrations higher than those at which intoxication developed.[10] In chronic alcoholics the tolerance may be great enough to permit sobriety

at blood concentrations well above 100 mg/dl. Urso and associates measured blood alcohol levels of 120 to 540 mg/dl (mean 268 mg/dl) in 65 sober alcoholic patients.[11] Thus, concentrations of alcohol that are lethal in nonalcoholics may fail to intoxicate alcoholics. Lethal blood alcohol concentrations are also higher in alcoholics, and blood levels of 730 to 780 mg/dl[12,13] and 1,127 mg/dl[14] have been measured in patients who later recovered from alcoholic coma.

Minor Withdrawal Syndrome

The characteristic symptoms of alcohol withdrawal described by Victor and Adams may follow abrupt cessation of drinking.[15] Tremulousness is the most common early symptom, becoming most marked 24 to 36 hours after the last drink. The tremor is generalized, resembles an accentuated physiological tremor, and is accompanied by signs of autonomic hyperactivity such as arousal, tachycardia, flushing, and hyperreflexia. These signs are associated with elevated blood and urinary catecholamine levels and increased levels of catecholamine metabolites in the cerebrospinal fluid (CSF).[16]

Withdrawal Seizures

Victor and Adams found that seizures occurred in 12 percent of 266 hospitalized alcoholic patients.[15] Alcohol withdrawal seizures, as characterized by Victor and Brausch,[17] are usually associated with a history of daily alcohol consumption, but briefer drinking sprees may also culminate in seizures. Generalized tonic-clonic seizures are most common; focal seizures occur in fewer than 5 percent of cases and suggest an etiology other than alcohol withdrawal. More than 90 percent of seizures occur within 7 to 48 hours after cessation of drinking. Approximately 60 percent of patients have more than one seizure, but fewer than 15 percent have more than four. Status epilepticus is unusual and occurs in only 3 percent of cases, but alcohol withdrawal was responsible for approximately 15 percent of all cases of status in one series.[18] The period of risk for withdrawal seizures is short: less than 6 hours in 85 percent of cases and less than 12 hours in 95 percent. About one-half of patients manifest photomyoclonic and photoconvulsive responses on the electroencephalogram (EEG) during the convulsive period.

Status epilepticus due to alcohol withdrawal is a medical emergency and should be treated with anticonvulsants in the same fashion as status due to any other etiology. It is important to recognize that alcoholics are at risk for a variety of other treatable conditions that may cause status epilepticus, including occult head trauma, meningitis, hypoglycemia, hyponatremia, and other drug ingestions. For patients without status epilepticus, anticonvulsant therapy is usually not required, as the convulsive period is brief.

The use of anticonvulsant drugs for the prevention of alcohol withdrawal seizures is controversial. Sampliner and Iber reported that 300 mg of phenytoin per day prevented withdrawal convulsions in 78 alcoholic patients despite low serum levels of the drug (3 to 4 μg/ml).[19] However, these patients also received sedative doses of chlordiazepoxide, which may have influenced their outcome. A more recent study[20] showed that phenytoin fails to prevent alcohol withdrawal seizures. Rothstein reported that among 200 patients withdrawing from alcohol, no seizures occurred in those receiving sedative doses of chlordiazepoxide alone or in combination with 400 mg of phenytoin per day.[21] He concluded that chlordiazepoxide is sufficiently effective against withdrawal seizures that additional anticonvulsants are unnecessary. Lidocaine,[22] valproic acid,[23] and carbamazepine[24] have attenuated alcohol withdrawal seizures in laboratory animals, but controlled studies in humans are lacking.

Delirium Tremens

Approximately 16 percent of patients become delirious 2 to 5 days after ethanol withdrawal, and one-third of these patients may develop the syndrome of delirium tremens with marked confusion, hallucinations, tremor, hyperpyrexia, and sympathetic hyperactivity.[15] The risk of developing delirium tremens is higher in alcoholics with withdrawal seizures; as many as one-third of these patients may develop this life-threatening syndrome after the cessation of seizures.[17] The major threat to life is from associated illnesses or injuries, hyperthermia, dehydration, and hypotension.[15,25] A variety of sedatives, anticonvulsants, sympatholytics, and neuroleptics have been administered to patients with delirium and delirium tremens, usually in uncontrolled trials.[16,26] Several double-blind studies have suggested that benzodiaze-

pines are effective in controlling the symptoms of alcohol withdrawal.[16,27,28] A typical regimen is to administer 5 to 10 mg of diazepam intravenously every 10 to 15 minutes until the patient is calm, followed by 5 to 10 mg every few hours as needed to control delirium and agitation. Shorter-acting benzodiazepines such as oxazepam or lorazepam may be safer in patients with liver disease.[29] Fluid and electrolyte abnormalities can be severe and require prompt therapy. Dehydration accompanying delirium tremens may lead to circulatory collapse requiring replacement of up to 4 to 10 liters of fluid during the first 24 hours.[30] Hypomagnesemia is common; it should be treated with magnesium sulfate (2 g intravenously or intramuscularly every 6 hours during the first day in persons with adequate renal function). Potassium should be included in intravenous solutions, as hypokalemia may be exacerbated by glucose administration and cause cardiac arrhythmias.

DEMENTIA

Several disorders may cause dementia in alcoholic patients. With these conditions, cognitive function is impaired in a diffuse and nonspecific fashion.

Pellagra

Pellagra, which results from deficiency of nicotinic acid (niacin) or its amino acid precursor, tryptophan, may produce dementia in alcoholics.[30] The disorder is uncommon in developed countries because of fortification of processed foods with niacin. Neuropathological changes[30,31] involve mainly the large neurons of motor cortex, although changes are also seen elsewhere in the cortex, in large neurons of the basal ganglia, in cranial motor and deep cerebellar nuclei, and in anterior horn cells. Affected neurons appear swollen and rounded, with eccentric nuclei and loss of Nissl substance. Axonal damage is too minor to account for the chromatolysis, which is more likely related to metabolic effects on nerve cell bodies.[31]

Systemic manifestations of pellagra include diarrhea, glossitis, anemia, and erythematous cutaneous lesions that appear in sun-exposed areas. Early mental symptoms of irritability, depression, fatigue, insomnia, and inability to concentrate are nonspecific and suggest a psychiatric disorder. However, the later development of confusion, hallucinosis, or paranoid ideation confirms the presence of an encephalopathy, and is usually accompanied by spastic weakness and Babinski signs. Tremor, rigidity, polyneuropathy, optic neuritis, and deafness may also be present. Pellagra responds readily to administration of niacin, although cerebral symptoms may not be completely reversible. Further details are given in Chapter 15.

Marchiafava-Bignami Disease

Marchiafava-Bignami disease was first described in 1903 in wine-drinking Italian men but has since been observed among persons of many nationalities and with consumption of all types of alcoholic beverages.[30,32] In this disorder there is destruction of myelin mainly in the corpus callosum and anterior commissure. Exceptionally, lesions extend laterally to involve the centrum semiovale, and in some instances the middle cerebellar peduncles are demyelinated. Neurons in layer 3 of cerebral cortex may be replaced by gliosis, possibly due to disruption of callosal fibers. Many histological features are similar to those found in central pontine myelinolysis (see below), and both disorders have occurred in the same patient, which could suggest a common pathogenetic mechanism.[33] The disorder is usually diagnosed postmortem, as the clinical signs are nonspecific. Most patients are alcoholics of longstanding, and many have associated malnutrition or liver disease. Symptoms may present acutely with seizures and coma or may follow a subacute course. Irritability, aggressiveness, and confusion are common early features and are often followed by abulia, prominent frontal release signs, and spasticity or rigidity. Symptoms may respond somewhat to abstinence from alcohol and improved nutrition, but patients usually remain demented.[30]

Acquired Hepatocerebral Degeneration

Alcoholic liver disease may be accompanied by acquired hepatocerebral degeneration, as described by Victor and co-workers.[34] Neuropathological lesions in this disorder consist of diffuse, patchy necrosis with microcavitation at the junction of cerebral gray and white matter, and a loss of neurons and myelinated fibers in the basal ganglia and cerebellum. Proto-

plasmic type II (Alzheimer) astrocytes are increased in number, and Opalski cells may be present. Most patients are demented and show reduced attentiveness and diminished ability to concentrate on problems, retain new facts, and sustain mental activity. Motor signs always accompany the dementia and include cerebellar ataxia, dysarthria, tremor, and choreoathetosis. Mild corticospinal tract deficits may also be present, and occasional patients have myoclonus or show signs of a myelopathy. In some cases the neurological findings precede recognition of liver disease by several years. The deficits are irreversible, the rate of progression is variable, and the course is often punctuated by superimposed episodes of reversible hepatic encephalopathy. Death usually occurs as a complication of advanced liver disease or intercurrent infection rather than from the neurological disorder.

Alcoholic Dementia

Dementia unrelated to the foregoing disorders has been recognized in alcoholics for several years. Numerous psychometric studies have shown cognitive impairment to be common in alcoholics.[35,36] Parker and colleagues found performance on tests of abstraction ability to also be impaired in social drinkers, and the degree of impairment was correlated with the amount of alcohol consumed per drinking occasion.[37] Some investigators[30,38,39] have argued that unrecognized Korsakoff's syndrome (see below) accounts for most cases of cognitive impairment among alcoholics, whereas others[40,41] claim that alcohol is directly toxic to the brain and induces structural nervous system pathology that accounts for dementia.

In rodents, chronic alcohol consumption can lead to learning deficits, altered dendritic morphology, and neuronal loss.[41,42] However, in humans the histological evidence for alcohol-induced dementia is controversial. Courville first described several neuropathological findings in patients with alcoholic dementia,[43] including cortical atrophy, especially in frontal regions; thickening and opacification of the meninges; enlargement of the anterior horns of the lateral ventricles; swelling, pyknosis, and pigmentary atrophy of neurons; loss of pyramidal cells in superficial and intermediate cortical laminae; and degeneration of cortical nerve fibers. Although the lesions were attributed to a direct toxic effect of alcohol, detailed clinicopathological correlation was not provided. Victor and Adams have questioned the specificity of many of these findings, as ventricular dilatation, meningeal opacification, and pigmentary change are commonly found in patients with other diseases, as well as in normal, aged persons.[30] Lynch also examined the brains of 11 alcoholics and noted a patchy loss of cortical nerve cells and fibers in the rolandic gyrus.[44] However, 5 of these patients had died with delirium tremens and 3 from bleeding esophageal varices, and clinical data in these cases were insufficient to eliminate factors such as anoxia and hepatic disease that may have influenced the pathological findings.[30]

Other postmortem studies have attempted to document the existence of alcohol-induced dementia by quantifying changes in brain weight and size, and the number of cortical neurons in alcoholics. Torvik and associates compared the brain weights of 545 male alcoholics and 586 age-matched controls and found that the brains of alcoholics weighed an average of 31 g less.[39] Skullerud found a 70- to 90-g reduction in brain weight in alcoholics that was independent of the presence of liver disease or malnutrition.[45] Harper and Kril compared brains from 25 alcoholics and 44 control patients and found that there was a statistically significant loss of brain tissue in chronic alcoholics, which was worse in patients with associated thiamine deficiency or liver disease.[46] Harper and associates also found that the number of neurons in the frontal cortex was significantly reduced in chronic alcoholics.[47]

Computed tomographic (CT) and magnetic resonance imaging (MRI) studies have also shown decreased brain size in alcoholics.[48–56] In the CT studies the incidence of atrophy ranged from 7 to 100 percent among alcoholics and heavy social drinkers,[52] and atrophy tended to be greater in alcoholics than in nonalcoholics.[36,50–54] Neuropsychiatric abnormalities are also more common in nondemented alcoholics but correlate poorly with CT scan abnormalities.[36,51,53,54] Neither variable correlates well with the duration or pattern of drinking.[36,51,53,55] CT and neuropsychiatric abnormalities are partly reversible during abstinence.[40,53,56] However, Carlen and colleagues[56] found that improving CT parameters correlated better with improvement in physical than in cognitive abnormalities and correlated poorly with changes in psychometric test performance. Therefore, although CT changes and neuropsychiatric abnormalities are present in alcoholics, it has been difficult to substantiate a cause-and-effect relation between them.[36]

Most radiographic and psychometric examinations have been performed within the first 2 to 4 weeks of abstinence, yet several biochemical and physiological abnormalities require many weeks to resolve following alcohol withdrawal. In chronic alcoholics, CSF acidosis may persist for weeks following the last drink,[57] and evoked response abnormalities may require up to 3 weeks to resolve.[58,59] CT and psychometric abnormalities during the first month of abstinence might therefore be related to alcohol withdrawal rather than permanent brain damage due to alcohol. Thus, it is not certain that radiological and neuropsychiatric abnormalities observed in alcoholics result from a direct toxic and dementing effect of alcohol.

WERNICKE'S ENCEPHALOPATHY

Wernicke's encephalopathy is an acute disorder manifested by ophthalmoplegia, gait ataxia, and a confusional state.[60–62] Neuropathological findings include demyelination, glial and vascular proliferation, hemorrhage, and necrosis, which particularly affect gray matter regions of the thalamus, hypothalamus, brainstem, and cerebellum. An underlying disorder that predisposes to malnutrition appears to be common to all cases. Alcoholism is the most frequent predisposing factor, but persistent vomiting due to a variety of causes, starvation, and malignancy or other chronic systemic diseases have also been implicated. A detailed account of its clinical features is provided in Chapter 15.

The link between malnutrition and Wernicke's encephalopathy is a deficiency of vitamin B_1 (thiamine). With chronic alcoholism decreased dietary intake of thiamine may be compounded by alcohol-induced defects in intestinal absorption, metabolism, and hepatic storage of thiamine. However, the manner in which thiamine depletion produces neurological dysfunction is unknown. Thiamine pyrophosphate is a required cofactor for at least four enzymes involved in intermediary metabolism: pyruvate dehydrogenase, α-ketoglutarate dehydrogenase, transketolase, and branched-chain α-ketoacid dehydrogenase. Several investigators have reported heterogeneity of transketolase affinity for thiamine or variant forms of transketolase,[63–67] which could provide a basis for preferential vulnerability of certain alcoholic patients to thiamine deficiency. Thiamine phosphates have also been suggested to have a role in axonal conduction or synaptic transmission. Experimental thiamine deficiency is characterized by widespread depression of glucose metabolism in gray matter regions,[68–71] which may be accompanied by enhanced metabolism in white matter tracts[70]; a later phase of gray matter hypermetabolism may precede the onset of histological lesions.[71]

Ocular abnormalities in Wernicke's encephalopathy may take a variety of forms.[60] The most common is nystagmus, which almost always exhibits a horizontal component; vertical nystagmus is less common, and rotatory nystagmus is rare. Ocular palsies are also frequent, particularly lateral rectus palsy, which is usually bilateral. Horizontal or horizontal and vertical gaze palsies are often seen. Ptosis and internuclear ophthalmoplegias are rare, and loss of pupillary reactivity does not occur.

Ataxia results from pathology in the superior cerebellar vermis and vestibular nuclei. Consequently, the gait is most severely affected. Only a few patients exhibit limb ataxia, such as is revealed by finger-to-nose or heel-knee-shin testing; dysarthria is unusual.

The acute confusional state is nonspecific. As with other metabolic encephalopathies, there is typically sedation, disorientation, and inattention, and the level of consciousness may fluctuate. The ability to incorporate new memories is severely impaired.

Most patients with Wernicke's encephalopathy have an associated polyneuropathy at the time of presentation. Hypothalamic involvement occasionally leads to hypothermia or hypotension. Coma may occur.

The diagnosis of Wernicke's encephalopathy is established by the clinical findings and the response to thiamine (discussed below). However, acute, reversible MRI abnormalities have also been described[72,73] and may be helpful for diagnosing mild cases or those with atypical clinical features. In patients who present with ophthalmoplegia, ataxia, and confusion, the differential diagnosis includes sedative drug intoxication and structural lesions in the posterior fossa.

Wernicke's encephalopathy is, at least in theory, a preventable disorder. One widely discussed approach is the fortification of alcoholic beverages with thiamine.[74] Although thiamine hydrochloride is stable in alcoholic beverages, it is poorly absorbed by alcoholic patients; thiamine propyldisulfide, which is well absorbed, is unstable. Thus, new analogues combining the desirable properties of these two compounds will have to be developed before this approach is technically feasible. Prevention of iatrogenically induced Wernicke's encephalopathy is more easily achievable. Iatrogenic conditions associated with Wernicke's disease include digitalis intoxication leading to persistent vomiting,[75] inadequate parenteral nutrition,[76] kidney dialysis,[77] and the administration of large amounts of glucose[78] or oral hypoglycemic agents[79] to severely malnourished patients. Such patients at risk for nutritional deficiency should receive thiamine regardless of whether clinical signs of Wernicke's encephalopathy are present.

Treatment of Wernicke's encephalopathy is by repletion of thiamine. Patients should be hospitalized and receive 100 mg of thiamine intravenously daily for several days. Outpatient therapy with 50 mg of oral thiamine per day should follow, although in alcoholic patients absorption of the vitamin is likely to be impaired.

The prognosis of Wernicke's encephalopathy depends on the prompt institution of appropriate treatment. The overall mortality is high, with figures in the range of 10 to 20 percent commonly cited. Following the institution of treatment, ocular and gaze palsies begin to improve within hours to days and nystagmus, gait ataxia, and confusion within days to weeks. Long-term sequelae include residual nystagmus or gait ataxia (alcoholic cerebellar degeneration; see below) in about 60 percent of patients and a chronic memory disorder (Korsakoff amnestic syndrome; see below) in more than 80 percent.

KORSAKOFF'S AMNESTIC SYNDROME

Korsakoff's syndrome is a selective disorder of memory (amnestic syndrome) that typically arises in chronic alcoholics in the wake of one or more episodes of Wernicke's encephalopathy. The distribution of histopathological lesions is identical to that seen in acute Wernicke's disease.[60,80] Memory impairment is thought to be related to involvement of the dorsomedial nucleus of the thalamus or the mamillary bodies.

A causal relation between (acute) Wernicke's encephalopathy due to thiamine deficiency and (chronic) Korsakoff syndrome is generally assumed. However, this issue is not resolved. For example, Korsakoff's syndrome was rarely a consequence of Wernicke's disease in malnourished prisoners of war in the Pacific theater during World War II. This may be because the duration of malnutrition was briefer than is usually the case with chronic alcoholics or because alcohol itself contributes to the risk of developing the syndrome. In addition, although treatment with thiamine reverses most of the manifestations of Wernicke's encephalopathy, it is relatively ineffective in preventing Korsakoff's syndrome.

Although considerable progress has been made toward understanding the biological basis of memory,[81–85] how the Korsakoff syndrome produces a disorder of memory is unknown. Some authors have proposed that memory impairment in Korsakoff's syndrome is due to selective damage to ascending noradrenergic pathways by brainstem and diencephalic lesions,[86] whereas others have found no such abnormality.[87]

The disability afflicting patients with Korsakoff's syndrome is among the most striking in clinical neurology. There is both impaired retrieval of previously established, especially recent, memories (retrograde amnesia) and inability to incorporate new memories (anterograde amnesia). Immediate recall, tested by having patients immediately repeat what is said to them, is intact. Patients are typically disoriented to time and place. Hospitalized patients are characteristically unaware of their room numbers or hospital floor, how long they have been in the hospital, what they had for their last meal, or who visited them. At the same time, very distant memories may be preserved in detail. Some patients appear to be stuck in time, insisting that the year is one decades past. Patients with Korsakoff's syndrome appear to be unaware of their deficit and commonly attempt to reassure the examiner that nothing is seriously wrong. Confabulation, the invention of material to fill in gaps in memory, is often but not invariably seen. Other aspects of cognitive function may exhibit subtle impairment,[60] but alertness and language are intact.

Patients with Korsakoff's syndrome may show evidence of other alcohol-related neurological disorders. Nystagmus and gait ataxia related to past bouts of Wernicke's disease are common, as are signs of a peripheral neuropathy.

The Korsakoff amnestic syndrome is a clinical diagnosis. This relatively selective memory disorder must be distinguished from the more global cognitive impairment that occurs in dementia due to a variety of causes. The differential diagnosis of a chronic amnestic syndrome resembling Korsakoff's syndrome includes pancerebral hypoxia or ischemia, bilateral posterior cerebral artery strokes, herpes simplex virus encephalitis, paraneoplastic limbic encephalitis, and brain tumors in the vicinity of the third ventricle.

Although acute Wernicke's disease should always be treated with thiamine, the effectiveness of thiamine in preventing the subsequent development of the chronic amnestic syndrome is uncertain. Neither has thiamine been shown to be effective for the treatment of established Korsakoff's syndrome, although patients with this disorder may improve spontaneously.

ALCOHOLIC CEREBELLAR DEGENERATION

Some alcoholic patients develop a chronic cerebellar syndrome that, like the Korsakoff amnestic syndrome, may represent a long-term sequela of Wernicke's encephalopathy.[88] In common with the Wernicke and Korsakoff syndromes, alcoholic cerebellar degeneration is generally attributed to nutritional deficiency and specifically to depletion of thiamine.[88,89] However, it has also been suggested that the disorder may result from a direct toxic effect of alcohol on the cerebellum or from electrolyte abnormalities associated with alcoholism.[90]

The neuropathology of alcoholic cerebellar degeneration consists of loss of cerebellar cortical neurons, especially Purkinje cells, with particular predilection for the anterior and superior vermis; the anterior and superior cerebellar hemispheres are affected less often.[88] This distribution of cerebellar pathology is strikingly similar to that seen in Wernicke's encephalopathy,[60,80] providing an important clue that the two disorders may be pathophysiologically linked.

The natural history of alcoholic cerebellar degeneration is variable.[88] The syndrome usually occurs in the setting of chronic alcoholism of 10 years' or more duration. The most frequent mode of onset is with cerebellar ataxia that progresses steadily for weeks to months. A more gradually progressive disorder that evolves over years is also common. Less often, a mild and stable deficit that has been present for years may become suddenly worse.

Although gait ataxia is the most prominent manifestation of both alcoholic cerebellar degeneration and Wernicke's encephalopathy,[60,88] the pattern of involvement in the two disorders may otherwise differ. Limb ataxia, which is absent in most patients with Wernicke's syndrome, is usually detectable in alcoholic cerebellar degeneration. Examination of such patients typically discloses severe involvement of the legs, with milder involvement of the arms. Dysarthria, which is usually mild, is also more frequent in alcoholic cerebellar degeneration. In contrast, nystagmus is present far less often than in Wernicke's encephalopathy.

Uncommon manifestations of alcoholic cerebellar degeneration include hypotonia, ocular dysmetria, and postural tremor.[88] Patients with alcoholic cerebellar degeneration may also exhibit signs of a polyneuropathy (see below).

Alcoholic cerebellar ataxia is a clinical diagnosis. The CT scan or MRI may show cerebellar cortical atrophy, but laboratory findings are generally helpful only for excluding other causes of ataxia. Conditions that must be considered in the differential diagnosis of subacute or chronic cerebellar ataxia in middle life include multiple sclerosis, hypothyroidism, paraneoplastic cerebellar degeneration, idiopathic cerebellar or olivopontocerebellar atrophies, Creutzfeldt-Jakob disease, and posterior fossa tumors. Like alcoholic cerebellar degeneration, many of these disorders can produce ataxia preferentially affecting the gait.

Ataxia due to alcoholic cerebellar degeneration often stabilizes or improves with cessation of drinking and improved nutritional status,[88,91] although the relative importance of these two factors is uncertain. Patients with this condition should receive parenteral thiamine.

CENTRAL PONTINE MYELINOLYSIS

Central pontine myelinolysis is a disorder manifested by rapidly evolving paraparesis or quadriparesis, pseudobulbar palsy, and impaired consciousness. Certain aspects of the disorder are discussed in Chapter 17. A history of alcoholism is present in most

of the patients,[92] but the disorder has also been described in patients with severe electrolyte disorders, liver disease, malnutrition, Wilson's disease, burns, and cancer.[93,94] Central pontine myelinolysis, like Wernicke's disease, does not appear to be caused directly by alcohol. The disorder was first described in 1959 by Adams and associates,[95] and its appearance coincided with the widespread use of intravenous therapy for correction of fluid and electrolyte disorders.[92] Virtually all cases have occurred in a hospital setting, suggesting that central pontine myelinolysis may be an iatrogenic disorder.[92]

Hyponatremia frequently precedes central pontine myelinolysis, and aggressive correction of hyponatremia appears to be a precipitating factor.[94, 96–98] Norenberg and colleagues retrospectively studied the records of 12 patients with autopsy-proved pontine myelinolysis.[98] All had been hyponatremic, and their serum sodium levels had been raised by more than 20 mEq/L over 1 to 3 days. Eleven patients became hypernatremic (serum sodium level of more than 147 mEq/L) during treatment. Signs of central pontine myelinolysis developed 3 to 10 days after correction of the serum sodium. In a control group of nine hyponatremic patients without pontine myelinolysis at autopsy, the serum sodium had increased more slowly or to lower maximal levels.

Studies in rats[99,100] and dogs[101] also indicate a causal relation between correction of hyponatremia and central pontine myelinolysis. Kleinschmidt-De-Masters and Norenberg found that rats treated with hypertonic saline after 3 days of vasopressin-induced hyponatremia developed ataxia, diminished hind leg extension, and adduction of forepaws.[99] At autopsy there were demyelinative lesions in corpus striatum, cerebral cortex, cerebral white matter, thalamus, hippocampal fimbria, brainstem tegmentum, and cerebellum. Ayus and co-workers treated hyponatremic rats with hypertonic saline or water restriction to achieve normal serum sodium levels within 24 hours.[100] All but 2 of the 20 rats that survived the hyponatremic period developed ataxia and spasticity after correction of the serum sodium, and at autopsy all 18 of these rats had severe necrotic and demyelinative brain lesions. Laureno found pontine and extrapontine myelinolysis in five of ten dogs that survived vasopressin-induced hyponatremia and were treated with water restriction and hypertonic saline.[101] The dogs deteriorated neurologically 2 to 3 days after correction of the serum sodium. All showed leg weakness and were unable to stand; four had intermittent flexor spasms; and two developed ataxia. Six dogs treated with water restriction alone so that the serum sodium never surpassed 130 mEq/L recovered completely, and only one dog in this group had extrapontine myelinolysis at autopsy. In all of these studies, neither hyponatremia by itself nor administration of hypertonic saline to normal animals caused myelinolysis. Thus it appears that rapid correction of hyponatremia can cause myelinolysis in laboratory animals.

In humans, rapid correction of hyponatremia is frequently accomplished without the development of central pontine myelinolysis,[102] although the true incidence of the disorder is unknown. Interspecies differences may account for differences in susceptibility to myelinolysis between humans and rats or dogs and may also account for differences in lesion topography between the human and animal diseases. The existence of well-documented cases of central pontine myelinolysis in patients with hypernatremia or normal serum sodium levels[92,103,104] suggests that rapid correction of hyponatremia is not the only cause of this neurological disorder in humans.

The characteristic pathological lesion in central pontine myelinolysis is bilaterally symmetrical, focal destruction of myelin in the ventral pons, although pathology is occasionally limited to one side or may be multifocal. In about 10 percent of cases, characteristic lesions also are present outside the basis pontis. In these cases, myelinolysis has been observed in the pontine tegmentum, thalamus, cerebellum, basal ganglia, deep layers of cerebral cortex and adjacent white matter, anterior commissure, subthalamic nucleus, and corpus callosum.[93,96,105] Histologically, there is severe loss of myelin, and oligodendroglia are reduced in number. Neurons and axons are relatively spared, although axonal swelling and neuronal shrinkage or acidophilia may occur, particularly in the center of lesions. There is no inflammation, and blood vessels are normal.

Coexistent illnesses often influence the clinical manifestations of central pontine myelinolysis, making it difficult to diagnose this disorder. Furthermore, small lesions detected postmortem can be asymptomatic.[95] Thus it is often not recognized before death.[92,93,97] Nevertheless, certain clinical features are typical of reported cases. Central pontine myelinolysis often evolves over several days to weeks in a severely ill patient, and mental confusion is a prominent feature in almost all cases.[93] Demyelination of pontine corticobulbar fibers leads to dysarthria or mutism, dysphagia, facial and neck weakness, and impaired lingual movement. Conjugate gaze palsies may also occur. Spastic or flaccid weakness of the limbs is common, often with Babinski signs. Although cerebellar demyelination is found in 10 percent of cases, cerebellar signs are usually obscured by weakness. Sensory abnormalities are seldom described. Progressive demyelination of corticospinal and corticobulbar tracts in the basis pontis may produce a locked-in syndrome.[92] Hypotension, seizures, and coma are occasionally noted[93] and may reflect associated metabolic disorders.

The CSF is normal in 50 to 72 percent of patients.[93,106] Elevated CSF pressure, increased protein concentration, and mononuclear pleocytosis occur in a few. Immunoglobulins are normal, but myelin basic protein may be elevated.[107] The EEG is either normal or shows generalized slowing, corresponding to depression of consciousness.[93] Brainstem auditory evoked potentials may show prolongation of the I–V or III–V interpeak latencies[108–110] or absence of waves IV or V.[111] CT brain scans may be normal[92] or may show nonenhancing pontine[97,109,111–113] and extrapontine[109] lucencies. Clinical recovery can precede resolution of CT findings by as much as 18 months.[112] MRI may demonstrate marked prolongation of T_1 and T_2 relaxation times in myelinolytic regions.[110] Because MRI allows better visualization of the brainstem, it is preferable to CT for imaging central pontine myelinolysis.

Because most cases are diagnosed at autopsy, the disorder appears to carry a poor prognosis. Several patients, however, have shown symptomatic improvement after 1 to 4 weeks.[97,107,108,111–114] Therefore patients with suspected central pontine myelinolysis should be supported aggressively because improvement may occur after a few weeks.

Prevention of central pontine myelinolysis remains a controversial issue. Severe hyponatremia (less than 120 mEq/L) is a life-threatening condition that demands prompt treatment,[115] whereas central pontine myelinolysis occurs only rarely. In a study by Ayus and co-workers, factors contributing to myelinolysis in treated hyponatremic patients included an increase in serum sodium to normal or hypernatremic levels during the first 48 hours, a change in serum sodium of more than 25 mEq/L during the first 48 hours, an episode of cerebral hypoxia, or an elevation of serum sodium to hypernatremic levels in patients with hepatic encephalopathy.[116] Therefore the risk of central pontine myelinolysis may be minimized by increasing the serum sodium to mildly hyponatremic levels by no more than 25 mEq/L during the first 48 hours.[116]

ALCOHOLIC NEUROPATHY

Neuropathy is the most frequently encountered chronic neurological disorder related to alcohol abuse. Although both nutritional deficiency[117] and a direct, toxic effect of alcohol[118] have been invoked as etiologies, neither hypothesis has been conclusively validated.[119] Axonal degeneration appears to be the principal pathogenetic process.[118] Segmental demyelination also occurs and may be secondary to the primary axonal disorder or a consequence of concomitant nutritional deficiency.[2]

Alcoholic neuropathy usually presents as a distal, symmetrical, sensorimotor polyneuropathy that is typically gradual in onset. Symptoms include weakness, pain, paresthesias, muscle cramps, numbness, gait ataxia, and burning dysesthesias.[119] Neurological examination may reveal any combination of reflex, sensory, and motor abnormalities, with predominant involvement of the legs. Absent or decreased reflexes and impaired vibration sense are virtually universal findings. Defective appreciation of light touch and weakness are also seen in most patients. Pain and temperature sensation are affected less often, and autonomic dysfunction and cranial nerve involvement are comparatively rare. In addition to the neurological abnormalities, affected limbs may exhibit edema, hyperpigmentation or ulceration of the skin, and bony deformities.[119]

Nerve conduction studies are useful for documenting the presence of neuropathy and for demonstrating the predominantly axonal pathology.[118] Laboratory studies on blood and CSF can exclude other causes of polyneuropathy—for example, diabetes, chronic inflammatory polyradiculoneuropathy, uremia, dysproteinemia, and vasculitis.

Abstinence from alcohol and vitamin (especially thiamine) supplementation can often arrest the progression of alcoholic polyneuropathy and in some cases lead to clinical improvement. Neuropathic pain may respond to anticonvulsants or tricyclic antidepressants.

ALCOHOLIC MYOPATHY

Chronic alcoholism has adverse effects on both skeletal and cardiac muscle, although the manner in which these effects are produced is controversial.[120] Two distinct clinical presentations of alcoholic myopathy are recognized, one acute and the other chronic.[119]

Acute Necrotizing Myopathy

An acute, necrotizing myopathy may develop over the course of 1 to 2 days in the setting of heavy binge drinking. Symptoms include muscle pain and weakness, which may be asymmetrical or focal in nature. Neurological examination shows tender, swollen muscles in the affected areas. Weakness is a prominent finding, is commonly proximal in distribution, and may be associated with dysphagia. Signs of congestive heart failure may be present.

Laboratory abnormalities include moderate to severe elevation of serum creatine kinase (CK) and in some cases myoglobinuria. The electrocardiogram may reveal arrhythmias or conduction defects. Electromyography (EMG) discloses myopathic changes as well as fibrillations. The muscle biopsy shows necrosis of muscle fibers.

Acute alcoholic myopathy must be distinguished from other causes of acute weakness in alcoholic patients (e.g., hypokalemia and hypophosphatemia). In the former condition, weakness is not accompanied by muscle pain, and myoglobinuria does not occur. Hypophosphatemia closely reproduces the clinical features of acute alcoholic myopathy and may contribute to its pathogenesis.[121] Consequently, serum potassium and phosphorus concentrations should always be measured in acutely weak alcoholic patients.

Complications of acute alcoholic myopathy, such as cardiac disturbances and renal compromise due to myoglobinuria, should be treated urgently. Electrolyte abnormalities should be carefully monitored and corrected if necessary. Muscle pain and tenderness may improve with analgesics. Abstinence from alcohol appears to be important for recovery, as resumption of intake during convalescence can cause symptoms to recur.[119] The role of nutritional factors in promoting recovery is less clear, but a nutritionally adequate diet should be ensured. Recovery within weeks to months is the rule, but some patients exhibit residual weakness and cardiac conduction abnormalities.

Chronic Myopathy

A chronic myopathy, which develops insidiously over weeks to months, is also seen in alcoholic patients. This syndrome is characterized by proximal leg weakness with relative preservation of the reflexes. In contrast to the acute, necrotizing alcoholic myopathy discussed above, muscle pain is inconspicuous or absent. Where the clinical diagnosis is uncertain, chronic alcoholic myopathy can be distinguished from polyneuropathy by EMG or by a muscle biopsy showing selective atrophy of type II muscle fibers.[122] Cessation of drinking and an improved diet are associated with clinical improvement over several months in most cases.

ALCOHOL AND STROKE

Epidemiological studies suggest that alcohol consumption influences the risk of stroke.[123,124] For intracerebral and subarachnoid hemorrhage, the risk increases linearly with increasing daily alcohol intake. Possible explanations for this association include disorders of coagulation or fibrinolysis, thrombocytopenia or impaired platelet function, and acute or chronic hypertension. Heavy alcohol consumption may also influence the outcome after aneurysmal subarachnoid hemorrhage adversely by increasing the risk of rebleeding or of vasospasm.[125] In contrast, the relation between daily alcohol intake and ischemic stroke is biphasic, at least in some (e.g., white) populations. Thus, moderate drinking—fewer than about three drinks per day—appears to reduce ischemic stroke risk compared to that observed in nondrinkers, while less temperate drinking patterns predispose to ischemic stroke. The protective effect of small amounts of alcohol has been attributed to elevated levels of prostacyclin, enhanced fibrinolysis, or changes in the relative concentrations of circulating high- and low-density lipoproteins. Mechanisms that could be responsible for an increased risk for ischemic

stroke include alcohol-related cardiomyopathy or arrhythmias, the increased incidence of cigarette smoking in heavy drinkers, rebound thrombocytosis occurring with alcohol withdrawal, and hypercoagulable states.[126,127]

Because not all episodes of focal cerebral ischemia culminate in permanent deficits, the acute pharmacological effects of alcohol could contribute to reducing the risk of stroke by protecting ischemic but still viable neural tissue. In this regard, several studies have shown that ethanol protects cultured cerebral neurons from injury induced by excitotoxic amino acid neurotransmitters, such as glutamate, that have been implicated in ischemic neuronal death.[128–130] Conversely, chronic exposure to high concentrations of ethanol may upregulate excitatory amino acid receptors on cerebral neurons, as has been demonstrated in cultured cerebral cortical cells,[131] and thereby increase neuronal susceptibility to infarction.

ACKNOWLEDGMENTS

The authors' work is supported in part by grants NS01151 (R.O.M.), AA08117 (R.O.M.), NS14543 (D.A.G.), and AA07031 (D.A.G.) from the U.S. Public Health Service, and a grant from the Alcoholic Beverage Medical Research Foundation (R.O.M.).

REFERENCES

1. Charness ME, Simon RP, Greenberg DA: Ethanol and the nervous system. N Engl J Med 321:442, 1989
2. Messing RO, Diamond I: Molecular biology of alcohol dependence. p. 129. In Rosenberg RN, Prusiner SB, DiMauro S, et al (eds): The Molecular and Genetic Basis of Neurologic Disease. Butterworth-Heinemann, Boston, 1993
3. Samson HH, Harris RA: Neurobiology of alcohol abuse. Trends Pharmacol Sci 13:206, 1992
4. Gonzales RA, Hoffman PL: Receptor-gated ion channels may be selective CNS targets for ethanol. Trends Pharmacol Sci 12:1, 1991
5. Leslie SW, Brown LM, Dildy JE, et al: Ethanol and neuronal calcium channels. Alcohol 7:233, 1990
6. Estrin WJ: Alcoholic cerebellar degeneration is not a dose-dependent phenomenon. Alcohol Clin Exp Res 11:372, 1987

7. Cloninger CR: Neurogenetic adaptive mechanisms in alcoholism. Science 236:410, 1987

8. Schenker S: Effects of alcohol on the brain: clinical features, pathogenesis, and treatment. p. 480. In Lieber CS (ed): Medical Disorders of Alcoholism: Pathogenesis and Treatment. WB Saunders, Philadelphia, 1982

9. Goldberg L: Quantitative studies on alcohol tolerance in man. Acta Physiol Scand 5, Suppl 16:1, 1943

10. Mirsky IA, Piker P, Rosenbaum M, Lederer H: Adaptation of the central nervous system to varying concentrations of alcohol in the blood. J Stud Alcohol 2: 35, 1941

11. Urso T, Gavaler JS, Van Thiel DH: Blood ethanol levels in sober alcohol users seen in an emergency room. Life Sci 28:1053, 1981

12. Hammond KB, Rumack BH, Rodgerson DO: Blood ethanol: a report of unusually high levels in a living patient. JAMA 226:63, 1973

13. Watanabe A, Kobayashi M, Hobara N, et al: A report of unusually high blood ethanol and acetaldehyde levels in two surviving patients. Alcohol Clin Exp Res 9:14, 1985

14. Berild D, Hasselbalch H: Survival after a blood alcohol of 1127 mg/dl. Lancet 2:363, 1981

15. Victor M, Adams RD: The effect of alcohol on the nervous system. Res Publ Assoc Nerv Ment Dis 32: 526, 1953

16. Gessner PK: Drug therapy of the alcohol withdrawal syndrome. p. 375. In Majchrowicz E, Nobel EP (eds): Biochemistry and Pharmacology of Ethanol. Vol. 2. Plenum, New York, 1979

17. Victor M, Brausch C: The role of abstinence in the genesis of alcoholic epilepsy. Epilepsia 8:1, 1967

18. Aminoff MJ, Simon RP: Status epilepticus: causes, clinical features, and consequences in 98 patients. Am J Med 69:657, 1980

19. Sampliner R, Iber FL: Diphenylhydantoin control of alcohol withdrawal seizures. JAMA 230:1430, 1974

20. Alldredge BK, Lowenstein DH, Simon RP: Placebo-controlled trial of intravenous diphenylhydantoin for short-term treatment of alcohol withdrawal seizures. Am J Med 87:645, 1989

21. Rothstein E: Prevention of alcohol withdrawal seizures: the roles of diphenylhydantoin and chlordiazepoxide. Am J Psychiatry 130:1381, 1973

22. Freund G: The prevention of alcohol withdrawal seizures in mice by lidocaine. Neurology 23:91, 1973

23. Hillbom ME: The prevention of ethanol withdrawal seizures in rats by dipropylacetate. Neuropharmacology 14:755, 1975

24. Chu N: Carbamazepine: prevention of alcohol withdrawal seizures. Neurology 29:1397, 1979

25. Tavel ME, Davidson W, Batterton TD: A critical analysis of mortality associated with delirium tremens. Am J Med Sci 242:18, 1961

26. Moskowitz G, Chalmers TC, Sacks HS, et al: Deficiencies of clinical trials of alcohol withdrawal. Alcohol Clin Exp Res 7:42, 1983

27. Kaim SC, Klett CJ, Rothfeld B: Treatment of the alcohol withdrawal state: a comparison of four drugs. Am J Psychiatry 125:1640, 1969

28. Thompson WL, Johnson AD, Maddrey WL: Diazepam and paraldehyde for treatment of severe delirium tremens. Ann Intern Med 82:175, 1975

29. Miller WC Jr, McCurdy L: A double-blind comparison of the efficacy and safety of lorazepam and diazepam in the treatment of the acute alcohol withdrawal syndrome. Clin Ther 6:364, 1984

30. Victor M, Adams RD: The alcoholic dementias. p. 335. In Vinken PJ, Bruyn GW, Klawans HL (eds): Handbook of Clinical Neurology. Vol. 46. Elsevier, Amsterdam, 1985

31. Duchen LW, Jacobs JM: Nutritional deficiencies and metabolic disorders. p. 581. In Hume J, Corsellis JAN, Duchen LW (eds): Greenfield's Neuropathology. John Wiley & Sons, New York, 1984

32. Allen IG: Demyelinating diseases. p. 369. In Hume J, Corsellis JAN, Duchen LW (eds): Greenfield's Neuropathology. John Wiley & Sons, New York, 1984

33. Ghatak NR, Hadfield G, Rosenblum WI: Association of central pontine myelinolysis and Marchiafava-Bignami disease. Neurology 28:1295, 1978

34. Victor M, Adams RD, Cole M: The acquired (non-Wilsonian) type of chronic hepatocerebral degeneration. Medicine (Baltimore) 44:345, 1965

35. Wilkinson DA, Carlen PL: Chronic organic brain syndromes associated with alcoholism: neuropsychological and other aspects. p. 107. In Israel Y, Glase FB (eds): Research Advances in Alcohol and Drug Problems. Vol. 3. Plenum, New York, 1981

36. Parsons OA, Leder WR: The relationship between cognitive dysfunction and brain damage in alcoholics: causal, interactive, or epiphenominal? Alcohol Clin Exp Res 5:326, 1981

37. Parker ES, Parker DA, Brody JA, Schoenberg R: Cognitive patterns resembling premature aging in male social drinkers. Alcohol Clin Exp Res 6:46, 1982

38. Lishman WA: Alcoholic dementia: a hypothesis. Lancet 1:1184, 1986

39. Torvik A, Lindboe CF, Rogde S: Brain lesions in alcoholics: a neuropathologic study with clinical correlations. J Neurol Sci 56:233, 1982

40. Carlen PL, Wortzman G, Holgate RC, et al: Reversible cerebral atrophy in recently abstinent chronic alcoholics measured by computed tomography scans. Science 200:1076, 1978

41. Walker DW, Barnes DE, Zornetzer SF, et al: Neuronal loss in hippocampus induced by prolonged ethanol consumption in rats. Science 209:711, 1980

42. Riley JN, Walker DW: Morphological alterations in hippocampus after long-term alcohol consumption in mice. Science 201:646, 1978

43. Courville CB: Effects of Alcohol on the Nervous System of Man. San Lucas Press, Los Angeles, 1955

44. Lynch MJG: Brain lesions in chronic alcoholism. Arch Pathol 69:342, 1960

45. Skullerud K: Variations in the size of the human brain: influence of age, sex, body length, body mass index, alcoholism, Alzheimer changes, and cerebral atherosclerosis. Acta Neurol Scand Suppl 102:61, 1985

46. Harper C, Kril J: Brain atrophy in chronic alcoholic patients: a quantitative pathological study. J Neurol Neurosurg Psychiatry 48:211, 1985

47. Harper C, Kril J, Daly J: Are we drinking our neurones away? Br Med J 294:534, 1987

48. Pfefferbaum A, Lim KO, Zipursky RB, et al: Brain gray and white matter volume loss accelerates with aging in chronic alcoholics: a quantitative MRI study. Alcohol Clin Exp Res 16:1078, 1992

49. Cala LA, Mastaglia FL: Computerized tomography in chronic alcoholics. Alcohol Clin Exp Res 5:283, 1981

50. Bergman H, Borg S, Hindmarsh T, et al: Computed tomography of the brain and neuropsychological assessment of male alcoholic patients and a random sample from the general population. Acta Psychiatr Scand Suppl 286:77, 1980

51. Carlen PL, Wilkinson DA, Wortzman G, et al: Cerebral atrophy and functional deficits in alcoholics without clinically apparent liver disease. Neurology 31: 377, 1981

52. Ishii T: A comparison of cerebral atrophy in CT scan findings among alcoholic groups. Acta Psychiatr Scand Suppl 309:7, 1983

53. Ron MA, Acker W, Shaw GK, Lishman WA: Computerized tomography of the brain in chronic alcoholism: a survey and follow-up study. Brain 105:497, 1982

54. Bergman H, Borg S, Hindmarsh T, et al: Computed tomography of the brain, clinical examination and neuropsychological assessment of a random sample of men from the general population. Acta Psychiatr Scand Suppl 286:47, 1980

55. Jacobson R: Female alcoholics: a controlled CT brain scan and clinical study. Br J Addict 81:661, 1986

56. Carlen PL, Wilkinson DA, Wortzman G, Holgate R: Partially reversible cerebral atrophy and functional improvement in recently abstinent alcoholics. Can J Neurol Sci 11:441, 1984

57. Carlen PL, Kapur B, Huszar LA, et al: Prolonged cerebrospinal fluid acidosis in recently abstinent chronic alcoholics. Neurology 30:956, 1980

58. Chu NS, Squires KC, Starr A: Auditory brain stem potentials in chronic alcohol intoxication and alcohol withdrawal. Arch Neurol 35:596, 1978

59. Porjesz B, Begleiter H: Human evoked brain potentials and alcohol. Alcohol Clin Exp Res 5:304, 1981

60. Victor M, Adams RD, Collins GHP: The Wernicke-Korsakoff Syndrome and Related Neurologic Disorders Due to Alcoholism and Malnutrition. FA Davis, Philadelphia, 1989

61. Greenberg DA, Diamond I: Wernicke-Korsakoff syndrome. p. 295. In Tarter RE, Van Thiel DH (eds): Alcohol and the Brain: Chronic Effects. Plenum, New York, 1985

62. Reuler JB, Girard DE, Cooney TG: Wernicke's encephalopathy. N Engl J Med 312:1035, 1985

63. Blass JP, Gibson GE: Abnormality of a thiamine-requiring enzyme in patients with Wernicke-Korsakoff syndrome. N Engl J Med 297:1367, 1977

64. Leigh D, McBurney A, McIlwain H: Erythrocyte transketolase activity in the Wernicke-Korsakoff syndrome. Br J Psychiatry 139:153, 1981

65. Nixon PF, Kaczmarek MJ, Tate J, et al: An erythrocyte transketolase isoenzyme pattern associated with the Wernicke-Korsakoff syndrome. Eur J Clin Invest 14:278, 1984

66. Jeyasingham MD, Pratt OE, Burns A, et al: The activation of red blood cell transketolase in groups of patients especially at risk from thiamine deficiency. Psychol Med 17:311, 1987

67. Mukherjee AB, Svoronos S, Ghazanfari A, et al: Transketolase abnormality in cultured fibroblasts from familial chronic alcoholic men and their male offspring. J Clin Invest 79:1039, 1987

68. Hakim AM, Pappius HM: The effect of thiamine deficiency on local cerebral glucose utilization. Ann Neurol 9:334, 1981

69. Sharp FR, Bolger E, Evans K: Thiamine deficiency limits glucose utilization and glial proliferation in brain lesions of symptomatic rats. J Cereb Blood Flow Metab 2:203, 1982

70. Sharp FR, Evans K, Bolger E: Local cerebral glucose utilization in the symptomatic thiamine-deficient rat: increases in fornix and pyramidal tract. Neurology 32: 808, 1982

71. Hakim AM, Pappius HM: Sequence of metabolic, clinical, and histological events in experimental thiamine deficiency. Ann Neurol 13:365, 1983

72. Gallucci M, Bozzao A, Splendiani A, et al: Wernicke encephalopathy: MR findings in five patients. AJNR 155:887, 1990

73. Donnal JF, Heinz ER, Burger PC: MR of reversible thalamic lesions in Wernicke syndrome. AJNR 155: 893, 1990

74. Bishai DM, Bozzetti LP: Current progress toward the prevention of the Wernicke-Korsakoff syndrome. Alcohol Alcohol 21:315, 1986

75. Richmond J: Wernicke's encephalopathy associated with digitalis poisoning. Lancet 1:344, 1959

76. Kramer J, Goodwin JA: Wernicke's encephalopathy: complication of intravenous hyperalimentation. JAMA 238:2176, 1977

77. Jagadha V, Deck JHN, Halliday WC, Smyth HS: Wernicke's encephalopathy in patients on peritoneal dialysis or hemodialysis. Ann Neurol 21:78, 1987

78. Drenick EJ, Joven CB, Swendseid ME: Occurrence of acute Wernicke's encephalopathy during prolonged starvation for the treatment of obesity. N Engl J Med 274:937, 1966

79. Kwee IL, Nakada T: Wernicke's encephalopathy induced by tolazamide. N Engl J Med 309:599, 1983

80. Malamud N, Skillicorn SA: Relationship between the Wernicke and the Korsakoff syndrome. Arch Neurol Psychiatry 76:586, 1956

81. Squire LR: Mechanisms of memory. Science 232: 1612, 1986

82. Thompson RF: The neurobiology of learning and memory. Science 233:941, 1986

83. John ER, Tang Y, Brill AB, et al: Double-labeled maps of memory. Science 233:1167, 1986

84. Smith SJ: Progress on LTP at hippocampal synapses: a post-synaptic Ca^{2+} trigger for memory storage? Trends Neurosci 10:142, 1987

85. Bear MF, Cooper LN, Ebner FF: A physiological basis for a theory of synapse modification. Science 237:42, 1987

86. McEntee WJ, Mair RG, Langlais PJ: Neurochemical pathology in Korsakoff's psychosis: implications for other cognitive disorders. Neurology 34:648, 1984

87. Martin PR, Weingartner H, Gordon EK, et al: Central nervous system catecholamine metabolism in Korsakoff's psychosis. Ann Neurol 15:184, 1984

88. Victor M, Adams RD, Mancall EL: A restricted form of cerebellar cortical degeneration occurring in alcoholic patients. Arch Neurol 76:586, 1956

89. Mancall EL, McEntee WJ: Alterations of the cerebellar cortex in nutritional encephalopathy. Neurology 15: 303, 1965

90. Kleinschmidt-DeMasters BK, Norenberg MD: Cerebellar degeneration in the rat following rapid correction of hyponatremia. Ann Neurol 10:561, 1981

91. Diener HC, Dichgans J, Bacher M, Guschlbauer B: Improvement of ataxia in alcoholic cerebellar atrophy through alcohol abstinence. J Neurol 231:258, 1984

92. Messert B, Orison WW, Hawkins MJ, Quaglieri CE: Central pontine myelinolysis: consideration on etiology, diagnosis, and treatment. Neurology 29:147, 1979

93. Goebel HH, Herman-BenZur P: Central pontine myelinolysis. p. 285 In Vinken PJ, Bruyn GW (eds): Handbook of Clinical Neurology. Vol. 28. Elsevier, Amsterdam, 1976

94. Brucar PJ, Norenberg MD, Yarnell PR: Hyponatremia and central pontine myelinolysis. Neurology 27:223, 1977

95. Adams RD, Victor M, Mancall EL: Central pontine myelinolysis: a hitherto undescribed disease occurring in alcoholic and malnourished patients. Arch Neurol Psychiatry 81:154, 1959

96. Wright D, Laureno R, Victor M: Pontine and extrapontine myelinolysis. Brain 102:361, 1979

97. Telfer RB, Miller EM: Central pontine myelinolysis following hyponatremia, demonstrated by computerized tomography. Ann Neurol 6:455, 1979

98. Norenberg MD, Leslie KO, Robertson AS: Association between rise in serum sodium and central pontine myelinolysis. Ann Neurol 11:128, 1982

99. Kleinschmidt-DeMasters BK, Norenberg MD: Rapid correction of hyponatremia causes demyelination: relation to central pontine myelinolysis. Science 211: 1068, 1981

100. Ayus JC, Krothapalli RK, Armstrong DL: Rapid correction of severe hyponatremia in the rat: histopathological changes in the brain. Am J Physiol 248:F711, 1985

101. Laureno R: Central pontine myelinolysis following rapid correction of hyponatremia. Ann Neurol 13: 232, 1983

102. Ayus JC, Olivero JJ, Frommer JP: Rapid correction of severe hyponatremia with intravenous saline solution. Am J Med 72:43, 1982

103. Tampi R, Alexander WS: Wernicke's encephalopathy with central pontine myelinolysis presenting with hypothermia. NZ Med J 95:342, 1982

104. Finlayson MH, Snider S, Olivia LA, Gualt MH: Cerebral and pontine myelinolysis: two cases with fluid and electrolyte imbalance and hypotension. J Neurol Sci 18:399, 1973

105. Goldman JE, Horoupian DS: Demyelination of the lateral geniculate nucleus in central pontine myelinolysis. Ann Neurol 9:185, 1981

106. Fishman RA: Cerebrospinal Fluid in Diseases of the Nervous System. 2nd Ed. WB Saunders, Philadelphia, 1992

107. Kandt RS, Heldrich FJ, Moser HW: Recovery from probable central pontine myelinolysis associated with Addison's disease. Arch Neurol 40:118, 1983

108. Stockard JJ, Rossiter VS, Wiederholt WC, Kobayashi RM: Brain stem auditory-evoked responses in suspected central pontine myelinolysis. Arch Neurol 33: 726, 1976

109. Thompson DS, Hutton JT, Stears JC, et al: Computerized tomography in the diagnosis of central and extrapontine myelinolysis. Arch Neurol 38:243, 1981

110. DeWitt LD, Buonanno FS, Kistler JP, et al: Central pontine myelinolysis: demonstration by nuclear magnetic resonance. Neurology 34:570, 1984

111. Yufe RS, Hyde ML, Terbrugge K: Auditory evoked responses and computerized tomography in central pontine myelinolysis. Can J Neurol Sci 7:297, 1980

112. Gerber O, Geller M, Stiller J, Yang W: Central pontine myelinolysis: resolution shown by computed tomography. Arch Neurol 40:116, 1983

113. Anderson TL, Moore RA, Grinnell VS, Itabashi HH: Computerized tomography in central pontine myelinolysis. Neurology 29:1527, 1979

114. Wiederholt WC, Kobayashi RM, Stockard JJ, Rossiter VS: Central pontine myelinolysis: a clinical reappraisal. Arch Neurol 34:220, 1977

115. Arieff AI, Llach F, Massry SG: Neurological manifestations and morbidity of hyponatremia: correlation with brain water and electrolytes. Medicine (Baltimore) 55:121, 1976

116. Ayus JC, Krothapalli RK, Arieff AI: Treatment of symptomatic hyponatremia and its relation to brain damage. N Engl J Med 317:1190, 1987

117. Victor, M: Polyneuropathy due to nutritional deficiency and alcoholism. p. 1899. In Dyck PJ, Thomas PK, Lambert EH, Bunge R (eds): Peripheral Neuropathy. 2nd Ed. WB Saunders, Philadelphia, 1984

118. Behse F, Buchthal F: Alcoholic neuropathy: clinical, electrophysiological, and biopsy findings. Ann Neurol 2:95, 1977

119. Layzer RB: Neuromuscular Manifestations of Systemic Disease. FA Davis, Philadelphia, 1985

120. Rubin E: Alcoholic myopathy in heart and skeletal muscle. N Engl J Med 301:28, 1979

121. Knochel JP: Hypophosphatemia. West J Med 134:15, 1981

122. Mills KR, Ward K, Martin F, Peters TJ: Peripheral neuropathy and myopathy in chronic alcoholism. Alcohol Alcohol 21:357, 1986

123. Camargo CAJ: Moderate alcohol consumption and stroke: the epidemiologic evidence. Stroke 20:1611, 1989

124. Gorelick PB: The status of alcohol as a risk factor for stroke. Stroke 20:1607, 1989

125. Juvela S: Alcohol consumption as a risk factor for poor outcome after aneurysmal subarachnoid haemorrhage. Br Med J 304:1663, 1992

126. Wolf PA: Cigarettes, alcohol, and stroke. N Engl J Med 315:1087, 1986

127. Hillbom M, Kaste M, Rasi V: Can ethanol intoxication affect hemocoagulation to increase the risk of brain infarction in young adults? Neurology 33:381, 1983

128. Takadera T, Suzuki R, Mohri T: Protection by ethanol of cortical neurons from N-methyl-D-aspartate-induced neurotoxicity is associated with blocking calcium influx. Brain Res 537:109, 1990

129. Lustig HS, Chan J, Greenberg DA: Ethanol inhibits excitotoxicity in cerebral cortical cultures. Neurosci Lett 135:259, 1992

130. Lustig HS, von Brauchitsch KL, Chan J, et al: Ethanol and excitotoxicity in cultured cortical neurons: differential sensitivity of N-methyl-D-aspartate and sodium nitroprusside toxicity. J Neurochem 59:2193, 1992

131. Ahern K von B, Lustig HS, Greenberg DA: Enhancement of NMDA toxicity and calcium responses by chronic exposure of cultured cortical neurons to ethanol. Neurosci Lett 165:211, 1994

31

Neurological Complications of Drugs of Abuse

George A. Ricaurte
J. William Langston

Recreational drug abuse, which has reached epidemic proportions in the United States and abroad, has been associated with numerous neurological disorders. Some are easily recognized, others defy ready diagnosis. Although many of the neurological syndromes stemming from drug abuse mimic naturally occurring disorders, some do not. Unfortunately, in many cases the history of drug abuse is not readily apparent, and in some instances it is deliberately concealed. Furthermore, with the proliferation of new synthetics, or "designer drugs," the number of perplexing neurological presentations is likely to increase because the toxicity of such novel compounds is largely uncharacterized and often difficult to predict.

The purpose of this chapter is to describe various neurological complications arising from nonmedical use of psychoactive drugs and to discuss therapeutic strategies that can be employed. Given the wide array of such substances, it would be beyond the scope of this chapter to deal with the effects of each of these drugs in detail. As such, this chapter focuses on neurological complications associated with the use of the more popular recreational drugs, including cocaine, methamphetamine, marijuana, heroin, phencyclidine (PCP), solvent inhalants, and a few of the new synthetic drugs, of which 1-methyl-4-phenyl-1,2,3,6-tetrahydropyridine (MPTP) and 3,4-methylenedi-

oxymethamphetamine (MDMA, "ecstasy") are perhaps the best known. Particular emphasis is given to diagnostic clues that should alert the clinician to the fact that he or she is dealing with a complication of substance abuse.

COCAINE

Cocaine is one of the most widely abused illicit drugs in the United States.[1] It is derived from the leaves of *Erythroxylon coca,* a shrub that grows on the eastern slopes of the Andes Mountains. Cocaine is found in the coca leaf with approximately 13 other alkaloids.[2] To what extent these other alkaloids contribute to the psychoactive effects of the coca leaf is not clear. For centuries, South American Indians have used coca leaves for their stimulant, anorectic, and possibly thirst-reducing effects. The leaves are chewed, placed inside one cheek, and there exposed to some alkali such as lime, which helps extract cocaine along with the other alkaloids from the leaves. Used in this manner, cocaine has been remarkably free of untoward effects.[3]

In contradistinction, cocaine use in the United States seems fraught with problems.[4] It seems largely related to the tendency of North Americans to use cocaine intranasally or intravenously rather than orogastrically. In addition, cocaine preparations in the United States are much more potent than those used by South American natives. Coca leaves used in the Andes rarely contain more than 0.5 percent cocaine.[2] By contrast, some samples in the United States approach 100 percent purity (Irwin, personal communication). On the street, cocaine is sold as a powder that goes by the names "coke," "snow," "gold dust," "toot," or "lady." More recently, the terms "rock" and "crack" have also come into usage; they refer to a hardened type of cocaine that is in the free base form. This cocaine preparation is usually self-administered by means of smoke inhalation rather than by being sniffed up the nose, or "snorted."

Health problems associated with use of cocaine in the United States range from perforated nasal septa to deaths from overdose.[4] Cocaine acts principally by augmenting neurotransmission across monoaminergic synapses, primarily by blocking the reuptake inactivation of dopamine, norepinephrine, and serotonin.[5] In this regard, cocaine can be viewed as a fast, indirectly acting sympathomimetic agent. In addition, cocaine possesses local anesthetic effects. In general, the acute toxic effects of cocaine represent extensions of its pharmacological actions. In moderate doses, cocaine increases alertness, raises blood pressure, causes a mild hyperthermia, reduces appetite and thirst, and induces a euphoric sense of well-being.[6] In high doses cocaine can produce hyperpyrexia, hypertension, respiratory depression, cardiac arrhythmias, and sudden death.[7] Cocaine intoxication can also lead to the development of a psychotic state that in some regards resembles paranoid schizophrenia.

Common neurological complications associated with cocaine abuse are seizures, headache, tremor, and various types of cerebrovascular accidents.[8-14] In recent years, stroke has emerged as a particularly common complication of cocaine abuse.[15-19] Subarachnoid hemorrhage,[20] intracerebral hemorrhage,[21,22] cerebral infarction,[23,24] and transient ischemic attacks[10,11] have all been reported. There is some indication that cerebrovascular complications (particularly hemorrhage) may be more frequent with the "crack" form of cocaine,[18,19] but the basis for this is unclear. In the majority of cases, individuals who suffer a neurovascular complication of cocaine are found to have some predisposing factor, such as aneurysm or an arteriovenous malformation.[19] In addition, some biopsy proven cases of vasculitis associated with cocaine abuse have been reported.[14,25] Other neurological complications associated with cocaine abuse include dystonic reactions,[26,27] exacerbation of movement disorders,[13,28] cerebrospinal fluid rhinorrhea,[29] fungal cerebritis,[4] and agitation and other alterations in mental status.[11] Neurological complications associated with cocaine abuse may be increasing, but it is not known if this is due to increased use of cocaine, use of other forms of cocaine ("crack") by different routes of administration ("snorting"), or improved recognition of cocaine-related syndromes.

Treatment of acute cocaine intoxication should be with a potent dopamine receptor blocking agent such as haloperidol. Such drugs are helpful in ameliorating the agitation and confusion often seen following cocaine overdose. When seizures pose the main problem, diazepam is the drug of choice, although phenytoin and phenobarbital are also effective.[7] Hypertension can be counteracted with diazoxide or hydralazine. Standard antiarrhythmic agents are indicated in the patient with ventricular dysrhythmia.

METHAMPHETAMINE

Unlike cocaine, methamphetamine is a synthetic stimulant drug that was first elaborated by Ogata in 1919. Along with amphetamine, it was introduced into the United States during the early part of this century as a nasal decongestant. Since then, methamphetamine has been tried in the treatment of narcolepsy, childhood hyperkinesis, obesity, and mild forms of depression.[30] Structurally, methamphetamine is closely related to both dopamine and norepinephrine. In fact, these neurotransmitters are believed to mediate many of methamphetamine's effects. Methamphetamine acts by promoting release of dopamine and norepinephrine and by blocking the reuptake of these transmitter substances from the synaptic cleft. In this regard, methamphetamine is similar to cocaine, but its duration of action is considerably longer.

In the illicit drug market, racemic methamphetamine is known as "speed," "crystal meth," or "crank." Street samples that are said to contain amphetamine ("uppers," "dex," "bennies") usually consist primarily of methamphetamine. Nonmedical use of methamphetamine has been recognized almost since its first synthesis. During the era following World War II, epidemics of methamphetamine abuse occurred in Japan, Great Britain, Sweden, and the United States.[32] To this day, methamphetamine abuse continues to be a problem. Indeed, in recent years, a new illicit dosage form of methamphetamine has appeared. It is referred to as "ice" and consists of pure dextro-methamphetamine that has been crystallized and is usually inhaled or smoked.[33] By contrast, racemic methamphetamine is most often taken orally at a dose of 10 to 20 mg. However, some individuals ("speed freaks") take higher doses of the drug intravenously. Typically, these individuals go on "runs" of methamphetamine use that may last 3 or 4 days, during which time they do not sleep, eat, or drink as they would normally.

By enhancing catecholaminergic neurotransmission in the periphery and in the brain, methamphetamine produces many of the same pharmacological effects as cocaine, including tachycardia, hyperthermia, mydriasis, anorexia, and a sense of physical well-being.[31] The toxic effects of methamphetamine also parallel those of cocaine. Hyperpyrexia, seizures, cardiac arrhythmias, and psychotic states have all been noted.[6]

One of the better-known complications of methamphetamine use is intracranial hemorrhage.[34] Most commonly, it occurs in the setting of vascular abnormalities, which are said to be part of an "amphetamine-induced vasculitis."[35–37] It should be noted, however, that hemorrhagic[38–40] as well as ischemic[41] strokes in the absence of vascular abnormalities have been reported following methamphetamine use. In addition, intracranial hemorrhage and vasculitis have been reported after other central stimulant drugs such as ephedrine.[42] Therefore, the exact relation between methamphetamine and intracranial hemorrhage is unclear. The hypertensive effects of methamphetamine have been thought to play a role, but not all of the patients have elevated blood pressure at the time of admission.[38] Moreover, blood pressure may be elevated secondary to intracranial bleeding.

The relation between methamphetamine and vasculitis is a complicated one. Adulterants in methamphetamine preparations have been implicated,[10] but vasculitis has been observed in patients taking pure

methamphetamine.[40] Infectious agents injected during the intravenous administration of nonsterile drug solutions have also been suggested to play a role in the etiology of amphetamine-induced vasculitis.[43] However, vasculitis has been observed in subjects who have taken the drug orally and have not had any signs or symptoms of infection.[40] Central nervous system (CNS) vasculitis has also been noted following use of other psychomotor stimulant drugs, such as ephedrine.[42] Therefore it has been suggested that methamphetamine and related compounds should be suspected in any young adult presenting with unexplained intracranial hemorrhage or CNS vasculitis.

Another notable complication of methamphetamine abuse is a choreiform movement disorder.[44,45] Typically, this complication occurs in individuals using the drug repeatedly and at high dosage. The movement disorder generally resolves within days after cessation of drug intake. The involuntary movements are probably related to excessive stimulation of postsynaptic dopamine receptors.

Recent studies indicate that repeated administration of high doses of methamphetamine to a variety of experimental animals causes prolonged depletion of dopamine and serotonin in various regions of the CNS.[46] These depletions are related to the destruction of dopaminergic and serotonergic nerve terminals, with cell bodies in the substantia nigra and the raphe nuclei remaining unaffected. No functional consequences of this toxicity have yet been identified. Whether humans abusing methamphetamine develop these complications is not yet known. Certainly, a parkinsonian syndrome (resulting from destruction of the nigrostriatal dopamine system) as a consequence of methamphetamine abuse has not been well documented. Nonetheless, the possibility that these individuals have subclinical damage of the nigrostriatal system deserves consideration. One might predict that such individuals would display enhanced sensitivity to haloperidol and other dopamine receptor blockers and might be at an increased risk for developing Parkinson's disease at an earlier age; but, at the current time, data to substantiate these suggestions are lacking.

Clinical management of methamphetamine intoxication involves the use of a dopamine receptor blocking agent, such as chlorpromazine or haloperidol, to counteract methamphetamine's catecholaminergic effects. In addition, a peripheral alpha receptor blocking agent such as phentolamine can be used to combat the drug's hypertensive effects. Acidification of the urine with ammonium chloride is indicated to promote renal excretion of methamphetamine. Measures should also be taken to lower body temperature, as the hyperthermic effects of methamphetamine are considerable and potentially lethal.[6,32]

MARIJUANA

Marijuana is a dried mixture of all parts of the hemp plant *Cannabis sativa*. For thousands of years, marijuana has been used in the Middle and Far East. It was introduced into the United States by Mexican migrant workers shortly after World War I. Marijuana did not become a popular recreational drug until the 1960s and today is probably the most widely used of all illegal drugs. Popular street names include "grass," "weed," or "pot." There are numerous psychoactive alkaloids in marijuana, but the most potent is trans-Δ9-tetrahydrocannabinol (THC). THC content of marijuana ranges from 1 to 2 percent.[2] Marijuana is generally smoked but can also be taken orally. Absorption from the gastrointestinal tract is slower and more erratic.

The main organ systems affected by marijuana are the brain and the cardiovascular system. Central effects vary depending on dose and route of administration, but typically moderate doses of marijuana produce changes in mood, impair motor coordination, alter cognitive abilities, and engender a different sense of time.[47] Psychopharmacologically, marijuana is perhaps best characterized as a mild psychedelic, but its effects clearly differ from those of true hallucinogens. Cardiovascular effects most commonly noted after marijuana are a mild increase in heart rate and a reddening of the conjunctiva.[47] Effects on the endocrine and immune systems have also been reported, but the significance of these effects is as yet unclear.[48]

Neurologically, low doses of marijuana impair coordination and gait.[49] High doses of marijuana cause disorientation, confusion, and, if doses are sufficiently high, a frank toxic psychosis. More commonly, this complication occurs after oral ingestion. Typically, the sensorium clears entirely within days, and therapeutic intervention is not required. At present, there is no evidence that chronic marijuana use produces any long-term deleterious effects on the CNS. A thinning of the cerebral cortex along with enlargement of the ventricles was reported in an earlier study utilizing pneumoencephalography.[50] However, these findings have not been confirmed with computed tomography.[51] At the ultrastructural level, changes in synaptic morphology in the limbic system have been reported in nonhuman primates.[52] This finding awaits validation.[53]

In recent years, THC has found a place in the medical pharmacopoeia for the treatment of glaucoma and intractable nausea and vomiting.[6]

HEROIN

Heroin is perhaps the best-known and most widely abused of the opiate narcotics. Originally, these drugs were perceived as depressing brain function, hence their designation as *narcotic*, a term derived from the Greek word meaning "stupor." Opium is the parent compound for all narcotics. It is found in the opium poppy *Papaver somniferum*. Opium is typically smoked or taken by mouth. Although the main active ingredient in opium is morphine (named after Morpheus, the Greek god of dreams), opium also contains more than 20 other active alkaloids.[2] Unlike opium, which is a gummy solid, morphine is a white crystalline powder that can be injected directly into the bloodstream.

Heroin, the diacetyl derivative of morphine, is three to five times more potent than morphine, has a shorter duration of action, and is the most popular street opiate.[54] It can be smoked, sniffed up the nose, or injected subcutaneously ("skin popping"). When taken intravenously, heroin produces a warm flushing of the skin along with an intense sensation in the lower abdomen that is said to be more pleasurable than orgasm. Other pharmacological effects of heroin result principally from actions of the drug on the central nervous and gastrointestinal systems. Through its actions on the CNS, heroin relieves pain, suppresses cough, depresses respiration, and clouds the sensorium.[6] In the gut, heroin interferes with intestinal motility and can thereby cause constipation. Another well-known effect of heroin is pupillary constriction. This effect is probably at the level of the autonomic portion of the oculomotor complex.[55]

The hallmarks of heroin intoxication are coma, respiratory depression, and pinpoint pupils. These untoward effects are readily reversed by naloxone, a specific opiate antagonist. It is important to bear in mind that naloxone has a relatively short half-life, approximately 40 minutes.[56] As such, repeated doses may be required, because most narcotics have a longer duration of action.

Neurological complications arising from heroin abuse can be subdivided into those that stem from infectious sources and those that are of noninfectious origin.[57,58] Those of noninfectious origin arise mostly from hypoxia and hypotension produced by heroin overdose. They include postanoxic encephalopathy, cerebral infarction, unilateral parkinsonism, hemiballistic movements, bilateral deafness, acute transverse myelitis involving primarily the cervical and thoracic levels, and a stroke-like syndrome that occurs in the absence of endocarditis or mycotic aneurysms.[59–62] Interestingly, a syndrome of delayed postanoxic encephalopathy has also been described[63] along with a progressive ventral pontine syndrome.[64] The mechanisms underlying either of these syndromes are not well understood. Neurological complications observed in heroin abusers and related to infection are meningitis, cerebral abscess, and, in patients with endocarditis, embolic infarcts.[44,65] Not infrequently, cerebral emboli in these patients are associated with mycotic aneurysms. Intravenous drug abuse has also become an important vector for the transmission of the acquired immunodeficiency syndrome (see Ch. 38).

Peripheral nerve disorders have also been noted in heroin abusers. Usually they can be attributed to prolonged compression of nerves during periods of stupor or to direct trauma from injection.[66] A number of brachial and lumbosacral plexopathies, however, have been difficult to explain on this basis. In these cases, local infections and autoimmune processes have been implicated as etiological factors.[64] However, precise mechanisms underlying these plexopathies are still poorly understood.

Another major neurological complication of heroin abuse is addiction. It is characterized by compulsive craving for the drug, tolerance, and physical dependence. The latter becomes evident when signs and symptoms of withdrawal appear upon discontinuing the drug.

Heroin addiction or dependence can be managed in one of three ways: (1) substitution of an opiate agonist that can be given orally and is long-acting (e.g., methadone); (2) treatment with an opiate antagonist (e.g., naltrexone); or (3) gradual detoxification, often with the aid of an opiate agonist such as methadone or a nonopiate drug such as clonidine.[58,67]

PHENCYCLIDINE

PCP, known on the street as "angel dust" or the "peace pill," was first synthesized during the 1950s. Initially it was marketed as a surgical anesthetic, but this use was quickly discontinued after patients complained of untoward mental effects. Along with ketamine, PCP is characterized as a "dissociative anesthetic" because individuals taking it feel removed from their environment. PCP first appeared on the illicit drug market during the 1960s. However, by this time it had become known as an animal tranquilizer because of its introduction into veterinary medicine as an anesthetic. PCP can be ingested orally, taken intranasally, or used by smoking. The inhalation route is generally preferred because it allows better titration of effects.

The mechanism of action of PCP is both unique and complex. It produces a mixture of stimulant, depressant, anesthetic, and hallucinogenic effects.[68] Neurochemically, PCP affects virtually every neurotransmitter system studied to date, including the dopamine and acetylcholine systems.[69] Pharmacological effects include decreased pain sensation, tachycardia, raised blood pressure, flushing and sweating, and altered perception.[68] In higher doses, PCP produces nystagmus (either horizontal or vertical), ataxia, dysarthria, and an acute confusional state that may progress to stupor and coma.[70] The combination of nystagmus and hypertension in an individual with an abrupt behavioral change should alert the clinician to the possibility of PCP intoxication. Remarkably, some patients intoxicated with PCP are vigilant but unresponsive and can be mistaken for being catatonic or in a state of akinetic mutism. Other neurological complications include major motor seizures, focal dystonias, and athetoid movements.[70] It is important to remember that PCP exerts anesthetic effects and that patients may therefore complain of numbness. It is generally thought that the combination of anesthesia and mental status changes accounts for cases of self-mutilation, some of which are severe.

Toxic effects may persist for days, as the half-life of PCP after overdose may be prolonged for as long as 3 days.[71] It can be shortened by acidifying the urine with ammonium chloride. However, this measure should not be taken if rhabdomyolysis is an intercurrent problem. Instead, aggressive hydration and diuretics are indicated. Control of psychotic behavior can generally be accomplished with haloperidol. Phenothiazines should be avoided because their anticholinergic effects may aggravate those of PCP.[72] When seizures occur, diazepam is the drug of choice.[73]

Whether chronic PCP abuse can lead to long-lasting neurological complications is not clear. Memory and language disturbances have been reported but are not well documented.[68] Abrupt lapses into confusional states occurring weeks or months after PCP ingestion have also been noted. These behavioral alterations may have the flavor of schizophrenic behavior. The possibility that PCP acts as a precipitant in an individual already at risk has not been excluded.

ORGANIC SOLVENTS

Abuse of volatile organic solvents has become increasingly popular over the last two decades. In part, this may be related to their ready availability. Common household products containing organic solvents include some glues, paint thinner, varnish, lighter fluid, and spot removers, to name just a few. Some people breathe the fumes of these organic solvents directly from containers; others put organic solvents on rags or in plastic bags, which they then place over the nose or head. The principal active ingredients in organic solvents are simple carbon-based molecules (e.g., toluene, hexane, and benzene).[74]

Acute behavioral effects of organic solvents include lightheadedness, giddiness, and a hot, flushed, exhilarated feeling.[75] Auditory and visual hallucinations are also reported. With repeated and prolonged exposure, toxic effects become manifest, including nausea and vomiting, tinnitus, diplopia, and impaired cognitive function. Ataxia, dysarthria, hyporeflexia, and nystagmus may also be observed. Later, respiratory depression may occur, along with increasing disorientation and confusion that may evolve to loss of consciousness. Confusional states related to solvent inhalation may persist for days.[75]

One early and well known neurological complication of *n*-hexane organic solvent abuse is a distal symmetrical sensorimotor polyneuropathy.[76,77] Typi-

cally, it stabilizes and partially resolves after solvent abuse has been curtailed, but it may persist for months. Generally, the more extensive the abuse has been, the longer it takes for the neuropathy to resolve, and even then resolution may be incomplete. Neurological complications seen in later stages of chronic organic solvent abuse are cerebellar ataxia, corticospinal tract dysfunction, oculomotor abnormalities, and dementia,[75] depending on the solvent to which exposure occurred. It is of note that cerebral and cerebellar degeneration have been observed after inhalation of toluene and house paint fumes. It therefore appears that some of the neurotoxic effects of organic solvent inhalation are not reversible.

Treatment of acute solvent inhalant intoxication can be difficult, as no specific antidotes are available. In the agitated patient, diazepam can be used for sedation. Aside from this measure, only routine supportive respiratory and cardiovascular measures can be provided.

NEW SYNTHETICS ("DESIGNER DRUGS")

The "designer drugs" pose a growing health threat to society. They are analogues of controlled substances synthesized by clandestine chemists attempting to circumvent the law. By structurally redesigning scheduled drugs, illicit chemists strive to create compounds that are legal and meet the individual tastes of their consumers.[78] Until recently, it was possible to manufacture these substances because drug enforcement legislation in the United States required that any controlled substance be designated specifically by name and structure. As these analogues had not been so designated, they could be manufactured, distributed, and sold without fear of legal sanction. Although extraordinarily profitable, controlled substance analogues are potentially hazardous. The reason is twofold. First, illicit chemists rarely have the capability for carrying out the kind of quality control required to ensure that no dangerous contaminants or by-products are present in their samples. Second, these newly designed drugs do not undergo testing in experimental animals; accordingly, little is known about their potency or side effects. Given these conditions, the "designer drug" industry is likely to spawn human tragedy.

Two such tragedies have already been recorded. The first resulted from the proliferation of fentanyl analogues. Fentanyl is a widely used but controlled surgical anesthetic (Sublimaze). It is five to ten times more potent than morphine. Taking its potency as a clue, illicit chemists set out to create a more potent yet legal fentanyl analogue. Thus seven fentanyl analogues have surfaced in the black market. One of these, 3-methylfentanyl ("China white"), is approximately 6,000 times more potent that morphine. Predictably, use of this analogue by unsuspecting addicts has resulted in more than 100 overdose deaths in the state of California alone. Recently, 3-methylfentanyl was also identified in overdose deaths in the northeastern United States.[79,80]

The second tragedy also occurred in California. It grew out of a clandestine chemist's attempt to elaborate an uncontrolled analogue of meperidine. The desired product was 1-methyl-4-phenyl-4-propionoxypiperidine (MPPP). Unbeknownst to the chemist, however, a by-product of this synthesis was 1-methyl-4-phenyl-1,2,3,6-tetrahydropyridine (MPTP). The latter turned out to be a potent neurotoxin that destroys dopamine-containing cells in the pars compacta of the substantia nigra,[81] the chief site of pathology in Parkinson's disease. Not surprisingly, soon after addicts began using what they believed was a new synthetic heroin, a number of them developed a striking neurological syndrome that had all the elemental features of Parkinson's disease, including marked bradykinesia, rigidity, loss of postural reflexes, and tremor at rest.[82] These patients responded to standard dopamine replacement therapies. Indeed, they also developed the typical complications of levodopa therapy, including peak dose dyskinesias and on-off phenomena.[83] Moreover, there is recent evidence that some of the individuals who were exposed to MPTP but did not develop immediate signs or symptoms of parkinsonism are now (almost 10 years later) beginning to show evidence of extrapyramidal motor dysfunction.[84] Thus, MPTP has revitalized research on Parkinson's disease, but it has also taught a sobering lesson regarding the dangers of new synthetics.

With continued production of synthetic analogues, recurrence of such tragedies would not be unexpected. Already, a number of novel amphetamine analogues have been identified on the street. Two of them, 3,4-methylenedioxymethamphetamine (MDMA) and 3,4-methylenedioxyethylamphetamine (MDEA), are proving toxic to serotonin-containing neurons in the CNS of experimental animals[85–87] and possibly humans.[88,89] This finding raises concern regarding the potential long-term effects of these compounds. As the function of serotonergic cells in the human brain is not well understood, it is difficult to anticipate what types of neuropsychiatric disturbances may develop with time in individuals abusing these novels analogues.

However, some individuals have already been identified who, following MDMA intoxication, developed problems in behavioral domains in which serotonin has been implicated (e.g., mood regulation, memory), and later responded to treatment with serotonin reuptake blockers.[90] Should such subjects present to physicians in the future, their history of drug abuse may hold the key for unraveling what otherwise may be a puzzling clinical presentation.

Most recently, several new synthetic analogs have appeared in the illicit drug market, including 4-methylaminorex ("euphoria"), paramethoxymethamphetamine (PMMA), and methcathinone ("cat"), and there is preclinical evidence that at least two of these (PMMA[91] and methcathinone; Ricaurte, unpublished observation) are toxic to serotonin and dopamine neurons, respectively, in rodents. The neurotoxic potential of these drugs in humans is unknown, but emergency room visits after methcathinone use have already occurred.

CONCLUDING COMMENT

This chapter has detailed neurological problems frequently encountered in the patient with a history of substance abuse and has outlined suggestions regarding effective modes of therapy. Particular emphasis has been placed on the most popular illicit drugs, and attention has been drawn to the growing threat posed to public health by the rapidly expanding number of new synthetic drugs. It can be stated with some certainty that, in the years ahead, physicians will be increasingly challenged by the patient whose neurological problems are directly related to either recent or past abuse of an illicit drug. Unfortunately, the growing number of synthetic "designer drugs" is making this already difficult task even more so.

ACKNOWLEDGMENTS

Preparation of this work was supported by grants DA05707, DA05938, DA06275, and DA00206 from the National Institute on Drug Abuse to G.A.R.

REFERENCES

1. Johnson LD, O'Malley PM, Bachman JG: National Survey Results on Drug Use. National Institute on Drug Abuse. NIH Publication No. 93-3597. US Government Printing Office, Washington, DC, 1993
2. Weil A, Rosen W: Chocolate to Morphine: Understanding Mind-Active Drugs. Houghton Mifflin, Boston, 1983
3. Van Dyke C, Byck R: Cocaine. Sci Am 246:128, 1982
4. Cregler LL, Mark H: Medical complications of cocaine abuse. N Engl J Med 315:1495, 1986
5. Galloway MP: Neurochemical modulation of monoamines by cocaine. p. 163. In Lakowski JM, Galloway MP, White FJ (eds): Cocaine: Pharmacology, Physiology and Clinical Strategies. CRC Press, Boca Raton, FL, 1992
6. Jaffe JH: Drug addiction and drug abuse. p. 532. In Gilman AG, Goodman LS, Rall TW, Murad F (eds): Goodman and Gilman's The Pharmacological Basis of Therapeutics. Macmillan, New York, 1985
7. Gay GR: Clinical management of acute and chronic cocaine poisoning. Ann Emerg Med 11:562, 1982
8. Pascual-Leone A, Dhuna A, Altafullah I, Anderson DC: Cocaine-induced seizures. Neurology 40:404, 1990
9. Alldredge BK, Lowenstein DH, Simon RP: Seizures associated with recreational drug use. Neurology 39:1037, 1989
10. Mody CK, Miller BL, McIntyre HB, et al: Neurologic complications of cocaine abuse. Neurology 38:1189, 1988
11. Lowenstein DH, Massa SM, Rowbotham MC, et al: Acute neurologic and psychiatric complications associated with cocaine abuse. Am J Med 83:841, 1987
12. Spivey WH, Euerle B: Neurologic complications of cocaine abuse. Ann Emerg Med 19:1422, 1990
13. Van Viet H, Chevalier P, Sereni C, et al: Neurologic complications of cocaine abuse. Presse Med 19:1045, 1990
14. Case records of the Massachusetts General Hospital: Case 27-1993. A 32 year-old-man with the sudden onset of a right-sided headache and left hemiplegia and hemianesthesia. N Engl J Med 329:117, 1993
15. Sloan MA, Kittner SJ, Rigamonti D, Price TR: Occurrence of stroke associated with use/abuse of drugs. Neurology 41:1358, 1991
16. Kaku DA, Lowenstein DH: Emergence of recreational drug abuse as a major risk factor for stroke in young adults. Ann Intern Med 113:821, 1990
17. Levine SR, Washington JM, Jefferson MF, et al: "Crack" cocaine-associated stroke. Neurology 37:1849, 1987
18. Levine SR, Brust JC, Futrell N, et al: Cerebrovascular complications of the use of the "crack" form of alkaloidal cocaine. N Engl J Med 323:699, 1990
19. Levine SR, Brust JC, Futrell N, et al: A comparative study of the cerebrovascular complications of cocaine: alkaloidal versus hydrochloride—a review. Neurology 41:1173, 1991
20. Lichtenfeld PJ, Rubin DB, Feldman RS: Subarachnoid hemorrhage precipitated by cocaine snorting. Arch Neurol 41:223, 1984
21. Caplan LR, Hier DB, Banks G: Current concepts of cerebrovascular disease–stroke: stroke and drug abuse. Stroke 13:869, 1982
22. Wojak JC, Flamm ES: Intracranial hemorrhage and cocaine use. Stroke 18:712, 1987
23. Golbe LI, Merkin MD: Cerebral infarction in a user of free-base cocaine ("crack"). Neurology 36:1602, 1986
24. Rowley HA, Lowenstein DH, Rowbotham MC, Simon RP: Thalamomesencephalic strokes after cocaine abuse. Neurology 39:428, 1989
25. Krendel DA, Ditter SM, Frankel MR, Ross WK: Biopsy-proven cerebral vasculitis associated with cocaine abuse. Neurology 40:1092, 1990
26. Farrell PE, Diehl AK: Acute dystonic reaction to crack cocaine. Ann Emerg Med 20:322, 1991
27. Hegarty AM, Lipton RB, Merriam AE, Freeman K: Cocaine as a risk factor for acute dystonic reactions. Neurology 41:1670, 1991
28. Cardoso FE, Jankovic J: Cocaine-related movement disorders. Mov Disord 8:175, 1993
29. Sawicka EH, Trosser A: Cerebrospinal fluid rhinorrhea after cocaine sniffing. Br Med J 286:1476, 1983
30. Weiner N: Norepinephrine, epinephrine, and the sympathomimetic amines. p. 130. In Gilman AG, Goodman LS, Rall TW, Murad F (eds): Goodman and Gilman's The Pharmacological Basis of Therapeutics. Macmillan, New York, 1985
31. Seiden LS, Sabol KE, Ricaurte GA: Amphetamine: effects on catecholamine systems and behavior. Annu Rev Pharmacol Toxicol 33:639, 1993
32. Kalant OJ: The Amphetamines: Toxicity and Addiction. Charles C Thomas, Springfield, IL, 1966
33. Cho AK: Ice: a new dosage form of an old drug. Science 249:631, 1990
34. Brust JCM: Stroke and substance abuse. p. 875. In Bar-

nett HJ, Stein BM, Yatsu FM (eds): Stroke: Pathophysiology, Diagnosis, and Management. 2nd Ed. Churchill Livingstone, New York, 1992

35. Citron BP, Halpern M, McCarron M, et al: Necrotizing angiitis associated with drug abuse. N Engl J Med
283:1003, 1970

36. Olson ER: Intracranial hemorrhage and amphetamine
usage. Angiology 28:464, 1977

37. Bostwick DG: Amphetamine induced cerebral vasculitis. Hum Pathol 12:1031, 1981

38. Delaney P, Estes M: Intracranial hemorrhage with amphetamine abuse. Neurology 30:1125, 1980

39. D'Souza T, Shraberg D: Intracranial hemorrhage associated with amphetamine use. Neurology 31:922, 1981

40. Harrington H, Heller A, Dawson D, et al: Intracerebral
hemorrhage and oral amphetamine. Arch Neurol 40:
503, 1983

41. Rothrock JF, Rubenstein R, Lyden PD: Ischemic stroke
associated with methamphetamine inhalation. Neurology 38:589, 1988

42. Nadeau SE: Intracerebral hemorrhage and vasculitis related to ephedrine abuse. Ann Neurol 15:114, 1984

43. Koff RS, Widrich WC, Robbins AH: Necrotizing angiitis in a methamphetamine user with hepatitis B—angiographic diagnosis, five-month follow-up results and
localization of bleeding site. N Engl J Med 288:946,
1973

44. Richter RW: Drug abuse. p. 730. In Rowland LP (ed):
Merrit's Textbook of Neurology. 7th Ed. Lea & Febiger, Philadelphia, 1984

45. Rhee KJ, Albertson TE, Douglas JC: Choreoathetoid
disorder associated with amphetamine-like drugs. Am
J Emerg Med 6:131, 1988

46. Ricaurte GA, Schuster CR, Seiden LS: Long-term effects of repeated methamphetamine administration on
dopamine and serotonin neurons in the rat brain: a regional study. Brain Res 193:153, 1980

47. Petersen RC (ed): Marijuana Research Findings: NIDA
Research Monograph Series. DHSS Publ. No. (ADM)
80-1001. US Government Printing Office, Washington, DC, 1980

48. Braude MC, Laufford JP (eds): Marijuana Effects on
the Endocrine and Reproductive Systems. NIDA Research Monograph Series. DHSS Publ. No. (ADM)
84-1278. US Government Printing Office, Washington, DC, 1984

49. Fehr KO, Kalant H (eds): Cannabis and Health Hazards. The Addiction Research Foundation, Toronto,
1983

50. Campbell AMG, Evans M, Thomson JLG, et al: Cerebral atrophy in young cannabis smokers. Lancet 2:
1219, 1971

51. Co BT, Goodwin DW, Gado M, et al: Absence of

cerebral atrophy in chronic cannabis users: evaluation
by computerized transaxial tomography. JAMA 237:
1229, 1977

52. Heath RG, Fitzjarrell RE, Garey RE, Meyers WA:
Chronic marijuana smoking: its effect on function and
structure of the primate brain. p. 657. In Nahas GG,
Paton WAM (eds): Marijuana: Biologic Effects. Pergamon Press, New York, 1979

53. Landfield PW: Delta-9-tetrahydrocannabinol-depen-
dent alterations in brain structure. p. 52. In Friedman
DP, Clouet DH (eds): The Role of Neuroplasticity in
the Response to Drugs. NIDA Research Monograph
No. 78. US Government Printing Office, Washington,
DC, 1987

54. Ashley R (ed): Heroin. St. Martins Press, New York,
1972

55. Lee HK, Wang SC: Mechanism of morphine induced
miosis in the dog. J Pharmacol Exp Ther 192:415, 1975

56. Lewis JW, Bentley KW, Cowan A: Narcotic analgesics
and antagonists. Annu Rev Pharmacol Toxicol 11:241,
1971

57. Pearson J, Richter RW: Addiction to opiates: neurologic aspects. p. 365. In Vinken PJ, Bruyn GW (eds):
Handbook of Clinical Neurology, Vol 37: Intoxications of the Nervous System, Part II. North Holland,
Amsterdam, 1979

58. Ricaurte GA, McCann UD: Opiate overdose and de-
pendence. p. 302. In Johnson RT, Griffin JW (eds):
Current Therapy in Neurologic Disease. 4th ed.
Mosby Year Book, St Louis, MO, 1993

59. Richter RW, Pearson J, Bruun B: Neurological complications of addiction to heroin. Bull NY Acad Med 49:
3, 1973

60. Krause GS: Brown-Sequard syndrome following heroin injection. Ann Emerg Med 12:581, 1983

61. Richter RW, Rosenberg RN: Transverse myelitis associated with heroin addiction. JAMA 206:1255, 1968

62. Brust JCM, Richter RW: Stroke associated with addiction to heroin. J Neurol Neurosurg Psychiatry 39:194,
1976

63. Protass LM: Delayed postanoxic encephalopathy after
heroin use. Ann Intern Med 74:738, 1971

64. Hall JH, Karp RH: Acute progressive ventral pontine
disease in heroin abuse. Neurology 23:6, 1973

65. Gilroy J, Andaya L, Thomas VJ: Intracranial mycotic
aneurysms and subacute bacterial endocarditis in heroin
addiction. Neurology 23:1193, 1973

66. Finelli PF, Taylor GW: Unusual injection neuropathy
in heroin addict: case report. Milit Med 142:704, 1977

67. Weddington WW: Use of pharmacologic agents in the
treatment of addiction. Psychiatr Ann 22:425, 1992

68. Aniline O, Pitts FN: Phencyclidine (PCP): a review
and perspectives. Crit Rev Toxicol 10:1045, 1982

69. Johnson KM: Phencyclidine: behavioral and biochemical evidence supporting a role for dopamine. Fed Proc 42:2579, 1983

70. McCarron MM, Schulze BW, Thompson GA, et al: Acute phencyclidine intoxication: incidence of clinical findings in 1000 cases. Ann Emerg Med 10:237, 1981

71. McCarron MM: Phencyclidine intoxication. p. 209. NIDA Research Monograph Series. DHHS Publ. No. (ADM) 86-1371. US Government Printing Office, Washington, DC, 1986

72. Burns RS, Lerner SE: Stroke associated with addiction to heroin. J Neurol Neurosurg Psychiatry 39:194, 1976

73. Rappolt RT, Gay GR, Farris RD: Emergency management of acute phencyclidine intoxication. J Am Coll Emerg Phys 8:35, 1979

74. Seppalainen AM: Organic solvent neurotoxicity. ISI Atlas Sci Pharmacol 1:151, 1987

75. Hormes JT, Filley CM, Rosenberg NL: Neurological sequelae of chronic solvent vapor abuse. Neurology 36:698, 1986

76. Korobkin R, Asbury AK, Sumner AJ, Nielsen SL: Glue sniffing neuropathy. Arch Neurol 32:158, 1975

77. Towfighi J, Gonatas NK, Pleasure D, et al: Glue sniffer's neuropathy. Neurology 26:238, 1976

78. Ziporyn T: A growing industry and menace: makeshift laboratory's designer drugs. JAMA 256:3061, 1986

79. Martin M, Hecker J, Clark R, et al: China White epidemic: an eastern United States emergency department experience. Ann Emerg Med 20:158, 1991

80. Hibbs J, Perper J, Winek CL: An outbreak of designer-drug related deaths in Pennsylvania. JAMA 265:1011, 1991

81. Langston JW: MPTP and Parkinson's disease. Trends Neurosci 8:79, 1985

82. Langston JW, Ballard PA, Tetrud JW, Irwin I: Chronic parkinsonism in humans due to a product of meperidine-analog synthesis. Science 219:979, 1983

83. Langston JW, Ballard P: Parkinsonism induced by 1-methyl-4-phenyl-1,2,3,6-tetrahydropyridine (MPTP): implications for treatment and the pathogenesis of Parkinson's disease. Can J Neurol Sci 11, suppl:160, 1984

84. Vingerhoets FJ, Snow BJ, Langston JW, et al: Evolution of subclinical dopaminergic lesions in MPTP exposed humans. Neurology 43:A389, 1993

85. Schmidt CJ: Neurotoxicity of the psychedelic amphetamine, methylenedioxymethamphetamine. J Pharmacol Exp Ther 240:1, 1987

86. Ricaurte GA, Finnegan KF, Nichols DE, et al: 3,4-Methylenedioxyethylamphetamine (MDE), a novel analogue of MDMA, produces long-lasting depletion of serotonin in the rat brain. Eur J Pharmacol 137:265, 1987

87. Ricaurte GA, Forno LS, Wilson MA, et al: (±)3,4-Methylenedioxymethamphetamine selectively damages serotonergic neurons in nonhuman primates. JAMA 260:51, 1988

88. Ricaurte GA, Finnegan KF, Irwin I, Langston JW: Aminergic metabolites in cerebrospinal fluid of humans previously exposed to MDMA: preliminary observations. Ann NY Acad Sci 600:699, 1990

89. McCann UD, Ridenour A, Shaham Y, et al: Serotonin neurotoxicity after MDMA ("Ecstasy"): a controlled study in humans. Soc Neurosci Abs 18:1169, 1993

90. McCann UD, Ricaurte GA: Lasting neuropsychiatric sequelae of (±)methylenedioxymethamphetamine ("ecstasy") in recreational users. J Clin Psychopharmacol 11:302, 1991

91. Steele TD, Katz JL, Ricaurte GA: Evaluation of the neurotoxicity of N-methyl-1-(4-methoxyphenyl)-2-aminopropane (para-methoxymethamphetamine, PMMA). Brain Res 589:349, 1992

32

Neurological Complications of Toxin Exposure in the Workplace

Gareth J. G. Parry

Only a few of the tens of thousands of chemicals used in industries in the United States have been shown to be neurotoxic.[1] Furthermore, even those with proven neurotoxic potential in the laboratory are rarely demonstrably toxic to humans in the workplace. This is a tribute as much to the resiliency of the human organism as to preventive measures taken by industry. Nonetheless, many cases of human neurotoxicity resulting from industrial exposure are documented each year and probably many more go unrecognized. There is probably a level of neurotoxic injury that is inevitable in industrial societies during the late twentieth century, and the chief weapon in limiting its spread is constant vigilance on the part of the medical and paramedical professions. In this chapter, discussion will be concentrated on those instances in which neurotoxicity has been proven by rigorous scientific investigation. This is not meant to imply that the many other postulated instances are factitious but only that no definite conclusions can be reached concerning them until more information is forthcoming.

BASIC TENETS OF NEUROTOXICOLOGY

Establishing that a particular chemical is neurotoxic or that a certain clinical syndrome is due to exposure to a neurotoxin is no easy task. Spencer and Schaumburg have proposed an evolving series of useful rules to follow in this regard (Table 32-1).[2-4] These serve only as a guide and should not be arbitrarily applied. For the purpose of further discussion, they can be considered in the form of the following questions, which should be posed when the possible neurotoxic basis of a neurological disorder is being evaluated:

1. Does the suspected neurotoxin produce a consistent pattern of neurological dysfunction in exposed humans? It is rare for only one or a few workers similarly exposed to a given toxin to develop symptoms and signs of intoxication. There will certainly be some variation in the severity of the clinical syndrome, based on age, sex, genetic makeup and the presence of coexisting disorders such as diabetes, renal disease, liver disease and

Table 32-1 Characteristic Features
of Neurotoxic Disorders

1. There is a consistent pattern of neurological dysfunction.
2. The neurotoxic syndrome can be reproduced in animals.
3. There are reproducible pathological or pathophysiological findings.
4. The demonstrable pathological and pathophysiological findings can account for the clinical findings.
5. There is a temporal relationship between intoxication and onset of the clinical syndrome.
6. The disorder is nonfocal.

preexisting neurological disease, but all workers will usually have some clinical evidence that they have been exposed to a neurotoxic chemical. Involvement of a single worker may have several explanations. First, the clinical syndrome may not be due to a toxin; the symptoms of intoxication are often so nonspecific that any of a large number of systemic, neurological, and psychological disorders may have identical symptoms. Second, if the illness is due to a toxin, the intoxication may not have taken place at work; abuse of drugs and alcohol is so ubiquitous that the development of a syndrome of neurointoxication may be due to recreational exposure. In addition, there is potential for exposure to others toxins from hobbies. Finally, the exposure may be the result of an unusual or unique work habit; a lone affected individual may not use a mask or may not wash after exposure to a neurotoxin. A visit to the workplace by an appropriately trained individual may be necessary to unearth a habit that is resulting in excessive exposure. While this first rule certainly should be rigorously applied, it is of limited usefulness in occupational intoxications. By far the most common effect of intoxication (real or imagined) on the nervous system is a rather stereotyped but entirely nonspecific syndrome of encephalopathy; patients complain of headache, dizziness, numbness, paresthesias, weakness, difficulty in concentrating, memory loss, and sleep disturbances. Such symptoms are common to a wide variety of neurological and psychological conditions. Furthermore, in outbreaks of proven intoxication, a syndrome of mass hysteria may result once the symptoms are publicized by the media, as they almost invariably are in such situations; large numbers of individuals may then develop identical symptoms even in the absence of exposure. This first rule, then, is useful primarily in evaluating objective findings rather than symptoms, and although it is sensitive, it is not specific. This rule also presumes an accurate knowledge of the range of clinical phenomena that may occur following exposure to a single neurotoxin. For example, massive, short-term exposure to acrylamide causes an encephalopathy with seizures, confusion, hallucinations, and cognitive impairment as well as a cerebellar ataxia, whereas a somewhat lower level of chronic exposure causes a sensory axonopathy with distal sensory loss.

2. Can the neurotoxic syndrome be reproduced in experimental animals under similar conditions of exposure? All too often, a substance is labeled neurotoxic based on animal data derived from exposure to much higher levels and for much longer periods of time than that likely to be experienced by humans. In human neurotoxicology, there is a very strong dose-response relationship, and the argument that there may be a form of neurological "allergy" to very low levels of toxic chemicals is unpersuasive and unsupported by experimental evidence.[5] The inability to reproduce similar neurotoxic disease experimentally in animals does not rule out neurotoxicity in humans, because differences in species susceptibility are well documented. Moreover, the cognitive and functional disturbances that are so common in humans are hard to reproduce in animals.[6] It is important also to be aware that mixtures of chemicals may produce a neurotoxic syndrome at concentrations of individual chemicals that are harmless. This enhancement of neurotoxicity by chemicals which may not themselves be neurotoxic is best exemplified by the mixture of n-hexane and methyl ethyl ketone.[7] When an attempt was made to reduce the toxicity of a mixed organic solvent by lowering the concentration of the known neurotoxin n-hexane with the addition of methyl ethyl ketone, which is not neurotoxic, there was an outbreak of neuropathy. Subsequent experimental studies conclusively demonstrated that methyl ethyl ketone markedly potentiated the neurotoxicity of n-hexane.[8]

3. Are there reproducible pathological or pathophys-

iological findings in the nervous system in either humans or animals? This stringent requirement, if applied arbitrarily, would eliminate the many neurotoxic syndromes for which the pathological or pathophysiological basis is unknown.

4. Can demonstrable pathological or pathophysiological abnormalities of the nervous system account for the observed neurological or behavioral syndrome? Demonstration that a substance is neurotoxic does not necessarily mean that it accounts for the observed clinical syndrome. For example, electrodiagnostic demonstration of an unequivocal peripheral neuropathy obviously does not provide a satisfactory explanation for a disturbance of cognitive function.

5. Is there a temporal relationship between exposure to the neurotoxin and the suspected neurotoxic illness? Neurotoxic illnesses almost always occur at the time of exposure or very shortly thereafter. A number of toxic neuropathies (arsenic, thallium, organophosphates) occur after a delay, but this is only of 2 to 3 weeks. Moreover, in many cases, improvement eventually occurs when the exposure is terminated, although it may be incomplete. It is well to be aware of the phenomenon of "coasting," in which continued deterioration occurs for a period of days to weeks following termination of exposure.[9–11] The temporal relationship between exposure and illness is much easier to establish with acute intoxications than with chronic ones, although, in some cases, improvement of symptoms over weekends or during a vacation may be an important clue to work-related exposure to a neurotoxin. Of course, psychological symptoms related to dissatisfaction with work or disputes with supervisors or co-workers and symptoms of malingering are also likely to improve over weekends and on vacations.

6. Is the clinical syndrome nonfocal? Most neurotoxic syndromes involve a functional depression or overt degeneration of neural elements or their supporting cells (glia, Schwann cells) that is diffusely distributed. Occasionally, a focal presentation may lead to the unearthing of an unsuspected diffuse condition, so it is well to be vigilant. For example, a toxic polyneuropathy may present with symptoms of carpal tunnel syndrome. Thus, neurotoxic diseases resemble many other meta-

bolic and degenerative diseases of the nervous system. A corollary to this is that neuroimaging studies are nearly always normal, and the results of electrodiagnostic studies, although often abnormal, are extremely nonspecific. These techniques of investigation are primarily used to rule out other disorders with similar clinical features.

These general considerations are important to bear in mind when evaluating patients with suspected neurotoxic illnesses.

CLINICAL SYNDROMES OF NEUROTOXICITY

Neurotoxic syndromes can reflect dysfunction of either the central or peripheral nervous systems.

Acute Encephalopathy

The most common clinical neurological syndrome that results from intoxication is an acute but nonspecific encephalopathy. In its mildest form the main symptoms are headache and an associated sense of lightheadedness; these resolve within minutes to hours after the exposure is terminated. Neurological examination is usually normal, even during the period of maximal symptoms. In a more severe form, there may also be confusion and irritability, impaired judgment, alteration in the level of consciousness, rotatory dysequilibrium, tinnitus, numbness and paresthesias, ataxia, a sense of weakness, and nausea and vomiting; recovery may take 24 hours or more but is usually complete.

Standard clinical neurological examination is often normal, although there may be nystagmus and ataxia. Neuropsychological examination, which is more sensitive, is likely to be abnormal but, because recovery is rapid and complete, is seldom performed. If exposure continues, alteration in the level of consciousness supervenes and may progress to coma; seizures may also occur. If this stage is reached, morbidity and mortality increase sharply. Any recovery that occurs is often more protracted and sometimes incomplete. This acute neurological syndrome usually provides little diagnostic challenge, at least in workplace exposures, since the history of exposure is promptly forthcoming. Often many workers are affected and there may be a variety of nonneurological manifestations, such as irritation of the eyes, mucous membranes, and skin, as well as shortness of breath; with severe encephalopathy, concomitant systemic effects may also be severe and include such manifestations as pulmonary edema and circulatory collapse. These complications, which in themselves cause severe neurological dysfunction independent of the neurotoxicity of the chemical or chemicals involved, contribute significantly to morbidity and mortality.

Chronic Encephalopathy

The encephalopathy that results from chronic exposure to neurotoxins is not well characterized. In fact, there is no incontrovertible evidence of a chronic neurotoxic encephalopathy. The most commonly cited symptoms are mild and nonspecific. They include headache, dizziness or light-headedness, difficulty in concentrating, memory impairment, irritability, sleep disturbances (both insomnia and hypersomnolence), loss of libido, depression, paresthesias, and weakness.

Although these symptoms are generally mild and may sound relatively innocuous, they are often disproportionately disabling. Such symptoms may be caused by any of a number of medical diseases unrelated to toxin exposure or by exposure to toxins unrelated to the workplace (such as alcohol and many other drugs of abuse). Furthermore, identical symptoms may occur with primary psychological diseases and may easily be claimed by malingerers. The routine neurological examination in these patients is invariably normal. Laboratory investigation is not much more rewarding. The electroencephalogram (EEG) may be mildly abnormal but the results are as nonspecific as the symptoms.[12] Evoked potentials (EPs) have also reportedly been abnormal, but the changes are often minimal and of questionable significance. For example, in one study the reported abnormalities in visual evoked potentials (VEPs) involved only the amplitude of the responses, which are notoriously unreliable, and there was only a small group of control subjects.[13] A wide variety of neurobehavioral abnormalities has been described, but the findings are inconsistent and the interpretation of neuropsychological tests is, as yet, an inexact science. Moreover, premorbid testing has almost never been

performed. Despite the skepticism expressed by many, the presence of a wide variety of abnormalities of function, as manifest in the results of neuropsychological and electrodiagnostic studies, supports the existence of this syndrome but provides little insight into its pathogenesis. The pathological basis of this syndrome is obscure.

Structural Neurotoxic Diseases of the Central Nervous System

There is a remarkable paucity of proven neurotoxic diseases that affect the structure of the central nervous system (CNS). There are even fewer in which the intoxication is thought to result from exposure in the workplace. Nonetheless, the existence of definite pathological changes occurring as the result of massive exposure to toxins by accident, abusive use, or suicidal or homicidal intent provides further support for the concept that milder forms of these syndromes may occur with occupational exposure. For most of these disorders, final confirmation of the pathological nature of the intoxication is lacking, but there are either consistent objective clinical abnormalities or abnormalities of neuroimaging or electrodiagnostic studies.

TOLUENE ABUSE

Chronic toluene abuse gives rise to dementia—which may be overt or subclinical—ataxia, dysarthria, nystagmus, tremor, and spasticity.[14] The clinical syndrome to date has been confined to individuals who abuse toluene, and possibly other organic solvents or solvent mixtures, in very large doses. Magnetic resonance imaging (MRI) shows cerebral, cerebellar, and brainstem atrophy and widespread periventricular white matter lesions. Brainstem auditory evoked potentials (BAEPs) may be abnormal, even when there are no other clinical or neuroimaging abnormalities, prompting some to suggest that the BAEP may be useful for screening at-risk workers.[14] However, a similar syndrome has never been seen with occupational exposure to these same chemicals. This difference probably reflects the prolonged exposure to very large doses that occurs during abusive use, but contamination of the solvents with other toxins or the concomitant administration of other chemicals and drugs may also play an important role.

CARBON MONOXIDE INTOXICATION

Carbon monoxide intoxication also causes structural brain damage, but again this usually occurs after massive accidental or suicidal poisoning outside the workplace. The mechanism of the brain injury is ischemic; carbon monoxide competes with oxygen for binding sites on the hemoglobin molecule and has a much greater affinity for hemoglobin than oxygen. The oxygen-carrying capacity of blood is therefore greatly reduced and tissue hypoxia results. Chronic low-level exposure may cause the syndrome of chronic encephalopathy described above, but there are no documented pathological abnormalities. Acute high-level exposure leads to the various stages of acute encephalopathy described earlier. Severely intoxicated individuals may never recover consciousness, and at autopsy are found to have cerebral edema with focal or diffuse necrosis of the cerebral cortex and occasionally the cerebellum.[15] Bilateral necrosis of the globus pallidus is considered the pathological hallmark of carbon monoxide intoxication but also occurs with other ischemic-hypoxic cerebral insults. In approximately 10 percent of cases, usually those severely intoxicated, there is partial or complete recovery, followed days or even weeks later by a secondary deterioration. Patients develop delirium and multifocal neurological signs, often with spasticity or rigidity. Many patients progress to a mute akinetic state and ultimately die, but some recover partially or even completely after a period of weeks to months.[16] Pathological studies show, in addition to the widespread necrosis described above, extensive zones of demyelination in the subcortical white matter.

HEAVY METAL EXPOSURE

Prolonged exposure to certain heavy metals causes various well-characterized clinical syndromes for which a pathological substrate has been identified and has also been implicated in a number of others.

Manganese

Exposure to manganese, usually by inhalation during mining, results in the syndrome of "manganese madness," with hallucinations, emotional instability, and bizarre behavior. With continued exposure, patients develop weakness, dysarthria, ataxia, tremor, and later an extrapyramidal syndrome that can closely resemble Parkinson's disease, although dystonia and tremor may be its only features.[17] After exposure is terminated, patients may stabilize or improve, but progression of the extrapyramidal syndrome sometimes continues for years. Pathological studies show degeneration of the basal ganglia.[18]

Mercury

Exposure to both organic and inorganic mercury also causes characteristic neurological syndromes. Inorganic mercury causes a delirium that was well-recognized in the felt-hat industry of the last century and gave rise to the expression "mad as a hatter"; it is often accompanied by tremor ("hatter's shakes"), weakness, and paresthesias. This form of mercury poisoning has virtually disappeared and there are no pathological studies. Chronic organic mercury poisoning leads to paresthesias, ataxia, and visual loss. Pathological studies show degeneration of the cerebral and cerebellar gray matter, particularly involving the calcarine (visual) cortex.[19] Mercury has also been implicated in the pathogenesis of peripheral neuropathy, but there is no reliable electrodiagnostic or pathological confirmation, suggesting that the paresthesias have a central origin.[20]

Lead

Lead causes an encephalopathy with high-level exposure, but this is seldom seen in the workplace. The brain is congested and edematous, and there is variable neuronal degeneration. Chronic exposure to lead and mercury has been implicated in the pathogenesis of amyotrophic lateral sclerosis, and aluminum toxicity has been held to contribute to the pathogenesis of Alzheimer's disease, but the evidence is not persuasive.

NITROUS OXIDE

Chronic intoxication with nitrous oxide produces a myeloneuropathy that is clinically identical to subacute combined degeneration of the spinal cord due to vitamin B_{12} deficiency.[21] As with toluene encephalopathy, the clinical syndrome is almost always seen following recreational use of the drug in very large doses over prolonged periods. It has nevertheless been suggested that dentists and dental assistants may be intoxicated due to leakage of gas during dental anesthesia. The clinical syndrome consists of spastic paraparesis, sensory ataxia, and sphincter disturbances. It may result from interference by nitrous oxide with the normal utilization of vitamin B_{12}.

ORGANOPHOSPHATES

Some of the organophosphates produce a myeloneuropathy that results from their ability to inhibit an enzyme called neuropathy target esterase (NTE, discussed on p. 657). Patients develop a severe neuropathy but, as the neuropathy resolves, signs of spinal cord dysfunction appear.

Toxic Neuropathy

Perhaps the most widely studied and best understood of the clinical syndromes that result from toxin exposure in the workplace is peripheral neuropathy. As with encephalopathy, the best understood and characterized neuropathic syndrome is that which occurs as a delayed effect of massive single or short-term repeated exposure. Such exposure to certain heavy metals (most notably arsenic and thallium) and organophosphates is followed after 1 to 3 weeks by the subacute development of distal sensory loss and weakness. The metal neuropathies tend to be predominantly sensory, but the organophosphate neuropathy is predominantly motor and there is additional involvement of the pyramidal tracts. Autonomic functions are usually spared. In these disorders the predominant pathological effect of the toxin is to cause that portion of the axon farthest from the cell body to degenerate. The terms *distal axonal neuropathy*, *dying-back neuropathy*, *distal axonopathy*, and *central-peripheral distal axonopathy* are synonomous and will be referred to as distal axonopathy in this chapter.

As a result of this pattern of pathological involvement, symptoms and signs are initially confined to the distal legs and progress proximally to a degree determined by the severity of the intoxication. The primary sensory neuron sends axons not only into the periphery but also into the spinal cord, and both degenerate toward the cell body. The central exten-

sions of the sensory neurons enter the spinal cord, and some ascend in the posterior columns as far rostrally as the cuneate and gracile nuclei in the caudal brainstem; these distal but centrally directed axons, because of their great length, are often among the first to degenerate. For example, the earliest manifestation of acrylamide intoxication, at least in experimentally intoxicated primates, is degeneration of these central extensions.[22] This has important implications for recovery, because regeneration does not occur in the CNS; if the axonal degeneration is severe, recovery will be incomplete despite effective regeneration of the peripheral nerves.

Chronic exposure to many of these and other chemicals also causes neuropathy. For example, heavy metals, acrylamide, some organophosphates, and many organic solvents cause progressive axonal degeneration following chronic exposure. In addition, minor abnormalities of nerve conduction can be demonstrated in individuals who are chronically exposed to other neurotoxins in the workplace, but there is little evidence to support the concept that these inevitably progress to clinical neuropathy. Nonetheless, prudence dictates that a high level of vigilance should be maintained at all times to minimize risk.

SCREENING AT-RISK WORKERS FOR NEUROTOXICITY

There are three important reasons for screening workers who are or may have been exposed to neurotoxins. In the first instance, it may permit the prevention of further intoxication if early neurological dysfunction is detected at a time when clinical symptoms and signs are covert—measures could be taken to prevent further exposure by whatever means necessary. Second, at times of recognized outbreaks of a neurotoxic disorder, screening may permit the identification of individuals who have been exposed to lower levels of the neurotoxin than overtly affected workers. Finally, in instances in which intoxication is claimed, screening techniques may have a role in documenting neurological involvement in those workers claiming to have been affected as well as documenting any subclinical involvement of fellow workers similarly exposed. As indicated earlier, all similarly exposed workers should develop at least some of the symptoms and signs of intoxication. Therefore, screening of fellow workers may provide invaluable diagnostic information in a case of suspected exposure.

Each of the screening techniques to be discussed below has serious limitations; each is either insensitive, nonspecific, time-consuming, expensive, nonstandardized, or poorly tolerated by patients. However, they are all that is available: one of the greatest needs in neurotoxicology is a simple, inexpensive, and reliable method for objectively evaluating the nervous system in situations of minimal dysfunction.[23]

Clinical History

A detailed history is the cornerstone on which an accurate diagnosis of neurotoxic illness is based. In the clinical evaluation of any individual, a brief occupational history is an integral part of the complete medical history. This is especially important in the evaluation of patients with neurological diseases of obscure etiology. If exposure to toxins is suspected, a comprehensive and accurate list of chemicals used in the workplace should be obtained from the patient or employer. Exposure at past places of employment should also be considered as a cause of symptoms, at least if they are long-standing, although neurotoxic disease almost always appears in close temporal proximity to exposure. The situations in which exposure to any potential neurotoxin may have taken place should be explored.[23] This involves enquiry about (1) ventilation in the working environment; (2) the provision, use, cleaning, and discarding of protective clothing; (3) the provision and use of facilities for washing after exposure; and (4) the area in which food is stored and the likelihood of its contamination. The commonest routes of exposure in the working environment are inhalation and through the skin; ingestion is much less frequent.

It may be necessary to visit the workplace to clarify many of these issues, because the patient is often unaware of potentially hazardous habits. Contrary to popular belief, it is not the giant corporations that are most likely to expose their workers to risk of intoxication; smaller companies and cottage industries are more likely to be using hazardous techniques and procedures to the detriment of their workers, who are often poorly educated. It is also necessary to question co-workers of the patient, either in person or indirectly, to determine whether they have similar symptoms, and it may be necessary to examine those individuals who work in a closely similar environment. A detailed history is also important when co-workers without symptoms are being screened for possible exposure to a known neurotoxin. In such situations, questioning may be more focused, based on the symptoms in recognized cases; self-administered, standardized symptom questionnaires may be useful and time-saving.

Clinical Examination

Routine clinical examination of the nervous system is of limited utility as a screening technique. It is notorious for inter- and intraobserver variability, even for such apparently objective measures as the presence of tendon reflexes. The principal role of the examination is therefore to exclude other conditions. As mentioned above, neurotoxic disease is almost never focal, and the presence of focal neurological abnormalities should raise doubt about a diagnosis of intoxication. Other, coexisting nonneurological disorders may also be found during the routine medical examination.

There have been many attempts to quantitate neurological function for the purpose of screening individuals for subtle neurological dysfunction and following improvement or deterioration of patients with overt neurological deficits. Most of these have concerned quantitation of sensory function.[24] Many human toxic neuropathies preferentially affect large myelinated axons, which mediate vibratory and proprioceptive sensations, and attempts have concentrated on objectively and quantitatively evaluating vibration threshold. Arezzo and co-workers studied one such system in a group of acrylamide-exposed workers.[25] Testing was done by local nurses at each of two plants, and the results were highly reproducible both between and within subjects. The authors emphasized the simplicity and speed of the evaluation but, at least as described, the testing appears to have been neither; no details are given of the time taken for testing or for training the paraprofessional personnel, and a detailed protocol was followed to ensure reproducibility and accuracy. Nonetheless, the results of this study and of several others using similar technology and procedures[26,27] indicate that the method is accurate, noninvasive, and painless, and that it can be administered by paraprofessionals, unlike many other methods of evaluating function in large-diameter afferent fibers.

Quantitative methods of evaluating small-diameter fibers, using temperature threshold sensitivity, have also been developed, but these are both time-consuming and less reproducible and therefore less applicable to screening large populations of patients.[28,29] Fortunately, toxic neuropathies and other toxic neurological conditions are less likely to preferentially affect small rather than large fibers. Quantitative tests of motor function, including strength and coordination, have been developed but remain too cumbersome to apply to large populations as screening devices.

Electrodiagnostic Testing

There are several electrophysiological methods of evaluating the function of the nervous system, with varying degrees of sensitivity and specificity. The EEG and various types of EPs can be used to assess CNS function, while electromyography (EMG) and nerve conduction studies can be used similarly to evaluate the function of peripheral nerves. These techniques are important in evaluating individual patients with known or suspected neurotoxic disease.[30] They have also enabled a more thorough characterization of the pathophysiological basis for many neurotoxic disorders and have become an essential component in evaluating neurotoxic disorders in the experimental laboratory. However, they do have major limitations. First, each of these procedures is time-consuming, physician-intensive, and requires sophisticated electronic equipment that is expensive. Second, although EMG and nerve conduction studies can be performed in the field, the quality of the recordings may be poor; EEGs and EPs can be recorded only in the clinical laboratory. Third, EMG and nerve conduction studies are poorly tolerated by many patients because they are painful. Finally, a high level of expertise is needed to interpret many of the results; this is particularly true of EMG, in which there is often underreporting of abnormalities, and of EEG, where there is often overreporting of nonspecific changes.

ELECTROENCEPHALOGRAPHY

The EEG is abnormal in most patients with acute toxic/metabolic encephalopathy, commonly showing a diffuse slowing of background activity that may be continuous or intermittent. Focal slowing may occasionally be seen and does not exclude a toxic etiology. These changes are entirely nonspecific and do not distinguish between toxic and nontoxic forms of encephalopathy or between different toxic states. Furthermore, in patients with suspected chronic encephalopathy, where there is a major need for some objective means of establishing cerebral dysfunction, the EEG is much less likely to be abnormal. The EEG is therefore of little practical use in screening patients for possible neurotoxic injury.

EVOKED POTENTIALS

Sensory EPs provide some measure of the functional integrity of various afferent pathways in the CNS.[30] More complex polysynaptic pathways can be evaluated using event-related potentials of long latency, but these techniques have not been fully validated and their role in neurotoxic disease remains within the realm of the investigator. For the most part, sensory EPs can be regarded as measures of central conduction velocity; they provide a means of determining the speed of conduction (expressed as a latency) along different fiber tracts in the CNS. The amplitude of EPs varies so much in normal subjects that it cannot be relied upon to detect abnormalities. Most neurotoxins produce axonal degeneration, and this will cause changes in amplitude but little change in latency of responses; accordingly, EPs should be relatively insensitive to neurointoxication and this is, for the most part, true.

Rosenberg and co-workers found that some toluene abusers had prolonged BAEP latencies at a time when there were no other clinical or neuroimaging abnormalities; they suggested that the technique might be useful in screening for subclinical intoxication in the setting of occupational exposure.[14] However, there has been no validation of the technique in this situation. Seppalainen and co-workers found abnormalities in amplitudes but not the latencies of the electroretinogram and VEP in individuals chronically exposed to organic solvents.[13] Similarly, Estrin and co-workers reported abnormalities of the P300, one of the complex, polysynaptic, event-related potentials, in patients exposed to ethylene oxide, but they also showed abnormalities only of amplitude, not of latency,[31] and thus of questionable validity. These are intriguing examples of the role of EPs as a research tool but in no way support the use of EPs as a method of screening workers exposed to neurotoxins.

EMG AND NERVE CONDUCTION STUDIES

Nerve conduction studies remain the "gold standard" for evaluating peripheral nerve function, supplemented when necessary by needle EMG. The techniques, when used by experienced personnel, are quantitative, accurate, and reproducible. They can be used to evaluate both conduction velocity and amplitude of the bioelectric signals and are thus useful in situations of both axonal degeneration and demyelination; axonal degeneration results in reduced amplitudes of compound action potentials, whereas demyelination causes conduction slowing. These techniques do, however, have several drawbacks. First and foremost, they are painful and therefore are not always well accepted by individuals without symptoms of intoxication. Second, if the results are to be reliable, skilled personnel are required to both perform the studies and interpret the results. Third, they require expensive equipment. Nevertheless, it is clearly feasible to use these techniques when screening for neuropathy. Whether nerve conduction studies give better results than the less expensive, painless quantitative sensory testing, using the techniques outlined earlier, is unresolved. However, abnormalities detected by means of quantitative sensory testing should certainly be corroborated by traditional electrodiagnostic testing. Quantitative sensory testing can simply demonstrate that an abnormality exists, whereas electrodiagnostic evaluation can more clearly define the most likely underlying pathology and thus give invaluable information concerning etiology.

Psychometric Testing

There have been steady advances in the accuracy and reproducibility of psychometric testing in recent years, and these have improved its usefulness as a screening device. The tests are sensitive to subtle cognitive dysfunction but are highly nonspecific. Furthermore, it is still difficult to distinguish reliably between organic cerebral dysfunction, psychological disturbances, and malingering. Traditional psychometric testing takes about 3 hours per patient to perform, largely because the most important element is a detailed history, without which interpretation of the results is unreliable. Attempts have been made to speed up the process without sacrificing accuracy and sensitivity, by the use of self-administered questionnaires and computer-driven testing, but the process remains time-consuming. Baker and colleagues developed a computer-based system for evaluating memory, visual/motor function, vocabulary, and mood, which incorporated symptoms and history of exposure.[32,33] They described the technique as rapid, but the entire test took over an hour to administer. They found that the results compared favorably with other methods and that there was excellent stability of the results when applied to normal subjects over 4 to 6 months. Bowler and associates took portions of several widely used neuropsychological tests and developed a composite screening battery that could be administered in under an hour and yet retained good correlation with a more detailed analysis.[34] However, these tests are still time-consuming and, while useful for the evaluation of individual patients suspected of having neurotoxic exposure, they are less helpful in screening large numbers of individuals.

Other Laboratory Testing

The role of traditional laboratory testing in screening for neurotoxic disorders is minimal. The excretion of heavy metals in the urine or other tissues can be measured in workers with suspected exposure, but most other toxins are rapidly metabolized and difficult to detect. With organophosphate intoxication, the levels of certain enzymes may be affected, but this is of little use for screening purposes. Routine laboratory testing may reveal abnormalities of liver, renal, or bone marrow function, but these are nonspecific and, by the time they are abnormal, intoxication is already advanced. Nerve biopsy can demonstrate the highly specific changes of solvent-induced neuropathy but is very rarely indicated in the evaluation of individuals with neuropathy and is never indicated for screening purposes.

CLINICAL SYNDROMES ASSOCIATED WITH SPECIFIC OCCUPATIONAL NEUROTOXINS

Organic Solvents

Intoxication with organic solvents is a major public health problem because these chemicals are so ubiquitous. Individual solvents or mixtures of different solvents are used in some way in practically every workplace. They are used for cleaning and degreasing and for thinning other liquids, as well as in the manufacture of many other chemical products. Their neurotoxicity results almost entirely from their use as cleaners, degreasers, and thinners. A major problem in identifying solvent intoxication is that the composition of solvent mixtures is often unknown, particularly in smaller industries. This problem is compounded by ignorance of, or indifference to, the potential for intoxication of exposed workers.

Most organic solvents are highly volatile liquids with high lipid solubility. The major route of exposure is by inhalation, so the potential for exposure to toxic levels is greatest in poorly ventilated areas. Pulmonary absorption of these chemicals is greatly increased by exercise, which increases blood flow to the lungs, making lower environmental concentrations potentially toxic. Some absorption also takes place through the skin. Those chemical which are both lipid and water soluble and are somewhat less volatile have a greater potential for absorption by this route. Conversely, the most volatile solvents are less likely to be absorbed through the skin because most of the chemical will evaporate before significant amounts can be absorbed.

CNS EFFECTS OF ORGANIC SOLVENTS

Almost all organic solvents, because of their high lipid solubility, enter the brain rapidly, where they act as nonspecific CNS depressants. In fact, some industrial solvents were used in the past as general anesthetics for surgery. There is good correlation between the lipid solubility of a solvent and its action as a CNS depressant. Lipid solubility and therefore anesthetic potency also increases with the length of the carbon chain, the number of double bonds (i.e., the degree of unsaturation) and the number of halogen or alcohol substitutions. Acute exposure to practically any of the organic solvents can cause the syndrome of toxic/metabolic encephalopathy described above. Treatment entails removal of the individual from exposure; recovery occurs within minutes to hours, usually without sequelae, although headache may persist for several days. If acute exposure is of sufficient severity and duration to cause coma, recovery may be incomplete, probably because of hypoxic brain damage rather than a direct action of the chemical. Whether a syndrome of chronic encephalopathy results from long-term exposure to organic solvents is controversial, as has already been discussed. Several epidemiological studies have suggested that there is increased prevalence of neuropsychological dysfunction in spray painters, chronically exposed to solvents used as thinners, but the evidence is unconvincing.[35,36] Perhaps most persuasive is the chronic encephalopathy that has been described following long-term exposure to carbon disulfide, used primarily in the manufacture of cellophane and rayon.[37]

As discussed earlier, there have been many cases of incompletely reversible encephalopathy which have resulted from exposure to toluene or mixtures of chemicals containing toluene. All of the cases have resulted from massive exposure during recreational use rather than industrial exposure. However, it is possible that the syndrome of chronic encephalopathy described in spray painters could have been caused by toluene. Most of these individuals have been exposed to solvent mixtures, the composition of which is usually unknown or at least unreported, and toluene is commonly a constituent of mixed organic solvents. An argument against the existence of toluene encephalopathy is that no abnormalities have been seen in the brains of chronically exposed animals.[38]

The clinical syndrome consists of a neurobehavioral disorder with memory loss, attention deficits, and apathy, associated with cerebellar and pyramidal tract signs. Latencies of BAEP components are prolonged in about one-half of cases and are occasionally abnormal even when the neurological examination and MRI are normal. MRI is abnormal in about one-third of cases, showing cerebral atrophy, loss of gray/white contrast, and increased periventricular signal. Improvement occurs with prolonged abstinence, but some patients have been followed for almost a year of proven abstinence without completely returning to normal.

Methyl alcohol causes optic neuropathy, resulting in blindness, when ingested in large quantities, either acutely or over protracted periods of time. Almost all cases result from accidental or intentional ingestion of methanol in place of ethanol or of methanol-contaminated ethanol. Methyl acetate, which is metabolized to methanol, can also cause optic neuropathy. It has been suggested that the neurotoxic potential of methanol is related to its metabolism to formate, and the organic solvent, methyl formate, also causes optic neuropathy when ingested. It is doubtful that any cases of optic neuropathy have resulted from industrial exposure to these compounds.

ORGANIC SOLVENTS AND PERIPHERAL NEUROPATHY

Only a few of the hundreds of organic solvents or solvent mixtures used in industry have been shown to be toxic to peripheral nerves. The major culprits are *n*-hexane, methyl *n*-butyl ketone, and carbon disulfide. Trichlorethylene causes cranial neuropathy but not a diffuse neuropathy. There has been a single outbreak of neuropathy following exposure to the plastic-foaming catalyst 2-*t*-butylazo-2-hydroxy-5-methylhexane.[39] This discussion will concentrate on the hexacarbons, *n*-hexane and methyl *n*-butyl ketone (MnBK), because several outbreaks of neuropathy have been traced to their use. Furthermore, both are metabolized to 2,5-hexanedione, which is largely or entirely responsible for the neuropathic effect.

Neuropathy results from repetitive and prolonged exposure to *n*-hexane, usually in concentrations in inhaled air of greater than 100 ppm: the threshold limit value (TLV) for the workplace in the United States is 50 ppm. The TLV for MnBK is 5 ppm. Methyl ethyl ketone, a common constituent of organic solvent mixtures, is not neurotoxic in itself but clearly potentiates the neurotoxic properties of *n*-hexane and MnBK.[8] Neuropathy is also seen following inhalation of organic solvents, usually contained in glues, for recreational purposes (glue-sniffer's neuropathy).

Clinically, the hexacarbon neuropathies are quintessential distal axonopathies. The earliest symptoms are sensory; there is an insidious onset of symmetrical numbness in the toes and, later, the fingers. If exposure continues, the numbness migrates proximally; it may reach as far as the knees but rarely extends higher. There is less weakness, but in advanced cases mild foot drop and weakness and atrophy of the intrinsic hand muscles may develop. Rarely, the motor features predominate. The neuropathy has evolved slowly in all cases resulting from industrial exposure. With the much larger exposures occurring during recreational use, the neuropathy evolves more rapidly and may be more extensive, with proximal weakness; indeed, it may superficially resemble Guillain-Barré syndrome, although the evolution is over a period of weeks. Examination confirms that there is significant cutaneous sensory loss, with relative preservation of vibration sense and particularly of proprioception. Distal reflexes are usually absent or reduced, but more proximal reflexes are generally preserved. Autonomic dysfunction may occur when exposure relates to recreational use, and leads to hyperhidrosis and cold blue extremities; it has not been described with industrial cases.

The solvent neuropathies always improve when the exposure stops, but it is important to recognize that continued deterioration (coasting) for a period of weeks to months almost invariably occurs.[40] The degree and rapidity of recovery depend on the severity of the neuropathy. Recovery is by way of axonal regeneration, which is a slow and inefficient process, and patients with severe neuropathy may recover incompletely over 2 to 3 years. Milder cases return to normal within a few months.

Hexacarbon neuropathy is an example of a condition in which electrodiagnostic screening is useful in the detection of subclinical cases. In a major outbreak of MnBK neuropathy which occurred in Ohio, 43 percent of cases had characteristic electrophysiological abnormalities in the absence of symptoms and signs of neuropathy.[9] The most consistent abnormalities in all of the patients, regardless of severity, were found with needle EMG. There were fibrillation potentials and positive sharp waves, indicating active denervation, in distal leg muscles. Most patients, even those mildly involved, also had slowing of motor conduction velocity. Although the hexacarbon neuropathies are distal axonopathies, the slowing of conduction velocity is greater than is usually seen in axonal neuropathies, for reasons that are discussed below.

The pathology of the hexacarbon neuropathies has

been extensively studied in both humans and animals. In animals chronically intoxicated with *n*-hexane (or 2,5-hexanedione), there are many swollen axons, filled with maloriented neurofilaments, mitochondria, neurotubules, and smooth endoplasmic reticulum, as a result of a defect in axonal transport. These axonal enlargements are first seen on the proximal side of the nodes of Ranvier in the distal part of the axon. Because of this enlargement of the paranodal portion of the axon, there is retraction of myelin from the node and, ultimately, segmental demyelination. It is because of this secondary demyelination that the conduction velocity is disproportionately slowed. With time the axons degenerate distal to these enlargements. In keeping with the concept that these are distal axonopathies, similar changes are seen in the most rostral sensory axons in the spinal cord, which are the very distal extensions of the primary sensory neuron whose cell body is in the dorsal root ganglion. Identical changes are seen in sural nerve biopsies taken from humans and were also seen in the gracile fasciculus of the rostral spinal cord in autopsy tissue taken from a glue sniffer. The pathogenesis of these pathological changes is thought to be cross-linking of axonal neurofilament proteins, interfering with axonal transport.[41]

Neuropathy can also result from exposure to trichloroethylene and possibly also to perchloroethylene, organic solvents that are extensively used in the dry-cleaning industry as degreasing agents. The neuropathy was recognized decades ago when trichloroethylene was used as an anesthetic agent.[42] The neuropathy is extremely unusual in that it is confined to the cranial nerves. Initial involvement is restricted to the trigeminal nerve, with early onset of facial numbness or dysesthesias and later weakness of the muscles of mastication. The lower cranial nerves are occasionally involved, and optic neuropathy may also occur. Recovery occurs over a period of months, with the sensory deficit receding toward the center of the face until only the tip of the nose is involved,[43] indicating that this too is a distal axonopathy but one that is confined to cranial nerves. Patchy facial sensory loss and absent corneal reflexes may persist indefinitely.[44] Trigeminal neuropathy may develop after only a few minutes of exposure to high concentrations of trichloroethylene.[43] It is doubtful that exposure to pure trichloroethylene causes trigeminal neuropathy; rather, the neuropathy results from the spontaneous decom-

position product dichloroacetylene, which is formed when trichloroethylene is exposed to alkalis.

Heavy Metals

Many heavy metals have been shown to have neurotoxic potential. In contrast to the highly volatile organic solvents that are rapidly eliminated from the body and cause neurotoxicity primarily following ongoing, intensive exposure, the heavy metals tend to accumulate in the body tissues, particularly bone, over prolonged periods of low-level exposure. Toxicity may therefore result from many years of exposure to low levels in the working environment, and recovery may be extremely delayed because of the long time-course of elimination of the metal from the body. Accidental exposure to higher concentrations can also cause well-recognized syndromes of neurotoxicity, as discussed below. In addition to their well-documented neurotoxicity, the heavy metals produce a plethora of systemic effects, particularly on the hematopoietic and gastrointestinal systems. The heavy metals that have been documented to cause neurotoxicity and the clinical syndromes that result from intoxication are shown in Table 32-2. It should be emphasized that all of these intoxications are rare in the industrial setting, at least in their overt form. The heavy metals to which there is the greatest likelihood of exposure are lead and arsenic; the remaining discussion concentrates on these.

LEAD

Lead is toxic to the central and peripheral nervous systems in both its organic and inorganic forms. Industrial exposure is mainly to inorganic lead and is chiefly by way of inhalation of fine particulate matter, but lead may also be absorbed following ingestion. The latter is the main cause of poisoning of children who chew objects painted with lead-based paints. An increasing amount of lead is present in the air, released through the combustion of fossil fuel to which organic lead has been added to improve its combustion. It is estimated that almost one-half million metric tons of lead are dispersed into the atmosphere every year by this means. Industrial exposure to lead must be considered in this context.

Table 32-2 Metal Neurotoxicity

Metal	Neurotoxic Syndrome
Lead	Acute encephalopathy
	Chronic encephalopathy (?)
	Motor neuropathy (wrist drop)
Arsenic	Acute encephalopathy
	Chronic encephalopathy (?)
	Distal axonal neuropathy
Mercury	Organic psychosis
	Tremor
	Optic neuropathy
	Hearing loss
	Parasthesias (? distal axonal neuropathy)
Thallium	Acute encephalopathy
	Ataxia
	Dystonia
	Distal axonal neuropathy
	Autonomic instability
Manganese	Subacute organic psychosis
	Tremor, ataxia, dysarthria
	Dystonia
	Parkinsonism
Tin	Acute encephalopathy
	Papilledema
	Seizures

Lead Encephalopathy

Acute occupational exposure to lead results mainly in systemic effects involving the hematopoietic, gastrointestinal, and renal systems, and sparing the nervous system. Lead encephalopathy, with headache, seizures, stupor, and coma—related to increasing cerebral edema—is much more common in acutely or subacutely exposed children and is therefore beyond the scope of this review. Several studies have suggested that chronic encephalopathy may result from long-term exposure to low levels of lead.[45–47] The manifestations are mainly subclinical and consist of abnormalities of neuropsychological and neurophysiological testing. A number of nonspecific symptoms such as apathy, insomnia, loss of libido, memory loss, and difficulty in concentrating occur more commonly in the exposed cohorts. Whether these subtle findings translate into a significant long-term risk of developing clear-cut clinical dysfunction is not established.

Lead Neuropathy

Chronic exposure to lead causes neuropathy. The neuropathy develops only after several years of exposure in most cases. In the 16 patients with clinical neuropathy reported by Cullen and colleagues, only 2 had been exposed for less than 4 years.[48] However, Seppalainen and colleagues found that nerve conduction velocities were slower after only 2 years of exposure, although there is no evidence that those individuals progressed to overt neuropathy.[49] The slowing of conduction velocity increases with the duration of exposure and with the blood lead level,[50] but clinical neuropathy does not develop in individuals with blood lead level below 70 μg/dl[51,52]; the maximum allowable blood lead level in exposed workers in the United States is 60 μg/dl.

Clinical lead neuropathy is unique in its clinical manifestations. It is predominantly motor, affects the arms more than the legs, affects the extensors of the wrists and fingers much more than other muscles, and is often asymmetrical. In these characteristics, it differs from all other toxic neuropathies, which are distally accentuated and therefore affect the feet first, are almost always predominantly sensory, and are usually symmetrical. Weakness of the interossei and foot drop do occur occasionally with lead neuropathy, but these are unusual and late features. This throws considerable doubt on the contention that slowing of nerve conduction in lead-exposed individuals, which affects sensory conduction more than motor[53] and almost always involves the median and peroneal motor nerves selectively,[52] may predict the inevitable development of clinical neuropathy.

The clinical picture of lead neuropathy is so characteristic that the diagnosis is seldom difficult. Nonetheless, before a completely confident diagnosis is made, involvement of other organ systems should be demonstrated; lead neuropathy never occurs in isolation. Almost all individuals with lead neuropathy have a microcytic, hypochromic anemia. Basophilic stippling of red blood cells is not always present and is not specific for lead poisoning. Lead interferes with hemoglobin synthesis by inhibiting the enzyme delta-aminolevulinic acid (δALA) dehydrase and the enzyme substrate (δALA) begins to appear in the urine when the blood lead level reaches 40 to 50 μg/dl, which is below the level at which neuropathy results. Therefore, neuropathy should not be diagnosed if the urinary δALA is normal. An increased body lead load should also be demonstrated, either an increased blood lead level or increased 24-hour urinary excretion. None of these measures is useful if exposure to lead is no longer ongoing; they represent exposure to lead over the preceding weeks to months. Past excessive exposure to lead can be measured through its accumulation in teeth or bones, but this is seldom practicable. It has been suggested that lead excretion in response to a dose of the chelating agent EDTA can be used to establish an excessive body lead load, but this method has not been widely validated.[54]

The pathology of lead neuropathy in humans is unknown, primarily because the disease in its overt form has become rare since the advent of good methods for the morphological study of peripheral nerves. The problem is compounded by the fact that different laboratory animals react differently to lead poisoning. The early development of slowed conduction velocity might be taken to suggest that the primary pathology in humans is demyelination, as occurs in rats.[55] Indeed, there is a slight but statistically significant increase in paranodal and segmental demyelination in humans with lead poisoning, but not enough to account for the clinical findings.[56] The target for lead in the lower motor neuron is unknown and may be the perikaryon or the motor axon. The reason for the predilection for muscles innervated by the radial nerve or the C7 segment is quite obscure. All of these issues notwithstanding, it is clear that in overt neuropathy the predominant abnormality is motor axonal degeneration, as manifested by severe denervation of affected muscles.

The primary treatment of lead neuropathy, as with all intoxications, is to remove the individual from the toxic environment. All persons exposed to lead in the workplace should be regularly screened by determination of the blood lead level so that any individual with an increased level can be removed for the environment before overt neuropathy develops. It is currently recommended that individuals with a single blood level above 60 μg/dl or with three consecutive monthly levels above 50 μg/dl be removed from exposure. If the blood level is below 40 μg/dl, the level should be tested every 6 months; for levels above 40 μg/dl, monthly surveillance is recommended.[57] Chelation therapy with EDTA or penicillamine is effective in accelerating removal of lead from the body[58] and should be given to all patients with overt neuropathy. There is no consensus concerning the preferred treatment. Penicillamine has the advantage that it may be taken orally, but EDTA is slightly more effective in removing the lead.[59] The duration of treatment

is also controversial. Some recommend that treatment be continued until the blood lead and the urinary δALA levels have returned to normal,[60] whereas others have suggested that it should continue until a steady-state lead excretion has been achieved.[61]

ARSENIC

Arsenic may enter the body by inhalation during smelting of arsenic-containing ores or by ingestion of contaminated food or water. The principal effect of arsenic intoxication is peripheral neuropathy. Encephalopathy and a wide variety of systemic effects occur with both acute and chronic intoxication; as with all other industrial poisons, the role of arsenic in the pathogenesis of chronic encephalopathy is controversial and is therefore not addressed further. Arsenic neuropathy is in marked contrast to lead neuropathy. It is more typical of toxic neuropathies in general in that it is a predominantly sensory, distal axonopathy. It may occur following exposure to high concentrations of arsenic, usually by ingestion with suicidal or homicidal intent, or as a chronic complication of long-duration low-level exposure.[62]

Following acute intoxication there are usually prominent gastrointestinal symptoms which are followed, within 1 to 3 weeks, by the onset of neuropathy. The earliest symptoms are sensory, with numbness, burning, and tingling in the feet and later, as the symptoms migrate proximally, the legs, hands, and arms. Pain may be severe. In advanced cases there may be sensory ataxia, but cutaneous sensory symptoms generally predominate. Weakness is usually present but is overshadowed by the sensory symptoms, at least in milder cases. With more severe intoxication, there may be marked limb and truncal weakness, including respiratory failure. Autonomic instability may occur but is usually minor and of little consequence. Examination confirms the sensory loss and weakness, which, in contrast to lead neuropathy, is strikingly symmetrical and distally accentuated. This is the clinical picture of a distal axonopathy. With repeated lower-level exposure, the neuropathy may evolve somewhat more slowly. With chronic exposure, the sensory predominance is even more apparent and the neuropathy evolves in an insidious manner, over many weeks to months. With acute exposure, the neuropathy may continue to progress over 4 to 6 weeks, even after exposure is terminated.[63]

In addition to the gastrointestinal symptoms, other systemic effects are usually seen. Hyperkeratosis and desquamation of the skin, particularly of the palms and soles, or redness and swelling of the hands and feet are common. In chronic poisoning, there may be patchy areas of both increased and decreased skin pigmentation. Transverse gray lines in the nails (Mees' lines) are common with acute or repeated exposure but are not specific for arsenic. Proteinuria or more severe renal failure may also develop. Anemia is common and there may be a more severe pancytopenia. As with lead neuropathy, there may be basophilic stippling of red blood cells.

If the history of arsenic exposure is not forthcoming, the acutely evolving form of the neuropathy may be mistaken for Guillain-Barré syndrome, with the initial gastrointestinal symptoms being mistaken for a prodromal illness.[64] The confusion may be compounded by the fact that the cerebrospinal fluid protein is often elevated without an increase in cells, the albuminocytologic dissociation which is so characteristic of Guillain-Barré syndrome. The electrodiagnostic findings in acute arsenic neuropathy superficially resemble those of Guillain-Barré syndrome as well. The predominant abnormality reflects the underlying axonal degeneration, but there is also an element of toxic demyelination that results in electrodiagnostic abnormalities characteristic of an acute demyelinating neuropathy. Clues to the correct diagnosis include desquamation of the skin, depression of the bone marrow, and development of Mees' lines in the nails, although the latter appear only after a delay of several weeks.

The diagnosis of arsenic neuropathy requires the demonstration of arsenic in blood, urine, or tissues. Arsenic is rapidly cleared from the blood and measurement of blood levels is seldom diagnostically helpful unless very recent acute exposure is suspected. Urine excretion of arsenic is elevated for weeks or even months after a single dose.[65] With chronic intoxication, the urine excretion usually exceeds 25 μg/24 h and this is the most reliable means for monitoring exposure in at-risk occupations. In individuals with a diet extremely high in fish, much higher levels may be found because of the accumulation of arsenic in the flesh of fish. Arsenic is cleared from blood into tissues and in particular is bound to keratin of growing hair or nails. Since these tissues are slowly turned over, arsenic may be found there for months or even years. This is particularly true for slow-growing hair, such as pubic or axillary hair. This is important if exposure is not suspected until long after the event. Arsenic does not appear in these tissues for 4 to 6 weeks after a single exposure,[66] so levels may be useful in timing the exposure.

Treatment of arsenic neuropathy primarily consists of removing the individual from exposure. Hastening the excretion of arsenic from the body by chelation has a theoretical role, but it has not been shown to increase the rate of recovery from neuropathy; it probably should be reserved for the treatment of severely intoxicated individuals with marked systemic effects. Recovery from arsenic neuropathy is protracted, occurring over months to years. Prognosis is directly related to the severity of the neuropathy; mild cases recover completely, but a residual deficit is common with severe neuropathy.

OTHER NEUROTOXIC METALS

Mercury

Mercury may cause toxicity in both its organic and inorganic forms. Organic mercury intoxication usually results from ingestion of methyl mercury and causes a syndrome characterized by optic neuropathy with constriction of visual fields, hearing loss, cerebellar signs, and dementia or organic psychosis. There are also prominent parasthesias which may be due to peripheral nerve or dorsal root ganglion involvement,[67] although LeQuesne and colleagues suggested that these too are central in origin.[20] Inorganic mercury is poorly absorbed from the gastrointestinal tract and is mainly absorbed by way of inhalation of the vapor during smelting; this is the major source of occupational exposure. Inorganic mercury can also cause a toxic encephalopathy whose major features are toxic psychosis and tremor. Peripheral neuropathy, resembling acute or chronic inflammatory polyneuropathy, has been linked to both forms of mercury, but the evidence is scanty. Mercury has also been implicated in the pathogenesis of some cases of motor neuron disease, but the evidence for this is even less persuasive.

Thallium

Thallium intoxication closely resembles arsenic intoxication. Acute intoxication causes a toxic encephalopathy with psychosis, convulsions, and cerebellar and extrapyramidal effects.[68] There is also a neuropathy (distal axonopathy) whose onset is delayed for 3 to 7 days.[69] Autonomic instability is common and may be so severe as to be life-threatening; it may have a peripheral or central basis. The systemic features of thallitoxicosis are also closely similar to arsenic poisoning, with the added common occurrence of diffuse alopecia as a late manifestation.[69] Thallitoxicosis as a result of occupational exposure has disappeared, but occasional cases of accidental ingestion still occur.

Manganese

Manganese intoxication results from inhalation of dust or vapor; this may occur during the mining or smelting of manganese.[70] The earliest manifestation is a toxic psychosis with later development of headache, weakness, dysarthria, tremor, and incoordination. Finally an extrapyramidal syndrome characterized by dystonia or parkinsonism may develop. A recent report emphasized that progression may continue even after exposure is terminated.[17]

Tin

Tin, in its organic form, may cause intoxication through inhalation or ingestion.[71] The major manifestations are those related to the marked elevation of intracranial pressure. There is headache, often accompanied by nausea and vomiting, visual disturbances related to papilledema, convulsions, and coma. Focal neurological signs sometimes develop. The symptoms develop rather suddenly after a latent period of 4 to 7 days after acute exposure. Recovery is slow and often incomplete except in the mildest cases. Tin causes severe interstitial cerebral edema as well as intramyelinic edema in the central and peripheral nervous system.

Organophosphates

Organophosphates are neurotoxic by virtue of their ability to inhibit acetylcholinesterase (AChE), which accounts for their central neurotoxicity, and neuropathy target esterase (NTE, formerly known as neurotoxic esterase), which accounts for the delayed neuropathy that occurs following exposure to many of these compounds. The ability to inhibit NTE is used to screen new organophosphates for potential neurotoxicity. However, although inhibition of NTE is es-

sential for the development of peripheral neurotoxicity, not all organophosphates that inhibit NTE cause neuropathy. The other factors that determine which NTE-inhibiting organophosphates are neurotoxic are unknown. Different organophosphates have differing potencies against these enzymes, although almost all have some anticholinesterase effects. Those that are used as insecticides and rodenticides have most activity against AChE and relatively weak activity against NTE. The quintessential NTE inhibitor is triorthocresyl phosphate (TOCP), an additive to gasoline, mineral oil, and plastics, which has minimal activity against AChE; several pesticides also have NTE-inhibiting properties. Most organophosphates are readily absorbed through the skin as well as by inhalation and ingestion. Neurotoxicity usually results from acute exposure, either as a single event or following repeated short-term exposure.

NEUROTOXICITY FROM INHIBITION OF ACETYLCHOLINESTERASE

Exposure to organophosphates which are AChE inhibitors results in a clinical syndrome that reflects increased activity of acetylcholine at cholinergic synapses, both centrally and peripherally. Because AChE is inhibited at these sites, acetylcholine released from the presynaptic nerve terminal is not degraded normally and its action at the postsynaptic membrane is prolonged. The earliest manifestations represent inhibition of CNS cholinergic receptors and postganglionic parasympathetic receptors (muscarinic). The CNS effects begin with behavioral changes, mainly agitation, and progress to convulsions. The peripheral muscarinic effects include miosis, diarrhea or even involuntary defecation, urinary urgency or incontinence, and increased salivation and lacrimation. The nicotinic (neuromuscular junction) effects include muscle fasciculations and weakness. In severe intoxications, death from respiratory paralysis may occur. The combination of convulsions with weakness of respiratory muscles is particularly dangerous. The cholinergic effects of organophosphate poisoning usually begin within hours of exposure, although in mild cases they may be delayed for 2 to 3 days. The earliest signs are muscarinic (type I or early syndrome)[72] whereas the nicotinic effects (type II or intermediate syndrome) may be delayed for 1 to 2 days after exposure.[73]

Recognition of AChE inhibition seldom presents a diagnostic dilemma except in the mildest cases, at least in the workplace. There is usually a clear history of exposure and the clinical syndrome is highly characteristic. There are even more characteristic electrophysiological abnormalities associated with inhibition at the nicotinic receptor.[74] The earliest sign is repetitive firing of the compound muscle action potential in response to a single electrical stimulus delivered to a motor nerve.[75] A little later there is a decremental response of the muscle to repetitive stimulation of the motor nerve. AChE activity can be measured in plasma or red cells, preferably the latter, since this most closely reflects neurotoxicity, to confirm suspected intoxication and to monitor exposure in at-risk occupations.

Primary treatment of AChE-related intoxications is with agents that block the action of acetylcholine at postsynaptic receptors. The quintessential muscarinic receptor blocker is atropine, which can be given intravenously. A test dose of 0.5 mg is given; this would cause tachycardia and mydriasis in normal persons but has virtually no effect in an organophosphate-intoxicated individual. Atropine can then be given repeatedly in doses of 1 to 2 mg intravenously until signs of atropine toxicity develop. Because atropine can precipitate cardiac arrhythmias, an effect potentiated by hypoxemia, treatment should always be given in the intensive care unit with the patient intubated and monitored. Unfortunately, atropine has no effect on the nicotinic neuromuscular receptors so is ineffective treatment for weakness and respiratory paralysis. Neither does it moderate the CNS effects of agitation and convulsions. It is useful only for controlling the diarrhea, incontinence, and excessive salivation and lacrimation. If intoxication is recognized early, administration of pralidoxime chloride may be effective.[76] Pralidoxime acts by accelerating the cleavage of the bond between the organophosphate and AChE and restoring AChE activity to normal. Therefore, effectiveness is independent of receptor type, and the drug may also cross the blood-brain barrier and have a beneficial central effect.[77] The complex that forms between the organophosphate and cholinesterase is initially reversible, but with time irreversible configurational changes take place that have been termed *aging*.[78] Once the complex has "aged," the enzyme is permanently deactivated and pralidoxime is ineffective. It should be emphasized that the most important treatment of organophosphate intoxication is supportive care, including artificial ventilation and anticonvulsant medication if necessary.

NEUROTOXICITY FROM INHIBITION OF NEUROPATHY TARGET ESTERASE

NTE inhibition causes a distal axonal neuropathy following acute or repeated exposure to some organophosphates. The onset of the neuropathy is typically delayed for 1 to 3 weeks after exposure.[79,80] Preceding cholinergic symptoms may be mild or even absent. The earliest symptoms are cramping calf pain and burning or tingling in the distal extremities, mainly the feet. Weakness develops early and is unusually severe, in contrast with most toxic neuropathies. It also involves distal muscles initially but progresses proximally; occasionally truncal muscles are involved, including the respiratory muscles. There may be ataxia out of proportion to the weakness, suggesting particular involvement of proprioception. Distal reflexes are absent and more proximal reflexes are usually depressed. Cranial nerves are not involved and autonomic function is spared. With time, severe distal muscle atrophy develops. The neuropathy evolves in a subacute fashion and the nadir is usually reached within 2 to 3 weeks of the onset of symptoms. Thereafter, patients improve slowly but steadily; the extent of improvement of the neuropathy is directly related to the severity of the neuropathic deficit at the nadir. Unfortunately, there is always CNS involvement in patients with organophosphate-induced neuropathy, although this is usually obscured by the severe peripheral neuropathy in the early stages. As the neuropathy improves, the CNS signs are unmasked and the overall prognosis usually depends on the severity of CNS injury.[81,82] Most commonly there is significant spasticity and often there is also ataxia. There is no treatment.

Diagnosis of organophosphate-induced neuropathy is not difficult if a history of exposure is forthcoming. Intoxication should be considered in any acutely evolving distal axonopathy even in the absence of a history of exposure. Unfortunately there are no pathognomonic signs of organophosphate intoxication. Clinically and electrophysiologically, the neuropathy is little different from any other distal axonopathy, although there is an unusual degree of motor involvement. Electrodiagnostic studies confirm distal axonal degeneration, and there is also some slowing of conduction velocity, but these features are nonspecific. By the time the neuropathy develops and the patient comes to medical attention, red blood cell cholinesterase levels have returned to normal and all clinical and electrophysiological signs of AChE inhibition have resolved. Levels of NTE in lymphocytes can be measured, but the technique is not widely available.[83] Measurement of lymphocyte NTE levels has been suggested as a means of monitoring for chronic excessive exposure.[84]

Acrylamide

Acrylamide in its nontoxic polymeric form is widely used as a grouting agent and flocculator. It is the acrylamide monomer that is neurotoxic, and most cases of poisoning occur during the manufacture of the monomer or during the polymerization process at the work site.[85,86] Although the polymer is not neurotoxic, it usually does contain traces of the monomer, but no instances of neurotoxicity have been traced to exposure to the polymerized product alone. Acrylamide may be absorbed by inhalation or ingestion and through the skin. The latter is probably the major route of absorption in the workplace. Clinically apparent intoxication in the workplace usually arises as the result of either single massive accidental exposure or repeated exposure over short periods. However, administration of small amounts of acrylamide to animals over long periods of time produces an identical, albeit more slowly evolving, neurological disorder.[87] It is therefore prudent to consider the possibility that chronic low-level exposure may also be harmful to humans. Unlike almost all the other toxins discussed in this chapter, there are few systemic toxic effects of acrylamide. It may produce a mild exfoliative dermatitis and some weight loss, but its serious toxicity is confined to the nervous system. Furthermore, the only meaningful toxicity is to the peripheral nervous system, causing a distal axonopathy. There is a mild encephalopathy with acute exposure,[88] and the ataxia that accompanies the neuropathy has prompted some to suggest a cerebellar disorder, although a sensory ataxia is a more plausible explanation. Nonetheless, there is Purkinje cell degeneration in animals experimentally exposed to high concentrations of acrylamide.[89]

Like most toxic neuropathies, acrylamide neuropathy is a predominantly sensory neuropathy and is strikingly length-dependent. Initial complaints are of numbness and hyperhidrosis of the distal extremities, particularly the feet, associated with unsteadiness of gait. The ataxia of gait is out of proportion to the weakness and probably reflects the predilection of acrylamide for the large myelinated proprioceptive fibers in peripheral nerves. There is also a disproportionate loss of reflexes, further indicating involvement of large-diameter afferent fibers from muscle spindles. Distal weakness is present but is not as severe as the sensory involvement. Cranial nerves are spared. Apart from the hyperhidrosis, there are no signs of autonomic instability, despite clear evidence of involvement of sympathetic and parasympathetic nerves in experimentally intoxicated animals.[90] There are no specific diagnostic tests to establish acrylamide as the cause of the neuropathy. If no history of exposure is forthcoming, the diagnosis is essentially impossible to establish; the key to diagnosis is a high index of suspicion and a thorough occupational history. There is no treatment for acrylamide intoxication other than removal from the toxic environment. Once exposure is terminated, there is steady improvement; functional recovery is complete in mild cases, although some reflex loss may be permanent.

It is difficult to monitor for acrylamide exposure in the workplace. Acrylamide is rapidly eliminated from the circulation, metabolized to incompletely characterized end products, and eliminated from the body in the urine. Monitoring by means of measuring urinary metabolites has been unsuccessful. Since its entire meaningful toxicity is to peripheral nerves, excessive exposure can be monitored by testing peripheral nerve function. This task is made easier because of the preferential involvement of large myelinated fibers whose function can be accurately and reproducibly monitored with nerve conduction studies or quantitative measures of vibration threshold. Both have been used to monitor for excessive exposure in the workplace.

Toxic Gases

Any gas that is present in sufficient concentration in the inhaled air can have a narcotizing effect. Perhaps the most common gas to cause problems in the workplace in this regard is carbon dioxide. As discussed already, carbon monoxide is a more potent poison because of its high affinity for hemoglobin, which results in its accumulation in the circulation and a prolonged recovery phase. The early symptoms of both carbon dioxide and carbon monoxide poisoning are headache, irritability, difficulty in concentrating, and defects in judgment, all of which are signs of a mild encephalopathy. Recovery is usually rapid and complete except when there is progression to coma and convulsions, which is rare with occupational exposure. Toxicity of nitrous oxide is discussed above (p. 645). Whether chronic unintentional exposure in the workplace can result in myeloneuropathy has not been established but seems unlikely. A variety of other gases have been suggested to have primary toxicity to the CNS, independent of the level of hypoxia produced, but the evidence remains scanty.[91] Further comment will therefore be confined to ethylene oxide.

Ethylene oxide is a gas that acts as an alkylating agent; it is therefore useful for sterilizing heat-sensitive objects. It is established as being toxic to the peripheral nervous system following high-level (i.e., greater than 250 ppm) single or intermittent exposure. There have also been suggestions that much lower levels of exposure for prolonged periods may be toxic to both peripheral nerves and the CNS. Hospital sterilization workers exposed to low levels for many years with occasional exposure to much higher concentrations have been reported to have an increased prevalence of neurobehavioral abnormalities[92,93] and some neurophysiological abnormalities,[31] although these contentions have not gone unchallenged.[94] On a firmer footing is the issue of neuropathy.[95,96] Humans and animals chronically exposed to ethylene oxide develop a predominantly sensory, distal axonal neuropathy, typical in every way of a toxic neuropathy. As with acrylamide, there seems to be a predilection for involvement of large myelinated axons, so that vibration and position sense are particularly affected, and there is widespread reflex loss, which may be permanent. The human neuropathy is usually mild and recovery is excellent once exposure is terminated. No other treatment is available or necessary.

REFERENCES

1. Estrin WJ, Parry GJ: Neurotoxicology. p. 267. In LaDou J (ed): Occupational Medicine. Appleton & Lange, East Norwalk, CT, 1990

2. Spencer PS, Schaumburg HH: An expanded classification of neurotoxic responses based on cellular targets of chemical agents. Acta Neurol Scand 70, suppl 100: 9, 1984

3. Spencer PS, Schaumburg HH: Organic solvent neurotoxicity: facts and research needs. Scand J Work Environ Health 11, suppl 1:53, 1985

4. Schaumburg HH, Spencer PS: Recognizing neurotoxic disease. Neurology 37:276, 1987

5. Brodsky CM: 'Allergic to everything': a medical subculture. Psychosomatics 24:731, 1983

6. Becker CE, Lash A: Detecting subtle human CNS dysfunction: challenge for toxicologists in the 1990's. J Toxicol Clin Toxicol 28:7, 1990

7. Altenkirch H, Mager J, Stoltenburg G, Helmbrecht J: Toxic polyneuropathies after sniffing a glue thinner. J Neurol 214:137, 1977

8. Altenkirch H, Stoltenburg G, Wagner HM: Experimental studies on hydrocarbon neuropathies induced by methyl-ethyl-ketone (MEK). J Neurol 219:159, 1978

9. Allen N, Mendell JR, Billmaier DJ, et al: Toxic polyneuropathy due to methyl n-butyl ketone: an industrial outbreak. Arch Neurol 32:209, 1975

10. Le Quesne PM: Neurological disorders due to toxic occupational hazards. Practitioner 223:40, 1979

11. Berger AR, Schaumburg HH, Schroeder C, et al: Dose response, coasting, and differential fiber vulnerability in human toxic neuropathy: a prospective study of pyridoxine neurotoxicity. Neurology 42:1367, 1992

12. Seppalainen AM: Neurotoxic effects of industrial solvents. Electroencephalogr Clin Neurophysiol 34:702, 1973

13. Seppalainen AM, Raitta C, Huuskonen MS: n-Hexane-induced changes in visual evoked potentials and electroretinograms of industrial workers. Electroencephalogr Clin Neurophysiol 47:492, 1979

14. Rosenberg NL, Spitz MC, Filley CM, et al: Central nervous system effects of chronic toluene abuse—clinical, brainstem evoked resonse and magnetic resonance imaging studies. Neurotoxicol Teratol 10:489, 1988

15. Schochet SS Jr: Exogenous toxic-metabolic diseases including vitamin deficiency. p. 372. In Davis RL, Robertson DM (eds): Textbook of Neuropathology. Williams & Wilkins, Baltimore, 1985

16. Ginsberg MD: Carbon monoxide. p. 374. In Spencer PS, Schaumburg HH (eds): Experimental and Clinical Neurotoxicology. Williams & Wilkins, Baltimore, 1980

17. Huang C-C, Lu C-S, Chu N-S, et al: Progression after chronic manganese exposure. Neurology 43:1479, 1993

18. Barbeau A, Inoue N, Cloutier T: Role of manganese in dystonia. Adv Neurol 14:339, 1976

19. Chang LW: Mercury. p. 508. In Spencer PS, Schaumburg HH (eds): Experimental and Clinical Neurotoxicology. Williams & Wilkins, Baltimore, 1980

20. Le Quesne PM, Damluji SF, Rustam H: Electrophysiological studies of peripheral nerves in patients with organic mercury poisoning. J Neurol Neurosurg Psychiatry 37:333, 1974

21. Blanco G, Peters HA: Myeloneuropathy and macrocytosis associated with nitrous oxide abuse. Arch Neurol 40:416, 1983

22. Schaumburg HH, Spencer PS, Arezzo JC: Studies of the primate somatosensory system in experimental acrylamide intoxication. Neurotoxicology 6:3, 1985

23. Becker CE: Key elements of the occupational history for the general physician. West J Med 137:581, 1982

24. Dyck PJ, Zimmerman IR, O'Brien PC, et al: Introduction of automated systems to evaluate touch-pressure, vibration, and thermal cutaneous sensation in man. Ann Neurol 4:502, 1978

25. Arezzo JC, Schaumburg HH, Peterson CA: Rapid screening for peripheral neuropathy: a field study with the Optacon. Neurology 33:626, 1983

26. Lipton RB, Galer BS, Dutcher JP, et al: Quantitative sensory testing demonstrates that subclinical sensory neuropathy is prevalent in patients with cancer. Arch Neurol 44:944, 1987

27. Arezzo JC, Schaumburg HH: The use of the Optacon as a screening device. J Occup Med 22:461, 1980

28. Arezzo JC, Schaumburg HH, Laudadio C: Thermal sensitivity tester: device for quantitative assessment of thermal sense in diabetic neuropathy. Diabetes 35:590, 1986

29. Jamal GA, Hansen S, Weir AI, Ballantyne JP: An improved automated method for measurement of thermal thresholds: I. Normal subjects. J Neurol Neurosurg Psychiatry 48:354, 1985

30. Aminoff MJ: Electrophysiologic recognition of certain occupation-related neurotoxic disorders. Neurol Clin 3:687, 1985

31. Estrin WJ, Bowler RM, Lash A, Becker CE: Neurotoxicological evaluation of hospital sterilizer workers exposed to ethylene oxide. J Toxicol Clin Toxicol 28:1, 1990

32. Baker EL, Letz R, Fidler A: A computer-administered neurobehavioral evaluation system for occupational and environmental epidemiology. J Occup Med 27:206, 1985

33. Baker EL, Letz RE, Fidler AT, et al: A computer-based neurobehavioral evaluation system for occupational and environmental epidemiology: methodology and validation studies. Neurobehav Toxicol Teratol 7:369, 1985

34. Bowler RM, Thaler CD, Becker CE: California neuropsychological screening battery (CNS/B I&II). J Clin Psychol 42:946, 1986

35. Fidler AT, Baker EL, Letz RE: Neurobehavioural effects of occupational exposure to organic solvents among construction painters. Br J Ind Med 44:292, 1987

36. Gregersen P, Klausen H, Elsnab CU: Chronic toxic encephalopathy in solvent-exposed painters in Denmark 1976–1980: clinical cases and social consequences after a 5-year follow-up. Am J Ind Med 11:399, 1987

37. Aaserud O, Hommeren OJ, Tvedt B, et al: Carbon disulfide exposure and neurotoxic sequelae among viscose rayon workers. Am J Ind Med 18:25, 1990

38. Spencer PS: Experimental evaluation of selected petrochemicals for subchronic neurotoxic properties. p. 249. In MacFarland HN, Holdsworth CE, MacGregor JA, et al (eds): The Toxicity of Petroleum Hydrocarbons. American Petroleum Institute, Washington, DC, 1982

39. Spencer PS, Beaubernard CM, Bischoff-Fenton MC, Kurt TL: Clinical and experimental neurotoxicity of 2-t-butylazo-2-hydroxy-5-methylhexane. Ann Neurol 17:28, 1985

40. Korobkin R, Asbury AK, Sumner AJ, Nielsen SL: Glue-sniffing neuropathy. Arch Neurol 32:158, 1975

41. Genter St Clair MB, Amarnath V, Moody MA, et al: Pyrrole oxidation and protein cross-linking as necessary steps in the development of gamma-diketone neuropathy. Chem Res Toxicol 1:179, 1988

42. Humphrey JH, McClelland M: Cranial nerve palsies with herpes following general anesthesia. Br Med J 1:315, 1944

43. Feldman RG, Mayer RM, Taub A: Evidence for peripheral neurotoxic effect of trichloroethylene. Neurology 20:599, 1970

44. Feldman RG, White RF, Currie JN, et al: Long-term follow-up after single toxic exposure to trichloroethylene. Am J Ind Med 8:119, 1985

45. Valciukas JA, Lilis R, Singer R, et al: Lead exposure and behavioral changes: comparisons of four occupational groups with different levels of lead absorption. Am J Ind Med 1:421, 1980

46. Jeyaratnam J, Devathasan G, Ong CN, et al: Neurophysiological studies on workers exposed to lead. Br J Ind Med 42:173, 1985

47. Pasternak G, Becker CE, Lash A, et al: Cross-sectional neurotoxicology study of lead-exposed cohort. J Toxicol Clin Toxicol 27:37, 1989

48. Cullen MR, Robins JM, Eskenazi B: Adult inorganic lead intoxication: presentation of 31 new cases and a review of recent advances in the literature. Medicine (Baltimore) 62:221, 1983

49. Seppalainen AM, Hernberg S, Vesanto R, Kock B: Early neurotoxic effects of occupational lead exposure: a prospective study. Neurotoxicology 4:181, 1983

50. Seppalainen AM, Hernberg S, Kock B: Relationship between blood lead levels and nerve conduction velocities. Neurotoxicology 1:313, 1979
51. Nielsen CJ, Nielsen VK, Kirkby H, Gyntelberg F: Absence of peripheral neuropathy in long-term lead-exposed subjects. Acta Neurol Scand 65:241, 1982
52. Ehle AL: Lead neuropathy and electrophysiological studies in low level lead exposure: a critical review. Neurotoxicology 7:203, 1986
53. Singer R, Valciukas JA, Lilis R: Lead exposure and nerve conduction velocity: the differential time course of sensory and motor nerve effects. Neurotoxicology 4:193, 1983
54. Reiders F: Current concepts in the therapy of lead poisoning. p. 143. In Seven MJ (ed): Metal Binding in Medicine. JB Lippincott, Philadelphia, 1960
55. Windebank AJ, McCall JT, Hunder HG, Dyck PJ: The endoneurial content of lead related to the onset and severity of segmental demyelination. J Neuropathol Exp Neurol 39:692, 1980
56. Buchthal F, Behse F: Electrophysiology and nerve biopsy in men exposed to lead. Br J Ind Med 36:135, 1979
57. Lewis R: Metals. p. 297. In LaDou J (ed): Occupational Medicine. Appleton & Lange, East Norwalk, CT, 1990
58. Windebank AJ: Metal neuropathy. p. 1549. In Dyck PJ, Thomas PK, Griffin JW, et al (eds): Peripheral Neuropathy. 3rd Ed. WB Saunders, Philadelphia, 1993
59. Harris CEC: A comparison of intravenous calcium disodium versenate and oral penicillamine in promoting elimination of lead. Can Med Assoc J 79:664, 1958
60. Goldberg A, Smith JA, Lochhead AC: Treatment of lead-poisoning with oral penicillamine. Br Med J 1: 1270, 1963
61. Selander S, Cramer K, Hallberg L: Studies in lead poisoning. Oral therapy with penicillamine: relationship between lead in blood and other laboratory tests. Br J Ind Med 23:282, 1966
62. Feldman RG, Niles CA, Kelly-Hayes M, et al: Peripheral neuropathy in arsenic smelter workers. Neurology 29:939, 1979
63. LeQuesne PM, McLeod JG: Peripheral neuropathy following a single exposure to arsenic. Clinical course in four patients with electrophysiological and histological studies. J Neurol Sci 32:437, 1977
64. Donofrio PD, Wilbourn AJ, Albers JW, et al: Acute arsenic intoxication presenting as Guillain-Barré-like syndrome. Muscle Nerve 10:114, 1987
65. Mealey J, Brownwell GL, Sweet WH: Radioarsenic in plasma, urine, normal tissues, and intracranial neoplasms: distribution and turnover after intravenous injection in man. Arch Neurol Psychiatry 81:310, 1959
66. Murphy MJ, Lyon LW, Taylor JW: Subacute arsenic neuropathy: clinical and electrophysiological observations. J Neurol Neurosurg Psychiatry 44:896, 1981
67. Takeuchi T: Neuropathology of Minamata disease in Kumamoto, especially in the chronic stage. p. 235. In Roizin L, Shiraki H, Grcevik N (eds): Neurotoxicology. Raven Press, New York, 1977
68. Cavanagh JB, Fuller NH, Johnson HRM, Rudge P: The effects of thallium salts, with particular reference to the nervous system changes. Q J Med 43:293, 1974
69. Bank WJ, Pleasure DE, Suzuki K, et al: Thallium poisoning. Arch Neurol 26:456, 1972
70. Smyth LT, Ruhf RC, Whitman NE, Dugan T: Clinical manganism and exposure to manganese in the production and processing of ferromanganese alloy. J Occup Med 15:101, 1973
71. Watanabe I: Organotins (triethyltin). p. 545. In Spencer PS, Schaumburg HH (eds): Experimental and Clinical Neurotoxicology. Williams & Wilkins, Baltimore, 1980
72. Wadia RS, Sadagopan C, Amin RB, Sardesai HV: Neurological manifestations of organophosphorous insecticide poisoning. J Neurol Neurosurg Psychiatry 37: 841, 1974
73. Senanayake N, Karalliedde L: Neurotoxic effects of organophosphorus insecticides. An intermediate syndrome. N Engl J Med 316:761, 1987
74. Wadia RS, Chitra S, Amin RB, et al: Electrophysiological studies in acute organophosphate poisoning. J Neurol Neurosurg Psychiatry 50:1442, 1987
75. Besser R, Gutmann L, Dillmann U, et al: End-plate dysfunction in acute organophosphate intoxication. Neurology 39:561, 1989
76. Rosenberg J: Pesticides. p. 401. In LaDou J (ed): Occupational Medicine. Appleton & Lange, East Norwalk, CT, 1990
77. Lotti M, Becker CE: Treatment of acute organophosphate poisoning: evidence of a direct effect on central nervous system by 2-PAM (pyridine-2-aldoxime methyl chloride). J Toxicol Clin Toxicol 19:121, 1982
78. Johnson MK: The target for initiation of delayed neurotoxicity by organophosphorus esters: biochemical studies and toxicological applications. Rev Biochem Toxicol 4:141, 1982
79. Lotti M, Becker CE, Aminoff MJ: Organophosphate polyneuropathy: pathogenesis and treatment. Neurology 34:658, 1984
80. Senanayake N, Johnson MK: Acute polyneuropathy after poisoning by a new organophosphate insecticide. N Engl J Med 306:155, 1982
81. Senanayake N: Tri-cresyl phosphate neuropathy in Sri Lanka: a clinical and neurophysiological study with a three year follow up. J Neurol Neurosurg Psychiatry 44:775, 1981

82. Morgan JP, Penovich P: Jamaica ginger paralysis: forty-seven year follow-up. Arch Neurol 35:530, 1978

83. Osterloh J, Lotti M, Pond SM: Toxicologic studies in a fatal overdose of 2,4-D, MCPP, and chlorpyrifos. J Anal Toxicol 7:125, 1983

84. Lotti M, Becker CE, Aminoff MJ, et al: Occupational exposure to the cotton defoliants DEF and merphos: a rational approach to monitoring organophosphorous-induced neurotoxicity. J Occup Med 25:517, 1983

85. Auld RB, Bedwell SF: Peripheral neuropathy with sympathetic overactivity from industrial contact with acrylamide. Can Med Assoc J 96:652, 1967

86. Garland TO, Patterson MWH: Six cases of acrylamide poisoning. Br Med J 4:134, 1967

87. Schaumburg HH, Arezzo JC, Spencer PS: Delayed onset of distal axonal neuropathy in primates after prolonged low-level administration of a neurotoxin. Ann Neurol 26:576, 1989

88. Igisu H, Goto I, Kawamura Y, et al: Acrylamide encephaloneuropathy due to well water pollution. J Neurol Neurosurg Psychiatry 38:581, 1975

89. Cavanagh JB, Gysbers MF: Ultrastructural features of the Purkinje cell damage caused by acrylamide in the rat: a new phenomenon in cellular neuropathology. J Neurocytol 12:413, 1983

90. Post EJ, McLeod JG: Acrylamide autonomic neuropathy in the cat: Part 2. Effects on mesenteric vascular control. J Neurol Sci 33:375, 1977

91. Wald PH, Becker CE: Toxic gases used in the microelectronics industry. Occup Med 1:105, 1986

92. Crystal HA, Schaumburg HH, Grober E, et al: Cognitive impairment and sensory loss associated with chronic low-level ethylene oxide exposure. Neurology 38:567, 1988

93. Klees JE, Lash A, Bowler RM, et al: Neuropsychologic "impairment" in a cohort of hospital workers chronically exposed to ethylene oxide. J Toxicol Clin Toxicol 28:21, 1990

94. Katzenstein AW: Ethylene oxide and CNS dysfunction. J Toxicol Clin Toxicol 29:285, 1991

95. Gross JA, Haas ML, Swift TR: Ethylene oxide neurotoxicity: report of four cases and review of the literature. Neurology 29:978, 1979

96. Kuzuhara S, Kanazawa I, Nakanishi T, Egashira T: Ethylene oxide polyneuropathy. Neurology 33:377, 1983

33

Acute Bacterial Infections of the Central Nervous System

Vincent G. Pons

The critical nature of bacterial infections of the central nervous system (CNS) has traditionally provoked a sense of urgency in establishing the diagnosis and in the necessity to initiate therapy promptly. Bacterial meningitis, brain abscess, subdural empyema, and epidural abscess continue to be important causes of morbidity and mortality in all age groups and in all hosts, despite the availability of potent antibiotics. Some of the more common bacterial infections of the CNS are discussed here with emphasis on the advances that have been made in understanding these important infectious diseases.

BACTERIAL MENINGITIS

Bacterial meningitis is an acute inflammation of the leptomeninges and the subarachnoid space caused by invading bacteria from the bloodstream or from a contiguous focus of infection or local trauma. Descriptions of fulminant meningitis can be traced back to the writings of Hippocrates. The uniformly poor outcome of this disease remained unchanged until the discovery and use of antibiotics in the 1940s. Despite the development of more effective antibiotics, the mortality rates for bacterial meningitis (which range from 5 to 40 percent) have not changed in the last 40 years. Significant morbidity, especially deafness in

children, also remains unacceptably high (approximately 10 to 15 percent). Recent advances in understanding the pathophysiology of this disease and new therapeutic regimens may reduce these morbidity and mortality rates.

Epidemiology

The important factors that define the epidemiology of bacterial meningitis include age, the status of the host immune system, colonization of the nasopharynx with potential pathogens, climatic and seasonal conditions, bacterial antimicrobial resistance patterns, and bacterial virulence factors. Table 33-1 summarizes the relationship of age with bacterial causes of meningitis.

Neonates (up to 1 month of age) have the highest incidence of meningitis. The risk is particularly great in infants of low birthweight or with premature rupture of the membranes more than 24 hours prior to delivery.[1] The unique list of likely pathogens in neonatal meningitis includes group B streptococcus, *Escherichia coli,* other gram-negative enteric bacteria (i.e., *Enterobacter, Citrobacter*) and *Listeria. Enterococcus* and *Staphylococcus aureus* are also included in this list but occur less frequently.

In children between 1 month and 6 years of age, *Hemophilus influenzae* type b (Hib) and *Neisseria men-*

Table 33-1 Epidemiology of Bacterial Meningitis and Associated Mortality

Age or Circumstance	Etiological Agent	Incidence (Percent)	Mortality (Percent)
Neonates	*Escherichia coli*	40	30–40
	Other Enterobacteriaceae	20	40–60
	Group B streptococcus	20	40
	Listeria	3–5	40
	Enterococcus	2	40
	Staphylococcus species	2	60
Infants and children, 2 months to 5 years	*Hemophilus influenzae*	60[a]	5–10
	Neisseria meningitidis	25	5
	Streptococcus pneumoniae	15	10–25
Adults	*Streptococcus pneumoniae*	50	30–40
	Neisseria meningitidis	10	10
	Escherichia coli	10	50
	Listeria	5–10	50
	Hemophilus influenzae	2–5	5
Skull fracture with CSF leak	*Streptococcus pneumoniae*	80[b]	5–10
	Hemophilus influenzae, other gram-negative organisms	10	5
	Other (*Staphylococcus, Streptococcus*)	10	5
Postneurosurgical	*Escherichia coli*	20	
	Klebsiella, Enterobacter, Serratia	50	
	Acinetobacter	5	
	Staphylococcus aureus	10–20	
	Staphylococcus epidermidis[c]	5–50	
	Streptococcus species	5–10	

[a] Data from prevaccine era.
[b] Within the first 3 days after injury.
[c] Most common organism in CSF shunt–related meningitis.

ingitidis predominate as the cause of meningitis. *H. influenzae* has been the most common cause of bacterial meningitis in the United States, with an estimated 10,000 cases per year and peaks in the summer and fall.[2] There is a higher incidence in nonwhites. *H. influenzae* meningitis is uncommon in the first few months of life, reflecting the placental transfer of protective maternal anticapsular antibody to Hib, and most common in the age bracket of 4 months to 2 years. Up to 50 percent of household contacts of a case of *H. influenzae* meningitis will be colonized asymptomatically with Hib. Subsequent increased risk of developing serious *H. influenzae* disease may occur in these "carrier" contacts, especially those with immunoglobulin or complement deficiencies, immunodeficient states, or splenectomy. Programs of *H. influenzae* vaccination and chemoprophylaxis have reduced those risks.

N. meningitidis causes approximately 2,500 cases of meningitis per year in the United States, occurring mostly in the late winter months and early spring. Epidemic outbreaks of meningococcal meningitis usually reflect crowding conditions, concurrent respiratory infection, the susceptibility of the host, and other as yet poorly defined factors.[3] As described for Hib, meningococcal meningitis is a disease of children; but unlike Hib, it affects also young adults, as evidenced by the numerous reported outbreaks in military recruit camps. Close contacts of infected patients have an increased risk of colonization and subsequent serious infection with meningococci. The immune status of the host is an important factor that determines whether a contact or carrier of this organism will go on to invasive clinical disease. Both specific serum antibodies and serum complement protect the host. Recurrent bouts of meningococcal meningitis in an individual should prompt an evaluation for a complement deficiency (late components of complement C5, C6, C7, or C8). Once a close contact becomes colonized with meningococci, the time frame for the expression of clinical disease is short, usually within 1 week. Attempts to avert the development of clinical disease in close contacts, therefore, can be successful only through prompt use of chemoprophylaxis to eradicate the carrier state. Among patients with meningococcal meningitis, 50 percent are children under 5 years of age. Epidemics are caused by any of the serogroups of meningococcus but most commonly by group A and less often by group B, C, or Y.

Streptococcus pneumoniae is an important cause of meningitis, mostly in adults and especially in patients with sickle cell disease, other hemoglobinopathies, splenectomy, cirrhosis, and nephrotic syndrome. Nasopharyngeal colonization with a virulent strain in an immunologically naive host initiates the process leading to infection and clinical disease. It is the most common cause of bacterial meningitis occurring in the first 3 days after closed head trauma with basilar skull fracture and cerebrospinal fluid (CSF) leaks. Pneumococcal pneumonia, sinusitis, or otitis are found as antecedent illnesses in a significant percentage of patients (15 to 30 percent) who subsequently develop meningitis. As with *H. influenzae* and meningococcus, the capsule of the pneumococcus is an important component of the bacterium that resists phagocytosis and defines the capsular serotype and its virulence. Pneumococci can be part of the normal flora of the nasopharynx in 5 to 50 percent of the population, depending on age and crowding conditions.

Etiology

In addition to the major pathogens discussed above, almost any bacteria that enter the CSF can cause meningitis, including anaerobes, higher bacteria (i.e., *Nocardia, Actinomyces*), mycobacteria, spirochetes, and others (*Salmonella* species, corynebacteria, group A streptococcus, enteric gram-negative bacilli). The leading causes of meningitis in the United States have been reviewed by the National Bacterial Meningitis Surveillance Study.[4] *H. influenzae* meningitis is the most common, approaching 50 percent of all cases of bacterial meningitis. *S. pneumoniae* (10 to 15 percent) and *N. meningitides* (20 percent) are also common. Group B streptococcus, *E. coli*, *Listeria mo-*

nocytogenes, and enterococcus species account for 10 to 15 percent of cases, usually those at the extremes of age (the neonate and the elderly).

Staphylococcus epidermidis is a rare cause of meningitis overall, but it is the most common organism found in CSF shunt–related meningitis, with *S. aureus* a close second in this setting. *S. aureus* meningitis is also described as a consequence of postoperative neurosurgical procedures, penetrating head wound injury, endocarditis, sinusitis, CNS abscess, or a paraspinal infection with this organism.

Aerobic gram-negative bacteria are also notable causes of meningitis in postoperative neurosurgical patients and the elderly.[5] Organisms like *Klebsiella, Pseudomonas, Proteus* species, *Enterobacter,* and *Serratia* species (in addition to the already mentioned *E. coli*) are an important albeit infrequent cause of bacterial meningitis in patients who are severely immunocompromised or neutropenic. Anaerobes *(Bacteroides, Fusobacterium, Peptostreptococcus, Clostridium)* are rare causes of bacterial meningitis. These organisms have been associated with polymicrobial infection of the CSF, reflecting either rupture of a polymicrobial brain abscess into the subarachnoid space, head trauma, or extension of infection into the CSF from sinusitis or another parameningeal focus of infection.[6,7]

Pathogenesis and Pathophysiology

Bacteria enter the CSF by one of several possible routes. Hematogenous seeding of the subarachnoid space from a distal focus of infection or spontaneous bacteremia from nasopharyngeal colonization with the pathogen is the most common. A contiguous spread or direct extension of invading bacteria into the subarachnoid space (e.g., from rupture of a parameningeal abscess) and traumatic or surgical events to the CNS that allow direct implantation of bacteria into the subarachnoid space reflect the other pathways of entry for bacteria.

The precise sequence of events in the process of developing bacterial meningitis is not fully understood, but much has been learned in the past decade. For the most common cause of meningitis, the bacteria must first attach to epithelial cells in the nasopharynx. *H. influenzae* and *N. meningitidis* have pili, which are the elements of the bacteria that attach to the specific receptors on host mucosal cells.[8–11] In order to bind to receptors on host cells, the bacteria must evade the local secretary mucosal IgA antibody. All the major bacterial pathogens causing meningitis have IgA proteases that disarm IgA, thereby clearing the path to attachment.[12] The bacteria must pass through these cells and access the bloodstream. The precise mechanism involved is not known; processes like endocytosis, with bacterial transport via cell vacuoles, or passage through an intercellular route have been proposed.[13] Once in the blood, bacteria must survive the immune system (i.e., circulating complement and phagocytosis by leukocytes) and eventually arrive at CNS capillaries. The most common organisms causing bacterial meningitis are able to avoid these host defenses in the bloodstream by virtue of the antiphagocytic and anticomplement nature of their polysaccharide capsules. *E. coli* may also avoid destruction in the bloodstream by the outer membrane proteins that protect the bacteria from phagocytosis and lysis.

From the CNS capillaries, the bacteria must penetrate the blood-brain barrier and cross into the subarachnoid space. CNS vascular endothelial cells are unique in their microanatomy (i.e., they are bound by "tight junctions," which effectively serve as a screening barrier to circulating substances). These tight junctions define the blood-brain barrier. Bacteria enter the CSF via capillaries in the choroid plexus of the lateral ventricles. The mechanism enabling certain bacteria to do this remains largely unknown. Once in the CSF, bacteria can multiply freely because the CSF is virtually devoid of complement, antibody, and phagocytic cells. Even with the emergence of inflammation and the ingress of cells, complement, and antibody into the CSF, the infection generally continues to progress.

Brain injury as the ultimate clinical expression of bacterial meningitis arises from the immune inflammatory response to the presence of components of the bacterial cell wall. Endotoxin (lipid A moiety of the gram-negative bacterial cell wall) and teichoic acid fragments of the gram-positive bacterial cell wall are instrumental in provoking the CNS endothelial cells and other glial cells to release proinflammatory cytokines, notably tumor necrosis factor (TNF) and interleukin-1α and β (IL-1). Thereafter a cascade of events follows and includes a more complex interaction of these cytokines—including IL-6, platelet-activating factor, and leukotrienes—to break down the blood-brain barrier. Disruption of this barrier allows ingress of leukocytes and complement and movement of albumin into the subarachnoid space, which is important in the development of vasogenic brain edema. Animal models of bacterial meningitis have indicated that it is the cytokines directly that induce inflammation and disrupt the blood-brain barrier.[14] The leukocytes and mediators then interact to cause further pathological changes, including thrombosis of veins and vasculitis, with resultant ischemic damage to the CNS and direct cytotoxic swelling of CNS cells (cytotoxic brain edema). The intense inflammatory response also inhibits the reabsorption of CSF in the arachnoid granulations, prompting further increase in intracranial pressure by increasing interstitial brain edema. Brain edema can be further induced by the presence of arachidonic acid and its metabolites, which are released from damaged cells of the CNS, and by the fatty acids released from polymorphonuclear leukocytes. The metabolites of the cyclo-oxygenase pathway of arachidonate create alterations in vascular endothelial cell permeability. The leukocyte attracted to CNS endothelial cells in bacterial meningitis exhibits a specific adhesion molecule that causes adherence to those endothelial cells and further provokes disruption of the blood-brain barrier. Monoclonal antibodies to this leukocyte adhesion receptor have been developed; they prevent CSF leukocytosis and protect against the development of brain edema in an animal model of bacterial meningitis.[15] All of these factors ultimately lead to an increase in brain edema and a decrease in the perfusion of the brain due to increased intracranial pressure and endothelial cell vasculitis and thrombosis. The final common pathway of these processes is ischemic damage to the CNS.[16,17]

THERAPEUTIC IMPLICATIONS

The implication of the pathophysiology summarized above is that potent bactericidal antibiotics that cause rapid lysis of bacterial cell walls in the CSF may promote cytokine release and thereby worsen brain edema, vasculitis, and thrombosis; the resulting increase in intracranial hypertension can be severe enough to cause herniation[18] and, ultimately, CNS ischemia that is associated with brain injury and neuronal cell death. This may well be the explanation for the unchanging mortality statistics despite the development of newer antibiotics that are more potent against bacterial pathogens and penetrate well into the CSF. It may also help to explain the poorer results obtained in the treatment of bacterial meningitis in infants by direct instillation of aminoglycosides into the ventricular space.[19]

The attraction of interfering with or inhibiting the inflammatory response as a therapy for bacterial meningitis has been intensified by the understanding of this pathophysiology. Recent clinical studies to evaluate the use of corticosteroids, cyclo-oxygenase inhibitors, and monoclonal antibodies to leukocyte adhesion receptors, TNF, and endotoxin, and to define the effect of different antibiotics on the production of cell-wall lysis and subsequent release of these inflammatory mediators[20] in the treatment of bacterial meningitis are a direct result of advances made in the elucidation of the pathophysiology.[21] The use of dexamethasone and pentoxifylline has been shown to inhibit the release of TNF and IL-1 (two of the most implicated proinflammatory cytokines) from microglial cells[22] and mononuclear cells.[23] The use of corticosteroids in the treatment of bacterial meningitis has received the most attention. Original observations of its benefit in animal models of meningitis[24-26] prompted clinical studies in humans. Corticosteroids (dexamethasone 0.15 mg/kg every 6 hours for 4 days) were used as adjunct therapy with antibiotics in the treatment of bacterial meningitis in children in several studies. The patients receiving dexamethasone fared better than the placebo groups by measured laboratory and clinical parameters. Lower CSF protein and lactate levels, lower interleukin-1β and TNF concentrations, lower CSF pressures, and significantly less neurological impairment and hearing loss were seen in the corticosteroid-treated groups. Nevertheless, none of the studies showed a significant difference in overall mortality.[27-29] Moreover, critical analysis of these studies reveals limitations that should temper enthusiasm for the use of corticosteroids in the treatment of all patients with bacterial meningitis. Most of the benefits derived from corticosteroids were demonstrated in infants and children, with the use of ceftriaxone as the antibiotic and *H. influenzae* as the pathogen. Studies in the adult population and in children with bacterial meningitis caused by other pathogens are needed in order to confirm the benefit of dexamethasone.

DIAGNOSTIC IMPLICATIONS

Another benefit derived from recent advances in defining the pathophysiology of bacterial meningitis is the use of CSF concentrations of cytokines as diagnostic tools. Elevated CSF levels of TNF-α were found in 42 of 51 patients with purulent bacterial meningitis and in only 5 of 78 patients with nonbacterial meningitis. The CSF levels of TNF were elevated in seven of eight patients in whom the diagnosis of bacterial meningitis was probable but not definite.[30] Similar observations of elevated CSF concentrations of TNF-α and IL-1β in bacterial meningitis (but not in viral or other forms of aseptic meningitis[31]) and the correlation of elevated levels of TNF and platelet-activating factor with the severity of disease[32] have stimulated interest in using CSF cytokine levels for establishing the diagnosis of bacterial meningitis. The clinical context in which these CSF cytokine levels may be most useful includes "culture-negative" bacterial meningitis and the postoperative neurosurgical "posterior fossa meningitis syndrome." In the latter disorder, intradural neurosurgery is followed by a postoperative aseptic meningeal syndrome clinically indistinguishable from bacterial meningitis and with a similar CSF formulation (low CSF glucose and high protein levels, accompanied by a CSF pleocytosis with predominantly polymorphonuclear leukocytes). The syndrome is commonly noted at the time of corticosteroid taper and resolves quickly when the corticosteroids are increased. The traditional CSF parameters do not reliably differentiate aseptic from bacterial meningitis in most of these patients.[33] Recent analysis of the CSF concentration of cytokines in patients with the neurosurgical aseptic meningitis syndrome and those with postoperative bacterial meningitis has suggested that this may indeed be diagnostically useful—elevated CSF levels of TNF and IL-1 were noted in bacterial but not aseptic meningitis.[34]

MEDICOLEGAL IMPLICATIONS

In patients with clinically overt meningitis and fulminant infections, it has generally been held that the first dose of an antibiotic should not be delayed for more than 30 minutes.[35] Although no one would support the purposeful delay of therapy in established bacterial meningitis, it is not clear that the ultimate outcome and sequelae of bacterial meningitis, including death, are altered by short delays in the initiation of antibiotic therapy. It is provocative to think that the first doses of antibiotics correlate with bacterial cell-wall lysis, release of endotoxin or teichoic acid, and the subsequent burst release of the cytokines that are responsible for the ultimate damage to the CNS in bacterial meningitis. These initial pathophysiological events occur over a period of several hours. It is unlikely that the timing of antibiotic therapy will influence the outcome of a patient presenting with clinically fulminant meningitis, who is likely to die within a short period of time (several hours). In theory, interference and modulation of the inflammatory response may have a more important role in the therapy and ultimate outcome of bacterial meningitis than the immediate administration of antibiotics.

Several reviews of bacterial meningitis have failed to show any differences in mortality or neurological sequelae among patients with an abrupt presentation with overt meningitis or a more prolonged presentation with several days' duration of illness.[36] Available data from clinical studies in bacterial meningitis do not indicate that the longer the duration of symptoms, the worse the outcome; nor do they show that a short delay in the initiation of antibiotics affects the outcome, particularly in the fulminant case.[37] The medicolegal implications of this are obvious.

Clinical Manifestations

The clinical presentation of bacterial meningitis can be abrupt (within 24 hours) or more insidious (developing over several days). The classic review by Carpenter and Petersdorf describes the clinical spectrum of bacterial meningitis.[38] In the acute presentation, headache, fever, and altered mental status are seen within 24 hours and there is usually no other focus of infection; in the insidious presentation of bacterial meningitis, the illness develops over several days to a week and pneumonia, sinusitis, or otitis media is present more commonly. The common and classic triad of fever, headache, and stiff neck have always suggested the diagnosis. Depending on the age group (Table 33-2) and the virulence of the bacteria, however, the clinical presentation can be quite variable. The factors other than age that determine some of the clinical manifestations include the degree of meningeal infection and inflammation (stiff neck); the pres-

ence of increased intracranial pressure (headache, vomiting, bulging fontanelle, papilledema); the occurrence of vasculitis or venous thrombosis (hemiparesis, other focal neurological deficits, seizures); and the development of subdural effusions (hemiparesis, seizures).

In the neonate with early-onset infection (i.e., when the child is only several days old), fever, abdominal distention, and respiratory distress are the likely presenting features; in later-onset disease (at the age of several weeks), fever, seizures, irritability, meningismus, and bulging fontanelle are more likely to be observed. In one large review of bacterial meningitis in children less than 2 years of age, meningeal signs were present in more than 90 percent, and fever was consistently present. The diagnosis of bacterial meningitis in the few who had no signs of meningeal irritation was suggested by other signs and symptoms of CNS infection.[39]

Bacterial meningitis in children and young adults usually presents with the classic signs and symptoms of fever, headache, photophobia, nausea, vomiting, and meningismus. Fever is almost always present. Meningeal irritation may be suggested by the presence of a positive Brudzinski sign (flexion of the neck producing flexion of the hip and knee) and Kernig sign (extension of the knee, with the patient recumbent and the leg flexed at the hip, causing pain and resistance to the movement). These signs of meningeal irritation are seen in up to 50 percent of older children and 90 percent of adults. Lethargy and confusion are more common in bacterial than viral meningitis, and the altered mental status is a consistent finding in older children and adults. Headache is usually present and is intense, severe, and unremitting in quality. With pneumococcal meningitis, an associated pulmonary, ear, or sinus infection is often found. Focal neurological deficits (including cranial neuropathies, seizures, and hemiparesis) may relate to cerebritis or CNS infarction secondary to large vessel vasculitis or dural sinus thrombosis. Localizing neurological deficits should prompt investigation for brain abscess, subdural effusion, or empyema.

Seizures occur in approximately 20 percent of adult patients, usually within 1 day of admission and especially with pneumococcal meningitis. Of the focal neurological deficits other than seizures, the more common are gaze preferences, aphasia, visual field defects, and hemiparesis. In children, ataxia can be a

Table 33-2 Frequency of Signs and Symptoms of Bacterial Meningitis

Age	Symptom	Percent	Sign	Percent
Children[a]	Fever	80–90	Stiff neck	50
	Nausea/vomiting	70	Seizure	30
	Irritability	30–40	Petechiae or purpura[b]	20
	Lethargy	20	Focal neurological deficit[c]	10–15
	Headache	10–15		
	Coma	5		
Adult	Headache	90	Stiff neck	80–90
	Fever	80–90	Pneumonia[d]	30
	Lethargy/confusion	70–80	Otitis media[e]	20–30
	Nausea/vomiting	50	Seizures	15
			Focal neurological deficits	15
Elderly	Fever	90	Disorientation	90
	Lethargy/confusion	90	Stiff neck	50
	Headache	20–30	Sinusitis/pneumonia	30–50
			Seizures	5–15

[a] Percentages vary between infants and older children.
[b] Seen mostly with meningococcemia.
[c] Includes palsy of cranial nerves IV, VI, VII or hemiparesis.
[d] Seen with pneumococcal meningitis.
[e] Seen with *H. influenzae* meningitis and pneumococcal meningitis.

presenting feature often associated with *H. influenzae* meningitis and is probably due to inflammation of the vestibular cranial nerve. It is linked to the development of hearing loss in these children.[40]

In the elderly, bacterial meningitis may frequently present with an abnormal mental status. Most patients develop disorientation or confusion.[41] Fever may be absent and meningeal irritation can be dismissed as reflecting cervical osteoarthritic stiffness. The elderly may be misdiagnosed as having a stroke, organic brain syndrome, or drug intolerance and toxicity. Bacterial meningitis due to gram-negative enteric bacteria can present in the elderly with a subtle disturbance that subsequently evolves into a rapidly fulminant sepsis leading to coma and death.[42]

Most patients with meningococcal meningitis will have cutaneous manifestations of the systemic infection, characteristically described as petechiae or purpura. However, pneumococcal and staphylococcal meningitis may also cause this rash.[43]

One of the more difficult clinical situations in the diagnosis of CNS infections is to distinguish postoperative neurosurgical changes from true bacterial meningitis. Fever, stiff neck, altered mental status, and coma are frequently encountered after major intradural CNS surgery, regardless of the occurrence

of bacterial meningitis. Fevers that emerge with the tapering of corticosteroids in patients who are otherwise clinically improving after CNS surgery suggest the aseptic meningitis syndrome. *E. coli* and other aerobic gram-negative bacteria predominate as the cause of nosocomial neurosurgical bacterial meningitis. This form of gram-negative bacterial meningitis is frequently benign in its initial clinical presentation, with fevers and headache as the manifestation of the infection. As mentioned earlier, the gram-positive bacteria, notably *S. epidermidis,* predominate as the cause of bacterial meningitis complicating CSF shunt placement.

Other clinical syndromes can mimic bacterial meningitis and prompt a lumbar puncture. Brain abscess, subdural empyema, or intracranial epidural abscess are CNS infections that may present like bacterial meningitis. Fever is less common, and headache and seizures more common in these other infections; focal neurological deficits evolve over several days. A change in the level of consciousness indicates increasing intracranial pressure. The decision to perform a lumbar puncture in these circumstances should be made with caution and is best delayed until the results of a computed tomography (CT) scan or magnetic resonance imaging (MRI) are known. The risk of provoking cerebral herniation with a lumbar puncture in patients with intracranial mass lesions has been well described.[44–48]

Delay in the treatment of bacterial meningitis may be inappropriately long if the results of neuroimaging studies and analysis of the CSF are awaited. The validity of CSF culture and Gram stain is unlikely to be altered for several hours after antibiotic therapy is started. Most cultures of the CSF will remain positive for several hours after the first dose of an antibiotic; about 50 percent are negative after 8 to 12 hours, and by 24 hours most CSF cultures are negative.[49–53] The most reasonable recommendation in most circumstances requiring exclusion of a mass lesion is to initiate antibiotics empirically before sending the patient for imaging studies and before the results of the CSF analysis can be determined.

Infection with the spirochete *Borrelia bergdorferi* can lead to a form of meningitis, as discussed in Chapter 34. The diagnosis is established by serological markers in the serum and CSF. Rocky Mountain spotted fever and other rickettsial infections may present with fever and severe headache. The rash is characteristic, beginning at the distal extremities (palms and soles) and spreading centrally to the trunk. Initially it is usually a macular rash, but it subsequently becomes petechial and purpuric. Approximately one-third of patients will have a CSF pleocytosis. The diagnosis is made on clinical and epidemiological grounds (tick bite) as well as by serology.

Laboratory Diagnosis

Once the diagnosis of meningitis is suspected and mass lesions of the CNS have been excluded, a lumbar puncture must be done. Gram stain and culture of the CSF will result in identification of bacteria in most cases of bacterial meningitis (90 percent or more). Prior antibiotic therapy may reduce the yield of Gram stain and culture of the CSF by between 4 and 41 percent.[54] Ideally, then, CSF and blood should be cultured before initiating antibiotics, because the identity of the responsible bacterium is important in guiding treatment. Table 33-3 shows the typical CSF findings in bacterial meningitis. The CSF is usually cloudy and contains several hundreds to thousands of white blood cells, predominantly polymorphonuclear leukocytes. However, when the CSF white cell count is low (less than 1,000/mm³), the CSF pleocytosis may initially be predominantly lymphocytic in up to

one-third of patients with documented bacterial meningitis.[55] A CSF pleocytosis with lymphocyte predominance may falsely suggest a viral meningitis. In such circumstances the lumbar puncture should be repeated after several hours if the clinical situation does not become clear. A polymorphonuclear predominance is usually then found, and CSF cultures and Gram stain provide supporting evidence of bacterial meningitis. CSF leukocytosis greater than 10,000 cells/mm³ should suggest the presence of a brain abscess or parameningeal abscess with rupture into the subarachnoid space.

CSF glucose concentration is usually low in bacterial meningitis (i.e., less than 50 percent of the simultaneous serum concentration), with levels ranging from less than 10 mg/dl to 50 mg/dl. The ratio of CSF/serum glucose in bacterial meningitis should be less than 0.3 but no higher than 0.5. CSF protein concentrations are elevated (usually greater than 100 mg/dl); if the protein exceeds or approaches 1,000 mg/dl, however, a subarachnoid block of CSF flow should be suspected. Changes in CSF glucose and protein levels are less pronounced in viral than bacterial meningitis (Table 33-3).

The development of rapid tests of CSF for the detection of specific bacterial antigens or the presence of endotoxin from gram-negative bacteria has helped in establishing the diagnosis of bacterial meningitis. In addition to their rapidity, these assays aid in the detection of bacteria when CSF cultures and Gram stains are negative due to prior use of antibiotics or poor technique in the collection and culture of the CSF. The available diagnostic tests include latex particle agglutination (LPA) kits that contain antisera directed against the specific capsular antigens of *H. influenzae, S. pneumoniae,* and *N. meningitidis.* Coagglutination tests (CoA) and counter-immune electrophoresis (CIE) tests are also available. The accuracy of these diagnostic kits varies with the organism and with the timing of the sample of CSF if obtained after antibiotic treatment. Nonetheless, they have a sensitivity and specificity of between 50 and 90 percent.[56,57]

The limulus lysate test on CSF can detect the presence of endotoxin and thereby support a diagnosis of gram-negative bacterial meningitis,[58] but it is rarely used in clinical practice. The detection of specific cytokines (TNF, IL-1α) and of C-reactive protein in CSF may be the best nonspecific tests for the diagno-

Table 33-3 CSF Characteristics in Meningitis

Characteristics	Bacterial	Viral	Normal
CSF leukocytosis (cells/mm^3)	PMNs^a predominate; range >5 to 10,000	Lymphocytes predominate; usually <2,000	0–5 (no PMNs)
CSF glucose	<10 to 50 mg/dl	Usually normal	Greater than 50% serum glucose
CSF/serum ratio	0.3 to 0.5	Usually normal	
CSF protein	100 to 500 mg/dl	Normal to mildly elevated	<50 mg/dl
CSF Gram stain/culture	90% positive	Negative	

^{a} PMN, polymorphonuclear leukocytes.

sis of bacterial infections, but further studies are needed to establish their role in clinical practice.

Neuroradiology

Inflammation of the meninges can be demonstrated with contrast CT scans or gadolinium-enhanced MRI, but this information plays no role in the management of the patient with bacterial meningitis. The role of CT scan or MRI in meningitis is to exclude other CNS lesions or sequelae of bacterial meningitis. These imaging studies may reveal the presence of brain abscess, subdural effusions, hydrocephalus, or CNS infarction secondary to vasculitis or dural sinus thrombosis. MRI may be more sensitive than CT in defining these sequelae of bacterial meningitis.

Treatment

Therapy of bacterial meningitis depends on several factors. Knowledge of the underlying pathophysiology and the role of the proinflammatory cytokines, coupled with the clinical studies published to date, prompts the use of dexamethasone prior to the initiation of antibiotics in the treatment of bacterial meningitis. Knowledge of the epidemiology of meningitis in certain populations helps to direct antibiotic choices depending on the patient's age and circumstance. The pharmacokinetic and bactericidal activity of different antibiotics against the targeted pathogens is also an important factor in antibiotic choice. The ideal antibiotic for a bacterial pathogen causing meningitis (1) penetrates the blood-brain barrier and achieves CSF concentrations at least 10 times greater than the minimal bactericidal concentration for the organism, (2) is nontoxic to the patient, (3) is bactericidal but not bacteriolytic, (4) does not promote the

emergence of resistance, and (5) sterilizes the CSF quickly. Tables 33-4, 33-5, and 33-6 summarize the antibiotic approach to the treatment of bacterial meningitis. The antimicrobial regimen is usually initiated by covering the likely pathogens and then tailored to be more specific after cultures of the CSF have defined the organism and its sensitivities to various antibiotics.

In neonatal bacterial meningitis the list of likely pathogens is well covered with a regimen of ampicillin and gentamicin. The use of ampicillin alone lacks sufficient bactericidal capacity to treat enterococcus, *Listeria,* and some group B streptococci. Ampicillin alone is not broad enough to cover all the *E. coli* strains and other Enterobacteriaceae. Likewise, the use of the newer "third-generation" cephalosporins alone (i.e., cefotaxime, ceftizoxime, ceftriaxone), while sufficient for some of the gram-negative bacteria and group B streptococci, does not adequately treat the enterococcus or *Listeria.* Therefore the use of a combination of ampicillin and gentamicin is appropriate until the infecting pathogen has been defined by cultures. Since the blood-brain barrier has not fully formed at this age, aminoglycosides (gentamicin, tobramycin, amikacin) enter the CSF in adequate concentration via the intravenous route alone. Only in unresponsive and severe ventriculitis is intraventricular administration of gentamicin indicated, and then only if the gram-negative bacteria are resistant to the newer cephalosporins. For the most part the role of the aminoglycoside is to provide a synergistic effect in the killing of certain pathogens (*Listeria,* enterococcus, and group B streptococcus). The routine and direct instillation of aminoglycosides intraventricularly should be avoided in neonatal meningitis because of the worse morbidity and mortality associated with that route of administration.[59] The duration

Table 33-4 Antibiotic Therapy in Bacterial Meningitis

Clinical/Epidemiological Factors	Empirical Regimen	Etiological Agents	Directed Antibiotic of Choice[a]	Alternative
Neonate	Ampicillin + gentamicin	E. coli	Ampicillin	Cephalosporin[b]
		Group B streptococcus	Ampicillin + gentamicin	Cephalosporin[b]
		Listeria	Ampicillin + gentamicin	TMP/SMZ[d]
		Enterococcus	Ampicillin + gentamicin	Vancomycin + gentamicin
		Staphylococcus species[c]	Nafcillin	Vancomycin
Age 2 months to 5 years	Cephalosporin[b]	H. influenzae	Ampicillin (if sensitive)	Cephalosporin[b] or chloramphenicol
		N. meningitidis	Penicillin G	Cephalosporin[b] or chloramphenicol
		S. pneumoniae	Penicillin G	Cephalosporin[b] or vancomycin
Adult	Cephalosporin[b]	S. pneumoniae	Penicillin G	Cephalosporin[b] or vancomycin
		N. meningitidis	Penicillin G	Cephalosporin[b] or chloramphenicol
Elderly/Immunosuppressed (as above for adults)	Ampicillin + cephalosporin[b]	E. coli[e]	Ampicillin	Cephalosporin[b] or TMP/SMZ[d]
		H. influenzae	Ampicillin	Cephalosporin[b] or chloramphenicol
		Listeria	Ampicillin + gentamicin	TMP/SMZ[d]
Skull fracture with CSF leak				
Within 3 days	Cephalosporin[b]	S. pneumoniae	Penicillin G	Cephalosporin[b] or chloramphenicol or vancomycin
After 3 days	See postsurgical or penetrating head injury, below			
After neurosurgery or penetrating CNS injury	Vancomycin IV and IT + cephalosporin[b] + aminoglycoside IV and IT	Staphylococcus aureus	Nafcillin	Vancomycin
		Staphylococcus epidermidis	Vancomycin	
		E. coli	Ampicillin or cephalosporin	Aminoglycoside IV and IT
		Pseudomonas	Ceftazidime plus aminoglycoside[f] IV and IT	Piperacillin + aminoglycoside

[a] Sensitivity data known. Dosing regimen in Table 33-5.
[b] Cefotaxime, ceftriaxone, or ceftizoxime (ceftazidime only if *Pseudomonas* or resistant gram-negative organism present).
[c] Consider *Staphylococcus* species with neurosurgery or shunt-related infection.
[d] Trimethoprim/sulfamethoxazole.
[e] Chloramphenicol not recommended in enteric gram-negative meningitis.
[f] Aminoglycoside: gentamicin, tobramycin, amikacin. IV, intravenous; IT, intrathecal.

Table 33-5 Antibiotic Dosing—Children

Drug	Total Daily Dose	Hourly Dose Interval
Penicillin G	300,000 U/kg	4
Ampicillin	100–300 mg/kg	4–6
Ceftriaxone	50–100 mg/kg	12
Cefotaxime	100–200 mg/kg	6–8
Ceftizoxime	100–200 mg/kg	6–8
Ceftazidime	100–200 mg/kg	6–8
Vancomycin	40 mg/kg	6
Gentamicin/ tobramycin	5 mg/kg	8
Amikacin	15 mg/kg	12
Trimethoprim/ sulfamethoxazole (TMP/SMZ)	10–15 mg/kg (as TMP)	8–12

of antibiotic treatment for neonatal meningitis has traditionally been 2 to 3 weeks. If intraventricular antibiotics are used, a daily dose for 3 to 5 days is usually sufficient to sterilize the CSF compartment.

In older children and adults, use of the newer third-generation cephalosporins (Tables 33-4, 33-5, and 33-6) is recommended in the initial empiric regimen. These antibiotics are established in the therapy of *H. influenzae, S. pneumoniae,* and *N. meningitidis* disease. When the pathogen has been defined and its antibiotic sensitivities are known, therapy may be simplified. Penicillin G is the drug of choice for the pneumococcus and meningococcus. *H. influenzae* may be resistant to ampicillin (hence the initial use of cephalosporin); when sensitive, ampicillin should be used. In the patient with severe penicillin/β-lactam antibiotic al-

lergy, chloramphenicol can be used for these three common pathogens. Recent documentation of penicillin-resistant pneumococci has prompted a reevaluation of the optimal antibiotic alternative. Failure of chloramphenicol therapy in penicillin-resistant pneumococcal meningitis has been described.[60] Moreover these strains of pneumococci may also be resistant to cephalosporins. The optimal antibiotic regimen in this situation appears to be vancomycin plus a third-generation cephalosporin.[61] If the percentage of pneumococci that are resistant to penicillin and cephalosporins continues to increase, future recommendations for the initial empiric antimicrobial regimens in children and adults will have to include vancomycin.

In the elderly patient or the severely immunocompromised host, the additional pathogen to cover in bacterial meningitis is *Listeria.* Since none of the third-generation cephalosporins is adequate for the treatment of *Listeria* infection, ampicillin or trimethoprim/sulfamethoxazole should be added to the cephalosporin until the culture results are known. If *Listeria* is the cause of meningitis, trimethoprim/sulfamethoxazole may be the antibiotic of choice because of its excellent bactericidal activity against this organism and its superb penetration into the CSF.

The postoperative neurosurgical patient who develops bacterial meningitis as a complication of surgery poses a special problem. Although staphylococci and aerobic gram-negative bacteria are the common causes in this setting, any of the nosocomial pathogens associated with the hospital and its environment can be responsible. Methicillin-resistant staphylococci, *Pseudomonas* species, *Enterobacter* species, enterococci, and even fungi have been described as causes

Table 33-6 Antibiotic Dosing—Adults

Drug	Total Daily Dose	Hourly Dose Interval	Intrathecal Dose
Penicillin G	24 million units	4	
Ampicillin	12 g	4	
Ceftriaxone	4 g	12	
Cefotaxime	12 g	6	
Ceftizoxime	12 g	6	
Ceftazidime	9 g	8	
Vancomycin	2 g	6	4–15 mg/d for 3–5 days
Gentamicin/tobramycin	5 mg/kg	8	1–8 mg/d for 3–5 days
Amikacin	15 mg/kg	12	
Trimethoprim/sulfamethoxazole (TMP/SMZ)	10–15 mg/kg (as TMP)	8–12	

of postneurosurgical meningitis, and polymicrobial infections are also possible. The empiric initial antimicrobial regimen therefore must be quite broad and reflect the nosocomial flora of the hospital. When the clinical suspicion of postcraniotomy bacterial meningitis prompts lumbar puncture (or ventricular tap if necessary), I recommend that intrathecal vancomycin (10 mg) and gentamicin (5 mg) be available to be given at the completion of the spinal tap. Initial intravenous antibiotic therapy should include vancomycin, ceftazidime or piperacillin, and aminoglycoside. Metronidazole can be added if the suspicion of anaerobic infection is high. This regimen can be continued for 24 to 48 hours, until a clearer definition of the cause of bacterial meningitis is made. Vancomycin via the intravenous route is usually adequate for therapy of most cases of gram-positive bacterial meningitis, but intrathecal administration may be required if the CSF does not become sterile within 48 hours or the clinical picture does not improve. Daily intrathecal vancomycin for 3 to 5 days is usually sufficient as adjunctive therapy to the intravenous route.

The duration of antimicrobial therapy, given via the intravenous route, for the treatment of most cases of bacterial meningitis is 7 to 10 days. Longer durations of therapy (2 to 3 weeks) have traditionally been recommended for staphylococcal and gram-negative bacillary meningitis.

The use of dexamethasone as adjunctive therapy in pediatric bacterial meningitis has been widely embraced.[62] The use of dexamethasone in adult bacterial meningitis is more controversial because of the lack of convincing, well-controlled clinical trials.

Treatment of Complications

Sepsis, hypotension, hypoxemia, and increased intracranial pressure all contribute to a reduction in perfusion of the CNS. Supportive measures to maintain an adequate circulation to the CNS should include reversal of hypoxemia and hypercarbia; intubation and ventilatory support may be necessary for this purpose. Increased $PaCO_2$ causes cerebral vasodilatation and thereby may worsen intracranial pressure. Hyperventilation may be beneficial by causing vasoconstriction and thus reducing cerebral blood volume and decreasing intracranial pressure. Fluid restriction during the first several days in bacterial meningitis has been recommended as a management of the syndrome of inappropriate antidiuretic hormone secretion (SIADH). However, if this is done too vigorously, hypotension and decreased CNS perfusion may result. A reasonable approach is to give approximately two-thirds of the daily fluid maintenance volume (about $1 L/m^2/d$ in adults). Mannitol can be used to decrease cerebral edema by osmotic movement of fluid from edematous brain tissue to the intravascular compartment. The dose of mannitol is 0.5 g/kg given intravenously over 30 minutes; it can be given repeatedly over a 24-hour period to a total maximum dose of 2 g/kg. Dexamethasone (not prednisone) may reduce vasogenic brain edema by a direct effect on vascular endothelial cells.[63]

Subdural effusions develop in 15 to 30 percent of patients with bacterial meningitis who are less than 2 years old. These effusions are usually benign and need not be surgically drained unless they are causing a clinically significant increase in intracranial pressure or they become infected. CT scan or MRI can readily identify subdural effusions. Diagnostic needle aspiration of the effusion is indicated in the clinical setting of prolonged fevers, bulging fontanelles, or focal neurological deficits occurring as a consequence of increased intracranial pressure.

Outcome and Prognosis

The morbidity and mortality associated with bacterial meningitis are clearly related to the host (age, immune status), the organism (virulence factors), and the adequacy of therapy. Untreated bacterial meningitis is usually fatal. Mortality rates for children in the modern antibiotic era indicate that up to 50 percent or more of newborns with gram-negative bacillary meningitis will die. Recent analysis of data on the most common causes of meningitis in children in developed countries show mortality rates of 3 to 5 percent for *H. influenzae,* 7 to 8 percent for *N. meningitidis,* and 15 percent for *S. pneumoniae.* The important residual deficits of mental retardation, spasticity or paresis, and deafness continue to occur in about 10 to 30 percent of children.[64] Pneumococcal meningitis carries a greater risk for death and permanent neurological sequelae than meningitis due to *N. meningitidis* or *H. influenzae.*

Recent controlled trials using adjunct therapy with dexamethasone in bacterial meningitis in children have revealed a lowering in incidence of sensorineural hearing loss (16 percent in the placebo group and 3 percent in the dexamethasone group)[27] and overall fewer neurological sequelae (38 percent and 14 percent, respectively).[29]

In adults the mortality rates have been reported to range from 10 to 40 percent in general. Worse outcome is related to advanced age and to presentation with seizures or obtundation. A higher risk of death is associated with the absence of nuchal rigidity.[65] Mortality rates appear highest in meningitis caused by mixed organisms (39 percent) and *S. aureus* (28 percent). Meningitis resulting from pneumococcus or enterococcus has a mortality of about 25 percent, and that from gram-negative bacilli a mortality of about 20 percent. The lowest mortality rate is seen with *N. meningitidis* (10 percent).[66] In adults overall, about 25 percent of patients will have focal neurological deficits, including ocular nerve palsies, blindness, and deafness.

Prevention

CHEMOPROPHYLAXIS AND VACCINES FOR *HAEMOPHILUS INFLUENZAE*

Household contacts of an index patient with *H. influenzae* meningitis are at significantly increased risk of acquiring *H. influenzae* and developing *H. influenzae* disease. This increased risk of secondary spread is related to the age of the contact in the family—the younger the individual, the greater the risk. Those family members less than 1 year of age are most likely to develop *H. influenzae* disease. If illness occurs, it will develop within 1 month (usually within the first week) after exposure to the index case. After age 6, the increased risk to the contact is no longer present. Rifampin is the drug of choice to eradicate the nasopharyngeal colonization of *H. influenzae* and thereby prevent infection from developing. The dose is 600 mg/d for adults and 20 mg/kg/d for children; it should be given for 4 days. Adults are treated not to prevent disease expression in them but to eradicate the organism and thus prevent spread to younger family members. The index child with *H. influenzae* meningitis also needs a course of rifampin after successful treatment of the acute disease, to ensure that nasopharyngeal colonization is eradicated. Pregnant mothers of a child with *H. influenzae* disease should not take rifampin prophylaxis, however, because the potential toxicity to the developing fetus from rifampin is not known. Formal recommendations for contacts that occur in day care centers have not been fully established.

Over the past decade, several vaccines against *H. influenzae* have been developed for use in children. Recent attempts have focused on developing conjugate *H. influenzae* vaccines that are more immunogenic and can produce protective antibody responses in younger children. Several are available for use.[67] Since 1988, the use of these vaccines has markedly decreased the incidence of Hib disease (see Ch. 42). Indeed, the elimination of this disease in children by 1996 has been projected.

CHEMOPROPHYLAXIS AND VACCINES FOR *NEISSERIA MENINGITIDIS*

An increased risk of developing meningococcal disease occurs in young children who are household contacts of an index case of meningococcal meningitis.[68] However, individuals of any age are at increased risk if they have been close contacts of the index case. If contacts develop meningococcal disease, it usually occurs within the first week after exposure. Rifampin is recommended for chemoprophylaxis although it is not as effective in meningococcal contacts as it is in *H. influenzae* contacts. The dose of rifampin is 600 mg by mouth twice daily for 2 days in adults and 10 mg/kg by mouth twice daily for 2 days in children (5 mg/kg in infants). Alternatives to rifampin include sulfadiazine (1 g orally twice daily for 2 days) if the organism is known to be sensitive to sulfa drugs. Minocycline (100 mg twice daily for 5 days) in adults is also effective. Recent studies with the use of ciprofloxacin in adults (750 mg orally in a single dose) showed excellent results in the eradication of the carrier state.[69–71] The index case of meningococcal meningitis should also receive chemoprophylaxis after therapy for the meningitis, since penicillin G is not sufficient to eradicate fully the nasopharyngeal colonization. Ceftriaxone, 250 mg intramuscularly, is effective in that situation, however.[72]

Vaccination for protection against meningococcal disease has been developed for adults with a multivalent vaccine containing the four capsular serotype antigens A, B, C, and Y. This quadrivalent vaccine is recommended for high-risk groups such as the specific immunocompromised host with complement deficiency or asplenia, military recruits at high risk in endemic areas, or during outbreaks of disease. Routine immunization of all children and adults is not recommended.

BRAIN ABSCESS

In 1893 Sir William Macewen published his classic treatise *Pyogenic Infective Diseases of the Brain and Spinal Cord* and described the successful management of brain abscess by surgical drainage.[73] This established him as the "father" of modern CNS abscess therapy.

With recent advances of neurosurgical technique (i.e., development of the operating microscope and of stereotactic CT-guided aspiration or biopsy), the development of more potent antimicrobials, and, most important, the use of CT scan and MRI for the diagnosis and management of brain abscess, the mortality and morbidity due to this disease have improved. The advent of CT scanners alone has been accompanied by reduction in the mortality associated with brain abscess from 40 to 4 percent.[74]

Pathogenesis

A brain abscess may develop as a consequence of the entry of bacteria into the CNS from a contiguous focus of infection, by hematogenous seeding of the CNS, or by direct implantation of organisms secondary to penetrating head trauma or neurosurgical procedures. The most common cause is by local extension of infection from sinusitis, mastoiditis, or dental infections. Bacteria from sinusitis and adjacent otitis may enter the CNS by retrograde migration through the diploic veins toward the frontal lobe (frontal, ethmoid sinusitis) or temporal lobe (maxillary sinusitis). Otitis media and mastoiditis are associated with temporal lobe and cerebellar abscesses respectively. Spread of infection from the temporal lobe to the posterior fossa may occur by the retrograde spread of septic thrombophlebitis of emissary veins. Earlier reviews of brain abscesses revealed that up to 45 percent were due to a contiguous focus of infection and that one-third of these were from an otic infection. More recent reviews suggest a decreasing role of otic infec-

tions as a cause of brain abscess (10 to 15 percent).[74,75] CNS abscesses developing from contiguous sites of infection are usually single and adjacent to the focus. The peak incidence of brain abscesses reflects the underlying etiology. For example, abscesses secondary to otitis are seen more often in children, whereas those that are a consequence of sinusitis occur in persons between 10 and 30 years of age.[76,77]

Brain abscesses arising hematogenously from a remote site of infection are typically multiple "metastatic" lesions that lie in the gray and white matter junction in the distribution of the middle cerebral artery. Most often the bacteremic seeding of the CNS occurs from endocarditis or primary pulmonary infections and in patients with congenital heart disease or pulmonary arteriovenous malformations with right-to-left shunting that allows bacteria in the bloodstream to bypass the filtering system of the pulmonary capillary bed.[78,79] Endocarditis is the cause in up to 5 percent of all brain abscesses.

Head trauma and neurosurgery may cause brain abscess. Clearly a penetrating head injury with a dirty foreign body contaminates the surrounding, injured brain parenchyma with bacteria. Brain abscess is uncommon as a postoperative wound infection in clean neurosurgical procedures; it is associated with craniotomy bone-flap infections or with radioactive CNS implants for the local treatment of brain cancer.

Despite all the technical advances in the ability to find a primary focus of infection, the source remains cryptogenic in up to 20 percent of brain abscesses.

The evolution of a brain abscess has been well described from animal models of brain abscess.[80] The "early cerebritis" stage (days 1 to 3) encompasses acute inflammation, recruitment of macrophages, and development of perivascular leukocytic infiltrates with marked edema around the inciting focus. The "late cerebritis" stage occurs between days 4 to 9 and is characterized by the development of a necrotic center surrounded by active fibroblast activity with reticulin formation. New vessel formation occurs around the developing abscess. Early (days 10 to 13) and late capsule formation (day 14 and after) features a decrease in size of the necrotic center and formation of a mature collagen capsule. The development of the capsule is less pronounced on the ventricular side of the abscess; this may explain the intraventricular rupture that occurs in a small percentage of brain abscesses. Corticosteroids may be harmful by inhibiting capsule formation and impairing the recruitment of leukocytes to the infected area.[81] Corticosteroids also affect the penetration of some antibiotics into the abscess and CNS by restoring the integrity of the blood-brain barrier.

text. Anaerobes, in general, are found in 50 to 90 percent of all brain abscesses if carefully looked for in the microbiology laboratory. *Nocardia* brain abscess is highly associated with a primary pulmonary infection in the immunocompromised host.

Etiology

The bacteria that cause a brain abscess reflect those responsible for the original primary focus of infection. Table 33-7 summarizes the bacteriology of brain abscesses in relation to their site and the original focus of infection. Of note is the absence of the pneumococcus as a cause of brain abscess despite its frequency in sinusitic, otic, and pulmonary infections. Likewise, *H. influenzae* is an uncommon pathogen in this con-

Clinical Presentation

The most common signs and symptoms of a brain abscess are related to the anatomical location of the lesion or lesions and any mass effect. Hence, headache (75 percent), focal or lateralizing neurological deficits (65 percent), and a change in mental status (60 percent) are most common.[74] There may be few indicators of systemic infection; many patients with brain abscess have no fever. If the brain abscess has arisen

Table 33-7 Brain Abscess

Predisposing Source of Infection	Location of Brain Abscess	Common Organisms
Contiguous spread		
Otitis/mastoiditis	Temporal lobe, cerebellum	*Streptococcus* *Bacteroides* Gram-negative bacilli
Sinusitis		
Frontal/ethmoid	Frontal lobe	*Streptococcus* *Bacteroides* *Hemophilus influenzae* *Staphylococcus aureus* Gram-negative bacilli
Sphenoid/maxillary	Frontal/temporal lobe	As above
Dental/periodontal infections	Frontal lobe	*Fusobacterium* *Streptococcus* *Bacteroides*
Trauma/neurosurgery	At the site of the wound infection	*Staphylococcus aureus* *Streptococcus* Gram-negative bacilli
Hematogenous seeding		
Endocarditis	Multiple abscesses in distribution of middle cerebral artery	*Streptococcus viridans* *Staphylococcus aureus*
Pulmonary	As above	*Streptococcus* Microaerophilic streptococci *Staphylococcus* Gram-negative bacilli *Actinomyces* *Nocardia*
Other sites (osteomyelitis, cutaneous infection)	As above	Depends on the organism at the primary source

from a contiguous site of infection, symptoms of otitis, sinusitis, or dental infection may be present. Seizures (40 percent of patients) may be the presenting clinical feature. Nausea and vomiting and papilledema are seen in 20 to 30 percent of cases and reflect the increased intracranial pressure. Nuchal rigidity may also be present.[82,83] Focal neurological deficits are directly related to the anatomical location of the abscess.[84–86]

The presentation of brain abscess is usually semiacute, with most patients having symptoms over a period of 1 to 2 weeks before the diagnosis is established. Less often, patients present with an indolent illness over several weeks to months.

Diagnosis

The routine blood tests indicative of infection are not helpful in the diagnosis of brain abscess. A peripheral leukocytosis is seen in only a minority of patients and the erythrocyte sedimentation rate is usually normal. Skull radiographs may suggest a mass lesion if the calcified pineal gland is shifted. Spinal fluid analysis is neither diagnostic nor helpful (unless rupture of a brain abscess into the ventricle occurs) and is contraindicated in patients with increased intracranial pressure because of the risk of brainstem herniation. The most important advance in diagnosis has been the ability to detect, localize, and follow the course

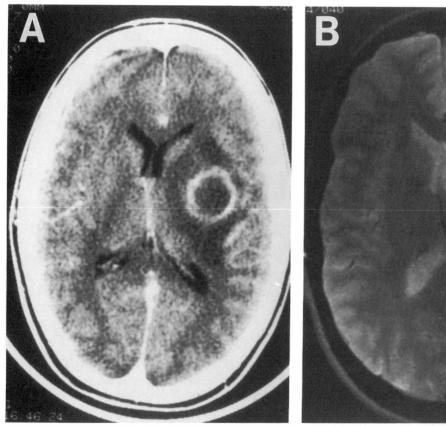
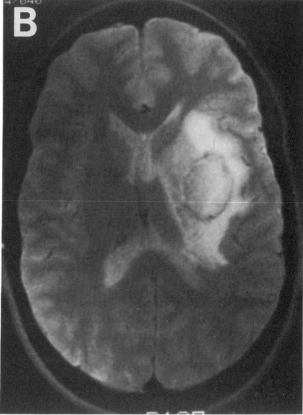

Fig. 33-1 (A) CT scan with contrast, demonstrating ring-enhancing lesion in the deep left parietal lobe with a moderate amount of surrounding edema. The smooth inner margin is typical of pyogenic abscess, in contrast to neoplasms which often (but not always) have irregular inner margins. **(B)** T_2-weighted MRI at the same level again demonstrates ring-type lesion. Note thin and regular wall. The abscess capsule is low in signal intensity, which again is frequently reported in pyogenic abscess.

of brain abscesses by CT scan or MRI. These noninvasive imaging studies have replaced the use of arteriography and technetium 99 brain scans; they have been responsible for the decrease in mortality from this infection.[87]

The typical appearance of a brain abscess by contrast-enhanced CT scan and by MRI is depicted in Figure 33-1. The abscess appears as a circular, smooth, thin-walled lesion with decreased density in the center; it is surrounded by edema. The presence of gas in the lesion or of marked ventricular or meningeal enhancement provides additional support for the diagnosis of abscess. However, CNS tumors, infarctions, hematomas, and radiation necrosis may have a CT appearance indistinguishable from that of brain abscess.[81] CT scan alone, therefore, cannot be the definitive diagnostic test, and a diagnostic and therapeutic neurosurgical intervention (aspiration, biopsy, excision) is almost always required. Indium[111]–labeled leukocyte scans can be of some value in helping to distinguish CNS abscess from tumor.[88]

MRI may be superior to CT scan in its ability to detect early cerebritis, edema, and disruption of the blood-brain barrier and may detect lesions not seen on CT scan.[89–92]

Gadolinium-enhanced MRI scans may also allow more valid analysis of the degree of resolution of an abscess with therapy, because abnormalities on enhanced CT scans may remain for months after successful treatment. Indeed, the findings on CT scan have, in many instances, prolonged antibiotic therapy unnecessarily.

Treatment and Management

The factors that guide the approach to the treatment of brain abscess include the size, number, and location of the lesions, the need for bacteriological definition, the host's status and degree of risk of the surgery, and the response to the initial antibiotic therapy.

SURGICAL ISSUES

The treatment of brain abscess almost always involves neurosurgical intervention. Excision of an abscess is indicated for patients with single, encapsulated, accessible lesions that are not located in eloquent areas of the brain. Large abscess (greater

than 3 cm in diameter) usually do not respond to antibiotic therapy and require drainage: either excision or aspiration. Small abscess (less than 2 cm) may respond to antibiotics alone,[93] but even in this situation a stereotactic CT-guided needle aspiration should be performed for diagnostic and bacteriological confirmation. A causative organism can be cultured from brain abscess aspirates in up to 90 percent of patients. Prior use of antibiotics can lessen this yield. In one series, 30 percent of patients receiving antibiotics preoperatively had sterile cultures, whereas only 4 percent were sterile in the group who did not receive antibiotics.[74] A reasonable approach when a diagnostic procedure is contemplated on a suspected brain abscess is to give a single-dose prophylactic antibiotic either just prior to surgery or intraoperatively after the specimen is obtained; a regimen of antibiotics (see below) is then continued if abscess is present and while awaiting definitive culture data. Nonsurgical management of brain abscess has been successful but limited to small numbers of patients with multiple deep-seated lesions in delicate areas of the brain or with mild and stable neurological deficits, or who are extremely poor surgical candidates and in whom the etiological cause may be presumed based on blood or other tissue cultures. In this setting repeated neurological evaluation and CT scans are required while antibiotics are given empirically. If there is no change or an increase in size of the lesion on CT scan after 4 weeks of therapy in a neurologically stable patient, brain biopsy or aspiration must be reconsidered.

In most cases of multiple brain abscess, at least one of the lesions is reasonably accessible for a CT-guided needle aspiration.

ANTIBIOTIC ISSUES

The choice of antibiotics in the treatment of brain abscess should be based on the results of culture and sensitivity studies. In general, the factors that determine the success of any antibiotic therapy for brain abscess include the potency of the drug in killing the putative organisms, the penetration and concentration of the drug at the site of infection, the influence of the pH and leukocytic enzymes in the abscess on the antibiotic, and the duration of therapy. However, there are no clinical studies or observations correlating the degree of penetration and concentration of an antibiotic into brain abscess with the efficacy of therapy.

In many cases antibiotics are started empirically. Because most abscesses are caused by streptococci, staphylococci, anaerobes, and gram-negative organisms, a broad-spectrum regimen of antimicrobials seems sensible. In cases with no bacteriological definition, this approach has to be followed. When culture data are available, the antibiotic regimen can be tailored to the specific organisms. Regimens that include penicillin, a third-generation cephalosporin (cefotaxime, ceftizoxime, ceftriaxone), and metronidazole are attractive.[94]

The duration of antibiotic therapy has been 6 to 8 weeks in most of the published cases in the literature. It is not necessary to treat with antibiotics until the CT scan is normal, because CT abnormalities may persist for months after successful therapy. Whether MRI will be a more useful tool in determining the end point of antibiotic therapy has yet to be defined. Antibiotics should always be given via the intravenous route except for the exceptional antibiotics whose predictable absorption from the gastrointestinal tract equals the achievable blood and tissue levels attained with the intravenous route (e.g., metronidazole).

Outcome and Prognosis

Major improvements in the mortality rate of brain abscess occurred when antibiotics (specifically penicillin) were developed in the 1940s and then again when CT scanning became available in the 1970s. The mortality rate in the preantibiotic era ranged between 50 and 80 percent and in the antibiotic era from 30 to 50 percent; at present it is between 5 and 25 percent.[74,95–98] The prognosis depends on the clinical status at initial presentation. Patients in coma have the worst prognosis. Permanent neurological sequelae are described in 30 to 50 percent of cases.[85,99,100] Children with brain abscess are more likely to have permanent cognitive deficits or hemiparesis.[101,102] Seizures occur as a persistent consequence of treated brain abscess in 30 to 50 percent of patients.[103,104]

SUBDURAL EMPYEMA

A subdural empyema is an acute suppurative infection in the subdural space between the dura and the arachnoid membrane. This infection accounts for up to 25 percent of all focal intracranial infections and is life-threatening.[105] Subdural empyema commonly occurs over the convexity of the cerebral hemispheres. The barriers to the spread of infection in this space include the falx cerebri, tentorium cerebelli, base of the brain, and foramen magnum. It is unusual to find a subdural empyema below the tentorium.

Pathogenesis

Most subdural empyemas occur as a consequence of contiguous spread from sinusitis, otitis, or mastoiditis, or from direct trauma to the skull or surgery involving it. Sinusitis with concomitant osteomyelitis accounts for 50 to 80 percent of cases, otic infections for 10 to 20 percent, and trauma for less than 5 percent. Occasionally subdural hematomas will become infected. Uncommonly, subdural empyema occurs as an extension of infection from a brain abscess or bacterial meningitis. Hematogenous seeding of the subdural space is a much less common cause, accounting for less than 5 percent of cases. The mechanism of direct spread of bacteria from sinus infection to the subdural space involves the retrograde passage of organisms through the emissary veins and consequent septic thrombophlebitis. The cerebral parenchyma beneath the empyema is usually ischemic and accounts for the seizures associated with this focal infection.

It is rare for subdural empyema to extend into the subarachnoid space and cause meningitis, or vice versa, although the arachnoid membrane and pia mater may be infiltrated with inflammatory cells, and leukocytes are present in the CSF.

Etiology

The bacteria most commonly found reflect the site of the original infection. Sinusitis and otitis-associated subdural empyema is usually due to streptococci or *S. aureus*. Other anaerobes and gram-negative organisms are less common. Postoperative neurosurgical and traumatic cases are due to *S. aureus* and gram-negative bacteria *(E. coli, Klebsiella, Enterobacter, Pseudomonas).*[106] In infants, subdural effusions occur as a consequence of bacterial meningitis, and a small percentage (2 percent) of those effusions become infected with the meningitic pathogen.[107] Therefore *H. influenzae,* pneumococcus, group B streptococcus, *E.*

coli, and meningococcus have been described as causes of subdural empyema in this population. The etiological agent is determined from cultures taken at the time of surgical drainage in 70 percent of cases. The 30 percent of "sterile" cultures are partially explained by the prior use of antibiotics. Subdural empyema is due to single pathogens in most cases.

Clinical Presentation

Most patients present acutely ill with headache, fever, focal neurological deficit, and stiff neck. There is frequently a history of preceding sinusitis or otitis before the rapid development of acute neurological dysfunction. The headache is intense and begins focally at the origin of the sinusitis or otitis but later becomes generalized.[108]

Periorbital or frontal edema is often present and is associated with sinusitis, reflecting thrombosis of the superficial veins draining the sinuses. Focal neurological signs (e.g., hemiplegia) and progressive deterioration of mental status is seen in 80 to 90 percent of patients. Obtundation and coma can evolve rapidly. Rapid diagnosis and urgent surgical drainage are imperative for successful management. Table 33-8 summarizes the common clinical signs and symptoms.

Diagnosis

Spinal tap is not helpful and is contraindicated. The CSF will almost always be sterile (except in infants) and the abnormal pleocytosis is not helpful.

CT scan and MRI are the methods of choice for establishing the diagnosis and defining the location of the empyema, and MRI is emerging as the superior approach.

Table 33-8 Symptoms and Signs of Subdural Empyema at Presentation

Symptoms and Signs	Percent
Headache	80–90
Fever	80–90
Altered mental status	60–75
Nuchal rigidity	60–80
Focal neurological deficit	40–50
Seizures	40–60
Papilledema	20–40
Edema of orbit/forehead	10–30

Purulent fluid obtained at surgery should immediately be evaluated with a Gram stain and be submitted for aerobic and anaerobic cultures.

Treatment

The best therapy is urgent surgical drainage of the infected space and appropriate intravenous antibiotic therapy. Antibiotics should be started based on the presumed likeliest pathogens and then tailored to the specific organisms identified in culture. Regimens should include coverage for streptococci, staphylococci, and gram-negative bacilli. Vancomycin or nafcillin plus a third-generation cephalosporin (cefotaxime, ceftizoxime, ceftriaxone) is a reasonable regimen. The addition of metronidazole is appropriate when mixed infections or anaerobes are suspected. After culture data are obtained, this aggressive empiric antibiotic regimen can be simplified. In cases where the empyema is "sterile," continuation of prior antibiotics (if any) is appropriate. If no antibiotics were given previously, a regimen of penicillin or a third-generation cephalosporin with metronidazole should be prescribed. The duration of antibiotic treatment ranges from 3 to 6 weeks depending on size of the empyema, the adequacy of drainage, the presence of osteomyelitis, and the clinical response.

Drainage is accomplished either through a burr hole or a formal craniotomy. Controversy exists as to which method is superior. A craniotomy affords a more aggressive opportunity to drain the empyema fully, especially if loculations occur, but it is a major surgical undertaking compared to a burr-hole procedure. Inadequate drainage with reaccumulation of pus is more commonly associated with the burr-hole procedure; repeat MRI or CT scan is indicated when fevers persist and neurological deficits worsen. The placement of drains in the space for postoperative irrigations with antibiotics is of uncertain value. If seizures have occurred, the instillation of antibiotics locally over ischemic or traumatized areas of the brain directly contiguous to the empyema may worsen seizures or provoke more of them.

Treatment of the predisposing infection should also be addressed and the need for drainage or debridement of sinusitis or mastoiditis should be determined at that time.

If brain edema and increased intracranial pressure

are clinically significant, corticosteroids may be used in high dose for a short period of time.

Outcome

The mortality rate continues to be high (25 to 40 percent) due to the rapid clinical progression that has been described. Prompt and aggressive diagnostic and therapeutic surgical drainage procedures are imperative for optimal outcome. Adjacent brain may be damaged by septic venous thrombosis and consequent ischemic damage. Infarction and necrosis, with the development of brain abscess, may occur as a consequence in up to 10 percent of cases.[109–112]

EPIDURAL ABSCESS

Cerebral epidural abscess is a suppurative infection in the space between the dura and the inner surface of the cranial bone. The dura is usually quite adherent; therefore the infection is not able to progress rapidly through this space (in contrast to subdural empyema). The pathogenesis and etiology are similar to those described for subdural empyema, with sinusitis the most frequently described predisposing cause. Extension of infection from osteomyelitis of the sinuses, orbits, or mastoid bone proceeds into the epidural space. Subdural empyema may coexist with the epidural infection. Streptococci and staphylococci are the most frequently cultured pathogens. Hematogenous seeding of cranial epidural abscess is extremely rare.

The clinical presentation includes headache and fever. The predisposing source of infection (i.e., the sinusitis, orbital infection, facial cellulitis, or otic infection) causes most of the clinical complaints. Because of the tight adherence of the dura, the process of infection is characteristically insidious and focal neurological deficits are uncommon. Symptoms of fever and headache can persist for months before a diagnosis is established.

Uncommon complications include retrograde spread of infection to cause meningitis or brain abscess, increasing intracranial pressure with the enlarging abscess mass, and seizures. The diagnostic method of choice is the CT scan or MRI with contrast enhancement. The approach to therapy is similar to that for subdural empyema except that, in most cases, the urgency to drain the lesion is not as great. The

outcome and prognosis are good and most patients who receive appropriate surgical drainage and antibiotic therapy recover fully with few or no sequelae.[106]

SPINAL EPIDURAL ABSCESS

Spinal epidural abscess is an acute suppurative infection in the space external to the dura in the spinal canal. It occurs most commonly in the lower thoracic and lumbar areas. Hematogenously seeded abscesses are usually situated posteriorly and with more axial extension than abscesses located anteriorly (the adherent dura to bone anteriorly inhibits the axial spread). Posterior abscesses involve four to six or more vertebral levels, whereas anterior ones encompass one or two levels less. Anterior lesions are associated with contiguous spread from vertebral osteomyelitis, retropharyngeal abscess, or peritonsillar abscess. In the past, abscesses were more commonly posterior than anterior. Recent reviews suggest an equal frequency.[113] The incidence of spinal epidural abscess is approximately 1 case per 10,000 hospital admissions.

Pathogenesis

Bacteria can enter the epidural space either by direct spread of contiguous infection or by hematogenous seeding from a remote focus of infection. Contiguous spread may occur from vertebral osteomyelitis, infected decubitus ulcerations, retropharyngeal abscesses, and after surgical procedures on the spine (laminectomy, corticosteroid injections). Hematogenous spread is frequently associated with bacteremias from cutaneous (furunculosis), pulmonary, or genitourinary infections and intravenous drug abuse.[114–116]

Approximately 30 percent of cases have no identifiable primary source of infection. Local trauma to the spine has been described in 20 to 30 percent of patients, implicating injured soft tissue or small hematomas as a nidus for bacteremic seeding.[117] The damage to the spinal cord that causes the devastating neurological deficits is a consequence either of direct mechanical compression from the expanding epidural mass or of ischemic injury due to vascular occlusion with thrombosis of the intra- and extramedullary veins. Both mechanisms probably occur; the degree of neurological deficit does not correspond to the size and extent of the lesion as defined neuroradiologically.

Etiology

S. aureus is the predominant pathogen, accounting for up to 60 to 90 percent of all epidural abscesses. Streptococci are also frequently found (10 to 20 percent). Recent studies have noted the importance of aerobic gram-negative bacilli as the cause in 15 to 30 percent of cases.[114,118] This reflects the increasing number of patients in whom intravenous drug abuse leads to primary infection and of older patients with primary genitourinary infections. Postoperative spinal wound infections complicated by epidural abscess are associated mostly with *S. aureus* but also with *S. epidermidis*.[119,120]

Clinical Manifestations

Most patients have a predisposing condition that indicates the source of hematogenous infection (e.g., furunculosis, pneumonia, pyelonephritis, or intravenous drug abuse) or a history of vertebral spine disease or trauma. Back pain and fever are the most common clinical features. They have usually been present for a week or so in most patients. However, acute presentations of 1 to 2 days are described, as are more insidious presentations with symptoms of several weeks' duration. The ultimate outcome and progression of neurological deficits is not predictable or related to the mode of clinical presentation.[114,121,122] The implication is that the manner of presentation (i.e., acute or chronic) should not influence the urgent and aggressive approach to management. Clinical progression has been divided into four stages.[117]

Stage 1: Focal spinal back pain, tenderness, or ache at the level of infection

Stage 2: Nerve root pain, with radiating pain from the spinal level of involvement

Stage 3: Weakness and/or sensory deficits, including neurogenic bowel or bladder

Stage 4: Paralysis

The time it takes to progress from one stage to the next is not predictable in any given patient. Progression may occur over several days or to complete paralysis within hours.[114,121,123–125]

Diagnosis

The peripheral white blood count is frequently elevated. Blood cultures are useful and have been reported to be positive in 50 to 90 percent of cases. The culture of the epidural pus obtained at surgery or by needle aspiration will yield the etiological agent in 90 percent or more of patients. Lumbar puncture is unnecessary and contraindicated in most cases. The possibility of entering the epidural abscess at lumbar puncture is real, and neurological deterioration following lumbar puncture has been described. Lumbar puncture may lead to subdural infection or meningitis if performed through the epidural abscess; it may also create a change in CSF pressure around the spinal cord. The CSF, when obtained, usually has a mild pleocytosis and elevated protein content. Extremely high protein concentrations can reflect complete spinal block. CSF glucose levels are usually normal. Cultures and Gram strains of the CSF rarely yield the diagnosis.

Routine radiographs of the spine cannot establish the diagnosis but may indicate the presence of a predisposing factor like vertebral osteomyelitis. CT scans are helpful in diagnosis in approximately 50 to 70 percent of patients, but CT myelograms are more useful in most cases. With complete spinal block, it may be necessary to do CT myelography both above and below the lesion in order to define the extent of the infection. MRI with gadolinium enhancement is also very useful and may ultimately be the method of choice in defining the lesion. MRI has the advantage of not requiring a lumbar puncture, and it can visualize and characterize the nature and extent of the abscess directly[126] (Fig. 33-2). It is important to emphasize that a CT scan with contrast (but without myelography) may be normal.

Treatment

The optimal approach to management involves the aggressive use of appropriate bactericidal antibiotics for a prolonged period of time combined with urgent surgical intervention to decompress the abscess.

Antibiotics are usually chosen empirically while the results of blood cultures and cultures of the abscess obtained at surgery are awaited. Regimens should be aimed at covering at least *S. aureus* but should also contain antibiotics that cover the aerobic gram-nega-

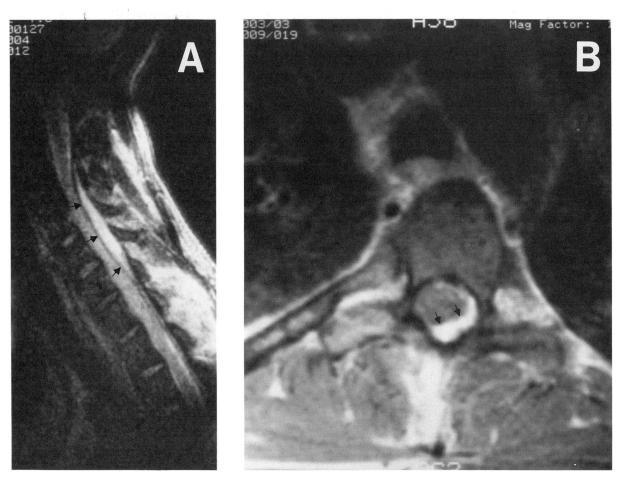

Fig. 33-2 (A) T₂-weighted sagittal image (gradient echo technique) of the cervical spine demonstrates high-signal dorsal epidural collection *(arrows).* The thin low-signal line represents the dura. The high signal reflects proteinaceous material. Note anterior displacement and compression of the cervical cord. **(B)** T₁-weighted contrast-enhanced axial scan demonstrates marked enhancement, again with anterior displacement and compression of the cord.

tive bacilli, especially in those patients with a predisposing factor that is associated with gram-negative bacterial infections (pyelonephritis, the elderly, intravenous drug abusers). Therefore combinations of vancomycin or nafcillin plus a third-generation cephalosporin (i.e., cefotaxime, ceftriaxone, ceftizoxime, *or* ceftazidime, aztreonam, cefoperazone if *Pseudomonas* is suspected) are appropriate initial antimicrobials. After cultures define the etiological agent, the antibiotic regimen should be simplified and directed at the pathogen. The duration of antibiotic treatment is usually 4 to 6 weeks or longer, especially in the presence of a vertebral osteomyelitis.

Almost all patients with spinal epidural abscesses should be considered medical and surgical emergencies. In the presence of neurological deficits (stage 3 or 4) or if progression is occurring, it is imperative that surgical intervention be performed on an emergency basis. The exceptions to this directive are few. In cases where the neurological deficit at stage 4 (paralysis) has been present and unchanging for more than 72 hours, it is unlikely that surgical decompression of the abscess will result in any recovery of function. In this situation, surgery may be indicated to drain the abscess on clinical grounds (pain, persistent fever, sepsis, and leukocytosis).

When patients present with acutely progressive and changing neurological deficits, the need for surgery is urgent. Recovery from these deficits has been observed when surgery is done within 24 hours. Close analysis of individual cases reported in published series indicates that neurogenic weakness or sensory deficits that have been present and stable for 48 hours or more in patients receiving appropriate intravenous antibiotics may nonetheless progress acutely to paralysis. Such observations have prompted some to recommend surgical decompression of all spinal epidural abscesses.

The nonsurgical approach to these lesions has been well described in the literature.[122,127-129] Reasonable criteria that may be used for nonsurgical management of patients include the following:

1. The diagnosis is established before any neurological deficits have occurred.
2. The etiological agent has been identified by blood culture or needle aspiration and the appropriate intravenous antibiotic therapy has been given.
3. The patient has been observed in hospital for at least 2 weeks with no evidence of any neurological change and with no evidence of increasing spinal cord compression or complete block by MRI or CT myelography, and
4. Close expert neurological monitoring is available.

In patients with already established neurological weaknesses or sensory deficits that have been stable for longer than 24 hours and in whom clinical and radiographic improvement has been documented, nonsurgical management may be reasonable.

The use of corticosteroids in the treatment of spinal epidural abscess has not been carefully studied. Anecdotal experiences have indicated its usefulness especially if compression of the cord or the surrounding vascular channels is due to edema and inflammation surrounding the abscess. Dramatic reversal of neurological deficits within 12 to 24 hours has been associated with the administration of dexamethasone (M. B. Edwards, personal communication) and cannot be explained by the effect of antibiotic therapy. It is reasonable to administer dexamethasone for the first 24 to 48 hours of therapy, especially in patients who are being considered for nonsurgical management, who have some neurological deficits to follow, and who have significant edema defined on MRI.

Outcome and Prognosis

From the descriptions above, it is clear that a delay in diagnosis can be associated with a worse outcome, because it may allow progression of neurological deficits and thereby lessen the potential for any recovery that might have been achieved by earlier surgical intervention (less than 24 hours after the onset of the neurological deficit). The clinical stage at presentation correlates with outcome. If paralysis is already present at initial evaluation and has been present for more than 3 days, the prognosis for recovery is grim. Mortality rates of 20 to 30 percent have been reported and are related to several host factors, including underlying disease, age, immune status, and the severity of the predisposing clinical factor.

REFERENCES

1. Niswander KR, Gordon M: The women and their pregnancies: The collaborative perinatal study of the National Institute of Neurological Diseases and Stroke. DHEW Publ. No. NIH 73-379. US Government Printing Office, Washington, DC, 1972
2. Sherry B, Emanuel I, Kronmal RA, et al: Interannual variation of the incidence of Haemophilus influenzae type b meningitis. JAMA 261:1924, 1989
3. Schwartz B, Moore PS, Broome CV: The global epidemiology of meningococcal disease. Clin Microbiol Rev 2:S118, 1989
4. Schlech WF III, Ward JI, Band JD, et al: Bacterial meningitis in the United States, 1978 through 1981: the national bacterial meningitis surveillance study. JAMA 253:1749, 1985
5. Cherubin CE, Marr JS, Sierra MF: Listeria and gram-negative bacillary meningitis in adults. Am J Med 71:199, 1981
6. Heerema MS, Ein ME, Musher DM, et al: Anaerobic bacterial meningitis. Am J Med 67:219, 1979
7. Downs NJ, Hodges GR, Taylor SA: Mixed bacterial meningitis. Rev Infect Dis 9:693, 1987
8. Guerina NG, Langermann S, Clegg HW, et al: Adherence of piliated Haemophilus influenzae type b to human oropharyngeal cells. J Infect Dis 146:564, 1982
9. Stephens DS, McGee ZA: Attachment of Neisseria meningitidis to human mucosal surfaces: influence of pili and type of receptor cell. J Infect Dis 143:525, 1981
10. Stephens DS, Hoffman LH, McGee ZA: Interaction of Neisseria meningitidis with human nasopharyngeal mucosa: attachment and entry into columnar epithelial cells. J Infect Dis 148:369, 1983

11. McGee ZA, Stephens DS, Hoffman LH, et al: Mechanisms of mucosal invasion by pathogenic Neisseria. Rev Infect Dis 5:708S, 1983

12. Plant AG: The IgA 2 proteases of pathogenic bacteria. Annu Rev Microbiol 37:603, 1983

13. Stephens DS, Farley MM: Pathogenic events during infection of the human nasopharynx with Neisseria meningitidis and Hemophilus influenzae. Rev Infect Dis 13:22, 1991

14. Sharief MK, Ciardi M, Thompson EJ: Blood-brain barrier damage in patients with bacterial meningitis: association with tumor necrosis factor-α but not interleukin-1β. J Infect Dis 166:350, 1992

15. Tuomanen E, Saukkonen K, Sande S, et al: Reduction of inflammation, tissue damage, and mortality in bacterial meningitis in rabbits treated with monoclonal antibodies against adhesion-promoting receptors of leukocytes. J Exp Med 170:959, 1989

16. Chan PH, Fishman RA: Brain edema: induction in cortical slices by polyunsaturated fatty acids. Science 201:358, 1978

17. Tureen JH, Stella FB, Clyman RI, et al: Effect of indomethacin on brain water content, cerebrospinal fluid white blood cell response and prostaglandin E_2 levels in cerebrospinal fluid in experimental pneumococcal meningitis in rabbits. Pediatr Infect Dis J 6, suppl: 1151, 1987

18. Horwitz SJ, Boxerbaum B, O'Bell J: Cerebral herniation in bacterial meningitis in childhood. Ann Neurol 7:524, 1980

19. Mustafa MM, Mertsola J, Ramilo O, et al: Increased endotoxin and interleukin-1β concentrations in cerebrospinal fluid of infants with coliform meningitis and ventriculitis associated with intraventricular gentamicin therapy. J Infect Dis 160:891, 1989

20. Friedland IR, Jafari H, Ehrett S, et al: Comparison of endotoxin release by different antimicrobial agents and the effect on the inflammation in experimental E. coli meningitis. J Infect Dis 168:657, 1993

21. Quagliarello V, Scheld WM: Bacterial meningitis: pathogenesis, pathophysiology and progress. N Engl J Med 327:864, 1992

22. Chao CC, Hu S, Close K, et al: Cytokine release from microglia: differential inhibition by pentoxifylline and dexamethasone. J Infect Dis 166:847, 1992

23. Sullivan GW, Carper HT, Novick WJ Jr, Mandell Gl: Inhibition of the inflammatory action of interleukin-1 and tumor necrosis factor (alpha) on neutrophil function by pentoxifylline. Infect Immun 56:1722, 1988

24. Scheld WM, Dacey RC, Wimm HR, et al: Cerebral spinal fluid outflow resistance in rabbits with experimental meningitis: alterations with penicillin and methylprednisolone. J Clin Invest 66:243, 1980

25. Tauber MG, Khayam-Baslir H, Sande MA: Effects of ampicillin and corticosteroids on brain water content, cerebrospinal fluid pressure and cerebrospinal fluid lactate levels in experimental pneumococcal meningitis. J Infect Dis 151:528, 1985

26. Mustafa MM, Ramilo O, Mertsola J, et al: Modulation of inflammation and cachectin activity in relation to treatment of experimental H. influenzae type b meningitis. J Infect Dis 160:818, 1989

27. Lebel MH, Freij BJ, Syrogiannopoulos GA, et al: Dexamethasone therapy for bacterial meningitis: results of two double-blind, placebo controlled trials. N Engl J Med 319:964, 1988

28. McCracken GH Jr, Lebel MH: Dexamethasone therapy for bacterial meningitis in infants and children. Am J Dis Child 143:287, 1989

29. Odio CM, Faingezicht I, Paris M, et al: The beneficial effects of early dexamethasone administration in infants and children with bacterial meningitis. N Engl J Med 324:1525, 1991

30. Glimaker M, Kragsbjerg P, Forsgren M, Olcen P: Tumor necrosis factor-α (TNFα) in cerebrospinal fluid from patients with meningitis of different etiologies: high levels of TNFα indicate bacterial meningitis. J Infect Dis 167:882, 1993

31. Lopez-Cortes LF, Cruz-Ruiz M, Gomez-Mateos J, et al: Measurement of levels of tumor necrosis factor-α and interleukin-1β in the CSF of patients with meningitis of different etiologies: utility in the differential diagnosis. Clin Infect Dis 16:534, 1993

32. Arditi M, Manogue KR, Caplan M, Yogev R: Cerebrospinal fluid cachectin/tumor necrosis factor-α and platelet-activating factor concentrations and severity of bacterial meningitis in children. J Infect Dis 162: 139, 1990

33. Ross D, Rosegay H, Pons V: Differentiation of aseptic and bacterial meningitis in post-operative neurosurgical patients. J Neurosurgery 69:669, 1988

34. Denlinger SL, Obana WG, Ross DA, et al: Cerebrospinal fluid interleukin-1, tumor necrosis factor, and lactate levels in neurosurgical postoperative aseptic and bacterial meningitis. Presented at the annual meeting, American Association of Neurosurgeons, Boston, 1993

35. McGee ZA, Baringer JR: Acute meningitis. p. 742. In Mandell GL, Douglas RG, Bennett JE (eds): Principles and Practice of Infectious Disease. 3rd. Ed. Churchill Livingstone, New York, 1990

36. Kilpi T, Antilla M, Kallio M, et al: Length of prediagnostic history related to the course and sequelae of childhood bacterial meningitis. Pediatr Infect Dis J 12: 184, 1993

37. Radetsky M: Duration of symptoms and outcome in

bacterial meningitis: an analysis of causation and the implications of a delay in diagnosis. Pediatr Infect Dis J 11:694, 1992

38. Carpenter RR, Petersdorf RG: The clinical spectrum of bacterial meningitis. Am J Med 33:262, 1962

39. Geiseler PJ, Nelson KE: Bacterial meningitis without clinical signs of meningeal irritation. South Med J 75: 448, 1982

40. Kaplan SL, Geigin RD: Clinical presentations, prognostic factors and diagnosis of bacterial meningitis. p. 83. In Sande MA, Smith AL, Root RK (eds): Bacterial Meningitis. Churchill Livingstone, New York, 1985

41. Gorse GJ, Thrupp LD, Nudleman KL, et al: Bacterial meningitis in the elderly. Arch Intern Med 144:1603, 1984

42. Lefrock JL, Smith BR: Gram-negative bacillary meningitis in adults. p. 103. In Vinken PJ, Bruyn GW, Klawans HL, Harris AA (eds): Handbook of Clinical Neurology. Vol 52. Elsevier, Amsterdam, 1988

43. Durand ML, Calderwood SB, Weber DJ, et al: Acute bacterial meningitis in adults: a review of 493 episodes. N Engl J Med 328:21, 1993

44. Duffy GP: Lumbar puncture in the presence of raised intracranial pressure. Br Med J 1:407, 1969

45. Duffy GP: Lumbar puncture in spontaneous subarachnoid haemorrhage. Br Med J 285:1163, 1982

46. Garfield J: Management of supratentorial intracranial abscess: a review of 200 cases. Br Med J 2:7, 1969

47. Carey ME, Chou SN, French LA: Experience with brain abscesses. J Neurosurg 36:1, 1972

48. Korein J, Cravisto H, Leicach M: Reevaluation of lumbar puncture: a study of 129 patients with papilledema or intracranial hypertension. Neurology 9: 290, 1959

49. Wilson HD, Haltalin KC: Ampicillin in Haemophilus influenzae meningitis: clinicopharmacologic evaluation of intramuscular vs. intravenous administration. Am J Dis Child 129:208, 1975

50. Feldman WE: Concentrations of bacteria in cerebrospinal fluid of patients with bacterial meningitis. J Pediatr 88:549, 1976

51. Overturf GD, Steinberg EA, Underman AE, et al: Comparative trial of carbenicillin and ampicillin therapy for purulent meningitis. Antimicrob Agents Chemother 11:7420, 1977

52. Barson WJ, Miller MA, Brady MT, Powell DA: Prospective comparative trial of ceftriaxone vs. conventional therapy for treatment of bacterial meningitis in children. Pediatr Infect Dis 4:362, 1985

53. Del Rio MA, Chrane D, Shelton S, et al: Ceftriaxone versus ampicillin and chloramphenicol for treatment of bacterial meningitis in children. Lancet 1:1241, 1983

54. Talan DA, Hoffman JR, Yoshikawa TT, Overturf

GD: Role of empiric parenteral antibiotics prior to lumbar puncture in suspected bacterial meningitis: state of the art. Rev Infect Dis 10:365, 1988

55. Powers WJ: Cerebrospinal fluid lymphocytosis in acute bacterial meningitis. Am J Med 79:216, 1985

56. Kaplan SL: Antigen detection in cerebrospinal fluid—pros and cons. Am J Med 75:109, 1983

57. Hoban DJ, Witwicki E, Hammond GW: Bacterial antigen detection in cerebrospinal fluid of patients with meningitis. Diagn Microbiol Infect Dis 3:373, 1985

58. Dwelle TL, Dunkle LM, Blair L: Correlation of cerebrospinal fluid endotoxinlike activity with clinical and laboratory variables in gram-negative bacterial meningitis in children. J Clin Microbiol 25:856, 1987

59. McCracken GH Jr, Mize SG, Threlkeld N: Intraventricular gentamicin therapy in gram-negative bacillary meningitis of infancy. Lancet 1:787, 1980

60. Friedland I, Klugman K: Failure of chloramphenicol therapy in penicillin-resistant pneumococcal meningitis. Lancet 339:405, 1992

61. Freidland I, Paris M, Ehrett S, et al: Evaluation of antimicrobial regimens for treatment of experimental penicillin-and-cephalosporin-resistant pneumococcal meningitis. Antimicrob Agents Chemother 37:1630, 1993

62. Klass P, Klein J: Therapy of bacterial sepsis, meningitis and otitis media in infants and children: 1992 poll of directors of programs in pediatric infectious diseases. Pediatr Infect Dis 11:702, 1992

63. Fishman RA: Brain edema and disorders of intracranial pressure. p. 262. In Rowland LP (ed): Merritt's Textbook of Neurology. 8th Ed. Lea & Febiger, Philadelphia, 1989

64. Baraff LJ, Lee SI, Schriger DL: Outcomes of bacterial meningitis in children: a meta-analysis. Pediatr Infect Dis 12:389, 1993

65. Hodges GR, Perkins RL: Acute bacterial meningitis: an analysis of factors influencing prognosis. Am J Med Science 270:427, 1975

66. Durand ML, Calderwood SB, Weber DJ, et al: Acute bacterial meningitis in adults: a review of 493 episodes. N Engl J Med 328:21, 1993

67. Wenger JD, Ward JI, Broome CV: Prevention of Haemophilus influenzae type b disease: vaccines and passive prophylaxis. Curr Clin Top Infect Dis 10:306, 1989

68. Scheld WM: Meningococcal diseases. p. 798. In Warren KS, Mahmoud AAF (eds): Tropical and Geographical Medicine. 2nd Ed. McGraw-Hill, New York, 1990

69. Pugsley MP, Dworzack DL, Roccaforte JS, et al: An open study of the efficacy of a single dose of ciprofloxacin in eliminating the chronic nasopharyngeal car-

riage of Neisseria meningitidis. J Infect Dis 157:852, 1988

70. Gaunt PN, Lambert BE: Single-dose ciprofloxacin for the eradication of pharyngeal carriage of Neisseria meningitidis. J Antimicrob Chemother 21:489, 1988

71. Lefrock JL, Smith BR: Gram-negative bacillary meningitis in adults. p. 103. In Vinken PJ, Bruyn GW, Klawans HL, Harris AA (eds): Handbook of Clinical Neurology. Vol 52. Elsevier, Amsterdam, 1988

72. Schwartz B, Al-Tobaiqi A, Al-Ruwais A, et al: Comparative efficacy of ceftriaxone and rifampicin in eradicating carriage of group A Neisseria meningitidis. Lancet 1:1239, 1988

73. Macewen W: Pyogenic infective diseases of the brain and spinal cord. J Maclehose & Sons, Glasgow, 1893

74. Mampalam TJ, Rosenblum ML: Trends in the management of bacterial brain abscesses: a review of 102 cases over 17 years. Neurosurgery 23:451, 1988

75. Schliamser SE, Backman K, Norrby SR: Intracranial abscesses in adults: an analysis of 54 consecutive cases. Scand J Infect Dis 20:1, 1988

76. Small M, Dale BAB: Intracranial suppuration 1968–1982—a 15-year review. Clin Otolaryngol 9: 315, 1984

77. Bradley PJ, Manning KPP, Shaw MDM: Brain abscess secondary to paranasal sinusitis. J Laryngol Otol 98:719, 1984

78. Pruitt AA, Rubin RH, Karchmer AW, Duncan GW: Neurologic complications of bacterial endocarditis. Medicine (Baltimore) 57:329, 1978

79. Fischbein CA, Rosenthal A, Gischer EG, et al: Risk factors for brain abscess in patients with congenital heart disease. Am J Cardiol 34:97, 1974

80. Britt RH: Brain abscess. p. 1928. In Wilkins RH, Rengachary SS (eds): Neurosurgery. McGraw-Hill, New York, 1985

81. Rosenblum ML, Mampalam TJ, Pons VG: Controversies in the management of brain abscess. Clin Neurosurg 33:603, 1986

82. Morgan H, Wood M, Murphey F: Experience with 88 consecutive cases of brain abscess. J Neurosurg 38: 698, 1973

83. Samson DS, Clark K: A current review of brain abscess. Am J Med 54:201, 1973

84. Garfield J: Brain abscess and focal suppurative infection. p. 107. In Vinken PJ, Bruyn GW (eds): Handbook of Clinical Neurology. Vol 33. North-Holland, Amsterdam, 1979

85. Chun CH, Johnson JD, Hofstetter M, Raff MJ: Brain abscess: a study of 45 consecutive cases. Medicine (Baltimore) 65:415, 1986

86. Shaw MDM, Russell JA: Cerebellar abscess—a review of 47 cases. J Neurol Neurosurg Psychiatry 38: 429, 1975

87. Rosenblum ML, Hoff JT, Norman D, et al: Decreased mortality from brain abscesses since advent of computerized tomography. J Neurosurg 49:658, 1978

88. Rehncrona S, Brismar J, Holtas S: Diagnosis of brain abscesses with indium-111-labeled leukocytes. Neurosurgery 16:23, 1985

89. Runge VM, Clanton JA, Price AC, et al: Evaluation of contrast-enhanced MR imaging in a brain-abscess model. AJNR 6:139, 1985

90. Grossman RI, Joseph PM, Wolf G, et al: Experimental intracranial septic infarction: magnetic resonance enhancement. Radiology 155:649, 1985

91. Zimmerman RD, Haimes AB: The role of MR imaging in the diagnosis of infections of the central nervous system. Curr Clin Top Infect Dis 10:82, 1989

92. Davidson MD, Steiner RE: Magnetic resonance imaging in infections of the central nervous system. AJNR 6:499, 1985

93. Rosenblum ML, Hoff JT, Norman DA, et al: Nonoperative treatment of brain abscess in selected high risk patients. J Neurosurg 52:217, 1980

94. Sjolin J, Eriksson N, Arneborn P, Cars O: Penetration of cefotaxime and desacetylcefotaxime into brain abscesses in humans. Antimicrob Agent Chemother 35: 2606, 1991

95. Beller AJ, Sahar A, Praiss I: Brain abscess: review of 89 cases over 30 years. J Neurol Neurosurg Psychiatry 36:757, 1973

96. Morgan H, Wood M, Murphy F: Experience with 88 consecutive cases of brain abscess. J Neurosurg 38: 698, 1973

97. Samson DS, Clark K: A current review of brain abscess. Am J Med 54:201, 1973

98. Ballantine HJ, White JC: Brain abscess: influence of the antibiotic on therapy and morbidity. N Engl J Med 248:14, 1953

99. Alderson D, Strong AJ, Ingham HR, et al: Fifteen year review of the mortality of brain abscess. Neurosurgery 8:1, 1981

100. Gruszkiewicz J, Doron Y, Peyser E, et al: Brain abscess and its surgical management. Surg Neurol 18: 7, 1982

101. Carey ME, Chow SN, French LA: Experience with brain abscesses. J Neurosurg 36:1, 1972

102. Carey ME, Chou SN, French LA: Long-term neurological residua in patients surviving brain abscess with surgery. J Neurosurg 34:652, 1971

103. Jooma OV, Pennybacker JB, Tutton GK: Brain abscess: aspiration, drainage, or excision? J Neurol Neurosurg Psychiatry 14:308, 1951

104. Legg NJ, Gupta PC, Scott DF: Epilepsy following cerebral abscess: a clinical and EEG study of 70 patients. Brain 96:259, 1973

105. Ariza J, Casanova A, Viladrich F, et al: Etiological agent and primary source of infection in 42 cases of focal intracranial suppuration. J Clin Microb 24:899, 1986

106. Silverberg AL, DiNubile MJ: Subdural empyema and cranial epidural abscess. Med Clin North Am 69:361, 1985

107. Jacobson Pl, Farmer TW: Subdural empyema complicating meningitis in infants: improved prognosis. Neurology 31:190, 1981

108. Helfgott DC, Weingarten K, Hartman BJ: Subdural empyema. p. 490. In Scheld WM, Whitley RJ, Durack DT (eds): Infections of the Central Nervous System. Raven Press, New York, 1991

109. Mauser HW, Tulleken CA: Subdural empyema. Clin Neurol Neurosurg 86:255, 1984

110. Khan M, Griebel R: Subdural empyema: a retrospective study of 15 patients. Can J Surg 27:283, 1984

111. Coonrod JD, Dans PE: Subdural empyema. Am J Med 53:85, 1972

112. Kaufman DM, Miller MH, Steigbigel NH: Subdural empyema: analysis of 17 recent cases and review of the literature. Medicine (Baltimore) 54:485, 1975

113. Hlavin ML, Kaminski HJ, Ross JS, Ganz E: Spinal epidural abscess: a ten year perspective. Neurosurgery 27:177, 1990

114. Darouiche RO, Hamill RJ, Greenberg SB, et al: Bacterial spinal epidural abscess: review of 43 cases and literature survey. Medicine (Baltimore) 71:369, 1992

115. Kaufman DM, Kaplan JG, Litman N: Infectious agents in spinal epidural abscess. Neurology 30:844, 1980

116. Baker AS, Ojemann RG, Swartz MN, et al: Spinal epidural abscess. N Engl J Med 293:463, 1975

117. Heusner AP: Nontuberculous spinal epidural infections. N Engl J Med 239:845, 1948

118. Jabbari B, Pierce JF: Spinal cord compression due to Pseudomonas in a heroin addict. Neurology 27:1034, 1977

119. Brian JE Jr, Westerman GR, Chadduck WM: Septic complications of chemonucleolysis. Neurosurgery 15:730, 1984

120. Loarie DJ, Fairley HB: Epidural abscess following spinal anesthesia. Anesth Analg 57:351, 1978

121. Danner RL, Hartman BJ: Update of spinal epidural abscess: 35 cases and review of the literature. Rev Infect Dis 9:265, 1987

122. Wheeler D, Keiser P, Rigamonti D, Keay S: Medical management of spinal epidural abscesses: case report and review. Clin Infect Dis 15:22, 1992

123. Baker AS, Ojemann RG, Swartz MN, Richardson EP Jr: Spinal epidural abscess. N Engl J Med 293:463, 1975

124. Phillips GE, Jefferson A: Acute spinal epidural abscess: observations from fourteen cases. Postgrad Med J 55:712, 1979

125. Simpson RK Jr, Azordegan PA, Sirbasku DM, et al: Rapid onset of quadriplegia from a panspinal epidural abscess. Spine 16:1002, 1991

126. Post MJD, Sze G, Quencer RM, et al: Gadolinium-enhanced MR in spinal infection. J Comput Assist Tomogr 14:721, 1990

127. Leys D, Lesoin F, Viaud C, et al: Decreased morbidity from acute bacterial spinal epidural abscesses using computed tomography and nonsurgical treatment in selected patients. Ann Neurol 17:350, 1985

128. Hanigan WC, Asner NG, Elwood PW: Magnetic resonance imaging and the nonoperative treatment of spinal epidural abscess. Surg Neurol 34:408, 1990

129. Mampalam TJ, Rosegay H, Andrews BT, et al: Nonoperative treatment of spinal epidural infections. J Neurosurg 71:208, 1989

34

Neurological Manifestations of Spirochetal Infections

Andrew R. Pachner

[The spirochetes] . . . may live in the body as long as the host is alive . . . they cause the production of antibodies in the tissues and it seems possible that with time a strain of spirochetes may result with greater resistance but perhaps less power of reproduction. The infection then does not cause any active symptoms, but may persist indefinitely in a latent form to resume activity after a long interval of quiescence.

Osler and McCrae: *The Principles and Practice of Medicine,* 9th ed., 1923, p. 269

The study of neurological manifestations of spirochetal infections continues to be an exercise in speculation and wonderment. Much has occurred in the field over the past 70 years, such as the development of antibiotics and the recognition of Lyme disease, but our understanding of the neurotropism of spirochetes and the latency of spirochetal infections has changed little. In fact, instead of the picture becoming more simplified and straightforward, the occurrence of new intercurrent chronic infections, such as acquired immunodeficiency syndrome (AIDS), the widespread use of antibiotics, and the rising incidence of Lyme disease are increasing the complexity of the neurological presentations of spirochetal infections. This chapter reviews the well-established and the changing features of neurosyphilis and summarizes current knowledge concerning neurological involvement in Lyme disease. In many ways these two diseases be-

have similarly, and these similarities are noted. Spirochetal infections such as relapsing fever and leptospirosis that are rare in the United States are not discussed.

NEUROSYPHILIS

. . . clear-cut classic forms of the disease are increasingly uncommon, and atypical or mixed manifestations are often seen.[1]

The universal fear and respect for syphilis felt by physicians during the first half of the twentieth century has disappeared in today's era of powerful antibiotics. Yet the incidence of syphilis has actually increased since 1958. It is estimated that there are currently more than one-half million untreated cases (all stages of the disease) in the United States. The incidence of new cases has risen particularly among homosexual men.[2]

Etiology and Pathogenesis

Treponema pallidum belongs to the family Treponemataceae, which includes *Treponema, Borrelia,* and *Leptospira.* This group of organisms shares the attribute of being able to propel themselves by spinning around their longitudinal axis. The lack of success thus far in finding a suitable culture medium for *T. pallidum* has significantly hindered our progress in understanding this organism.

The spirochete is known from both animal experiments and clinical experience to be highly neurotropic. Approximately 20 percent of patients with symptomatic primary syphilis have an increase in cells in the cerebrospinal fluid (CSF),[3] and the number of persons with an abnormal CSF is even higher among those who are asymptomatic during the first 2 years after infection. Thus, because fewer than 10 percent of untreated luetics develop neurosyphilis, most individuals with *T. pallidum* invasion of the brain must somehow clear the infection spontaneously. In those who develop tertiary syphilis, the long latency of infection dictates that the organisms lie dormant for years prior to "activation." The factors that control susceptibility, resistance and latency, and activation are unknown but probably have an immunogenetic basis.

It has been stressed that all forms of neurosyphilis begin as meningitis, and some believe that all the subsequent damage to the nervous system is due to the chronic meningitis and its effects on the vessels.[4] The meningitis is usually asymptomatic but can result in symptoms similar to those of other subacute meningitides—for example, headache, stiff neck, and cranial nerve palsies (see Syphilic Meningitis, below). The pathology of some chronic meningitic processes (e.g., tuberculosis, cryptococcosis) sometimes mimics the findings in neurosyphilis, with thrombotic endarteritis, meningomyceloencephalitis, and ependymitis. Of course, with tertiary parenchymal neurosyphilis, there is significant infection of brain with spirochetes,[5] and it seems probable that this infiltration with organisms and the subsequent inflammation lead to impaired function. The proportional contribution in any particular case of parenchymal inflammation due to infection as opposed to chronic vascular changes due to the basilar meningitis is difficult to determine.

Thus the "early" syndromes of symptomatic syphilitic meningitis and meningovascular syphilis can merge, as can the latter process with the "late" syndromes of general paresis and tabes dorsalis. Of course, asymptomatic neurosyphilis can be found at any point after infection. In the summary of these syndromes below, clinical findings are described for each type of neurosyphilis, and CSF and serological evaluation of each is reviewed.

Clinical Manifestations

ASYMPTOMATIC NEUROSYPHILIS

The identification of asymptomatic neurosyphilis usually derives from the presence of another manifestation of syphilis or a positive serology. The importance of obtaining CSF for analysis in cases of untreated or inadequately treated syphilis cannot be overly stressed, as most patients with untreated asymptomatic neurosyphilis progress to later symptomatic neurological involvement. Reports in the literature have questioned the adequacy of some of the current therapeutic regimens for primary and secondary syphilis; thus the most aggressive approach to detect asymptomatic neurosyphilis would be to perform a lumbar puncture on all patients with a history of syphilis, regardless of whether treated. This matter remains controversial because the chances of inadequacy with currently recommended treatment as well as the risks of lumbar puncture are low. Perhaps an appropriate compromise is to perform a lumbar puncture on those patients "adequately" treated for primary or secondary syphilis only if they are more likely to be treatment failures, such as those with human immunodeficiency virus (HIV) infection (see below).

SYPHILITIC MENINGITIS

Syphilitic meningitis is often classified as "early" neurosyphilis because it usually occurs within the first few years after infection. Symptoms consist of headache, stiff neck, cranial nerve palsies, and occasionally confusion. Fever is unusual. Usually this meningitis is self-limited, lasting weeks to months, with no apparent sequelae except for the rare occurrence of hydrocephalus. As is true for other spontaneously regressing stages of this illness, the active infection with *T. pallidum*, if not treated, continues and reexpresses itself as another form of neurosyphilis.

MENINGOVASCULAR SYPHILIS

The stage known as meningovascular syphilis classically appears 1 to 10 years after infection. It probably represents the clinical manifestation of the involvement of arteries that occurs in all patients with the chronic meningitis of syphilis. Symptoms of cerebral and spinal involvement may coexist in the same patient. Cerebral involvement may be localized or diffuse. It may lead to seizures, intellectual changes, isolated or multiple cranial neuropathies, or the sudden onset of a focal neurological deficit such as a hemiplegia. Spinal involvement may lead to pyramidal deficits, sensory disturbance, or rarely an anterior spinal artery syndrome. The pathology in this stage of the disease includes not only inflammation of the vessels but also significant fibrosis, with narrowing and occlusion, a combination called *Heubner's arteritis*. The vessel most commonly involved is the middle cerebral artery.[6]

Some investigators believe that neurosyphilis more commonly presents with meningovascular involvement today than it did 50 years ago[7]; certainly neurosyphilis, because it can be treated, must always be considered in the differential diagnosis of vascular disease in the young. For example, a recent report documented the occurrence of basis pontis infarction causing pure motor hemiplegia in two young men with meningovascular syphilis.[8]

GENERAL PARESIS

General paresis and tabes dorsalis are considered late manifestations because the time between initial infection and these stages is usually one to three decades. Although the two can and do occur together, they are different enough to be considered separately. Pathologically, general paresis is a chronic, progressive frontotemporal encephalitis in which there is meningeal thickening, gliosis, cortical atrophy, perivascular inflammation, and occasionally meningeal fibrosis. Although its incidence does not approach that in the preantibiotic era, during which it accounted for about 10 percent of psychiatric admissions, new cases continue to appear in community mental health clinics.[9] The symptoms frequently are not different from those of patients with Alzheimer's disease, and examination does not generally add distinguishing characteristics except for the common occurrence in general paresis of pupillary disturbances and tremor. Other clinical accompaniments may include focal or generalized seizures, dysarthria, optic atrophy, and pyramidal deficits, especially at an advanced stage of the disease. However, the primary clinical manifestation of general paresis is a progressive dementia, often with emotional lability and changes in affect.

TABES DORSALIS

The clinical hallmark of tabes dorsalis is the symptom of lightning pains. These pains often occur in bouts, resulting in jabbing, lancinating pain, frequently in the legs. Sometimes the involvement is visceral, leading to the mistaken diagnosis of an acute abdomen. The primary area of involvement is probably the posterior nerve root as it enters the spinal cord. The neurological findings, as one might predict, are the loss of peripheral sensation and occasionally loss of sensory aspects of bladder and genital function. Sensory ataxia can also occur and is one of the symptom triad of lightning pains, dysuria, and ataxia that is associated with a classical triad of signs (Argyll-Robertson pupils, areflexia, ataxia). The combination is of diagnostic importance.

FORMES FRUSTES

In recent years some clinicians have thought that the clinical manifestations of neurosyphilis have changed and that the probable cause of this change has been the widespread use of oral antibiotics. In a study of 241 patients published in 1972,[10] patients most often came to the attention of neurologists because of an incidental finding of a positive fluorescent treponemal antibody absorption test (FTA-ABS) in blood during evaluation for a problem unrelated to the nervous system. In another review of "postantibiotic era" experience with neurosyphilis in Copenhagen,[11] two points of particular importance emerged: (1) The most common presentation was with personality changes, dementia, or both; and (2) a significant percentage of patients who subsequently developed neurosyphilis had received recommended doses of antibiotics for treatment of their primary lesions. By contrast, Wolters studied retrospectively two groups of patients with neurosyphilis admitted to the University of Amsterdam Hospital, one between 1920 and 1940 and the other between 1970 and 1984, and found no marked differences in clinical manifestations between the two groups.[12]

COMBINED *TREPONEMA PALLIDUM* AND HIV INFECTION AND THE ROLE OF CELL-MEDIATED IMMUNITY IN SYPHILIS

Another cause of a change in the usual presentation of neurosyphilis in some patients has been the concomitant presence of infection with the HIV virus, which results in impaired cell-mediated immunity. The contribution of cell-mediated immunity in protection against spirochetal infection is unknown. Four cases of neurosyphilis in anti-HIV antibody-positive patients were treated at the Massachusetts General Hospital in 1985 and 1986; they were notable for the development of neurosyphilis in an accelerated fashion or after recommended treatment for secondary syphilis.[13] Similarly, a case of meningovascular syphilis in a 26-year-old anti-HIV antibody-positive man occurred 5 months after recommended treatment for secondary syphilis.[14] Recent work by Berger and his colleagues has emphasized that the course of neurosyphilis is more aggressive and that syphilitic meningitis and ophthalmic disease are more common in HIV-infected patients than non-HIV-infected controls.[15–19]

On the basis of this clinical experience, the prediction might be that, in an experimental system, interference with T-cell function produces a more malignant form of syphilis. This has, in fact, not proved uniformly to be the case. In an interesting experimental study, Pavia found that guinea pigs depleted of T cells by thymectomy, irradiation, and replacement with syngeneic bone marrow cells did not have increased susceptibility to the development of syphilitic skin lesions.[20] A number of recent studies in experimental animals have documented that *T. pallidum*-immune immunoglobulin G is protective against reinfection,[21–23] although the presence of high-titer antibody does not seem to affect the spread or number of organisms in regional lymph nodes. There is thus a discrepancy between the human and experimental situations in the effects of defects in cell-mediated immunity. It is most likely due to the difference between activation of latent central nervous system (CNS) infection (human neurosyphilis) and the primary lesions resulting from a new induced infection (the experimental models), but it may also be due to fundamental differences in the way that humans and animals mount immune responses to treponemes.

Diagnosis

CEREBROSPINAL FLUID

Although a number of authors have suggested that lumbar punctures are done too often,[24,25] it is impossible to care for a patient with suspected neurosyphilis without having the CSF findings. The abnormalities found in the CSF of patients with neurosyphilis are as follows:

1. Elevated number of white blood cells (WBCs), predominantly lymphocytes or monocytes
2. Elevated protein concentration
3. Positive VDRL

The presence of abnormal CSF in a seropositive patient with neurological involvement essentially mandates treatment for neurosyphilis. It is unclear if the diagnosis should be made in the presence of normal CSF. For instance, in a study of 30 patients with neurosyphilis at the University of Michigan Hospital,[7] the diagnosis was made on the basis of a positive FTA-ABS and at least one of the abnormalities of the CSF listed above. The authors excluded from the study three patients with neurological problems but normal CSF. It is of interest that these authors commented on the benignity of the CSF in their patients compared with syphilitic patients during the preantibiotic era. For instance, 62 percent of the modern syphilitics had normal cell counts, whereas in previous times patients typically had 25 to 2,000 WBCs/mm^3. In addition, CSF protein concentrations now seem be much lower in neurosyphilis, with most being in the range of 46 to 100 mg/dl. The CSF VDRL was once thought to be almost universally positive in neurosyphilis, but a negative test definitely does not exclude the diagnosis. A positive CSF VDRL, however, does aid in confirmation.[26]

Thus a number of forces have combined to change the way in which neurosyphilis is diagnosed. Prior to 1920, the diagnosis was made clinically on the basis of a history of previous stages of the illness and a characteristic neurological syndrome accompanied by evidence in the CSF of inflammation. The advent of reaginic tests helped, particularly in the diagnosis of primary and secondary syphilis but less so in neurosyphilis. The advent of both antibiotics and specific serological tests (e.g., FTA-ABS or *T. pallidum* immobilization—TPI) has led to dramatic changes in the diagnosis and management of the disease. Because late neurosyphilis generally appears at least 10 years after initial infection, the full impact of these changes on diagnosis and treatment cannot yet be assessed. Needless to say, it is desirable to eradicate the illness as soon as possible, without waiting for characteristic clinical findings or even CSF abnormalities. Thus specific serology has attained great diagnostic importance in this disease, in which the means of diagnosis usually used for bacterial illness (i.e., culture and visualization on biopsy) have proved unsuccessful. Because serology can remain positive for years after eradication of the infection either spontaneously (only a few cases of untreated syphilis progress to neurosyphilis) or with antibiotics, it cannot be used as a means of diagnosing active infection. Thus the activity of the infection must be assessed clinically or by CSF analysis. These criteria are not flawless, as a number of disease processes other than neurosyphilis that are difficult to diagnose can cause neurological involvement and CSF abnormalities in seropositive patients. In addition, the situation is made even more complex by the perceived risk of missing treatable illness by relying on "classic" clinical and CSF findings, given that clinical manifestations of neurosyphilis may be changing and the CSF may be less abnormal than previously. Because the risk of treatment with intravenous antibiotics is low, it is reasonable to treat seropositive patients who have neurological findings that may be consistent with neurosyphilis, especially if the patient has not previously been treated with antibiotics. Some investigators require the presence of CSF abnormalities for the diagnosis,[2] whereas others do not. Clearly, the diagnosis is optimally made in the presence of clinical findings consistent with the disease and CSF abnormalities in a seropositive patient. Resolution with appropriate treatment also confirms the diagnosis.

More accurate diagnostic tests of neurosyphilis have recently been a subject of intense laboratory investigation. The CSF of patients with active neurosyphilis contains spirochetes that, when injected into experimental animals, transfer the infection. The rabbit infectivity test (RIT), in which CSF from patients with presumed neurosyphilis is injected into rabbit testicles, has come to be considered a "gold standard" for the diagnosis of neurosyphilis, since its specificity is great for detection of the presence of live, infective spirochetes.[27] Another diagnostic assay recently developed is the polymerase chain reaction (PCR) assay,

in which the small amount of specific *T. pallidum* DNA present in the CSF is amplified, using bacterial DNA polymerase, and detected, usually using either gel electrophoresis or hybridization with a specific probe.[28] A recent study of congenital syphilis compared a variety of assays of the CSF to RIT and PCR and found that RIT and PCR correlated quite well.[29] However, in infants in whom CNS invasion might have been predicted (i.e., positive serum IgM antibody with pleocytosis and raised protein concentration in the CSF), RIT and PCR were negative. Neither of these assays is available at this time to most clinicians, and their sensitivity and specificity for a broad range of specimens have not yet been determined. However, these approaches are very important in that they represent a new class of assays for neurosyphilis that test specifically for the presence of the organism rather than antibody.

Treatment

Many clinicians will accept nonstringent criteria for the diagnosis of neurosyphilis, since treatment is relatively benign and the risk of progression and permanent injury without treatment is significant. However, there continues to be no standard, well-accepted therapy for neurosyphilis. Ideally, treatment would result in treponemicidal levels of drug within the CSF. One of the schedules recommended by the US Public Health Service, 0.6 million units of procaine penicillin, has been found to be unsuccessful in achieving treponemicidal levels in the CSF, even when probenecid was added.[30] By contrast, there is evidence that intravenous penicillin 0.15 million IU/kg/d for 15 days results in continuous treponemicidal levels in the CSF.[31,32] Because 20 million U/d is tolerated well in most adults, it is frequently the dose employed, for both neurosyphilis and Lyme disease. Cephalosporins with good penetration into the brain, such as ceftriaxone, may also have a role.

LYME NEUROBORRELIOSIS

Lyme disease was initially described in 1977 as Lyme arthritis by Steere and associates.[33] The characteristic feature of this arthritis was a relapsing-remitting oligoarticular inflammation, usually involving the knee or the hip, signaled in all cases by the previous appearance of a characteristic rash, erythema chronicum migrans. The spectrum of the disease was soon broadened to include neurological and cardiac involvement.[34] Since the identification of the causative organisms in 1982[35,36] and the development of a serological assay for the presence of antibodies to the organism shortly thereafter,[37] it has become clear that a number of syndromes in Europe are due to Lyme disease. The most common of these syndromes is a painful radiculoneuritis, called Garin-Bujadoux meningopolyneuritis or Bannwarth's syndrome, described in 1922 in France and 1941 in Germany. Erythema chronicum migrans, the characteristic acute skin rash, had first been described in Sweden by Afzelius in 1909. A chronic skin lesion that sometimes lasts for decades, called acrodermatitis atrophicans and first described in 1883 in Germany, is also due to Lyme disease, but it seems to be much less common in the United States than in Europe. These syndromes are described in depth below, but their presence for decades in Europe prior to the description of Lyme disease suggests that the organism was originally in Europe and made its way secondarily to the United States.

Causative Organism

Borrelia burgdorferi is a spirochete that was first described by Burgdorfer in 1982. The finding of the organism in the midgut of the tick *Ixodes dammini* was serendipitous.[38] Burgdorfer was actually investigating this insect as a possible vector of Rocky Mountain spotted fever, because the usual vector, *Dermacentor variabilis,* on Long Island was negative for *Rickettsia rickettsii.* Irregularly coiled spirochetes were found in 75 of 124 ticks dissected. Burgdorfer immediately speculated that these organisms might be the causative agent of erythema chronicum migrans and Lyme disease, as the association between ixodid ticks and these illnesses was known. It has since become clear that Lyme disease and its European counterparts, Bannwarth's syndrome and acrodermatitis, are caused by the same organism.

The organism is a *Borrelia* by DNA homology and by morphological and biochemical criteria and is antigenically related to treponemes. Strains differ in respect to DNA homology, plasmid content, and to some extent serology. Forty-five isolates from ticks, infected animals, and patients from three European countries (Switzerland, West Germany, and Sweden) and six states in the United States (Connecticut, New Jersey, New York, Minnesota, California, and Texas) were recently analyzed for reactivity by immunofluorescence with three monoclonal antibodies.[39] There were five patterns of reactivity. Simple sodium dodecyl sulfate (SDS) polyacrylamide gel electrophoresis of 23 strains from southern Germany revealed nine patterns.[40] There are also considerable ultrastructural differences among various isolates of *Borrelia burgdorferi;* 11 strains were examined, and there were significant differences in length, wavelength, width, and number of flagella in the organisms.[41] Thus there seems to be considerable heterogeneity in the major surface proteins expressed by *B. burgdorferi;* this may reflect not only a variety of strains of the spirochete but also the ability of a strain within an infected animal to change its surface proteins in a manner similar to that demonstrated for *Borrelia hermsii.*[42] If further studies show that this organism can undergo antigenic variation, this phenomenon may explain its ability to remain alive and latent within humans who have high specific antibody titers.

Experimental models of Lyme borreliosis have been established in a variety of animals, with the best ones being in mice, rats, and hamsters.[43–49] In murine Lyme borreliosis, infection intradermally with 10 to 100 spirochetes from infective strains results in chronic infection of the skin, heart, and bladder and development of specific antibody and positive Western blot. PCR has been found to be more sensitive than culture for detection of the spirochete in infected tissue.[45] Interestingly, PCR can detect persistent *Borrelia* in culture-negative brain of infected mice for months after infection, although the spirochete load in heart and bladder is greater than in brain. It is conceivable that the PCR positivity represents relatively transient infection; alternatively, brain infection could be chronic, as in the mouse heart, in which the organism remains for the life of the animal. Murine Lyme borreliosis is an excellent model for human Lyme disease in that infection and inflammation are chronic and the *Borrelia* antigens recognized during the development of the antibody response are similar.

In the murine model of Lyme borreliosis, the spirochete has a predilection for blood vessels and interstitium and is frequently found wrapped in collagen fibrils.[50,51] In animals infected for more than a few months, the spirochete is commonly found within cardiac myocytes.[51] The finding of *B. burgdorferi* within cells during infection in vivo and in vitro[52] indicates that antibiotics or specific antibody circulating in the blood may have difficulty completely clearing spirochetes in chronic infection.

Clinical Manifestations

It is likely that most humans bitten by a tick infected with *B. burgdorferi* do not get Lyme disease. The explanation for this fact may lie in the presence of spirochetocidal activity in normal serum from uninfected humans, as has been reported for syphilis; thus individuals who become infected after exposure may have less of such activity in their serum. Alternatively, the difference may lie in the individual-to-individual variation of the potency of the antispirochete immune response in dealing with the infection, an attribute probably controlled by immune response genes. Finally, the differences in probability of infection may relate not to immunity to *B. burgdorferi* at all, but to immunity to the tick vector. Thus most patients who present with a history of a tick bite have not been infected with *B. burgdorferi,* even in areas highly endemic for Lyme disease.

Lyme disease has been divided into three stages, depending on type of clinical manifestation and time after initial infection. These stages can be thought of as occurring days to weeks (first stage), weeks to months (second stage) and months to years (third stage) after the infecting bite by the *Ixodes* tick. The stages can overlap, and later stages may occur without the occurrence of earlier stages. For instance, Lyme arthritis, a third-stage manifestation, can occur without any previous symptom or sign of Lyme disease.

First stage. This stage occurs almost exclusively during the warm weather months, mostly July and August. There is a "flu-like" illness frequently accompanied by the characteristic skin rash, erythema chronicum migrans. In about one-half to two-thirds of patients with this rash, a tick or tick bite is found. The rash can be cured and progression of the disease halted with oral tetracycline. Erythromycin and penicillin are also successful, but a small percentage (2 to 6 percent) of patients treated with these antibiotics develop Lyme meningitis.[53]

Second stage. The most common neurological manifestation occurs during the second stage of the disease, a few weeks to a few months after the initial infection,

and consists of a subacute or chronic meningitis.[54] Because infection with *B. burgdorferi* generally occurs during the late spring or summer, Lyme meningitis usually is a disease of summer or early fall. The first symptoms frequently occur when the rash is still present, although there is often an asymptomatic hiatus between the first and second stages. The most common symptoms are headache and stiff neck, although they are often mild. "Encephalitic" symptoms such as poor memory, irritability, difficulty concentrating, and emotional lability are common. Because these symptoms are often mild, and because Lyme meningitis usually clears spontaneously on its own, it is probable that a significant number of patients do not recognize their illness as serious and thus do not seek medical attention. Because patients with untreated Lyme meningitis are at risk for developing later complications of *B. burgdorferi* infection, it is crucial to identify the infection at this stage even in patients whose symptoms are minimal.

Cranial nerve palsies are common in Lyme meningitis, and it is almost always the seventh nerve that is involved, either unilaterally or bilaterally. Among 951 patients with Lyme disease, 124 cases of seventh nerve palsy were identified and retrospectively evaluated.[55] Almost all presented during the summer or early fall months. A few patients had facial palsy without meningitis, but in those patients undergoing lumbar punctures, most (84 percent) had a lymphocytic pleocytosis in the CSF. The erythrocyte sedimentation rate was increased in 77 percent of these patients. Treatment did not affect the time to resolution of the paralysis, with both treated and untreated patients experiencing return of function within a mean of 3 to 4 weeks after diagnosis. Of 38 patients with Lyme meningitis, 19 had a seventh nerve palsy, which in 7 was bilateral.[54]

Involvement of the peripheral nervous system is common, being seen in about one-third of patients. The extent and type of peripheral nerve manifestations of this illness are controversial. For instance, some authors find a predominantly demyelinating neuropathy, with slowed conduction velocities and prolonged distal latencies,[56] whereas others describe an axonal neuropathy on the basis of nerve biopsies and the electrophysiological findings.[57] Clinically, especially in European *B. burgdorferi* infections, the predominant symptom is often not sensory disturbances or motor weakness but severe radicular pain, indicating probable root involvement. The radicular pain may occur in the distribution of any root and may be unilateral or bilateral. This "radiculitis" is the major symptom of Bannwarth's syndrome, also called Garin-Bujadoux syndrome, the predominant European form of neurological Lyme borreliosis. The pathogenesis of the radiculitis may be similar to that of tabes dorsalis, although as yet there are no pathological studies available.

Lumbar puncture in patients with Lyme meningitis reveals a lymphocytic pleocytosis in the CSF and frequently an elevated protein concentration. Some patients with only cranial nerve findings may have a normal CSF.[55,58] Other laboratory abnormalities of the CSF indicative of inflammatory disease within the subarachnoid space are frequently also present—for example, oligoclonal bands and an elevated immunoglobulin G (IgG)/albumin ratio. Some investigators have claimed that selective concentration of specific anti-B. burgdorferi antibody is particularly helpful for confirming CNS involvement in Lyme meningitis[59,60]; our experience has been that although there is usually some selective concentration, especially in Lyme meningitis, there is enough of an overlap with normal values that the test cannot be used diagnostically. With late CNS involvement, when there is little inflammatory response in CSF obtained by lumbar puncture, there is frequently no evidence of selective concentration.

Third stage. Arthritis, dermatitis, or CNS disease[61] may occur many months to years after the initial infection. The ability of B. burgdorferi to live for prolonged periods in the human has been demonstrated by culturing organisms from 10-year-old acrodermatitis lesions. Although the organism has been detected in joints and brain, it is not clear whether most of the involvement is due to direct infection or parainfectious immune events. The positive response of some patients with arthritis and CNS involvement to intravenous antibiotics is some evidence for an infectious etiology of these manifestations. Neurological manifestations of the third stage include chronic or subacute encephalitis, symptoms of "psychiatric" disease, or clinical evidence of focal disease of the brain that can have a demyelinative basis.[62] Six patients with these manifestations of CNS disease have been described in detail.[63]

The organization of Lyme disease into three stages is helpful as a general framework for learning about the infection and for comparison of the infection to syphilis. However, for any particular patient with neurological manifestations, this division may not be useful. Facial palsy can occur very early or very late in the infection. The meningoradiculitis ("second stage") frequently occurs at the same time as arthritis ("third stage"). Therefore, some investigators choose to divide Lyme disease into "localized" (skin) disease and "disseminated" disease with involvement of organs other than the skin.

Diagnosis and Serology and the Question of Latent Infection

Diagnostic criteria for Lyme neurological disease are not yet clear. B. burgdorferi, like T. pallidum, can almost never be cultured from CSF or blood, and biopsies are often dangerous and unrevealing. In patients from endemic areas who have meningitis, radiculoneuritis, and/or cranial neuritis during the summer or early fall, with characteristic CSF profiles and positive serologies, the diagnosis is clear. Many patients, particularly those with third-stage involvement, do not have clear-cut presentations, especially as little is known about the disease spectrum. When neurological disease without known etiology occurs in areas endemic for Lyme disease in patients with positive serologies for B. burgdorferi, the diagnosis of Lyme neurological involvement must be strongly suspected. Helpful confirmatory evidence is a history of erythema chronicum migrans, previous meningitis, or arthritis. A response to parenteral antibiotics is also helpful diagnostically.

Thus the assay for antibodies to the organism is important when diagnosing this disease, whose clinical manifestations are still being delineated. The two most common methods for identifying antibodies to B. burgdorferi are the immunofluorescence assay (IFA) and the enzyme-linked immunosorbent assay (ELISA). The former is similar to the FTA-ABS; visual examination for the binding of fluorescence-labeled second antibodies to the organisms is required. The ELISA is a much easier test and lends itself to automated screening of a large number of samples. The two methods have been found by many investigators to yield similar information.[37,64]

The measurement of antibody to B. burgdorferi in the blood suffers from both false negativity and false positivity. False negativity usually occurs for one of three reasons. First, the blood is drawn from a patient very early in the infection before a significant antibody response has been mounted. Since the antibody titer increases gradually during the first few months of infection, this problem can be addressed by testing twice: during the initial clinical presentation and 1 to 2 months later. Second, some laboratories, in an effort to increase diagnostic specificity, adjust the cutoff of the assay to a higher level, thus decreasing sensitivity. Our laboratory adjusts the assay to be sensitive, but considers low positive serologies as indeterminate and requiring further analysis in an end-point analysis. Third, many laboratories, especially those using commercially available kits, do not perform the test well and do not have adequate sensitivity.[65] This problem is currently being addressed by the Centers for Disease Control, which are developing quality assurance testing for Lyme serology. For a patient in whom Lyme neuroborreliosis is high in the differential diagnosis, negative Lyme serology from a laboratory of questionable accuracy should prompt reevaluation in a university-based laboratory that performs research on Lyme disease. Such a secondary reference laboratory is most likely to perform a reliable assay.

False positivity in the serology of Lyme borreliosis is also a major diagnostic problem. False-positive ELISAs or IFAs are usually accompanied by a negative Western blot and can also occur for three reasons. First and most commonly, in patients with other infections, inflammatory processes such as rheumatoid arthritis or systemic lupus, and malignancies, false positivity can occur on the basis of cross-reactivity between borrelial antigens and the antigens recognized by antibodies in these illnesses.[66] Second, patients may have had previous exposure unrelated to their current illness (i.e., a transient clinical infection, usually localized to skin) that cleared but resulted in the development of antibody to *B. burgdorferi*. Third, a patient may be latently infected with the organism without clinical manifestations,[67] and the symptoms prompting the blood test may be unrelated to this latent infection. The combined incidence of these three forms of false positivity in an asymptomatic population is generally 5 to 10 percent,[68,69] but this number may be higher for symptomatic patients with a variety of illnesses.

The distinction between these three possibilities and active Lyme neuroborreliosis may be difficult.

For these reasons, a positive serology in a neurologically ill patient without other characteristic clinical manifestations of Lyme borreliosis should be interpreted with caution and should prompt further testing, including a Western blot and CSF analysis.

Most patients with Lyme neuroborreliosis who have had symptoms for more than 1 month without treatment have a well-developed antibody response, with a positive Western blot (i.e., reactivity to multiple *B. burgdorferi* antigens). The Western blot is thus a very helpful aid to diagnosis in Lyme neuroborreliosis[70]; a negative Western blot should prompt a careful search for other causes of the patient's symptoms.

The CSF is usually abnormal in patients with Lyme neuroborreliosis. There is commonly a lymphocytic or monocytic pleocytosis or an elevated protein concentration. Patients with active inflammation in the subarachnoid space generally have elevated levels of antibody in the CSF. Finally, PCR testing of the CSF may be very helpful.[71–74] The PCR sometimes detects *B. burgdorferi* DNA in the CSF when all other assays in the CSF are negative.

Because infection with the organism can go unnoticed and early stages of the disease can be subclinical, individuals who are asymptomatic but have high titers of anti-*B. burgdorferi* antibodies should be considered at risk for developing late manifestations of Lyme disease, and should undergo lumbar puncture. If the CSF is abnormal, they should be treated; if it is normal they should be carefully followed.

Treatment

The first stage of Lyme disease is optimally treated by oral antibiotics. From a study comparing the efficacy of tetracycline, penicillin, and erythromycin, tetracycline was the most effective in preventing progression to meningitis or arthritis.[53] Oral antibiotics also clear the rash and treat the flu-like symptoms associated with the first stage.

Treatment of Lyme meningitis during the second stage of the disease has been successful in ameliorating the symptoms, decreasing CNS inflammation, and preventing progression of disease. The largest study has been that of 12 patients treated with intravenous penicillin compared to 15 patients treated with prednisone alone.[75] The most dramatic difference between the two groups was the duration of symptoms after initiation of treatment, which was 29 weeks for the prednisone group and 1 week for the group receiving intravenous penicillin. The mean WBC count and protein concentration in the CSF dropped from 153 cells/mm^3 and 70 mg/dl, respectively, to 54 cells/mm^3 and 53 mg/dl by the end of therapy with 20 million units of penicillin G intravenously per day for 10 days. This treatment regimen must be considered the treatment of choice, although other antibiotics (e.g., ceftriaxone) have been used.

Treatment of the third stage is more problematic. Some patients with third-stage manifestations have progressed despite high-dose intravenous penicillin; such outcomes are consistent with either inadequate treatment or a "parainfectious" etiology (or both) for some of the manifestations of this stage.

OTHER SPIROCHETES CAUSING NEUROLOGICAL DISEASE IN THE UNITED STATES

There is no definite evidence that spirochetes other than *Treponema pallidum* and *Borrelia burgdorferi* (and to a much lesser extent *Leptospira interrogans* and *Borrelia* of relapsing fever) cause neurological disease. However, there is an underlying suspicion among many investigators that the reactivation of interest in spirochetes generated by the discovery of Lyme disease and the subsequent increase in our knowledge about these organisms will lead to finding other spirochetal infections of humans. A disease of cattle, epizootic bovine abortion, has been found to be spirochetal in origin[76] using methodology developed for research into Lyme disease. The situation can be compared to that in areas of New England during the 1960s and 1970s, when patients who developed classic Lyme meningitis were thought to have "viral" or "aseptic" meningitis. Thus it is not overly speculative to predict that during the next decades more spirochetoses will be found, some with neurological manifestations.

REFERENCES

1. Rudolph AH: Syphilis. p. 517. In Hoeprich P (ed): Infectious Diseases, 2nd Ed. Harper & Row, Hagerstown, MD, 1977
2. Simon RP: Neurosyphilis. Arch Neurol 42:606, 1985
3. Gilroy J, Meyer JS: Medical Neurology, 2nd ed. Macmillan, New York, 1975
4. Adams RD, Victor M: Principles of Neurology. McGraw-Hill, New York, 1977
5. Noguchi H, Moore JW: A demonstration of Treponema pallidum in the brain in cases of general paresis. J Exp Med 17:648, 1913
6. Merritt H, Adams RD: Neurosyphilis. Oxford University Press, New York, 1946
7. Burke JM, Schaberg DR: Neurosyphilis in the antibiotic era. Neurology 35:1368, 1985
8. Johns DR, Tierney M, Parker SW: Pure motor hemiplegia due to meningovascular neurosyphilis. Arch Neurol 44:1062, 1987
9. Gomez EA, Aviles M: Neurosyphilis in community health clinics: a case series. J Clin Psychiatry 45:127, 1984
10. Hooshmand H, Escobar MR, Kopf SW: Neurosyphilis, a study of 241 patients. JAMA 219:726, 1972
11. Nordenbo AM, Sorensen PS: The incidence and clinical presentation of neurosyphilis in greater Copenhagen, 1974–8. Acta Neurol Scand 63:237, 1981
12. Wolters E: Neurosyphilis: a changing diagnostic problem. Eur Neurol 26:23, 1987
13. Johns DR, Tierney M, Felsenstein D: Alteration in the natural history of neurosyphilis by concurrent infection with the human immunodeficiency virus. N Engl J Med 316:1569, 1987
14. Berry CD, Hooton TM, Collier AC, Lukehart SA: Neurologic relapse after benzathine penicillin therapy for secondary syphilis in a patient with HIV infection. N Engl J Med 316:1587, 1987
15. Berger JR: Spinal cord syphilis associated with human immunodeficiency virus infection: a treatable myelopathy. Am J Med 92:101, 1992
16. Berger JR, Waskin H, Pall L, et al: Syphilitic cerebral gumma with HIV infection. Neurology 42:1282, 1992
17. Katz DA, Berger JR, Duncan RC: Neurosyphilis: a comparative study of the effects of infection with human immunodeficiency virus. Arch Neurol 50:243, 1993
18. Katz D, Berger JR: Neurosyphilis in acquired immunodeficiency syndrome. Arch Neurol 46:895, 1989
19. Berger JR: Neurosyphilis in human immunodeficiency virus type 1-seropositive individuals: a prospective study. Arch Neurol 48:700, 1991
20. Pavia CS: Enhanced primary resistance to Treponema pallidum infection and increased susceptibility to toxoplasmosis in T-cell depleted guinea pigs. Infect Immun 53:305, 1986
21. Azadegan AA, Schell RF, Steiner BM, et al: Effect of immune serum and its immunoglobulin fractions on hamsters challenged with Treponema pallidum ssp. pertenue. J Infect Dis. 153:1007, 1986

22. Blanco DR, Miller JN, Hanff PA: Humoral immunity in experimental syphilis: the demonstration of IgG as a treponemicidal factor in immune rabbit serum. J Immunol 133:2693, 1984

23. Pavia CS, Niederbuhl CJ: Acquired resistance and expression of a protective humoral immune response in guinea pigs infected with Treponema pallidum Nichols. Infect Immun 50:66, 1985

24. Marton KI, Gean AD: The spinal tap: a new look at an old test. Ann Intern Med 104:840, 1986

25. Wiesel J, Rose DN, Silver AL, et al: Lumbar puncture in asymptomatic late syphilis: an analysis of the benefits and risks. Arch Intern Med 145:465, 1985

26. Dans PE, Cafferty L, Otter SE, Johnson RJ: Inappropriate use of the cerebrospinal fluid Venereal Disease Research Laboratory (VDRL) test to exclude neurosyphilis. Ann Intern Med 104:86, 1986

27. Lukehart SA, Hook EW, Baker-Zander SA, et al: Invasion of the central nervous system by Treponema pallidum: implications for diagnosis and treatment. Ann Intern Med 109:855, 1988

28. Burstain JM, Grinprel E, Lukehart SA, et al: Sensitive detection of Treponema pallidum by using the polymerase chain reaction. J Clin Microbiol 29:62, 1991

29. Sanchez PJ, Wendel GD, Grimprel E, et al: Evaluation of molecular methodologies and rabbit infectivity testing for the diagnosis of congenital syphilis and neonatal central nervous system invasion by *Treponema pallidum.* J Infect Dis 167:148, 1993

30. Goh BT, Smith GW, Samarasinghe L, et al: Penicillin concentrations in serum and cerebrospinal fluid after intramuscular injection of aqueous procaine penicillin 0.6 MU with and without probenecid. Br J Vener Dis 60:371, 1984

31. Schoth PE, Wolters EC: Penicillin concentrations in serum and CSF during high-dose intravenous treatment for neurosyphilis. Neurology 37:1214, 1987

32. Faggi L, Citterio A, Frigo GM, et al: Penicillin CSF levels following intravenous therapy in syphilitic patients. Ital J Neurol Sci 4:423, 1983

33. Steere AC, Malawista SE, Snydman DR, et al: Lyme arthritis: an epidemic of oligoarticular arthritis in children and adults in three Connecticut communities. Arthritis Rheum 20:7, 1977

34. Steere AC, Malawista SE, Hardin JA, et al: Erythema chronicum migrans and Lyme arthritis: the enlarging clinical spectrum. Ann Intern Med 86:685, 1977

35. Steere AC, Grodzicki RL, Kornblatt AN, et al: The spirochetal etiology of Lyme disease. N Engl J Med 308:733, 1983

36. Benach JL, Bosler EM, Hanrahan JP, et al: Spirochetes isolated from the blood of two patients with Lyme disease. N Engl J Med 308:740, 1983

37. Craft JE, Grodzicki RL, Steere AC: The antibody response in Lyme disease: evaluation of diagnostic tests. J Infect Dis 149:789, 1984

38. Burgdorfer W: Discovery of the Lyme disease spirochete: a historical review. Zentralbl Bakteriol Mikrobiol Hyg [A] 263:7, 1987

39. Barbour AG, Schrumpf ME: Polymorphisms of major surface proteins of Borrelia burgdorferi. Zentralbl Bakteriol Mikrobiol Hyg [A] 263:83, 1987

40. Wilske B, Preac-Mursic V, Schierz G, Busch KV: Immunochemical and immunological analysis of European Borrelia burgdorferi strains. Zentralbl Bakteriol Mikrobiol Hyg [A] 263:92, 1987

41. Hovind-Hougen K, Asbrink E, Stiernstedt G, et al: Ultrastructural differences among spirochetes isolated from patients with Lyme disease and related disorders, and from Ixodes ricinus. Zentralbl Bakteriol Mikrobiol Hyg [A] 263:103, 1987

42. Stoenner HG, Dodd T, Larsen C: Antigenic variation of Borrelia hermsii. J Exp Med 156:1297, 1982

43. Pachner AR, Itano A: Borrelia burgdorferi infection of the brain: characterization of the organism and response to antibiotics and immune sera in the mouse model. Neurology 40:1535, 1990

44. Pachner AR, Delaney E, Ricalton NS: Murine Lyme borreliosis: route of inoculation determines immune response and infectivity. Reg Immunol 4:345, 1992

45. Pachner AR, Ricalton N, Delaney E: Comparison of polymerase chain reaction with culture and serology for diagnosis of murine experimental Lyme borreliosis. J Clin Microbiol 31:208, 1993

46. Armstrong AL, Barthold SW, Persing DH, Beck DS: Carditis in Lyme disease susceptible and resistant strains of laboratory mice infected with Borrelia burgdorferi. Am J Trop Hyg 47:249, 1992

47. Barthold SW, Beck DS, Hansen GM, et al: Lyme borreliosis in selected strains and ages of laboratory mice. J Infect Dis 162:133, 1990

48. Barthold SW, Moody KD, Terwilliger GA, et al: An animal model for Lyme arthritis. Ann NY Acad Sci 539:264, 1988

49. Johnson RC, Marek N, Kodner C: Infection of Syrian hamsters with Lyme disease spirochetes. J Clin Microbiol 20:1099, 1984

50. Barthold SW, Persing DH, Armstrong AL, Peeples RA: Kinetics of Borrelia burgdorferi dissemination and evolution of disease after intradermal inoculation of mice. Am J Pathol 139:263, 1991

51. Pachner AR, Basta J, Hulinska D: Localization by electron microscopy of Borrelia burgdorferi in internal organs of infected mice. Submitted for publication

52. Montgomery RR, Nathanson MH, Malawista SE: The fate of Borrelia burgdorferi, the agent for Lyme disease, in mouse macrophages. J Immunol 150:909, 1993

53. Steere AC, Hutchinson GJ, Rahn DW, et al: Treatment of the early manifestations of Lyme disease. Ann Intern Med 99:22, 1983

54. Pachner AR, Steere AC: The triad of neurological manifestations of Lyme disease: meningitis, cranial neuritis, and radiculoneuritis. Neurology 35:47, 1985

55. Clark JR, Carlson RD, Sasaki CT, et al: Facial paralysis in Lyme disease. Laryngoscope 95:1341, 1985

56. Graf M, Kristofferitsch W, Baumhackl U, et al: Electrophysiologic findings in meningopolyneuritis of Garin-Bujadoux-Bannwarth. Zentralbl Bakteriol Mikrobiol Hyg [A] 263:324, 1986

57. Lubeau M, Vallat JM, Hugon J, et al: Tick bite meningoradiculitis. Zentralbl Bakteriol Mikrobiol Hyg [A] 263:321, 1986

58. Pohl P, Schmutzhard E, Stanek G: Cerebrospinal fluid findings in neurological manifestations of Lyme diseases. Zentralbl Bakteriol Mikrobiol Hyg [A] 263:314, 1986

59. Henriksson A, Link H, Cruz M, Stiernstedt G: Immunoglobulin abnormalities in cerebrospinal fluid and blood over the course of lymphocytic meningoradiculitis. Ann Neurol 20:337, 1986

60. Hofstad H, Matre R, Nyland H, et al: Bannwarth's syndrome: serum and CSF IgG antibodies against Borrelia burgdorferi examined by ELISA. Acta Neurol Scand 75:37, 1987

61. Pachner AR, Steere AC: CNS manifestations of third stage Lyme disease. Zentralbl Bakteriol Mikrobiol Hyg [A] 263:301, 1987

62. Reik L, Smith L, Khan A, Nelson W: Demyelinating encephalopathy in Lyme disease. Neurology 35:267, 1985

63. Pachner AR, Duray P, Steere AC: Central nervous system manifestations of Lyme disease. Arch Neurol 46:790, 1989

64. Magnarelli L, Meegan JM, Anderson JP, et al: Comparison of an indirect fluorescent antibody test with an enzyme-linked immunosorbent assay for serological studies of Lyme disease. J Clin Microbiol 20:181, 1984

65. Bakken LL, Case KL, Callister SM, et al: Performance of 45 laboratories participating in a proficiency testing program for Lyme disease serology. JAMA 268:891, 1992

66. Pachner AR, Delaney E, Ricalton NS: The frequency of false positive B. burgdorferi ELISAs as assessed with end-point dilution, quantitative Western blotting, and clinical followup. Proc Vth Int Conf Lyme Borreliosis, A24, 1992

67. Steere AC, Taylor E, Wilson ML, et al: Longitudinal assessment of the clinical and epidemiological features of Lyme disease in a defined population. J Infect Dis 154:295, 1986

68. Ross AH, Benach JL: The significance of controls in Lyme arthritis of children. Zentralbl Bakteriol Mikrobiol Hyg [A] 263:400, 1986

69. Mertz LE, Wobig GH, Duffy J, Katzmann JA: Ticks, spirochetes, and new diagnostic tests for Lyme disease. Mayo Clin Proc 60:402, 1985

70. Pachner AR, Ricalton NS: Western blotting in evaluating Lyme seropositivity and the utility of a gel densitometric approach. Neurology 42:2185, 1992

71. Pachner AR, Ricalton NS, Delaney E: Detection of Borrelia burgdorferi DNA in the cerebrospinal fluid by polymerase chain reaction: sensitivity and use of nonradioactive probes. Ann Neurol 32:284, 1992

72. Pachner AR, Delaney E: The polymerase chain reaction in the diagnosis of Lyme neuroborreliosis. Ann Neurol 34:544, 1993

73. Lebech AM, Hansen K: Detection of Borrelia burgdorferi DNA in urine and cerebrospinal fluid samples from patients with early and late Lyme neuroborreliosis by polymerase chain reaction. J Clin Microbiol 30:1646, 1992

74. Keller TL, Halperin JJ, Whitman M: PCR detection of Borrelia burgdorferi DNA in cerebrospinal fluid of Lyme neuroborreliosis patients. Neurology 42:32, 1992

75. Steere AC, Pachner AR, Malawista SE: Neurologic abnormalities of Lyme disease: successful treatment with high-dose intravenous penicillin. Ann Intern Med 99:767, 1983

76. Osebold JW, Spezialetti R, Jennings MB, et al: Congenital spirochetosis in calves: association with epizootic bovine abortion. J Am Vet Med Assoc 188:371, 1986

35

Tuberculosis of the Central Nervous System

John M. Leonard
Roger M. Des Prez

Tuberculosis in all its forms remains a challenging clinical problem and a public health issue of considerable magnitude. The World Health Organization estimates that 8 to 10 million new cases occur in the world each year. Incidence rates vary widely from country to country in relation to socioeconomic conditions; for example, the incidence is about 9 cases per 100,000 population per year in the United States compared to rates of 110 to 165 cases per 100,000 in the developing countries of Asia and Africa.[1]

The incidence of tuberculosis in the United States declined steadily from 1953 to 1985. The expected yearly decline was not seen in 1985 and has since been followed by a slight rise. This has been attributed to several factors: the expanding human immunodeficiency virus (HIV) epidemic, the increase in the prevalence of poverty and homelessness, and the influx of persons from Asia and the Pacific Islands—a group that accounts for approximately 20 percent of cases in the United States.[2–4]

Tuberculosis of the central nervous system (CNS) accounts for approximately 15 percent of extrapulmonary cases or about 0.7 percent of all clinical tuberculosis in the United States.[5] Although pulmonary tuberculosis has been on the decline over the past 35 years, the incidence of CNS disease, as well as other forms of extrapulmonary tuberculosis, has remained almost constant, and the case: fatality ratio is still relatively high (15 to 40 percent).[5–7] The increased longevity of the population and the impact of technology on western culture and medical care have expanded the pool of individuals rendered susceptible to progression of tuberculous infection by chronic disease, immunosuppressive therapies, and alcoholism. The growing number of persons with acquired immunodeficiency syndrome (AIDS) also constitutes a significant subset of the population at risk.[8] Clearly, CNS tuberculosis will continue to be an important and challenging problem for the neurologist, internist, and pediatrician.

At the present time, CNS tuberculosis may be considered as comprising three clinical categories: meningitis, intracranial tuberculoma, and spinal tuberculous arachnoiditis. The clinical presentation and character of illness within each category are highly variable and nonspecific; they overlap with other infections of the CNS as well as with vascular syndromes and space-occupying lesions.

MENINGITIS

Pathogenesis

The now classic studies of Rich and McCordock demonstrated that tuberculous meningitis originates from the discharge of bacilli into the cerebrospinal fluid (CSF) from adjacent older, caseous foci of infection situated within the substance of the brain, meninges, or adjacent bone. A single such discharging focus was found by careful search in 77 of 82 cases of tuberculous meningitis in their meticulous autopsy series.[9] These critically located tuberculous foci (tubercles) may be established in the brain and other tissues during the bacillemia that follows primary infection or late-reactivation tuberculosis elsewhere in the body. The number, character, and location of lesions in the brain vary from case to case. Their destiny is determined by proximity to the surface of the brain, the rapidity of progression, and the rate at which encapsulation follows acquired immune resistance. *The chance occurrence and progression of a suitably located subependymal tubercle is the critical event in the development of tuberculous meningitis.*

The widespread and dense distribution of infectious foci in progressive miliary tuberculosis greatly increases the chance that a juxtaependymal tubercle will be established and from this critical location will break down to contaminate the subarachnoid space. Such is the case in most infants and young children presenting with meningitis, as the very young are especially susceptible to progressive hematogenous tuberculosis following primary infection.[10,11] Adults may also acquire CNS infection in association with clinically apparent progressive miliary disease, or meningitis may develop from other, less apparent or entirely hidden foci of chronic organ tuberculosis as well. Reactivation of such foci with resultant secondary hematogenous dissemination may be intermittent or chronic and progressive. In either case, bacilli are spread to distant organs, producing scattered tubercles of varying size and encapsulation, including some adjacent to the subarachnoid space with the potential for subsequent breakdown. Subependymal foci arising in this manner may remain quiescent, harboring bacilli for months or years, but always with the potential to destabilize and contaminate the subarachnoid space as a result of local conditions or general depression in host immunity.

Conditions such as advanced age, use of immunosuppressant drugs, lymphoma, alcoholism, and HIV infection may compromise cellular immunity in persons with smoldering chronic organ tuberculosis, leading to reactivation of latent infection and progression of the clinical syndrome of late generalized tuberculosis. In a recent excellent summary of this syn-drome, careful postmortem examination revealed meningeal involvement in 54 percent of patients studied.[12] Finally, it must be emphasized that a significant proportion of cases of tuberculous meningitis occurs in the absence of any clinically demonstrable extracranial infection or apparent defect in host immune function. The frequently noted association between head trauma and the development of tuberculous meningitis suggests that intracranial caseous foci may be destabilized by physical factors as well.

Pathology

The pathological changes observed in the CNS result from a hypersensitivity reaction induced by the presence of organisms and associated antigenic material within the substance of the brain or the subarachnoid space. Regardless of where the discharging tuberculous focus may be, the resultant exudative inflammatory reaction is always most marked at the base of the brain.[9] Three features dominate the pathology and explain the clinical manifestations of tuberculous meningitis: (1) proliferative, inflammatory, predominantly basilar, meningeal exudate; (2) vasculitis of arteries and veins traversing this exudate; and (3) disturbance of CSF circulation or resorption.[9,13]

Proliferative arachnoiditis is most marked at the base of the brain and, in cases of more than a few days' duration, may become thick, gelatinous, and mass-like, extending from the pons to the optic nerves but most prominent in the area of the optic chiasm.[13] As the process of optochiasmic arachnoiditis becomes more chronic, it may come to resemble a fibrous mass involving and compromising the function of cranial nerves. Uncommonly, a similar gelatinous or fibrous process can surround the spinal cord, producing various symptoms by encroaching on exiting spinal nerves.

Vasculitis with resultant thrombosis and hemorrhagic infarction may develop in vessels that traverse the basilar or spinal exudate or within the brain substance itself.[14,15] The vascular inflammatory reaction is initiated by direct invasion of the adventitia by mycobacteria or by secondary extension of the adjacent arachnoiditis. An early polymorphonuclear reaction followed by infiltration of lymphocytes, plasma cells, and macrophages leads to progressive destruction of the adventitia, disruption of elastic fibers, and extension of the inflammatory process to involve the intima. Eventually, fibrinoid degeneration within small arteries and veins produces aneurysms, multiple thrombi, and focal hemorrhage in some combination. Depending on the location and extent of the vasculitis, a variety of stroke syndromes may result. Involvement of perforating vessels to the basal ganglia and pons can produce movement disorders or simulate lacunar infarcts. Multiple lesions are common, and areas of ischemic injury most frequently involve the basal ganglia, cerebral cortex, pons, and cerebellum. In a review of the pathological features of intracranial tuberculous vasculitis, Poltera found phlebitis in 22 cases and varying degrees of arteritis in 20 of 27 cases studied, including 8 patients with an obstructive tuberculous thrombophlebitis associated with hemorrhagic cerebral infarction.[16,17] Intracranial vasculitis is a common feature of autopsy studies and a major determinant of residual neurological deficits in those recovering after therapy.

Extension of the inflammatory process to the basilar cisterns may impede CSF circulation and resorption, leading to *communicating hydrocephalus* in the majority of cases that have been symptomatic for more than 2 to 3 weeks.[18] Less frequently, obstruction of the aqueduct develops from contraction of exudate surrounding the brainstem, inflammation of the ependymal lining of the ventricles, or a strategically placed brainstem tuberculoma.[19] In far advanced cases, increased intracranial pressure can cause brainstem compression and tentorial herniation.

Clinical Presentation

SYMPTOMS AND SIGNS

Tuberculous meningitis has been divided into prodromal, meningitic, and paralytic stages. Usually there will be a subacute prodrome of insidious onset characterized by vague ill health, malaise, lassitude, personality change, intermittent headache, and low-grade fever. This phase is followed usually within 2 to 3 weeks by more prominent neurological findings, including meningismus, protracted headache, vomiting, confusion, cranial nerve palsies, and long tract signs.[20] The pace of illness may accelerate rapidly at this stage; confusion gives way to stupor and coma, seizures may occur, and hemiparesis or hemiplegia sometimes develops. In the majority of untreated cases, death supervenes within 5 to 8 weeks of the onset of illness, although the occasional patient will follow a more indolent, slowly progressive course over weeks or months. The symptoms and signs compiled in a well-studied series are presented in Table 35-1. In children, irritability, loss in interest in play, restlessness, and anorexia are early symptoms. Headache is less common and vomiting often much more prominent, especially in the very young.[5,21] Generalized seizures are more common in children and are apt to be an early or presenting symptom.

Table 35-1 Preadmission Symptoms and Admission Clinical Signs

Symptoms and Signs	No. of Cases	%
Symptoms		
General		
Respiratory problems	16	31
Pains	16	31
Fever	10	19
Weight loss	10	19
Fatigue	9	17
Irritability	9	17
Gastrointestinal		
Vomiting	37	70
Anorexia	26	50
Constipation	19	37
Neurological		
Headache	38	73
Drowsiness	14	27
Confusion	9	17
Diplopia	6	12
Convulsions	5	10
Signs		
General		
Pharyngitis	11	21
Lung adventitial sounds	9	17
Lymphadenopathy	8	15
Neurological		
Meningeal irritation	47	90
Drowsiness	23	44
Confusion	15	29
Stupor	6	12
Coma	2	4
Papilledema	16	31
Extensor plantar responses	13	25
Cranial nerve palsies	10	19
Hemiparesis	2	4
Choroidal tubercle	1	2

(From Kennedy DF, Fallon RJ: Tuberculous meningitis. JAMA 241:264, 1979, with permission.)

For purposes of prognosis, it is helpful to categorize patients into clinical stages. *Stage 1* comprises patients who are conscious and rational, with or without meningismus but with no focal neurological signs or evidence of hydrocephalus; *stage 2* patients are confused or have focal neurological signs such as cranial nerve palsies or hemiparesis; in *stage 3,* disease is more advanced, with coma, delirium, or dense hemiplegia or paraplegia.[7] The clinical stage on presentation is related to duration of illness, although some patients progress rapidly to advanced stages within a few days. The response to treatment is much influenced by the clinical stage at the time therapy is initiated, as discussed below.

ATYPICAL FEATURES

In some adults, the prodrome may be a slowly progressive dementia over months or even years, characterized by personality change, social withdrawal, loss of libido, and memory deficits. At the other end of the spectrum, patients may present with an acute, rapidly progressive meningitic syndrome indistinguishable from pyogenic bacterial meningitis. At times this accelerated form is superimposed on a chronic dementing illness. Seizures and focal neurological disturbances such as cranial nerve palsy or hemiparesis may occur early and dominate the clinical presentation. Of the cranial nerves, the sixth is the most commonly involved, followed by the third and the fourth. Instances of internuclear ophthalmoplegia have been observed, characterized by adduction paresis of one or both eyes on lateral gaze, often with nystagmus of the abducting eye and failure of convergence.[22] Occasionally the symptoms and signs of hydrocephalus (headache, papilledema, diplopia, and visual disturbance) precede the signs of meningeal irritation.

Udani and Dastur have described an encephalitic course in children characterized by stupor, coma, and convulsions without signs of meningitis.[23] The CSF may show a mild pleocytosis and protein elevation or may be entirely normal. This syndrome of "tuberculous encephalopathy" also occurs occasionally in adults.[24]

TUBERCULOUS MENINGITIS AND HIV INFECTION

Extrapulmonary tuberculosis is common in patients with AIDS, and coinfection with HIV has recently been reported in 21 percent of patients with extrapulmonary tuberculosis in the United States.[25] Although CNS tuberculosis has not yet become a widespread problem in AIDS patients, two centers have reported an unusual frequency of tuberculous meningitis in HIV-infected intravenous drug users with AIDS and AIDS-related complex.[26,27] Among 52 patients with tuberculosis seen by Bishburg and associates over a 3-year period, 10 had CNS disease. The clinical spectrum included meningitis, tuberculoma, and cerebral abscess.[26] Berenguer and co-workers reported that 10 percent of 455 patients with both tuberculosis and HIV infection had meningitis. HIV-infected patients accounted for 59 percent of cases of tuberculous meningitis seen during the study period. In contrast, only 2 percent of HIV-negative patients with tuberculosis had meningitis. Superficial, intrathoracic, and intra-abdominal lymphadenopathy was much more frequent in HIV-positive patients.[27] Dube and colleagues compared the clinical features, laboratory findings, and in-hospital mortality in patients having tuberculous meningitis with or without HIV infection. Intracerebral tuberculomas were more common in the HIV-infected group (60 percent compared to 14 percent); otherwise, coinfection with HIV did not alter the clinical manifestations, CSF findings, or response to therapy.[28]

Diagnosis

Few problems in medicine so critically challenge the physician's diagnostic acumen and clinical judgment as the patient with CNS tuberculosis. Once the possibility of tuberculosis meningitis has been considered, the central task is rapid and thorough assessment of supporting evidence followed by a prompt decision regarding treatment. Clues to the diagnosis include a positive family history of tuberculosis, recent exposure to others with active tuberculosis, especially in cases involving children and immunosuppressed adults, a history of recent head trauma, and alcoholism. Evidence of active tuberculosis elsewhere in the body, observed in 20 to 70 percent of cases, provides the most reliable basis for the presumptive diagnosis in patients with CNS disease. A meticulous physical examination with careful attention to abnormal findings is essential. Significant but easily overlooked clues include lymphadenopathy, spinal and other joint lesions, splenomegaly, scrotal mass, and draining fistulas. Abnormalities on chest x-ray, including miliary infiltrate and less commonly hilar adenopathy or upper lobe nodular infiltrates, occur in most childhood cases and in about 50 percent of adults. These often provide the basis for diagnosis.

LABORATORY STUDIES

Patients with tuberculous meningitis may exhibit mild anemia and leukocytosis, but often the complete blood count and even the erythrocyte sedimentation rate are entirely normal. Hyponatremia and other biochemical features of inappropriate secretion of antidiuretic hormone have been observed in some cases of miliary tuberculosis complicated by meningitis.[29,30]

A positive tuberculin skin test has been reported in up to 80 percent of patients in recent series and is of greatest diagnostic importance in very young children.[10,11] A negative test is of no help, as false negatives occur commonly in all forms of tuberculosis.

CEREBROSPINAL FLUID EXAMINATION

Lumbar puncture and careful examination of the CSF are the keys to diagnosis in most instances. The opening pressure is usually elevated, the fluid is clear or "ground glass" in appearance, and, on standing, a delicate web-like clot often forms. Classically, the CSF formula shows elevated protein and low glucose concentrations as well as mononuclear pleocytosis.[30] The CSF protein concentration ranges from 100 to 500 mg/dl in most patients, is less than 100 mg/dl in 25 percent, and is more than 500 mg/dl in 10 percent. Patients with subarachnoid block may exhibit extremely high protein concentrations, in the range of 2 to 6 g/dl, associated with xanthochromia and a poor prognosis. The CSF glucose concentration is typically low, being less than 45 mg/dl in about 80 percent of cases. The CSF cell count is between 100 and 500/mm^3 in most patients, under 100 cells/mm^3 in approximately 15 percent, and between 500 and 1,500 cells/mm^3 in 20 percent. The predominant cellular reaction is lymphocytic; however, early in the course of active infection the cellular reaction is often atypical, with only very few cells or a tendency for polymorphonuclear cells to predominate. The initial inflammatory reaction has been conceptualized as essentially allergic, analogous to a tuberculin reaction.

It consists of a transient polymorphonuclear reaction that is replaced by the typical mononuclear cellular response characteristic of subacute or chronic tuberculosis. Thus the common observation has been that CSF fluids with an atypical cellular reaction at the onset evolve in the direction of more typical findings with repeated lumbar punctures. Misinterpretation of this sequence as improvement or as response to antibacterial therapy when an erroneous diagnosis of pyogenic meningitis is being entertained can have serious consequences. On occasion, an initial mononuclear pleocytosis may briefly change in the direction of polymorphonuclear predominance when therapy is initiated, a change that may be associated with clinical deterioration. Smith has stated that such a "therapeutic paradox" is almost pathognomonic of tuberculous meningitis.[31]

Specific diagnosis rests on the demonstration of *Mycobacterium tuberculosis* in the CSF by either direct smear or culture. Cultures are positive in about 75 percent of cases but require 6 weeks for detectable growth. Consequently, the preparation and careful examination of CSF for acid-fast organisms is of obvious and critical importance for reaching a rapid diagnosis and therapeutic decision. The utility of the smear for acid-fast bacilli is directly related to the care and attention given by medical and laboratory personnel. *The importance of repeated, careful examination and culture of CSF specimens cannot be overemphasized.* In one carefully defined series, the incidence of a positive smear was 37 percent on examination of the first specimen but increased to 87 percent when up to four serial CSF specimens were examined, even though some patients had already received antituberculous therapy before the first smear was positive.[7] Other series using multiple samples have reported equally good results.[32,33] We recommend that a minimum of three lumbar punctures be performed at daily intervals, bearing in mind that one need not delay treatment, as the yield remains good for several days after the institution of therapy. To achieve optimum benefit from this important diagnostic procedure, it seems prudent to heed the experience and recommendation of those in whose hands it has been most successful. Merritt and Fremont-Smith, in their classic treatise on CSF,[34] provided guidelines for the preparation and examination of CSF specimens for acid-fast organisms. The following points[7,34] are noteworthy:

1. Acid-fast organisms can be demonstrated most readily in a smear of the clot or sediment.

2. It is best to use the last fluid removed at lumbar puncture, taking 10 to 15 ml.

3. If no clot forms, the addition of 2 ml of 95 percent alcohol (so that the alcohol mixes with only the upper portion of the CSF) gives a heavy protein precipitate which, on centrifuging, carries bacilli to the bottom of the tube.

4. Of the centrifuged deposit of CSF, 0.02 ml should be applied to a glass slide in an area not exceeding 1 cm in diameter and stained by the standard Kenyon or Ziehl-Neilsen method.

5. Between 200 and 500 high-power fields should be examined (about 30 minutes), preferably by more than one observer.

The use of fluorescent staining as a rapid screening device is advantageous, but simultaneous staining with the Ziehl-Neilsen or Kenyon stain is also advisable in view of the importance of diagnostic accuracy.

New methods for the rapid diagnosis of tuberculous meningitis are under investigation.[35] Highly sensitive assays have been developed for detecting specific antibodies to myocbacterial antigens and specific enzymes derived from T lymphocytes in the CSF of patients with tuberculous infection. Unfortunately, these assays lack specificity and are currently of limited value. A more promising approach has been the use of enzyme-linked immunosorbent assay (ELISA) and latex-particle agglutination assays of CSF to detect mycobacterial antigen. Early results indicate that this approach may yield a rapid and sensitive diagnostic test with high specificity. The polymerase chain reaction (PCR) has also been used effectively to detect mycobacterial DNA sequences.[36] Further confirmation and simplification of these various techniques are necessary before they can be widely utilized. Direct examination of CSF smear by conventional staining techniques remains the principal clinical tool for diagnosing CNS infection.

NEURORADIOLOGICAL EVALUATION

Older neuroradiological techniques (e.g., brain scan, angiography, and air contrast ventriculography) have now been replaced by computed tomography (CT) and magnetic resonance imaging (MRI). These methods have enlarged concepts of pathogenesis as well as facilitated clinical assessment. CT can define the presence and extent of basilar arachnoiditis, the presence of cerebral edema and infarction, and the presence and course of hydrocephalus.[18,37–39] Serial CT studies have demonstrated that hydrocephalus alone is uncommon and carries a good prognosis. On the other hand, hydrocephalus combined with marked basilar enhancement is indicative of advanced tuberculous meningitis and implies a poor prognosis. Marked basilar enhancement, an indicator of extensive basilar meningitis, is often associated with vasculitis and portends serious risk for basal ganglia infarction.[38] CT has been used to monitor the effectiveness of adjunctive therapy, such as corticosteroids and neurosurgical shunting procedures. In one series of 60 patients reported from India, CT demonstrated hydrocephalus in 83 percent, cerebral infarct in 28 percent, and tuberculomas in 10 percent. Hydrocephalus was associated with a longer duration of symptoms before treatment and was seen more often in children than in adults. Importantly, it was the authors' opinion that CT findings were of prognostic significance: those with an entirely normal scan recovered completely on antituberculous therapy; those with mild or moderate basilar exudate showed some improvement with early ventriculoatrial shunting; and those with a severe degree of basilar exudate did not do well even with shunt surgery.[18] In another series of 37 patients, a poor prognosis was associated with CT evidence of "basilar edema," a finding attributed to infarction in the area of the basal ganglia.[40]

The degree to which MRI is superior to or will supplant CT is not yet clear. In a careful prospective study of 27 childhood cases, including clinical, radiological, and pathological findings, Schoeman and co-workers found MRI superior to CT in delineating focal infarcts of the basal ganglia and diencephalon and in defining the presence and extent of associated lesions in the brainstem.[41] The character and severity of brainstem abnormality, as defined by MRI, correlated well with clinical evidence of brainstem disease. In the unusual patient with suspected spinal tuberculosis, either epidural or intradural in location, MRI is the preferred diagnostic modality.

DIFFERENTIAL DIAGNOSIS

Differential diagnosis of CNS tuberculosis includes a variety of inflammatory, vascular, and neoplastic

Table 35-2 Differential Diagnosis
of Tuberculous Meningitis

Fungal meningitis (cryptococcosis, histoplasmosis, blasto-
mycosis, coccidioidal mycosis)
Viral meningoencephalitis (herpes simplex, mumps)
Partially treated bacterial meningitis
Neurosyphilis
Focal parameningeal infection
Pyogenic brain abscess
CNS toxoplasmosis
Neoplastic meningitis (lymphoma, carcinoma)
Cerebrovascular accident
CNS sarcoidosis

conditions of the CNS. The classic clinical presentation of granulomatous meningitis—fever, encephalopathy, meningeal signs, and a CSF formula characterized by lymphocytic pleocytosis, lowered glucose
concentration, and high protein content—can be
caused by tuberculosis, fungal infection, syphilis, and
brucellosis. The syndrome is also encountered among
patients with parameningeal suppurative foci related
to sphenoid sinusitis, brain abscess, and endocarditis.
Patients with herpes simplex and mumps encephalitis
pose the greatest challenge, as they may present with
fever, rapid neurological deterioration, and mild lowering of the CSF glucose concentration, as discussed
in Chapter 37. Careful evaluation for tuberculosis is
warranted in every patient suspected of any of the
other diagnoses listed in Table 35-2.

Error or delay in diagnosis may result from atypical
CSF findings, such as minimal abnormalities of glucose and protein concentration or predominance of
neutrophils.[42] Repeat examination of the CSF will
frequently show a falling glucose level, a rising protein concentration, and a shift to mononuclear predominance. It is helpful to bear in mind that CSF
protein concentrations in excess of 150 mg/dl are
rarely seen in viral meningitis and should always raise
suspicion of tuberculous or fungal infection.[43]

TUBERCULOMA

Tuberculomas are conglomerate caseous foci
within the substance of the brain that develop from
deep-seated tubercles acquired during a recent or remote episode of hematogenous dissemination. Cen-

trally located, active lesions may reach considerable
size without producing meningitis.[9,44] Under conditions of poor host resistance, this process may result
in focal areas of cerebritis or frank abscess formation,
but the more usual course is coalescence of caseous
foci and fibrous encapsulation (tuberculoma). If they
are defined radiologically as lesions apparent on CT
scanning, then clinically silent single or multiple enhancing granulomata are observed in a significant minority of cases of tuberculous meningitis and also in
some cases of miliary tuberculosis without meningitis.[45] The characteristic CT finding is a nodular enhancing lesion with a central hypodense region.[46,47]
Their frequency suggests that macroscopic parenchymal lesions are more common in miliary tuberculosis
and tuberculous meningitis than previously suspected. These lesions usually disappear with medical
therapy, although cases have been reported in which
tuberculomas developed and progressed early during
the course of antituberculous therapy.[48–50]

In contrast to lesions evident on CT but producing
no symptoms, clinical tuberculomas presenting as intracranial mass lesions are distinctly uncommon in
the West. However, in India and other parts of Asia,
especially among children, intracranial tuberculomas
account for 20 to 30 percent of all intracranial space-
occupying lesions.[51] The usual clinical picture is simply that of a space-occupying lesion in the brain;
symptoms of systemic illness and meningeal inflammation are usually lacking. About 30 percent have
evidence of tuberculosis outside the CNS.[51–53]

The diagnosis and management of intracranial tuberculoma have been greatly advanced by the availability of CT scanning. Contrast enhancement is essential. Early stages are characterized by low-density
or isodense lesions, often with edema out of proportion to the mass effect and little encapsulation. At a
later stage, well-encapsulated tuberculomas appear as
isodense or hyperdense lesions with peripheral ring
enhancement.[47,51,54] CT is especially helpful in assessing the presence of cerebral edema and the risk of
herniation and for monitoring response to medical
therapy.[51]

In areas of the world where intracranial tuberculoma is a common cause of space-occupying lesions
of the brain, the diagnosis is often made on clinical
and radiographic grounds or by needle biopsy. Surgical removal of tuberculomas in the prechemotherapy
era was often complicated by severe, fatal meningitis.

Although this can now be prevented by antituberculous chemotherapy, recent series have emphasized that conservative medical management is superior to surgical intervention.[51,53,55] Surgery for purposes other than diagnosis may be required when lesions are critically located so as to produce obstructive hydrocephalus or compression of the brainstem. Corticosteroids are helpful in selected cases where cerebral edema out of proportion to the mass effect contributes to altered mental status or focal neurological deficits.[51]

SPINAL TUBERCULOUS ARACHNOIDITIS

Outside the developed countries of Europe and America, cases of tuberculous meningitis, intracranial tuberculomas, and spinal tuberculosis are seen with approximately equal frequency.[56,57] Tuberculous arachnoiditis or tuberculoma may arise at any level of the spinal cord in association with breakdown of a "Rich" focus within the cord or meninges, or by extension from an adjacent area of inapparent spondylitis. The inflammatory process is usually confined locally, gradually producing partial or complete encasement of the spinal cord in a gelatinous or fibrous exudate.[44] In other cases tuberculomas of the extradural, intradural, or intramedullary space may produce symptoms of a local tumor. Patients usually present with some combination of nerve root and cord compression signs secondary to impingement by the advancing arachnoiditis. Wadia and Dastur, in an exhaustive analysis, have employed the term *radiculomyelopathy,* emphasizing that the clinical manifestations are more neurological than infectious, protean in nature, and associated with an ascending or transverse radiculomyelopathy of variable pace at single or multiple levels.[58] The majority of their cases evolved within 2 months; some reached maximum severity within 2 to 5 days and others developed over years. Symptoms include pain, hyperesthesia, or paresthesias in the distribution of the nerve root; a lower motor neuron paralysis; and bladder or rectal sphincter incontinence. On occasion, the granulomatous mass or abscess may be confined largely to the epidural space, producing symptoms of cord compression with no evidence of meningeal inflammation. An associated vasculitis may result in thrombosis of the anterior spinal artery and infarction of the cord. Whether localized to the epidural, meningeal, or extramedullary levels, all forms of tuberculous spinal arachnoiditis may cause subarachnoid block characterized by high concentrations of protein in the CSF with or without a cellular response.[14,42,59]

The diagnosis of spinal tuberculous arachnoiditis should be considered in the patient with any combination of the following clinical and laboratory features: subacute onset of spinal or nerve root pain; rapidly ascending transverse myelopathy or multiple-level myelopathy; increased CSF protein concentration and cell count; extensive filling defects on myelography or signs of arachnoiditis or epidural space infection by MRI, usually with a spinal block; and evidence of tuberculosis elsewhere in the body. Surgical intervention and tissue biopsy are often required for diagnosis. Some patients progress from an initial spinal syndrome to tuberculous cranial meningitis terminally.

THERAPY

Antituberculous Chemotherapy

The most important principle of therapy is that it should be initiated when the disease is suspected and not delayed until proof has been obtained. Much more harm results from delay, even of only a few days, than from inappropriate therapy so long as efforts are continued to confirm the diagnosis.

The prognosis for tuberculous meningitis was radically improved by the advent of isoniazid.[60] In contrast to pulmonary tuberculosis, the availability of rifampin or pyrazinamide has not further improved prognosis to an appreciable degree. There are no reliable clinical trials of the chemotherapy of tuberculous meningitis of the sort that are available with respect to pulmonary tuberculosis, nor will there be, given the incidence of the disease. In meningeal tuberculosis the number of organisms is small, and the challenge to chemotherapy is delivery of drugs to the site of infection, beginning as promptly as possible so as to forestall the damage that can result from the host response to infection. On theoretical grounds there is reason to expect that combination drug therapy should enhance sterilization of the CSF; however, in a practical sense, the main purpose of multiple drug therapy is to cover the possibility of drug resistance, to reduce the risk of emerging resistance during treatment, and to treat more effectively any non–CNS foci of disease, particularly in the lungs.

Isoniazid is the cornerstone of treatment. It diffuses readily into CSF and achieves concentrations many times that required for bactericidal activity in the presence or absence of meningeal inflammation.[61] A dosage of 10 mg/kg daily in adults and children is advisable until a favorable course has been established, at which time the dose should be adjusted to 5 mg/kg. Pyridoxine in a dose of 50 mg should be given concurrently so as to avoid the neurological complications of isoniazid-induced pyridoxine deficiency. An injectable form of isoniazid is available when this drug cannot be administered by mouth or nasogastric tube. It may be administered by intramuscular injection or intravenous bolus infusion (300 mg over 5 to 10 minutes).[62]

Rifampin penetrates the CSF poorly except in the presence of meningeal inflammation; CSF concentrations then exceed the inhibitory concentration of sensitive strains.[63] The contribution of rifampin to the treatment of meningitis is a matter of controversy, but it is always included in current treatment regimens because of its contribution to the resolution of infection elsewhere in the body.[64] An intravenous formulation of rifampin is available on a "compassionate use" basis from the manufacturer. It is administered at usual dosage (600 mg in adults) in 500 ml saline.[62]

Studies of pulmonary tuberculosis have demonstrated that the addition of *pyrazinamide* (25 to 35 mg/kg) to regimens that include isoniazid and rifampin produces a more powerful antituberculous effect without increasing the incidence of hepatotoxicity when the duration of pyrazinamide therapy is restricted to 2 months or less.[65] Because of good CSF penetration and bactericidal activity, pyrazinamide is added to treatment regimens for meningitis during the first 2 months of therapy.

With the advent of other effective, less toxic agents there is less dependence on *streptomycin* than in the past, when its addition to isoniazid was designed to enhance sterilization and reduce the risk of clinical relapse from resistant organisms. Even in the presence of inflamed meninges, streptomycin penetrates the CSF poorly and is most efficacious when intramuscular (1 g daily) is combined with intrathecal (50 mg in 10 to 15 ml saline) administration.[66] Although there is controversy on this point, many hold that streptomycin is not indicated for most cases of tuberculous meningitis. It does merit consideration in selected situations, such as limited access to alternative drugs, suspicion of multidrug resistance, management of patients in whom other combinations are obviated by hepatotoxicity, and when clinical deterioration (stage 2 to stage 3) proceeds rapidly despite therapy with a more conventional regimen (see below).

Ethambutol is a weak drug that reaches the subarachnoid space in moderate concentration. Its major toxicity, optic neuritis, occurs in as many as 3 percent of patients receiving 25 mg/kg but is very rare at a dosage of 15 mg/kg. This complication limits the use of ethambutol in young children because of the difficulty of monitoring visual function in the very young, and for the same reason limits its use in patients with an altered sensorium.[67] When ethambutol is used, it is advisable to check visual acuity, red-green color vision, and visual fields if possible.[68] Its advantages are too slight and its toxic potential often too confounding to warrant routine use of ethambutol for tuberculous meningitis.

Ethionamide is a second-line antituberculous agent which readily penetrates the CSF and accordingly should be considered in cases of suspected or known isoniazid-resistant infection.

Chemotherapy Regimens

On the basis of an extensive clinical experience in Britain, physicians at Oxford utilize the regimen of isoniazid, rifampin, pyrazinamide and streptomycin, including intrathecal streptomycin, 50 mg daily for the first week and on alternate days during the second week. The Oxford group is also unique in that intrathecal purified protein derivative (PPD) is used to prevent the formation of basilar exudate. Although these recommendations for intrathecal streptomycin and PPD have not been accepted widely, Oxford physicians have the distinct impression that this approach has been highly efficacious in some cases which had responded poorly to more conventional therapy.[66]

In Hong Kong and Bangkok, major centers for the study of tuberculous meningitis in Asia, four drugs are given routinely because of the high prevalence of isoniazid resistance. Isoniazid 10 mg/kg and rifampin 10 mg/kg form the mainstay of therapy; pyrazinamide 35 mg/kg and streptomycin 20 mg/kg with a maximum dose of 1 g daily are added for the first 2 months of treatment, when the meninges are inflamed and CSF penetration by streptomycin is maximal.[64,69]

RECOMMENDED REGIMEN

There is general agreement that in populations with little isoniazid resistance, like most groups in the United States, streptomycin may be omitted. At present the usual recommended regimen is isoniazid, rifampin, and pyrazinamide for 2 months; then isoniazid and rifampin for an additional 7 months. For patients in whom drug-resistant infection is suspected (e.g., Third World origin, history of previous treatment, homeless individuals, exposure to source patients harboring drug-resistant organisms), a fourth drug—either streptomycin or ethambutol—should be added, and consideration given to the use of ethionamide as well.[70] The inherent variability of cases of tuberculous meningitis and the absence of numerically valid clinical studies makes each drug-resistant case a clinical experiment of itself.

Toxicity

The rate of hepatotoxicity in adults receiving isoniazid is on the order of 1 percent; it doubles with the addition of rifampin. This increased hepatotoxicity of regimens containing both drugs has been attributed by some to the induction by rifampin of the hepatic P-450 oxidated enzymes which accelerate the conversion of isoniazid to toxic metabolites.[71,72] Administration of other inducers of the P-450 oxidase pathway, notably phenobarbital and phenytoin but also halothane, to persons receiving isoniazid and rifampin has been associated with fulminant and fatal hepatic necrosis. Alcoholic liver disease does not modify the indications for isoniazid and rifampin. When hepatitis develops on isoniazid-rifampin, it is possible to reintroduce both drugs successfully in serial fashion in more than 70 percent of patients after a period of time has elapsed.[73]

Rifampin accelerates the metabolism of a number of important pharmacological agents (cortisol, cyclosporine, coumadin, theophylline, methadone, phe-

nytoin, ketoconazole, and oral contraceptives), with clinically important results. Other important but uncommon side effects of rifampin include interstitial nephritis and, rarely, autoimmune phenomena such as thrombocytopenia or hemolytic anemia.

Pyrazinamide, as mentioned, does not add to the hepatotoxicity of isoniazid and rifampin. It may cause arthralgia associated with hyperuricemia and, rarely, frank gout.

Adjunctive Therapy

CORTICOSTEROIDS

The role of corticosteroids in the management of tuberculous meningitis has long been a matter of great clinical interest and some uncertainty. Studies bearing on this issue have been flawed by small patient numbers and failure to stratify the severity of illness groups according to specific neurological manifestations. In one early controlled trial in children presenting with tuberculous encephalopathy, dramatic improvement in the inflammatory quality of the CSF formula was observed, but there was no apparent improvement in survival.[74] Although large-scale controlled data supporting their use are lacking, the results of limited trials and recent clinical experience favor the selective use of corticosteroids for preventing and, in some cases, treating the neurological complications of meningitis. This is the practice in most major clinical centers of Europe and of countries in Asia and Africa, where corticosteroids are administered routinely to patients with clinical stage 2 and 3 disease. Humphries, analyzing an extensive (199 patients) and well-studied experience from China, reported mortality figures of 11 percent and 61 percent for stage 2 and 3 patients treated without corticosteroids and of 5 percent and 30 percent respectively in corticosteroid-treated patients.[64] Girgis and associates reported, from Egypt, a reduction in mortality in drowsy patients from 50 percent to 15 percent with corticosteroid treatment ($p < 0.04$) and from 33 percent to 14 percent ($p < 0.02$) in those who lived long enough to receive 10 days of treatment.[75]

Complications for which corticosteroids are felt to be most beneficial are raised intracranial pressure, cerebral edema, stupor, focal neurological signs, and spinal block. To this list we would add evidence of either hydrocephalus or basilar optochiasmic pachymeningitis on CT scanning. The recommended daily dose of prednisone is 60 mg in adults and 1 to 3 mg/kg in children. Clinical improvement should become evident in a matter of days, following which the dose should be tapered gradually over 3 to 4 weeks. Patients without significant neurological compromise (stage 1) have such an excellent prognosis that adjunctive corticosteroid therapy is unwarranted.

The decision to employ corticosteroids should rest on a strong presumptive or positive diagnosis. Their use in a patient with an uncertain diagnosis can be especially devastating if the patient has, for example, fungal meningitis. Consequently, the benefit of corticosteroids must be judged against this possibility, and where fungal infection has not been confidently excluded, the addition of systemic antifungal therapy is advisable.

SURGERY

Surgical intervention is important for management of increased intracranial pressure resulting from hydrocephalus, which, if left untreated, may lead to permanent neurological damage. In patients with clinical stage 2 disease, the combination of serial lumbar punctures and corticosteroid therapy is a useful temporizing measure while the early response to chemotherapy is being assessed by serial CT scans. However, surgical decompression of the ventricular system should not be delayed in the very ill and in those with progressive neurological impairment in spite of conservative management.[76]

Paradoxical Worsening on Therapy

In a widely quoted article, Teoh and co-workers reported 10 patients and collected 12 more from the literature who developed symptomatic new tuberculomas, with neurological deterioration, during the course of effective drug therapy for tuberculous meningitis.[50] The latent period between the initiation of treatment and onset of neurological deterioration ranged from 2 weeks to 18 months. Watson and associates reported 5 more cases of paradoxical tuberculoma development in a series of 22 cases of CNS tuberculosis.[77] Although several of the patients reported had initially been treated with corticosteroids, it is not possible from the details to determine

Table 35-3 Clinical Stage of Tuberculous Meningitis and Outcome of Treatment

	No. of Patients by Stage of Disease		No. of Patients by Category of Outcome[a]			
Stage	At Admission	At Start of Treatment	1	2	3	4
1	16[b]	10	9	1	0	0
2	28	30	21	5	1	3
3	8	11	5	0	1	5
Total	52	51	35	6	2	8

[a] 1 = normal; 2 = minor neurological sequelae; 3 = major neurological sequelae; 4 = death.
[b] One patient was not treated (patient recovered).
(From Kennedy DH, Fallon RJ: Tuberculous meningitis. JAMA 241:264, 1979, with permission.)

whether or not these complications had developed on full dose or following discontinuation of corticosteroid therapy. Most patients improved with continued conservative management including reinstitution or increase in the dose of corticosteroid therapy.

Prognosis and Outcome

The clinical outcome in any individual case is greatly influenced by age, duration of illness, clinical stage at the time that treatment is instituted, and the extent and character of optochiasmic arachnoiditis and vascular complications. The influence of initial clinical stage on outcome is illustrated in Table 35-3. In general, when the treatment regimens outlined above, combined with adjunctive corticosteroid therapy, have been administered before patients progress beyond stage 1 or early stage 2 disease, they have resulted in cure rates of 85 to 90 percent.[7,69] Age below 5 and over 50 years is associated with a poorer prognosis. In general, the observed mortality exceeds 50 percent in patients over 50 years and in those with stupor and coma.[20,78] The incidence of residual neurological deficits after recovery from tuberculous meningitis varies from 10 to 30 percent in recent series. Late sequelae include cranial nerve deficits, gait disturbance, hemiplegia, blindness, deafness, learning disability, dementia, and various syndromes of hypothalamic or pituitary dysfunction.[7,13,79]

CONCLUDING COMMENTS

CNS tuberculosis is an uncommon, potentially devastating, but eminently treatable disorder. Current drugs are highly effective when treatment is initiated early, before the onset of altered mentation or focal neurological deficits. Early recognition is of paramount importance because clinical outcome depends greatly on the stage at which therapy is initiated. Patients with a meningitic syndrome and CSF findings of low glucose concentration, elevated protein, and pleocytosis should be treated immediately if there is evidence of tuberculosis elsewhere in the body or if prompt evaluation fails to establish an alternative diagnosis. Serial examination of the CSF is the best diagnostic approach; with sufficient diligence, smears and cultures for acid-fast bacilli will usually yield positive results, even days after therapy has been started. In a patient with compatible clinical features, CT evidence of basilar meningeal enhancement combined with any degree of hydrocephalus is strongly suggestive of tuberculous meningitis. Serial CT is useful for following the course of hydrocephalus and tuberculoma, particularly in reference to the need for, or response to, adjunctive therapy with corticosteroids and surgery.

Corticosteroids should be administered to patients with focal neurological abnormalities, deterioration of mental status, or evidence of spinal block. Surgical shunting should be considered early in the patient with hydrocephalus and symptoms of increased intracranial pressure. Tuberculomas are best treated medically. The recommended treatment regimen for drug-sensitive tuberculous meningitis is isoniazid and rifampin in all patients, together with pyrazinamide for the first 2 months.

REFERENCES

1. Gracey DR: Tuberculosis in the world today. Mayo Clin Proc 63:1251, 1988
2. Barry MA, Wall C, Shirley L, et al: Tuberculosis screening in Boston's homeless shelters. Public Health Rep 101:487, 1986
3. Centers for Disease Control, U.S. Department of Health and Human Services: Diagnosis and management of mycobacterial infection and disease in persons with human immunodeficiency virus infection. Ann Intern Med 106:254, 1987
4. Reider HL, Cauthen GM, Kelly GD, et al: Tuberculosis in the United States. JAMA 262:385, 1989
5. Farer LS, Lowell AM, Meador MP: Extrapulmonary tuberculosis in the United States. Am J Epidemiol 109:205, 1979
6. Snider DE: Extrapulmonary tuberculosis in Oklahoma, 1965 to 1973. Am Rev Respir Dis 111:641, 1975
7. Kennedy DH, Fallon RJ: Tuberculous meningitis. JAMA 241:264, 1979
8. Pons VG, Jacobs RA, Hollander H: Nonviral infectious of the central nervous system in patients with acquired immunodeficiency syndrome. p. 275. In Rosenblum ML, Levy RM, Bredesen DE (eds): AIDS and the Nervous System. Raven Press, New York, 1988
9. Rich AR, McCordock HA: Pathogenesis of tuberculous meningitis. Bull Johns Hopkins Hosp 52:5, 1933
10. Idriss ZH, Sinno AA, Kronfol NM: Tuberculous meningitis in childhood: forty-three cases. Am J Dis Child 130:364, 1976
11. Smith AL: Tuberculous meningitis in childhood. Med J Aust 1:57, 1975
12. Slavin RE, Walsh TJ, Pollack AD: Late generalized tuberculosis: a clinical pathologic analysis and comparison of 100 cases in the preantibiotic and antibiotic eras. Medicine (Baltimore) 59:352, 1980
13. Auerbach A: Tuberculous meningitis: correlation of therapeutic results with pathogenesis, pathologic changes, general considerations and pathogenesis. Am Rev Tuberc 64:408, 1951
14. Dastur DK, Lalitha VS: The many facets of neurotuberculosis: an epitome of neuropathology. p. 103. In Zimmerman HM (ed): Progress in Neuropathology. Vol 2. Grune & Stratton, Orlando, FL, 1973
15. Goldzieher J, Lisa J: Gross cerebral hemorrhage and vascular lesions in acute tuberculous meningitis and meningo-encephalitis. Am J Pathol 23:133, 1946
16. Poltera AA: Vascular lesions in intracranial tuberculosis. Pathol Microbiol 43:192, 1975
17. Poltera AA: Thrombogenic intracranial vasculitis in tuberculous meningitis: a 20 year "post mortem" survey. Acta Neurol Belg 77:12, 1977
18. Bhargava S, Gupta AK, Tandon PN: Tuberculous meningitis: a CT study. Br J Radiol 55:189, 1982
19. Lorber J: Studies of the cerebrospinal fluid circulation in tuberculous meningitis in children: II. A review of 100 pneumonencephalograms. Arch Dis Child 26:28, 1951
20. Hinman AR: Tuberculous meningitis at Cleveland Metropolitan General Hospital 1959 to 1963. Am Rev Respir Dis 95:670, 1967
21. Molavi A, LeFrock JL: Tuberculous meningitis. Med Clin North Am 69:315, 1985
22. Sandyk R, Brennan MJW: Internuclear ophthalmoplegia in tuberculous meningitis. Eur Neurol 23:148, 1984
23. Udani PM, Dastur DK: Tuberculous encephalopathy with and without meningitis: clinical features and pathological correlations. J Neurol Sci 10:541, 1970

24. Taylor KB, Smith HV, Vollum RL: Tuberculous meningitis of acute onset. J Neurol Neurosurg Psychiatry 18:165, 1955

25. Braun MN, Byers RH, Heyward WL, et al: Acquired immunodeficiency syndrome and extrapulmonary tuberculosis in the United States. Arch Intern Med 150: 1913, 1990

26. Bishburg E, Sunderam G, Reichman LB, Kapila R: Central nervous system tuberculosis with the acquired immunodeficiency syndrome and its related complex. Ann Intern Med 105:210, 1986

27. Berenguer J, Moreno S, Laguna F, et al: Tuberculous meningitis in patients infected with the human immunodeficiency virus. N Engl J Med 326:668, 1992

28. Dube MP, Holtom PD, Larsen RA: Tuberculous meningitis in patients with and without human immunodeficiency virus infection. Am J Med 93:520, 1992

29. Munt PW: Miliary tuberculosis in the chemotherapy era: with a clinical review in 69 American adults. Medicine (Baltimore) 51:139, 1972

30. Karandanis D, Shulman JA: Recent survey of infectious meningitis in adults: review of laboratory findings in bacterial, tuberculous, and aseptic meningitis. South Med J 69:449, 1976

31. Smith HV: Tuberculous meningitis. Int J Neurol 4:134, 1975

32. Illingsworth RS: Miliary and meningeal tuberculosis: difficulties in diagnosis. Lancet 2:646, 1956

33. Stewart SM: The bacteriologic diagnosis of tuberculous meningitis. J Clin Pathol 6:241, 1953

34. Merritt HH, Fremont-Smith F: The Cerebrospinal Fluid. WB Saunders, Philadelphia, 1938

35. Daniel TM: New approaches to the rapid diagnosis of tuberculous meningitis. J Infect Dis 155:599, 1987

36. Kaneko K, Onodera O, Miyatake T, Tsuji S: Rapid diagnosis of tuberculous meningitis by polymerase chain reaction (PCR). Neurology 40:1617, 1990

37. Artopoulos J, Chalemis Z, Christopoulos S, et al: Sequential computed tomography in tuberculous meningitis in infants and children. Comput Radiol 8:271, 1984

38. Kingsley DPE, Hendrickse WA, Kendall BE, et al: Tuberculous meningitis: role of CT in management and prognosis. J Neurol Neurosurg Psychiatry 50:30, 1987

39. Price HI, Danziger A: Computed tomography in cranial tuberculosis. AJR 130:769, 1978

40. Bullock MRR, Welchman JM: Diagnostic and prognostic features of tuberculous meningitis on CT scanning. J Neurol Neurosurg Psychiatry 45:1098, 1982

41. Schoeman J, Hewlett R, Donald P: MR of childhood tuberculous meningitis. Neuroradiology 30:473, 1988

42. Kocen RS, Parsons M: Neurological complications of tuberculosis: some unusual manifestations. Q J Med 39:17, 1970

43. Lepow ML, Coyne N, Thompson LB: A clinical, epidemiologic, and laboratory investigation of aseptic meningitis during the 4-year period, 1955–1958. N Engl J Med 266:1188, 1962

44. Dastur DK: Neurosurgically relevant aspects of pathology and pathogenesis of intracranial and intraspinal tuberculosis. Neurosurg Rev 6:103, 1983

45. Stevens DL, Everett ED: Sequential computerized axial tomography in tuberculous meningitis. JAMA 239: 642, 1978

46. Weisberg LA: Granulomatous diseases of the CNS as demonstrated by computerized tomography. Comput Radiol 8:309, 1984

47. Whelan MA, Stern J: Intracranial tuberculoma. Radiology 138:75, 1981

48. Lees AJ, MacLeod AF, Marshall J: Cerebral tuberculomas developing during treatment of tuberculous meningitis. Lancet 1:1208, 1980

49. Pauranik A, Behari M, Mehashwari MC: Appearance of tuberculoma during treatment of tuberculous meningitis. Jpn J Med 26:332, 1987

50. Teoh R, Humphries MJ, O'Mahony G: Symptomatic intracranial tuberculoma developing during treatment of tuberculosis: a report of 10 patients and review of the literature. Q J Med 63:449, 1987

51. Harder E, Al-Kawi MZ, Carney P: Intracranial tuberculoma: conservative management. Am J Med 74:570, 1983

52. Bagga A, Kalra V, Ghai OP: Intracranial tuberculoma. Clin Pediatr 27:487, 1988

53. Traub M, Colchester ACF, Kingsley DPE, Swash M: Tuberculosis of the central nervous system. Q J Med 53:81, 1984

54. Van Dyk A: CT of intracranial tuberculomas with specific reference to the "target sign." Neuroradiology 30: 329, 1988

55. Tandon PN, Bhargava S: Effect of medical treatment on intracranial tuberculoma: a CT study. Tubercle 66: 85, 1985

56. Al-Deeb SM, Yaqub BA, Sharif HS, Motaery KR: Neurotuberculosis: a review. Clin Neurol Neurosurg 94, suppl:S30, 1992

57. Bahemuka M, Murungi JH: Tuberculosis of the nervous system: a clinical, radiological and pathological study of 39 consecutive cases in Riyadh, Saudi Arabia. J Neurol Sci 90:67, 1989

58. Wadia NH, Dastur DK: Spinal meningitides with radiculo-myelopathy. J Neurol Sci 8:239, 1969

59. Rahman NU: Atypical forms of spinal tuberculosis. J Bone Joint Surg [Br] 62:162, 1980

60. Falk A: U.S. Veterans Administration–Armed Forces cooperative study on the chemotherapy of tuberculosis: XIII. Tuberculous meningitis in adults with special ref-

erence to survival, neurologic residuals, and work status. Am Rev Respir Dis 91:823, 1965

61. Des Prez R, Boone IU: Metabolism of C^{14} isoniazid in humans. Am Rev Respir Dis 84:42, 1961

62. Koestner JA, Jones LK, Polk WH, Sawyers JL: Prolonged use of intravenous isoniazid and rifampin. DICP 23:48, 1989

63. Sippel JE, Mikhail IA, Girgis NI, Youssef HH: Rifampin concentrations in cerebrospinal fluid of patients with tuberculous meningitis. Am Rev Respir Dis 109: 579, 1974

64. Humphries M: The management of tuberculous meningitis. Thorax 47:577, 1992

65. British Thoracic Association: A controlled trial of six months chemotherapy in pulmonary tuberculosis. Br J Dis Chest 75:141, 1981

66. Parsons M: The treatment of tuberculous meningitis. Tubercle 70:79, 1989

67. Citron KM: Ethambutol: a review with special reference to ocular toxicity. Tubercle 50, suppl:32, 1969

68. Chatterjee VKK, Buchanan DR, Friedmann AI, Green M: Ocular toxicity following ethambutol in standard dosage. Br J Dis Chest 80:288, 1986

69. Phuapradit P, Vejjajiva A: Treatment of tuberculous meningitis: role of short-course chemotherapy. Q J Med 62:249, 1987

70. Hughes IE, Smith HV, Kane PO: Ethionamide and its passage into the cerebrospinal fluid in man. Lancet 1: 616, 1962

71. Gangadharam PRJ: Isoniazid, rifampin, and hepatotoxicity. Am Rev Respir Dis 133:963, 1986

72. Lauterburg BM, Smith CV, Todd EL, Mitchell JR: Oxidation of hydrazine metabolites formed from isoniazid. Clin Pharmacol Ther 38:566, 1985

73. Parthasarathy R, Sarma GR, Janardhanam B, et al: Hepatic toxicity in South Indian patients during treatment of tuberculosis with short-course regimens containing isoniazid, rifampin, and pyrazinamide. Tubercle 67:99, 1986

74. O'Toole RD, Thornton GF, Mukherjee MK, Nath RL: Dexamethasone in tuberculous meningitis: relationship of cerebrospinal fluid effects to therapeutic efficacy. Ann Intern Med 70:39, 1969

75. Girgis NI, Farid Z, Kilpatrick ME, et al: Dexamethasone adjunctive treatment for tuberculous meningitis. Pediatr Infect Dis J 10:179, 1991

76. VanBeusekom GT: Complications in hydrocephalus shunting procedure. p. 28. In Wellenbur R, Brock M, Klinger M (eds): Advances in Neurosurgery. 6th Ed. Springer-Verlag, New York, 1968

77. Watson JDG, Shnier RC, Seale JP: Central nervous system tuberculosis in Australia: a report of 22 cases. Med J Aust 158:408, 1993

78. Ogawa SK, Smith MA, Brennessel DJ, Lowy FD: Tuberculous meningitis in an urban medical center. Medicine (Baltimore) 66:317, 1987

79. Udani PM, Parekh UC, Dastur DK: Neurological and related syndromes in CNS tuberculosis: clinical features and pathogenesis. J Neurol Sci 14:341, 1971

36

Neurological Complications of Leprosy

Thomas D. Sabin
Thomas R. Swift

The acid-fast organism *Mycobacterium leprae,* the cause of leprosy, was the first pathogen conclusively linked to a human disease, a discovery made by Dr. G. Armauer Hansen in 1874.[1] Leprosy affects over 10 million people worldwide.[2] A recent study reports 5.5 million active cases.[3] About 6,000 cases are in the United States, making the disease much more common than the rare neuropathies frequently discussed.[4]

The leprosy bacillus is unique in two ways: it is the only bacterial pathogen that regularly resides in peripheral nerves, and it multiplies at temperatures 7° to 10° lower than the core body temperature of 37°C.[5] These two factors account for several important clinical features of the disease. All patients with leprosy have some degree of nerve involvement, making leprous neuritis undoubtedly the commonest cause of treatable neuropathy in the world. Deformities from involvement of facial structures, eyes, nerves, bone, and skin result in stigmatization and social ostracism. The diagnosis of leprosy is often missed by physicians in the United States, leading to delay of treatment during which progressive neuropathy, visual loss, and deformity may occur.

GENERAL MANIFESTATIONS

Leprosy may be spread by aerosol or skin-to-skin contact[4]; fortunately, over 95 percent of individuals are naturally immune.[4] In susceptible patients the organisms rapidly gain access to dermal tissues, primarily cutaneous and subcutaneous nerves and nerve networks, skin appendages, sweat glands, and erector pili muscles. Leprosy occurs in three major forms: tuberculoid, borderline, and lepromatous.[4] The type of leprosy that develops depends on the degree of host resistance rather than the bacterium, which is the same for all three types.[6]

In patients with high resistance, the leprosy that develops is called tuberculoid or TT. A single patch of skin is involved by a granulomatous infiltrate, often with enlargement of underlying nerve trunks, but systemic dissemination does not occur, bacterial organisms are few, and self-healing is the rule. The skin lesions have raised edges and may have one or more satellite lesions (Fig. 36-1). Within these lesions, nerves are destroyed in an epithelioid granulomatous reaction. Often a superimposed inflammatory re-

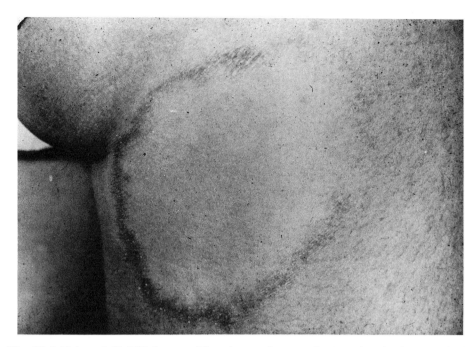

Fig. 36-1 Tuberculoid (TT) leprosy. There is complete anesthesia within this lesion, which has a raised, erythematous border and a pale dry center. (Photo courtesy of Gillis W. Long Hansen's Disease Center, Carville, LA.)

sponse, known as a reversal reaction, occurs within the lesion either spontaneously or in response to drug treatment. Such a reaction reflects altered immunological responsiveness by the host to the organism and often results in bacteriological clearing of the lesions.

In contrast, patients with multibacillary leprosy (called lepromatous or LL) have little or no resistance, and bacilli are disseminated throughout the body through a continuous bacteremia,[7] multiplying to extremely high numbers. There is little histological evidence of host resistance; histiocytes are literally stuffed with huge numbers of organisms that proliferate in cool areas of the body: the skin, upper respiratory tract, anterior one-third of the eye, superficial nerves, testes, and other tissues. Beading of corneal nerves may be seen.[6] While bacilli may be deposited passively in the deeper, and therefore warmer, vital organs such as lung, heart, liver, kidney, and brain, there is little evidence of bacterial proliferation or pathological tissue reaction at those sites. Clinically, patients present with skin infiltration, particularly prominent in the cool areas such as facial promontories, dorsal forearms, legs, nasal mucosa, and scrotum

(Fig. 36-2). Biopsy or skin scrapings of such tissues reveal innumerable acid-fast organisms. Without treatment, lepromatous leprosy continues to progress, eventually leading to severe deformities in most cases. At times spontaneously, but more often in response to antibacterial treatment, a reaction known as erythema nodosum leprosum occurs. Clinically, this is a very severe form of erythema nodosum and is a result of the deposition of antigen-antibody complexes in the walls of small arteries. Erythema nodosum leprosum occurs in areas where large amounts of mycobacterial antigen are present; the resulting inflammatory lesions can be devastating to the cornea and anterior eye, peripheral nerves, testes, and skin, producing multiple painful erythematous nodules, leading to frank ulceration in some cases (Fig. 36-3. During the course of erythema nodosum leprosum, iritis, neuritis, and orchitis occur and may be more damaging than the underlying leprosy itself. Erythema nodosum leprosum is a complex immunological reaction occurring with the production of cytokines such as tumor necrosis factor–α.[9,10] It is ironic that the circulating antibodies to mycobacterial disease becoming more like lepromatous (BL) disease (downgrading reaction), or evolving more toward the tuberculoid (BT) form (reversal reaction). Such shifts on the spectrum may occur spontaneously or in response to drug treatment or intercurrent medical conditions such as underlying neoplasms or secondary infections.

NEUROPATHOLOGY

In tuberculoid leprosy, the few organisms present in peripheral nerve evoke a strong granulomatous response with early and severe nerve damage, fortunately limited to the few nerves involved. It is not clear how the organisms present in peripheral nerve in lepromatous leprosy produce nerve damage. Whereas the overwhelming majority of organisms are present in Schwann cells (Fig. 36-5), most of the neuropathological and electrophysiological data suggest a preponderance of axonal destruction with relatively little demyelination,[13] and the demyelinating lesions themselves may be secondary to axonal changes.[14] While the nerve lesions of leprosy tend to be permanent, prompt treatment of reactions may improve neurological deficits.[13,15] It is also unclear to what extent or by what mechanisms erythema nodosum leprosum produces nerve damage, but it is likely that cytokines released by immunocompetent cells are important. Exogenous interferon gamma used in an attempt to treat leprosy has caused erythema nodosum leprosum in patients who then have increased release of tumor necrosis factor.[9] Thalidomide, which controls erythema nodosum leprosum, reduces tumor necrosis factor secretion.[9] Thalidomide also reduces elevated numbers of CD4+ lymphocytes in the blood of patients with erythema nodosum leprosum.[16] In lepromatous leprosy, during erythema nodosum leprosum, there is a loss of suppressor cell function and increase in interleukin-2 production.[16] Cyclosporine suppresses erythema nodosum leprosum and restores suppressor cell activity, possibly by its effect on macrophages.[17,18]

LEPROUS NEURITIS

A meticulous neurological examination will reward the clinician with definitive diagnostic information for this common and treatable neuropathy. The

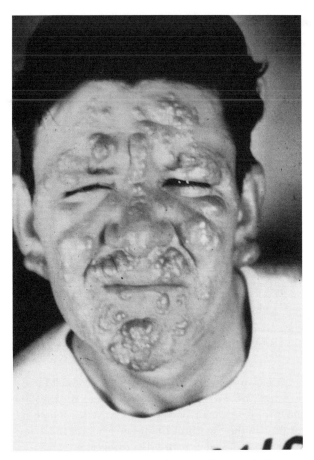

Fig. 36-2 Lepromatous (LL) leprosy. There is infiltration of the cooler facial promontories—i.e., ears, upper lip, chin, supraorbital and malar areas. (Photo courtesy of Gillis W. Long Hansen's Disease Center, Carville, LA.)

antigen, constituting the host's only immunological responsiveness to the offending organism, should paradoxically result in additional tissue damage.

In the third type of leprosy, called borderline leprosy (or BB), there occurs a spectrum of disease depending upon the degree of host resistance, which is variable. In patients having low resistance the disease resembles lepromatous disease (BL), whereas in those with higher resistance it resembles tuberculoid disease (BT). Patients with borderline leprosy have less skin involved than lepromatous cases and may have more circumscribed skin lesions, but they have more skin lesions than tuberculoid cases (Fig. 36-4). A form of "pure neuritic" leprosy occurs without visible skin lesions.[11,12] In the spectrum of borderline leprosy immunity may change, with patients worsening, their

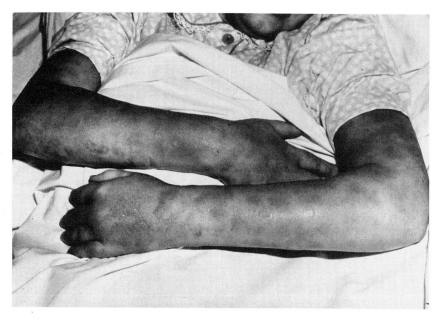

Fig. 36-3 Erythema nodosum leprosum. Painful subcutaneous nodules cover the face, trunk, and extremities. (Photo courtesy of Gillis W. Long Hansen's Disease Center, Carville, LA.)

diagnosis is based on the recognition of two interplaying themes which, although they produce limitless combinations in individual cases, capture the unique nature of this neuropathy once they are discerned. These themes both rest upon the fact that *M. leprae* is the only bacterium that consistently invades peripheral nerves.

The first of the two diagnostic themes is based upon another biological feature of *M. leprae*—that is, a highly thermosensitive growth rate which is optimal at 27° to 30°C.[5,19,20] The organism does not reproduce at all at core body temperature. This feature limits leprosy to involvement of only superficial nerves. The distinction between the superficial neuropathy of leprosy and a distal polyneuropathy is vital for correct diagnosis. This has been a source of confusion, because long nerves tend to innervate cooler parts of the body. In leprosy, nerve damage is limited to intracutaneous nerve endings and networks and to the named nerves of gross anatomy at certain segments along their length where they course closest to the cooler surface of the body.[21] Since *M. leprae* cannot proliferate at core body temperature, peripheral nerves that are situated in deep tissues under muscles, nerve roots, and the central nervous system are not actively involved.

The second diagnostic theme relates to host factors that determine the immune resistance to the invasion and proliferation of bacilli. This host resistance has resulted in the classification of leprosy into three subtypes and is the other major determinant of the clinical features of nerve damage.

Lepromatous Leprosy

There is very little evidence of tissue-mediated immune responses to *M. leprae* in lepromatous leprosy, and lepromin skin testing is negative. The organism proliferates most rapidly in the coolest tissues and there is a constant bloodstream dissemination of organisms.[7] In untreated cases, this type of leprosy becomes widespread and symmetrical within superficial tissues and may involve large areas of the skin, the anterior chamber of the eye, the upper respiratory tract, and the testes, as well as superficial nerves. Sensory loss is largely due to destruction of intracutaneous nerve endings and first appears in cool areas such as the dorsal surfaces of the hands, dorsal medial surfaces of the forearms, dorsal surfaces of the feet, and anterolateral aspects of the legs, as well as in the pinnae of the ears, especially the helices and ear-

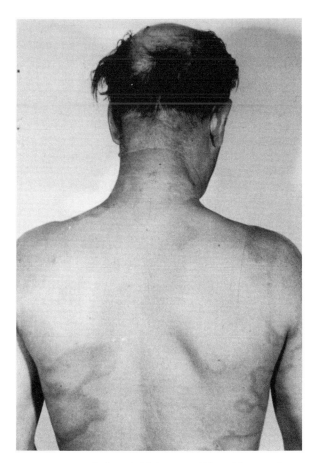

Fig. 36-4 Borderline (BB) leprosy. The widespread symmetrical skin lesions are hypesthetic. (Photo courtesy of Gillis W. Long Hansen's Disease Center, Carville, LA.)

lobes[22,23] (Fig. 36-6). The tip of the nose, malar areas, breasts, central abdomen, and buttocks are often the next to show intracutaneous sensory loss (Fig. 36-7). There is a stage with sparing of the soles of the feet and palms of the hands, which may be in part due to the insulating effect of the thickened corium in these areas. If the patient is examined at the right stage, a distinct change in sensation at the cuticular border can sometimes be found in the hands or feet. When the intracutaneous pattern has evolved to this point, nerve trunk deficits supervene. Involvement of a 10- to 15-cm segment of the ulnar nerve proximal to the olecranon groove is most common, but the segment just proximal to the wrist may also be affected. Further paralysis is seen with damage to the median nerve in the segment where it assumes a superficial position

just proximal to the transverse carpal ligament (Fig. 36-8), to the peroneal nerve where it courses around the fibular head, and to the branch to extensor digitorum brevis and posterior tibial nerve at the level of the ankle.[21] There is also a unique patchy paralysis of the most superficial facial nerve twigs, causing lagophthalmos as well as paralysis of some segments of the orbicularis oris and of the medial aspects of the corrugators of the forehead.[24]

With progression of the intracutaneous sensory loss, this pattern is more easily recognized by the areas of sparing that include the intergluteal fold, the perineum, the anterior neck, under the scalp hair, in the posterior creases at the attachment of the ears to the head, the axillae, the sternal area, and the center of the back where skin lies closest to the paraspinal muscles. Sparing may be found in the webs of the toes or fingers and the antecubital and popliteal fossae (Fig. 36-9). A careful search may reveal unique features such as sparing under constantly worn items of clothing (e.g., under a watchband or at a belt line) and even in small cutaneous vascular malformations.[25] Examination of the distal extremities alone may result in confusion with a distal sensory neuropathy; therefore the search must include the ears, nose, malar areas, and other proximal but "cooler" areas in order to detect the pattern of temperature-linked sensory loss. This differential diagnosis is also suggested by the preservation of deep tendon reflexes. Even severe destruction of the mixed sensorimotor nerves at the sites outlined above would fail to disrupt the arcs for the usually elicited tendon reflexes. Despite the appearance of an extensive sensorimotor neuropathy with clawed toes, foot drop, and clawed hands, intact reflexes are the rule. Rarely, radial nerve involvement affects the segment that emerges from under the triceps, 4 to 6 cm proximal to the elbow. There is paralysis and atrophy in the wrist and finger extensors, whereas the triceps, brachioradialis, and anconeus muscles tend to be spared. The differential diagnosis of leprous neuritis is provided in Table 36-1.

A variety of cutaneous lesions are associated with lepromatous leprosy, and they are most abundant and prominent in the areas where bacilli are most common in the cooler tissues. There is no precise linkage between those skin lesions and the intracutaneous sensory loss. Because the tissue immune response to the bacilli in lepromatous leprosy is very indolent, the neuropathy evolves over many years. Nerves that

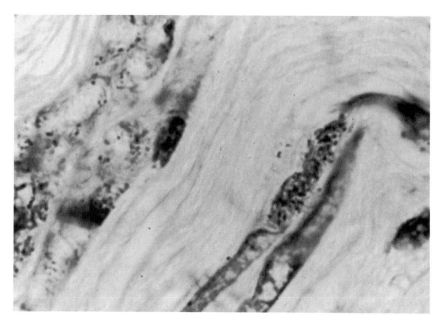

Fig. 36-5 Sural nerve biopsy, lepromatous leprosy (LL). This acid-fast stain reveals numerous organisms in endoneurial vacuoles. (Photo courtesy of Gillis W. Long Hansen's Disease Center, Carville, LA.)

are grossly enlarged and infiltrated with abundant bacilli may still function well. These enlarged nerves are more liable to recurrent trauma, and measures must occasionally be taken to prevent the addition of mechanical damage to these already vulnerable nerves.

Tuberculoid Leprosy

At the other end of the spectrum of host response to infection with *M. leprae* is tuberculoid leprosy. There is a vigorous tissue-mediated immune response to the invasion of bacilli which greatly limits spread and proliferation of *M. leprae*.[4] Only rare organisms are found in the resulting epithelioid granuloma, and nerve damage occurs as the lesion develops. This means that the neurological picture is generally one of a clearly demarcated patch of sensory loss and absent sweating corresponding with a visible skin lesion that is usually hypopigmented, with an elevated border (Fig. 36-1). Bacteria have often been cleared from the center of these lesions but are still detectable in biopsies at the perimeter. Lepromin skin testing is positive in this form of the disease. Temperature has only a "permissive" role, in the sense that the lesions must occur in a region where the bacilli can reproduce; tissue temperature does not otherwise determine the precise nature of the neuropathy, as it does in lepromatous disease. Local bacillary invasion of nerves and the immediate immune tissue response are the two factors that result in focal, limited, and asymmetrical disease. There is a tendency for self-healing in this variety of leprosy. A named mixed, motor, or sensory nerve near a solitary tuberculoid patch may also be affected. These observations have suggested that *M. leprae* can travel from the intracutaneous endings back to the major nerve supplying the area of anesthetic skin. The major mixed nerves that are most commonly affected are the ulnar, median, peroneal, and facial. Subcutaneous sensory nerves near the tuberculoid patch are most likely to be enlarged, but one should also palpate for enlargement of distant nerves such as the superficial cutaneous radial, digital, sural, and posterior auricular nerves. The tissue response within nerves may be so intense that there is necrosis and formation of a "cold" abscess. Intense local pain results, requiring surgical drainage of the abscess.[26] Calcification resulting in radiographically detectable linear streaks within nerves may also occur, and enlarged nerves may be demonstrable on computed tomographic scans.[27] Anhidrosis is always

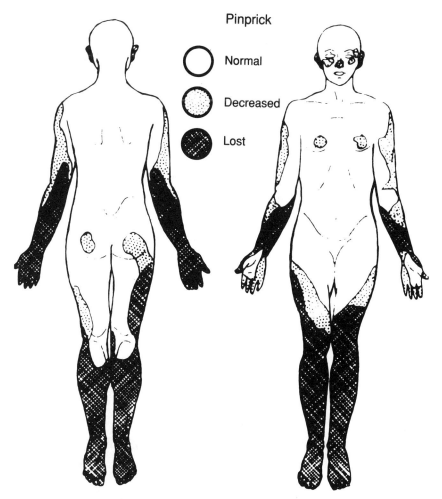

Pinprick

◯ Normal

◔ Decreased

⬤ Lost

Fig. 36-6 Lepromatous leprosy (LL). Sensation is diminished in cool zones of face, trunk, and extremities.

present within tuberculoid lesions; injections or iontophoresis of cholinergic agents into the area may be helpful in establishing the diagnosis.[28]

Borderline Leprosy

Many patients have clinical and pathological features that fall between polar tuberculoid and lepromatous leprosy and are classified as borderline leprosy.[4] Such patients demonstrate unending permutations in the roles of tissue temperatures and host resistance in the pathogenesis of their nerve dysfunction. The neurologist experienced in leprosy can place patients along a spectrum paralleling a pathological classification, where the letters T, B, and L stand for *tuberculoid, borderline,* and *lepromatous*. TT represents pure tuberculoid and LL represents pure lepromatous disease. TB, BB, BL are the intermediate borderline varieties. The borderline cases near tuberculoid disease (TB) have several skin lesions that tend to be larger and less distinctly demarcated than in the pure tuberculoid cases. As one moves away from the tuberculoid end of the spectrum, there is less superimposition of the sensory deficit with the visible skin lesion. In the midrange of borderline leprosy (BB), lesions many be quite large and begin to coalesce with insensitivity, covering a large area of the body, but they retain geographical borders that do not closely reflect

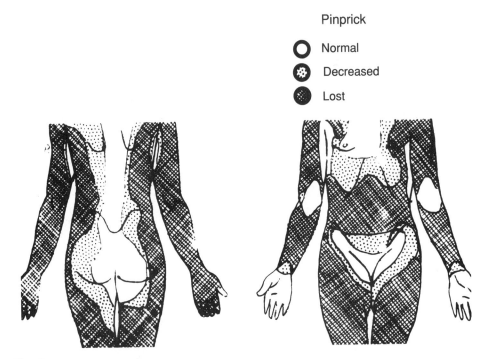

Fig. 36-7 Lepromatous leprosy (LL). Sensation is preserved in warm areas: axillae, palms, antecubital fossae, inguinal region, gluteal cleft, center of back and chest.

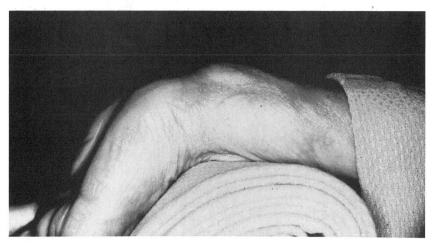

Fig. 36-8 Lepromatous leprosy (LL). Enlargement of the median nerve proximal to the carpal tunnel. (Photo courtesy of Dr. Paul Brand and Gillis W. Long Hansen's Disease Center, Carville, LA.)

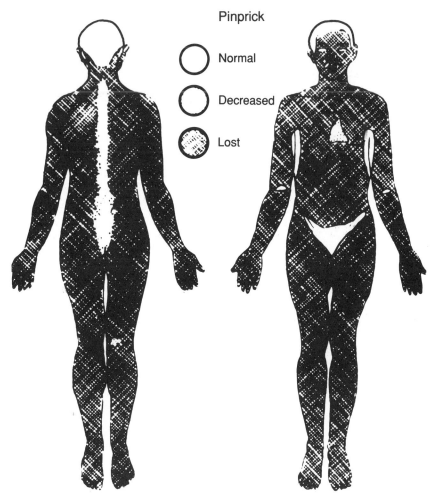

Pinprick

◯ Normal

◯ Decreased

◉ Lost

Fig. 36-9 Lepromatous leprosy (LL). Sensory sparing under scalp, in axillae and groin, in the center of back and chest, and in the antecubital fossae and nasolabial folds.

tissue temperature gradients beyond a general tendency to spare the warmest parts of the body (Fig. 36-10). Sensory maps in such cases may show extensive intracutaneous loss which does not conform to the disruption of named peripheral nerves, nerve roots, or any known neuropathy. Further movement toward lepromatous disease (BL) is revealed by symmetry of neural deficits and the loss of linkage between the perimeters of skin lesions and areas of sensory loss. A definite tendency toward temperature-linked patterns of sensory loss emerges, but these are not as perfectly symmetrical and graduated as in pure lepromatous disease (LL).

In addition to the damage to nerves done by the invasion of *M. leprae,* there are several types of leprosy reactions in which there is a sudden and often sustained increase in immune response to bacilli or products released by dead bacilli. Erythema nodosum leprosum occurs only in lepromatous leprosy and appears to be a clinical example of the Arthus phenomenon, with consumption of complement and an intense vasculitis.[29] The vasculitis is most severe in the regions of greatest bacterial density and therefore may result in a devastating acute neuritis. Thalidomide or high doses of corticosteroids are required to treat erythema nodosum leprosum. In tuberculoid and bor-

Table 36-1 Differential Diagnosis of Leprous Neuritis

Neurological Disorder	Clinical Features			
	Paralysis Confined to Major Nerve Trunks	Deep Tendon Reflexes Preserved	Enlarged Nerves	Pattern of Sensory Loss
Peripheral nerve diseases				
"Superficial" neuropathy				
Lepromatous leprosy	+	+	+	Unique—superficial loss beginning over coolest body surfaces and certain nerve trunks
Tuberculoid leprosy	+	+	+	Coterminous with skin lesion and certain nerve trunks
Peripheral neuropathies				
Most toxic, metabolic, and nutritional neuropathies	0	0	0	"Stocking-glove"
Rare types with nerve enlargement (primary amyloidosis, Refsum's, Dejerine-Sottas' interstitial hypertrophic)	0	0	+	"Stocking-glove"
Mononeuropathy and mononeuropathy multiplex Patients with arteritis (lupus, polyarteritis), diabetes, serum neuritis, lead neuropathy, Lyme disease	+	+	0	In distribution of affected nerve trunks
Multifocal motor (and sensory) neuropathy	+	+	0	Localized, e.g., digit or single sensory nerve
Chronic pressure palsies	+	+	0	Nerve trunks
Types with nerve enlargement				
von Recklinghausen's neurofibromatosis	+(& roots)	+	+	Roots or trunks
Sarcoidosis	+(& roots)	+	+/0	Roots or trunks
Radiculoneuropathies				
Guillain-Barré syndrome and similar syndrome in diabetes, AIDS, porphyria, and arteritides	0	0	0	Sensation often spared; deep sensibility loss may be present
Chronic inflammatory demyelinating polyneuropathy	0	0	+/0	Sensory loss often involving hands, feet, mouth, genitalia
Relapsing form of Austin	0	0	0	Deep sensation most affected
Diseases confused with leprosy because of painless injuries, with trophic ulcers and absorption of digits (not classified above)				
Syringomyelia	0	0	0	"Forequarter" or "cape" dissociated sensory loss
Universal insensitivity to pain	0	+	0	Pain loss only, whole body affected
Tabes dorsalis	0	0	0	Patchy thermoanalgesia with profound loss of deep sensation

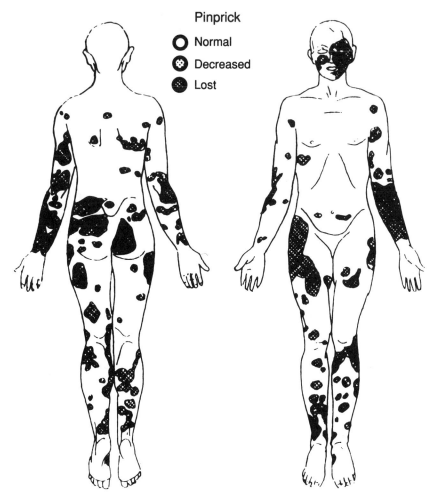

Pinprick
○ Normal
◉ Decreased
● Lost

Fig. 36-10 Borderline leprosy (BB). Sensory loss occurs in the skin lesions. Skin lesions tend to affect cooler areas.

derline leprosy, reactions consist of sudden increase in tissue-mediated immunity, with flaring of the skin lesions and acute neuritis. Corticosteroids (but *not* thalidomide) are effective in these reactions.

TREATMENT

The treatment of leprosy is threefold: (1) drug treatment aimed at the eradication of *M. leprae;* (2) drug treatment of leprosy reactions; and (3) rehabilitation, cosmetic and restorative procedures, and prevention of further deformity consequent to loss of sensation.

The drug treatment of leprosy is changing. Since 1940, sulfones have been the mainstay of treatment, replacing chaulmoogra oil, which had only limited antimycobacterial action. However, with sulfones, many patients developed recurrent disease after periods of apparent bacterial negativity by organisms which were demonstrated in the mouse footpad test to be sulfone-resistant.[30]

In addition, sulfones themselves may produce peripheral neuropathy and other idiopathic and dose-related side effects, such as hemolysis and, rarely, agranulocytosis.[31] Another useful drug is clofazimine (Lamprene, B663), a rimino phenazine dye, and this drug may be helpful in suppressing erythema nodosum leprosum.[4] However, it discolors the skin and is therefore unacceptable to many patients, and its hepatotoxicity is a major side effect.

In patients with tuberculoid or high-resistance borderline disease, current guidelines of the World Health Organization suggest a combination of dapsone and rifamycin.[4] With low resistance disease (low resistance borderline, and lepromatous leprosy) double or triple therapy with dapsone, rifamycin and clofazimine is advocated. Doses for paucibacillary cases are dapsone 100 mg/d and rifamycin 600 mg/d for 6 months, followed by dapsone for 3 to 5 years. Multibacillary patients are given the same regimen for 3 years rather than 6 months, followed by dapsone monotherapy for 10 years to life. Clofazimine may be added if dapsone resistance is suspected. Other regimens have also been recommended, and the field is changing. For the most recent treatment recommendations, biopsy interpretation, patient referrals, or suggestions for management, the reader is urged to call the Gillis W. Long Hansen's Disease Center in Carville, Louisiana.

The treatment of leprosy reactions is important because of the threat that such reactions pose to the patient. Leprosy reactions are of three types. Erythema nodosum leprosum is treated with high-dose corticosteroids (prednisone 60 to 80 mg or more daily), particularly if accompanied by neuritis, or by thalidomide, 300 to 400 mg/d. Thalidomide is available in the United States at no charge through arrangements with the Gillis W. Long Hansen's Disease Center. (Female patients receiving thalidomide must take absolute precautions to prevent pregnancy because the drug induces phocomelia.) Thalidomide reduces the secretion of tumor necrosis factor α by monocytes[9,10] and causes a decrease in the ratio of CD4+ to CD8+ lymphocytes.[16] When erythema nodosum leprosum is controlled, the dose is tapered to 100 mg/d. Long-term thalidomide treatment may also cause or worsen peripheral neuropathy.[32,33] Reversal reactions, which may be very intense, are treated with high-dose corticosteroids as necessary. Clofazimine in a dose of 200 to 300 mg/d is also of value in treating reactions, in addition to being antibacterial. After the reaction is controlled, the dose can be tapered to 100 mg/d.

Rehabilitation of leprosy patients is difficult because the associated stigma makes patients reluctant to come forward for treatment. Many such patients who have cosmetic and crippling deformities involving face, eyes, eyelids, eyebrows, ears, nose, hands, and feet may benefit from surgical restorative procedures. The attendant peripheral neuropathy (with loss of temperature and pain sensation and of sweating but with preservation of motor function) creates the risk of progressive damage to hands and feet from painless injury followed by ulceration, infection, osteomyelitis, and eventually bone resorption. Such patients must be instructed in the care of hands, feet, and eyes to prevent secondary disability attendant upon the neuropathy, similar to patients with other neurological conditions where pain sensation is lost but power is retained, such as syringomyelia, hereditary sensory and autonomic neuropathies, amyloid neuropathy, certain cases of diabetic neuropathy involving small fibers, and other conditions. In fact, patients with these neurological conditions can often be found in leprosariums, where they are mistakenly believed to have leprosy because the mutilating deformities are so similar.

REFERENCES

1. Hansen GA: Umder sogeiser angaende spedalskhedens arsager tiedels ud forte sammen med forstander Hartwig. Norske Mag Laegevidensk, suppl 4:1, 1874
2. World Health Organization: A Guide to Leprosy Control. 2nd Ed. World Health Organization, Geneva, 1988
3. Nordeen SK, Lopez Bravo L, Sundaresan TK: Estimated number of leprosy cases in the world. Bull WHO 70:7, 1992
4. Sabin TD, Swift TR, Jacobson RR: Leprosy. p. 1354. In Dyck PJ, Thomas PK, Griffin JW, et al (eds): Peripheral Neuropathy. 3rd Ed. WB Saunders, Philadelphia, 1993
5. Shepard CC: Temperature optimum of Mycobacterium leprae in mice. J Bacteriol 90:1271, 1965
6. Sehgal VN, Joginder, Sharma VK: Immunology of leprosy, a comprehensive survey. Int J Dermatol 28:574, 1989
7. Powell CS, Swan LL: Leprosy: pathologic changes in 50 consecutive necropsies. Am J Pathol 31:1131, 1955
8. Prendergast JJ: Ocular leprosy in the United States. Arch Ophthalmol 23:112, 1940
9. Sampaio EP, Moreira AL, Sarno EN, et al: Prolonged treatment with recombinant interferon gamma induces erythema nodosum leprosum in lepromatous leprosy patients. J Exp Med 175:1729, 1992
10. Barnes PF, Chatterjee D, Brennan PJ, et al: Tumor

necrosis factor production in patients with leprosy. Infect Immun 60:1441, 1992

11. Jacob M, Mathai R: Diagnostic efficacy of cutaneous nerve biopsy in primary neuritic leprosy. Int J Lepr Other Mycobact Dis 56:56, 1988

12. Uplekar MW, Antia NH: Clinical and histopathological observations on pure neuritic leprosy. Indian J Lepr 48:513, 1986

13. Naafs B, Pearson JMH, Baar AJM: A follow-up study of nerve lesions in leprosy during and after reaction using motor nerve conduction velocity. Int J Lepr Other Mycobact Dis 44:188, 1976

14. Jacobs JM, Shetty VP, Antia NH: Teased fibre studies in leprous neuropathy. J Neurol Sci 79:301, 1987

15. Becx-Bleumink M, Berhe D: Occurrence of reactions, their diagnosis and management in leprosy patients treated with multidrug therapy: experience in the leprosy control program of the All Africa Leprosy and Rehabilitation Training Center (ALERT) in Ethiopia. Int J Lepr Other Mycobact Dis 60:173, 1992

16. Shannon EJ, Ejigu M, Haile-Mariam HS, et al: Thalidomide's effectiveness in erythema nodosum leprosum is associated with a decrease in CD4+ cells in the peripheral blood. Lepr Rev 63:5, 1992

17. Miller RA, Shen JY, Rea TH, Harnisch JP: Treatment of chronic erythema nodosum leprosum with cyclosporine A produces clinical and immunohistologic remission. Int J Lepr Other Mycobact Dis 55:441, 1987

18. Uyemura K, Dixon JF, Wong L, et al: Effect of cyclosporine A in erythema nodosum leprosum. J Immunol 137:3620, 1986

19. Brand PW: Temperature variation and leprosy deformity. Int J Lepr 27:1, 1959

20. Hastings RC, Brand PW, Mansfield RE, Ebner JD: Bacterial density in the skin in lepromatous leprosy as related to temperature. Lepr Rev 39:71, 1968

21. Sabin TD, Hackett ER, Brand PW: Temperatures along the course of certain nerves affected in leprosy. Int J Lepr Other Mycobact Dis 42:38, 1974

22. Sabin TD: Temperature-linked sensory loss: a unique pattern in leprosy. Arch Neurol 20:257, 1969

23. Sabin TD, Ebner JE: Patterns of sensory loss in lepromatous leprosy. Int J Lepr Other Mycobact Dis 37:239, 1969

24. Monrad-Krohn GH: The Neurological Aspect of Leprosy. Jacob Dybward, Christiana, 1923

25. Sabin TD: Preservation of sensation in a cutaneous vascular malformation in lepromatous leprosy. N Engl J Med 282:1084, 1970

26. Enna CD, Brand PW: Peripheral nerve abscess in leprosy. Lepr Rev 41:175, 1970

27. Barbancon O, Rath S, Alqubati Y: Hansen's disease: computed tomography findings in peripheral nerve lesions. Ann Radiol (Paris) 32:579, 1989

28. MacMillian AL, Spalding JMK: Human sweating response to electrophoresed acetylcholine. J Neurol Neurosurg Psychiatry 32:155, 1969

29. Wemambu SNC, Turk JL, Wates MFR, Rees RJW: Erythema nodosum leprosum: a clinical manifestation of the Arthus phenomenon. Lancet 2:933, 1969

30. Shepard CC: Experimental chemotherapy in leprosy, then and now. Int J Lepr Other Mycobact Dis 41:307, 1973

31. Sirsat AM, Lalitha VS, Pandya SS: Dapsone neuropathy—report of three cases and pathologic features of a motor nerve. Int J Lepr Other Mycobact Dis 55:23, 1987

32. Awofeso N: Thalidomide peripheral neuropathy. Trop Doct 22:139, 1992

33. Gunzler V: Thalidomide in human immunodeficiency virus (HIV) patients. A review of safety considerations. Drug Saf 7:116, 1992

37

Nervous System Complications of Systemic Viral Infections

Larry E. Davis

The brain should be an easy target for viral infections because it is an immunoprivileged organ. The brain lacks a lymphatic system, and it has few immunological cells migrating through the brain parenchyma. Normal cerebrospinal fluid (CSF) has fewer than 5 lymphocytes/mm^3 and has only about 1/200 the amount of antibody that is present in serum.[1] Many viruses replicate in the central nervous system (CNS) when directly inoculated into the brain. The resulting brain infection is usually severe, whereas the same viral infection of other organs may be mild. For example, herpes simplex virus infection in labial skin causes a localized small blister, but infection in brain causes a severe encephalitis.

Despite the potential vulnerability of the CNS, most systemic viral infections do not cause CNS disease. To reach the CNS, a virus must overcome several major protective systems. First, viruses entering the body do not have the opportunity to infect nerves directly. With the exception of the olfactory nerves, the nervous system does not come into direct contact with the environment. To reach the CNS, all viruses must first establish a primary site of replication. Viruses that enter the gastrointestinal tract (e.g., poliovirus) establish a primary site of replication in the oral pharynx and gastrointestinal tract.[2] Viruses that enter via the respiratory system (e.g., mumps virus) establish local replication in the upper respiratory tract and regional lymph nodes.[3] Viruses that enter the body via inoculation (e.g., arboviruses) establish local replication in vascular endothelium and regional lymph nodes.[4,5] To date, viruses have not been shown to reach the CNS through primary infection of olfactory nerves. During the primary viral infection, the host's normal defense system comes into play to counteract the local infection. The few viruses that do successfully reach the CNS do so by two major routes: blood and peripheral nerves. Hematogenous spread is the most common. Following primary viral replication, a viremia often develops that allows secondary tissues to become infected and results in a systemic illness. Despite the viremia, most viruses still do not reach the CNS because of several factors. Virus particles, like other colloidal particles in the blood, are efficiently cleared by the reticuloendothelial system. For example, the reticuloendothelial system can clear more than 90 percent of an arbovirus viremia within 1 hour.[6] Within days, the host humoral immune system—immunoglobulin M (IgM) antibodies against the virus—and cellular immune system (macrophages and lymphocytes) actively participate in clearing the virus from infected tissues and blood.

The blood-brain barrier also prevents viruses from entering the CNS. The morphological blood-brain barrier consists of cerebral capillaries that have tight junctions between cells to prevent egress of plasma and white blood cells.[7] These tight junctions prevent viral particles from escaping the capillary lumen. In addition, cerebral capillaries and endothelial cells have few pinocytotic vesicles, and the vessels are surrounded by tight astrocytic footplates. The occasional viral infection that does bridge the blood-brain barrier appears to do so by either infecting and replicating within capillary endothelial cells with release of progeny virions into the brain or by infecting choroid plexus epithelial cells.[2] Capillaries in the choroid plexus have fenestrations, but the adjacent choroid epithelial cells have tight junctions. Thus viruses such as mumps appear to reach the CSF by infecting choroid plexus epithelial cells with subsequent release of progeny virions into the CSF.[8]

The efficiency with which these defense systems prevent viruses from infecting the CNS is remarkable. Fewer than 1 percent of nonimmune children infected with wild poliovirus develop poliomyelitis,[9] and fewer than 5 percent of individuals infected with St. Louis encephalitis virus develop encephalitis.[4]

A few viruses are transported to the CNS via peripheral nerves. With rabies, there is local virus replication in muscle following inoculation from the animal bite. As the muscle infection spreads, virus eventually reaches synapses at the neuromuscular junction or muscle spindle.[10] After viral attachment to presynapic membranes, the virus is transported via retrograde axoplasmic flow to the brainstem, spinal cord, or dorsal root ganglion, where it then spreads throughout the CNS. There is some evidence that herpes simplex encephalitis may be the result of exacerbation of latent virus in the trigeminal ganglion and spread to the brain via branches of the trigeminal nerve.[11] This unusual neural route circumvents the reticuloendothelial system and blood-brain barrier.

Should a virus infect the CNS, the cellular immune system appears to play an important role in clearance of the virus. With experimental viral meningitis, the meningeal infection elicits an inflammatory response that contains mainly T lymphocytes[12] that are specifically immune-mediated.[13] Likewise, with experimental viral encephalitis, the inflammatory response is one of specifically immune-mediated lymphocytes.[14]

The brain is not a homogeneous organ, such as the liver. Viral infections directed toward different brain locations or cell types in the CNS result in differing signs and symptoms. Viruses that infect leptomeningeal cells cause a meningitis, whereas viruses that infect neurons and glia cause an encephalitis.[15] Even subtypes of neurons (e.g., those of the motor system) can be preferentially infected by viruses such as poliovirus, giving rise to an illness in which muscle weakness predominates. The time course of spread of the viral infection varies from virus to virus. Some viruses, such as echovirus, give rise to a brief (about 1 week) infection of the leptomeninges and are cleared promptly by the immune system.[16] Other viruses, such as measles (rubeola virus), occasionally cause a chronic infection, subacute sclerosing panencephalitis, that slowly progresses over months to years.[17] Some viruses, such as varicella–zoster virus, can escape immune surveillance by becoming latent in dorsal root ganglion neurons following the primary chickenpox infection.[18] Decades later they can reactivate to cause shingles, an acute neuritis involving a dermatome.

In summary, most viruses that cause systemic illnesses in humans do not reach the CNS. When they occasionally do, they cause a variety of diseases with differing signs and symptoms and varying time courses.

This chapter focuses on the common and important nervous system syndromes that occur with or following systemic viral infections. Table 37-1 lists the major viruses that infect humans and estimates the frequency (per 100,000 systemic viral infections) of a variety of nervous system syndromes that can develop.

VIRAL MENINGITIS

Viral meningitis, the most common viral infection of the CNS, is due to a viral infection of leptomeningeal cells. Viral meningitis is often discussed along with aseptic meningitis. *Aseptic meningitis* includes viral meningitis plus transient meningeal inflammation from other causes such as bacteria that do not grow in routine cultures (*Leptospira icterohaemorrhagiae, Treponema pallidum, Mycoplasma pneumoniae*),

Table 37-1 Frequency of Neurological Syndromes with Systemic Viral Infections

Virus	Meningitis	Encephalitis	Transverse Myelitis	Poliomyelitis	Chronic Nervous System Infection	Postviral Encephalomyelitis	Guillain-Barré Syndrome	Reye's Syndrome	Deafness and Vertigo	Optic Neuritis
Enterovirus	A	B	B	B	B[a]		B	C	C	
Poliovirus	A			A						
Hepatitis A	C	C	C				B		C	C
Reovirus	C									
Influenza	C	B	C			B	B	B	B	
Parainfluenza	C							B	B	
Mumps	A	B	C			B	C	C	B	C
Respiratory syncytial	C	C	C							
Measles (rubeola)	A	B	B		B	A	B	C	B	B
Rabies	A	A								
Human immunodeficiency	A	C	C		A		B		C	
Lymphocytic choriomeningitis	A	B	B							
Togavirus	A	A							C	
Dengue	B	B	C				C		C	C
Rubella, postnatal	C	B	B				C		C	C
Rubella, congenital	A	A			C				A	
Colorado tick fever	A	A			C					
Herpes simplex	B	B	B	C	A		B	C	B	
Varicella-zoster	B	B	B		A	B	B	B	B	B
Cytomegalovirus, postnatal	C					C	B	C		
Cytomegalovirus, congenital	A	A	A						A	
Epstein-Barr	C	B	B		C	C	B	C	B	
Adenovirus	B	B		B[a]					C	
Hepatitis B		B	B							
Papovavirus (JC)					B					
Creutzfeld-Jakob agent					A[b]					

A = >1 per 1,000 primary infections. B = <1 per 1,000 primary infections. C = Only few scattered case reports.

[a] In patients with agammaglobulinemia.

[b] Because the incidence of primary infection is unknown, the risk of CNS disease is unknown.

Table 37-2 Causes of Viral Meningitis

Virus	Frequency	Epidemiology	Associated Features	Common Diagnostic Procedures
Enteroviruses[19,20] (echo, coxsackie, polio)	Common	Occurs mainly in summer and fall	Occasional abdominal or chest pain; occasional rash	Viral isolation from throat and stool (rarely from CSF)
Mumps[21,22]	Common	Outbreaks	Often associated with parotid swelling	Viral isolation from CSF Serology
Herpes simplex type 2[23,24]	Uncommon	Sporadic Recent sexual exposure	Sometimes genital herpetic lesions	Isolation from CSF and genital lesion
Togaviruses[25] (arbovirus)	Common	Outbreaks in summer and fall	Myalgia	Serology
Human immuno-deficiency virus[26]	Uncommon	Increased in homosexuals and IV drug abusers	Fever, adenopathy, rash, mononucleosis-like syndrome	HIV antibodies during convalescence: virus isolation from CSF
Lymphocytic chorio-meningitis[27]	Uncommon	From infected pet; laboratory or wild mouse or hamster urine	High lymphocyte levels in CSF	Serology
Adenovirus[28]	Rare	Sporadic		Viral isolation from CSF

parasites (*Toxoplasma gondii*), and parameningeal infections.[16] However, most cases of aseptic meningitis are due to a variety of viruses (Table 37-2).

Each year more than 8,000 cases of aseptic meningitis are reported to the Centers for Disease Control (CDC) in Atlanta, Georgia.[29] The annual incidence of aseptic meningitis has varied from 11 to 27 cases per 100,000 individuals.[30,31] Most cases occur in children and young adults during summer and early fall.

Irrespective of the viral etiology, the clinical signs and symptoms are similar.[19,20] The illness is characterized by the abrupt onset of fever, headache, nuchal rigidity, and occasionally nausea, vomiting, and photophobia (Table 37-3). Patients may experience lethargy and irritability, but obtundation and coma should not occur. The headache is particularly intense and usually is the most dramatic feature. However, in young children and infants it may be less prominent.

The peripheral white blood cell (WBC) count may be normal or elevated. Lumbar CSF may have a normal or mildly elevated opening pressure. The CSF always contains a pleocytosis, usually ranging from 100 to 2,000 WBC/mm^3. On the first day with symptoms, the CSF may contain mainly neutrophils, but lymphocytes rapidly come to predominate.[32] The CSF glucose level is usually normal, but mildly depressed levels have occasionally been reported in patients with mumps, varicella zoster, herpes simplex type 2, and lymphocytic choriomeningitis viruses.[16] If the CSF glucose level is below 25 mg/dl, bacterial or fungal causes should be seriously considered. In patients with a viral meningitis, cultures of the CSF should not grow bacteria or fungi, which should also not be seen on Gram stain of the CSF sediment; bacterial or fungal antigens should not be detected in CSF. The electroencephalogram (EEG) is usually normal but occasionally shows mild background slowing. Marked asymmetries or seizure foci should not be seen. Computed tomography (CT) scans and magnetic resonance imaging (MRI) of the brain are typically normal.

Table 37-3 Signs and Symptoms of Viral Meningitis

Common
  Headache
  Stiff neck
  Fever
  Nausea, vomiting

Less common
  Lethargy, mild confusion, irritability
  Seizures
  Systemic signs including rash, diarrhea, pharyngitis, parotitis, myalgias, adenopathy

The clinical diagnosis of aseptic meningitis is thus based on the presence of typical clinical and laboratory features that may occur in association with a mild systemic illness (rashes, parotitis, orchitis, diarrhea, myalgia, herpangina, or pharyngitis). To determine the etiology of the viral meningitis, one must identify the specific virus by virus isolation or serological studies. CSF obtained early, preferably during the first day of illness, often contains a recoverable virus.[28,33] The virus may also be recovered from other body sites. Enteroviruses and mumps virus can be isolated from throat swabs or stool, herpes simplex virus type 2 from a genital herpetic lesion, and lymphocytic choriomeningitis (LCM) virus from urine. It is often possible to isolate these viruses during the first week of illness. Serological studies of acute and convalescent serum (obtained 3 to 6 weeks after the acute serum sample) may be useful for establishing meningitis due to mumps, arbovirus, human immunodeficiency virus (HIV), and LCM viruses. Serological studies to diagnose enterovirus infections are seldom done because of technical difficulties requiring the use of neutralization tests.

As a group, patients with viral meningitis generally make a complete recovery within 1 to 2 weeks. However, there have been occasional reports of permanent sequelae in small children, including mental retardation, deafness, cranial nerve palsies, and aqueductal stenosis.[19]

Enteroviruses

In the United States, enteroviruses account for up to 80 percent of cases of viral meningitis.[34] Enteroviruses belong to the picornavirus family and are small (30-nm diameter) RNA viruses.[35] Initially, enteroviruses were subdivided into echoviruses and coxsackieviruses. Newly isolated enteroviruses are now assigned numbers as enteroviruses (e.g., enterovirus 70, or EV 70). Enteroviruses have a worldwide distribution and often cause epidemics, primarily during the summer and early fall. The enterovirus subgroup is stable at room temperature, stable at acidic pH as low as 3.0, and resistant to lipid solvents because it lacks a lipid envelope. These viruses are thus well suited to survive in water and sewage and are transmitted by the fecal-oral or hand-to-mouth routes.

Enteroviruses initially replicate in the gastrointestinal tract.[35] This replication is asymptomatic or causes a mild gastroenteritis or pharyngitis. A secondary viremia then develops with subsequent tissue infections that may involve regional lymph nodes, skeletal muscle, myocardium, pericardium, brown fat, skin, lung, pancreas, and leptomeninges. Patients with enterovirus infections may develop rashes, pericarditis, myocarditis, myalgia, orchitis, herpangina, arthritis, polymyositis, hemolytic-uremic syndrome, nephritis, insulin-dependent diabetes mellitus, respiratory symptoms, and conjunctivitis.[35] When enteroviruses invade the CNS, most patients develop meningitis. However, occasional strains of enteroviruses have been reported to cause a poliomyelitis syndrome, meningoencephalitis, cerebellar ataxia, transverse myelitis, and Guillain-Barré syndrome. Children with X-linked hypogammaglobulinemia may develop a chronic meningitis and have difficulty in eradicating the enterovirus infection from CSF and stool.[36]

Mumps Virus

Worldwide, mumps virus is the most common cause of viral meningitis.[37] In the United States, however, the incidence of mumps meningitis is low, as a consequence of the widespread administration of mumps vaccine to children. Mumps virus is a large (100 to 600 nm in diameter), roughly spherical RNA paramyxovirus that spreads primarily via respiratory droplets.[3] Initial replication is within the upper respiratory tract and regional lymph nodes. A viremia disseminates the virus to parotid glands and occasionally to submaxillary glands, testes, ovaries, mammary glands, and the leptomeninges. The parotitis usually occurs 16 to 18 days after exposure to the virus. About one-half of all individuals with mumps parotitis develop a CSF pleocytosis.[21] In some the meningeal infection is asymptomatic, whereas in others a typical viral meningitis develops. The meningitis usually occurs 2 to 10 days after the onset of the parotitis, but it may rarely precede the parotitis or even occur without it.[22] In most patients the meningitis spontaneously resolves within 2 weeks, and full recovery occurs. Occasional individuals develop complications, including deafness[38] cortical blindness,[39] and aqueductal stenosis with obstructive hydrocephalus.[40] One to five percent of patients with a CNS mumps infection develop a meningoencephalitis.[22] Available pathological studies suggest that the meningoencephalitis may result from direct viral invasion of the brain[41] or from a postviral encephalitis with perivenous demyelination.[42] Although most of these individuals recover completely, occasional patients are left with permanent sequelae.

Herpes Simplex Virus, Type 2

In young, sexually active adults with viral meningitis, herpes simplex virus (HSV) type 2 should be considered. This virus accounts for 0.5 to 5.0 percent of all cases of viral meningitis. The meningitis develops in up to 25 percent of patients with a primary genital HSV infection[23] and occasionally occurs in individuals with recurrent genital herpes or without recognized genital lesions.[24]

Human Immunodeficiency Virus

Primary HIV meningitis should be considered in young adults with meningitis, particularly if they are homosexual or have a history of intravenous drug abuse and have a coexistent mononucleosis-like syndrome (see Ch. 38). It is of importance that these individuals usually do not have antibodies to HIV during the acute meningitis but develop antibody 1 to 3 months later during convalescence.[26]

Treatment of Viral Meningitis

Treatment of most cases of viral meningitis is symptomatic. Analgesics may be required for individuals with severe headaches and antiemetics for those with considerable nausea and vomiting.[16] Hospitalization is seldom required except when the vomiting is severe enough to cause dehydration or when bacterial meningitis cannot be completely ruled out. If an acutely ill patient has CSF containing hypoglycorrhachia or a pleocytosis in which neutrophils predominate, it may not be possible initially to rule out bacterial meningitis. In these cases it is often prudent to hospitalize the patient and treat the individual with antibiotics over the first day. By the second day, the patient usually feels better, the initial CSF bacterial cultures are sterile, and a repeat lumbar puncture shows that the CSF pleocytosis now contains mainly lymphocytes.[32] Treatment of patients with mild to moderately severe HSV meningitis is usually symptomatic. In severe cases, treatment with acyclovir (30

mg/kg divided into three doses per day) may be given slowly intravenously over 1 hour for 5 to 10 days.[43] This treatment should be given early in the illness to have maximal benefit. Oral acyclovir probably does not achieve high enough CSF levels to be beneficial in the treatment of the meningitis. Subsequent genital herpetic recurrences usually are not associated with recurrences of meningitis.

VIRAL ENCEPHALITIS

Viral encephalitis is due to a viral infection of the brain parenchyma. The viral infection causes widespread death of neurons and glia, with accompanying inflammation and edema. Each year in the United States between 1,000 and 5,000 cases are reported to the CDC. Most of the cases occur during the summer and early fall.[44] Viral encephalitis occurs worldwide, with a particularly high incidence in the tropics. Table 37-4 outlines the major viruses that cause encephalitis in the United States and lists some of their distinguishing characteristics.

The hallmark of encephalitis is the abrupt onset of mental obtundation, headaches, and fever (Table 37-5). Encephalitis differs from meningitis in that the patients have prominent mental symptoms and minimal signs of meningeal irritation. The mental changes may include confusion, delirium, lethargy, stupor, and even coma. Seizures often occur and may be generalized or focal.[25,47,56] On physical examination, patients often demonstrate hyperreflexia, spasticity, and Babinski signs. Papilledema may be present. Some patients develop focal neurological signs including hemiparesis, cranial nerve palsies, aphasia, ataxia, tremors, dysarthria, and cortical blindness.[47] Depending on a variety of factors including age (the very young and the elderly do worst) and strain of virus, the encephalitis may be mild or severe.

Many patients have a prodromal illness several days before the onset of the encephalitis. The prodrome may include parotitis (mumps) or fever, malaise, and myalgias (togavirus). However, no prodromal illness develops in herpes simplex virus encephalitis.

The leukocyte count is often elevated in the blood. Blood urea nitrogen, creatine kinase, and transaminase levels may be elevated (particularly with arbovirus encephalitis). Hyponatremia may occur from inappropriate secretion of antidiuretic hormone.[47] A

Table 37-4 Major Causes of Acute Viral Encephalitis

Virus	Vector	Geographic Distribution
Togavirus		
Western equine[45,46]	Mosquito	USA, Canada
St. Louis[25,47]	Mosquito	USA, Canada
Eastern equine[45,48]	Mosquito	Eastern USA, Caribbean
Venezuelan equine[45]	Mosquito	Central America, southwestern USA
California[49]	Mosquito	USA
Colorado tick fever[50]	Tick	USA, Canada
Japanese B[51,52]	Mosquito	Eastern Asia, Pacific Islands
Murray Valley[53]	Mosquito	Australia, New Guinea
Russian spring-summer[54]	Tick	Eastern Europe, Asia
West Nile[55]	Mosquito	Africa, India, Middle East
Mumps virus[22,41,42]		Worldwide
Herpes simplex virus[56–61]		Worldwide
Varicella-zoster virus[62]		Worldwide
Epstein-Barr virus[63]		Worldwide
Human immunodeficiency virus[64]	Human blood or semen	Worldwide
Rabies virus[65]	Dog, wolf, skunk, fox, bat, raccoon	Worldwide except certain islands, e.g., England and Japan

lumbar puncture shows a normal or elevated opening pressure. The CSF usually contains five to several hundred WBCs per cubic millimeter, which are mainly lymphocytes. In occasional cases the CSF is acellular or hemorrhagic.[57] The CSF glucose is usually normal, whereas the protein level is elevated in the range of 50 to 200 mg/dl. Bacterial cultures are sterile. Viruses are seldom isolated from CSF.[66] The EEG is always abnormal and typically shows diffuse background slowing with occasional epileptiform or electrographic seizure activity. If high-voltage periodic complexes develop in the temporal lobe area, the

possibility of HSV encephalitis is increased. Early in the illness MRI studies may show areas of increased signal on the T_2-weighted scan, particularly in the frontal or temporal lobes.[67] The CT scan is often normal early in the illness, but later shows areas of increased vascular permeability, necrosis, or hemorrhage.[57]

Diagnosis of Encephalitis

During an epidemic of encephalitis, the diagnosis of a classic case of encephalitis is not difficult. However, sporadic cases may be difficult to distinguish from patients with a metabolic encephalopathy. The presence of fever, headaches, fluctuating mental changes, focal neurological signs, or seizures (particularly if focal) favor encephalitis over encephalopathy.[16] Similarly, the presence of a blood leukocytosis, CSF pleocytosis, and focally abnormal areas on the EEG, brain scan, or MRI favor encephalitis over encephalopathy.

In years past, all cases of encephalitis were treated symptomatically, and the diagnosis was made during convalescence using serological tests.[51] With the advent of specific antiviral drugs, such as acyclovir to treat HSV or varicella-zoster encephalitis, there is

Table 37-5 Signs and Symptoms of Viral Encephalitis

Common
  Fever, headache
  Confusion, lethargy, stupor, delirium or coma
  Seizures, generalized or focal
  Hyperreflexia, Babinski signs
  Mild stiff neck

Less common
  Hemiparesis, spasticity
  Cranial nerve palsies
  Tremors
  Aphasia, ataxia, blindness

now a need to determine the etiology of the encephalitis rapidly. Several factors may be helpful for narrowing the list of possible viruses. In the United States, arbovirus encephalitis occurs predominantly during the summer and fall, when the vector (mosquito or tick) is present. Similarly, cases of arbovirus encephalitis usually cluster and may develop into epidemics. Occasionally the prodromal illness is of help. The presence of parotitis suggests mumps meningoencephalitis. Rashes may accompany Colorado tick fever, varicella zoster (dermatomal rash), or Rocky Mountain spotted fever (*Rickettsia*) infections. Thrombocytopenia may develop from Rocky Mountain spotted fever, lymphocytic choriomeningitis, and Colorado tick fever infections. Most serological tests for encephalitis require acute and convalescent serum and therefore are not helpful early in the illness.[66] Recently, an immunoglobulin M antibody capture enzyme-linked immunosorbent assay (MAC ELISA) has been developed to detect early antibody to arboviruses but not HSV.[52] This test is helpful for the early diagnosis of patients with arbovirus encephalitis.

Herpes Simplex Virus

Unfortunately, HSV encephalitis has no characteristics that easily distinguish it from other types of encephalitis.[57,58] HSV encephalitis occurs worldwide, during all seasons and at all ages. The encephalitis has no characteristic prodromal illness and no specific laboratory findings.[57] Isolation of the virus from the mouth is not helpful, as it commonly occurs in any individual with an acute febrile illness.

Attempts to develop early serological tests for HSV encephalitis have been difficult. Most individuals have previously been infected with HSV during childhood, and therefore most adults have serum antibodies to HSV. Serum or CSF HSV immunoglobulin M or G (IgM or IgG) antibody titer elevations, intrathecal HSV antibody synthesis, and low ratios of CSF/serum HSV antibody titers develop in patients with HSV encephalitis.[56,59] However, these serological changes develop over the first 10 to 12 days of the illness, making it impossible to use them reliably as an early serological test. Thus at present the only definite way to diagnose HSV encephalitis during the acute illness is by brain biopsy.[58,66]

Arguments in favor of performing a brain biopsy in cases of suspected HSV encephalitis include the following: (1) The biopsy firmly establishes the diagnosis. Immunofluorescence studies for the presence of HSV antigen in brain tissue can be done within hours of the brain biopsy. Viral cultures for HSV are usually positive within 1 to 3 days. (2) Knowledge of the specific diagnosis enables better treatment of the patient. Experience from the National Institute of Allergy and Infectious Diseases cooperative encephalitis studies has shown that only one-third to one-half of patients clinically suspected of HSV encephalitis actually had this disorder.[58] The brain biopsies frequently established other etiologies, such as cryptococcal, *Listeria,* or tuberculous meningitis, toxoplasmosis, CNS sarcoidosis, and brain abscesses, which were amenable to treatment. (3) Antiviral drugs are not innocuous. Although acyclovir has a relatively low toxicity, it can cause transient renal failure, liver enzyme abnormalities, and bone marrow suppression. Because this drug is useful only against HSV, Epstein-Barr virus, and varicella-zoster virus, it should not be used indiscriminately in all cases of viral encephalitis. (4) The risk of complications from brain biopsy when performed by experienced neurosurgeons is only about 2 percent.[58]

Arguments against routine brain biopsy include the following: (1) A craniotomy must be peformed, giving the patient a small but measurable risk of complications. (2) A virus diagnostic laboratory must be available to handle the biopsy specimen. (3) Not all patients with HSV encephalitis have a virus isolated from the biopsy. However, the rate of false-negative biopsies is about 2 percent if a positive culture at autopsy is compared to a negative culture at biopsy.[58]

Until better diagnostic tests are available, a brain biopsy should seriously be considered in any patient with encephalitis of unknown etiology if the patient is seen early in the illness, the patient has severe signs or symptoms or shows clinical progression, and the medical center has appropriate surgical facilities and a diagnostic virus laboratory. The brain biopsy specimen should be obtained from an area of suspected pathological involvement based on clinical examination and EEG, CT, or MRI studies. Brain tissue should be cultured for viruses, bacteria, and fungi, as well as examined histologically and immunohistochemically for HSV antigen. Acyclovir can probably be started up to 1 day before the biopsy surgery without significantly affecting the ability to isolate HSV from the biopsy specimen.

New diagnostic tests of CSF may eliminate the need for a brain biopsy to diagnose HSV encephalitis. An experimental assay has identified HSV glycoprotein antigens in the CSF of biopsy-proven encephalitis.[60] Another assay, the polymerase chain reaction (PCR), is an extremely sensitive test that can rapidly detect tiny amounts of specified nucleic acids in fluids or tissues. The PCR test has recently been adapted to detect fragments of HSV nucleic acid in CSF.[61] Using this test, it has been possible to accurately detect HSV nucleic acid in the CSF of patients with brain biopsy proven HSV encephalitis but not from the CSF of patients with other forms of encephalitis.[61] The PCR test for HSV or other viruses causing encephalitis is not yet commercially available.

Treatment of Viral Encephalitis

Treatment of all types of viral encephalitis requires excellent symptomatic care.[51] Patients should be placed in an intensive care unit early in the illness because the encephalitis may progress rapidly. If seizures develop, anticonvulsant drugs such as phenytoin should be given. Increased intracranial pressure often develops as a consequence of vascular engorgement and cerebral edema. Placement of an intracranial pressure monitor should therefore be considered to directly monitor the intracranial pressure. Treatment of increased intracranial pressure consists of nasotracheal intubation with hyperventilation from a mechanical ventilator. Arterial PCO_2 should be maintained between 25 and 30 mmHg. Mannitol, at a dose of 0.25 to 0.50 g/kg, may be given intermittently as a bolus intravenously to control pressure. Serum osmology should be monitored to ensure that it is maintained below 320 mOsm/L. Intravenous fluid initially should be restricted to about two-thirds the calculated daily requirement, but care should be taken to ensure that the patient does not become hypovolemic, because this can cause arterial hypotension and severely decrease cerebral blood perfusion. Use of corticosteroids is controversial, as much of the cerebral edema appears to be cytotoxic, and this type of

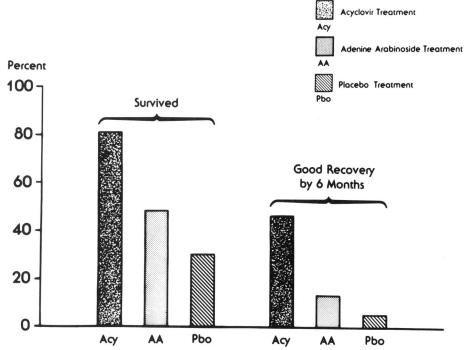

Fig. 37-1 Outcome of herpes simplex encephalitis following treatment with acyclovir, adenine arabinoside, or placebo. (From Davis LE: Acute viral meningitis and encephalitis. p. 156. In Kennedy PGE, Johnson RT (eds): Infections of the Nervous System. Butterworths, London, 1987, with permission.)

edema usually does not respond to corticosteroids. All patients should receive excellent nursing care to prevent decubitus ulcers, corneal abrasions, and contractures. Optimal oxygenation of the patient should be maintained. During convalescence, patients may require physical therapy and speech therapy. Neuropsychological testing is often needed to assess intellectual damage. The length of convalescence varies with the severity of the illness, but several months may be required.

There is now an effective antiviral treatment for HSV encephalitis. Both Swedish and American collaborative antiviral studies of HSV encephalitis have found acyclovir to be significantly better than adenine arabinoside (Fig. 37-1).[56,58] The earlier in the course of encephalitis that the acyclovir was given, the better was the outcome. Patients who were lethargic at the start of therapy did better than those who were comatose. Acyclovir not only increased the number of patients who survived but also improved the quality of survival. The acyclovir should be given as 30 mg/kg/d divided into three doses. The drug should be given intravenously slowly over 1 hour because rapid administration can cause renal toxicity, and it should be given for at least 10 days. If the biopsy is culture-negative for HSV after 5 days of culture and the clinical picture does not suggest HSV encephalitis, administration of the drug may be discontinued.

The prognosis of viral encephalitis depends on the etiological agent.[4,47,51] Rabies encephalitis is normally fatal. Eastern equine, Japanese B, Murray Valley, and Russian spring-summer encephalitides usually are severe, with mortality rates as high as 20 to 40 percent; permanent neurological sequelae are seen in up to 50 percent of survivors. These neurological sequelae include dementia, seizures, and focal neurological deficits such as hemiparesis, aphasia, cranial nerve palsies, and ataxia. Western equine encephalitis, St. Louis encephalitis, California encephalitis, and mumps encephalitis are moderately severe, with a 2 to 10 percent mortality rate; 5 to 10 percent of patients are left with permanent sequelae. Venezuelan encephalitis and Colorado tick fever viruses cause a mild encephalitis from which full recovery occurs.

PARALYTIC POLIOMYELITIS

Poliovirus does not infect all neurons and glia but selectively infects specific neuronal populations, mainly of the motor system.[68] Instead of developing encephalitis, patients develop an illness that has specific clinical characteristics: weakness and atrophy of skeletal muscles. Although most cases of paralytic poliomyelitis are due to infection with poliovirus, occasional cases have been reported due to echovirus and coxsackievirus. In the United States, paralytic poliomyelitis is rare, a direct consequence of widespread administration of polio vaccine.[9] However, in developing countries that do not widely administer the vaccine, poliomyelitis is still common. Although most poliovirus infections result in asymptomatic illness, approximately 1 in 1,000 young children who are infected develop paralysis. In adults the risk may be as high as 1 in 100 infections.[9]

In patients developing paralysis, the incubation period is 4 to 10 days. The illness begins with malaise, headaches, and fever followed 1 day later by neck and back stiffness.[9,69] Some 2 to 5 days later the weakness begins. Patients often complain of stiff, sensitive, painful muscles. A progressive asymmetrical flaccid weakness develops, typically with greater involvement of the proximal than the distal muscles. Legs are more often affected than arms. Atrophy begins in involved muscles about 5 to 7 days after the onset of weakness and progresses over several weeks. Muscles of the thorax and trunk occasionally are severely involved. About 10 to 15 percent of patients develop pharyngeal and laryngeal muscular weakness along with a facial diplegia. In rare patients there is involvement of the reticular formation, thalamus, and hypothalamus, with lethargy, respiratory difficulties, and autonomic instability.[68] The CSF typically contains 20 to 500 WBC/mm^3, mildly elevated protein concentration, and normal glucose.[9] Initially, neutrophils predominate in the CSF, but the fluid soon converts to contain predominantly lymphocytes.[69] Other routine laboratory tests are usually normal.

Poliomyelitis should be suspected in any patient with a rapidly progressive asymmetrical weakness and CSF with a lymphocytic pleocytosis. The diagnosis can be confirmed by isolating the poliovirus from throat or stool specimens or from the spinal cord at autopsy.[9] Poliovirus is rarely isolated from CSF. All poliovirus isolates from patients should be sent to reference laboratories to determine whether the virus is wild-like or vaccine-like. In the United States, one to five patients per year who received the live Sabin oral poliovirus vaccine develop poliomyelitis from the vaccine virus.[70]

There is no specific treatment for poliomyelitis. Patients should be hospitalized and watched carefully for respiratory complications.[69] If the vital capacity falls below 30 to 50 percent of predicted volume, if respirations become irregular or labored, or if arterial oxygen tension decreases, the patient should be placed on assisted ventilation. Patients with severe paralysis often experience rapid resorption of bone with increased serum and urinary calcium that can result in nephrolithiasis or bladder calculi. Adequate hydration and acidification of the urine should be ensured to prevent urinary stone formation. Patients with severe muscle weakness usually require extensive physical therapy during convalescence. Death occurs in about 8 percent of patients, usually from bulbar involvement. In survivors, strength begins to increase a few weeks after the acute illness ends. By 6 months, 80 percent of patients have made a good or full recovery.

Poliomyelitis can be effectively prevented through immunization with either killed (Salk) trivalent poliovirus vaccine[71] or live (Sabin) trivalent poliovirus vaccine.[72] However, an outbreak of type 3 poliomyelitis has occurred in Finland in individuals who had previously been vaccinated with killed virus vaccine.[73] Live poliovirus vaccine, on the other hand, should not be given to individuals with a possible immunodeficiency, as they are at increased risk of developing paralytic poliomyelitis.[74,75]

Postpolio Syndrome

It is now recognized that individuals with a past history of poliomyelitis years earlier are at risk for developing late complications.[76,77] Clinical features of the postpolio syndrome include progressive weakness, fatigue that does not correlate with the weakness, and muscle and joint pains. Joint problems include arthritis, tendinitis, bursitis, and ligament strain from incorrect posture and use of joints. Neurological signs may include new muscle weakness, fasciculations, cramps, respiratory insufficiency, sleep apnea, dysarthria, and dysphagia. Individuals at particular risk are those who were older at the onset of the acute poliomyelitis, had severe disease, and were very active after their recovery. Currently the diagnosis of postpolio syndrome requires a credible history of poliomyelitis, partial recovery, minimum of 10 years of stability, and progressive weakness that cannot be

explained otherwise. Multiple studies have failed to find any evidence of poliovirus persistence as the cause of the progressive weakness. Current hypotheses include premature exhaustion of previously damaged motor neurons due to excessive metabolic demand of enlarged motor units, and immune-mediated damage to motor neurons. At present there is no specific treatment for the syndrome, but careful physical therapy with exercise to strengthen weak muscles does not seem to accelerate disease progression. At times, splints and other orthopedic appliances may be of benefit.

CHRONIC VIRAL CNS INFECTIONS

Subacute Sclerosing Panencephalitis

Most cases of viral encephalitis have a brief duration, although occasional viral infections become chronic, persistent infections. Subacute sclerosing panencephalitis (SSPE) is an example of a chronic measles (rubeola) virus infection.[78] Primary measles is an exanthematous disease that occurs principally in children. In the developed countries, almost all of the children recover completely. Approximately one per million individuals infected with measles virus, however, develops SSPE. SSPE begins an average of 7 years after the primary measles.[74] Early symptoms include a subtle, progressive deterioration in school performance, irritability, and personality changes.[79,80] There are no associated systemic symptoms such as fever, adenopathy, or malaise. The dementia steadily worsens over several months. Speech becomes dysarthric, and myoclonic jerks, seizures, hyperkinesia, and ataxia often develop. A chorioretinitis is common. By 1 year after clinical onset, the individual usually is severely demented, blind, and quadriplegic.

The CSF usually has an elevated total protein and IgG level.[80] The EEG characteristically shows periodic bursts of stereotypical slow and sharp waves occurring at 3- to 10-second intervals.[79] The diagnosis of SSPE is made by finding markedly elevated serum and CSF antibody titers to measles.

Currently there is no effective antiviral treatment. Fortunately, SSPE can be prevented. Since the introduction of rubeola vaccination in the United States and other countries, there has been a marked decrease in cases of SSPE in those countries.[81]

Rubeola virus can cause another disease, progressive measles encephalitis, in immunocompromised individuals.[82,83] These patients usually develop a severe primary measles infection but recover. Some 4 to 5 months later, a progressive subacute encephalitis develops. Patients develop focal seizures, generalized seizures, and a rapidly progressive course characterized by dementia, spasticity, chorioretinitis, and quadriparesis. These individuals may not develop the characteristic EEG pattern or have elevated CSF and serum rubeola titers.

Progressive Rubella Panencephalitis

Progressive rubella panencephalitis is similar to SSPE and rarely develops in children following acquired or congenital rubella.[84,85] Typically, these children develop normally over the first 10 to 12 years of life before the fatal neurological syndrome begins. Patients have elevated CSF and serum rubella titers. No effective antiviral treatment is available.

Progressive Multifocal Leukoencephalopathy

Progressive multifocal leukoencephalopathy is a rare progressive demyelinating disease of the CNS white matter that usually develops in adults with impaired immune responses.[86,87] The disease appears to result from recrudescence of a previous childhood infection with a papovavirus (JC strain), and antibodies to the JC strain are found in most normal adults.[88] The initial signs and symptoms usually indicate multifocal lesions in cerebral hemispheres, but often the signs from one hemisphere predominate. The onset is insidious, often with a slowly progressive hemiplegia, dysarthria, personality change, or homonymous hemianopia. Fever, headache, and meningismus are not present. The disease steadily progresses to death over 6 months to several years. The CSF is normal, and the EEG usually shows nonspecific slowing. MRI and CT scans show multifocal areas of discrete white

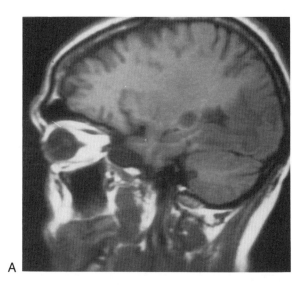

A

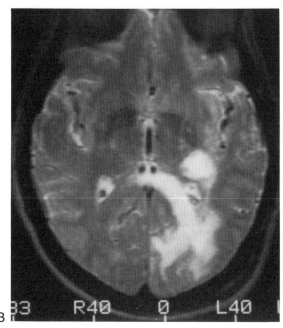

B

Fig. 37-2 Sagittal T_1-weighted (**A**) and axial T_2-weighted (**B**) MRI at the level of the occipital lobes, showing multifocal areas of discrete white matter change in a patient with progressive multifocal leukoencephalopathy.

matter damage (Fig. 37-2). No laboratory or serological test is diagnostic,[89] and the definite diagnosis must be made by brain biopsy, with electron microscopic identification of intranuclear inclusions within oligodendrocytes or of papovavirus virions within oligodendrocytes. Virus can be isolated from brain biopsy by inoculation onto human fetal glial tissue culture cells.[86,89] No effective treatment is available.

HERPES ZOSTER

Varicella-zoster virus, a member of the herpes family of viruses, causes herpes zoster (shingles). Herpes zoster typically develops in patients who decades earlier had a primary infection with varicella-zoster virus as chickenpox. Following the primary infection, the virus becomes latent within neurons of the sensory ganglia.[90] The incidence of herpes zoster ranges from 1.3 to 4.8 cases per 100,000 person-years.[91,92] Most cases are seen in patients older than 50 years. The precipitating cause for herpes zoster is unknown in most cases. However, systemic cancer, irradiation of the vertebrae, immunodeficiency, spinal trauma, and old age are recognized as precipitants.

The patient usually experiences a sharp, burning discomfort in a dermatomal distribution for 2 to 5 days before the onset of the rash. A localized redness with red macules that become vesicles develops in the same dermatomal pattern.[92] New vesicles usually appear over the first 2 days, but occasionally new vesicles continue to appear over the first week. The vesicles evolve to pustules and form crusts in 2 weeks. Often the regional lymph nodes become swollen. The distribution of herpes zoster is usually unilateral and involves a single dermatome. The rash appears on the trunk in 50 percent, on the head in 20 percent, on the arms in 15 percent, and on the legs in 15 percent of cases. Over the next month the dermatomal pain slowly disappears, leaving a residual hypo- or hyperalgesia.

Treatment of acute herpes zoster depends on the severity and location of the dermatomal rash and immunocompetence of the individual. Individuals with a mild rash may require only symptomatic treatment with nonnarcotic analgesics. Individuals with trigeminal nerve involvement or who are suspected of being immunodeficient should be treated with acyclovir. Acyclovir 7.5 mg/kg should be given slowly intravenously over 1 hour three times per day for a total of 7 days.[93] This drug has been shown to shorten the period of acute dermatomal pain, to accelerate cutaneous healing of the rash, and to prevent virus dissemination. However, acyclovir has not been shown to reduce the incidence or severity of postherpetic neuralgia. Use of zoster immune globulin has not been shown to be beneficial. Use of prednisone (40 to 60 mg/d for 10 days) during the acute rash is controversial, but some authors believe it decreases acute pain and may help prevent postherpetic neuralgia.

Complications from acute herpes zoster develop from spread of the virus to the eye (herpes zoster ophthalmicus),[94] the anterior roots or motor nerves, spinal cord (myelitis),[95] brain (encephalomyelitis),[62] and the entire body (disseminated zoster).[96] Herpes zoster auricularis or Ramsay Hunt syndrome, with involvement of motor fibers of the facial nerve, causes marked peripheral facial weakness, with pain and vesicles appearing over the skin of the external pinna and external auditory canal.[97] Occasional individuals with herpes zoster ophthalmicus develop contralateral hemiparesis up to 2 months after the acute rash.[98] Studies suggest that a necrotizing granulomatous angiitis involves the ipsilateral carotid artery and some of the small and medium-sized meningeal vessels. The angiitis results in arterial stenosis and occlusion with cerebral infarction.

Postherpetic neuralgia is a dreaded complication of shingles and occurs in 9 to 14 percent of patients with herpes zoster.[99,100] In one-third of these individuals the pain persists for a year or more. The incidence of postherpetic neuralgia increases with age. Over the age of 60, about one-half of patients develop postherpetic neuralgia. Two types of pain occur—a steady, burning, boring or tearing aching pain and one that is paroxysmal, jabbing, lancinating, and tic-like. They may occur together and may be aggravated by contact of involved skin with clothing. The pathogenesis of postherpetic neuralgia is unknown, and the pain is difficult to treat. Amitriptyline (50 to 100 mg/d in divided doses) often reduces the severity of the burning pain. Carbamazepine (200 to 600 mg/d in divided doses) often helps the lancinating pain. Use of transcutaneous electrical nerve stimulators may also help.

POSTVIRAL ENCEPHALOMYELITIS

It is apparent that some viruses appear capable of damaging the nervous system by mechanisms other than conventional viral replication (viral encephalitis)

Table 37-6 Postviral Complications of the Nervous System[a]

Encephalomyelitis
  Measles (rubeola)[101–104]
  Varicella-zoster (chickenpox)[101,104–106]
  Rubella[101,105–107]
  Mumps[42,101,105,106]
  Infectious mononucleosis[108]
  Influenza[109]
  Measles vaccine[110]
  Smallpox vaccine[111,112]
  Influenza vaccine[109]
  Rabies vaccine[113,114]

Cerebellar ataxia
  Varicella-zoster (chickenpox)[115]
  Measles (rubeola)[101,105,106]
  Mumps[101,105,106]
  Measles vaccine[110]
  Epstein-Barr[116]

Myelitis
  Measles (rubeola)[117]
  Mumps[118]
  Influenza[119]
  Epstein-Barr[120]
  Rabies vaccine[113,114,121]
  Herpes simplex[122]
  Varicella-zoster (shingles)[95,123]
  Dengue[124]
  Rubella[107,125]
  Smallpox vaccine[117,126]
  Hepatitis[126]
  Enteroviruses[127]

Optic neuritis
  Measles (rubeola)[103,128]
  Rubella[107]
  Mumps[128]
  Varicella-zoster[128]
  Infectious hepatitis[15]
  Infectious mononucleosis[15]
  Rabies vaccine[15]

Guillain-Barré syndrome or cranial nerve palsies
  Measles (rubeola)[129,130]
  Cytomegalovirus[131–133]
  Epstein-Barr[133,134]
  Enteroviruses[135,136]
  Mumps[137]
  Varicella-zoster (chickenpox)[129,138]
  Herpes simplex[139,140]
  Rubella[141]
  Hepatitis A virus[142,143]
  Human immunodeficiency virus[144]

Guillain-Barré syndrome (*continued*)
  Influenza viruses A + B[145]
  Rabies vaccine[113,114]
  Influenza A/New Jersey 1976 vaccine[146]
  Smallpox vaccine[147]
  Rubella vaccine[148]

Deafness and vertigo
  Mumps[38]
  Cytomegalovirus[149,150]
  Rubeola[151]
  Rubella[152]
  Herpes simplex[153]
  Varicella-zoster[154]
  Epstein-Barr[155]
  Hepatitis[156]
  Adenovirus[157]
  Influenza[158]
  Parainfluenza[153]
  Enteroviruses[159]
  Encephalomyocarditis[160]
  Yellow fever[161]
  Western equine encephalitis[162]
  Tick-borne encephalitis[163]
  St. Louis encephalitis[164]
  Lymphocytic choriomeningitis[165]

Aqueductal stenosis with hydrocephalus
  Mumps[166]

Reye's syndrome
  Adenovirus[167]
  Coxsackie virus[168]
  Cytomegalovirus[169]
  Dengue[170]
  Epstein-Barr[171]
  Herpes simplex[172]
  Influenza A[173]
  Influenza B[174]
  Mumps[175]
  Parainfluenza[176]
  Poliovirus vaccine[177]
  Reovirus[178]
  Respiratory syncytial[179]
  Rotavirus[180]
  Rubeola[181]
  Varicella-zoster[182]

Parkinson's disease
  Von Economo's encephalitis[183]
  Measles (rubeola)[184]
  Japanese B[184]
  Western equine encephalitis[184]

[a] In some instances, the relation between viral infection or immunization procedure and subsequent neurological complication may be fortuitous.

(Table 37-6). Measles (rubeola), mumps, varicella-zoster, influenza, rubella, and Epstein-Barr viruses are reported to cause postviral encephalomyelitis.[101,104–106] Vaccination with live virus vaccines (measles, rubella, vaccinia) or killed virus vaccines (influenza, rabies) also occasionally has been reported to cause a similar postvaccinal encephalopathy or encephalomyelitis (see Ch. 42). Although associated with a variety of viruses, postviral encephalomyelitis has several features in common. The neurological symptoms typically begin during the late stages of the primary illness; the neurological illness is monophasic, and the clinical disease is characterized by depressed levels of consciousness and multifocal neurological signs.[104]

Measles is thought to have the highest rate of postviral encephalomyelitis (100 cases per 100,000 primary infections).[102,104] Varicella-zoster virus has an incidence of about 10 cases per 100,000 primary infections, but some of these cases may be of Reye's syndrome, which has a different pathological picture. Rubella has an incidence of about 5 cases per 100,000 primary infections. Neurological complications following influenza virus and Epstein-Barr virus appear to be rare.

Measles

Uncomplicated measles frequently has neurological manifestations. Many children complain of headache, myalgia, lethargy, and photophobia. An abnormal EEG, demonstrating pathological slowing of background activity, occurs in about 50 percent of individuals.[185] In 10 percent, lumbar puncture demonstrates a CSF pleocytosis. Behavioral disturbances are thought by some to occur more frequently during the months immediately following uncomplicated measles.[186,187] However, other studies have found no significant increase in mental retardation or minor neurological signs following measles.[188,189] The etiology of the acute neurological manifestations of measles is unknown, and rubeola virus has not been isolated from CSF or brain.

About 1 per 1,000 individuals develop encephalomyelitis associated with measles. This neurological illness begins 2 to 7 days after the onset of rash, usually when the rash is fading and the child is recovering from the primary measles.[101–106] Older children and adults are disproportionately affected. Common clinical signs include depressed levels of consciousness, seizures, and focal neurological signs including hemiparesis, paraparesis, and ataxia. Less common signs include cranial nerve palsies, choreoathetosis, and myoclonus. The EEG is abnormal, showing diffuse slowing of activity. The CSF typically shows a mononuclear cell pleocytosis with protein elevation. However, the CSF is normal in approximately one-third of patients. Contrast-enhanced CT scans are usually normal. However, MRI may demonstrate focal areas of increased signal intensity, primarily in cerebral white matter and the brainstem.

Pathological studies have shown multiple focal areas of perivenous mononuclear cell cuffing and demyelination.[104] In more severe cases perivenous hemorrhage, edema, and adjacent nerve cell damage may occur. Viruses have only rarely been isolated from CSF or brain in these patients,[190] and viral antigen was not found in the brains of 10 patients who died with postmeasles encephalomyelitis.[191] Intrathecal synthesis of rubeola virus antibody rarely occurs.[102] Thus the pathology, virology, and immunology of postmeasles encephalomyelitis differ considerably from the findings in more conventional viral encephalitis and from two other CNS complications of measles, subacute sclerosing panencephalitis and progressive measles encephalitis.

Because the clinical and pathological picture of postviral encephalitis may follow vaccination with killed viruses, many investigators have postulated that the encephalomyelitis results from an aberrant immune response.[5,102,104] In favor of this hypothesis is the observation that about one-half of these patients have CSF antibody to myelin basic protein and blood lymphocytes that demonstrate an in vitro lymphoproliferative response to myelin basic protein.[102]

Chickenpox

Varicella-zoster virus causes uncomplicated chickenpox in most children. Occasional children, however, develop CNS symptoms as they are recovering from chickenpox, most commonly acute cerebellar ataxia.[101,105,106,115] Limb and gait ataxia appear an average of 21 days after the onset of the rash. The CSF usually contains a mononuclear pleocytosis and increased protein concentration. The pathology of acute cerebellar ataxia is unknown.

Management of Postviral Encephalomyelitis

Patients with severe postviral encephalomyelitis should be hospitalized in an intensive care unit. There is no specific treatment, and hyperimmune γ-globulin is not beneficial. Corticosteroids (prednisone 40 to 60 mg/d for 10 days) are frequently given during the acute illness. However, in one randomized study[192] and another nonrandomized study,[193] corticosteroid treatment was not shown to be beneficial. Symptomatic treatment to control body temperature, seizures, and intracranial pressure should be undertaken. Use of intracranial pressure monitoring may be helpful. If intracranial pressure is elevated, use of hyperventilation and intravenous mannitol (0.25 to 0.5 g/kg) in boluses may be helpful.

The prognosis of patients with mild encephalomyelitis, mild transverse myelitis, or acute cerebellar ataxia is good, with recovery typically occurring over several months.[101,105,106] Individuals with severe encephalomyelitis, particularly from measles, carry a worse prognosis. The mortality rate has been reported to be about 25 percent.[105] Most of those who survive have permanent neurological sequelae, including mental retardation, behavior problems, spasticity, ataxia, hemiparesis, and paraparesis.

TRANSVERSE MYELITIS AND MYELOPATHY

Transverse myelitis is a clinically recognized entity that follows viral infections in a few patients.[117,124,126] The disease affects all ages, but the incidence appears somewhat increased during the second decade of life.[124,126] Transverse myelitis has been reported to occur following several viral infections (Table 37-6).

The initial symptoms usually include fever, pain in the back and legs, muscle weakness, sensory disturbances, and sphincter dysfunction. The tendon reflexes are usually decreased or absent during the acute stage, and the affected limbs are flaccid. Over the next several weeks, most patients develop hyperactive reflexes, spasticity, and extensor plantar responses. The interval between the first symptom and maximal neurological deficit ranges from hours to 1 to 2 weeks. Usually a sensory level is identified in the patient, most often in the thoracic segments but occasionally

in the cervical or lumbar segments.[126] The findings in the CSF are variable. Most patients present with a CSF pleocytosis and elevated protein concentration. The pleocytosis may have a predominance of either neutrophils or lymphocytes. CSF protein levels may be as high as 500 mg/dl. However, about one-fourth of patients present with normal CSF. Myelography is normal, but MRI of the spinal cord may demonstrate focal areas of increased signal.

Most patients do not die during the acute illness. Consequently, pathological studies are few, but the ones available have tended to show focal areas of necrosis, inflammation, or perivenous demyelination.[194] Lymphocytes from patients with acute transverse myelitis have been shown to undergo a specific and significant transformation when cultured in vitro in the presence of either CNS myelin basic encephalitogenic protein or the peripheral nerve myelin P_2 protein.[194]

Criteria for the diagnosis usually include the following: (1) an acutely developing paraparesis, affecting motor and sensory systems as well as sphincters; (2) spinal segmental levels of sensory disturbances; (3) a stable, nonprogressive clinical course after the acute phase; (4) no evidence of spinal cord compression; and (5) the absence of other known neurological diseases that affect the spinal cord, such as syphilis, severe back trauma, encephalitis, or malignant disease with spinal metastases.[126]

Patients should be hospitalized and placed in the intensive care unit. Catheterization of the bladder is usually necessary. Corticosteroids are often given, but their efficacy is unknown. About one-third of patients make a good recovery, one-third make a moderate recovery, and one-third do poorly.[124,126] Rarely, in adults the acute transverse myelitis is the first episode of multiple sclerosis.

OPTIC NEURITIS

Several viral infections, including measles, mumps, Epstein–Barr virus, and varicella-zoster virus, have been associated with optic neuritis.[195] As the primary viral infection is subsiding, the patient develops a rapidly progressive loss of central vision with decreased visual acuity.[128] The visual loss is unilateral in about 75 percent of patients. Patients may complain of drabness or desaturation of colored objects and decreased appreciation of brightness (Marcus-Gunn phenomenon). Retrobulbar pain may be present. The retina and optic disc may appear normal or show evidence of papillitis. With papillitis the disc is edematous with blurred margins, and the retina is edematous, often with flame hemorrhages. Visual evoked potentials may be unobtainable, attenuated, or prolonged in latency. CT scan and skull radiographs are usually normal but may be required to rule out paranasal sinus infections or tumor. The CSF is usually normal. Prednisone (40 to 60 mg/d for 10 days) is often given. Most patients make a good recovery, but some individuals are left with a relative central visual defect or a pericentral visual defect and slightly decreased color vision. Visual acuity usually returns to better than 20/40. Some of the adult patients subsequently develop multiple sclerosis.[196]

DEAFNESS AND VERTIGO

Mumps, measles, varicella-zoster, influenza, and HSV infections have been those most often associated with acquired deafness and vertigo.[197] During the primary infection or as it is subsiding, patients experience the abrupt onset of unilateral sensorineural hearing loss, vertigo, or both. Patients may complain of tinnitus, nausea, and vomiting, which may be severe. Otitic pain is uncommon. On examination, the patient usually exhibits deafness or a high-frequency sensorineural hearing loss, often with hypoactive caloric responses on the involved side. The vertigo typically resolves over weeks, but the hearing loss may be permanent. The inner ear damage may result from direct viral invasion of the inner ear or possibly from an immune-mediated process. Rubella and cytomegalovirus can cause congenital hearing loss, which may suddenly worsen 5 to 20 years later.[149,152]

REYE'S SYNDROME

First recognized in 1963,[198] the incidence of Reye's syndrome rapidly increased during the 1960s and 1970s to become second to viral encephalitis as the most common fatal virus-related disease of the childhood nervous system.[199] Although most cases occur in children, adults can also develop the disease.[200]

During the 1980s the incidence of Reye's syndrome declined,[201] and it has remained low in the 1990s.

The pathogenesis of Reye's syndrome is unknown. Epidemiological studies have strongly implicated influenza B virus, influenza A virus, and varicella zoster viruses as being associated with this illness.[202,203] A variety of other viruses have also occasionally been associated with it (Table 37-6). In addition, the consumption of aspirin during the prodromal illness increases the risk of developing Reye's syndrome.[204]

Usually there is a prodromal illness that may be an upper respiratory tract infection, chickenpox, or gastroenteritis. As symptoms of the primary illness begin to remit, the child abruptly undergoes a period (6 to 72 hours) of severe vomiting. The child then becomes lethargic and mildly confused (stage 1). Following this phase the patient may develop delirium, acute confusion, restlessness, irritability, and seizures (stage 2). The encephalopathy may then progress to a light coma (stage 3), which may become deeper (stages 4 and 5). The illness may spontaneously stop at any stage or relentlessly progress to death.[198,205]

The CSF usually shows a normal cell count and normal protein and glucose concentrations. The CSF pressure may be normal early in the hospitalization but become markedly elevated at later stages of the disease. Viruses are only rarely isolated from CSF. Liver function studies indicate hepatocellular disease, with an elevated serum aspartate transaminase (AST) or serum glutamic oxaloacetic transaminase (SGOT) and elevated serum alanine transaminase (ALT) or serum glutamic pyruvic transaminase (SGPT).[206,207] Bilirubin levels are normal. Arterial ammonia levels are markedly elevated. There may be other evidence of liver dysfunction, including hypoglycemia, abnormal serum levels of amino acids, elevated short-chain fatty acids, and prolongation of prothrombin time.

The diagnosis of Reye's syndrome as defined by the CDC is an acute, noninflammatory encephalopathy documented by the clinical picture of alteration in the level of consciousness and liver dysfunction. The CSF should contain no more than 8 leukocytes/mm^3. Histological sections of brain, when available, should demonstrate cerebral edema without perivascular or meningeal inflammation. The encephalopathy must be associated with either (1) fatty metamorphosis of the liver diagnosed by biopsy or autopsy or (2) a threefold or greater increase in the levels of either ALT, AST, or serum ammonia. There must be no other reasonable explanation for the cerebral or hepatic abnormalities.[208]

Treatment of Reye's syndrome to date has been symptomatic because the etiology and pathogenesis are poorly understood.[205,207] Treatment to correct liver dysfunction is usually successful and includes administration of vitamin K and glucose. Over the next week the microvesicular fatty metamorphosis slowly disappears without significant residual hepatic necrosis. Treatment of the increased intracranial pressure is more difficult and may not be successful. Placement of an intracranial pressure monitor aids in hour-to-hour management. Methods to reduce increased intracranial pressure often include intubation and hyperventilation, intravenous boluses of mannitol (0.25 to 0.5 g/kg), and release of CSF (if an intraventricular pressure monitor is used). The goal of therapy is to keep the intracranial pressure below 20 mmHg and to maintain mean cerebral perfusion pressure (mean arterial blood pressure minus intracranial pressure) at 60 to 90 mmHg.[209]

The mortality of patients who progress to coma ranges as high as 40 percent, with morbidity rates ranging to 34 percent. Permanent neurological sequelae include mental retardation, hyperactive behavior, focal neurological deficits, and seizures.

GUILLAIN-BARRÉ SYNDROME

Viral infections have been associated with syndromes involving the peripheral nervous system as well as the CNS. The best recognized is acute idiopathic polyneuritis, or Guillain-Barré syndrome. This illness occurs during all seasons, affects both children and adults, and equally involves both sexes.[210–212] Guillain-Barré syndrome commonly follows a viral infection. About one-half of the patients experience an upper respiratory tract or gastrointestinal tract infection 1 to 3 weeks before the onset of polyneuritis.[210] Several viruses,[211] including Epstein-Barr virus,[133,134] infectious hepatitis,[142] cytomegalovirus,[131–133] and influenza A/New Jersey vaccination,[146] have received particular attention. Viruses have not been successfully isolated from involved peripheral nerves. However, herpes-like viral particles have been found within intranuclear inclusion bodies typical of cytomegalovirus in lumbar dorsal roots and retroperitoneal peripheral nerves of two

patients with Guillain-Barré syndrome.[131] Patients characteristically complain of leg and foot paresthesias and weakness at the onset of the illness. Over the next 10 days the patient develops a progressive flaccid weakness.[210–212] In most patients the weakness begins in the legs and ascends proximally, although it occasionally begins in the face and bulbar muscles. Initially, tendon reflexes are somewhat depressed, and they typically disappear as the illness progresses. Objective sensory loss is usually minor, involving vibration and position sense in the feet. Mentation is normal. In about 25 percent of patients the weakness may progress, and respiration is sufficiently impaired that assisted ventilation is required. As discussed in Chapter 8, autonomic disturbances are common and may be life-threatening, particularly cardiac arrhythmias and marked fluctuations in blood pressure.[213,214] Fever, lymphadenopathy, and splenomegaly are usually absent.

The CSF is under normal pressure and is acellular, usually with an elevated protein concentration.[210] Infectious agents are not isolated from CSF. Initially, motor nerve conduction velocities are normal or slightly depressed, and F waves may be abnormal.[215] Over the next several weeks, marked slowing of motor nerve conduction velocities and abnormalities of sensory conduction usually develop.

Most patients with this clinical picture have Guillain-Barré syndrome. However, diphtheria polyneuropathy, poliomyelitis, HIV-associated chronic inflammatory neuropathy, tick paralysis, and acute toxic neuropathies must be considered in the differential diagnosis.

Pathological studies have shown that involved peripheral nerves develop an inflammatory segmental demyelination.[216,217] Perivascular lymphocytic infiltrates are scattered throughout cranial nerves, the ventral and dorsal roots, and along the peripheral nerves. Focal areas of segmental demyelination are usually seen throughout the peripheral nerves.

The etiology of Guillain-Barré syndrome is unknown, but current evidence suggests that several factors, including surgery, immunization, and infections, can trigger the illness.[211,212] In animals, experimental allergic neuritis (EAN) has similar clinical and pathological features.[218] EAN follows immunization of animals with whole or components of peripheral nerves and suggests that Guillain-Barré syndrome may have similar immune features.[212] It should be noted, however, that Guillain-Barré syndrome can occur in individuals who are partially immunosuppressed.[219]

Patients with Guillain-Barré syndrome should be hospitalized, usually in an intensive care unit. Because the weakness may progress rapidly to involve respiratory muscles, the patient's respiratory status must be assessed frequently. Respiratory assistance should be instituted at the first signs of dyspnea, usually when the vital capacity falls below 800 ml or a decrease in blood oxygen saturation occurs. Nasotracheal intubation should be the first step, but prolonged respiratory failure may require a tracheostomy. Cardiac monitoring should be undertaken, as life-threatening cardiac arrhythmias may occur, particularly during nasotracheal suction or when the patient is moved about in bed.[213,214] Treatment with plasmapheresis has been shown to significantly decrease the time a patient is on a respirator and to shorten the time to ambulation.[220] A series of plasmaphereses should be started within the first 2 weeks of onset for maximal benefit. If these are performed carefully, patients do not appear to be at increased risk of complications. Use of corticosteriods has been shown not to be beneficial.

Prognosis is generally excellent if the patient survives the acute illness.[210] Excellent recovery occurs in more than 75 percent of patients, but occasional patients are left with some residual weakness. Recovery begins after a plateau phase of several weeks and may continue for up to 24 months. Children tend to make a faster and better recovery than older adults. Histological studies have shown that remyelination of involved peripheral nerves occurs during recovery. Recurrences of Guillain-Barré syndrome are rare.

CREUTZFELDT-JAKOB DISEASE

It is now recognized that Creutzfeldt-Jakob disease (CJD) results from a newly recognized class of infectious agents called unconventional agents, slow viruses, spongiform encephalopathy agents, or proteinaceous infectious particles (PRIONS).[221,222] This class of infectious agents causes CJD, kuru, and the Gerstmann-Straussler syndrome in humans, and scrapie in sheep.

CJD has a worldwide distribution with an occurrence rate of one to two cases per million population per year. The age of onset ranges from 35 to 65 years. Most cases are sporadic, but 12 percent appear to cluster in families. Both sexes are equally involved.

The clinical features broadly fall into three phases.[223,224] The *onset* is insidious, with the development of mental deterioration. The patient typically becomes forgetful and nervous, with a decline in work performance. A relentless, slowly progressive dementia then develops. Progressive memory loss, parietal lobe dysfunction, and dysphasia often develop. Behavioral disturbances include the appearance of personality change, apathy, irritability, depression, and paranoia. Systemic signs such as fever, meningismus, adenopathy, and splenomegaly do not develop. Headaches are rare. In the *second phase,* more than 85 percent of patients develop myoclonic jerks—involuntary, repetitive muscular contractions that are quick, shock-like, and of sufficient severity to cause visible displacement of limbs. They may be stimulus-sensitive. Some patients develop spasticity with Babinski signs, whereas others develop cortical blindness, severe ataxia, or amyotrophy. In the *third phase,* the patient develops severe dementia, wasting, and spasticity. The clinical course to death usually ranges from 6 months to 2 years.

The CSF is acellular with a normal protein content. CSF and serum immunoglobulin levels are normal. The EEG is distinctly abnormal in 75 percent of cases, usually in the later stages of the illness. The tracing is characterized by repetitive, periodic, stereotyped, bilaterally synchronous sharp waves, usually occurring at a frequency of 1 to 2 per second.[225] They are often associated with myoclonic jerks. The CT scan and MRI are often normal early in the disease but later show diffuse cerebral atrophy. The diagnosis of CJD is usually made on the basis of a rapidly progressive dementia, the presence of myoclonic jerks, and a characteristic EEG. Promising marker proteins have been identified in the CSF of patients with CJD.[226] However, although these marker proteins appear to be present in most patients with CJD, they have also been found in the CSF of patients with herpes simplex encephalitis, multiple sclerosis, and Parkinson's disease.

The pathology appears to be confined to the CNS.[227] There is diffuse atrophy of the brain. Histologically, there is extensive loss of neurons, prominent astrocytic gliosis, conspicuous absence of inflammatory changes, and a characteristic spongiform change. This spongiform appearance is due to vacuoles located in the cytoplasm of neurons and astrocytes. To date, electron microscopy has failed to identify infectious particles in the brain.

The characteristics of the infectious particle are still unclear. It is of small molecular weight, hydrophobic, and tightly bound to membranes. The particle appears to replicate within the cytoplasm.[221,222] There is some doubt as to whether the particle contains a nucleic acid.[222] The infectious agent appears not to stimulate a humoral or cellular immune response. Infectivity of the agent is not destroyed by common virucidal agents such as ultraviolet light, formalin, β-propiolactone, and 100°C heat. However, it is destroyed by autoclaving for 1 hour at 125°C at 20 pounds per square inch or by soaking infected tissues for at least 1 hour in 2M sodium hydroxide. The natural transmission of this disease is unknown. Experimental evidence suggests that the agent may be transmitted through direct inoculation and rarely through the gastrointestinal tract. Iatrogenic spread of CJD has been documented via infected corneal grafts, dural grafts, and growth hormone prepared from human pituitary glands.[228,229] Thus patients who die from unexplained dementia should not be organ donors. The infectious agent does not appear to be in saliva, urine, or stool. Therefore spouses or individuals caring for the patient are not at increased risk of contracting the disease. The patient does not require isolation, but needles, blood, and CSF should be considered infectious and autoclaved before being discarded.[230] At present, no effective treatment exists.

ACKNOWLEDGMENT

Supported by the Neurology Service, Veterans Administration Medical Center, and the Departments of Neurology and Microbiology, University of New Mexico School of Medicine, Albuquerque, New Mexico.

REFERENCES

1. Fishman RA: Cerebrospinal Fluid in Diseases of the Nervous System. WB Saunders, Philadelphia, 1980
2. Johnson RT: Viral Infections of the Nervous System. Raven Press, New York, 1982
3. Wolinsky JS, Server AC: Mumps virus. p. 1255. In Fields BN, Knipe DM, Chanock RM, et al (eds): Virology. Raven Press, New York, 1985
4. Monath TP: Flaviviruses. p. 955. In Fields BN, Knipe DM, Chanock RM, et al (eds): Virology. Raven Press, New York, 1985
5. Johnson RT: The pathogenesis of acute viral encephalitis and postinfectious encephalomyelitis. J Infect Dis 155:359, 1987
6. Mims CA: Aspects of the pathogenesis of virus diseases. Bacteriol Rev 28:30, 1964
7. Oldendorf WH: Overview of blood-brain barrier transport. In Pardridge WM (moderator): Blood-brain barrier: interface between internal medicine and the brain. Ann Intern Med 105:82, 1986
8. Wolinsky JS, Baringer JR, Margolis G, Kilham L: Ultrastructure of mumps virus replication in a newborn hamster's central nervous system. Lab Invest 31:403, 1974
9. Price RW, Plum F: Poliomyelitis. p. 93. In Vinken PJ, Bruyn GW (eds): Handbook of Clinical Neurology. Vol 34. North Holland, Amsterdam, 1978
10. Murphy FA, Bauer SP, Harrison AK, Winn WC: Comparative pathogenesis of rabies and rabies-like viruses: viral infection and transit from inoculation site to the central nervous system. Lab Invest 28:361, 1973
11. Davis LE, Johnson RT: An explanation for the localization of herpes simplex encephalitis? Ann Neurol 5:2, 1979
12. Fryden A: B and T lymphocytes in blood and cerebrospinal fluid in acute aseptic meningitis. Scand J Immunol 6:1283, 1977
13. Berger ML: Immunologic requirements for adoptive transfer of ectromelia virus meningitis. J Neuropathol Exp Neurol 41:18, 1982
14. McFarland HF, Griffin DE, Johnson RT: Specificity of the inflammatory response in viral encephalitis. J Exp Med 136:216, 1972
15. Davis LE, Reed WP: Infections of the nervous system. p. 301. In Rosenberg RG (ed): The Clinical Neurosciences. Churchill Livingstone, New York, 1983
16. Davis LE: Acute viral meningitis and encephalitis. p. 156. In Kennedy PGE, Johnson RT (eds): Infections of the Nervous System. Butterworths, London, 1987
17. Haddad FS, Risk WS, Jabbour JT: Subacute sclerosing panencephalitis in the Middle East: report of 99 cases. Ann Neurol 1:211, 1977
18. Kennedy PGE: Neurological complications of varicella-zoster virus. p. 177. In Kennedy PGE, Johnson RT (eds): Infections of the Nervous System. Butterworths, London, 1987
19. Lepow ML, Coyne N, Thompson LB, et al: A clinical, epidemiologic and laboratory investigation of

aseptic meningitis during the four-year period, 1955–1958. N Engl J Med 266:1188, 1962

20. Wilfert CM, Lehrman SN, Katz SL: Enteroviruses and meningitis. Pediatr Infect Dis 2:333, 1983

21. Bang HO, Bang J: Involvement of the central nervous system in mumps. Acta Med Scand 113:487, 1943

22. Johnstone JA, Ross CAC, Dunn M: Meningitis and encephalitis associated with mumps infection—a 10-year survey. Arch Dis Child 47:647, 1972

23. Corey L, Adams HG, Brown ZA, Holmes KK: Genital herpes simplex virus infections: clinical manifestations, course, and complications. Ann Intern Med 98:958, 1983

24. Stalder H, Oxman MN, Dawson DM, Levin MJ: Herpes simplex meningitis: isolation of herpes simplex virus type 2 from cerebrospinal fluid. N Engl J Med 289:1296, 1973

25. Southern PM, Smith JW, Luby JP, et al: Clinical and laboratory features of epidemic St. Louis encephalitis. Ann Intern Med 71:681, 1969

26. Ho DD, Sarngadharan MG, Resnick L, et al: Primary human T-lymphotropic virus type III infection. Ann Intern Med 103:880, 1985

27. Farmer TW, Janeway CA: Infections with the virus of lymphocytic choriomeningitis. Medicine (Baltimore) 21:1, 1942

28. Kelsey DS: Adenovirus meningoencephalitis. Pediatrics 61:291, 1978

29. Centers for Disease Control: Reported morbidity and mortality in the United States: annual summary 1984. MMWR 32:17, 1986

30. Beghi E, Nicolosi A, Kurland LT, et al: Encephalitis and aseptic meningitis, Olmsted County, Minnesota, 1950–1981: I. Epidemiology. Ann Neurol 16:283, 1984

31. Ponka A, Pettersson T: The incidence and aetiology of central nervous system infections in Helsinki in 1980. Acta Neurol Scand 66:529, 1982

32. Varki AP, Puthuran P: Value of second lumbar puncture in confirming a diagnosis of aseptic meningitis. Arch Neurol 36:581, 1979

33. Sullivan JR, Davis LE, Chin TDY: Viral aseptic meningitis: twelve years experience in the Missouri area. Mo Med 68:693, 1971

34. Centers for Disease Control: Annual summary 1976: aseptic meningitis surveillance. CDC, Atlanta, 1979.

35. Melnick JL: Enteroviruses: polioviruses, coxsackieviruses, echoviruses, and newer enteroviruses. p. 739. In Fields BN, Knipe DM, Chanock RM, et al (eds): Virology. Raven Press, New York, 1985

36. Wilfert CM, Buckley RH, Mohanakumar T, et al: Persistent and fatal central-nervous-system echovirus infections in patients with agammaglobulinemia. N Engl J Med 296:1485, 1977

37. Tardieu M, Dussaix E, Lebon P, Landrieu P: Prospective study of 59 cases of viral meningitis in children: clinical and neurologic diagnosis, epidemiology and physiopathology. Arch Fr Pediatr 43:9, 1986

38. Vuori M, Lahikaimen EA, Peltonen T: Perceptive deafness in connection with mumps: a study of 298 servicemen suffering from mumps. Acta Otolaryngol (Stockh) 55:231, 1962

39. Davis LE, Harms AC, Chin TDY: Transient cortical blindness and cerebellar ataxia associated with mumps. Arch Ophthalmol 85:366, 1971

40. Thompson JA: Mumps: a cause of acquired aqueductal stenosis. J Pediatr 94:923, 1979

41. Bistrian B, Phillips CA, Kaye IS: Fatal mumps meningoencephalitis—isolation of virus premortem and postmortem. JAMA 222:478, 1972

42. Schwarz GA, Yang DC, Noone EL: Meningoencephalomyelitis with epidemic parotitis. Arch Neurol 11:453, 1964

43. Levy DM, Sagar HJ: Herpes simplex type 2 meningitis treated with acyclovir. Postgrad Med J 60:282, 1984

44. Centers for Disease Control: Enterovirus Surveillance Report, 1970–1979. pp. 1–74. CDC, Atlanta, 1980

45. Shope RE: Alphaviruses. p. 931. In Fields BN, Knipe DM, Chanock RM, et al (eds): Virology. Raven Press, New York, 1985

46. Finley KH, Fitzgerald LH, Richter RW, et al: Western encephalitis and cerebral ontogenesis. Arch Neurol 16:140, 1967

47. Brinker KR, Monath TP: The acute disease. p. 503. In Monath TP (ed): St. Louis Encephalitis. American Public Health Association, Washington, DC, 1980

48. Howitt BR, Bishop LK, Gorrie RH, et al: An outbreak of equine encephalomyelitis, eastern type, in southwestern Louisiana. Proc Soc Exp Biol Med 68:70, 1948

49. Johnson KP, Lepow ML, Johnson RT: California encephalitis: I. Clinical and epidemiological studies. Neurology 18:250, 1968

50. Goodpasture HC, Poland JD, Francy DB, et al: Colorado tick fever: clinical, epidemiologic, and laboratory aspects of 228 cases in Colorado in 1973–74. Ann Intern Med 88:303, 1978

51. Booss J, Esiri MM: Viral Encephalitis—Pathology, Diagnosis and Management. Blackwell Scientific Publications, Oxford, 1986

52. Burke DS, Nisalak A, Ussery MA: Antibody capture immunology detection of Japanese encephalitis immunoglobulin M and G antibodies in cerebrospinal fluid. J Clin Microbiol 16:1034, 1982

53. Bennett N McK: Murray Valley encephalitis, 1974: clinical features. Med J Aust 2:446, 1976

54. Gresikova M, Beran GW: Tick-borne encephalitis. p.

201. In Beran GW (ed): CRC Handbook Series in Zoonoses, Section B: Viral Zoonoses. Vol 1. CDC Press, Boca Raton, FL, 1981

55. Marberg K, Goldblum N, Sterk VV, et al: The natural history of West Nile fever: I. Clinical observations during an epidemic in Israel. Am J Hyg 64:259, 1956

56. Skoldenberg B, Forsgren M, Alestig K, et al: Acyclovir versus vidarabine in herpes simplex encephalitis: randomised multicenter study in consecutive Swedish patients. Lancet 2:707, 1984

57. Whitley RJ, Soong S, Linneman C, et al: Herpes simplex encephalitis. JAMA 247:317, 1982

58. Whitley RJ, Alford CA, Hirsch MS, et al: Vidarabine versus acyclovir therapy in herpes simplex encephalitis. N Engl J Med 314:144, 1986

59. Vandvik B, Vartdal F, Norrby E: Herpes simplex virus encephalitis: intrathecal synthesis of oligoclonal virus-specific IgG, IgA and IgM antibodies. J Neurol 228:25, 1982

60. Lakeman FD, Koga J, Whitley RJ: Detection of antigen to herpes simplex virus in cerebrospinal fluid from patients with herpes simplex encephalitis. J Infect Dis 155:1172, 1987

61. Rowley A, Lakeman F, Whitley R, Wolinsky S: Diagnosis of herpes simplex encephalitis by DNA amplification of cerebrospinal fluid cells. Lancet 335:440, 1990

62. Jemsek J, Greenberg SB, Taber L, et al: Herpes zoster-associated encephalitis: clinicopathologic report of 12 cases and review of the literature. Medicine (Baltimore) 62:81, 1983

63. Lange BJ, Berman PH, Bender J, et al: Encephalitis in infectious mononucleosis: diagnostic considerations. Pediatrics 58:877, 1976

64. Price RW, Navia BA, Cho ES: AIDS encephalopathy. Neurol Clin 4:285, 1986

65. Anderson LJ, Nicholson KG, Tauxe RV, et al: Human rabies in the United States, 1960 to 1979: epidemiology, diagnosis and prevention. Ann Intern Med 100:728, 1984

66. Rubin SJ: Detection of viruses in spinal fluid. Am J Med 75:124, 1983

67. Schroth G, Gawehn J, Thron A, et al: Early diagnosis of herpes simplex encephalitis by MRI. Neurology 37:179, 1987

68. Bodian D: Histopathologic basis of clinical findings in poliomyelitis. Am J Med 6:563, 1949

69. Baker AB: Poliomyelitis. DM 1:1, 1955

70. Schonberger LB, Sullivan-Bolyai JZ, Bryan JA: Poliomyelitis in the United States. Adv Neurol 19:217, 1978

71. Salk D: Eradication of poliomyelitis in the United States: II. Experience with killed poliovirus vaccine. Rev Infect Dis 2:243, 1980

72. Sabin AB: Oral poliovirus vaccine: history of its development and use and current challenge to eliminate poliomyelitis from the world. J Infect Dis 151:420, 1985

73. Hovi T, Cantell K, Huovilaninen A, et al: Outbreak of paralytic poliomyelitis in Finland: widespread circulation of antigenically altered poliovirus type 3 in a vaccinated population. Lancet 1:1427, 1986

74. Modlin JF, Jabbour JT, Witte JJ, et al: Epidemiologic studies of measles, measles vaccine, and subacute sclerosing panencephalitis. Pediatrics 59:505, 1979

75. Davis LE, Bodian D, Price D, et al: Chronic progressive poliomyelitis secondary to vaccination of an immunodeficient child. N Engl J Med 297:241, 1977

76. Dalakas MC, Elder G, Hallett M, et al: A long-term follow-up study of patients with post-poliomyelitis neuromuscular symptoms. N Engl J Med 314:959, 1986

77. Salazar-Grueso EF, Siegel I, Roos RP: Post-polio syndrome: evaluation and treatment. Compr Ther 16:24, 1990

78. Payne FE, Baublis JV, Itabashi HH: Isolation of measles virus from cell cultures of brain from a patient with subacute sclerosing panencephalitis. N Engl J Med 281:585, 1969

79. Ohya T, Martinez AJ, Jabbour JT, et al: Subacute sclerosing panencephalitis. Neurology 24:211, 1974

80. Dyken PR: Subacute sclerosing panencephalitis. Neurol Clin 3:179, 1985

81. Zilber N, Rannon L, Alter M, Kahana E: Measles, measles vaccination, and risk of subacute sclerosing panencephalitis (SSPE). Neurology 33:1558, 1983

82. Aicardi J, Goutieres F, Arsenio-Nunes ML, et al: Acute measles encephalitis in children with immunosuppression. Pediatrics 59:232, 1977

83. Agamanolis DP, Tan JS, Parker DL: Immunosuppressive measles encephalitis in a patient with a renal transplant. Arch Neurol 36:686, 1979

84. Townsend JJ, Baringer JR, Wolinsky JS, et al: Progressive rubella panencephalitis: late onset of congenital rubella. N Engl J Med 292:990, 1975

85. Weil ML, Itabashi HH, Cremer NE, et al: Chronic progressive panencephalitis due to rubella virus simulating subacute sclerosing panencephalitis. N Engl J Med 292:994, 1975

86. Padgett BL, Walker DL, ZuRhein GM, et al: JC papovavirus in progressive multifocal leukoencephalopathy. J Infect Dis 133:686, 1976

87. Berger JR, Kaszovitz B, Post JD, Dickinson G: Progressive multifocal leukoencephalopathy associated with human immunodeficiency virus infection. Ann Intern Med 107:78, 1987

88. Padgett BL, Walker DL: Prevalence of antibodies in

human sera against JC virus, an isolate from a case of progressive multifocal leukoencephalopathy. J Infect Dis 127:467, 1973

89. Padgett BL, Walker DL: Virologic and serologic studies of progressive multifocal leukoencephalopathy. p. 107. In Sever JL, Madden DL (eds): Polyomaviruses and Human Neurological Diseases. Alan R Liss, New York, 1983

90. Weller TH: Varicella and herpes zoster. N Engl J Med 309:1361, 1983

91. Hope-Simon RE: The nature of herpes zoster: a long-term study and a new hypothesis. Proc R Soc Med 58:9, 1965

92. Burgoon CF, Burgoon JS, Baldridge GD: The natural history of herpes zoster. JAMA 164:265, 1957

93. Bean B, Braun C, Balfour HH Jr: Acyclovir therapy for acute herpes zoster. Lancet 2:118, 1982

94. Edgerton AE: Herpes zoster ophthalmicus. Arch Ophthalmol 34:40, 1945

95. Hogan EL, Krigman MR: Herpes zoster myelitis. Arch Neurol 29:309, 1973

96. Dolin R, Reichman RC, Mazur MH, et al: Herpes zoster varicella infections in immunosuppressed patients. Ann Intern Med 89:375, 1978

97. Aleksic SN, Budzilovich GN, Lieberman AN: Herpes zoster oticus and facial paralysis (Ramsay Hunt syndrome). J Neurol Sci 20:149, 1973

98. Reshef E, Greenberg SB, Jankovic J: Herpes zoster ophthalmicus followed by contralateral hemiparesis: report of two cases and review of literature. J Neurol Neurosurg Psychiatry 48:122, 1985

99. Watson PN, Evans RJ: Postherpetic neuralgia: a review. Arch Neurol 43:836, 1986

100. Portenoy RK, Duma C, Foley KM: Acute herpetic and postherpetic neuralgia: clinical review and current management. Ann Neurol 20:651, 1986

101. Siriam S, Steinman L: Postinfectious and postvaccinal encephalomyelitis. Neurol Clin 2:341, 1984

102. Johnson RT, Griffin DE, Hirsch RL, et al: Measles encephalomyelitis—clinical and immunologic studies. N Engl J Med 310:137, 1984

103. Tyler HR: Neurological complications of rubeola (measles). Medicine (Baltimore) 36:147, 1951

104. Johnson RT, Griffin DE: Postinfectious encephalomyelitis. p. 209. In Kennedy PGE, Johnson RT (eds): Infections of the Nervous System. Butterworths, London, 1987

105. Miller HG, Stanton JB, Gibbons JL: Para-infectious encephalomyelitis and related syndromes. Q J Med 25:427, 1956

106. Scott TFM: Postinfectious and vaccinal encephalitis. Med Clin North Am 51:701, 1967

107. Connolly JH, Hutchinson WM, Allen IV, et al: Ca-

rotid artery thrombosis, encephalitis, myelitis and optic neuritis associated with rubella virus infections. Brain 95:583, 1975

108. Ambler M, Stoll J, Tzamaloukas A, Albala MM: Focal encephalomyelitis in infectious mononucleosis. Ann Intern Med 75:579, 1971

109. Hoult JG, Flewett TH: Influenzal encephalopathy and post-influenzal encephalitis: histological and other observations. Br Med J 1:1847, 1960

110. Landrigan PJ, Witte JJ: Neurologic disorders following live measles-virus vaccination. JAMA 223:1459, 1973

111. Angulo JJ, Pimenta-De-Campos E, De Salles-Gomes LF: Postvaccinal meningoencephalitis. JAMA 187:151, 1964

112. DeVries E: Postvaccinal Perivenous Encephalitis. Elsevier, Amsterdam, 1960

113. Hemachudha T, Griffin DE, Giffels JJ, et al: Myelin basic protein as an encephalitogen in encephalomyelitis and polyneuritis following rabies vaccination. N Engl J Med 316:369, 1987

114. Hemachudha T, Phanuphak P, Johnson RT, et al: Neurological complications of Semple-type rabies vaccine: clinical and immunological studies. Neurology 37:550, 1987

115. Peters ACB, Versteeg J, Lindeman J, Bots GTAM: Varicella and acute cerebellar ataxia. Arch Neurol 35:769, 1978

116. Cleary TG, Henle W, Pickering LK: Acute cerebellar ataxia associated with Epstein-Barr virus infection. JAMA 243:148, 1980

117. Paine RS, Byers RK: Transverse myelopathy in childhood. Am J Dis Child 85:151, 1953

118. Lightwood R: Myelitis from mumps. Br Med J 1:484, 1946

119. Owen NL: Myelitis following type A₂ influenza. JAMA 215:1986, 1971

120. Grose C, Feorino PM: Epstein-Barr virus and transverse myelitis. Lancet 1:892, 1973

121. Harrington RB, Olin R: Incomplete transverse myelitis following rabies duck embryo vaccination. JAMA 216:2137, 1971

122. Klastersky J, Cappel R, Snoeck JM, et al: Ascending myelitis in association with herpes-simplex virus. N Engl J Med 287:182, 1972

123. Rose FC, Brett EM, Burston J: Zoster encephalomyelitis. Arch Neurol 11:155, 1964

124. Altrocchi PH: Acute transverse myelopathy. Arch Neurol 9:111, 1963

125. Morris MH, Robbins A: Acute infectious myelitis following rubella. J Pediatr 23:365, 1943

126. Berman M, Feldman S, Alter M, et al: Acute transverse myelitis: incidence and etiologic considerations. Neurology 31:966, 1981

127. Bell EJ, Russell SJM: Acute transverse myelopathy and Echo-2 virus infection. Lancet 2:1226, 1963

128. Kennedy C, Carroll FD: Optic neuritis in children. Trans Am Acad Ophthalmol Otolaryngol 64:700, 1960

129. Glaze DG: Guillain-Barré syndrome. p. 507. In Feigin RD, Cherry JD (eds): Textbook of Pediatric Infectious Diseases. Vol 1. WB Saunders, Philadelphia, 1987

130. Drueke TB, Pujade-Lauraine E, Poisson M, et al: Measles virus and Guillain-Barré syndrome during long-term hemodialysis. Am J Med 60:444, 1976

131. Bishopric G, Bruner J, Butler J: Guillain-Barré syndrome with cytomegalovirus infection of peripheral nerves. Arch Pathol Lab Med 109:1106, 1985

132. Mozes B, Pines A, Sayar Y, et al: Guillain-Barré syndrome associated with acute cytomegalovirus mononucleosis syndrome. Eur Neurol 23:237, 1984

133. Dowling PC, Cook SD: Role of infection in Guillain-Barré syndrome: laboratory confirmation of herpesviruses in 41 cases. Ann Neurol 9, suppl:44, 1981

134. Glaser R, Brennan R, Berlin CM: Guillain-Barré syndrome associated with Epstein-Barr virus in a cytomegalovirus-negative patient. Dev Med Child Neurol 21:787, 1979

135. Parker W, Wilt JC, Dawson JW, Stackiw W: Landry-Guillain-Barré syndrome—the isolation of an echovirus type 6. Can Med Assoc J 82:813, 1960

136. Estrada-Gonzales R, Mas P: Virological studies in acute polyradiculoneuritis—Landry-Guillain-Barré syndrome: various findings in relation to coxsackie A4 virus. Neurol Neurocir Psiquiatr 18, suppl 2–3: 527, 1977

137. Collens WS, Rabinowitz MA: Mumps polyneuritis: quadriplegia with bilateral facial paralysis. Arch Intern Med 41:61, 1928

138. Boucharlat J, Groslambert R, Chateau R: Polyradiculoneuritis as a symptom of varicella (a case report). J Med Lyon 49:1443, 1968

139. Menonna J, Goldschmidt B, Haidri N, et al: Herpes simplex virus IgM specific antibodies in Guillain-Barré syndrome and encephalitis. Acta Neurol Scand 56:223, 1977

140. Siebert DG, Seals JE: Polyneuropathy after herpes simplex type 2 meningitis. South Med J 77:1476, 1984

141. Saeed AA, Lange LS: Guillain-Barré syndrome after rubella. Postgrad Med J 54:333, 1978

142. Berger JR, Ayyar R, Sheremata WA: Guillain-Barré syndrome complicating acute hepatitis B. Arch Neurol 38:366, 1981

143. Feutren G, Gerbal JL, Allinquant B, Schuller E: Association of Guillain-Barré syndrome and B-virus hepatitis: simultaneous presence of anti-DS-DNA antibodies and HBs antigen in cerebrospinal-fluid. J Clin Lab Immunol 11:161, 1983

144. Hagberg L, Malmvall BE, Svennerholm L, et al: Guillain-Barré syndrome as an early manifestation of HIV central nervous system infection. Scand J Infect Dis 18:591, 1986

145. Wells CEC, James WRI, Evans AD: Guillain-Barré syndrome and virus of influenza A (Asian strain): report of two fatal cases during the 1957 epidemic in Wales. Arch Neurol Psychiatry 81:699, 1959

146. Schonberger LB, Hurwitz ES, Katona P, et al: Guillain-Barré syndrome: its epidemiology and associations with influenza vaccination. Ann Neurol 9, suppl: 31, 1981

147. Kisch AL: Guillain-Barré syndrome following smallpox vaccination: report of a case. N Engl J Med 258: 83, 1958

148. Gunderman JR: Guillain-Barré syndrome: occurrence following combined mumps-rubella vaccine. Am J Dis Child 125:834, 1973

149. Stagno S, Reynolds DW, Amos CS, et al: Auditory and visual defects resulting from symptomatic and subclinical congenital cytomegaloviral and Toxoplasma infections. Pediatrics 59:669, 1977

150. Davis LE, Johnsson LG, Kornfeld M: Cytomegalovirus labyrinthitis in an infant: morphological, virological, and immunofluorescent studies. J Neuropathol Exp Neurol 40:9, 1981

151. Davey P: Deafness associated with measles and other virus diseases. J Otolaryngol Soc Aust 2:80, 1966

152. Menser MA, Forrest JM: Rubella—high incidence of defects in children considered normal at birth. Med J Aust 1:123, 1974

153. Jaffe BF: Clinical studies in sudden deafness. Adv Otorhinolaryngol 20:221, 1973

154. Byl FM, Adour KK: Auditory symptoms associated with herpes zoster or idiopathic facial paralysis. Laryngoscope 87:372, 1977

155. Beg JA: Bilateral sensorineural hearing loss as a complication of infectious mononucleosis. Arch Otolaryngol 107:620, 1981

156. Martynenko II, Ladyzhenskaya EA, Musabaev IK, Tuparov MT: Involvement of the eighth pair of nerves in viral hepatitis. Vestn Otorinolaringol 33:97, 1971

157. Maassab HF: The role of viruses in sudden deafness. Adv Otorhinolarygngol 20:229, 1973

158. Berg M, Pallasch H: Sudden deafness and vertigo in children and juveniles. Adv Otorhinolaryngol 27:70, 1981

159. Rowson KEK, Hinchcliffe R, Gamble DR: A virological and epidemiological study of patients with acute hearing loss. Lancet 1:471, 1975

160. Dick GWA, Best AM, Haddow AJ, et al: Mengo encephalomyelitis: a hitherto unknown virus affecting man. Lancet 2:286, 1948

161. Jaffe BF: Viral causes of sudden inner ear deafness. Med Clin North Am 11:63, 1978

162. Earnest MP, Goolishian HA, Calverley JR, et al: Neurologic, intellectual and psychologic sequelae following western encephalitis: a follow-up study of 35 cases. Neurology 21:969, 1971

163. Vaneeva GG: The state of auditory and vestibular functions in tick-borne encephalitis. Zh Nevropatol Psikhiatr 70:48, 1970

164. Bredeck JE, Brown GO, Hempelmann TC, et al: Follow-up studies of the 1933 St. Louis epidemic of encephalitis. JAMA 111:15, 1938

165. Hirsch E: Sensorineural deafness and labyrinth damage due to lymphocytic choriomeningitis: report of a case. Arch Otolaryngol 102:499, 1976

166. Timmons GD, Johnson KP: Aqueductal stenosis and hydrocephalus after mumps encephalitis. N Engl J Med 283:1505, 1970

167. Edwards KM, Bennett SR, Garner WL, et al: Reye's syndrome associated with adenovirus infections in infants. Am J Dis Child 139:343, 1985

168. Linneman CC, Ueda K, Hug G, et al: Reye's syndrome: epidemiologic and viral studies, 1963–1974. Am J Epidemiol 101:517, 1975

169. Tang TT, Siegesmund KA, Sedmak GV, et al: Reye syndrome: a correlated electron-microscopic, viral, and biochemical observation. JAMA 232:1339, 1975

170. Terry SI, Golden MHN, Hanchard B, Bain B: Adult Reye's syndrome after dengue. Gut 21:436, 1980

171. Fleisher G, Schwartz J, Lennette E: Primary Epstein-Barr virus infection in association with Reye syndrome. J Pediatr 97:935, 1980

172. Chalhub EG, DeVivo DC, Keating JP, et al: Reye syndrome complicated by a generalized herpes simplex type 1 infection. J Pediatr 98:73, 1981

173. Partin JC, Schubert WK, Partin JS, et al: Isolation of influenza virus from liver and muscle biopsy specimens from a surviving case of Reye's syndrome. Lancet 2:599, 1976

174. Norman MG, Lowden JA, Hill DE, Bannatyne RM: Encephalopathy and fatty degeneration of the viscera in childhood: II. Report of a case with isolation of influenza B virus. Can Med Assoc J 99:549, 1968

175. Roe CR, Schonberger LB, Gelbach SH, et al: Enzymatic alterations in Reye's syndrome: prognostic implications. Pediatrics 55:119, 1975

176. Powell MC, Rosenberg RN, McKellar B: Reye's syndrome: isolation of parainfluenza virus. Arch Neurol 29:135, 1973

177. Brunberg JA, Bell WE: Reye syndrome: an association with type 1 vaccine-like poliovirus. Arch Neurol 30:304, 1974

178. Joske RA, Keall DD, Leak PJ, et al: Hepatitis-encephalitis in humans with reovirus infection. Arch Intern Med 113:811, 1964

179. Griffin N, Keeling JW, Tomlinson AH: Reye's syndrome associated with respiratory syncytial virus infection. Arch Dis Child 54:74, 1979

180. Salmi TT, Arstila P, Koivikko A: Central nervous system involvement in patients with rotavirus gastroenteritis. Scand J Infect Dis 10:29, 1978

181. Cullity GJ, Kakulas BA: Encephalopathy and fatty degeneration of the viscera: an evaluation. Brain 93:77, 1970

182. Hurwitz ES, Goodman RA: A cluster of cases of Reye syndrome associated with chickenpox. Pediatrics 70:901, 1982

183. Von Economo C: Die Encephalitis Lethargica. Urban & Schwarzenberg, Vienna, 1929

184. Duvoisin RC, Yahr MD: Encephalitis and parkinsonism. Arch Neurol 12:227, 1965

185. Hanninen P, Arstila P, Lang H, et al: Involvement of the central nervous system in acute, uncomplicated measles virus infection. J Clin Microbiol 11:610, 1980

186. Miller DL: Frequency of complications of measles. Br Med J 2:75, 1964

187. Abruzzi W: Measles: a serious pediatric disease. J Pediatr 64:750, 1964

188. Wilner E, Cannon J, Brody JA: Measles, minor neurological signs and intelligence. Dev Med Child Neurol 11:449, 1969

189. Black FL, Fox JP, Elveback L, Kogon A: Measles and readiness for reading and learning: I. Background, purpose and general methodology. Am J Epidemiol 88:333, 1968

190. terMeulen V, Kackell Y, Muller D, et al: Isolation of infectious measles virus in measles encephalitis. Lancet 1:1172, 1972

191. Gendelman HE, Wolinsky JS, Johnson RT, et al: Measles encephalomyelitis: lack of evidence of viral invasion of the central nervous system and quantitative study of the nature of demyelination. Ann Neurol 15:353, 1984

192. Ziegra SR: Corticosteroid treatment for measles encephalitis. J Pediatr 59:322, 1961

193. Boe J, Solberg CO, Saeter T: Corticosteroid treatment of acute meningoencephalitis: a retrospective study of 346 cases. Br Med J 1:1094, 1965

194. Abramsky O, Teitelbaum D: The autoimmune features of acute transverse myelopathy. Ann Neurol 2:36, 1977

195. Bradley WG, Whitty CWM: Acute optic neuritis: its clinical features and their relation to prognosis for recovery of vision. J Neurol Neurosurg Psychiatry 30:531, 1967

196. Cohen MM, Lessell S, Wolf PA: A prospective study

of the risk of developing multiple sclerosis in uncomplicated optic neuritis. Neurology 29:208, 1979

197. Davis LE, Johnsson LG: Viral infections of the inner ear: clinical, virologic, and pathologic studies in humans and animals. Am J Otolaryngol 4:347, 1983

198. Reye RDK, Morgan G, Baral J: Encephalopathy and fatty degeneration of the viscera: a disease entity in childhood. Lancet 2:749, 1963

199. Corey L, Rubin RJ: Reye's syndrome 1974: an epidemiological assessment. p. 179. In Pollack JD (ed): Reye's Syndrome. Grune & Stratton, Orlando, FL, 1975

200. Davis LE, Kornfeld M: Influenza A virus and Reye's syndrome in adults. J Neurol Neurosurg Psychiatry 43:516, 1980

201. Arrowsmith JB, Kennedy DL, Kuritsky JN, Faich GA: National patterns of aspirin use and Reye syndrome reporting, United States, 1980 to 1985. Pediatrics 79:858, 1987

202. Sullivan-Bolyai JZ, Corey L: Epidemiology of Reye syndrome. Epidemiol Rev 3:1, 1981

203. Corey L, Rubin RJ, Hattwick MAW, et al: A nationwide outbreak of Reye syndrome. Am J Med 61:615, 1976

204. Hurwitz ES, Barrett MJ, Bregman D, et al: Public Health Service study of Reye's syndrome and medications: report of the main study. JAMA 257:1905, 1987

205. Davis LE: Reye's syndrome. p. 149. In McKendall R, Vinken PJ, Bruyn GW (eds): Handbook of Clinical Neurology: Vol 56. Elsevier, Amsterdam, 1989

206. Brown RE, Forman DT: The biochemistry of Reye's syndrome. CRC Crit Rev Clin Lab Sci 17:247, 1982

207. Devivo DC, Keating JP: Reye's syndrome. Adv Pediatr 22:175, 1976

208. Rogers MF, Schonberger LB, Hurwitz ES, Rowley DL: National Reye syndrome surveillance, 1982. Pediatrics 75:260, 1985

209. Ropper AH: Raised intracranial pressure in neurologic disease. Semin Neurol 4:397, 1984

210. Andersson T, Sidén A: A clinical study of the Guillain-Barré syndrome. Acta Neurol Scand 66:316, 1982

211. Ropper AH: The Guillain-Barré syndrome. N Engl J Med 326:1130, 1992

212. Arnason BGW: Acute inflammatory demyelinating polyradiculoneuropathies. p. 2050. In Dyck PJ, Thomas PK, Lambert EH, Bunge R (eds): Peripheral Neuropathy. 2nd Ed. WB Saunders, Philadelphia, 1984

213. Greenland P, Griggs RC: Arrhythmic complications in the Guillain-Barré syndrome. Arch Intern Med 140: 1053, 1980

214. Truax BT: Autonomic disturbances in the Guillain-Barré syndrome. Semin Neurol 4:462, 1984

215. McLeod JG: Electrophysiological studies in the Guillain-Barré syndrome. Ann Neurol 9, suppl:20, 1981

216. Asbury AK, Arnason BG, Adams RD: The inflammatory lesion in idiopathic polyneuritis: its role in pathogenesis. Medicine (Baltimore) 48:173, 1969

217. Prineas JW: Pathology of the Guillain-Barré syndrome. Ann Neurol 9, suppl:6, 1981

218. Lampert PW: Mechanisms of demyelination in experimental allergic neuritis. Lab Invest 20:127, 1969

219. Lisak RP, Mitchell M, Zweiman B, et al: Guillain-Barré syndrome and Hodgkin's disease: three cases with immunological studies. Ann Neurol 1:72, 1977

220. Guillain-Barré Syndrome Study Group: Plasmapheresis and acute Guillain-Barré syndrome. Neurology 35: 1096, 1985

221. Gajdusek DC: Unconventional viruses and the origin and disappearance of kuru. Science 197:943, 1977

222. Prusiner SB: Prions and neurodegenerative diseases. N Engl J Med 317:1571, 1987

223. Brown P, Cathala F, Castaigne P, Gajdusek C: Creutzfeldt-Jakob disease: clinical analysis of a consecutive series of 230 neuropathologically verified cases. Ann Neurol 20:597, 1986

224. Roos R, Gajdusek DC, Gibbs CJ: The clinical characteristics of transmissible Creutzfeldt-Jakob disease. Brain 96:1, 1973

225. Chiofalo N, Fuentes A, Galvez S: Serial EEG findings in 27 cases of Creutzfeldt-Jakob disease. Arch Neurol 37:143, 1980

226. Harrington MG, Merril CR, Asher DM, Gajdusek DC: Abnormal proteins in the cerebrospinal fluid of patients with Creutzfeldt-Jakob disease. N Engl J Med 315:279, 1986

227. Manuelidis EE: Creutzfeldt-Jakob disease. J Neuropathol Exp Neurol 44:1, 1985

228. Duffy P, Wolf J, Collins G: Possible person-to-person transmission of Creutzfeldt-Jakob disease. N Engl J Med 290:692, 1974

229. Norrby E: Pituitary growth hormone and Creutzfeldt-Jakob disease. Acta Paediatr Scand 325:116, 1986

230. Gajdusek DC, Gibbs CJ, Asher DM: Precautions in medical care of, and in handling materials from, patients with transmissible virus dementia (Creutzfeldt-Jakob disease). N Engl J Med 297:107, 1977

38

AIDS and the Nervous System

Joseph R. Berger

Clinically apparent and frequently debilitating neurological disease is common with infection by human immunodeficiency virus type 1 (which will be referred to simply as HIV), the etiological agent of the acquired immunodeficiency syndrome (AIDS). In excess of 50 percent of persons infected with HIV will develop symptomatic neurological disease. Early studies[1,2] detected an incidence of neurological complications with AIDS of approximately 40 percent, but these studies were retrospective in nature and performed at a time in the course of this pandemic when life expectancies were considerably shorter and many of the neurological illnesses associated with the infection were unrecognized. Subsequent studies demonstrated significantly higher rates of neurological disease.[3] Although neurological disease typically occurs with advanced disease and profound immunosuppression, it is not infrequently the harbinger of AIDS. The frequency with which neurological disease heralds AIDS ranges from 10 to 20 percent.[3,4] Perhaps 100,000 HIV-infected persons develop neurological disease annually in the United States. Furthermore, the frequency with which neurological disease is observed at the time of autopsy is substantially higher, with some series demonstrating neuropathological abnormalities in more than 90 percent of patients dying with AIDS.[5,6] It is not surprising that careful neurological examination, even in the absence of specific complaints by the HIV-infected patient, frequently reveals evidence of central nervous system (CNS) or peripheral dysfunction.

Not only is the spectrum of neurological disorders that complicate HIV infection extremely broad (Table 38-1), but any part of the neuraxis may be affected. In general, the illnesses affecting the nervous system can be classified into those that are believed to be the direct result of HIV, although the precise mechanism by which HIV results in the pathogenesis of these neurological disorders remains uncertain, and those that result from other identifiable etiologies. Among the disorders in the former category are encephalopathy, myelopathy, peripheral neuropathy, and inflammatory myopathy. Their relative frequencies are depicted in Table 38-2. The illnesses in the latter category are chiefly a consequence of the severe abnormalities of cellular immunity accompanying AIDS. Infectious complications, particularly, cerebral toxoplasmosis and cryptococcal meningitis, are among the most common complications (Table 38-3). As a rule, these opportunistic neurological infections are the consequence of a dissemination or recrudescence of a latent or persistent infection rather than a recently acquired one. Often these infections relapse after initially successful therapy. Therefore, secondary antibiotic prophylaxis is warranted in certain infections, such as *Toxoplasma* encephalitis and cryptococcal meningitis. Other causes of neurological disease seen in association with the immunosuppression of HIV infection include primary and metastatic neoplasms, metabolic–nutritional disorders, and cerebrovascular complications.

In evaluating and treating the HIV-infected patient with neurological disease, the physician must remain aware of the fact that the severely immunocompromised patient with AIDS often has two or more dif-

Table 38-1 Spectrum of Neurological Disorders Associated With HIV Infection

Disorders postulated to be directly related to HIV
  Meningitis
    Acute meningitis occurring at the time of seroconversion
    Chronic meningitis
  Encephalopathy
    HIV-associated minor cognitive/motor abnormalities
    HIV-associated major cognitive/motor abnormalities (AIDS dementia complex)
  Vacuolar myelopathy
  Peripheral neuropathy
    Predominantly sensory peripheral neuropathy
    Sensorimotor peripheral neuropathy
    Autonomic peripheral neuropathy
  Cranial neuropathy
    Bell's palsy
  Inflammatory myopathy

Disorders indirectly related to HIV
  Opportunistic infections (see Table 38-3)
  Neoplasms
    Primary CNS lymphoma
    Primary brain neoplasms
    Metastatic disease, including lymphoma and Kaposi's sarcoma
  Vascular disease
    CNS hemorrhage secondary to thrombocytopenia, vasculitis, or other causes
    CNS ischemic stroke
    CNS vasculitis due to HIV or herpes zoster
    Aspergillosis and mucormycosis
  Nutritional and metabolic disorders
    Wernicke's encephalopathy
    Vitamin B_{12} deficiency
    Other vitamin deficiency
  Drug toxicity
    Peripheral neuropathy secondary to antiretroviral agents
    Mitochondrial myopathy secondary to zidovudine
    Neuroleptic malignant syndrome

Table 38-2 Incidence of Clinically Recognized HIV-Related Complications[a]

Aseptic meningitis	<5%
AIDS dementia complex	33%
Vacuolar myelopathy	10%
Polyneuropathy	10–35%
Myopathy	<10%

[a] The frequency with which these disorders are recognized at the time of autopsy is substantially higher than the frequency of their clinical recognition.
(Modified from Berger JR, Portegies P: The neurological complications of human immunodeficiency virus infection. p. 376. In Weiner WJ, Goetz CG (eds): Neurology for the Non-neurologist. 3rd Ed. JB Lippincott, Philadelphia, 1993, with permission).

ferent illnesses responsible for neurological impairment. Furthermore, the neurological disease observed in the HIV-infected person is not always the consequence of disease related to the infection. Common neurological problems, such as migraines and herniated intervertebral discs with associated radiculopathies, may also occur. A high degree of vigilance is warranted, but these ordinary problems should not be overlooked.

MENINGITIS

Headache, meningismus, cranial nerve palsies, and other neurological symptoms with or without fever generally herald more ominous disorders resulting from a broad array of microbial pathogens or from lymphomatous infiltration of the meninges. Radiographically, meningitis may be suspected by contrast enhancement of the subarachnoid space on computed tomography (CT) or magnetic resonance imaging (MRI). This enhancement of the subarachnoid cisterns may be either diffuse or focal, but its absence does not preclude the diagnosis. Other radiographic features of meningitis include communicating hydrocephalus, arterial or venous infarctions due to vasculitis, sinus thrombosis, and brain abscesses. The diagnosis of meningitis necessitates cerebrospinal fluid (CSF) examination. In HIV-infected patients with suspected meningitis, the CSF examination is incomplete without thorough microbiological studies including fungal and mycobacterial cultures and stains, India ink and cryptococcal antigen studies, and the Venereal Disease Research Laboratory (VDRL) test.

Table 38-3 Frequency of CNS Opportunistic Infection at the Time of Autopsy

Organism	Percent
Cytomegalovirus	15.8
Toxoplasma	13.6
Cryptococcus	7.6
JC virus	4.0
Herpes simplex virus	1.6
Candida	1.1
Varicella-zoster virus	0.6
Histoplasma	0.4
M. tuberculosis	0.3
Aspergillus	0.3

(From Kure K, Llena JF, Lyman WD, et al: Human immunodeficiency virus-1 infection of the nervous system: an autopsy study of 268 adult, pediatric, and fetal brains. Hum Pathol 22:700, 1991, with permission.)

Viral cultures, particularly for cytomegalovirus, should also be considered. Cytological investigation is also essential in light of the relative frequency of lymphomatous meningitis.

Viral Meningitis

HIV MENINGITIS

The frequency of clinically apparent HIV meningitis is substantially lower than is suggested by the observation of an otherwise unexplained CSF pleocytosis or the findings of meningeal inflammation at the time of autopsy. In a minority of individuals, an acute meningitis may accompany primary infection with HIV. This acute viral illness, indistinguishable from many other viral illnesses, is characterized by fever, generalized lymphadenopathy, pharyngeal injection, splenomegaly and splenic tenderness, maculopapular rash, and urticaria. It typically develops within 3 to 6 weeks of infection,[7,8] before seroconversion to HIV, an event that averages 8 to 12 weeks after exposure. With this acute infection, a meningitis[7,9] or meningoencephalitis[10] may supervene, with headache, meningismus, photophobia, generalized seizures, and altered mental state. CSF examination reveals an increased protein concentration (greater than 100 mg/dl), mononuclear pleocytosis (more than 200 cells/mm³) and normal glucose content.[9] HIV may be isolated from the blood and CSF.

Routine examination of the CSF in asymptomatic individuals infected with HIV commonly reveals abnormal CSF parameters, including a sterile pleocytosis. A study of HIV-infected US Air Force personnel (80 percent entirely asymptomatic clinically) revealed some CSF abnormality in 63 percent.[11] Among the CSF abnormalities frequently detected were mononuclear pleocytosis, increased protein concentration, increased IgG, and the presence of oligoclonal bands.[11] The presence of myelin basic protein is unexpected. The CSF abnormalities do not appear to be predictive of the subsequent development of neurological disease,[11] and their interpretation requires caution.

Bacterial Meningitis

MYCOBACTERIAL INFECTIONS

Infection with *Mycobacterium tuberculosis, Mycobacterium avium-intracellulare,* and, rarely, other atypical mycobacteria occurs frequently in AIDS and is often extrapulmonary.[12] The frequency of CNS involvement varies with the organism and the population studied. Haitians, American blacks, and intravenous drug abusers[13] appear to be the risk groups that have the highest incidences of mycobacterial infection. In Miami, 2.4 percent of HIV-infected patients with CNS disease had CNS tuberculosis.[3]

In addition to meningitis, the clinical spectrum of CNS tuberculosis associated with HIV infection includes cerebral abscesses and tuberculomas[14] and spinal cord abscess.[15] The most common clinical manifestations of tuberculous meningitis in AIDS include seizures, altered mental status, fever, and meningismus.[14] Although HIV infection increases the risk for meningitis with *M. tuberculosis,* it may not alter the clinical manifestations or response to therapy.[16] In contrast to *M. tuberculosis,* which most often presents as meningitis, *M. avium-intracellulare* typically causes single or multiple mass lesions. Ring-enhancing lesions and hypodense areas are seen with CT scan. The CSF may, on occasion, be normal[14] or acellular,[17] emphasizing the value of brain biopsy in establishing the diagnosis in some patients.

All HIV-seropositive patients should be skin-tested for tuberculosis and, if positive, should be treated. In those with active tuberculosis, a regimen involving three or more drugs is required for a minimum of 9 months. Recent descriptions of multidrug-resistant

M. tuberculosis raise concerns about the adequacy of this treatment regimen, and sensitivities should be performed in all cases. In regions where multidrug-resistant organisms have been isolated, a more extensive regimen is probably required. Atypical mycobacterial infection requires a four-drug regimen[18] and may necessitate experimental antimicrobials, such as rifabutyn and clofazimine.[19]

TREPONEMA PALLIDUM

Neurosyphilis must always be considered in patients with HIV infection, even in the absence of neurological disease. In some populations, between 1 to 6 percent of all HIV-infected patients have neurosyphilis as defined by a positive VDRL test in the CSF[20-23]; this is probably an underestimate of the true incidence of neurosyphilis in AIDS because of the relative insensitivity of this test.[24] An acute, symptomatic, syphilitic meningitis during the course of secondary syphilis is not uncommon. A decrease in the latent period for the development of certain neurosyphilitic manifestations, such as meningovascular syphilis and general paresis, has been suggested. Johns and colleagues noted the development of meningovascular syphilis within 4 months of primary infection[25] despite the administration of accepted penicillin regimens. Relapse of neurosyphilis in HIV-infected individuals after appropriate doses of benzathine penicillin for secondary syphilis has also been noted.[26] Other unusual manifestations of syphilis that have been reported in association with HIV infection include unexplained fever,[27] bilateral optic neuritis with blindness,[28] Bell's palsy and severe bilateral sensorineural hearing loss,[29] syphilitic meningomyelitis,[30] syphilitic polyradiculopathy,[31] and syphilitic cerebral gumma presenting as a mass lesion.[32] Although still controversial, concomitant HIV infection appears to alter the natural course of syphilis.[33-35]

Treatment of syphilis requires the administration of intravenous, high-dose aqueous penicillin G (12 million or more U/d) for 10 to 14 days. Successful therapy of neurosyphilis with doxycycline 100 mg twice daily for 21 days in an HIV-infected person has been reported.[29] CSF examinations following treatment should be repeated at 6-month intervals over the succeeding 2 years. Ideally, the CSF cell count should be normal and the protein concentration lower, but the presence of concomitant HIV infection may alter the expected CSF resolution in successfully treated patients. The CSF VDRL titer should decline, but the CSF VDRL may remain reactive in low titer.

LISTERIA MONOCYTOGENES

Despite a profound impairment of cellular immunity, the incidence of *Listeria monocytogenes* infection appears to be less with AIDS than with other causes of impaired cell-mediated immunity. *Listeria* infection may result in meningitis[36] or brain abscess[37] and appears to have a predilection for the brainstem. In any case of meningitis of unknown cause occurring in a patient with AIDS the antibiotic regimen should include agents effective against *L. monocytogenes*,[38] such as ampicillin, high-dose penicillin, or trimethoprim/sulfamethoxazole.

OTHER BACTERIAL MENINGITIDES

Both infections that are typically associated with cellular immunodeficiency, such as *Salmonella,* and those more commonly seen with humoral immunodeficiency, such as *Streptococcus pneumoniae,* are seen with increased frequency in patients with AIDS.[39] These less common causes of meningitis must be considered in any AIDS patient presenting with meningitis.

Fungal Meningitis

CRYPTOCOCCAL MENINGITIS

The estimated incidence of cryptococcosis in patients with AIDS varies between 1.9[40] and 11 percent.[1] Blacks and intravenous drug abusers appear to have higher rates of this illness than other people. Cryptococcal meningitis, the chief clinical consequence of cryptococcal infection in patients with AIDS, may be the heralding illness or may occur simultaneously with other opportunistic infections.[3,41,42] In some communities, cryptococcal meningitis is more common than toxoplasmosis as the presenting neurological illness associated with HIV infection.[36] Symptomatically, headache is almost universally noted in patients with cryptococcal meningitis. Other frequently observed clinical features include nausea and vomiting, photophobia, blurred vision, fever, mental status changes, and meningismus. Cranial nerve palsies, hemiparesis, language disturbances, seizures, cerebellar findings, and psychosis occur with lesser frequencies. In one series of 25 patients with AIDS and cryptococcal meningitis, headache was present in 88 percent, fever in 84 percent, meningeal signs in 36 percent, mental status changes in 12 percent, and other neurological findings (cranial nerve palsies, papilledema, ataxia, and seizures) in 10 percent.[36] Though unusual, focal neurological findings may be observed with cryptococcal disease.[2,43,44]

Pathological examination reveals a basilar, chronic meningitis that is typically neither particularly thick nor exudative. Diffuse or focal opacifications of the leptomeninges and brain edema may be noted by gross examination. Small (2- to 3-mm) nodules may be observed studding the meninges, particularly in the interpeduncular fossa and in the sulci. Cystic lesions composed of clusters of budding yeast and displaying little surrounding inflammation or reactive gliosis may be seen throughout the brain, chiefly in the superficial layers of the cerebral cortex. When macroscopic in size, they are referred to as cryptococcomas.

Lumbar puncture typically reveals an elevated opening pressure, mononuclear pleocytosis, increased protein content, and depressed glucose level. However, two or three of the standard CSF parameters (protein, glucose, cell count) may be normal in up to 50 percent of these individuals.[36] India ink study is positive in over 70 percent[43,45] and the positivity rate of CSF cryptococcal antigen, CSF culture, and serum cryptococcal antigen exceeds 90 percent.[43] When cryptococcal meningitis is suspected, blood should be cultured and serum assayed for the presence of cryptococcal antigen. Cultures of other extraneural sites, such as bronchoalveolar lavage fluid, may also be positive.[45] Radiographic imaging is typically unremarkable. More often than not, brain CT scan does not reveal evidence of the pathological process.[46–49] In one series, mass lesions (cryptococcomas) and hydrocephalus were each observed in approximately 10 percent of patients and diffuse cerebral edema in another 3 percent.[50]

The mortality of cryptococcal meningitis is about 30 percent.[43] Many of the factors that predict a poor prognosis (positive India ink, a low CSF leukocyte count, a positive blood culture, the presence of *Cryptococcus neoformans* at extraneural sites, high CSF cryptococcal antigen titers, CSF hypoglycorrhachia, and an increased CSF opening pressure)[46] are present in AIDS. One study found that the most important predictor of poor outcome was an abnormal mental status at the time of diagnosis.[51] There remains considerable controversy, however, regarding the importance of these predictors of survival.[45]

The standard treatment of cryptococcal meningitis consists of intravenous amphotericin B (0.6 to 1 mg/kg/d) for a minimum of 6 weeks. However, a comparative study of amphotericin B (0.4 mg/kg) intravenously with or without flucytosine to oral fluconazole 200 mg/d showed similar rates of treatment success (40 versus 34 percent).[51] No benefit of flucytosine was detected.[51] Although oral fluconazole appears to be the equivalent of intravenous amphotericin B in the treatment of uncomplicated cryptococcal meningitis,[51] there remains considerable debate regarding the use of fluconazole as initial therapy. The current recommendation regarding treatment of cryptococcal meningitis is to use amphotericin B (0.7 mg/kg/d) with or without flucytosine (100 to 150 mg/kg/d). At the completion of 2 or more weeks, this therapy may be supplanted by oral fluconazole at 400 mg/day for 8 to 10 weeks. If at the end of this time the CSF culture is negative for *C. neoformans*, the fluconazole dose may be reduced to 200 mg/d and continued indefinitely as secondary prophylaxis to prevent relapse.

Half of the patients who are not treated with maintenance therapy following completion of their initial therapy relapse.[43] The prostate has been suggested as the site for redissemination of infection, as at least 20 to 30 percent of AIDS patients who have completed successful treatment for cryptococcal meningitis have positive urine cultures for *C. neoformans*.[52] Oral fluconazole is better tolerated than intravenous amphotericin and is the preferred agent for secondary prophylaxis.[53]

OTHER FUNGAL MENINGITIDES

Other fungal infections may also result in meningitis in the AIDS patient, including *Candida*. Although more than 50 percent of AIDS patients develop oropharyngeal or esophageal candidiasis, it is rarely observed in the brain at autopsy. Meningitis secondary to mucormycosis has been observed in parenteral drug abusers with AIDS[54,55] in the absence of the classic triad of ophthalmoplegia, necrotic nares, and diabetes insipidus. Large intracerebral lesions with associated vascular involvement are hallmarks of this typically fatal disease. Similarly, CNS *Aspergillus fumigatus* has been seen in AIDS,[56] but brain abscesses requiring surgical excision are a more common form of presentation than meningitis. Other fungal meningitides rarely observed with AIDS include histoplasmosis and coccidiomycosis.[36]

Lymphomatous Meningitis

Among patients with AIDS, 5 percent ultimately develop systemic lymphoma; approximately one-third of the latter have a neurological presentation.[57] The most common form of neurological illness occurring in association with AIDS-related systemic lymphoma is lymphomatous leptomeningitis, which may be either asymptomatic or symptomatic. The frequency of unsuspected lymphomatous meningitis occurring in AIDS-related lymphoma approaches 20 percent.[57] Accordingly, lumbar puncture is mandated in all AIDS patients with systemic lymphoma. Of these patients, 5 to 10 percent will also have cranial or peripheral nerve involvement and paraspinal masses.[58] The clinical features of symptomatic lymphomatous leptomeningitis include headache, altered mental status, seizures, cranial neuropathies, and radiculopathies. Cranial neuropathies are not infrequent in association with HIV infection, but the potential etiologies of cranial neuropathy occurring with AIDS are extremely diverse (Table 38-4).

The most likely mode of entry of the lymphomatous cells into the CNS is direct spread from contiguous extraneural sites.[59] The high frequency of lymphomatous bone marrow infiltration argues for dissemination from the medullary cavity through the dura and into the subarachnoid space.[59] The neurological manifestations of AIDS-associated lymphomatous meningitis, particularly cranial neuropathy, may be exquisitely responsive to the administration of corticosteroids. Appropriate treatment requires intrathecal chemotherapy.

GLOBAL ENCEPHALOPATHY

Both an alteration in cognitive abilities and a decline in level of consciousness may occur in the setting of HIV infection. The former, currently attributed to a direct effect of HIV infection, is usually insidious

Table 38-4 The Etiologies of Cranial Nerve Palsies With HIV Infection

Infectious meningitis
  Fungal
    Cryptococcosis
    Histoplasmosis
    Aspergillosis
    Mucormycosis
  Bacterial
    Mycobacterium tuberculosis
    Listeria monocytogenes
    Treponema pallidum
    Other
  Viral
    Varicella-zoster
    Cytomegalovirus
    HIV

Neoplastic meningitis
  Lymphoma
  Other

Compression from mass lesion
  Neoplastic
    Brain lymphoma
    Other
  Infectious
  Toxoplasmosis
  Cryptococcoma
  Tuberculoma

Vasculitis

Inflammatory neuropathy
  Guillain-Barré syndrome
  Chronic inflammatory polyradiculoneuropathy
  Other

Miscellaneous
  Malignant otitis externa
  Other

(From Berger JR, Flaster M, Schatz N, et al: Cranial neuropathy heralding otherwise occult AIDS-related large cell lymphoma. J Clin Neuro Ophthalmol 13:113, 1993, with permission.)

in nature but on occasion may present in precipitous fashion. Alterations in level of consciousness are often associated with focal neurological abnormalities and typically result from mass lesions of the brain, usually opportunistic infections or lymphoma. The evaluation of a global encephalopathy complicating HIV infection requires a thorough physical and neurological examination; laboratory studies that assess electrolytes, and renal, liver, and thyroid function; syphilis serologies; vitamin B$_{12}$ and folate levels; cranial MRI, preferably with gadolinium or, alternatively, CT with a double dose of contrast and delayed scanning; and CSF analysis (unless contraindicated) with recording of opening pressure, measurement of total cell and differential counts, determination of protein and glucose levels, detailed microbiological studies, and cytology.

Viral Encephalopathy

HIV ENCEPHALOPATHY (AIDS DEMENTIA COMPLEX)

Several appellations have been attached to the unique, progressive, dementing illness recognized shortly after the initial description of AIDS,[1,60] including subacute encephalitis, AIDS dementia complex, HIV encephalopathy, and, more recently, HIV-associated major cognitive/motor disorder.[61] The exact incidence of this encephalopathy in HIV-infected individuals is unknown. Of 144,184 persons with AIDS reported to the Centers for Disease Control (CDC) between September 1, 1987, and August 31, 1991, there were 10,553 (7.3 percent) reported to have HIV encephalopathy: in 2.8 percent of the adult patients with AIDS and 5.3 percent of children with AIDS,[61] HIV encephalopathy was the initial manifestation of the disease. In other studies, HIV encephalopathy was the initial AIDS-defining illness in 0.8 to 2.2 percent[2,3] of adult AIDS patients, and it has been detected in 4.0 percent of patients at the time of diagnosis of AIDS.[62] The annual incidence in AIDS patients has been reported to be between 7 and 14 percent.[62,63] By the time of death, approximately one-third of AIDS patients will exhibit this dementia,[61] although estimates in excess of 50 percent have been suggested.[64] An apparent decline in the incidence of this disorder may, in part, be the result of the widespread use of zidovudine.[63,65] The incidence of pathological features concordant with HIV encephalopathy that have been observed at autopsy has varied in different series but in general is substantially higher than the estimates based on clinical data.[5,66–71]

Considerable controversy has surrounded the issue of whether lesser degrees of cognitive impairment accompany HIV infection in its earlier stages. In general, large prospective longitudinal studies that have employed limited screening batteries have suggested that the occurrence of these abnormalities is no more frequent than in a suitably matched, control population without HIV infection. However, smaller studies that have employed more extensive neuropsychological screening measures and electrophysiological tests suggest an increased prevalence over the control population. Whether the presence of these cognitive abnormalities predicts the development of AIDS dementia complex remains uncertain.

Brain atrophy characterized by sulcal widening and ventricular dilatation is commonly observed at autopsy in patients with HIV encephalopathy. Meningeal fibrosis may also be present. Histologically, the most common and distinctive feature of this illness is pallor of the white matter, chiefly seen in a paravascular distribution and often accompanied by an astrocytic reaction.[72] The favored location for this demyelination is the periventricular and central white matter. Multinucleate giant cells, the pathological hallmark of the disease, probably result from direct virus-induced cell fusion.[64] Other microscopic features include microglial nodules, diffuse astrocytosis, and perivascular mononuclear inflammation. Thinning of the neocortex[73] and neuronal loss on quantitative assessment in specific brain regions[74] have also been noted.

HIV encephalopathy typically occurs in the context of advanced immunosuppression and coexistent systemic disease,[64,75–80] but it may be the presenting or even sole manifestation of HIV infection before the infected individual exhibits any other illnesses characteristic of impaired immunity.[81–83] The encephalopathy is characterized by an insidious onset of disturbed intellect. Fatigue and malaise, headaches, increasing social isolation, and loss of sexual drive are noted. On rare occasion the disorder begins abruptly and progresses rapidly. Symptoms include forgetfulness, difficulty in concentrating and reading, and a slowness in thinking, with an accompanying decline in job performance. Depression is frequently considered, but dysphoria is typically absent.[64] Sleep disturbance are not uncommon[84] and both focal and generalized seizures have been described.[85–87]

The hallmarks of advanced AIDS—namely wasting, alopecia, seborrheic dermatitis, and generalized lymphadenopathy—are typically apparent. The mental status examination reveals a slowing of mental processing (bradyphrenia) and other features consistent with a subcortical dementia. Abnormalities of both saccadic and pursuit eye movements are common.[88-92] Facial expression is diminished and the voice is often hypophonic and monotonous. Coordination is impaired, consistent with involvement of the basal ganglia.[93] Fine movements are performed slowly and imprecisely. Bradykinesia, postural instability, slow and clumsy gait, and altered muscle tone are noted.

CSF studies show a mononuclear pleocytosis in one-fifth of individuals, with counts usually less than 50 cells/mm³.[81] An increased protein concentration, but usually less than 200 mg/dl, is observed in two-thirds.[94] Intrathecal synthesis of HIV-specific antibody and oligoclonal bands are frequently present[95] but are not predictive of the development of CNS disease.[96] Potential surrogate markers in the CSF for HIV encephalopathy include an elevated HIV p24 antigen[97,98] and elevated levels of β_2-microglobulin, neopterin, and quinolinic acid. The isolation of HIV from CSF is not a useful marker for HIV-related neurological disease.[99]

The most important aspect of radiographic imaging of the brain in patients with suspected HIV encephalopathy is to rule out other neurological disorders.[100] The most commonly reported abnormality on CT scan of the brain is cerebral atrophy (Fig. 38-1).[2,93,101,102] MRI may show widespread involvement of large areas of white matter or smaller "patchy" or "punctate" lesions.[103] Neither the electroencephalogram (EEG) nor other electrophysiological studies are particularly useful diagnostic tools in HIV-infected individuals with HIV encephalopathy, despite assertions to the contrary. Detailed neuropsychological batteries, however, are often invaluable in determining whether there is an associated depression and in gauging the extent of the impairment and the response to therapy.

The initial anecdotal clinical reports[104,105] of improvement in HIV encephalopathy with zidovudine administration have been confirmed in controlled trials in adults[106,107] and in children.[108] The response appears to require higher doses of zidovudine than are routinely used.[109] Treatment should be with levels of zidovudine of 1,000 mg or more daily. If hematological toxicity supervenes, the use of erythropoietin or granulocyte colony stimulating factor may permit its use at these doses. If zidovudine cannot be administered or is ineffective, dideoxyinosine (600 mg daily) is usually employed.

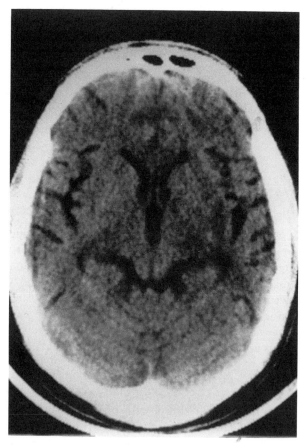

Fig. 38-1. CT scan of the brain in HIV encephalopathy. Considerable brain atrophy is evidenced by the sulcal widening and the ventricular and cisternal enlargement.

CYTOMEGALOVIRUS ENCEPHALITIS

Cytomegalovirus (CMV) not infrequently results in retinitis, pneumonitis, gastroenteritis, hepatitis, or encephalitis in the person with advanced immunosuppression due to AIDS.[110] Pathological evidence of its presence in the brains of AIDS patients with neurological disease was found in 36 percent of patients in one study.[1] Evidence for this involvement included neuropathological findings (i.e., microglial nodules, cytomegaly, and typical CMV inclusions), disseminated CMV infection, or serological evidence of prior CMV infection.

Despite histopathological and virological evidence implicating CMV in the etiology of an HIV-associated encephalitis, the clinical features of CMV encephalitis in the AIDS population remain poorly characterized and clinical recognition is difficult. Indeed,

CMV may localize to CNS tissues without significant clinical sequelae.[111,112] Although imaging studies and analysis of CSF may reveal abnormalities in many patients, none has been specific enough to allow a definitive diagnosis of CMV encephalitis. Kalayjian and colleagues argue that CMV ventriculoencephalitis in AIDS has sufficiently distinct clinical and pathological features to allow identification.[113] These features include prior or concomitant CMV retinitis or other serious CMV infection; altered mental status; nystagmus; cranial neuropathies; ventriculomegaly on neuroimaging; periventricular enhancement on CT scan; increased periventricular signal intensity on T_2-weighted MRI; CSF pleocytosis (up to 18,666 cells/mm^3, often with substantial numbers of polymorphonuclear cells); increased CSF protein (exceeding 50 mg/dl) and hypoglycorrhachia (less than 40 mg/dl). A multifocal CNS disorder[114] and isolated brainstem dysfunction[115] have been observed with CMV encephalitis. Other clinical syndromes associated with CMV in AIDS are polyradiculoneuropathy, vasculitic neuropathy, myelopathy, and adrenal insufficiency with concomitant hyponatremia.[113] Typically these illnesses occur after the onset of other AIDS-defining illnesses and in the presence of low CD4 lymphocyte counts.[113] Anecdotal reports support the use of ganciclovir, a selective guanosine analog, and foscarnet for CMV encephalitis.

FOCAL NEUROLOGICAL DYSFUNCTION OF CENTRAL ORIGIN

Focal neurological disturbances—such as hemianopia, hemiparesis, and hemianesthesia—occurring with HIV infection may result from a variety of lesions affecting the cerebrum. These lesions can be broadly classified in their order of frequency as opportunistic infections, tumors, and cerebrovascular disease. The most common opportunistic infections in this category are *Toxoplasma* encephalitis and progressive multifocal leukoencephalopathy. With rare exception, brain tumors occurring with AIDS are primary CNS lymphomas, although other primary CNS tumors and metastatic tumors have been reported. In the HIV-infected patient with focal neurological signs, either a cranial MRI with gadolinium or a double-dose, delayed brain CT scan is mandated.

The presence or absence of mass effect on radiographic imaging is extremely helpful in determining the etiology of the lesions.

Brain Disease With Mass Effect

Toxoplasma encephalitis is the most common cause of focal intracranial mass lesion in HIV infection, followed in frequency by lymphoma. An approach to the management of intracranial mass lesions occurring with HIV infection is found in the algorithm shown in Figure 38-2. Less common causes of intracranial lesions with mass effect are pyogenic abscess, syphilitic gumma, *Candida* abscess, *Nocardia* abscess, cryptococcoma and cryptococcal pseudocysts, other fungal and parasitic diseases, and vascular-occlusive lesions.

TOXOPLASMA GONDII

Approximately 20 to 30 percent of AIDS patients will develop *Toxoplasma* encephalitis. Usually, these patients present with focal neurological symptoms and signs often superimposed on a global encephalopathy. A prodrome of fever and malaise may occur for several days to weeks before the onset of the neurological illness. Mild hemiparesis is the most common focal finding.[116] Confusion, lethargy, brainstem and cerebellar disorders, and seizures are not rare.[116] The appearance of chorea in AIDS patients is believed to be virtually pathognomonic of toxoplasmosis.[117]

CT scan of the brain usually reveals multiple nodular or ring-enhancing lesions with edema and mass effect.[116,118,119] Occasionally the CT scan is normal or reveals only a hypodense lesion that fails to enhance with contrast. Most lesions occur in the basal ganglia[119,120] and the cerebral hemispheres, particularly the frontoparietal lobes.[116] MRI reveals discrete areas of increased signal intensity on T_2-weighted images.[121] The CT scan is probably the best radiographic method to judge the response to therapy. Although generally abnormal, the CSF findings in these patients are nonspecific. An elevation of CSF protein concentration (50 to 200 mg/dl) is seen in the majority, and one-third show a mononuclear pleocytosis (usually not exceeding 100 cells/mm^3). Cells counts in excess of 100 cells/mm^3 suggest the presence of another disease. Serological studies for toxoplasmosis

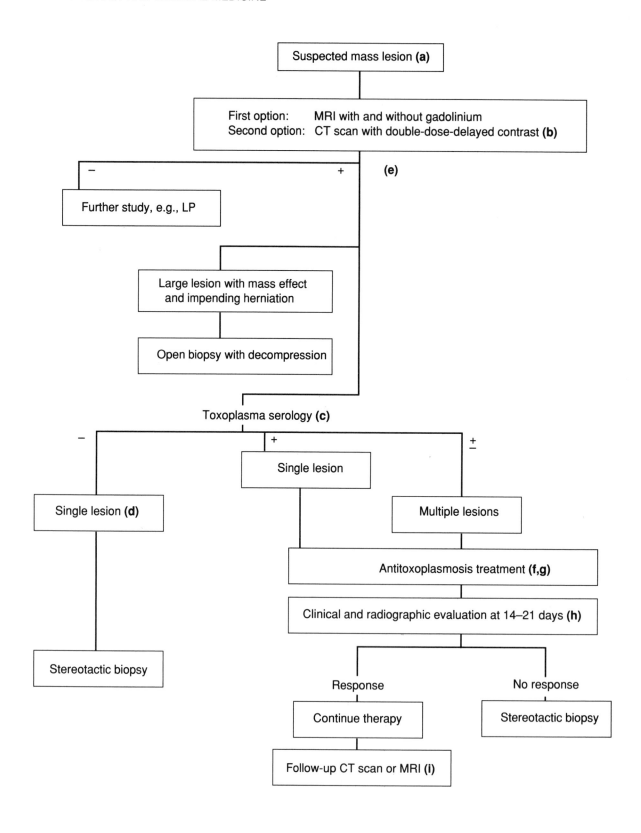

are typically elevated,[122] but this is not invariable.[123,124] A presumptive diagnosis is made on the basis of response to antitoxoplasmosis therapy, but brain biopsy is the only unequivocal means to establish the diagnosis. Excisional biopsies usually show tachyzoites on routine histology, particularly in the periphery of the necrotic lesion.[125]

A trial of antitoxoplasmosis therapy of 2 to 3 weeks' duration in those patients with suspected *Toxoplasma* encephalitis is recommended. These patients should be carefully monitored clinically and radiographically for resolution of their lesions. If the therapy fails to effect clinical and radiographic improvement, brain biopsy should be performed. The use of corticosteroids may confuse the interpretation of this therapeutic trial and their use should be avoided in this context.

The current recommended therapy of *Toxoplasma* encephalitis is combination therapy of sulfadiazine and pyrimethamine, a dihydrofolate reductase inhibitor. The pyrimethamine is administered orally in an initial loading dose of 200 mg, followed by 50 to 75 mg/d, and the sulfadiazine is administered as 4 to 6 g daily divided into four equal doses.[126] Folinic acid, 5 to 10 mg daily, is needed to diminish bone marrow suppression. Side effects of these medications are common, occurring in as many as 60 percent of patients.[127] If sulfadiazine is unavailable, an alternative preparation is sulfisoxazole. In patients not tolerating sulfa medications, clindamycin 2.4 g/d may be substituted. The risk of relapsing *Toxoplasma* encephalitis is high, warranting the use of secondary prophylaxis. Agents employed for prophylaxis of *Pneumocystis carinii* pneumonia, namely trimethoprim-sulfamethoxa-

---

Fig. 38-2. Algorithm for the management of intracranial mass lesions occurring with HIV infection. **(a)** The presence of an intracranial mass lesion is implied by the development of headache, altered mental status, or focal neurological findings. In addition to radiographic studies, CT scan, and MRI, other studies may be warranted to exclude infectious diseases other than toxoplasmosis (e.g., syphilis, tuberculosis, cryptococcosis), metabolic/nutritional disorders (e.g., vitamin B_{12} deficiency), and drug side effects.
(b) The technique of double-dose delayed (DDD) CT scan is performed by utilizing approximately 78 g of iodinated intravenous contrast via bolus and drip infusion followed 1 hour later by high-resolution CT scan. This technique has proved to be more sensitive in detecting lesions than a standard contrast CT scan.[48]
(c) Toxoplasmosis serology may be negative in the presence of established CNS toxoplasmosis. Thirteen of 80 (16 percent) patients with clinical toxoplasmosis and 4 of 18 (22 percent) with pathologically proved toxoplasmosis had undetectable plasma antitoxoplasma IgG antibody titers by indirect immunofluorescence assay.[124] The prevalence of falsely negative antibody titers for toxoplasmosis may increase with advanced immunosuppression.
(d) In one large study,[124] 28 of 103 (27 percent) patients with toxoplasmosis had single lesions on CT scan and 3 of 21 (14 percent) had single lesions on MRI.
(e) Opportunistic infections of the CNS, including toxoplasmosis, are rarely observed in children, in contrast to adults. Therefore, in HIV-infected children, proceeding directly to stereotactic biopsy may be a consideration to eliminate other diagnostic possibilities.
(f) The therapy of *Toxoplasma* encephalitis is oral pyrimethamine (an initial loading dose of 50 to 200 mg followed by 25 to 50 mg daily) and 6 to 8 g of sulfadiazine daily divided into four equal doses. In children, pyrimethamine 2 mg/kg/d is administered in divided doses every 12 hours for 1 to 3 days, then as 1 mg/kg daily or as divided doses every 12 hours to a maximum of 25 mg daily. It is administered in conjunction with sulfadiazine 120 mg/kg/d in divided doses every 6 hours in doses not to exceed the adult dose. Both drugs cross the blood-brain barrier. Folinic acid, 5 to 10 mg daily, is needed to diminish bone marrow suppression.
(g) Caution should be exercised in the evaluation of a seemingly therapeutic response to antitoxoplasmosis therapy if corticosteroids have also been administered. Re-evaluation on continued antibiotic therapy in the absence of corticosteroids is mandated within 2 weeks.
(h) Some authorities prefer a shorter period of time (10 to 14 days) in which unresponsiveness to treatment is demonstrated before resorting to stereotactic biopsy.
(i) Follow-up CT scan or MRI is warranted every 4 to 6 weeks until the lesions have regressed in their entirety or demonstrate no further change.
(Based upon preliminary recommendations of a working group of the American Academy of Neurology on Mass Lesions in AIDS.)

zole and pyrimethamine-sulfadoxine, significantly reduce the risk of developing *Toxoplasma* encephalitis.[128]

OTHER INFECTIOUS DISEASES

Nocardia asteroides, a gram-positive, weakly acidfast bacillus, may occasionally result in brain abscess in the AIDS patient. Treatment is often unsuccessful. Mass lesions associated with brain abscesses due to mixed bacterial flora, *Aspergillus,* and mucormycosis, tuberculous abscesses and tuberculomas due to *M. tuberculosis* or *M. avium-intracellulare,* cryptococcomas and cryptococcal pseudocysts, and syphilitic gummas are other causes of cerebral mass lesions of infectious origin seen in AIDS.

PRIMARY CNS LYMPHOMAS

In the setting of HIV infection, the incidence of primary CNS lymphomas increases dramatically. Up to 0.6 percent of patients will present with these tumors concurrent with the diagnosis of AIDS, and ultimately 2.0 percent develop the disease.[129] Estimates suggest that its incidence currently exceeds that of low-grade astrocytomas.[130] These tumors are mostly of B-cell origin and both large-cell immunoblastic and small noncleaved lymphomas are seen.[131] Of potential etiological significance is the observation that Epstein-Barr virus expression can be demonstrated in virtually all cases of AIDS-related primary CNS lymphomas.[132]

Primary CNS lymphoma typically presents with confusion, lethargy, memory loss, hemiparesis, speech and language disorders, seizures, and cranial nerve palsies, in descending order of frequency.[133] The lesions are often multiple, and involvement of the meninges is frequently demonstrated by cytological examination or at the time of postmortem examination. On CT scan, most lymphomas are either hyperdense or isodense, round or oval masses with homogeneous contrast enhancement and variable surrounding edema (Fig. 38-3).[134] These tumors respond both clinically and radiographically to whole-brain irradiation. A regimen of 4,000 rads administered over 3 weeks has been successfully employed,[130] and regimens employing chemotherapy have been reported.[135] The average survival is less than 4

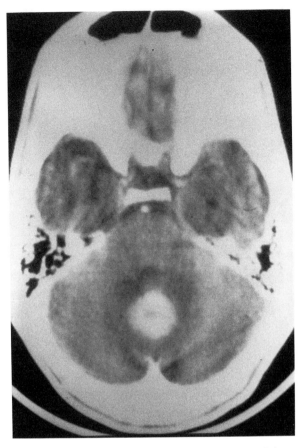

Fig. 38-3. CT scan of the brain in primary CNS lymphoma. Following contrast administration, there is an enhancing round mass lesion in the cerebellar vermis with surrounding edema. (From Berger JR, Post MJD, Levy RM: AIDS. In Greenberg J (ed): Neuroimaging: A Companion to Adams and Victor's Principles of Neurology. McGraw-Hill, New York, 1994, with permission.)

months,[135] with death often due to concurrent illnesses related to the immunodeficiency.

CEREBROVASCULAR DISEASE

The spectrum of cerebrovascular disease that has been reported in association with AIDS is broad (Table 38-5) and includes both ischemic and hemorrhagic disorders. In autopsy series, rates as high as 19 percent have been reported.[136] In a case-control autopsy series,[137] cerebrovascular disease was detected at autopsy in 8 percent of HIV-infected individuals but did not appear to occur significantly more frequently in

Table 38-5 Etiologies of Stroke Occurring With HIV Infection

Ischemic stroke
  Embolic
    Cardiac disease
      Nonbacterial endocarditis (marantic endocarditis)
      Bacterial endocarditis
      Other
  Thrombotic
    Vasculitis
      HIV-related
      Non-HIV infectious etiologies
        Herpes zoster
        T. pallidum
        Aspergillus
        Others
    Hematological conditions
      Lupus anticoagulant
      Disseminated intravascular coagulation
      Hyperviscosity syndrome
    Cerebral venous thrombosis with cachexia and dehydration
Intracranial hemorrhage
    Thrombocytopenia
      Autoimmune
      Drug-induced
      Disseminated intravascular coagulation
      Other
    Intracranial malignancy
    Vasculitis
    Ruptured mycotic aneurysm

(From Berger JR, Harris JO, Gregorios J, Norenberg M: Cerebrovascular disease in AIDS: a case control study. AIDS 4:239, 1990, with permission.)

HIV-infected persons than in age- and sex-matched controls with other terminal illnesses. Concomitant heart disease, particularly nonbacterial thrombotic (marantic) endocarditis, was frequent in both groups. Infectious vasculitis, especially meningovascular syphilis, must always be considered in the differential diagnosis of these disorders.

Brain Disease Without Mass Effect

The most common causes of intracranial lesions without mass effect in HIV-infected patients are progressive multifocal leukoencephalopathy, HIV encephalopathy, and CMV encephalitis. Of these disorders, only progressive multifocal leukoencephalopathy typically presents with focal neurological disturbances. MRI is the imaging study of choice, due to its superior contrast resolution and marked sensitivity in detecting lesions that affect the white matter.

PROGRESSIVE MULTIFOCAL LEUKOENCEPHALOPATHY

Progressive multifocal leukoencephalopathy is the result of infection of the brain with JC virus, a papovavirus. Before the AIDS pandemic it was a rare disease, almost invariably occurring in association with the

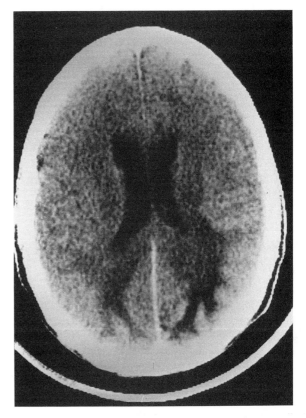

Fig. 38-4. CT scan of the brain in a patient with progressive multifocal leukoencephalopathy. This CT scan shows an extensive hypodense lesion without associated mass effect that involves both parieto-occipital regions. (From Berger JR, Post MJD, Levy RM: AIDS. In Greenberg J (ed): Neuroimaging: A Companion to Adams and Victor's Principles of Neurology. McGraw-Hill, New York, 1994, with permission.)

immunosuppression associated with lymphoproliferative disorders. Current estimates suggest that 2 to 5 percent of all patients with AIDS will develop it.[6,138]

In approximately one-quarter of AIDS patients with progressive multifocal leukoencephalopathy, the illness is the presenting manifestation of their immunosuppression. Limb weakness is the most common initial manifestation, followed in frequency by cognitive dysfunction, visual loss, gait disturbance, limb incoordination, speech or language disturbance, and headache. CT scan of the brain typically, although not invariably, reveals nonenhancing, hypodense white matter lesions without mass effect (Fig. 38-4). These lesions are chiefly located in the centrum semiovale, predominantly in the parieto-occipital region and the cerebellum.[138] T_2-weighted spin-echo MRI is highly sensitive in detecting these lesions (Fig. 38-5).[139] The CSF is usually normal, although a mild increase in protein concentration, the presence of myelin basic protein, an increase in IgG, and a pleocytosis (9 to 25 mononuclear cells mm³) have all been reported.[138] The presence of an increased opening pressure or significant CSF pleocytosis should raise serious concerns about the diagnosis. Diagnostic confirmation requires brain biopsy. The disorder is characterized pathologically by demyelination; giant astrocytes with pleomorphic, hyperchromatic nuclei; and altered oligodendrocytes containing enlarged nuclei that stain abnormally densely with hematoxylin and harbor ill-defined inclusion bodies. JC virus can be directly demonstrated by electron microscopy or by in situ hybridization. In a large series of patients with progressive multifocal leukoencephalopathy and AIDS, the mean survival was 4 months, ranging from 0.3 to 18 months.[138] However, perhaps 5 to 10 percent will have a prolonged survival (exceeding 1 year) and partial or complete neurological recovery.[139] At present no treatment strategy has proven effective, but anecdotal reports and in vitro data suggest that cytosine arabinoside may be useful.

SPINAL CORD DISEASE

Spinal cord disease is frequent in HIV infection. A unique HIV-associated vacuolar myelopathy is the chief cause of myelopathy. The diagnosis of this disorder, like that of HIV encephalopathy, is one of exclusion. A number of other myelopathies may also

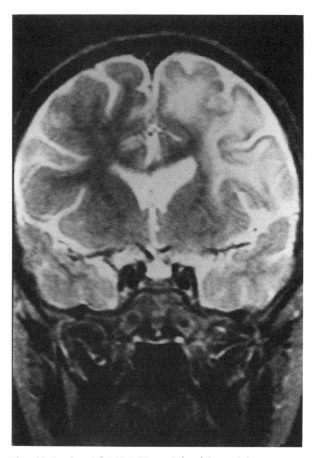

Fig. 38-5. Cranial MRI (T_2-weighted image) in progressive multifocal leukoencephalopathy shows a hyperintense signal involving the subcortical white matter of the left frontal lobe. (From Berger JR, Post MJD, Levy RM: AIDS. In Greenberg J (ed): Neuroimaging: A Companion to Adams and Victor's Principles of Neurology. McGraw-Hill, New York, 1994, with permission.)

occur with HIV infection, including infectious myelopathies (cytomegalovirus, herpes simplex type 2, herpes zoster, human T-lymphotropic virus type I (HTLV-I), mycobacteria, *Treponema pallidum*, and epidural abscesses), vascular myelopathies, epidural and intramedullary tumors, and a demyelinating myelopathy (Table 38-6).

For diagnostic and therapeutic purposes, it is useful to categorize spinal diseases occurring with HIV infection into two major groups, those that are the result of a mass lesion and those occurring in the absence of a mass lesion. The most common mass lesion affecting the spinal cord is lymphoma. Spinal lym-

Table 38-6 Diseases of the Spinal Cord Associated With HIV Infection

Infectious
  Virus
    HIV
      Chronic progressive myelopathy
      Acute transient myelopathy
      Relapsing and remitting myelitis
      Spinal myoclonus
    Cytomegalovirus
    Herpes simplex types 1 and 2
    Varicella-zoster
    HTLV-I
    HTLV-II[a]
    Adenovirus[a]
    Measles
  Bacteria
    Epidural abscesses
      M. tuberculosis
      Mixed infection
    Syphilitic meningomyelitis
  Fungi
    Nocardia
    Cryptococcus
    Other
  Parasitic
    T. gondii

Malignant
  Primary CNS lymphoma
  Metastatic lymphomas
  Astrocytoma/glioma
  Plasmacytoma

Vascular
  Necrotizing vasculitis
  Disseminated intravascular coagulation

Toxic/metabolic
  Vitamin B_{12} deficiency

[a] Possible etiologies
(From Berger JR, Levy RM: The neurological complications of human immunodeficiency virus infection. Med Clin North Am 77:1, 1993, with permission.)

phoma may present as (1) an intramedullary lesion, (2) meningeal lymphomatosis, (3) an epidural mass lesion, (4) bony metastases, and (5) some combination of these presentations. Other causes of mass lesions affecting the spinal cord are epidural and intramedullary nonlymphomatous tumors, intramedullary infections, and epidural abscesses. Epidural abscesses are most often seen in parenteral drug abusers and the most common organism isolated is *Staphylococcus aureus*.

HIV-Associated Myelopathy

This unique degeneration of the spinal cord is seen at autopsy in over 20 percent of patients dying with AIDS.[140] Usually, it begins insidiously and is characterized by leg weakness, gait impairment, paresthesias and vague leg discomfort, and bladder and bowel incontinence. Like HIV encephalopathy, HIV-associated myelopathy generally occurs with advanced immunosuppression. Casual recordings of the patient's symptoms often result in their being attributed to intercurrent illnesses and associated debilitation. However, neurological examination reveals spastic paraparesis, lower extremity hyperreflexia (except when diminished as a result of concomitant peripheral neuropathy), gait ataxia, and impaired sensation, with vibratory and position sense being disproportionately affected. Lower extremity involvement may be asymmetrical. A discrete sensory level is distinctly unusual. HIV-related vacuolar myelopathy is seldom associated with abnormalities on MRI but, on rare occasion, cord atrophy and hyperintense signals on T_2-weighted images may be observed.

Although gross examination of the spinal cord in this disorder is normal, histological examination reveals loss of myelin and spongy degeneration with relative axonal preservation, particularly affecting the dorsal and lateral columns.[140,141] Microglial nodules and HIV-laden multinucleate giant cells can be detected. No treatment has demonstrated unequivocal value in HIV-related vacuolar myelopathy. Other spinal cord disorders attributed to HIV include an acute myelopathy occurring at the time of primary infection,[140] spinal myoclonus,[142] and a relapsing-remitting myelopathy that may accompany optic neuritis.[143,144]

HTLV-I Associated Myelopathy

HTLV-I is recognized with increasing frequency in the HIV-infected population. It is transmitted in the same fashion as HIV. Coinfection has been associated with an HTLV-I associated myelopathy[145-147] A similar myelopathy has been observed in a person co-infected with HIV and HTLV-II.[148] HTLV-I-associated myelopathy is discussed further in Chapter 39.

PERIPHERAL NEUROPATHY

HIV infection is associated with a diverse group of peripheral neuropathies (Table 38-7). The exact role of HIV in the etiopathogenesis of these neuropathies remains obscure, and other factors such as concomitant infections, nutritional deficiencies, metabolic disorders, and side effects of drugs may be responsible for some of them. Prospective neurological evaluation may reveal evidence of peripheral neuropathy in up to 50 percent of patients with advanced HIV infection.

Although other types of peripheral neuropathy may be observed, the peripheral neuropathies associated with HIV infection can be divided into three major groups: a distal, symmetrical peripheral neu-

Table 38-7 Peripheral Nerve and Root Disease Associated With HIV Infection

Presumably HIV-mediated
Predominantly sensory neuropathy
Sensorimotor neuropathy
Autonomic neuropathy

Immune-mediated
Acute demyelinating polyradiculoneuropathy (Guillain-Barré syndrome)
Chronic inflammatory demyelinating polyradiculoneuropathy
Mononeuritis multiplex
Ataxic dorsal radiculopathy

Infectious
CMV polyradiculomyelopathy
Herpes zoster radiculitis
Syphilitic polyradiculopathy
M. avium-intracellulare

Nutritional
Vitamin B_{12} deficiency
Folate deficiency
Other nutritional disturbances

Toxic neuropathies
Dideoxyinosine (ddI)
Dideoxycytosine (ddC)
Foscarnet
Isoniazid

ropathy, an inflammatory demyelinating peripheral neuropathy, and mononeuritis multiplex. The most common is a symmetrical, distal, sensorimotor neuropathy that typically develops in the late stages of the disease. Patients complain of often debilitating, painful dysesthesias and numbness of the feet. When present, distal weakness is generally mild; muscle stretch reflexes are depressed or absent. The sensory loss is greatest for vibratory perception, but other sensory modalities may be affected. Nerve conduction velocities are usually slightly decreased and sensory action potentials are either absent or of low amplitude, suggesting an axonal neuropathy, although features of demyelination may also be seen. Nerve biopsy may reveal epineural and endoneural perivascular inflammation with axonal degeneration or demyelination.[149] Symptomatic therapy with carbamazepine, diphenylhydantoin, tricyclic antidepressants, mexitiline, and topical capsaicin may help the dysesthesias.

Both acute Guillain-Barré syndrome and a chronic, relapsing polyradiculoneuropathy may occur as a consequence of HIV infection.[150,151] Nerve conduction studies are compatible with a demyelinating neuropathy. CSF examination reveals a normal to increased protein concentration (but usually less than 200 mg/dl) with a mild mononuclear pleocytosis (usually no more than 50 cells/mm³) or, more rarely, a normal cell count. Therefore, in contradistinction to typical Guillain-Barré syndrome, a CSF albuminocytological dissociation occurs in only a minority of affected individuals. Plasmapheresis has been reported to be beneficial in those patients with chronic relapsing polyradiculoneuropathy,[151] and high-dose intravenous immunoglobulin may be associated with striking improvement.

On rare occasion, mononeuritis multiplex may be observed with HIV infection. Cranial, peripheral, or spinal nerves may be affected.[150] The disorder has been attributed to immune complex deposition resulting in a necrotizing vasculitis. Other causes of mononeuropathy—such as herpes zoster, cytomegalovirus, and lymphomatous nerve root infiltration—must be excluded.

Progressive polyradiculomyelopathy due to CMV[152,153] presents a striking picture. This illness is characterized at onset by lower extremity and sacral paresthesias. Progressive paraparesis ensues rapidly, with concomitant areflexia, ascending sensory loss, and sphincter dysfunction. Although reported rarely as an early manifestation of HIV infection,[154] it generally occurs with advanced immunodeficiency. An important clue to the presence of this potentially treatable illness is a polymorphonuclear pleocytosis. CMV can be detected in the CSF by culture, immunohistochemistry, and in situ hybridization.[153] Rarely, cytomegalic cells may be seen in the CSF.[153] A painful neuropathy has been attributed to a CMV-associated dorsal root ganglionitis, and CMV may also result in a disorder like the Guillain-Barré syndrome.[155] Ganciclovir or foscarnet are the treatment modalities for these CMV-related conditions, but favorable reports have been anecdotal.

MYOPATHY

Several forms of myopathy have been recognized in association with HIV infection. Among the most common is a polymyositis clinically indistinguishable from idiopathic polymyositis. This disorder is characterized by proximal muscle weakness, myalgias, excessive fatigability, and an increase in serum creatine kinase.[156,157] Weight loss and wasting, particularly of gluteal muscles, is often evident. Electromyographic features mirror those seen with idiopathic polymyositis. Muscle biopsy reveals fibrous tissue proliferation, necrosis, and phagocytosis of muscle fibers accompanied by an intense inflammatory infiltrate.[157] Another form of myopathy has been attributed to zidovudine therapy. This illness is chiefly characterized by muscle wasting and proximal weakness and tends to occur in individuals who have been treated with high doses of the drug for 6.5 to 17 months.[158] Compelling evidence suggests that this myopathy is the result of a toxic effect on muscle mitochondria. Some investigators have suggested that HIV polymyositis predisposes to the development of zidovudine-related myopathy.[156]

REFERENCES

1. Snider WD, Simpson DM, Nielsen S, et al: Neurological complications of the acquired immunodeficiency syndrome: analysis of 50 patients. Ann Neurol 14:403, 1983
2. Levy RM, Bredesen DE, Rosenblum ML: Neurological manifestations of the acquired immunodeficiency syndrome (AIDS): experience at UCSF and review of the literature. J Neurosurg 62:475, 1985
3. Berger JR, Moskowitz L, Fischl M, Kelley RE: Neurologic disease as the presenting manifestation of acquired immunodeficiency syndrome. South Med J 80: 683, 1987
4. Bredesen DE, Messing R: Neurological syndromes heralding the acquired immunodeficiency syndrome. Ann Neurol 14:141, 1983
5. Gray F, Gherardi R, Scaravilli F: The neuropathology of the acquired immune deficiency syndrome (AIDS). Brain 111:245, 1988
6. Kure K, Llena JF, Lyman WD, et al: Human immunodeficiency virus-1 infection of the nervous system: an autopsy study of 268 adult, pediatric, and fetal brains. Hum Pathol 22:700, 1991
7. Ho DD, Sarngadharan MG, Resnick L, et al: Primary human T-lymphotropic virus type III infection. Ann Intern Med 103:880, 1985
8. Cooper DA, Gold J, Maclean P, et al: Acute AIDS retrovirus infection: definition of a clinical illness associated with seroconversion. Lancet 1:537, 1985
9. Hollander H, Stringari S: Human immunodeficiency virus-associated meningitis: clinical course and correlations. Am J Med 83:813, 1987
10. Carne CA, Tedder RS, Smith A, et al: Acute encephalopathy coincident with seroconversion for anti-HTLV-III. Lancet 2:1206, 1985
11. Marshall DW, Brey RL, Cahill WT, et al: Spectrum of cerebrospinal fluid findings in various stages of human immunodeficiency virus infection. Arch Neurol 45: 954, 1988
12. Pumarola-Sune T, Navia BA, Cordon-Cardo C, et al: HIV antigen in the brains of patients with the AIDS dementia complex. Ann Neurol 21:490, 1987
13. Chaisson RE, Schecter GF, Theuer CP, et al: Tuberculosis in patients with the acquired immunodeficiency syndrome: clinical features, response to therapy, and survival. Am Rev Respir Dis 136:570, 1987
14. Bishburg E, Sunderam G, Reichman LB, Kapila R: Central nervous system tuberculosis with the acquired immunodeficiency syndrome and its related complex. Ann Intern Med 105:210, 1986
15. Doll DC, Yarbro JW, Phillips K, Klott C: Myocbacterial spinal cord abscess with an ascending polyneuropathy. Ann Intern Med 106:333, 1987
16. Berenguer J, Moreno S, Laguna F, et al: Tuberculous meningitis in patients infected with the human immunodeficiency virus. N Engl J Med 326:668, 1992
17. Laguna F, Adrados M, Ortega A, Gonzalez-Lahoz JM: Tuberculous meningitis with acellular cerebrospinal fluid in AIDS patients. AIDS 6:1165, 1992

18. Kemper CA, Meng TC, Nussbaum J, et al: Treatment of Mycobacterium avium complex bacteremia in AIDS with a four-drug oral regimen: rifampin, ethambutol, clofazimine, and ciprofloxacin. Ann Intern Med 116:466, 1992

19. Centers for Disease Control: Diagnosis and management of mycobacterial infection and disease in persons with human immunodeficiency virus infection. Ann Intern Med 106:204, 1987

20. Berger JR: Neurosyphilis in human immunodeficiency virus type 1-seropositive individuals: a prospective study. Arch Neruol 48:700, 1991

21. Holtom PD, Larsen RA, Leal ME, Leedom JM: Prevalence of neurosyphilis in human immunodeficiency virus-infected patients with latent syphilis. Am J Med 93:9, 1992

22. Appleman ME, Marshall DW, Brey RL, et al: Cerebrospinal fluid abnormalities in patients without AIDS who are seropositive for the human immunodeficiency virus. J Infect Dis 158:193, 1988

23. Livramento JA, Machado LR, Spina-Franca A: Cerebrospinal fluid abnormalities in 170 cases of AIDS. Arq Neuropsiquiatr 47:326, 1989

24. Berger JR: Diagnosing neurosyphilis: the value of the cerebrospinal fluid VDRL or lack thereof. J Clin Neuro Ophthalmol 9:234, 1989

25. Johns DR, Tierney M, Felsenstein D: Alteration in the natural history of neurosyphilis by concurrent infection with the human immunodeficiency virus. N Engl J Med 316:1569, 1987

26. Berry CD, Hooton TM, Collier AC, Lukehart SA: Neurologic relapse after benzathine penicillin therapy for secondary syphilis in a patient with HIV infection. N Engl J Med 316:1587, 1987

27. Chung WM, Pien FD, Grekin JL: Syphilis: a cause of fever of unknown origin. Cutis 31:537, 1983

28. Zambrano W, Perez GM, Smith JL: Acute syphilitic blindness in AIDS. J Clin Neuro Ophthalmol 7:1, 1987

29. Fernandez-Guerrero ML, Miranda C, Cenjor C, Sanabria F: The treatment of neurosyphilis in patients with HIV infection. JAMA 259:1495, 1988

30. Berger JR: Spinal cord syphilis associated with human immunodeficiency virus infection: a treatable myelopathy. Am J Med 92:101, 1992

31. Lanska MJ, Lanska DJ, Schmidley JW: Syphilitic polyradiculopathy in an HIV-positive man. Neurology 38:1297, 1988

32. Berger JR, Waskin H, Pall L, et al: Syphilitic cerebral gumma with HIV infection. Neurology 42:1282, 1992

33. Katz DA, Berger JR: Neurosyphilis in acquired immunodeficiency syndrome. Arch Neurol 46:895, 1989

34. Musher DM, Hamill RJ, Baughn RE: Effect of human immunodeficiency virus (HIV) infection on the course of syphilis and on the response to treatment. Ann Intern Med 113:872, 1990

35. Katz DA, Berger JR, Duncan RC: Neurosyphilis: a comparative study of the effects of infection with human immunodeficiency virus. Arch Neurol 50:243, 1993

36. Pons VG, Jacobs RA, Hollander H: Nonviral infections of the central nervous system in patients with acquired immunodeficiency syndrome. p. 263. In Rosenblum ML, Levy RM, Bredesen DE (eds): AIDS and the Nervous System. Raven Press, New York, 1988

37. Harris JO, Marquez J, Swerdloff MA, Magana IA: Listeria brain abscess in the acquired immunodeficiency syndrome. Arch Neurol 46:250, 1989

38. Kales CP, Holzman RS: Listeriosis in patients with HIV infection: clinical manifestations and response to therapy. J Acquir Immune Defic Syndr 3:139, 1990

39. Whimbey E, Gold JWM, Polsky B, et al: Bacteremia and fungemia in patients with the acquired immunodeficiency syndrome. Ann Intern Med 104:511, 1986

40. Editorial: Cryptococcus in AIDS. Lancet 1:1434, 1988

41. Kovacs JA, Kovacs AA, Polis M, et al: Cryptococcosis in the acquired immunodeficiency syndrome. Ann Intern Med 103:533, 1985

42. Giberson TP, Kalyan-Raman K: Cryptococcal meningitis: initial presentation of acquired immunodeficiency syndrome. Ann Emerg Med 16:802, 1987

43. Zuger A, Louie E, Holzman RS, et al: Cryptococcal disease in patients with the acquired immunodeficiency syndrome. Ann Intern Med 104:234, 1986

44. Maayan S, Wormser GP, Hewlett D, et al: Acquired immunodeficiency syndrome (AIDS) in an economically disadvantaged population. Arch Intern Med 145:1607, 1985

45. Gal AA, Evans S, Meyer PR: The clinical laboratory evaluation of cryptococcal infections in the acquired immunodeficiency syndrome. Diagn Microbiol Infect Dis 7:249, 1987

46. Diamond RD, Bennett JE: Prognostic factors in cryptococcal meningitis: a study of 111 cases. Ann Intern Med 80:176, 1974

47. Kelly WM, Brant-Zawadzki M: Acquired immunodeficiency syndrome: neuroradiologic findings. Radiology 149:485, 1983

48. Post MJD, Kursunoglu SJ, Hensley GT, et al: Cranial CT in acquired immunodeficiency syndrome: spectrum of diseases and optimal contrast enhancement technique. AJR 145:929, 1985

49. Whelan MA, Kricheff II, Handler M, et al: Acquired immunodeficiency syndrome: cerebral computed tomographic manifestations. Radiology 149:477, 1983

50. Popovich MJ, Arthur RH, Helmer E: CT of intracranial cryptococcosis. AJR 154:603, 1990

51. Saag MS, Powderly WG, Cloud GA, et al: Comparison of amphotericin B with fluconazole in the treatment of acute AIDS-associated cryptococcal meningitis. N Engl J Med 326:83, 1992

52. Larsen RA, Bozette S, McCutchan JA, et al: Persistent Cryptococcus neoformans infection of the prostate after successful treatment of meningitis. Ann Intern Med 111:125, 1989

53. Powderly WG, Saag MS, Cloud GA, et al: A controlled trial of fluconazole or amphotericin B to prevent relapse of cryptococcal meningitis in patients with the acquired immunodeficiency syndrome. N Engl J Med 326:793, 1992

54. Cuadrado LM, Guerrero A, Garcia Asenjo JAL, et al: Cerebral mucormycosis in two cases of the acquired immunodeficiency syndrome. Arch Neurol 45:109, 1988

55. Micozzi MS, Wetli CV: Intravenous amphetamine abuse, primary cerebral mucormycosis, and acquired immunodeficiency. J Forensic Sci 30:504, 1985

56. Koppel BS, Wormser GP, Tuchman AJ, et al: Central nervous system involvement in patients with acquired immune deficiency syndrome (AIDS). Acta Neurol Scand 71:337, 1985

57. Levine AM: Epidemiology, clinical characteristics, and management of AIDS-related lymphoma. Hematol Oncol Clin North Am 5:331, 1991

58. Ziegler JL, Beckstead JA, Volberding PA, et al: Non-Hodgkin's lymphoma in 90 homosexual men. N Engl J Med 311:565, 1984

59. Levitt LJ, Dawson DM, Rosenthal DS, Moloney WC: CNS involvement in the non-Hodgkin's lymphomas. Cancer 45:545, 1980

60. Britton CB, Miller JR: Neurologic complications in acquired immunodeficiency syndrome. Neurol Clin 2:315, 1984

61. Janssen RJ, Cornblath DR, Epstein LG, et al: Nomenclature and research case definitions for neurologic manifestations of human immunodeficiency virus-tye 1 (HIV-1) infection. Neurology 41:778, 1991

62. McArthur JC: HIV-associated CNS syndromes. p. 140. In Belman A (director): AIDS and the Nervous System. Syllabus for American Academy of Neurology Course No. 140, April 25, 1993. American Academy of Neurology, New York, 1993

63. Day JJ, Grant I, Atkinson JH, et al: Incidence of AIDS dementia in a two-year follow-up of AIDS and ARC patients on an initial phase II AZT placebo-controlled study: San Diego cohort. J Neuropsychiatry Clin Neurosci 4:15, 1992

64. Price RW, Brew B, Sidtis J, et al: The brain in AIDS: central nervous system HIV-1 infection and AIDS dementia complex. Science 239:586, 1988

65. Portegies P, deGans J, Lange JMA, et al: Declining incidence of AIDS dementia complex after introduction of zidovudine treatment. Br Med J 299:819, 1989

66. de la Monte SM, Ho DD, Schooley RT, et al: Subacute encephalomyelitis of AIDS and its relation to HTLV-III infection Neurology 37:562, 1987

67. Nielsen SL, Petito CK, Urmacher CD, Posner JB: Subacute encephalitis in acquired immune deficiency syndrome: a postmortem study. Am J Clin Pathol 82:678, 1984

68. Gullotta F, Kuchelmeister K, Masini T, et al: Zur Morphologie der HIV-Encephalopathies. Zentralbl allg Pathol 135:5, 1989

69. Kato T, Hirano A, Llena JF, Dembitzer HM: Neuropathology of acquired immune deficiency syndrome (AIDS) in 53 autopsy cases with particular emphasis on microglial nodules and multinucleated cells. Acta Neuropathol (Berl) 773:287, 1987

70. Kleihues P, Leib SL, Strittmatter C, et al: HIV encephalopathy: incidence, definition and pathogenesis. Acta Pathol Jpn 41:197, 1991

71. Petito CK, Cho ES, Lemann W, et al: Neuropathology of acquired immunodeficiency syndrome (AIDS): an autopsy review. J Neuropathol Exp Neurol 45:635, 1986

72. Navia BA, Cho ES, Petito CK, Price RW: The AIDS dementia complex: II. Neuropathology. Ann Neurol 19:525, 1986

73. Wiley CA, Masliah E, Morey M, et al: Neocortical damage during HIV infection. Ann Neurol 29:651, 1991

74. Everall IP, Luthert PJ, Lantos PL: Neuronal loss in the frontal cortex in HIV infection. Lancet, 337:1119, 1991

75. Price RW, Brew BJ: The AIDS dementia complex. J Infect Dis 158:1079, 1988

76. Brew BJ, Rosenblum M, Price RW: AIDS dementia complex and primary HIV brain infection. J Neuroimmunol 20:133, 1988

77. Van Gorp WG, Miller EN, Satz P, Visscher B: Neuropsychological performance in HIV-1 immunocompromised patients: a preliminary report. J Clin Exp Neuropsychol 11:763, 1989

78. Selnes OA, Miller E, McArthur J, et al: HIV-1 infection: no evidence of cognitive decline during the asymptomatic stages. Neurology 40:204, 1990

79. Sinforiani E, Mauri M, Bono G, et al: Cognitive abnormalities and disease progression in a selected population of asymptomatic HIV-positive subjects. AIDS 5:1117, 1991

80. Stern Y, Marder K, Bell K, et al: Multidisciplinary

baseline assessment of homosexual men with and without human immunodeficiency virus infection: III. Neurologic and neuropsychological findings. Arch Gen Psychiatry 48:131, 1991

81. Navia BA, Jordan BD, Price RW: The AIDS dementia complex: I. Clinical features. Ann Neurol 19:517, 1986

82. Beckett A, Summergrad P, Manschreck T, et al: Symptomatic HIV infection of the CNS in a patient without clinical evidence of immunosuppression. Am J Psychiatry 144:1342, 1987

83. Chermann J-C: HIV-associated diseases: acute and regressive encephalopathy in a seropositive man. Res Virol 141:137, 1990

84. Norman SE, Chediak AD, Kiel M, Cohn MA: Sleep disturbances in HIV-infected homosexual men. AIDS 4:775, 1990

85. Holtzman DM, Kaku DA, So YT: New-onset seizures associated with human immunodeficiency virus infection: causation and clinical features in 100 cases. Am J Med 87:173, 1989

86. Parisi A, Strosselli M, Pan A, et al: HIV-related encephalitis presenting as convulsant disease. Clin Electroencephalogr 22:1, 1991

87. Wong B, Gold JWM, Brown AE, et al: Central-nervous-system toxoplasmosis in homosexual men and parenteral drug abusers. Ann Intern Med 100:36, 1984

88. Nguygen N, Rimmer S, Katz B: Slowed saccades in the acquired immunodeficiency syndrome. Am J Ophthalmol 107:356, 1989

89. Rosenhall U, Häkansson C, Löwhagen G-B, et al: Otoneurological abnormalities in asymptomatic HIV-seropositive patients. Acta Neruol Scand 79:140, 1989

90. Currie J, Benson E, Ramsden B, et al: Eye movement abnormalities as a predictor of the acquired immunodeficiency syndrome dementia complex. Arch Neurol 45:949, 1988

91. Friedman DI, Feldon SE: Eye movements in acquired immunodeficiency syndrome. Arch Neurol 46:841, 1989

92. Merrill PT, Paige GD, Abrams RA, et al: Ocular motor abnormalities in human immunodeficiency virus infection. Ann Neurol 30:130, 1991

93. Arendt G, Hefter H, Hoemberg V, et al: Early abnormalities of cognitive event-related potentials in HIV-infected patients without clinically evident CNS deficits. Electroencephalogr Clin Neurophysiol Suppl 41: 370, 1990

94. Price RW, Navia BA: Infections in AIDS and in other immunosuppressed patients. p. 248. In Kennedy PGE, Johnson RT (eds): Infections of the Nervous System. Butterworths, London, 1987

95. Resnick L, diMarzo-Veronese F, Schupbach J, et al:

Intra-blood-brain-barrier synthesis of HTLV-III-specific IgG in patients with neurologic symptoms associated with AIDS or AIDS-related complex. N Engl J Med 313:1498, 1985

96. Gotswami KK, Kaye S, Miller R, et al: Intrathecal IgG synthesis and specificity of oligoclonal IgG in patients infected with HIV-1 do not correlate with CNS disease. J Med Virol 33:106, 1991

97. Epstein LG, Goudsmit J, Paul DA, et al: Expression of human immunodeficiency virus in cerebrospinal fluid of children with progressive encephalopathy. Ann Neurol 21:397, 1987

98. Goudsmit J, de Wolf F, Paul DA, et al: Expression of human immunodeficiency virus antigen (HIV-Ag) in serum and cerebrospinal fluid during acute and chronic infection. Lancet 2:177, 1986

99. Buffet R, Agut H, Chieze F, et al: Virological markers in the cerebrospinal fluid from HIV-1-infected individuals. AIDS 5:1419, 1991

100. Post MJD, Berger JR, Hensley GT: The radiology of central nervous system disease in acquired immunodeficiency syndrome. p. 1. In Taveras JM, Ferrucci JT (eds): Radiology: Diagnosis-Imaging-Intervention. JB Lippincott, Philadelphia, 1988

101. Bursztyn EM, Lee BCP, Bauman J: CT of acquired immunodeficiency syndrome. AJNR 5:711, 1984

102. Levy RM, Rosenbloom S, Perrett LV: Neuroradiologic findings in AIDS: a review of 200 cases. AJR 147:977, 1986

103. Olsen WL, Longo FM, Mills CM, Norman D: White matter disease in AIDS: findings at MR imaging. Radiology 169:445, 1988

104. Yarchoan R, Klecker RW, Weinhold KJ, et al: Administration of 3′-azido-3′-deoxythymidine, an inhibitor of HTLV-III/LAV replication, to patients with AIDS or AIDS-related complex. Lancet 1:575, 1986

105. Hollweg M, Riedel R-R, Goebel F-D, et al: Remarkable improvement of neuropsychiatric symptoms in HIV-infected patients after AZT therapy. Klin Wocheschr 69:409, 1991

106. Price RW, Koch MA, Sidtis JJ, et al: Zidovudine (AZT) treatment of the AIDS dementia complex (ADC): results of a placebo-controlled multicenter therapeutic trial. Abstract No. 331. Fifth International Conference on AIDS. Montreal, 1988

107. Schmitt FA, Bigley JW, McKinnis R, et al: Neuropsychological outcome of zidovudine (AZT) treatment of patients with AIDS and AIDS-related complex. N Engl J Med 319:1573, 1988

108. Pizzo PA, Eddy J, Falloon J: Acquired immune deficiency syndrome in children: current problems and therapeutic considerations. Am J Med 85:195, 1988

109. Sidtis JJ, Gatsonis C, Price RW, et al: Zidovudine

treatment of AIDS dementia complex: results of a placebo-controlled trial. Ann Neurol 33:343, 1993

110. Drew WL: Cytomegalovirus infection in patients with AIDS. J Infect Dis 158:449, 1988

111. Vinters HV, Kwok MK, Ho HW, et al: Cytomegalovirus in the nervous system of patients with the acquired immune deficiency syndrome. Brain 112:245, 1989

112. Post MJ, Hensley GT, Moskowitz LB, Fischl M: Cytomegalic inclusion virus encephalitis in patients with AIDS: CT, clinical, and pathologic correlation. AJR 146:1229, 1986

113. Kalayjian RC, Cohen ML, Bonomo RA, Flanigan TP: Cytomegalovirus ventriculoencephalitis in AIDS: a syndrome with distinct clinical and pathologic features. Medicine (Baltimore) 72:67, 1993

114. Masdeu JC, Small CB, Weiss L, et al: Multifocal cytomegalovirus encephalitis in AIDS. Ann Neurol 23:97, 1988

115. Fuller GN, Guiloff RJ, Scaravilli F, Harcourt Webster JN: Combined HIV-CMV encephalitis presenting with brainstem signs. J Neurol Neurosurg Psychiatry 52:975, 1989

116. Navia BA, Petito CK, Gold JW, et al: Cerebral toxoplasmosis complicating the acquired immune deficiency syndrome: clinical and neuropathological findings in 27 patients. Ann Neurol 19:224, 1986

117. Nath A, Jankovic J, Pettigrew LC: Movement disorders and AIDS. Neurology 37:37, 1987

118. Post MJD, Chan JC, Hensley GT, et al: Toxoplasma encephalitis in Haitian adults with acquired immunodeficiency syndrome: a clinical-pathologic-CT correlation. AJNR 4:155, 1983

119. Post MJD, Chan JC, Hensley GT, et al: Toxoplasma encephalitis in Haitian adults with acquired immunodeficiency syndrome: a clinical-pathologic-CT correlation. AJR 140:861, 1983

120. McArthur JC: Neurologic manifestations of AIDS. Medicine (Baltimore) 66:407, 1987

121. Jarvik JG, Hesselink JR, Kennedy C, et al: Acquired immunodeficiency syndrome: magnetic resonance patterns of brain involvement with pathologic correlation. Arch Neurol 45:731, 1988

122. Farkash AE, Maccabee PJ, Sher JH, et al: CNS toxoplasmosis in acquired immunodeficiency syndrome: a clinical-pathological-radiological review of 12 cases. J Neurol Neurosurg Psychiatry 49:744, 1986

123. Luft BJ, Brooks RG, Conley FK, et al: Toxoplasmic encephalitis in patients with acquired immune deficiency syndrome. JAMA 252:913, 1984

124. Porter SB, Sande MA: Toxoplasmosis of the central nervous system in the acquired immunodeficiency syndrome. N Engl J Med 327:1643, 1992

125. Wanke C, Tuazon CU, Kovacs A, et al: Toxoplasma encephalitis in patients with acquired immunodeficiency syndrome: diagnosis and response to therapy. Am J Trop Med Hyg 36:509, 1987

126. Luft BJ, Remington JS: Toxoplasmic encephalitis in AIDS. Clin Infect Dis 15:211, 1992

127. Haverkos HW: Assessment of therapy for toxoplasma encephalitis: the TE study group. Am J Med 82:907, 1987

128. Koepper S, Gruenwald T, Ruf B, Pohle HD: Aerosolized pentamidine versus fansidar in the primary and secondary prophylaxis of Pneumocystis carinii pneumonia. Abstract No WB2212. Program and Abstracts of the Seventh International Conference on AIDS. Florence, 1991

129. Levy RM, Janssen RS, Bush TJ, Rosenblum ML: Neuroepidemiology of acquired immunodeficiency syndrome. p. 13. In Rosenblum ML, Levy RM, Bredesen DE (eds): AIDS and the Nervous System. New York, Raven Press, 1988

130. Baumgartner JE, Rachlin JR, Beckstead JH, et al: Primary central nervous system lymphomas: natural history and response to radiation therapy in 55 patients with acquired immunodeficiency syndrome. J Neurosurg 73:206, 1990

131. So YT, Beckstead JH, Davis RL: Primary central nervous system lymphoma in acquired immune deficiency syndrome: a clinical and pathological study. Ann Neurol 20:566, 1986

132. MacMahon EME, Glass JD, Hayward SD, et al: Epstein-Barr virus in AIDS-related primary central nervous system lymphoma. Lancet 338:969, 1991

133. Rosenblum ML, Levy RM, Bredesen DE, et al: Primary central nervous system lymphomas in patients with AIDS. Ann Neurol 23, suppl:S13, 1988

134. Lee Y-Y, Bruner JM, Van Tassel P, Libshitz HI: Primary central nervous system lymphoma: CT and pathologic correlation. AJR 147:747, 1986

135. Remick SC, Diamond C, Migliozzi JA, et al: Primary central nervous system lymphoma in patients with and without the acquired immunodeficiency syndrome: a retrospective analysis and review of the literature. Medicine (Baltimore) 69:345, 1990

136. Anders K, Steinsapir KD, Iverson DJ, et al: Neuropathologic findings in the acquired immunodeficiency syndrome (AIDS). Clin Neuropathol 5:1, 1986

137. Berger JR, Harris JO, Gregorios J, Norenberg M: Cerebrovascular disease in AIDS: a case control study. AIDS 4:239, 1990

138. Berger JR, Kaszovitz B, Post MJD, Dickinson G: Progressive multifocal leukoencephalopathy associated with human immunodeficiency virus infection: a review of the literature with a report of 16 cases. Ann Intern Med 107:78, 1987

139. Whiteman ML, Post MJD, Berger JR, et al: Progressive multifocal leukoencephalopathy in 47 HIV-seropositive patients: neuroimaging with clinical and pathologic correlation. Radiology 187:233, 1993

140. Petito CK, Navia BA, Cho ES, et al: Vacuolar myelopathy pathologically resembling subacute combined degeneration in patients with the acquired immunodeficiency syndrome. N Engl J Med 312:874, 1985

141. Goldstick L, Mandybur TI, Bode R: Spinal cord degeneration in AIDS. Neurology 35:103, 1985

142. Berger JR, Bender A, Resnick L, Perlmutter D: Spinal myoclonus associated with HTLV III/LAV infection. Arch Neurol 43:1203, 1986

143. Berger JR, Sheremata WA, Resnick L, et al: Multiple sclerosis-like illness occurring with human immunodeficiency virus infection. Neurology 39:324, 1989

144. Berger JR, Tornatore C, Major EO, et al: Relapsing and remitting human immunodeficiency virus-associated leukoencephalomyelopathy. Ann Neurol 31:34, 1992

145. McArthur JC, Griffin JW, Cornblath DR, et al: Steroid-responsive myeloneuropathy in a man dually infected with HIV-1 and HTLV-1. Neurology 40:938, 1990

146. Berger JR, Raffanti S, Svenningsson A, et al: The role of HTLV in HIV-1 neurological disease. Neurology 41:197, 1991

147. Rosenblum MK, Brw BJ, Hahn B, et al: Human T-lymphotropic virus type I-associated myelopathy in patients with the acquired immunodeficiency syndrome. Hum Pathol 23:513, 1992

148. Berger JR, Svenningsson A, Raffanti S, Resnick L: Tropical spastic paraparesis-like illness occurring in a patient dually infected with HIV-1 and HTLV-II. Neurology 41:85, 1991

149. Lipkin WI, Parry G, Kiprov D, Abrams D: Inflammatory neuropathy in homosexual men with lymphadenopathy. Neurology 35:1479, 1985

150. Simpson DM: Neuromuscular complications of human immunodeficiency virus infection. Semin Neurol 12:34, 1992

151. Cornblath DR, McArthur JC, Kennedy PGE, et al: Inflammatory demyelinating peripheral neuropathies associated with human T-cell lymphotropic virus type III infection. Ann Neurol 21:32, 1987

152. Eidelberg D, Sotrel A, Vogel M, et al: Progressive polyradiculopathy in acquired immune deficiency syndrome. Neurology 36:912, 1986

153. Miller RG, Storey JR, Greco CM: Ganciclovir in the treatment of progressive AIDS-related polyradiculopathy. Neurology 40:569, 1990

154. Mahieux F, Gray F, Fenelon G, et al: Acute myeloradiculitis due to cytomegalovirus as the initial manifestation of AIDS. J Neurol Neurosurg Psychiatry 52:270, 1989

155. Moskowitz LB, Gregorios JB, Hensley GT, Berger JR: Cytomegalovirus-induced demyelination associated with acquired immune deficiency syndrome. Arch Pathol Lab Med 108:873, 1984

156. Dalakas M, Illa I, Pezeshkpour GH, et al: Mitochondrial myopathy caused by long-term zidovudine therapy. N Engl J Med 322:1098, 1990

157. Dalakas MC, Pezeshkpour GH, Gravell M, Sever JL: Polymyositis associated with AIDS retrovirus. JAMA 256:2381, 1986

158. Bessen LJ, Greene JB, Louie E, et al: Severe polymyositis-like syndrome associated with zidovudine therapy of AIDS and ARC. N Engl J Med 318:708, 1988

39

HTLV-I Infection and the Nervous System

John W. Engstrom

Recognition of the importance of infection with human T-lymphotropic virus type I (HTLV-I) is growing for several reasons. First, diagnosis of the infection is clinically relevant because spread of the responsible virus can be prevented. Second, the infection causes human disease—a chronic progressive myelopathy unaccompanied by extrinsic spinal cord pathology on magnetic resonance imaging (MRI) studies. Third, HTLV-I myelopathy is a model for a chronic, progressive neurological illness caused by viral infection. It is the intent of this chapter to summarize current knowledge of the epidemiology, clinical and laboratory features, pathology, pathophysiology, and therapy of HTLV-I myelopathy. The HTLV-II virus may also be important in causing neurological disease and has genetic, structural and functional similarities to HTLV-I.

HISTORY

A heterogeneous group of patients from the tropics who had a progressive thoracic myelopathy was described in 1964; their disorder was labeled "tropical spastic paraparesis." In retrospect, these patients probably represent the earliest known cases of HTLV-I myelopathy.[1] HTLV-I infection was first associated with human disease in 1980, when the retrovirus was isolated from a patient with mycosis fungoides.[2] In 1985, Gessain and colleagues reported that 10 of 17 patients with tropical spastic paraparesis had antibodies to HTLV-I, compared with 13 of 303 controls. They suggested that HTLV-I or a related virus was contributing to the pathogenesis of tropical spastic paraparesis.[3] A similar myelopathy associated with HTLV-I antibodies in the serum and cerebrospinal fluid (CSF) of Japanese patients was named HAM (HTLV-I-associated myelopathy) in 1986 by Osame and colleagues.[4] In 1988, Roman and Osame recognized that tropical spastic paraparesis and HAM were the same disease.[5] The term *HTLV-I myelopathy* is used in preference to these other designations in this chapter.

EPIDEMIOLOGY

The average age of onset of the myelopathy is approximately 40 years, but symptomatic myelopathy may begin between the ages of 20 and 70 years.[6–8] Women are affected more often than men by about 1.5:1.[9]

Geographic Distribution

HTLV-I infection is endemic near the equator.[1,6,10,11] There are high-frequency pockets in the Caribbean, the Seychelles, Colombia, and equatorial Africa.[12] HTLV-I myelopathy is becoming a more significant public health problem in developing countries because of the lack of preventive, diagnostic, and supportive services for disabled individuals and asymptomatic carriers. In regions outside endemic areas, including the United States, the disease is sporadic.[13]

Japan is exceptional among among nonequatorial regions in exhibiting a high frequency of HTLV-I infection.[14] Among patients with HTLV-I myelopathy in Japan, 70 percent are from the islands of Kyushu or Okinawa.[9]

Incidence and Prevalence

The calculated annual incidence of the myelopathy ranges from 0.04 per 100,000 inhabitants on Kyushu to 6 per 100,000 in Tumaco, Colombia.[9,10] Calculated prevalence ranges from 8.6 per 100,000 inhabitants on Kyushu, Japan, to a high of 1.0 per 1,000 inhabitants in Tumaco and the Seychelles.[9,10] The available incidence and prevalence data probably underestimate the scope of the problem and must be interpreted with caution. Accurate estimates of the frequency of HTLV-I myelopathy are hindered by nonuniform reporting of the disease and the limited availability of neurological expertise in many endemic areas.

The incidence and prevalence figures of the myelopathy in Japan have been expressed per 100,000 HTLV-I seropositive persons per year. The annual incidence of HTLV-I myelopathy is 3 per 100,000 and the prevalence in 68 per 100,000.[9,10] The calculated lifetime risk of HTLV-I myelopathy among seropositive patients is only 2 to 3 per thousand.[15] The factors responsible for the restricted expression of the myelopathy in a small subset of infected individuals are unknown.

Transmission

The three known routes of HTLV-I virus transmission are via breast milk, sexual intercourse, and exposure to contaminated blood products. The most common situations involving exposure to contaminated blood products are blood transfusion, reuse of contaminated hypodermic needles, and transplacental infection.

Animals can acquire postnatal HTLV-I infection via breast milk.[14] Breast milk containing HTLV-I-infected lymphocytes has been found among seropositive human mothers.[16] A model of milk-borne oral transmission of the HTLV-I virus has been developed in monkeys.[17] Approximately 25 percent of breast-fed infants born to HTLV-I infected mothers acquire the infection, as opposed to 5 percent of non-breast-fed children of infected mothers.[18,19] The efficiency of transmission via breast milk appears to be approximately five times greater than the transplacental route.

A long-term study of married couples in Japan found that transmission by sexual contact is far more effective from men to women (60.8 percent over 10 years) than from women to men (less than 1 percent over 10 years).[20] The presence of HTLV-I-infected lymphocytes in semen may partially explain this dramatic difference. Approximately one-fourth of the sex partners of HTLV-I/II-seropositive blood donors were infected in the preliminary report of another study.[21]

Transmission of the virus via transfusion of contaminated blood products is a well-documented route of infection.[9,22,23] A study in the United States of the prevalence of HTLV-I antibodies among blood donors yielded a rate of 0.02 percent.[24] Patients have developed seroconversion and a spastic paraparesis in as little as 6 months following transfusion with contaminated blood products.[22,25] In one case, the nucleotide sequence of the viruses of the blood donor and recipient were identical at 32 positions in which published HTLV-I sequences demonstrate molecular heterogeneity. Furthermore, this donor and recipient possessed viruses with identical nucleotide sequences that were different from all other published sequences.[22] The median time to development of myelopathy following blood transfusion was estimated at 3.3 years among 134 patients with *both* a history of blood transfusion and HTLV-I myelopathy.[9] There may be a relatively short latency to the development of myelopathy among recipients of blood transfusions, but there are no prospective quantitative data for estimating the risk of myelopathy among asymptomatic, infected individuals who contracted infection through a blood transfusion. It has been speculated that a high viral load at the time of the transfusion may predispose patients to the more rapid development of the myelopathy. Blood banks now routinely screen prospective donors for the presence of HTLV-I antibodies.

Reuse of contaminated needles among intravenous drug users ia a major route of HTLV-I infection. Khabbaz and colleagues performed an epidemiological survey of HTLV-I/II seroprevalence in 1988 and 1989 among both intravenous drug users and patients seen in clinics for sexually transmitted diseases.[26] The seroprevalence of HTLV-I/II antibodies among drug addicts increased from zero for patients younger than 19 years to 32 percent among patients over the age of 45 years. There was a high rate of HTLV-I/II infection in Seattle and Los Angeles compared with New York City. Patients seen in clinics for sexually transmitted diseases were 10 times more likely to be infected with HTLV-I/II if they were also intravenous drug users. The increased frequency of infection with age is consistent with an adult-acquired infection, and the 10-fold higher prevalence among intravenous drug users compared with other patients attending clinics for sexually transmitted diseases suggests that intravenous drug use is an important vector for infection. Other studies support the importance of intravenous drug use in the transmission of HTLV-I/II infection.[27]

CLINICAL AND LABORATORY FEATURES

Symptoms and Signs

The most common initial symptoms in three large series of patients were either leg weakness or difficulty in walking (Table 39-1).[6–8] Other common symptoms were painful legs, paresthesias, and back pain, and there were occasional complaints of bladder dysfunction. The mean duration of symptoms at the time of data collection was 13 years in two of these series.

The most common neurological sign among these patients was a spastic paraparesis, which was asymmetrical in one-third of patients.[6–8] Bilateral hyperreflexia in the arms was present in most patients, but upper limb weakness was uncommon. All patients symptomatic for over 7 years required assistance with walking and 5 of 21 were wheelchair-bound by the seventh year of their disease.[8] The usual course of the gait disorder was slow deterioration to severe disability over 2 to 10 years. Some authors have the clinical

Table 39-1 Symptoms and Signs of HTLV-I Myelopathy

	Number of Patients	Percent Affected
Symptom		
Leg weakness	67/67	100
Backache	15/46	33
Painful legs	25/46	54
Paresthesias	8/26	31
Bladder complaints	"Occasional"	—
Sign		
Leg spasticity	67/67	100
Arm spasticity	"Majority"	—
Unable to walk	18/46	39
Needs cane/crutch	17/46	37
Urinary frequency or incontinence	62/67	93
Sensory loss	11/25	44

(Data from Vernant and colleagues,[6] Matsuo and colleagues,[7] and Cruickshank and colleagues.[8])

impression that deterioration of gait eventually reaches a plateau and stabilizes.[1]

Bladder dysfunction was present in 96 percent of patients, despite the relative infrequency of subjective complaints of sphincter dysfunction. Urodynamic studies on 14 patients with HTLV-I myelopathy and urinary symptoms of urgency, frequency, or retention provided evidence for a spastic bladder in 13 instances.[28]

Loss of touch and pain sensation was present (after an average duration of illness of 8 years) in 40 percent of the patients in one series.[6] None of these patients are known to have exhibited a sensory level, but it is unclear how aggressively a sensory level was routinely sought.

The frequency of specific symptoms and signs varies among clinical studies and must be interpreted with caution. Each clinical series represents only a cross-sectional snapshot in time for a disease that evolves over years. Although the frequency of any individual neurological sign early in the disease is uncertain, it is likely that motor involvement occurs first.

Other clinical presentations of HTLV-I infection have been described occasionally. Some patients have an inflammatory myopathy indistinguishable from polymyositis.[29–33] Patients exhibit proximal weakness, have an elevated serum creatine kinase (CK) concentration, show electromyographic changes suggestive of a myopathy associated with muscle membrane instability, and have an endomysial lymphocytic inflammatory infiltrate on muscle biopsy. One patient with polymyositis but no clinical evidence of cord involvement had evidence on muscle biopsy of direct infection of muscle fibers with HTLV-I.[32] Polyneuropathy has been mentioned in the literature, but many reports lack complete clinical and neurophysiological information.[11,34] There is a paucity of information regarding peripheral nerve pathology among these patients.[35]

Optic neuropathy (15 percent) and hearing loss (7 percent) were described among the original patients with tropical spastic paraparesis in 1964, but this patient population was probably heterogeneous.[1] A recent series of carefully examined patients from Japan who were seropositive did not reveal neuro-ophthalmological abnormalities of the retina, fundus, or visual fields.[36] The true frequency of optic neuropathy and hearing loss among patients with HTLV-I myelopathy is unknown, but a few cases of optic neuropathy have been documented among patients with definite HTLV-I infection.[37,38]

Systemic Manifestations of HTLV-I Infection

Occasional patients develop pulmonary infiltrates, arthralgias, or arthritis.[39] Bronchial washings and synovial fluid samples contain lymphocytes that express HTLV-I antigens.[40] HTLV-I myelopathy has been associated with monoclonal gammopathy, hepatitis, sarcoid, sicca syndrome, diabetes, uveitis, and conjunctivitis. The pathogenetic relationship of these associated conditions to the viral infection is unclear.

Clinical Neurophysiology

Lower limb somatosensory evoked potential (SEP) studies detect unilateral or bilateral sensory spinal cord lesions in many patients with HTLV-I myelopathy.[28,41,42] The latency of cortical components of the response may be delayed in the absence of sensory signs on clinical examination.[42] The delay is due to central pathology, since the latency of components recorded over the lower spine is normal.[28] Lower limb SEPs may be used to provide objective information regarding the involvement of spinal sen-

sory systems and perhaps to follow the response of clinical or subclinical lesions to experimental therapies.

The recording of visual evoked potentials (VEPs), brainstem auditory evoked potentials (BAEPs), and upper limb SEPs is of less certain value. The latency of the cortical components of the median-derived SEP was delayed in 3 of 19 patients in one study and in none of 28 patients in two other studies.[28,41,42] Central conduction time (N14–N20 interval) was increased in 5 of 19 patients in another series.[17] VEP testing revealed delayed responses in 10 of 19 patients in one series but usually has shown abnormalities in only a minority of patients.[8,20,36,42] Experience with BAEP testing has similarly been varied.[8,43]

The variability in frequency of electrophysiological abnormalities may have several causes. First, it may reflect simply the stage of the disease. Second, it will depend on the location of lesions in a disease that affects the central nervous system (CNS) in multifocal fashion. Third, the criteria used to define electrophysiological abnormalities differ between laboratories, and this will influence the diagnostic yield of such studies.

With regard to the peripheral nervous system, minor slowing of conduction velocities, prolonged minimum F-wave latencies, and mild prolongation of distal motor latencies have been reported in some series, but nerve conduction studies have been normal in other instances.[8,28,34,42,44]

Neuroimaging

MRI of the cervical and thoracic spinal cord is usually normal or shows nonspecific changes.[8] Reports of high-resolution MRI of the spinal cord with axial images and administration of gadolinium are lacking. Brain MRI frequently reveals multifocal high-signal-intensity lesions on T_2-weighted images in the subcortical and deep white matter. Periventricular lesions are common as well.[45]

Brain MRI revealed more than 10 white matter lesions in 8 of 22 patients with HTLV-I myelopathy in one series.[46] The patients with multifocal white matter lesions had a longer duration of disease and greater disability on the Kurtzke scale than patients without white matter lesions. The age of the two groups was not different. In a follow-up study of patients treated for 2 years with corticosteroids, clinical deterioration occurred and follow-up brain MRI showed larger and more numerous lesions regardless of corticosteroid therapy.[47] The frequency of MRI abnormalities in different series probably reflects differences in disease severity and duration among the patients.

Cerebrospinal Fluid

The CSF is often abnormal in patients with HTLV-I myelopathy. A lymphocytic pleocytosis and elevated protein concentration occurs in about 50 percent of patients.[7,8,28] Glucose concentration is normal.

Oligoclonal bands are often present.[8,28] The CSF in 10 of 13 patients exhibited intrathecal synthesis of oligoclonal IgG, including 8 patients with bands common to the CSF and serum.[8] Antibodies from the bands were directed against specific HTLV-I antigens among 5 patients in one series and in 19 of 22 patients in another.[48,49]

The presence of specific anti-HTLV-I antibodies in the CSF may have several explanations. First, the antibodies may be synthesized elsewhere and reach the CSF by transudation across the blood-brain barrier. Second, there may be activated B-cell clones within and outside the CSF-CNS compartment.[49] Third, there may be selective synthesis of antibody within the CSF-CNS compartment.

Both an elevated IgG index and HTLV-I antibody index have been found in patients with HTLV-I myelopathy.[48,50] The presence of an elevated IgG index provides indirect evidence for synthesis of IgG antibody within the CNS.[51]

Serology

The US Public Health Service first established serological testing guidelines for HTLV-I antibodies in 1988.[52] Serological testing has been hampered by the need for multiple assays to confirm seroreactivity and by the inability of standard supplementary serological assays to distinguish HTLV-I from HTLV-II infection.

Specimens initially positive by enzyme-linked immunosorbent assay (ELISA) are retested in duplicate. If one of the duplicate tests is positive, then reactivity is unlikely to be due to errors of technique. The serum must be further analyzed by radioimmunoprecipitation assay or Western blot for immunoreactivity to

the *gag* gene product p24 and an *env* gene product (gp46 or gp61/68) for the specimen to be considered seropositive.[52] Specimens meeting these criteria are always positive for HTLV-I or HTLV-II using viral amplification techniques such as the polymerase chain reaction (PCR).[53]

Indeterminate specimens are those that are positive by ELISA and duplicate testing but in which immunoreactivity can be found to only one gene product. Repeated serological testing of indeterminate cases shows that they rarely meet the criteria for seropositivity.[54–56] In persistently unclear circumstances, testing of indeterminate samples using PCR remains the standard.

Incidence and prevalence data regarding infection are based upon serological screening with available ELISAs. The sensitivity of ELISAs is unknown because there are no population-based screening studies performed with PCR techniques, which are more sensitive for detecting minute quantities of virus. If there is a high clinical suspicion for HTLV-I infection and the screening ELISA is negative, a request for PCR analysis may be necessary to detect the virus.

The sensitivity of the radioimmunoprecipitation and Western blot assays has been hampered by the inconsistent demonstration of anti-*env* activity. A recombinant transmembrane glycoprotein (*env* p21e) has been added recently to immunoblot assays. The sensitivity of the assay approaches 100 percent among infected persons.[57]

Recombinant proteins specific for HTLV-I and HTLV-II can be incorporated into the assays and offer the possibility of both confirming and differentiating HTLV-I from HTLV-II infection with a single serological test. Analysis of 158 HTLV I/II seropositive specimens allowed both confirmation and differentiation of HTLV-I from HTLV-II in 156 seropositive samples (98.7 percent sensitivity).[58] This test is not available in all hospitals. When it is unavailable or when serological results are unclear, PCR remains the standard for differentiating HTLV-I from HTLV-II infection.

Hematology

A common feature is the presence of atypical lymphocytes with convoluted nuclei (flower cells) in the blood of infected patients.[59] These cells normally constitute 0.1 to 2 percent of the lymphocytes in seropositive, asymptomatic carriers regardless of geographic origin.[60,61] Flower cells occur with higher frequency among patients with T-cell leukemia and HTLV-I myelopathy.[62] It has been speculated that the increased number of atypical lymphocytes may indicate the presence of a high proviral load among patients with HTLV-I myelopathy or an exuberant T-cell response to the infection.

DIFFERENTIAL DIAGNOSIS

The differential diagnosis of HTLV-I myelopathy includes disorders causing a chronic progressive spastic paraparesis. Intrinsic spinal cord lesions and extrinsic mass lesions producing spinal cord compression can be excluded with appropriate imaging studies of the cervical and thoracic spine. Sensory disturbances almost always predominate over motor abnormalities in the myelopathies associated with vitamin B_{12} deficiency, nitrous oxide abuse, syphilis, and hypothyroidism. Patients with amyotrophic lateral sclerosis (ALS) can present with a spastic paraparesis, but diffuse lower motor neuron signs will appear with follow-up. Furthermore, bladder dysfunction is prominent in HTLV-I myelopathy and absent in ALS. Ingestion of raw cassava or chick-peas can precipitate a subacute myelopathy, but this will be suggested by a careful history. The pure form of hereditary spastic paraplegia occurs without bladder involvement; cases with bladder involvement should be reviewed for possible vertical transmission of HTLV-I myelopathy.

A predominantly spinal presentation of chronic progressive multiple sclerosis (MS) or a spinal dural arteriovenous fistula may be difficult to distinguish from HTLV-I myelopathy. Clinical features favoring MS include spontaneous exacerbation and remission of symptoms and signs, abnormalities of vision or extraocular movements, and conspicuous sensory findings. Features supporting a diagnosis of HTLV-I myelopathy include a predominantly motor clinical deficit, atypical multilobed lymphocytes on the peripheral blood smear, multiple oligoclonal bands in the serum, positive HTLV-I serum antibodies, and elevated HTLV-I CSF antibody index. Systemic manifestations of HTLV-I infection such as polymyositis and lymphocytic alveolitis may also help to distinguish HTLV-I myelopathy from MS. A spinal

dural fistula may be missed by CT and MRI and detectable only by myelography or spinal angiography. The diagnosis of a dural arteriovenous fistula is very unlikely in the presence of features supportive of HTLV-I myelopathy but should be considered where HTLV-I antibodies are absent and the other diagnostic possibilities mentioned above have been excluded from further consideration.

PATHOLOGY AND PATHOGENESIS

Pathology

There are few autopsies from patients with HTLV-I myelopathy.[1,63–65] The largest group consists of 10 cases described before the availability of antibody testing.[1] The pathological similarities between those 10 cases and more recent, isolated case reports is striking.

The pathological findings indicate an active chronic meningomyelitis involving predominantly the thoracic spinal cord.[1] Similar changes are frequently present to a lesser extent in the cervical spinal cord and brain and correlate with the presence of hyperreflexia in the arms, abnormal brain MRI findings, and abnormal evoked potential studies.[1,6,8,42,66]

The most conspicuous thoracic spinal cord damage is located in the lateral corticospinal tracts and consists of a severe loss of myelin. Damage to the gray matter of the spinal cord is less conspicuous. The meninges are thickened and nerve roots are involved in the inflammatory process. Capillary proliferation is present in the white matter more than the gray matter of the spinal cord and brain. Perivascular cuffing with lymphocytes and perivascular demyelination is common and profuse within the thoracic spinal cord. More rostral structures may demonstrate milder perivascular cuffing. Severe inflammation appears to be more common in cases of short rather than long duration. Autopsied cases of very long duration show little active inflammation; this may explain the clinical observation that the myelopathy sometimes reaches a plateau and then stabilizes.[1,63,64]

Pathogenesis

The exact pathogenesis of HTLV-I myelopathy is unclear, but HTLV-I infection is a prerequisite. The conclusion that HTLV-I infection is the cause of the myelopathy is drawn from several lines of evidence. First, intrathecal synthesis of anti–HTLV-I antibody has been demonstrated among affected patients.[48,50] Second, antibodies derived from oligoclonal bands within the CSF react with HTLV-I viral antigens.[48,50] Third, the virus has been isolated from cultured mononuclear cells obtained from the peripheral blood and CSF.[2,59,62,67,68] Fourth, HTLV-I-specific nucleic acid sequences and viral antigens have been found in the CSF.[13,56] And fifth, infection of animal models with retroviruses can result in a spastic paraparesis.[8] The sequence of intracellular and viral biochemical events leading to the development of the myelopathy is less clear.

The provirus is known to contain several genes important to virus survival and replication.[39,69,70] The *gag* region encodes the polypeptides comprising the viral core-associated proteins. The *pol* region encodes for retroviral nucleic acid enzymatic genes. The *env* region encodes for a single precursor peptide that is glycosylated and cleaved into a transmembrane protein and a spike protein. The spike protein acts as a ligand and may contribute to cellular tropism.[69]

The transactivator *(tax)* gene is important in the induction of acute T-cell leukemia in some patients. The *tax* gene is responsible for inducing transcription of both viral and host nucleic acid. Activation by the *tax* gene of the host genome results in the production of interleukin-2 and interleukin-2 receptors that function to stimulate the clonal expansion of T cells, stimulate the synthesis of γ-interferon, activate B cells, and promote B-cell differentiation into antibody-forming cells.[71,72] The release of γ-interferon from the host T cell may play a role in the recruitment of antibody-producing B cells and natural killer cells. It has been speculated that host production and release of tumor necrosis factor may play a role in the demyelination associated with the myelopathy.

There are animal models of retrovirus-related disease reminiscent of HTLV-I myelopathy.[8] Visna, a retroviral disease of sheep, is transmitted through breast milk. Some visna-infected animals develop a progressive paraparesis associated with CNS demyelination and perivascular inflammation.[8,69] A noninflammatory myelopathy and leukemia is associated with murine leukemia virus infection.[73] The routes of disease transmission and tropism for both neural and hematological tissue among these retroviral animal diseases are strikingly similar to HTLV-I infec-

tion in humans. In one animal model, mutations in the *env* gene allow the virus to replicate preferentially in neural tissue and result in hindlimb paralysis.[73] Other factors contributing to tissue tropism are unknown.

There are at least three mechanisms through which, either alone or in combination, HTLV-I infection could result in spinal cord injury. First, the virus may directly infect glial cells. Second, cytotoxic T cells may recognize and lyse infected host cells. Third, an inflammatory process caused by the infection may produce spinal cord damage.

Direct infection of glial cells may result in CNS tissue damage. Astrocytes can be infected in vitro with the virus, but the efficiency of infection is low.[74] Infection efficiency is improved by a factor of 1,000 when transfecting fetal astrocytes in culture.[75] Expression of class I human leukocyte antigen (HLA) molecules has been demonstrated from spinal cord lesions in one patient with HTLV-I myelopathy.[76] These observations suggest that the three components necessary for CNS T-cell-mediated immune responses (presence of viral antigen, expression of HLA molecules, and presence of T cells) are present in some spinal cord lesions.[77]

Recent evidence suggests that cytotoxic T cells may contribute to the spinal cord injury. These cells are abundant in the peripheral blood and CSF of patients with HTLV-I myelopathy but not among HTLV-I seropositive, asymptomatic controls.[62,77] The majority of the cytotoxic T-cell lines recognize HTLV-I gene products encoded by the regulatory region pX.[78] These lymphocytes may cause direct lysis of infected spinal cord cells or represent a response to a high viral load in patients with HTLV-I myelopathy.[77]

The host and viral factors that determine which infected individuals develop HTLV-I myelopathy, acute T-cell leukemia, or no clinical disease are unknown. Moreover, the host or viral factors that explain the predilection of the disease for the thoracic spinal cord are unknown. Indeed, the presumed in vivo target cells for infection and replication of HTLV-I virus within the CNS have not been defined. The clinical and pathological evidence that demyelination is important in the disease suggests that oligodendrocytes may be one such target.

The genetic, structural, and functional similarities between HTLV-I and II viruses imply that HTLV-II may also be implicated in malignant, neurological, or immunological disease.[70] The possible role for HTLV-II infection in the production of human disease is important because of the known high seroprevalence rate among intravenous drug users, the lack of data on the distribution and prevalence of infection among other population subgroups, and the preventable nature of the infection.[26,79,80] HTLV-II has been isolated from patients with hairy cell leukemia, but the majority of patients with hairy cell leukemia do not harbor the virus.[81–85] The pathogenetic role of HTLV-II in the production of hairy cell leukemia remains tenuous. There are several recent reports of HTLV-II infection associated with a spastic myelopathy, including the demonstration of selective intrathecal synthesis of anti-HTLV-II antibodies.[86–88] More information is needed to assess the importance of HTLV-II infection in the production of human neurological disease.

PREVENTION AND TREATMENT

Prevention

The US Public Health Service has provided guidelines for physicians and patients to prevent the spread of the HTLV-I virus. Patients should be instructed that the virus does not cause acquired immunodeficiency syndrome (AIDS) but results in a lifelong infection. There should be discussion about the mode and efficiency of transmission, disease associations, and the probability of developing disease. Patients should be advised to share the information with their physicians, avoid sharing needles or syringes, avoid breast-feeding infants, use latex condoms to prevent sexual transmission, and avoid donation of blood, semen, body organs, or other tissues.[80]

Immunomodulation

Definitive therapy and controlled trials evaluating experimental therapy are lacking for HTLV-I myelopathy. Clinical trials using corticosteroids have yielded predominantly negative results.[8,45] The observed initial benefit of corticosteroids among Japanese patients disappeared with long-term follow-up.[89] Another study demonstrated progression of white matter lesions on follow-up brain MRI despite corticosteroid therapy.[47] An uncontrolled trial of plasma exchange, prednisolone, or a combination of the two modalities revealed dramatic improvement in gait and sensory function in 5 of 21 patients, which lasted for only 2 to 4 weeks.[90] Clinical improvement has also been reported with use of the anabolic steroid danazol.[91] Experimental trials using zidovudine or antibodies directed against the interleukin-2 receptor are ongoing.[72,92] Controlled multicenter trials are necessary to recruit adequate numbers of affected patients and to obtain useful data regarding the best approach to therapy.

Symptomatic Treatment

Symptomatic therapy is focused on the relief of spasticity and painful muscle spasms and assiduous care of the spastic bladder. Baclofen is useful for the relief of painful spasms and limb spasticity. Acidification of the urine with ascorbic acid and a low threshold for performing urine cultures is necessary given the increased risk of urinary tract infection. Ditropan (oxybutynin chloride) may help relieve urinary urgency and frequency. The intervention of rehabilitation specialists may be helpful to preserve ambulation and other functional skills as long as possible.

REFERENCES

1. Montgomery RD, Cruickshank EK, Robertson WB, McMenemey W: Clinical and pathological observations on Jamaican neuropathy. Brain 87:425, 1964
2. Poiez BJ, Ruscetti FW, Gazdar AF, et al: Detection and isolation of type C retrovirus particles from fresh and cultured lymphocytes of a patient with cutaneous T-cell lymphoma. Proc Natl Acad Sci USA 77:7415, 1980
3. Gessain A, Barin F, Vernant JC, et al: Antibodies to human T-lymphotropic virus type-I in patients with tropical spastic preparesis. Lancet 2:407, 1985
4. Osame M, Usuku K, Izumo S, et al: HTLV-I associated myelopathy, a new clinical entity. Lancet 1:1031, 1986
5. Roman GC, Osame M: Identity of HTLV-I-associated tropical spastic paraparesis and HTLV-1-associated myelopathy. Lancet 1:651, 1988
6. Vernant JC, Maurs L, Gessain A, et al: Endemic tropical spastic paraparesis associated with human T-lymphotropic virus type I: a clinical and seroepidemiological study of 25 cases. Ann Neurol 21:123, 1987

7. Matsuo H, Nakamura T, Tsujihata M, et al: Human T-lymphotropic virus type I (HTLV-I) associated myelopathy in Nagasaki: clinical features and treatment of 21 cases. Jpn J Med 28:328, 1989

8. Cruickshank JK, Rudge P, Dalgleish AG, et al: Tropical spastic paraparesis and human T cell lymphotropic virus type I in the United Kingdom. Brain 112:1057, 1989

9. Osame M, Janssen R, Kubota H, et al: Nationwide survey of HTLV-I-associated myelopathy in Japan: association with blood transfusion. Ann Neurol 28:50, 1990

10. Roman GC, Roman LN, Spencer PS, Schoenberg BS: Tropical spastic paraparesis: a neuroepidemiological study in Colombia. Ann Neurol 17:361, 1985

11. Roman GC, Spencer PS, Schoenberg BS, et al: Tropical spastic paraparesis in the Seychelles islands: a clinical and case-control neuroepidemiologic study. Neurology 37:1323, 1987

12. Román GC: The neuroepidemiology of tropical spastic paraparesis. Ann Neurol 23, suppl:113, 1988

13. Bhagavati S, Ehrlich G, Kula R, et al: Detection of human T-cell lymphoma/leukemia virus type I DNA and antigen in spinal fluid and blood of patients with chronic progressive myelopathy. N Engl J Med 318:1141, 1988

14. Kusuhara K, Sonoda S, Takahashi K, et al: Mother-to-child transmission of human T-cell leukemia virus type I (HTLV-I): A fifteen-year follow-up study in Okinawa, Japan. Int J Cancer 40:755, 1987

15. Kaplan JE, Osame M, Kubota H, et al: The risk of development of HTLV-I-associated myelopathy/tropical spastic paraparesis among persons infected with HTLV-I. J Acquir Immune Defic Syndr 3:1096, 1990

16. Kinoshita K, Hino S, Amagasaki T, et al: Demonstration of adult T-cell leukemia virus antigen in milk from three seropositive mothers. Gann 75:103, 1984

17. Yamanouchi K, Kinoshita K, Moriuchi R, et al: Oral transmission of human T-cell leukemia virus type-I into a common marmoset (Callithrix jacchus) as an experimental model for milk-borne transmission. Jpn J Cancer Res 76:481, 1985

18. Takahashi K, Takezaki T, Oki T, et al: Inhibitory effect of maternal antibody on mother-to-child transmission of human T-lymphotropic virus type I. Int J Cancer 49:673, 1991

19. Hino S, Yamaguchi K, Katamine S, et al: Mother-to-child transmission of human T-cell leukemia virus type-I. Jpn J Cancer 76:474, 1985

20. Kajiyama W, Kashiwagi S, Ikematsu H, et al: Intrafamilial transmission of adult T-cell leukemia virus. J Infect Dis 154:851, 1986

21. Kleinman S, Fitzpatrick L, Lee H: Transmission of HTLV-I/II from blood donors to their sexual partners. In: Program and Abstracts–International Society of Blood Transfusion/American Association of Blood Banks Joint Congress Meeting (Los Angeles). Arlington, VA: American Association of Blood Banks, 1990

22. Kaplan JE, Litchfield B, Rouault C, et al: HTLV-I-associated myelopathy associated with blood transfusion in the United States: epidemiologic and molecular evidence linking donor and recipient. Neurology 41:192, 1991

23. Saxton EH, Lee H, Swanson P, et al: Detection of human T-cell leukemia/lymphoma virus type I in a transfusion recipient with chronic myelopathy. Neurology 39:841, 1989

24. Centers for Disease Control: Human T-lymphotropic virus type-I screening in volunteer blood donors—U.S., 1989. MMWR 39:915, 1990

25. Gout O, Baulac M, Gessain A, et al: Rapid development of myelopathy after HTLV-I infection acquired by transfusion during cardiac transplantation. N Engl J Med 322:383, 1990

26. Khabbaz RF, Onorato IM, Cannon RO, et al: Seroprevalence of HTLV-I and HTLV-II among intravenous drug users and persons in clinics for sexually transmitted diseases. N Engl J Med 326:375, 1992

27. Lee H, Swanson P, Shorty VS, et al: High rate of HTLV-II infection in seropositive IV drug abusers in New Orleans. Science 244:471, 1989

28. Shibasaki H, Endo C, Kuroda Y, et al: Clinical picture of HTLV-I associated myelopathy. J Neurol Sci 87:15, 1988

29. Morgan OS, Rodgers-Johnson P, Mora C, Char G: HTLV-I and polymyositis in Jamaica. Lancet 2:1184, 1989

30. Goudreau G, Karpati G, Carpenter S: Inflammatory myopathy in association with chronic myelopathy in HTLV-I seropositive patients. Neurology 38, suppl:1206, 1988

31. Francis DA, Hughes RA: Polymyositis and HTLV-I antibodies. Ann Neurol 24:311, 1989

32. Wiley CA, Nerenberg M, Cros D, Soto-Aguilar MC: HTLV-I polymyositis in a patient also infected with the human immunodeficiency virus. N Engl J Med 320:992, 1989

33. Evans BK, Gore I, Harrell LE, et al: HTLV-I associated myelopathy and polymyositis in a US native. Neurology 39:1572, 1989

34. Ludolph AC, Hugon J, Román GC, et al: A clinical neurophysiologic study of tropical spastic paraparesis. Muscle Nerve 2:392, 1988

35. Said G, Goulon-Goran C, La Croix C, et al: Inflamma-

tory lesions of peripheral nerve in a patient with human T-lymphotropic virus type-I-associated myelopathy. Ann Neurol 24:275, 1988

36. Arimura Y, Arimura K, Osame M, Igata A: Neuro-ophthalmological abnormalities in HTLV-I associated myelopathy. Neuro-ophthalmology 7:243, 1987

37. Roman GC, Schoenberg BS, Madden DL, et al: HTLV-I antibodies in patients with tropical spastic paraparesis from the Seychelles. Arch Neurol 44:605, 1987

38. Bhigjee AI, Kelbe C, Haribhai HC, et al: Myelopathy associated with human T-cell lymphotropic virus type I (HTLV-I) in Natal, South Africa. Brain 113:1307, 1990

39. Gessain A, Gout O: Chronic myelopathy associated with human T-lymphotropic virus type I (HTLV-I). Ann Intern Med 117:933, 1992

40. Ijichi S, Matsuda T, Maruyama I, et al: Arthritis in a human T lymphotropic virus type I (HTLV-I) carrier. Ann Rheum Dis 49:718, 1990

41. Kakigi R, Shibasaki H, Kuroda Y, et al: Multimodality evoked potentials in HTLV-I associated myelopathy. J Neurol Neurosurg Psychiatry 51:1094, 1988

42. Castillo JL, Cartier L, Araya F, et al: Evoked potential abnormalities in progressive spastic paraparesis associated with HTLV-I. Acta Neurol Scand 83:151, 1991

43. Newton M, Cruickshank C, Miller D, et al: Antibody to human T-lymphotropic virus type I in West-Indian-born UK residents with spastic paraparesis. Lancet 1:415, 1987

44. Barkhaus PE, Morgan O: Jamaican neuropathy: an electrophysiological study. Muscle Nerve 11:380, 1988

45. Gout O, Gessain A, Bolgert F, et al: Chronic myelopathies associated with human T-lymphotropic virus type I. Arch Neurol 46:255, 1989

46. Kira J, Minato S, Itoyama Y, et al: Leuko-encephalopathy in HTLV-I-associated myelopathy: MRI and EEG data. J Neurol Sci 87:221, 1988

47. Kira J, Fujihara K, Itoyama Y, et al: Leukoencephalopathy in HTLV-I-associated myelopathy/tropical spastic paraparesis: MRI analysis and a two year follow-up study after corticosteroid therapy. J Neurol Sci 106:41, 1991

48. Grimaldi LME, Roos RP, Davare SG, et al: HTLV-I-associated myelopathy: oligoclonal immunoglobulin G bands contain anti-HTLV-I p24 antibody. Ann Neurol 24:727, 1988

49. Link H, Cruz M, Gessain A, et al: Chronic progressive myelopathy associated with HTLV-I. Neurology 39:1566, 1989

50. Gessain A, Caudie C, Gout O, et al: Intrathecal synthesis of antibodies to human lymphotropic virus type I and the presence of IgG oligoclonal bands in the cerebrospinal fluid of patients with endemic tropical spastic paraparesis. J Infect Dis 157:1226, 1988

51. Fishman RA: Composition of the cerebrospinal fluid. p. 207. In: Cerebropsinal Fluid in Diseases of the Nervous System. 2nd Ed. WB Saunders, Philadelphia, 1993

52. Centers for Disease Control: Licensure of screening tests for antibody to human T-lymphotropic virus type I. MMWR 37:736, 1988

53. Ehrlich GD, Glaser JB, LaVigne K, et al: Prevalence of human T-cell leukemia/lymphoma virus (HTLV) type II infection among high-risk individuals: type-specific identification of HTLVs by polymerase chain reaction. Blood 74:1658, 1989

54. Khabbaz RF, Heneine W, Grindon A, et al: Indeterminate HTLV serologic results in U.S. blood donors: Are they due to HTLV-I or HTLV-II? J Acquir Immune Defic Syndr 5:400, 1992

55. Hartley TM, Malone GE, Khabbaz RF, et al: Evaluation of a recombinant human T-cell lymphotropic virus type I (HTLV-I) p21E antibody detection immunoassay as a supplementary test in HTLV-I/II antibody testing algorithms. J Clin Microbiol 29:1125, 1991

56. Imamura J, Tsujimoto A, Ohta Y, et al: DNA blotting analysis of human retroviruses in cerebrospinal fluid of spastic paraparesis patients: the viruses are identical to human T-cell leukemia virus type-I (HTLV-I). Int J Cancer 42:221, 1988

57. Lillehoj EP, Alexander SS, Dubrule CJ, et al: Development and evaluation of a human T-cell leukemia virus type I serologic confirmatory assay incorporating a recombinant envelope polypeptide. J Clin Microbiol 28:2653, 1990

58. Roberts BD, Foung SKH, Lipka JJ, Kaplan JE: Evaluation of an immunoblot assay for serological confirmation and differentiation of human T-cell lymphotropic virus types I and II. J Clin Microbiol 31:260, 1993

59. Osame M, Matsumoto M, Usuku K, et al: Chronic progressive myelopathy associated with elevated antibodies to human T-lymphotropic virus type I and adult T-cell leukemia-like cells. Ann Neurol 21:117, 1987

60. Matutes E, Dalgleish AG, Weiss RA, et al: Studies in healthy human T-cell-leukemia/lymphoma virus (HTLV-I) carriers from the Caribbean. Int J Cancer 38:41, 1986

61. Yasuda K, Sei Y, Yokoyama MM, et al: Healthy HTLV-I carriers in Japan: the hematological and immunological characteristics. Br J Haematol 64:195, 1986

62. Gessain A, Saal F, Gout O, et al: High human T-cell lymphotropic virus type I proviral DNA load with

polyclonal integration in peripheral blood mononuclear cells of French West Indian, Guianese, and African patients with tropical spastic paraparesis. Blood 75:428, 1990

63. Akizuki S, Setoguchi M, Nakazato O, et al: An autopsy case of human T-lymphotropic virus type-I associated myelopathy. Hum Pathol 19:988, 1988

64. Sasaki S, Komori T, Maruyama S, et al: An autopsy case of human T lymphotropic virus type I-associated myelopathy (HAM) with a duration of 28 years. Acta Neuropathol (Berl) 81:219, 1990

65. Bhigee AI, Wiley CA, Wachsman W, et al: HTLV-I-associated myelopathy: clinicopathologic correlation with localization of the provirus to spinal cord. Neurology 41:1990, 1991

66. Arimura K, Rosales R, Osame M, Igata A: Clinical electrophysiologic studies of HTLV-I-associated myelopathy. Arch Neurol 44:609, 1987

67. Kwok S, Kellog D, Ehrlich G, et al: Characterization of a sequence of human T-cell leukemia virus type I from a patient with chronic progressive myelopathy. J Infect Dis 158:1193, 1988

68. Gessain A, Louie A, Gout O, et al: Human T-cell leukemia-lymphoma virus type I (HTLV-I) expression in fresh peripheral blood mononuclear cells from patients with tropical spastic paraparesis/HTLV-I-associated myelopathy. J Virol 65:1628, 1991

69. Ehrlich GD, Glaser JB, Bryz-Gornia V, et al: Multiple sclerosis, retroviruses, and PCR. Neurology 41:335, 1991

70. Rosenblatt JD: Human T-lymphotrophic virus types I and II. West J Med 158:379, 1993

71. Eisenberg RA, Cohen PL: The role of immunologic mechanisms in the pathogenesis of rheumatic diseases. p. 39. In Schumacher HR (ed): Primer on the Rheumatic Diseases. 9th Ed. Arthritis Foundation, Atlanta, 1988

72. Tendler CL, Greenberg SJ, Blattner WA, et al: Transactivation of interleukin 2 and its receptor induces immune activation in human T-cell lymphotropic virus type I-associated myelopathy: pathogenetic implications and a rationale for immunotherapy. Proc Natl Acad Sci USA 87:5218, 1990

73. Gardner MB: Neurotropic retroviruses of wild mice and macaques. Ann Neurol 23, suppl:S201, 1988

74. Watabe K, Saida T, Kim SU: Human and simian glial cells infected by human T-lymphotropic virus type I in culture. J Neuropathol Exp Neurol 48:610, 1989

75. Yamada M, Watabe K, Saida T, et al: Increased susceptibility of human fetal astrocytes to human T-lymphotropic virus type I in culture. J Neuropathol Exp Neurol 50:97, 1991

76. Jacobson S, Raine CS, Mingioli ES, McFarlin DE: Isolation of an HTLV-I-like retrovirus from patients with tropical spastic paraparesis. Nature 331:540, 1988

77. Jacobsen S, McFarlin DE, Robinson S, et al: HTLV-I-specific cytotoxic lymphocytes in the cerebrospinal fluid of patients with HTLV-I-associated neurological disease. Ann Neurol 32:651, 1992

78. Jacobson S, Hisatoshi S, McFarlin DE, et al: Circulating CD8+ cytotoxic T lymphocytes specific for HTLV-I pX in patients with HTLV-I associated neurologic disease. Nature 348:245, 1990

79. Maloney EM, Biggar RJ, Neel JV, et al: Endemic human T cell lymphotropic virus type II infection among isolated Brazilian Amerindians. J Infect Dis 166:100, 1992

80. Centers for Disease Control and Prevention and the USPHS working group: Guidelines for counseling persons infected with human T-lymphotropic virus type-I (HTLV-I) and type II (HTLV-II). Ann Intern Med 118:448, 1993

81. Kalyanaraman VS, Sarngadharan MG, Robert-Guroff M, et al: A new subtype of human T-cell leukemia virus (HTLV-II) associated with a T-cell variant of hairy cell leukemia. Science 218:571, 1982

82. Rosenblatt JD, Golde DW, Wachman W, et al: A second isolate of HTLV-II associated with atypical hairy cell leukemia. N Engl J Med 315:372, 1986

83. Cervantes J, Hussain S, Jensen F, Schwartz JM: T-prolymphocytic leukemia associated with human lymphotropic virus II. Clin Res 34:454A, 1986

84. Sohn CC, Blayney DW, Misset JL, et al: Leukopenic chronic T-cell leukemia mimicking hairy cell leukemia: association with human retroviruses. Blood 67:949, 1986

85. Rosenblatt JD, Gasson JC, Glaspy J, et al: Relationship between human T-cell leukemia virus-II and atypical hair cell leukemia: a serologic study of hairy cell leukemia patients. Leukemia 1:397, 1987

86. Murphy EL, Engstrom JW, Miller K, et al: HTLV-II associated myelopathy in 43-year-old woman. Lancet 341:757, 1993

87. Jacobson S, Lehky T, Nishimura M, et al: Isolation of HTLV-II from a patient with chronic, progressive neurological disease clinically indistinguishable from HTLV-I-associated myelopathy/tropical spastic paraparesis. Ann Neurol 33:392, 1993

88. Harrington WJ, Sheremata W, Hjelle B, et al: Spastic ataxia associated with human T-cell lymphotropic virus type II infection. Ann Neurol 33:411, 1993

89. Osame M, Igata A, Matsumoto M, et al: HTLV-I associated myelopathy (HAM): treatment trials, retrospective survey and clinical and laboratory findings. Hematol Rev 3:271, 1990

90. Matsuo H, Nakamura T, Tsujihata M, et al: Plasmapheresis in treatment of human T-lymphotropic virus type-I associated myelopathy. Lancet 2:1109, 1988
91. Harrington WJ Jr, Sheremata WA, Snodgrass SR, et al: Tropical spastic paraparesis/HTLV-I-associated myelopathy (HAM): treatment with an anabolic steroid danazol. AIDS Res Hum Retroviruses 7:1031, 1991
92. Sheremata WA, Squilcote DC, DeFreitas E: A safety study of high-dose retrovirus (AZT) in HTLV-I-associated myelopathy (HAM): evidence for safety and possible efficacy. Neurology 41:142, 1991

40

Fungal Infections and the Central Nervous System

Gary M. Cox
John R. Perfect
David T. Durack

Fungal infections of the central nervous system (CNS) are being recognized with increasing frequency due to both the growing population of immunocompromised patients and improvements in diagnostic techniques. Information on the diagnosis and treatment of this diverse group of infections ranges from limited to extensive. Therefore, a careful reading of the existing literature coupled with personal experience form the basis of knowledge on the management of these important infections. This chapter summarizes our current understanding of fungal infections involving the CNS.

PATHOGENS

Fungi that may invade the CNS and cause infection can be split into two general groups. The first group consists of primary pathogens and includes *Cryptococcus neoformans, Coccidioides immitis, Blastomyces dermatitidis, Paracoccidioides brasiliensis, Sporothrix schenckii, Histoplasma capsulatum, Pseudallescheria boydii*, and the dematiaceous fungi. CNS involvement with these fungi can occur in patients with intact immune systems but appears to be more commonly found in pa-

tients with some sort of immunosuppression. The second group consists of opportunists that cause CNS infection almost exclusively in patients with defective host defenses; this group includes *Candida* species, *Aspergillus* species, and the Zygomycetes. Table 40-1 shows some of the features of CNS fungal infections. Then there are some fungi for which there are case reports of involvement in CNS infections. These are mostly common environmental fungi and include *Rhodotorula*,[1] *Acremonium*,[2] *Blastoschizomyces*,[3,4] *Trichosporon*,[5] *Sepedonium*,[6] *Schizophyllum*,[7] *Paecilomyces*,[8] and *Ustilago*.[9] This grouping on the basis of host immune status is not absolute because exceptions will occur, but it is useful as a framework for further discussion.

CRYPTOCOCCUS NEOFORMANS

An encapsulated yeast, *C. neoformans* is the most common cause of fungal meningitis and is therefore more thoroughly reviewed than other fungi. The first report of cryptococcal infection in humans was provided by Busse and Buschke in 1894–1895[10]; the patient had bone infection. The first case of meningeal cryptococcal infection was reported 10 years later, in

Table 40-1 Features of CNS Fungal Infections

Pathogen	Risk Factors	CSF Cultures Positive	CSF Serologies	Major Pathological Manifestations		
				Meningitis	Infarct	Abscess or Mass
Aspergillus spp.	Neutropenia; corticosteroids	Rare	None	+	+ + + +	+ +
Blastomyces dermatitidis	None known	Rare	Ab	+	—	+ +
Candida spp.	Neutropenia; corticosteroids; CSF shunts; PMN defects; prematurity	50%	None	+ +	—	+ + +
Coccidioides immitis	AIDS; corticosteroids	25–45%	Ab	+ + + +	+	+
Cryptococcus neoformans	AIDS; corticosteroids	75–85%	An	+ + + +	+	+ +
Dematiaceous fungi	None	Rare	None	+	—	+ + + +
Histoplasma capsulatum	AIDS; corticosteroids	50%	Ab/An	+ +	+	+
Paracoccidioides brasiliensis	None	Rare	None	+ +	—	+
Pseudallescheria boydii	Corticosteroids; Aspiration	Rare	None	+ +	—	+ +
Sporothrix schenckii	Alcohol; AIDS?	Rare	Ab	+ +	—	—
Zygomycetes (Mucorales)	Diabetes; deferoxamine; IV drug use	Rare	None	+	+ + + +	+ + +

Abbreviations: Ab, antibody test; An, antigen test; PMN, polymorphonuclear leukocytes.

1905.[11] During this century, cryptococcosis has emerged as a significant CNS pathogen. A review of the incidence of systemic mycoses in selected hospitals in the United States showed an increase in infections during the 1960s and 1970s.[12] The number of human infections with *C. neoformans* has risen particularly high in the United States and certain African countries during the 1980s and 1990s as a result of the human immunodeficiency virus (HIV) epidemic.[13] Presently in the United States, cryptococcal meningitis will occur in approximately 6 to 13 percent of patients with acquired immunodeficiency syndrome (AIDS).

This ubiquitous encapsulated saprophytic yeast occupies a wide environmental niche. It can be found worldwide in bird excreta, soil, animals, and even humans. It is likely that most infections occur after inhalation of small yeasts. The yeast has a polysaccharide capsule that ranges in size from 1 to 30 μm. On inhalation of the yeasts, a primary pneumonia may develop, or the host may form a primary lung–lymph node complex in which organisms may remain dormant for long periods, perhaps until host defenses become weakened. The reason this organism has a particular tendency to spread to the CNS remains unexplained, but CNS infection usually manifests as a meningitis, although mass lesions can be seen. There are four serotypes (a, b, c, d) based on capsular polysaccharide, and these are divided into two varieties: *C. neoformans* var. *neoformans* (serotypes a and d) and *C. neoformans* var. *gatti* (serotypes b and c). All serotypes can cause meningitis, but there is some geographical variation in distribution of disease caused by these serotypes. Most patients with cryptococcal meningitis in the United States and Europe have been infected with a serotype a or d strain. Infection with the b and c strains is more common in southern California, Southeast Asia, Australia, and Africa; this distribution reflects the natural distribution of the river red gum tree (*Eucalyptus camaldulensis*), which is the likely environmental niche for *C. neoformans* var. *gatti*.[14]

COCCIDIOIDES IMMITIS

C. immitis is a dimorphic fungus with a natural habitat in semiarid soil, which explains its geographical distribution in the southwestern United States and in parts of Mexico and South America.[15] Because many tourists travel through these areas and may become infected, clinicians outside the organism's natural habitat occasionally encounter coccidioidomycosis.[16] This fungal infection begins as a primary pulmonary infection after inhalation of the organism. Most patients remain asymptomatic, and fewer than 0.2 percent of primary infections disseminate. Occasionally, this fungus reaches the meninges, either by hematogenous spread or by direct extension from osteomyelitis of the skull or vertebrae.

HISTOPLASMA CAPSULATUM

H. capsulatum is a dimorphic fungus which is endemic in certain areas within the Ohio and Central Mississippi valleys and Latin America. It can be found in bird and bat guano and soil contaminated with guano. Many outbreaks of the disease have been attributed to disturbing contaminated soil, thus allowing the conidia to become airborne.[17,18] Most infections develop after inhalation of the conidia form of the fungus, and infection in endemic areas is very common.[19] Recent skin test data indicate that in one endemic area up to 69 percent of the population had evidence of prior infection with this fungus.[20] Most infected people have minimal symptoms, and dissemination occurs only rarely. When dissemination does occur, it has been estimated that between one-tenth and one-fourth of patients develop CNS involvement. Although granulomas and other brain parenchymal lesions have been described, most patients with CNS lesions present with meningitis.

BLASTOMYCES DERMATITIDIS

B. dermatitidis is a dimorphic fungus which is endemic in Africa and in certain parts of the lower Mississippi Valley, North Central states, and mid-Atlantic states within the continental United States. It is presumed to be inhaled from a source in soil, but its natural location in the environment has rarely been found. Most people with infection have subclinical disease, and dissemination occurs rarely.[21] Disseminated blastomycosis is characterized by suppurating, granulomatous lesions of the lung, bone, and skin. In some series, blastomycosis has been reported to involve the brain in 6 to 33 percent of disseminated cases. Although patients with CNS blastomycosis generally

present with evidence of infection at other sites, occasionally meningitis is the initial presentation, without evidence of extraneural disease.[22] CNS involvement is not limited to meningitis; an occasional patient will have a mass lesion (blastomycoma) in the brain parenchyma.[23,24]

PARACOCCIDIOIDES BRASILIENSIS

P. brasiliensis is a dimorphic fungus endemic to subtropical areas of Mexico and Central and South America. The lung is the primary location for initial infection; a few patients have widely disseminated disease that involves the CNS, but rarely has the infection been reported to involve only the CNS.[25]

SPOROTHRIX SCHENCKII

S. schenckii has a worldwide distribution and is a saprophyte of vegetation, notably roses and sphagnum moss. Sporothricosis presents as a chronic infection of skin and subcutaneous lymphatics, developing after a primary inoculation such as a rose-thorn puncture. Pulmonary disease from inhalation of spores is uncommon. Dissemination beyond the skin, lung, and joints is rare; only about a dozen cases of *Sporothrix* meningitis have been reported. Most of the patients with meningitis did not have overt extraneural disease at presentation.

CANDIDA SPECIES

Candida species are part of the normal human microbial flora and rarely cause invasive disease unless host defenses have been altered. This yeast can gain access to the bloodstream and then the CNS via contaminated intravenous catheters or by illicit intravenous drug use. Neonates, neutropenic subjects, and patients recovering from major surgery are particularly susceptible to invasive candidiasis, including CNS involvement. Based on autopsy studies, *Candida* species are reported to be the most common fungi to invade the CNS.[26] *Candida* may cause meningitis,[27] ventriculitis,[28] or parenchymal lesions such as abscesses or granulomas, and *C. albicans* is the species implicated in the majority of CNS infections.

ASPERGILLUS SPECIES

Aspergillus species are ubiquitous in the environment and can be found in the air of most hospitals. Both neutrophils and macrophages are important host defense mechanisms directed against the spores and hyphae of *Aspergillus*. CNS infection with *Aspergillus* species can develop by direct extension from the paranasal sinuses; by direct inoculation after head trauma, surgery, or lumbar puncture; or by hematogenous spread in immunocompromised hosts, particularly those with prolonged neutropenia. A clinically important characteristic of *Aspergillus* infections is their predilection to invade arteries, causing thromboses. Thus cerebral infarctions due to invasion along cerebral arteries is a common presentation of *Aspergillus* infection in the CNS. Meningitis and meningoencephalitis can also occur.[29,30]

ZYGOMYCOSIS

Fungi of the class Zygomycetes, also known as the "mucormycoses," are found widespread in the environment, and infection is usually due to inhalation of spores. Infection of the CNS in compromised hosts can occur by direct extension from the paranasal sinuses or through hematogenous spread such as by illicit intravenous drug use. The genus *Rhizopus* is responsible for most infections caused by this group. The zygomycetes, like *Aspergillus* species, commonly invade arteries and cause thromboses with resulting infarction.[31,32] Disease limited to the meninges is unusual.

PSEUDALLESCHERIA BOYDII

Pseudallescheria boydii has worldwide distribution in soil and contaminated water. This fungus is also known as *Monosporium apiospermum* or *Scedosporium apiospermum* when it is in the asexual state. Infection can rarely result in brain abscesses or meningitis, and there is an association of CNS infection with aspiration of contaminated water during trauma or near drowning.[33–35]

PHAEOHYPHOMYCOSIS

The dematiaceous fungi are common environmental molds that have brown pigment in their walls. This group of fungi has occasionally caused CNS infec-

tion. *Cladosporium trichoides*, also known as *Xylohypha bantiana*, is the most common isolate of this class of fungi found in CNS infections and usually manifests as a brain abscess, although meningitis has been described.[36–39]

HOST

The CNS is an immunologically sequestered site, with anatomical barriers that tend to exclude not only invading microorganisms but also some components of the immune system. Host defenses normally are highly effective in excluding fungi from the CNS, but certain conditions can lead to failure of this function. Some patients with fungal infections of the CNS have no apparent immune defect or underlying disease, but most have some flaw in their immune response that allows invasion by fungi. Some of these defects are obvious, such as direct inoculation of organisms into the CNS following trauma or via indwelling catheters, whereas others are subtle and involve defects in the cell-mediated immune system.

The most important risk factor for the development of CNS fungal infections is the suppression of the host immune system, whether it be due to drugs or underlying disease. The mycology of these infections and the response to therapy are somewhat dependent on the type of immune suppression. Immunosuppressive drugs are major factors, and systemic administration of corticosteroids is a well-known risk factor for developing CNS fungal infection, especially with *C. neoformans* and *Aspergillus* species. Neutropenia due to cancer chemotherapy is associated with CNS infection due to *Aspergillus* and *Candida* species, and treatment with the drug deferoxamine predisposes to rhinocerebral zygomycete infections.[40]

Several underlying diseases are associated with an increased incidence of CNS fungal infection; the most important of these is probably AIDS. From 6 to 13 percent of patients with HIV infection will eventually develop cryptococcal meningitis, and this infection is the fourth most common opportunistic infection seen in patients with AIDS in the United States. There have also been several reports of patients infected with HIV who have developed CNS infections with *Aspergillus* species.[41,42] These infections have, so far, presented predominantly as cerebral mass lesions, although cerebral infarctions, meningitis, and spinal cord involvement have also been seen. Patients with AIDS may also present with disseminated histoplasmosis[43] or coccidioidomycosis[44] with CNS involvement.

Patients who undergo organ transplantation and receive concomitant immunosuppression are at significant risk for CNS fungal infection. The most common fungal pathogens in this setting are *C. neoformans, Aspergillus* species, and *Candida* species.[45] Infections with *C. neoformans* in organ transplant patients usually manifest as a chronic meningitis occurring 6 months or more after the transplant procedure. Infections with *Aspergillus* and *Candida* species, however, usually occur within the first 2 months after transplantation, and CNS involvement is usually manifest by brain abscesses. In fact, CNS aspergillosis may be underdiagnosed in organ transplant patients.[46,47] In one series of 44 brains examined at autopsy from liver transplant recipients, 9 cases of cerebral aspergillosis were identified, of which only 2 were diagnosed before death.[48] Other underlying diseases associated with CNS fungal infection include malignancies, diabetes mellitus, and prematurity. Diabetics in ketoacidosis are at risk for rhinocerebral zygomycete infections; premature infants are at risk for disseminated infections with *Candida,* and the CNS is involved in two-thirds of these cases.

Infections that arise from direct inoculation of fungi into the CNS are usually seen after head trauma or neurosurgical procedures or as complications of CNS shunts. In patients who have suffered open head injuries, fungi that are ubiquitous in the environment may contaminate the wounds and lead to meningitis and focal brain abscesses.[49] With cerebrospinal fluid (CSF) leaks, the initial infection may be bacterial, but during the use of broad-spectrum antibacterial drugs, a superinfection of the meninges with *Candida* can occur. Infection is a frequent occurrence associated with the presence of a CSF diverting shunt, but fungi are only occasionally implicated in these infections. The most common fungus associated with CSF shunt infections is *Candida albicans,* and it appears that infection occurs as a result of either contamination of the shunt apparatus (during insertion or subsequent manipulation) or hematogenous spread.[50,51] Of the 20 cases of CSF shunt infection with *C. albicans* in the literature, there appears to be an association with recent antibacterial therapy and colonization with *Candida* species at another body site. Other fungi that

have caused CNS infection in the setting of a CSF shunt include *C. neoformans, Trichosporon beigelii,*[52] *Torulopsis glabrata,*[53] and *Candida tropicalis.* There is controversy concerning cryptococcal shunt infections. Many of the patients with CSF shunts who were subsequently found to have infection with *C. neoformans* had their shunts originally placed for idiopathic hydrocephalus or for chronic culture-negative meningitis.[54,55] These patients probably had chronic CNS cryptococcal infection before their shunts were inserted, and the diagnosis was made only after the shunt was in place. Therefore, it is not clear if the presence of a CSF shunt places a patient at higher risk for developing CNS cryptococcal infection. There are rare reports of fungal infection associated with neurosurgical procedures; among these infections, *Aspergillus* species account for most of the pathogens.[56–58] Some of these patients were considered to have had direct extension of the fungus from the sinuses during surgery and some were thought to have had fungi introduced along with hardware inserted during an operative procedure. Many of these patients had additional predisposing conditions such as treatment with antibacterials or high-dose corticosteroids.

CANDIDA SPECIES

In the normal host, *Candida* rarely causes deep-seated infections. However, there are multiple factors that can encourage spread of *Candida* from mucosal surfaces into deeper tissue, including the subarachnoid space. These factors include prematurity, broad-spectrum antibacterial therapy, hyperalimentation, malignancies, indwelling catheters, treatment with corticosteroids, neutropenia, abdominal surgery, diabetes mellitus, burns, and intravenous drug use. Interestingly, *Candida* is a more common invader of brain tissue than of the subarachnoid space. *Candida* species are susceptible to the oxidative and nonoxidative antimicrobial mechanisms of professional phagocytes, cells that are undoubtedly important for control of infections with *Candida.* The importance of the host response has been further emphasized by reports of *Candida* meningitis in both acquired and congenital immunodeficiency syndromes. Patients with chronic granulomatous disease of childhood may present with *Candida* meningitis.[59,60] Therefore this specific underlying immune deficiency should be considered in any case of spontaneously occurring *Candida* meningitis.

Several cases of *Candida* meningitis have been reported in patients with the global immune defect called severe combined immune deficiency (SCID).[61] Patients with AIDS frequently have mucocutaneous forms of candidiasis, such as thrush and esophagitis, but involvement of the CNS has only rarely been reported in these patients.[62–64] *Candida* meningitis has been described as a superinfection of the CSF in patients recovering from bacterial meningitis.[65] Finally, *Candida* can involve the brain and subarachnoid space by direct extension through trauma, ventriculostomy placement, or ventricular shunts.

CRYPTOCOCCUS NEOFORMANS

The complex interactions of the immune system with *C. neoformans* remain incompletely understood.[66] However, multiple lines of evidence suggest that host factors are paramount in preventing these yeasts from seeding the subarachnoid space. Despite earlier reports that about 50 percent of patients with cryptococcal meningitis had no known immune deficiency, more recent experience suggests that a much higher proportion of patients have some identifiable form of immunosuppression. Most cases of cryptococcal meningitis occur in those with defective cell-mediated immunity due to corticosteroid treatment, reticuloendothelial malignancy, organ transplantation, sarcoidosis, collagen vascular diseases, and AIDS. In further support of the contention that immune suppression is usually necessary for meningitis to develop are findings that lymphocyte functions are abnormal in most patients with disseminated cryptococcosis and most patients with HIV infection have CD4 counts below 100/ml. Moreover, certain immune defects may persist after infection has been eliminated by treatment. It is likely that both humoral and cell-mediated immunity are important for the prevention of cryptococcal meningitis, but cellular functions are the primary immune agents.

Two exogenous factors have played a major role in making cryptococcal meningitis the most common fungal meningeal pathogen. The first factor is corticosteroid treatment, which causes multiple immune defects. Excess endogenous or exogenous corticosteroids greatly increase the patient's susceptibility to cryptococcal meningitis. The second factor is HIV infection, with resulting loss of CD4 cells.[67] These cells, which are central to so many immune responses, must be particularly important in the host response to *C. neoformans*. Most AIDS patients with cryptococcosis will present with a particularly high burden of organisms. India ink examinations of the CSF are positive in 80 percent of patients; extraordinarily high titers of cryptococcal polysaccharide antigen in CSF and serum are common. A remarkable feature of the AIDS patient's response to infection is the lack of a CSF leukocytosis. Approximately two-thirds of patients with AIDS and cryptococcal meningitis had fewer than 20 leukocytes/mm^3 in the CSF on presentation. This quantitative lack of an inflammatory response indicates a deficient immune system and ultimately a poor prognosis despite therapy.

COCCIDIOIDES IMMITIS

Many patients who develop CNS infection with *C. immitis* have no underlying disease, but immunosuppressed patients are more likely to have such infections. Corticosteroid treatment has been associated with more severe manifestations of primary infection as well as reactivation of latent disease and dissemination to the CNS. Interestingly, the natural history of coccidioidal meningitis shows that patients whose only extrapulmonary site of infection was the CNS lived significantly longer than patients with more diffuse disease.[68] It has also been shown that the white cell count in the CSF will decrease during the course of untreated infection. There have been many cases of CNS infections with *Coccidioides* in patients with AIDS.[69] The fact that several areas of high prevalence of HIV infection are also areas of endemicity for this fungus has tremendous implications for the health care system, since it is likely that the number of CNS infections with *C. immitis* will parallel the growing numbers of patients with AIDS.

BLASTOMYCES DERMATITIDIS

Immunocompromised patients are at increased risk for infection with *B. dermatitidis*. A review of 24 cases of infection with *Blastomyces* in a heterogenous population of immunocompromised patients showed 6 cases of disseminated disease, including 4 with CNS involvement.[70]

HISTOPLASMA CAPSULATUM

Although *Histoplasma* meningitis can occur in apparently normal hosts, it has been shown to occur in the immunocompromised host at a higher rate.[71] Patients with AIDS are at high risk to develop disseminated disease, and it appears that this is usually due to reactivation of latent infection.

PARACOCCIDIOIDES BRASILIENSIS

Meningitis is an unusual manifestation of infection with *P. brasiliensis* but occurs occasionally in normal hosts.[72] The host response against this microorganism remains poorly understood.

SPOROTHRIX SCHENCKII

Although meningitis with *S. schenckii* is so uncommon that risk factors cannot be defined accurately, there are certain groups that may be predisposed to dissemination from a local infection. Patients with myelodysplastic syndromes, who abuse ethanol, or who are on corticosteroids may be at increased risk for dissemination. Disseminated sporothricosis has also been described in patients with AIDS.[73,74]

ASPERGILLUS SPECIES

Most intracranial infections with *Aspergillus* have occurred in neutropenic patients. The risk of disseminated aspergillosis with subsequent brain parenchymal involvement or meningitis increases with the duration of neutropenia.[75] Most infections manifest as parenchymal lesions, but meningitis and spinal cord lesions[76] have been seen. Occasionally, *Aspergillus* infection involves the vertebrae and eventually the subarachnoid space in patients with chronic granulomatous disease of childhood. The pulmonary alveolar macrophage may be most important in initial control of this ubiquitous fungus, but the polymorphonuclear leukocyte is probably crucial in the defense against CNS invasion.

ZYGOMYCOSIS

Although the Zygomycetes generally invade blood vessels and cause infarcts, they occasionally invade the subarachnoid space. Patients with diabetes mellitus with or without ketoacidosis, malignancy, or on immunosuppressive therapy are at risk for disseminated infection. There have been reports of disseminated zygomycosis, including brain involvement, in dialysis patients receiving deferoxamine.[40] This iron chelating agent may interfere with the antifungal activity of transferrin within the sera, thus allowing for dissemination of the zygomycete.

PHAEOHYPHOMYCOSIS

Most patients diagnosed with brain abscesses due to one of the dematiaceous fungi have had no apparent underlying immune defect. The portal of entry for these fungi in most cases is not known, but because of a predilection for the abscesses to be in the frontal and parietal lobes, it can be hypothesized that some of these infections result through extension from the frontal sinuses.

DIAGNOSIS

The diagnosis of CNS fungal infections can be very difficult, even when involvement of the CNS occurs in the setting of disseminated fungal infection. This is due to many factors involving unusual clinical presentations of patients with CNS fungal infection, difficulty in culturing the organism, and the lack of sensitive serology tests for most of the fungi.

In cases of cerebral mass lesions due to fungi, most patients present with nonfocal neurological complaints and signs. Many patients present only with an altered sensorium or seizures but are found to have extensive CNS infection on imaging studies. Patients with fungal meningitis usually present with chronic signs and symptoms. Some combination of fever, headache, lethargy, confusion, nausea, vomiting, stiff neck, and neurological deficits is generally present. However, these markers of CNS infection may not always be present when the patient is first seen. In fact, fever and headache are occasionally absent, and patients may present with only subacute dementia. Cases of cryptococcal, coccidioidal, and *Histoplasma* meningitis may be indolent, with persistent symptoms present for months to years if untreated.[77–81] Fungal meningitis may not always present with chronic symptoms; some cases of cryptococcal meningitis present acutely. In particular, immunocompromised patients such as those receiving high doses of corticosteroids or with HIV infection can develop symptoms and signs over a few days.

Fungal meningitis is a primary consideration in the differential diagnosis of chronic meningitis. Ellner

Table 40-2 Differential Diagnosis
of Chronic Meningitis

Infectious Causes	Noninfectious Causes
Fungal infections	Chronic benign lymphocytic meningitis
Mycobacterial infections	
Parameningeal infections	Subarachnoid hemorrhage
Syphilis	Systemic lupus erythematosus
Lyme disease	
Brucellosis	Granulomatous arteritis
Toxoplasmosis	Carcinomatous meningitis
Nocardiosis	Sarcoidosis
Actinomycosis	Behçet's disease
Leptospirosis	
Helminthic meningitis	
Viral meningitis	

and Bennett have defined this group of patients as those with CNS abnormalities that fail to improve or progress during at least 4 weeks of observation.[82] The differential diagnosis of chronic meningitis includes both infectious and noninfectious causes (Table 40-2), but fungal etiologies are primary considerations that may be particularly difficult to distinguish from certain other pathogens such as mycobacteria.

The CSF findings in fungal meningitis are well described. Most cases have a mononuclear pleocytosis that ranges between 20 and 500 cells/mm^3. Eosinophilic pleocytosis of the CSF has been described in several cases of coccidioidal meningitis and rare cases of cryptococcal meningitis.[83] Very low CSF leukocyte counts (fewer than 10/mm^3) may occur if the patient is severely immunosuppressed. CSF protein levels are generally elevated, but if very high protein concentrations (1 g/dl or more) are present in CSF, a subarachnoid block should be considered. CSF glucose can vary from normal to low levels. The causes of hypoglycorrhachia are listed in Table 40-3. The presence of hypoglycorrhachia favors an infectious disorder and may have prognostic significance. It is very unusual to see fungi on stained preparations of CSF except in the case of cryptococcal meningitis. India ink preparations of CSF are positive in approximately 50 percent of all patients with cryptococcal meningitis, and the sensitivity is higher in patients with HIV infection.

Unfortunately, CSF cultures are not always positive in fungal meningitis and are only very rarely positive in patients presenting with cerebral mass lesions.

For example, only one-third to one-half of patients with coccidioidal meningitis have CSF cultures that are positive. Blastomycotic meningitis rarely yields positive CSF cultures, and even at necropsy it is difficult to find *Histoplasma* in the subarachnoid space. Cryptococcal meningitis has positive CSF cultures in approximately 75 percent of all patients, but patients with HIV infection show a higher burden of organism and cultures are positive in 75 to 90 percent of cases. Because of these difficulties in the diagnosis of fungal meningitis, large volumes of CSF (10 to 20 ml) should be obtained and sent for culture in suspected cases. The laboratory should centrifuge specimens and culture the sediment on appropriate fungal media. *Candida* can be identified by the laboratory within a few days, and, in an occasional difficult patient, hypertonic media may be helpful for growing the organism. Cryptococci should be identified in most cases in between 5 to 10 days, but classic dimorphic fungi (e.g., *Histoplasma* or *Coccidioides*) may require longer incubations. The lysis-centrifugation method for isolating *H. capsulatum* from blood has improved detection compared to routine or radiometric methods. This method has not been evaluated on CSF specimens from patients with fungal meningitis but could certainly be used. Blood cultures may be helpful for identifying the fungus which is causing meningitis in that particular host. Unfortunately, except for *Candida* and *Cryptococcus*, blood cultures are rarely positive in patients with fungal meningitis. CSF cultures can also be negative because samples are not taken

Table 40-3 Differential Diagnosis of Low CSF
Glucose Concentration

Acute bacterial meningitis
Mycobacterial meningitis
Fungal meningitis
Subarachnoid hemorrhage
Carcinomatous meningitis
Meningeal cysticercosis/trichinosis
Drug-induced meningitis (nonsteroidal anti-inflammatory agents)
Acute syphilitic meningitis
Chemical meningitis (direct intrathecal injections)
Viral meningitis
Hypoglycemia
Rheumatoid meningitis
Lupus myelopathy
Amebic meningitis

from the site of active infection. Fungi commonly cause a basilar meningitis, so it is not surprising that cisternal fluid may yield organisms when lumbar fluid is sterile, as may the ventricular fluid.[84] Diagnosis in a difficult case of chronic meningitis may require repeated examination of lumbar spinal fluid but may also necessitate examination of cisternal or ventricular fluid.

Positive cultures are the standard for diagnosis of fungal CNS infections, but they may be difficult to obtain or may take a long time to grow. Hence, despite some limitations, serological tests remain important in the diagnosis of these infections. The latex agglutination test for cryptococcal polysaccharide antigen is the single best serological test for diagnosis of fungal infections. It can be used equally well on serum or CSF.[85] When samples are heated to eliminate rheumatoid factor and proper controls for nonspecific agglutination and interfering substances are used, the test is more than 90 percent sensitive and specific for cryptococcal infection. If surface condensation from agar plates is added to the assay, false positives may result. False-positive results can also be seen with disseminated *T. beigelii* infections and paravertebral bacterial infections. If a positive antigen test occurs in a patient whose clinical presentation is not consistent with cryptococcal meningitis, the laboratory should repeat the test; if it is still positive, a repeat lumbar puncture is indicated. False-negative tests occur as well, and can be due to too few replicating yeasts at the site of infection, a prozone phenomenon due to antigen excess, or the use of certain manufacturers' antigen detection kits.[86] In summary, the cryptococcal polysaccharide antigen test using appropriate controls is an excellent diagnostic test if positive at any titer. The test is rapid and can be positive when the culture is negative. The value of using antigen titers as a guide to therapy is discussed further in the treatment section.

Detection of the histoplasma polysaccharide antigen in urine and serum has proven to be an excellent adjunct in the diagnosis of patients with disseminated infections due to *H. capsulatum,* and it is also useful in monitoring therapy and the early detection of relapsing infections in patients with AIDS. This assay has been tested in the diagnosis of patients with *Histoplasma* meningitis and detected antigen in the CSF of 5 out of 12 patients.[87] However, there may be false-positive results in patients with meningitis due to

other fungi. Tests detecting antibodies in the CSF against *Histoplasma* antigens are also useful in diagnosing CNS infection and are found in approximately 75 percent of cases. The antibody serological tests are not very specific and positive results can also be found in patients with other fungal infections or with bacterial meningitis. Perhaps the best way to diagnose CNS *Histoplasma* infections when cultures are negative is to do both of these tests, since at least one of the antigen and antibody assays were found to be positive in 13 of 14 episodes of *Histoplasma* meningitis in one study.[87] In the absence of any other positive cultures or serologies, empiric treatment for *Histoplasma* should be started in patients with chronic meningitis of uncertain etiology when the *Histoplasma* antigen or antibody assays of the CSF are positive.

In coccidioidomycosis, elevated serum complement fixing antibody (CFA) titers above 1:32 to 1:64 are the hallmark of disseminated disease.[88] However, patients with meningitis only may have low serum CFA titers. In patients with coccidioidal meningitis, CFA titers are present in the CSF of 70 percent initially and in almost 100 percent of patients as the infection progresses. CFA is absent from unconcentrated CSF in the presence of high serum titers due to extraneural disease unless there is a parameningeal lesion next to the dura. The CFA titers appear to parallel the course of meningeal disease and have been used to guide treatment. The titers should fall with successful therapy.

The ability to detect specific antibodies in CSF has been used in the diagnosis of meningitis with *S. schenckii.*[89] Meningitis due to this particular organism is very difficult to diagnose and delays can occur for up to 7 months from the onset of symptoms when diagnosis is based on the results of cultures. Latex agglutination and enzyme immunoassay now have been used successfully to detect CSF antibodies and to confirm the diagnosis of *Sporothrix* meningitis. When a titer of 1:8 or more was used, there was no cross reaction with other fungal, bacterial, or viral pathogens.

There is intense interest is developing serological tests for other fungal infections, especially infections due to *Candida* and *Aspergillus*. Detection of unique antigens or metabolic products from these fungi have so far not been extensively used in the clinical setting of meningitis.

Imaging studies can be helpful in the diagnosis of

CNS fungal infections.[90,91] Localization of mass lesions or areas of meningeal inflammation by computed tomography (CT) or magnetic resonance imaging (MRI) can guide the neurosurgeon to areas for biopsy in selected cases. It appears that MRI with gadolinium (Gd-DTPA) enhancement is more sensitive than contrast CT scans.[92,93] In cases of fungal meningitis, CT scans and MRI are usually unremarkable but may show meningeal enhancement, hydrocephalus, atrophy, edema, or mass lesions.[94,95]

TREATMENT

Experience in the treatment of the various forms of fungal CNS infection is varied. Cryptococcal meningitis is one of the most intensively studied of all infectious diseases, whereas many fungal CNS infections are so rare that only a few cases have been described. In the treatment of fungal infections of the CNS, an important adjunct to antifungal therapy is the reversal, if possible, of any immunocompromising conditions. This may include decreasing doses of corticosteroids or the use of colony stimulating factors to increase leukocyte counts. Here, a short review of currently available antifungal agents is followed by recommendations for specific organisms.

Specific Antifungal Agents

AMPHOTERICIN B

Despite serious toxicities, the polyene antibiotic amphotericin B has been the "gold standard" in the treatment of disseminated mycoses for more than three decades. Amphotericin B has been used successfully to treat many cases of fungal meningitis, which is remarkable inasmuch as amphotericin B levels in the CSF during treatment are low or even unmeasurable.[96] These observations indicate that the drug may accumulate in the meninges to provide direct antifungal activity. Alternatively, the known immune stimulatory properties of amphotericin B may improve the host's CNS immune response. Because amphotericin B is poorly delivered to the subarachnoid space from the blood, it has occasionally been administered by direct injection into the CSF via lumbar or ventricular catheters. In doses up to 0.25 or 0.50 mg/d, intrathecal amphotericin B has been used to suppress coccidi-

oidal meningitis, treat overwhelming cryptococcal meningitis, and eliminate yeast from the CSF when previous intravenous administration has failed. However, intrathecal administration of amphotericin B carries certain major risks including arachnoiditis, vasculitis, and secondary bacterial infection of CSF catheters. There have been studies concerning the use of amphotericin B in various lipid complexes as a way to decrease the toxicity of this drug. Animal models and studies in limited numbers of human patients have shown that when compared to amphotericin B alone, higher doses of amphotericin B complexed with lipids can be given before significant toxicity is seen. However, it appears that higher doses of the lipid-complexed forms are necessary to achieve comparable clinical response rates to amphotericin B alone.[97] Currently, amphotericin B complexed with lipids is not commercially available in the United States. It can be obtained on a compassionate-use basis, and it seems reasonable to use one of the lipid formulations of this drug when a patient must receive amphotericin B but has severe toxicity associated with its administration.

FLUCYTOSINE

Flucytosine has been used to treat infections due to *Candida, Cryptococcus,* and chromoblastomycosis. It penetrates well into the subarachnoid space, with drug concentrations in the CSF approaching 75 percent of simultaneous serum levels. Despite its excellent pharmacokinetics, a problem with flucytosine when given alone in the treatment of CNS fungal infections is that fungi often develop resistance to it, resulting in treatment failure. Therefore, this agent is generally not used alone in CNS infections but rather in combination with other antifungals. Flucytosine has significant toxicity for the bone marrow, liver, and gastrointestinal tract. Toxicity can manifest as diarrhea, hepatitis, or potentially life-threatening bone marrow suppression. Flucytosine toxicity, especially bone marrow suppression, is usually related to serum concentrations of greater than 100 μg/ml. With the availability of assays to determine serum concentrations of flucytosine, there should be less reluctance to use this drug in patients with decreased bone marrow reserves because toxicity can be minimized by monitoring serum levels at least once during therapy, with repeated monitoring if renal function deteriorates.[98] Serum flucytosine concentrations 2 hours after a dose should be maintained between 30 and 100 µg/ml.

FLUCONAZOLE

Fluconazole is a triazole antifungal that has shown itself to have great potential in the treatment of many CNS fungal infections.[99] It has a favorable pharmacokinetic profile, and penetration into the CSF is excellent, with levels reaching 60 to 70 percent of those of serum.[100,101] Experience in treating cryptococcal meningitis with fluconazole in patients with AIDS is extensive and is reviewed below. Fluconazole has also been used successfully in cases of CNS infection due to *Candida, B. dermatitidis, C. immitis,* and *H. capsulatum.*[102]

ITRACONAZOLE

Itraconazole is another new triazole drug with a broad spectrum of in vitro activity.[99] This agent has limited penetration into the CSF, but in animal models and in limited numbers of human infections itraconazole has shown efficacy in CNS infections. It is thought that this agent may bind to host cells and be transported to the CNS sites of infection.[103] One of the main differences between itraconazole and fluconazole is in the activity of these agents against *Aspergillus* species.[104] Itraconazole is much more potent against *Aspergillus* and has been used in limited numbers in the treatment of CNS infections due to *Aspergillus* species. There is variable absorption of this drug; therefore, drug levels should be measured to ensure adequate serum concentrations.

KETOCONAZOLE

Ketoconazole is effective in treating a variety of deep-seated mycoses, including histoplasmosis, blastomycosis, and paracoccidioidomycosis. Despite reasonable in vitro activity against many fungi causing meningitis, poor penetration into the subarachnoid space has limited its use. Treatment with ketoconazole alone and in standard doses has failed in fungal meningitis. However, its efficacy may be improved by increasing the dosage to 1,200 mg/day, thus obtaining higher CSF drug levels, although toxicity may be a problem at these doses.[105] Some improvement in pa-

tients with coccidioidal meningitis was achieved using these high doses. Experiments in animals indicate that ketoconazole combined with either amphotericin B or flucytosine provides greater fungicidal effect in the CSF than any of these agents alone. However, no significant experience with these agents in combination in humans with fungal meningitis has been reported. Ketoconazole is available only in oral form, and absorption is decreased in patients with decreased gastric acidity.

MICONAZOLE

Experience with intravenous miconazole is limited in most forms of deep-seated mycoses. However, occasional successes and failures of miconazole in the treatment of fungal meningitis have been reported. Because miconazole does not penetrate well into the subarachnoid space, intrathecal miconazole has been used with some success.[106]

INVESTIGATIONAL REGIMENS

Combinations of antifungal drugs have been studied for the treatment of CNS infections in an attempt to obtain better results, shorter courses of therapy, and reduced toxicity of amphotericin B. Rifampin in combination with amphotericin B has shown increased activity against multiple yeasts when compared to amphotericin B alone in vitro.[107] There are few clinical data in humans to judge its effectiveness in treating CNS fungal infections, but rifampin does penetrate well into the subarachnoid space. There has been some interest in treating CNS fungal infections with a combination of polyene and azole antifungals.[108] There are no clinical data to support such combined regimens, but animal data have shown some additive effect from using amphotericin B and an azole together in treating cryptococcal meningitis. Current experience has shown that when amphotericin B and azoles are used in sequence, there is no detectable antagonism. Because of the prolonged treatment courses that must be used in CNS fungal infections, it is desirable to have an effective oral regimen. The combination of flucytosine and fluconazole has been presented as an oral regimen that may have clinical efficacy comparable to that of amphotericin B.[109] So far, the published experience with this combination in treating systemic fungal infections is limited, and its utility in CNS fungal infections has not been established.

SURGICAL TREATMENT OF CNS FUNGAL INFECTIONS

Neurosurgical procedures can have a very important role in the diagnosis and treatment of some CNS fungal infections.[110,111] Obtaining appropriate CSF or tissue samples for diagnosis using neurosurgical procedures may be required in some instances. In terms of treatment, the placement of CSF diverting shunts may be needed in cases of hydrocephalus or increased intracranial pressure. The placement of reservoirs to allow for chronic intrathecal administration of antifungals is sometimes required in certain CNS infections such as coccidioidal meningitis. Surgical resection of parenchymal lesions has been done to reduce mass effect in cases of *Histoplasma* and cryptococcal infection, but the presence of parenchymal lesions alone does not usually require their surgical removal. An exception to this is in infections due to *Cladosporium* species and other dematiaceous fungi. When these fungi cause mass lesions in the CNS, surgical resection is required for cure. Also, rhinocerebral infections due to zygomycetes require prompt debridement of necrotic tissue.[112]

Fungal infection of CSF shunts and reservoirs are rare and usually due to *Candida* species. Shunt infections should be treated with removal of the shunt and systemic antifungal therapy when possible. However, there are cases where shunt removal is not possible or when shunt placement occurs during periods of active meningitis. In our experience, we have been able to treat some cases of cryptococcal meningitis with amphotericin B and flucytosine in the presence of CSF diverting shunts, but we have also seen cases where removal of the shunt apparatus was required for cure. We recommend that in the setting of CNS fungal infection, CSF shunts should be removed when possible.

Treatment of Specific Fungi in the CNS

CRYPTOCOCCAL MENINGITIS

Prior to the availability of amphotericin B, cryptococcal meningitis was uniformly fatal, although an occasional untreated patient lived for years. Effective therapy is now available, but the optimal regimen is unknown. From early treatment trials it was shown that immunosuppressed patients with cryptococcal meningitis had higher treatment failure rates than immunocompetent patients. This was also true in patients with AIDS, who were found to have low response rates to initial therapy and very high relapse rates once therapy was stopped. Because there is this dichotomy in the patient population with cryptococcal meningitis, the treatment for patients with AIDS and those without AIDS is discussed separately.

Amphotericin B used alone at doses of 0.4 to 0.8 mg/kg/d to a total dose of 250 mg/kg remains as effective therapy for patients without HIV infection who develop cryptococcal meningitis. The addition of flucytosine to this regimen was tried in an effort to decrease both the duration of therapy and the total dose of amphotericin B. A collaborative trial compared amphotericin B 0.4 mg/kg/d for 10 weeks with amphotericin B 0.3 mg/kg/d plus flucytosine 150 mg/kg/d for 6 weeks.[113] The final outcome was similar in the two groups, suggesting that the addition of flucytosine to amphotericin B allows for shorter courses of therapy with lower doses of amphotericin B. Since this trial, there has been much experience using amphotericin B plus flucytosine as primary therapy in cryptococcal meningitis.[114] This combination usually sterilizes the CSF by 2 weeks and cures many patients within 4 to 6 weeks with manageable amphotericin B toxicity. Patients with good prognostic features and no known immunosuppressive conditions can be successfully managed with as little as 4 weeks of combined therapy. However, this regimen requires the administration of an intravenous medication for prolonged periods of time. The use of an orally active antifungal in cryptococcal meningitis is obviously very attractive, and both itraconazole and fluconazole have been used in this regard. There have been no large trials comparing azole antifungals to amphotericin B in patients without HIV infection. However, personal experience and extrapolated data from the trials with AIDS patients suggest that fluconazole can be used successfully as sole therapy for patients with cryptococcal meningitis but that it may not be as effective as amphotericin B plus flucytosine. Itraconazole has also been used successfully in treating cryptococcal meningitis,[115] but there is more experience with fluconazole and many physicians consider this the preferred azole agent. A compromise can be reached in an effort to reduce the amount of time needed for an intravenous line by using an "induction phase" of amphotericin B plus flucytosine followed by prolonged maintenance therapy with fluconazole or itraconazole. A combined regimen such as this should use amphotericin B at a dose of 0.5 to 0.7 mg/kg/d plus flucytosine at a dose to keep serum levels below 100 μg/ml for a total of 2 weeks, at which time the patient is switched to fluconazole at a daily dose of 400 to 800 mg, assuming normal creatinine clearance. A lumbar puncture should also be done at this time; if the CSF cultures still grow *C. neoformans,* treatment with amphotericin B and flucytosine should be reinstituted. If the CSF is sterile at 2 weeks after amphotericin B/flucytosine therapy, fluconazole can be continued. The duration of fluconazole therapy is tailored to the individual patient, but at least 8 weeks of treatment should be administered. Additional therapy may be required in patients with brain parenchymal lesions, persistent symptoms, concomitant immunosuppressive therapy, or underlying immunosuppressing diseases. The need for intraventricular or intrathecal amphotericin B in cryptococcal meningitis remains controversial. Some investigators have used intraventricular amphotericin B with success in cases with a poor prognosis. However, our experience is that this route of administration is rarely necessary.

Once therapy is started, the frequency of lumbar punctures should be determined by clinical response. A lumbar puncture done after the second week of therapy should show that the CSF is sterile if the combination of amphotericin B and flucytosine was used. Once therapy is completed, lumbar punctures should be performed, depending on the patient's signs and symptoms. Most relapses occur during the first 3 to 6 months after primary therapy. Persistently elevated antigen titers and positive India ink examinations indicate failure of therapy only when the CSF culture is positive or the patient has neurological deterioration. There is probably no value in following serial cryptococcal polysaccharide antigen titers.

The management of cryptococcal meningitis in patients with AIDS presents a major problem. Response to initial therapy in this group is poor, and the relapse rate is so high that for all intents and purposes a patient with AIDS and cryptococcal meningitis can never be assumed to be cured of the infection with present medical therapy. Recurrence of symptomatic

cryptococcal meningitis in patients with AIDS has been shown to be due to the same strain that caused the original infection,[116] and it is thought that the prostate or brain parenchyma can serve as a site for persistent infection despite sterilization of the CSF. The high rate of relapse in these patients has led to the routine institution of lifelong suppressive therapy for all patients with AIDS who respond to initial treatment for cryptococcal meningitis.

The regimen of choice in treating cryptococcal meningitis in patients with HIV infection is still undecided. A large clinical trial bearing on this issue was recently published. There were 194 eligible patients with AIDS-associated cryptococcal meningitis assigned to treatment with either amphotericin B at a mean daily dose of 0.4 mg/kg or fluconazole 200 mg daily after a one-time loading dose of 400 mg.[117] The results showed that there was no significant difference between the two drugs in terms of overall mortality. There was, however, a trend toward faster sterilization of the CSF and lower acute mortality with amphotericin B treatment. In this study, significant pretreatment factors predictive of death during therapy included abnormal mental status, CSF cryptococcal antigen titers greater than 1:1024, and CSF white cell count less than 20/mm³. These results show that fluconazole is an alternative to amphotericin B alone in patients with HIV infection and cryptococcal meningitis, but these regimens are far from optimal. Successful treatment rates for patients receiving amphotericin B or fluconazole in this study were only 40 and 34 percent respectively. Further studies are needed to determine if higher doses of fluconazole[118] or the combination of amphotericin B and flucytosine can give better results, especially in those patients presenting with poor prognostic signs. Many physicians are reluctant to use flucytosine in patients with AIDS, especially if they are receiving concomitant zidovudine therapy. However, as stressed above, flucytosine can be used with minimal side effects as long as serum levels are monitored and the dose is adjusted appropriately. It is our impression that an excellent regimen for treating AIDS-associated cryptococcal meningitis may be combination therapy similar to that described above for non-HIV infected patients, where patients are treated with the combination of amphotericin B and flucytosine for an induction period until the CSF is sterile and then switched to fluconazole at a daily dose of 400 to 800 mg for at least an additional 10 weeks. Once initial therapy is completed, the patient should be placed on lifelong suppressive therapy. There has been a large, controlled trial comparing weekly intravenous amphotericin B to oral fluconazole at a daily dose of 200 mg for suppressive therapy.[119] Fluconazole was significantly more effective than amphotericin B in preventing symptomatic relapses of cryptococcal meningitis. Serious drug toxicity and bacterial infections were both seen in significantly higher frequency in patients receiving amphotericin B. These data suggest that fluconazole may be the drug of choice for chronic suppressive therapy in patients with AIDS-related cryptococcal meningitis who have successfully responded to initial therapy. It should be stressed that we still have very little data to guide the use of chronic suppressive therapy for more than 1 year after infection. The present conservative approach has been to continue suppression for the duration of the patient's life, but further investigations of this policy are needed.

Increased intracranial pressure is a well-described problem in patients who are being treated for cryptococcal meningitis.[120] Symptoms in such patients usually begin shortly after initiation of antifungal therapy and include systemic hypertension, impaired consciousness, visual impairment, and cranial nerve palsies. These symptoms can occur suddenly, and head CT scans usually show no evidence for hydrocephalus or mass lesions. The opening pressure during lumbar puncture can be extremely high (exceeding 800 mmH$_2$O). Clinical improvement in patients with impaired consciousness may be rapid after lumbar puncture, and this procedure should be tried provided that there is no cerebral mass lesions.[121] The pathophysiology of increased intracranial pressure in this setting is uncertain but is suggestive of an outflow obstruction.[120] Repeated lumbar punctures or the placement of a CSF diverting shunt should be considered.[122] Acetazolamide and corticosteroids have also been used in an effort to decrease intracranial pressure.[123] However, visual loss in cryptococcal meningitis may not respond to maneuvers aimed at decreasing intracranial pressure. Visual loss is usually not due to endophthalmitis and is often bilateral and permanent.[124] Many treatments have been tried in an effort to restore vision, including repeat lumbar punctures, treatment with corticosteroids, fenestration of the optic nerve sheath, and release of perioptic nerve arachnoidal adhesions. Unfortunately, none of these approaches has been shown to be very effective.

Prognostic factors for patients with cryptococcal meningitis have been extensively studied.[125] In patients without HIV infection, the following clinical features were found to be associated with failure to respond to therapy with amphotericin B: (1) an initial positive India ink test; (2) high CSF opening pressure; (3) CSF leukocyte count less than 20/mm^3; (4) cryptococci isolated from extraneural sites; (5) initial CSF or serum cryptococcal antigen titer of 1:32 or more; and (6) corticosteroid therapy. However, the most important prognostic factor is the patient's underlying disease. Patients with cryptococcal meningitis and underlying malignancies or HIV infection have very low survival rates despite therapy. One study showed that the median overall survival for patients with AIDS was 9 months from diagnosis, compared with 2 months for patients with malignancies.[126] For patients with HIV infection, one study has found that significant prognostic factors for death during therapy included an abnormal mental status at presentation, a CSF cryptococcal antigen titer exceeding 1:1024, and a CSF leukocyte count below 20/mm^3.[117]

CANDIDA MENINGITIS

Treatment of *Candida* meningitis has received less attention than that of cryptococcal infection. There are reports of spontaneous cures of meningitis due to *Candida* species, but experience suggests that treatment is indicated in all of these patients. There is no consensus on the best regimen, but the combination of amphotericin B and flucytosine has synergistic activity against *Candida* in vitro. This combination has resulted in a high cure rate in our experience and in cases reported in the literature.

COCCIDIOIDAL MENINGITIS

In contrast to meningitis due to other fungi, the primary mode of treatment for coccidioidal meningitis has not been systemic but intraventricular amphotericin B. In these infections, systemic amphotericin B in total doses of 0.5 to 1.0 g are given mainly to treat undetected foci outside the CNS. Control of the CNS infection is then achieved by intraventricular administration of amphotericin B. Therapy is begun with small doses (0.01 mg/d) and increased gradually, as tolerated, up to 0.5 mg/d. The drug can be administered into the lumbar, cisternal, or ventricular space; the latter is preferred. Arachnoiditis, neurotoxicity, and secondary bacterial infections of the CSF can complicate therapy. Recommendations for length of therapy are variable, and because of the poor prognosis for complete cure, some patients have been treated indefinitely. The CSF leukocyte count has been used to follow progress and to judge the need for further therapy. Lowering of the CSF antibody titer is a good prognostic sign. During treatment, the clinician must watch continually for the development of hydrocephalus or superimposed bacterial infection. There has been some clinical benefit from using azole drugs. Miconazole and ketoconazole have been tried, but response has been only fair. Recent experience has focused on using fluconazole and itraconazole as therapy for coccidioidal meningitis. One recent article reported on the treatment of 47 patients with coccidioidal meningitis who were treated with 400 mg/d of fluconazole.[127] Response to therapy was seen in 37 patients and appeared to be unrelated to the presence of hydrocephalus or infection with HIV. Toxicity was minimal in patients treated for long periods of time. With this new data, it is now reasonable to consider fluconazole as a first-line treatment in patients with coccidioidal meningitis. Fluconazole's ease of administration and lack of toxicity when compared with intrathecal amphotericin B are important considerations. However, several important issues remain. The optimal dose of fluconazole is not known, and some authorities feel that 800 mg/d should be used. The use of induction therapy with intrathecal amphotericin B followed by indefinite azole therapy has also been proposed as a possible treatment strategy. Itraconazole has also been reported to be effective in patients with relapsing coccidioidal meningitis, but it is unknown what role this drug will have in treatment. Present strategies in treatment consider coccidioidal meningitis to be only suppressed by therapy and thus to require lifelong therapy.

OTHER FUNGI

Meningitis due to *Histoplasma, Sporothrix,* or *Blastomyces* usually responds to prolonged courses of amphotericin B. The role of azole drugs in these infections is not known. Infections of the CNS with *Aspergillus* species is usually fatal despite therapy. However, there are cases of successful therapy with high-dose amphotericin B. Our personal experience shows that some patients with CNS aspergillosis have responded to courses of high-dose amphotericin B followed by prolonged therapy with itraconazole.

REFERENCES

1. Pore RS, Chen J: Meningitis caused by Rhodotorula. Sabouraudia 14:331, 1976
2. Papadatos C, Pavlatou M, Alexiou D: Cephalosporium meningitis. Pediatrics 44:749, 1969
3. Naficy AB, Murray HW: Isolated meningitis caused by Blastoschizomyces capitatus. J Infect Dis 161:1041, 1990
4. Girmenia C, Micozzi A, Venditti M, et al: Fluconazole treatment of Blastoschizomyces capitatus meningitis in an allogeneic bone marrow recipient. Eur J Clin Microbiol Infect Dis 10:752, 1991
5. Surmount I, Vergauwen B, Marcelis L, et al: First report of chronic meningitis caused by Trichosporon beigelii. Eur J Clin Microbiol Infect Dis 9:226, 1990
6. Mukerji S, Patwardhan JR, Gadgil RK: Bacterial and mycotic infection of the brain. Indian J Med Sci 25:791, 1971
7. Chaves-Batista A, Mala JA, Singer P: Basidioneuromycosis in Man. p. 53. Institute of Mycology Publication No. 42. University of Recife, Brazil, 1955
8. Fagerburg R, Suh B, Buckley HR, et al: Cerebrospinal fluid shunt colonization and obstruction by Paecilomyces varioti. J Neurosurg 54:257, 1981
9. Moore M, Russell WO, Sachs E: Chronic leptomeningitis and ependymitis caused by Ustilago, probably U. zeae (corn smut); ustilagomycosis, second reported instance of human infection. Am J Pathol 22:761, 1946
10. Busse O: Uber parasitare zelleinschlusse und ihre zuchtung. Zentralbl Bakteriol 16:175, 1894
11. Hansemann D: Uber eine bisher nicht beobachtete gehirner Krankung durch Hefe. Verh Dtsch Ges Pathol 9:21, 1905
12. Fraser DW, Ward JI, Ajello L, et al: Aspergillosis and systemic mycosis. JAMA 242:1631, 1979
13. Dismukes WE: Cryptococcal meningitis in patients with AIDS. J Infect Dis 157:624, 1988
14. Ellis D, Pfeiffer T: The ecology of Cryptococcus neoformans. Eur J Epidemiol 8:321, 1992
15. Bronnimann DA, Galgiani JN: Coccidioidomycosis. Eur J Clin Microbiol Infect Dis 8:466, 1989
16. Taylor GD, Boettger DW, Miedzinski LJ, Tyrrell DL: Coccidioidal meningitis acquired during holidays in Arizona. Can Med Assoc J 142:1388, 1990

17. Leznoff A: Histoplasmosis in Montreal during the fall of 1963, with observation on erythema multiforme. Can Med Assoc J 91:1154, 1964

18. Wheat LJ, Slama TG, Eitzer HE, et al: A large urban outbreak of histoplasmosis: clinical features. Ann Intern Med 94:331, 1981

19. Wheat LJ: Diagnosis and management of histoplasmosis. Eur J Clin Microbiol Infect Dis 8:480, 1989

20. Leggiadro RJ, Luedtke GS, Convey A, et al: Prevalence of histoplasmosis in a midsouthern population. South Med J 84:1360, 1991

21. Davies SF, Sarosi GA: Blastomycosis. Eur J Clin Microbiol Infect Dis 8:474, 1989

22. Gonyea EF: The spectrum of primary blastomycotic meningitis: a review of central nervous system blastomycosis. Ann Neurol 3:26, 1978

23. Buechner HA, Clawson C: Blastomycosis of the central nervous system: II. A report of nine cases from the Veterans Administration Cooperative Study. Am Rev Resp Dis 95:820, 1967

24. Pitrak DL, Andersen BR: Cerebral blastomycoma after ketoconazole therapy for respiratory tract blastomycosis. Am J Med 86:713, 1989

25. San-Blas G: Paracoccidioidomycosis and its etiologic agent Paracoccidioides brasiliensis. J Med Vet Mycol 31:99, 1993

26. Parker JC, McCloskey JJ, Lee RS: The emergence of candidosis: the dominant postmortem cerebral mycosis. Am J Clin Pathol 70:31, 1978

27. Buchs S, Pfister P: Candida meningitis: course, prognosis and mortality before and after introduction of the new antimycotics. Mykosen 26:73, 1983

28. Jamjoom A, Jamjoom ZA, Al-Hedaithy S, et al: Ventriculitis and hydrocephalus caused by Candida albicans successfully treated by antimycotic therapy and cerebrospinal fluid shunting. Br J Neurosurg 6:501, 1992

29. Lammens M, Robberecht W, Waer M, et al: Purulent meningitis due to aspergillosis in a patient with systemic lupus erythematosus. Clin Neurol Neurosurg 94:39, 1992

30. Murai H, Kira J, Kobayashi T, et al: Hypertrophic cranial pachymeningitis due to Aspergillus flavus. Clin Neurol Neurosurg 94:247, 1992

31. Escobar A, Del Brutto OH: Multiple brain abscesses from isolated cerebral mucormycosis. J Neurol Neurosurg Psychiatry 53:431, 1990

32. McLean CA, Lieschke GJ, Gonzales MF: Test and teach. Number 61. Diagnosis: Cerebral and cerebellar infarctions due to mucormycosis with secondary hydrocephalus. Pathology 21:279, 1989

33. Durieu I, Parent M, Ajana F, et al: Monosporium apiospermum meningoencephalitis: a clinico-pathological case. J Neurol Neurosurg Psychiatry 54:731, 1991

34. Hachimi-Idrissi S, Willemsen M, Desprechins B, et al: Pseudallescheria boydii and brain abscesses. Pediatr Infect Dis J 9:737, 1990

35. Kershaw P, Freeman R, Templeton D, et al: Pseudallescheria boydii infection of the central nervous system. Arch Neurol 47:468, 1990

36. Heney C, Song E, Kellen A, et al: Cerebral phaeohyphomycosis caused by Xylohypha bantiana. Eur J Clin Microbiol Infect Dis 8:984, 1989

37. Sekhon AS, Galbraith J, Mielke BW, et al: Cerebral phaeohyphomycosis caused by Xylohypha bantiana, with a review of the literature. Eur J Epidemiol 8:387, 1992

38. Tintelnot K, de Hoog GS, Thomas E, et al: Cerebral phaeohyphomycosis caused by an Exophiala species. Mycoses 34:239, 1991

39. Sides EH, Benson JD, Padhye AA: Phaeohyphomycotic brain abscess due to Ochroconis gallopavum in a patient with malignant lymphoma of a large cell type. J Med Vet Mycol 29:317, 1991

40. Boelaert JR, Fenves AZ, Coburn JW: Deferoxamine therapy and mucormycosis in dialysis patients: report of an international registry. Am J Kidney Dis 18:660, 1991

41. Carrazana EJ, Rossitch E, Morris J: Isolated central nervous system aspergillosis in the acquired immunodeficiency syndrome. Clin Neurol Neurosurg 93:227, 1991

42. Woods GL, Goldsmith JC: Aspergillus infection of the central nervous system in patients with acquired immunodeficiency syndrome. Arch Neurol 47:181, 1990

43. Ankobiah WA, Vaidya K, Powell S, et al: Disseminated histoplasmosis in AIDS. NY State J Med 90:234, 1990

44. Galgiani JN, Ampel NM: Coccidioides immitis in patients with human immunodeficiency virus infections. Semin Respir Infect 5:151, 1990

45. Tolkoff-Rubin NE, Rubin RH: Clinical approach to viral and fungal infections in the renal transplant patient. Semin Nephrol 12:364, 1992

46. Hagensee M, Bauwens JE: Etiology of brain abscesses in bone marrow transplant patients. Abstract No. 843. 32nd Interscience Conference on Antimicrobioal Agents and Chemotherapy, October 1992

47. Mohrmann RL, Mah V, Vinters HV: Neuropathologic findings after bone marrow transplantation: an autopsy study. Hum Pathol 21:630, 1990

48. Boon AP, Adams DH, Buckels J, McMaster P: Cerebral aspergillosis in liver transplantation. J Clin Pathol 43:114, 1990

49. Morwood DT, Nichter LS, Wong V: An unusual complication of an open-head injury: coccidioidal meningitis. Ann Plast Surg 23:437, 1989

50. Shapiro S, Javed T, Mealey J: Candida albicans shunt infection. Pediatr Neurosci 15:125, 1989

51. Gower DJ, Crone K, Alexander E, Kelly DL: Candida albicans shunt infection: report of two cases. Neurosurgery 19:111, 1986

52. Ashpole RD, Jacobson K, King AT, Holmes AE: Cysto-peritoneal shunt infection with Trichosporon beigelii. Br J Neurosurg 5:515, 1991

53. Walter EB, Gingras JL, McKinney RE: Systemic Torulopsis glabrata infection in a neonate. South Med J 83:837, 1990

54. Ingram CW, Haywood HB, Morris VM, et al: Cryptococcal ventriculo-peritoneal shunt infection: clinical and epidemiological evaluation of two closely associated cases. Infect Control Hosp Epidemiol 14:719, 1993

55. Yadav SS, Perfect JR, Friedman AH: Successful treatment of cryptococcal ventriculoatrial shunt infection with systemic therapy alone. Neurosurgery 23:372, 1988

56. Takeshita M, Izawa M, Kubo O, et al: Aspergillotic aneurysm formation of cerebral artery following neurosurgical operation. Surg Neurol 38:146, 1992

57. Komatsu Y, Narushima K, Kobayashi E, et al: Aspergillus mycotic aneurysm—case report. Neurol Med Chir (Tokyo) 31:346, 1991

58. Sharma RR, Gurusinghe NT, Lynch PG: Cerebral infarction due to aspergillus arteritis following glioma surgery. Br J Neurosurg 6:485, 1992

59. Cohen MS, Isturiz RE, Malech HL, et al: Fungal infection in chronic granulomatous disease. Am J Med 71:59, 1981

60. Fleischmann J, Church JA, Lehrer RI: Case report: primary Candida meningitis and chronic granulomatous disease. Am J Med Sci 291:334, 1986

61. Smego RA, Devoe PW, Sampson HA, et al: Candida meningitis in two children with severe combined immunodeficiency. J Pediatr 104:902, 1984

62. Snider WD, Simpson DM, Nielsen S, et al: Neurological complications of the acquired immune deficiency syndrome: analysis of 50 patients. Ann Neurol 14:403, 1983

63. Oleske J, Minnefor A, Cooper R, et al: Immune deficiency syndrome in children. JAMA 249:2345, 1983

64. Bruinsma-Adams IK: AIDS presenting as Candida albicans meningitis: a case report. AIDS 5:1268, 1991

65. Gelfand MS, McGee ZA, Kaiser AB, et al: Candidal meningitis following bacterial meningitis. South Med J 83:567, 1990

66. Kwon-Chung KJ, Kozel TR, Edman JC, et al: Recent advances in the biology and immunology of Cryptococcus neoformans. J Med Vet Mycol 30, suppl 1: 133, 1992

67. Zuger A, Louie E, Holzman RS: Cryptococcal disease in patients with acquired immunodeficiency syndrome. Ann Intern Med 104:234, 1986

68. Vincent T, Galgiani JN, Huppert M, Salkin D: The natural history of coccidioidal meningitis: VA–Armed Forces cooperative studies, 1955–1958. Clin Infect Dis 16:247, 1993

69. Ampel NM, Dols CL, Galgiani JN: Coccidioidomycosis during human immunodeficiency virus infection: results of a prospective study in a coccidioidal endemic area. Am J Med 94:235, 1993

70. Pappas PG, Dismukes WE: Blastomyces dermatitidis as an opportunistic pathogen: a review of 24 cases of blastomycosis in immunocompromised patients. Abstract No. 836. 32nd Interscience Conference on Antimicrobial Agents and Chemotherapy, October 1992

71. Kauffman CA, Israel KS, Smith JW, et al: Histoplasmosis in immunosuppressed patients. Am J Med 64: 923, 1978

72. Dantas AM, Yamane R, Camara AG: South American blastomycosis: ophthalmic and oculomotor nerve lesions. Am J Trop Med Hyg 43:386, 1990

73. Penn CC, Goldstein E, Bartholomew WR: Sporothrix schenckii meningitis in a patient with AIDS. Clin Infect Dis 15:741, 1992

74. Shaw JC, Levinson W, Montanaro A: Sporotrichosis in the acquired immunodeficiency syndrome. J Am Acad Dermatol 21:1145, 1989

75. Gerson SL, Talbot GH, Hurwitz S, et al: Prolonged granulocytopenia: the major risk factor for invasive pulmonary aspergillosis in patients with acute leukemia. Ann Intern Med 100:345, 1984

76. Cravens G, Robertson H, Banta C, et al: Spinal cord compression due to intradural extramedullary aspergilloma and cyst: a case report. Surg Neurol 31:315, 1989

77. Beeson PB: Cryptococcal meningitis of nearly sixteen years' duration. Arch Intern Med 89:797, 1952

78. Campbell GD, Currier RD, Busey JF: Survival in untreated cryptococcal meningitis. Neurology 31:1154, 1981

79. Rosen E, Belber JP: Coccidioidal meningitis of long duration: report of a case of four years and eight months duration with necropsy findings. Ann Intern Med 34:796, 1951

80. Norman DD, Miller ZR: Coccidioidomycosis of the central nervous system: a case of ten years' duration. Neurology 4:713, 1954

81. Gelfand JA, Bennett JE: Active Histoplasma meningitis of 22 years' duration. JAMA 233:1294, 1975

82. Ellner JJ, Bennett JE: Chronic meningitis. Medicine (Baltimore) 55:341, 1976

83. Weller PF: Eosinophilic meningitis. Am J Med 95: 250, 1993

84. Gonyea EF: Cisternal puncture and cryptococcal meningitis. Arch Neurol 28:200, 1973

85. Nelson MR, Bower M, Smith D, et al: The value of serum cryptococcal antigen in the diagnosis of cryptococcal infection in patients infected with the human immunodeficiency virus. J Infect 21:175, 1990

86. Currie BP, Freundlich LF, Soto MA, Casadevall A: False-negative cerebrospinal fluid cryptococcal latex agglutination tests for patients with culture-positive cryptococcal meningitis. J Clin Microbiol 31:2519, 1993

87. Wheat LJ, Kohler RB, Tewari RP, et al: Significance of Histoplasma antigen in the cerebrospinal fluid of patients with meningitis. Arch Intern Med 149:302, 1989

88. Pappagianis D, Zimmer BL: Serology of coccidioidomycosis. Clin Microbiol Rev 3:247, 1990

89. Scott EN, Kaufman L, Brown AC, Muchmore HG: Serologic studies in the diagnosis and management of meningitis due to Sporothrix schenckii. N Engl J Med 317:935, 1987

90. Shuper A, Levitsky HI, Cornblath DR: Early invasive CNS aspergillosis: an easily missed diagnosis. Neuroradiology 33:183, 1991

91. Wehn SM, Heinz ER, Burger PC, Boyko OB: Dilated Virchow-Robin spaces in cryptococcal meningitis associated with AIDS: CT and MR findings. J Comput Assist Tomogr 13:756, 1989

92. Chang KH, Han MH, Roh JK, et al: Gd-DTPA-enhanced MR imaging of the brain in patients with meningitis: comparison with CT. AJNR 11:69, 1990

93. Takasu A, Taneda M, Otuki H, et al: Gd-DTPA-enhanced MR imaging of cryptococcal meningoencephalitis. Neuroradiology 33:443, 1991

94. Terk MR, Underwood DJ, Zee C, Colletti PM: MR imaging in rhinocerebral and intracranial mucormycosis with CT and pathologic correlation. Magn Res Imaging 10:81, 1992

95. Mathews VP, Smith RR: Choroid plexus infections: neuroimaging appearances of four cases. AJNR 13: 374, 1992

96. Bindschadler DD, Bennett JE: A pharmacologic guide to the clinical use of amphotericin B. J Infect Dis 120: 427, 1969

97. Perfect JR, Wright KA: Amphotericin B lipid complex in the treatment of experimental cryptococcal meningitis and disseminated candidiasis. J Antimicrob Chemother, in press

98. Francis P, Walsh TJ: Evolving role of flucytosine in immunocompromised patients: new insights into safety, pharmacokinetics, and antifungal therapy. Clin Infect Dis 15:1003, 1992

99. Bodey GP: Azole antifungal agents. Clin Infect Dis 14, suppl 1:S161, 1992

100. Byers M, Chapman S, Feldman S, Parent A: Fluconazole pharmacokinetics in the cerebrospinal fluid of a child with Candida tropicalis meningitis. Pediatr Infect Dis J 11:895, 1992

101. Debruyne D, Ryckelynck JP: Clinical pharmacokinetics of fluconazole. Clin Pharmacokinet 24:10, 1993

102. Sugar AM, Anaissie EJ, Graybill JR, Patterson TF: Fluconazole. J Med Vet Mycol 30, suppl 1:201, 1992

103. Perfect JR, Savani DV, Durack DT: Uptake of itraconazole by alveolar macrophages. Antimicrob Agents Chemother 37:903, 1993

104. Denning DW, Tucker RM, Hanson LH, Stevens DA: Treatment of invasive aspergillosis with itraconazole. Am J Med 86:791, 1989

105. Craven PC, Graybill JR, Jorgensen JH, et al: High-dose ketoconazole for treatment of fungal infections of the central nervous system. Ann Intern Med 98: 160, 1983

106. Graybill JR, Levine HB: Successful treatment of cryptococcal meningitis with intraventricular miconazole. Ann Intern Med 138:814, 1978

107. Medoff G, Kobayashi GS, Kwan CN, et al: Potentiation of rifampicin and 5-fluorocytosine as antifungal antibiotics by amphotericin B. Proc Natl Acad Sci USA 69:196, 1972

108. Cosgrove RF, Beezer AE, Miles RJ: In vitro studies of amphotericin B in combination with the imidazole antifungal compounds clotrimazole and miconazole. J Infect Dis 138:681, 1978

109. Allendoerfer R, Marquis AJ, Rinaldi MG, Graybill JR: Combined therapy with fluconazole and flucytosine in murine cryptococcal meningitis. Antimicrob Agents Chemother 35:726, 1991

110. Young RF, Gade G, Grinnell V: Surgical treatment for fungal infection in the central nervous system. J Neurosurg 63:371, 1985

111. Chan KH, Mann KS, Yue CP: Neurosurgical aspects of cerebral cryptococcosis. Neurosurgery 25:44, 1989

112. Karam F, Chmel H: Rhino-orbital cerebral mucormycosis. Ear Nose Throat J 69:187, 1990

113. Bennett JE, Dismukes W, Duma R, et al: A comparison of amphotericin B alone and combined with flucytosine in the treatment of cryptococcal meningitis. N Engl J Med 301:126, 1979

114. Dismukes WE, Cloud G, Gallis HA, et al: Treatment of cryptococcal meningitis with combination amphotericin B and flucytosine in 194 patients with cryptococcal meningitis. N Engl J Med 317:334, 1987

115. Denning DW, Tucker RM, Hanson LH, et al: Itraconazole therapy for cryptococcal meningitis and cryptococcosis. Arch Intern Med 149:2301, 1989

116. Spitzer ED, Spitzer SG, Freundlich LF, Casadevall A: Persistence of initial infection in recurrent Cryptococcus neoformans meningitis. Lancet 341:595, 1993

117. Saag MS, Powderly WG, Cloud GA, et al: Comparison of amphotericin B with fluconazole in the treatment of acute AIDS-associated cryptococcal meningitis. N Engl J Med 326:83, 1992

118. Berry AJ, Rinaldi MG, Graybill JR: Use of high-dose fluconazole as salvage therapy for cryptococcal meningitis in patients with AIDS. Antimicrob Agents Chemother 36:690, 1992

119. Powderly WG, Saag MS, Cloud GA, et al: A controlled trial of fluconazole or amphotericin B to prevent relapse of cryptococcal meningitis in patients with the acquired immunodeficiency syndrome. N Engl J Med 326:793, 1992

120. Denning DW, Armstrong RW, Lewis BH, Stevens DA: Elevated cerebrospinal fluid pressures in patients with cryptococcal meningitis and acquired immunodeficiency syndrome. Am J Med 91:267, 1991

121. Van Gemert HMA, Vermeulen M: Treatment of impaired consciousness with lumbar puncture in a patient with cryptococcal meningitis and AIDS. Clin Neurol Neurosurg 93:257, 1991

122. Tang LM: Ventriculoperitoneal shunt in cryptococcal meningitis with hydrocephalus. Surg Neurol 33:314, 1990

123. Johnston SRD, Corbett EL, Foster O, et al: Raised intracranial pressure and visual complications in AIDS patients with cryptococcal meningitis. J Infect 24:185, 1992

124. Rex JH, Larsen RA, Bennett JE: Catastrophic visual loss due to Cryptococcus neoformans meningitis. Abstract No. 842. 32nd Interscience Conference on Antimicrobial Agents and Chemotherapy, October 1992

125. Diamond RD, Bennett JE: Prognostic factors in cryptococcal meningitis: a study of 111 cases. Ann Intern Med 80:176, 1974

126. White M, Cirrincione C, Blevins A, Armstrong D: Cryptococcal meningitis: outcome in patients with AIDS and patients with neoplastic disease. J Infect Dis 165:960, 1992

127. Galgiani JN, Catanzaro A, Cloud GA, et al: Fluconazole therapy for coccidioidal meningitis. Ann Intern Med 119:28, 1993

41

Parasitic Infections of the Central Nervous System

Robert A. Salata
Charles H. King
Adel A. F. Mahmoud

Protozoa and helminths are unique infectious agents which contribute significantly to human morbidity and mortality. Although these agents are referred to as parasites, implying a dependent way of life, they are in this context no different from other infectious agents such as bacteria or viruses. However, protozoa differ biologically from metazoa or helminths. Protozoa are single-cell, generally microscopic animals that characteristically undergo multiplication in the mammalian host. In contrast, helminths are multicellular, vary tremendously in size, and in general are not capable of multiplying within the mammalian or definitive host, although exceptions exist.

Protozoa and helminths have complex life cycles and have adapted to exist within the hostile environment of one and sometimes several hosts. The distribution of these infectious agents parallels the poor socioeconomic conditions in the developing world. Some infections, however, are now becoming clinically significant to immunosuppressed patients worldwide. Central to the approach to the patient with central nervous system (CNS) infection with a protozoan or helminthic organism is a thorough geographic history and an increased index of suspicion.

Once such an infection is suspected, appropriate diagnostic tests should be helpful.

The following descriptions are organized to include the disease entities summarized in Table 41-1.

PROTOZOAN INFECTIONS

Cerebral Malaria

During the past 15 years there has been a major resurgence of malaria,[1] and this mosquito-borne infection is the leading parasitic cause of death worldwide.[1-3] Of the four species of *Plasmodium* that infect humans, *P. falciparum* causes the most significant morbidity and mortality. More than 80 percent of the fatal cases of *P. falciparum* malaria are associated with cerebral involvement.[4-6]

Malaria is estimated to have a worldwide prevalence of more than 200 million cases per year and, in Africa alone, more than 1 million malaria-related deaths occur annually.[1-3] Infection is widely distributed (Fig. 41-1), with *P. falciparum* predominating in Africa, Haiti, New Guinea, Southeast Asia, South America, and Oceania. Cases of malaria in the United

Table 41-1 Parasitic Infections of the CNS

Organism	Geographic Distribution	Major CNS Syndromes	Mode of Infection	CNS Pathological Stage
Protozoa				
Plasmodium falciparum	Africa, Haiti, South America, SE Asia, Oceania	Encephalopathy, coma, seizures	Mosquito	Merozoite
Toxoplasma gondii	Cosmopolitan	Congenital: retinopathy, intracranial calcification, mental retardation, seizures Immunocompromised: encephalitis, meningoencephalitis, mass lesions	Fecal-oral	Tachyzoite
Trypanosoma brucei, T. gambiense, T. rhodesiense	Northern and western sub-Saharan Africa, Eastern Equatorial Africa	Personality changes, indifference, stupor and coma in late stages	Tsetse flies	Procyclic form
Naegleria fowleri, Acanthamoeba species	Southern US, Australia, Great Britain, Czechoslovakia	Acute, subacute, chronic meningoencephalitis	Fresh water	Trophozoite
Entamoeba histolytica	Africa, Mexico, South America, India, SE Asia	Brain abscess	Fecal-oral	Trophozoite
Helminths				
Taenia solium	Cosmopolitan	Neurocysticerosis seizures, hydrocephalus, chronic meningitis	Fecal-oral	Intermediate tissue cyst
Echinococcus granulosus	Cosmopolitan	CNS hydatidosis	Fecal-oral	Intermediate tissue cyst
Echinococcus multicocularis	Arctic	CNS hydatidosis	Fecal-oral	Intermediate tissue cyst
Spirometra species	Cosmopolitan	Sparganosis	Ingestion of uncooked meat	Intermediate tissue cyst
Strongyloides stercoralis	Tropics, subtropics	Polymicrobial meningitis, encephalitis	Autoinfection	Filariform larvae
Trichinella spiralis	Cosmopolitan	Seizures, meningoencephalitis	Uncooked meat	Cysts of immature larvae
Angiostrongylus cantonensis	Asia, Africa, Pacific, Cuba	Eosinophilic meningitis	Uncooked snails, crustacea	Developing adult
Gnatnostoma spingnerum	Asia, India, Israel	Eosinophilic meningitis	Uncooked fish, frog, bird, snake	Developing adult
Toxocara species	Cosmopolitan	Seizures, palsies, retinal mass	Fecal-oral	Developing adult
Onchocerca volvulus	Africa, South America, Central America, Yemen	Retinopathy, keratitis	Black fly	Microfilariae
Loa loa	Africa	Encephalopathy	Deerfly	Microfilariae
Schistosome species	Africa, Asia, Brazil	Seizures, cerebritis, tumor, spinal cord compression	Exposure to infected fresh water	Eggs
Paragonimus species	Asia, Central & South America	Meningitis, mass lesion, infarction	Uncooked crustacea	Maturing adult
Fasciola	Cosmopolitan	As per *Paragonimus* spp.	Uncooked water plants	Maturing adult

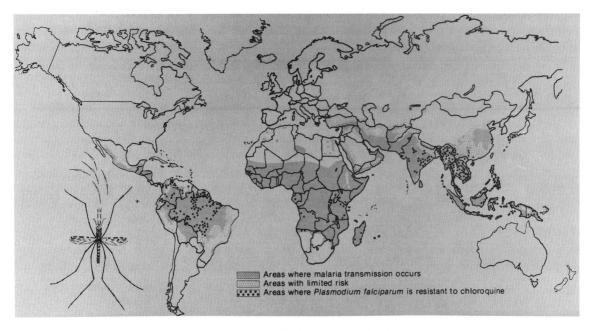

Fig. 41-1 Worldwide distribution of malaria.

States are either imported or transfusion-associated.[7-12] Currently, the growing number of cases of malaria seen in the United States is related to greater numbers of travelers to and immigrants from malarial areas.[7-10]

During this century, the history of malaria has been dominated by efforts directed at controlling the vector and developing antimalarial agents. In 1976, the World Health Organization abandoned a worldwide malaria eradication program because of the development of resistance to DDT by the vectors and resistance to chloroquine by *P. falciparum*.[1] Most recent efforts have been directed at seeking newer approaches, such as vaccines.[13]

Four species of malaria infect humans: *P. falciparum, P. vivax, P. ovale* and *P. malariae*.[2-3] The infective sporozoites are injected by female anopheline mosquitoes into subcutaneous tissue and thereafter circulate to the liver to invade hepatocytes. Parasites multiply and after 1 to 2 weeks schizonts rupture and release thousands of merozoites, which then enter the bloodstream to infect erythrocytes. All exoerythrocytic forms of *P. falciparum* rupture at about the same time, and none persist chronically in the liver.

Invasion of erythrocytes by merozoites requires specific surface receptors on the parasite and erythrocyte. *P. falciparum* requires glycoporin, the major surface glycoprotein on erythrocytes, for infection.[14,15] *P. falciparum* can develop in erythrocytes of all ages, and parasitemia can reach high levels; the magnitude of parasitemia relates to morbidity and mortality.[1-5,16,17]

Within the erythrocyte, merozoites develop eventually into schizonts, which rupture to release merozoites capable of infecting new erythrocytes. Only the asexual erythrocytic stages are directly deleterious to the host, and the mechanisms involved in the development of clinical manifestations are related to fever, anemia, tissue hypoxia, and immunopathological events (both humoral and cell-mediated).[1-3] A number of serious complications can occur in *P. falciparum* malaria, including acute renal failure, pulmonary edema, and cerebral malaria.[1-6,16-19] The exact mechanisms underlying these complications are unknown, but all are associated with tissue hypoxia.[16]

Cerebral malaria occurs in 0.5 to 1 percent of *P. falciparum* cases, and 20 to 50 percent of patients with cerebral malaria die.[20,21] Sequestration of parasitized erythrocytes within the capillaries of the central cortex is typically observed (Figs. 41-2 and 41-3).[4-6] Such sequestration may result from an interaction between vascular endothelial cells and protrusions

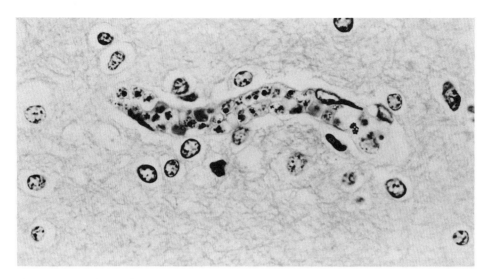

Fig. 41-2 Cerebral malaria: sequestration of parasitized erythrocytes in a cerebral capillary. (Hematoxylin and eosin; original magnification × 840.)

(knobs) of the parasitized erythrocytes due to specific receptors or possibly as a result of endothelial cell damage.[22,23] One mediator of endothelial cell damage is tumor necrosis factor (TNF).[24] In a murine model of cerebral malaria, TNF was essential for the histopathology and acute neurological manifestations.[25] It has been hypothesized that in human cases, erythrocyte sequestration may result subsequent to TNF-mediated vascular changes. Increased serum TNF levels have been measured in malaria patients.[25] There is some evidence that human cerebral malaria is related to the release of toxic products (such as nitrous oxide) and subsequent increased permeability of the blood-brain barrier. Few patients with cerebral malaria have cerebral edema on computed tomography (CT) scans[25] or increased intracranial pressure as measured

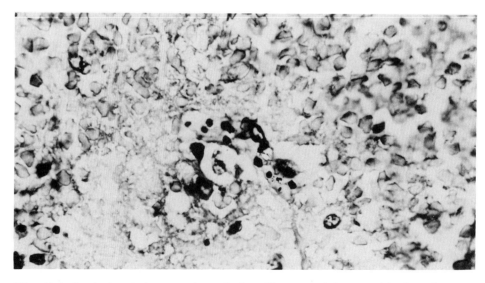

Fig. 41-3 Cerebral malaria: necrotic cerebral capillary containing parasitized erythrocytes and surrounded by a ring hemorrhage. (Hematoxylin and eosin; original magnification × 840.)

at lumbar puncture,[20,26–28] and no abnormalities in blood-brain barrier function have been identified.[29]

High fever and rigors are the hallmarks of acute malaria. A prodrome may occur with malaise, headache, myalgias, and fatigue that may mimic viral illness.[30] Other manifestations may include backache, arthralgia, abdominal pain, nausea, vomiting, cough, tachypnea, lethargy, and frank delirium. Fever commonly rises to 105°F and may remain elevated between paroxysms of P. falciparum infection. On examination, patients are frequently found to have splenomegaly and tender hepatomegaly. Lymphadenopathy is not a feature, and its presence should prompt investigation of an alternative etiology.[2,3,30]

Cerebral malaria occurring with P. falciparum infection may present with seizures, disturbances of consciousness, acute delirium, meningismus, and infrequently focal neurological findings, including pyramidal signs or movement disorders.[2,3,16,20] Other causes of encephalopathy must be excluded, and biochemical screening tests of the blood and examination of the cerebrospinal fluid (CSF) are mandatory. Hypoglycemia may occur as a complication of P. falciparum malaria, especially in pregnant patients or in association with severe disease, and may be responsible for deteriorating neurological status.[31]

The diagnosis of malaria rests primarily on the demonstration of parasites on peripheral blood smears.[2,3,32,33] Although a higher degree of parasitemia is expected during paroxysms, the time of obtaining blood smears is less important than that smears be collected several times daily and on several successive days. Efforts to quantify malarial forms are useful in assessing severity of disease and response to antimalarial therapy. A high degree of parasitemia, seen with P. falciparum malaria, is considered to exist when 5 percent of erythrocytes are infected.[2,3] Once parasites have been detected, species can be determined. Serological tests are not reliable in establishing the diagnosis of malaria.

A variety of abnormalities in laboratory tests may be observed in cases of malaria, including a normocytic, normochromic hemolytic anemia, leukopenia, monocytosis, thrombocytopenia, minimal proteinuria, mild azotemia, and elevated liver enzymes.[2,3] With severe P. falciparum malaria, renal failure, pulmonary edema, and hypoglycemia may be observed.[31]

In cases of P. falciparum cerebral malaria, CSF examination occasionally reveals elevated protein concentration or mild pleocytosis.[20,26,27] Hypoglycorrhachia is not a feature. There is no consistent CT pattern, and cerebral edema occurs in only a few cases.[26]

Delay in diagnosis of P. falciparum infection may prove to be fatal[1–5,8] because patients who appear clinically stable may deteriorate rapidly if not treated. If P. falciparum infection is suspected, the patient should be hospitalized. One should ascertain if the patient has traveled to or resided in an area with chloroquine-resistant P. falciparum[34–36] of if adequate prophylaxis has been taken. Patients with P. falciparum malaria that is suspected to be chloroquine-resistant or with transfusion-associated malaria, and who are not desperately ill, should be treated with oral quinine sulfate, pyrimethamine, and a sulfonamide.[2,3,36,37] Oral quinine may cause cinchonism, characterized by tinnitus, headache, nausea, and visual disturbances. In patients allergic to pyrimethamine or sulfonamides, or for those who have come from areas where resistance to the antifolates has been reported (especially Southeast Asia), quinine should be given with tetracycline.[2,3,37–40] Alternative oral agents for treatment include mefloquine or halofantrine. The special problems related to treating malaria in children and pregnant women have been reviewed elsewhere.[1–3,32,41,42]

In patients with suspected chloroquine-resistant P. falciparum malaria with high parasitemia or major complications, quinidine gluconate[37,41,43–45] may be administered by continuous intravenous infusion (10 mg/kg load, then 0.02 mg/kg/min). This infusion is continued for 72 hours or discontinued sooner if parasitemia decreases to 1 percent or less. Parenteral quinidine may be cardiotoxic, and appropriate monitoring must be performed.

In cases of malaria due to other species or in cases of P. falciparum malaria where chloroquine resistance is not a concern, chloroquine phosphate may be administered. A parenteral preparation of chloroquine has been used successfully in patients unable to take oral medications.[46] After initiation of antimalarial therapy, patients with P. falciparum infection must be closely monitored for complications and response to treatment.

Given the problems with resistance and toxicity among currently available antimalarials, there is a need for continued development and evaluation of alternative drugs.[47] Qinghaosu, from a traditional Chinese herbal remedy, is undergoing extensive controlled clinical trials.[1-3,32,47-50]

Symptomatic treatment of cerebral malaria should include fluid restriction and efforts aimed at minimizing nosocomial complications. High doses of corticosteroids, which have been administered traditionally, should be avoided because a double-blind, prospective trial demonstrated prolonged coma and a higher incidence of complications in dexamethasone-treated patients.[20] In fulminant cases of *P. falciparum* malaria, exchange blood transfusion has been used as a lifesaving adjunctive measure.[51-53]

Cerebral Toxoplasmosis

Infection due to *Toxoplasma gondii* may be acute or chronic, symptomatic or asymptomatic; and it may affect both normal and immunocompromised hosts.[54-57] Involvement of the CNS and retina primarily occurs in immunodeficient individuals or in congenital infection.[57,58]

Toxoplasma infects all orders of mammals; cats appear to be associated with disease transmission.[59] In humans, anti-*Toxoplasma* antibodies increase with advancing age: seropositivity may reach 90 percent by the fourth decade of life.[54,55] The two major routes of transmission to humans are through congenital and oral routes. The more frequent route of infection is probably through ingestion of meats, vegetables, and other food products that have been contaminated with oocysts.[54-59] Other routes of transmission of toxoplasmosis that have been recognized include self-inoculation of organisms in laboratory workers,[60] transfusion of whole blood or leukocytes with organisms,[61] and organ transplantation.[62-66]

After cysts or oocysts are ingested by cats. *T. gondii* invades the intestinal epithelial cells. Millions of non-infective oocysts may then be released daily, becoming infective for up to 1 year after sporulation. Upon entry into humans, the tachyzoite form of the parasite disrupts host cells and disseminates via the lymph and blood systems. Tachyzoite invasion is associated with focal necrosis and intense mononuclear cell infiltration. Both humoral and cell-mediated immune responses can limit tachyzoite invasion.[54-58] The lack of antibody transfer to the eye and CNS may allow more widespread proliferation in these areas. Cysts

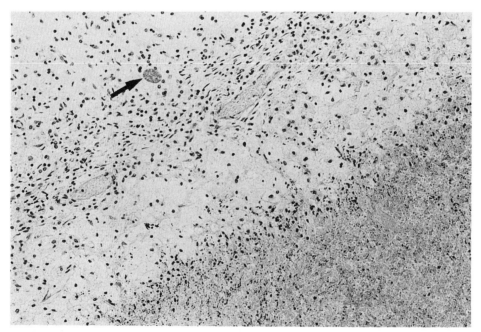

Fig. 41-4 Cerebral toxoplasmosis: a resolving lesion in a brain autopsy specimen from an AIDS patient. Mononuclear infiltrate is present, with the organism *(arrow)* visible at the periphery of the lesion. (Hematoxylin and eosin; original magnification × 140.)

that are established in numerous tissues and organs ordinarily elicit little or no inflammatory response but persist to serve as a potential reservoir for reactivation.[54-58] With congenital infection and in immunodeficient hosts, acute infection may produce severe and widespread necrosis and progress rapidly to involve the brain, lung, and heart, often resulting in death.[62-66]

Infection of the CNS may be associated with focal or diffuse necrotizing meningoencephalitis, with perivascular mononuclear cell proliferation that may or may not be associated with organisms (Fig. 41-4).[67] Infarction and hydrocephalus may result. Involvement of the eye with *Toxoplasma* may result in chorioretinitis characterized by severe inflammation and necrosis.[68,69]

Only 10 to 20 percent of adult cases of toxoplasmosis are symptomatic.[56] Nontender cervical adenopathy is most frequently seen, but generalized adenopathy may be present. In some cases adenopathy is accompanied by fever, night sweats, malaise, sore throat, rash, hepatosplenomegaly, and atypical lymphocytosis[70,71]; toxoplasmosis accounts for fewer than 1 percent of mononucleosis syndromes. In the immunocompetent individual, the course of toxoplasmosis is usually benign and self-limited. A form of the disease with persistent lymphadenopathy has been reported.[72] Rarely, normal individuals have progressive disseminated disease with CNS infection.

T. gondii is an important cause of chorioretinitis.[54,68,69,73,74] Most cases are a result of congenital infection, with occasional cases of reactivation disease seen in older individuals. The lesion is a focal, necrotizing retinitis with yellow-white patches. With healing, the lesions pale, atrophy, and often develop black pigment (Fig. 41-5).[75] Panuveitis may accompany chorioretinitis; papillitis is usually a sign of CNS involvement. There may be decreased visual acuity, scotoma, pain, photophobia, epiphora, and loss of central vision with macular involvement. Relapses of chorioretinitis are frequent, but they are rarely associated with systemic manifestations.[74]

Congenital infection results from asymptomatic infection of the mother during gestation. Infection developing in the mother prior to conception is not transmitted to the fetus.[58] Risk to the fetus increases with infection acquired later in pregnancy.[58] Signs and symptoms may be absent or may include chorioretinitis (bilateral), strabismus, blindness, epilepsy,

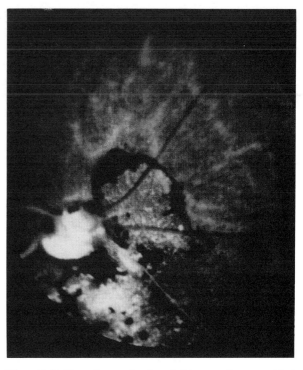

Fig. 41-5 *Toxoplasma* chorioretinitis: a pale, atrophied, black-pigmented lesion.

mental retardation, anemia, jaundice, rash, petechiae, encephalitis, pneumonitis, microcephaly, intracranial calcification, hydrocephalus, and hypothermia.[58] If clinical findings are apparent in the neonate, sequelae are usually severe. Most infants are without clinical evidence of infection at birth, and symptoms that develop later in life may be mild or severe.

Severe and often fatal toxoplasmosis has occurred in patients immunocompromised by treatment with corticosteroids or cytotoxic agents and in those with lymphoreticular malignancies, organ transplantation, or the acquired immunodeficiency syndrome (AIDS).[57,62-66,75-81] In these individuals, toxoplasmosis may be due to primary or reactivated disease. Most immunodeficient individuals with toxoplasmosis have disease of the CNS with encephalitis, meningoencephalitis, or mass lesions. Pneumonitis or myocarditis may also develop.[57,62-66,75-80]

In AIDS patients with cerebral mass lesions, toxoplasmosis is the most frequent etiology.[80] In AIDS patients, cerebral infection develops as a result of reactivation. In most instances, *Toxoplasma* encephalitis develops when the CD4 count falls below 100/mm³.

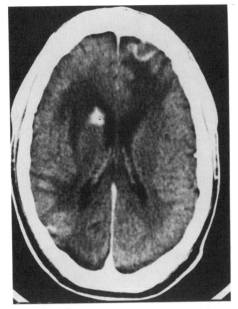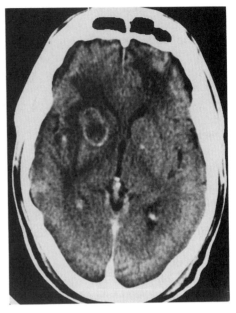

Fig. 41-6 Cerebral toxoplasmosis. CT scans from an AIDS patient demonstrate multiple, bilateral, enhancing hemispheric lesions with associated edema.

These patients most frequently have multifocal abscesses scattered throughout the cerebral hemispheres (Fig. 41-6) and present subacutely with focal neurological deficits.[79,80] The incidence of fever, new headache, seizures, and alterations in mental state has been variable.[75-80] Cerebral toxoplasmosis in AIDS patients is discussed further in Chapter 38.

The finding of *T. gondii* in blood or body fluids confirms acute infection. Most laboratories do not have the capacity to isolate *T. gondii*. The histological presence of tachyzoites also established the diagnosis of the acute form of toxoplasmosis.[58] The use of a peroxidase-antiperoxidase technique has been utilized with success to demonstrate tissue tachyzoites, particularly in the CNS of patients with AIDS.[80,82]

Serological testing for specific antibody against *T. gondii* is the primary means of diagnosis.[54,55] The Sabin-Feldman dye test, primarily measuring immunoglobulin G (IgG) antibodies, is both sensitive and specific.[83] Low titers may persist for life, and titers do not correlate with severity of infection.[83] The indirect fluorescent antibody test is easier to perform, safer, more economical than the dye test, and the most widely used. The indirect fluorescent antibody test measures the same antibodies as the dye test, but reliable quantitative titers are difficult to obtain.[58] Several

assays have been developed to measure IgM antibody, which appears earlier and declines faster than IgG.[84-86] Negative serological tests practically exclude the diagnosis of acute toxoplasmosis in immunocompetent individuals. Acute infection is documented with seroconversion or a twofold titer increase in acute and convalescent sera. Low titers of IgG antibody are usually present in patients with ocular toxoplasmosis; IgM titers are usually not present.[69] *Toxoplasma* chorioretinitis can usually be excluded if IgG serological tests are negative. Serological diagnosis of congenital infection depends on finding persistent or rising titers on the dye test or indirect fluorescent antibody test, or a positive IgM titer.[58]

The diagnostic criteria for serological testing in toxoplasmosis also apply to compromised hosts. However, serological diagnosis may be limited in these patients owing to depressed antibody responses. In AIDS cases, anti-*Toxoplasma* IgM or rising IgG levels are infrequently seen.[79,80,87] Although some reports have suggested that negative serology in AIDS patients excludes toxoplasmosis from consideration, other centers have not confirmed these observations[80] and seronegative patients are also at risk for developing acute toxoplasmosis.[76] It appears that *Toxoplasma* serology usually can neither confirm nor exclude the diagnosis of *T. gondii* in patients with AIDS.

The neuroradiographic features of toxoplasmosis of the CNS in AIDS patients have been extensively reviewed.[75–80,88] Neither the location, degree of enhancement, or associated edema on CT can necessarily distinguish toxoplasmosis from CNS lymphoma, which is the second most frequent etiology of intracranial mass lesions in AIDS patients.[79,80] Several investigators have now reported that magnetic resonance imaging (MRI) appears to be more sensitive than CT, often showing lesions or additional foci that were undetected by CT.[88,89] Pleocytosis (mononuclear), protein concentration elevation and normal glucose levels are most usually reported in the CSF[79,80]; these abnormalities are not specific, and lumbar puncture may be hazardous in patients with large mass lesions.

The greatest controversy regarding cerebral toxoplasmosis in AIDS patients relates to the necessity to perform invasive brain biopsy initially for diagnosis. Brain biopsies may be associated with hemorrhagic complications in AIDS patients.[80] Most authorities suggest that in an AIDS patient who has a consistent clinical and radiological presentation for cerebral toxoplasmosis, initial empirical therapy is reasonable.[80] Most patients respond to therapy within 2 to 3 weeks.[80,90] Biopsy should be reserved for those cases that are refractory to appropriate empirical therapy, for those with single lesions on MRI, or for presentations more suggestive of lymphoma or other processes.

Immunocompetent patients with lymphadenopathy are usually not treated unless there is evidence of visceral disease or when symptoms have persisted or are unusually severe. Normal individuals who have acquired the disease by laboratory accidents or via transfusions should be treated as having an infectious disease. In these circumstances infection is usually severe.[60] Normal patients should be treated for 2 to 4 months and then reassessed. Specific treatment of ocular toxoplasmosis has resulted in resolution of symptoms and improvement in vision.[55] Corticosteroids have been used with involvement of the macula or optic nerve, and photocoagulation has been used to treat active lesions or to prevent spread of lesions.[91]

Treatment of the infected pregnant woman decreases the incidence of fetal infection but does not completely eliminate it.[55] Results of uncontrolled human experience and animal studies suggest that postnatal treatment of infected infants may prevent the development of sequelae.[58] Guidelines for therapy of the pregnant patient and infected infant have been summarized elsewhere.[58]

Immunodeficient patients with toxoplasmosis should always be treated if the infection is acute. Treatment is continued for 4 to 6 weeks beyond the resolution of all signs and symptoms. Patients with AIDS and cerebral toxoplasmosis, in most cases, respond to specific therapy for *T. gondii*.[90] However, the prognosis in these patients is poor, with a median survival after diagnosis of 4 months. Toxicity associated with anti-*Toxoplasma* therapy has occurred in 60 percent and relapse of *Toxoplasma* encephalitis has been reported in 50 percent of cases.[90] It appears that lifelong suppression of toxoplasmosis is necessary after acute treatment in AIDS patients.

The most effective drugs for toxoplasmosis are pyrimethamine and the sulfonamides.[54,55] These antifolates are active against tachyzoites and are synergistic in combination. Pyrimethamine is lipid-soluble and readily absorbed from the gastrointestinal tract; 10 to 25 percent penetrates into the CSF. With severe infection, this drug is given in a dosage of 100 mg/d in two divided doses for 2 days and then as 25 to 50 mg daily or every other day based on the severity of illness. The most common adverse effect associated with pyrimethamine is bone marrow toxicity,[54,55] which theoretically can be reduced with the concurrent administration of folinic acid (10 mg/d). Less serious side effects have included headache, gastrointestinal symptoms, and rash. Sulfadiazine is administered as a loading dose of 75 mg/kg up to 4 g, followed by 100 mg/kg/d up to 8 g. Sulfamethazine and sulfamerazine have activity similar to that of sulfadiazine; all other sulfonamides have been inferior. Important adverse effects associated with the sulfonamides have included skin hypersensitivity reactions and bone marrow toxicity.[54,55]

Alternative agents for *Toxoplasma* infection have included spiramycin, clindamycin, and trimetrexate. Spiramycin is less toxic than standard therapy and has been used to treat infected pregnant women and infants.[58] No widespread experience of its use in immunocompromised patients or with cerebral toxoplasmosis has been reported. Clindamycin, which concentrates in the choroid, has been used successfully to treat ocular disease in uncontrolled animal and human studies.[92] It does not penetrate the blood-brain barrier and should not be used in cases of cerebral toxoplasmosis. Trimetrexate, a lipid-soluble antifolate, has been safe and effective when used alone or in combination with a sulfonamide in experimental models.[93] A trial of this agent, alone or in combination with sulfonamides, in humans is warranted. Preliminary and promising results have been seen with azithromycin, a new macrolide with a 72-hour half-life and increased tissue and intracellular penetration.[76]

African Trypanosomiasis

Known widely as sleeping sickness, African trypanosomiasis infects more than 12,000 Africans yearly[94,95] and remains a potential danger for travelers to endemic areas.[96] Two distinct forms of the disease in humans exist: western (chronic) due to infection by *Trypanosoma brucei gambiense* and eastern (acute) due to *Trypanosoma brucei rhodesiense*.[94,95]

African trypanosomiasis remains a risk for approximately 45 million people in endemic areas.[94,95] The cases of African sleeping sickness seen in US citizens have primarily been due to infection with *T. brucei rhodesiense*.[96]

T. brucei gambiense occurs mainly in the northern and western areas of sub-Saharan Africa.[94] This species is transmitted by blood-sucking *Glossina* flies (*G. palpalis* and related species), better known as tsetse flies. An important factor in the epidemiology of infection related to *T. brucei gambiense* is the chronic nature of the illness, with few incapacitating symptoms for many months.[94,95] Flies that feed on these individuals can easily become infected, thereby perpetuating epidemics.

East African trypanosomiasis is found in the eastern part of equatorial Africa.[94,95] This species is transmitted by *G. morsitans* and related species. These vectors are less fastidious, so that disease can occur in places not necessarily corresponding to the classic tropical forest. Wild animals are reservoirs of infection. Disease related to *T. brucei rhodesiense* is more acute and progressive, so that infected individuals do not usually serve as a source of continued infection as they are removed by treatment, hospitalization, or death.[97]

Tsetse flies become infected with trypanosomes after taking a blood meal from infected animals or humans. A complex set of developmental changes within the fly results in the formation of the infective metacyclic form.[95] When the fly bites humans, the parasites are injected into the bloodstream, where they develop into slender forms that rapidly divide. As infection progresses, the long, slender forms develop into short, stubby, nondividing forms. In the mammal, trypanosomes are restricted to extracellular spaces, including the bloodstream, lymphatics, tissue fluids, and, later in infection, the CSF.[98]

Antigenic variation by the long, slender forms accounts for the appearance of recurrent waves of parasites after antibody-mediated killing of earlier populations.[99,100] This cyclic phenomenon leads to ever-increasing immunoglobulin levels (mainly IgM) in the bloodstream and CSF.[94,95,101] In addition, there is the continued production of immune complexes.[102]

In African trypanosomiasis, significant lesions are demonstrable in the CNS and lymphatic system.[94] With infection due to *T. brucei rhodesiense,* there is less lymphatic involvement, and the findings in the heart and pericardium are often striking. In the CNS a meningoencephalitis occurs, with perivascular inflammation with lymphocytes, plasma cells, and pale-staining mononuclear cells called morular or Mott cells (Fig. 41-7).[94,95,103] These cells are believed to play an important role in the production of IgM.[103]

The earliest manifestation seen in both East and West African infections is a local, hard, painful lesion (chancre or trypanoma) developing at the site of the insect bite.[104] The second phase of the illness begins with widespread dissemination of the organism through the bloodstream and lymphatics, resulting in headache, fever, tachycardia, dizziness, and debility.[98] The systemic phase of trypanosomiasis occurs in recurrent fashion, with each episode lasting 1 to 6 days followed by an asymptomatic period of up to several weeks (Fig. 41-8). With progression of the disease, the systemic episodes decline in severity.

In Gambian disease, a frequent finding is lymphadenopathy, typically of the posterior cervical chain.[94,95] These nodes may be large, separated, and nontender; their consistency has been compared to that of ripe plums (Winterbottom's sign). The early systemic stage of Gambian trypanosomiasis lasts from 6 months to 1 year. Initial neurological changes in Gambian trypanosomiasis are often subtle and have included an indifferent attitude, aimless gazing, inversion of the sleep cycle, tremor, and hyperesthesia.

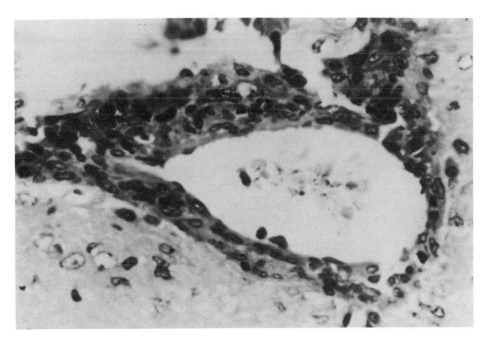

Fig. 41-7 African trypanosomiasis: perivascular cuffing with mononuclear cells. (Hematoxylin and eosin; original magnification × 1,000.)

In the late stage of disease there is progressive CNS involvement with somnolence alternating with insomnia, alterations in thermoregulation, incoordination, hypertonia, abnormal movements and gait, tremor, hyperreflexia, and, in the final stages, stupor and total indifference.[98] The disease is invariably fatal and undoubtedly contributed to by malnutrition, accidents, and concurrent infections.

With infection due to *T. brucei rhodesiense,* onset of symptoms occurs within a few days after a tsetse bite. The disease in travelers has often begun while journeying home or soon after return.[96,104,105] Lymphadenopathy is unusual. The clinical features of Rhodesian trypanosomiasis are similar to those seen with West African disease except that they are shorter in duration and more acute in presentation. Signs of

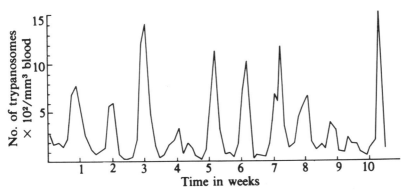

Fig. 41-8 African trypanosomiasis: periodicity of parasitemias, which correlates with systemic clinical features.

CNS invasion appear early, and neurological deterioration is very rapid. Death occurs in a matter of weeks to months after symptom onset, with the most common cause of death being cardiac failure.[95]

Examination of blood, CSF, and aspirate of a lymph node for trypanosomes are essential diagnostic steps. Buffy-coat samples of blood should be examined because of high sensitivity in parasite detection.[106] CSF has an increased protein concentration, pleocytosis (with morular cells), increased IgM levels, and occasional trypanosomes in centrifuged specimens. Other nonspecific laboratory abnormalities may include anemia, monocytosis, and increased serum IgM. Several immunodiagnostic tests developed for epidemiological surveys[107,108] are of limited usefulness in acute diagnosis.

The drugs traditionally used in the treatment of Africa trypanosomiasis are suramin, pentamidine, and the organic arsenicals.[109] Suramin, used for Rhodesian trypanosomiasis,[109] is given intravenously initially as 100 to 200 mg and increased as tolerated to 1 g on days 1, 3, 7, 14, and 21. Transient albuminuria is often observed; heavy proteinuria, shock, febrile reactions, and desquamative rash are less common side effects. Pentamidine, used for Gambian trypanosomiasis, is given intramuscularly at 3 mg/kg/d for 10 total doses. Hypotension, fever, rash, azotemia, liver enzyme abnormalities, and hypoglycemia may occur with pentamidine use.[110]

Neither suramin nor pentamidine penetrate the CNS adequately. Thus the more toxic arsenicals must be included in the regimen if infection of the CNS is suspected. Melarsopol is used most widely—in a series of three to four daily injections to a total dose of 3.6 mg/kg with a maximum of 200 to 500 mg per injection.[109,111] For patients with severe CNS involvement (higher CSF protein levels and pleocytosis),[94] up to four courses of arsenical therapy may be necessary. Toxic effects of the arsenicals include optic nerve atrophy, rash, and acute encephalopathy.

Treatment of trypanosomiasis is fraught with the difficulties of drug toxicity and the increasing emergence of trypanosomes resistant to arsenicals.[94] Studies have indicated that difluoromethylornithine, an inhibitor of polyamine biosynthesis, is curative for various trypanosome infections of laboratory animals.[112,113] Preliminary clinical studies have shown promising results in patients with CNS involvement, and with few side effects.[114] Extended clinical trials of this agent are now necessary to determine its place in treatment.

Primary Amebic Meningoencephalitis

Primary amebic meningoencephalitis is caused by the free-living amebas *Naegleria* and *Acanthamoeba*.[115,116] CNS infection may be acute, subacute, or chronic, but is generally fatal. Since this condition was first recognized in 1965 by Fowler and Carter,[117] more than 125 cases have been reported worldwide.

Primary amebic meningoencephalitis has been reported from 18 countries in both tropical and temperate areas.[115] Cases of infection with *Naegleria* have occurred primarily in the southern United States, Australia, Great Britain, and Czechoslovakia. In the United States, more than 50 cases from 14 states have occurred, primarily in children and young adults during summer months. The majority of cases (80 percent), caused by *N. fowleri,* are epidemiologically associated with fresh water contact.[118]

The epidemiology of infection related to *Acanthamoeba* is unknown, but because the natural habitat of this organism is soil and water a relationship to these elements is probably important. Because the primary meningoencephalitis due to *Acanthamoeba* occurs frequently in compromised individuals,[119,120] it is possible that this organism, which can be found in the oral pharynx, invades as an opportunist.[121]

The portal of entry for *Naegleria* is the nose, with invasion of the olfactory neuroepithelium. Organisms gain access to the CNS by being forced through the mucosa covering the cribriform plate.[122] *Acanthamoeba* may also invade the CNS in this manner but may secondarily involve the CNS after infection in other sites including the eye, lung, skin, or uterus.[115,123]

Naegleria initially involves the superficial gray matter and later the deep matter and cerebellum. Prominent involvement of the frontotemporal areas, olfactory bulbs, and subarachnoid space is observed.[122] Neutrophil invasion, extensive necrosis, and vascular invasion are typical (Fig. 41-9). Rarely, *Naegleria* infection disseminates from the CNS.[124] An acute, diffuse myocarditis has also occasionally been reported.[115,124] The pathogenesis of infection with free-living amebas is poorly understood but may involve

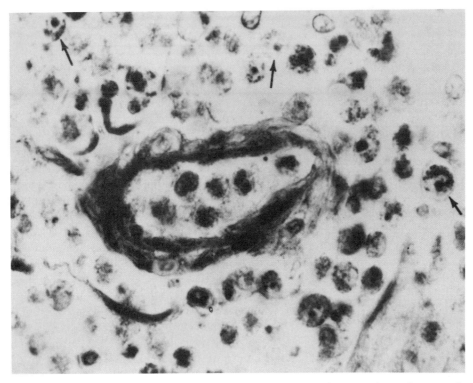

Fig. 41-9 Primary amebic meningoencephalitis: *Naegleria* trophozoites *(arrows)* surround a small blood vessel in autopsy brain. (Hematoxylin and eosin; original magnification × 1,000.)

phagocytosis, phospholipase A_2 activity,[125] or complement resistance.[126]

Acanthamoeba may also cause subacute or chronic encephalitis and multiple brain abscesses.[115] Granuloma formation occurs, with giant cells, vasculitis, mycotic aneurysms, and few neutrophils. With multiple brain abscesses, there is involvement of the midline deep structures and frontotemporal areas.[119]

Patients with acute amebic meningoencephalitis present with severe headache, fever, lethargy, nausea, and vomiting. Olfactory involvement, manifested as nasal stuffiness or changes in smell, may be clues to the etiology.[115,116,124] Seizures, nuchal rigidity, confusion, and then coma may develop within days. Focal neurological signs occur early. The course is one of rapid deterioration and death within 48 to 72 hours.[115] Pulmonary edema and heart failure may complicate the course. Death is usually the result of brainstem herniation.

Subacute or chronic syndromes caused by *Acanthamoeba* have a more insidious onset, with headache and focal findings as prominent features.[115,127] Focal findings predominate over signs of meningeal involvement. The course of these syndromes, lasting 2 to 3 weeks, is one of progressive deterioration ultimately leading to death.[127]

Examination of the CSF in patients with the acute syndrome reveals neutrophilic pleocytosis, hypoglycorrhachia, high protein concentration, and red blood cells.[115] In cases due to *Naegleria,* highly motile trophozoites are identified.[115,116,128] Cultures of the CSF may grow *Naegleria.*[129] In cases of acute disease related to *Acanthamoeba,* parasites are seldom identified.[129,130] With subacute or chronic presentations of *Acanthamoeba,* a moderate mononuclear pleocytosis is present along with increased protein and normal glucose concentrations[115]; amebas are usually not present in the CSF. CT may confirm the presence of multiple abscesses in deep midline areas.[115] Serological tests may be of value given the prolonged course. Histopathology or culture of brain biopsy may also yield the diagnosis.[115]

Only three survivors of acute primary amebic meningoencephalitis due to *Naegleria* have been reported.[115,131,132] The most effective agent for *Naegleria* infection is amphotericin B. Intravenous doses of amphotericin B should be increased as tolerated to as high as 1 mg/kg/d. Supplemental intrathecal, intracisternal, or intraventricular doses should be given. The most effective total dose of amphotericin B has not been determined, but therapy should be continued for at least 10 days.

At present, no effective therapy exists for CNS infection due to *Acanthamoeba*. In vitro sensitivity of this organism has been demonstrated to pentamidine, polymyxin B, 5-fluorocytosine, miconazole, paromomycin, acriflavine, and clotrimazole but not amphotericin B.[133] Attempts to treat *Acanthamoeba* CNS infection with 5-fluorocytosine in combination with polymyxin B and sulfonamides have failed.

Cerebral Amebiasis

Of the various extraintestinal sites of infection due to *Entamoeba histolytica,* brain abscess is a rare but generally fatal complication.[134–137] As of 1987, more than 150 cases of amebic brain abscess have been reported, but less than one-third have been confirmed parasitologically.

E. histolytica, the causative agent of amebiasis, has been reported to infect 10 percent of the world's population, accounting for 50 million symptomatic cases and 100,000 deaths per year.[138] Endemic areas include Africa, South and Central America, Mexico, India, and Southeast Asia.[138] In the United States, amebiasis, with a prelevance of 2 to 6 percent,[139] is seen most commonly in chronically institutionalized individuals, in homosexual men, and in lower socioeconomic groups in the Southeast.[140]

Humans are the primary reservoir of infection.[140,141] Infection is transmitted by ingestion of cysts in contaminated food or water, or unusually through fecal-oral contact. Excystation occurs in the small intestine, producing trophozoites. In the colon, where the parasite resides, encystation may occur with cysts passed in the stool. In a few cases, trophozoites invade the colonic mucosa, and symptoms result.[140,141] Once invasion of tissues occurs, significant necrosis of underlying host tissue is observed.[142]

Invasive disease most frequently presents as inflammatory colitis with the potential sequela of liver abscess.[140,141] Other extraintestinal complications, occurring less frequently, most often result from contiguous spread of infection from liver abscess into the pleural, pericardial, and peritoneal spaces. Hematogenous spread of infection has been recognized and may result in cerebral infection.[134–137]

In reported series, 0.6 to 8.1 percent of cases of fatal amebiasis have been complicated by brain abscess.[134–137] Lombardo and associates noted 17 cases of cerebral involvement in 210 autopsy cases of amebiasis from Mexico City.[135] Patients presented with focal neurological signs, seizures, and mental status changes.[135] Areas of the brain most frequently involved included the basal ganglia and frontal lobes. In the few cases where lumbar puncture was performed, a mild pleocytosis and increased protein concentration (as with pyogenic brain abscess) was observed.[134–137]

Most cases of cerebral amebiasis have occurred in the setting of hepatic abscess.[135] Diagnostically, 90 to 95 percent of cases of liver abscess are associated with positive serology.[140,141] Attempts to confirm the diagnosis of cerebral amebiasis by examination of CSF or stool for cysts and trophozoites have been largely unsuccessful. Thus, diagnosis of cerebral amebiasis largely lies in documenting extraintestinal sites of involvement, especially the liver, and serological confirmation.

Most cases of cerebral amebiasis have been fatal or found at autopsy.[135] Fatal outcome has been due in part to delay in diagnosis.[134–137] The early administration of metronidazole, an imidazole with exceptional tissue amebicidal activity and penetration into the CSF, provides the best chance of a successful outcome. A role for surgical drainage has not been established.

HELMINTHIC INFECTION

Because of their size (50 μm to 15 cm), multicellular (metazoan) parasites pose a distinct problem for host immunity.[143] The helminthic species that cause CNS disease are diverse; each parasite has a complex life cycle that involves human as well as nonhuman animal hosts in different stages of its development. To facilitate presentation of this section, the parasites under discussion have been grouped according to class—i.e., as cestodes (tapeworms), nematodes

Table 41-2 Helminths Causing CNS Disease

Class	Species
Cestodes (tapeworms)	*Taenia solium*
	Echinococcus granulosus
	Echinococcus multilocularis
	Spirometra species
Nematodes (roundworms)	*Strongyloides stercoralis*
	Trichinella spiralis
	Angiostrongylus cantonensis
	Toxocara species
	Onchocerca volvulus
	Loa loa
Trematodes (flukes)	*Schistosoma mansoni*
	Schistosoma japonicum
	Schistosoma haematobium
	Paragonimus species
	Fasciola hepatica

(roundworms), or trematodes (flukes)—for the reason that parasites of the same class share common features of development and often produce similar pathology in the CNS. As a reference, Table 41-2 summarizes the class distribution of the helminthic species discussed. Not included in this chapter, myiasis and pentastomiasis, which represent infestation with arthropods (insect larvae), may also involve invasion and encystment in CNS tissues and may also cause secondary bacterial infection of the CNS.[144]

Cestodes

CYSTICERCOSIS

Cysticercosis is perhaps the most common CNS helminthic infection in the United States,[145] and its manifestations are typical of many other metazoan parasite infections. The syndrome represents human infection with the immature or larval form of the tapeworm *Taenia solium*.[146] Because pigs are the usual intermediate host for *T. solium,* cysticercosis has a worldwide distribution in pork-producing countries: although rare in the United States, Canada, and western Europe, neurocysticercosis is common in Mexico, areas of Central and South America, Africa, the Cape Verde Islands, India, China, Thailand, Korea, the Philippines, and Indonesia.[146] Most US cases result from patient emigration from or travel to these

endemic areas.[145,147–149] Transmission within the United States has been documented among household contacts of tapeworm-infected immigrants from endemic areas.[150] Therefore, a careful exposure and travel history is essential in evaluating the potential for neurocysticercosis in symptomatic patients.

Typically, infection results from the accidental ingestion of tapeworm eggs via fecal contamination of foods. After ingestion, tapeworm eggs hatch within the gastrointestinal tract and penetrate the bowel wall. The organisms then migrate into host tissues, favoring muscle and subcutaneous tissue. Over the next 60 to 70 days, the early larval forms (oncospheres) mature to cysticerci measuring 0.5 to 3 cm in diameter.[146] Neurocysticercosis, discussed here, results from infection of the CNS or eye. Cysts may be found in any body tissue, however, including the heart, liver, lungs, and peritoneal cavity.[147–149]

After provoking an initial immune response by inflammatory white cells (neutrophils, eosinophils, and lymphocytes) within infected tissues, encysting *T. solium* larvae promote fibroblast proliferation and become surrounded by a thick fibrous capsule.[146–151] This encapsulation is associated with a waning of host inflammatory response. Later, when the parasite dies, the cysts begin to lose osmoregulation and may start to swell. In addition, local inflammation may recur due to parasite decomposition and the associated release of parasite antigens. It is frequently at this point that patients experience the onset of neurological symptoms. The reported onset of symptomatic neurocysticercosis ranges from 1 to 35 years after exposure,[152] although the average life-span of encysted cysticerci is estimated to be 4 to 5 years.

Clinical symptoms of neurocysticercosis become manifest by mass effect, by obstruction of ventricular outflow with hydrocephalus, or by chronic inflammation in the subarachnoid space. The latter syndrome mimics chronic meningitis and may lead to communicating hydrocephalus. As occurs with tuberculous meningitis, parasite-induced chronic inflammation at the base of the brain may entrap cerebral vessels, leading to angiitis, acute vascular compromise, and stroke. This presentation is particularly common in the "racemose" form of neurocysticercosis, in which multilobulated vesicles proliferate on the surface of the brain.[153] Both acute hydrocephalus and stroke may be associated with sudden death in the patient with neurocysticercosis[154,155]

With neurocysticercosis, the most common clinical presentation is epilepsy (30 to 92 percent of patients). Seizures may be focal or generalized and may vary in frequency. The onset of epilepsy may be associated with focal deficits corresponding to the location of the symptomatic cyst; if intracranial hypertension is present, papilledema may be noted. Hydrocephalus usually presents with headache and may be accompanied by nausea, vomiting, ataxia, visual disturbances, and confusion. Impairment of intellectual function may be significant; reported symptoms include amnesia, apathy, emotional lability, and hallucinations.[147–149] With acute heavy infections, a syndrome of cysticercotic encephalitis may develop, particularly in young women. Severe diffuse brain edema may ensue, leading to coma and death.[156] Spinal cord cysticercosis may lead to a compressive myelopathy or a radiculopathy due to chronic meningitis.

The specific diagnosis of neurocysticercosis may prove difficult, as history, physical examination, and laboratory studies may be nonspecific.[145,157] A history of exposure or residence in endemic areas adds weight to the diagnosis. Furthermore, a careful physical and radiographic search should be made for systemic cysticerci, which can be biopsied to confirm parasitic infection. CSF findings are suggestive of chronic meningitis, with most patients having a lymphocytic pleocytosis, hypoglycorrhachia, and elevated opening pressure.[147–149] Eosinophilic pleocytosis is less common (10 to 30 percent of patients) and is not specific to neurocysticercosis.[147–149]

Imaging studies, such as CT scanning or MRI, have proven to be the most useful tests in supporting the diagnosis of neurocysticercosis.[149,155] Multiple cysts up to 5 cm in diameter are frequently noted in the cortex and meninges as well as in the cerebral white matter. Most cases have 10 or fewer cysts evident. The parasites' appearance may vary depending on their stage of development and viability. Early lesions may appear solid, whereas older lesions appear cystic. With time, cysts may eventually calcify and regress into scars.[147–149] The appearance may be modified by surrounding inflammation, with some lesions becoming evident only on contrast-enhanced CT scans. The appearance of cysts may alter with therapy, with some cysts showing more marked contrast enhancement after drug treatment.[157,158] Ordinary CT scans may not demonstrate intraventricular or subarachnoid cysts well. In such cases, metrizamide contrast

cisternograms or MRI may prove useful.[158–160] Experience with MRI suggests that this modality may provide more sensitive and specific diagnosis of neurocysticercosis, particularly in cases where ventricular or subarachnoid cysts are involved.[159,160] Not only can degenerate and viable cysts be discriminated by T_1- and T_2-weighted MRIs, but it is frequently possible to discern the protoscolex of the viable tapeworm cyst.

Serological testing for cysticercosis is available from the Centers for Disease Control, Atlanta, Georgia. In large series, however, testing of serum *and* CSF by complement fixation, indirect hemagglutination, or enzyme-linked immunosorbent assay (ELISA) has proven of variable sensitivity and specificity.[147–149,161] Indirect hemagglutination or ELISA testing appears to provide the greatest sensitivity (60 to 90 percent), but false-positive reactions may occur in patients with echinococcosis, schistosomiasis, or other tapeworm infections. The constellation of suggestive CT scan or MRI, positive serology, and evidence of systemic cysticercosis strongly favors the diagnosis of neurocysticercosis. In the presence of a negative serology or with an ill-defined solitary cyst, the diagnosis is more tenuous; the differential diagnosis must include glioma or other CNS tumors, brain abscess, vasculitis, tuberculosis, cryptococcosis, echinococcosis (hydatidosis), or other parasitic infection. In some cases, stereotactic biopsy may be necessary to establish the diagnosis.

Specific antiparasitic therapy is not required in all cases of neurocysticercosis. In a series of CT-diagnosed disease, 90 percent of patients with hemispheric lesions and 92 percent of patients without hydrocephalus had benign outcomes without specific antiparasitic therapy.[149] Nonspecific therapy, including anticonvulsants for control of seizures, ventricular shunting for control of hydrocephalus, and corticosteroids for reduction of pericystic inflammation successfully controlled CNS symptoms in these patients. Nevertheless, the overall case fatality rate for neurocysticercosis is 10 percent, indicating that certain groups of patients with more aggressive or advanced disease require specific antiparasitic treatment to control their disease.[148]

In recent years, the antihelminthics praziquantel and albendazole have been accepted as effective antiparasitic treatment for patients with neurocysticercosis.[158,162–165] Clinical improvement is seen in the majority of patients given antihelminthics, although many untreated patients experience a benign course, as noted above. Initiation of antiparasitic treatment is often associated with exacerbation of neurological symptoms, requiring the addition of corticosteroid therapy.[158,162] Patients with basilar disease or arachnoiditis may not respond well to antiparasitic therapy.[163] Based on experience in treating 40 to 45 patients each, workers in Los Angeles[166] and Mexico City[164] have published guidelines for surgical and chemotherapeutic intervention. In view of the significant variation between patients in cyst number, location, and activity, the decision to use surgery or antiparasitic agents for treatment of neurocysticercosis must be individualized for each patient.

ECHINOCOCCOSIS (HYDATID DISEASE) AND SPARGANOSIS

Other cestodes (tapeworms) that can cause human CNS tissue injury include the canine tapeworms *Echinococcus granulosus* and *Echinococcus multilocularis* and the diphyllobothroid tapeworms of the *Spirometra* genus.[146,167] As in cysticercosis, humans serve as the unwilling intermediate host in the tapeworm life cycle. Echinococcosis is common in the Mideast, the Mediterranean basin, regions of Africa, Australia, and in the Arctic regions of Asia and North America.[168] With echinococcosis, migrating oncospheres rarely encyst in the CNS. However, echinococcal cysts that reach the CNS may produce symptoms by local inflammation, by mechanical obstruction of CSF flow (hydrocephalus), or by cortical irritation (with associated seizures).[167] In addition, when hydatid cysts form within vertebral bone, compression or spinal dislocation may lead to secondary spinal cord damage.[169] When found, CNS hydatid cysts are most frequently associated with cysts elsewhere in the body (Fig. 41-10). Eosinophilia or eosinophilic meningitis are inconstant findings, but serological testing (indirect hemagglutination or ELISA combined with immunoelectrophoresis) has proven fairly sensitive and specific for the diagnosis of echinococcosis.[167,170] Serological response tends to be weaker, however, in extrahepatic hydatid disease,[171] and excisional surgical biopsy, with precautions to prevent spread of the cyst, may be necessary to establish the diagnosis in the CNS. For symptomatic cysts, the approach to treatment involves chemotherapy with albendazole

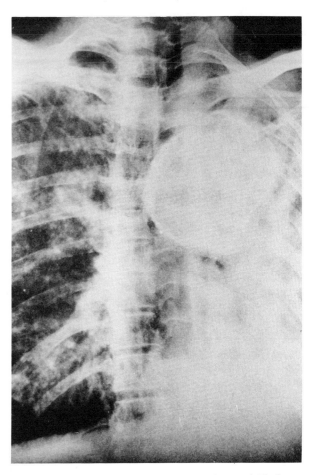

Fig. 41-10 Pulmonary echinococcosis: a large calcified cyst of the left lung.

or mebendazole,[172–176] combined with surgical resection where practical. Chemotherapy of vertebral hydatid cysts has not proved successful[172–174] and, when possible, surgical excision remains the treatment of choice for symptomatic CNS cysts.

Sparganosis, caused by *Spirometra* larvae, is rare. Humans acquire infection by ingesting procercoids in copepods found in pond water or by ingestion of, or cutaneous exposure to, meat from plerocercoid-infected animals.[146,177] Symptoms arise from mass effects from cysts found in the CNS or may result from cyst invasion in and around the eye, with secondary infection.[178,179] Surgery is the treatment of choice, although mebendazole and praziquantel therapy have been attempted.[180]

Nematodes

DISSEMINATED STRONGYLOIDIASIS

Strongyloides stercoralis is a gastrointestinal nematode parasite of humans that is endemic to many tropical and subtropical regions of the world as well as to southern areas of the United States.[181] Travel to or migration of patients from these areas accounts for most of the disease seen in temperate regions. It is of note that, after exposure, infection may persist for decades.[181] A second distinctive feature of *Strongyloides* (that contrasts it with the other enteric nematodes) is its release of living progeny instead of eggs within the gastrointestinal tract. Normally, these immature larvae are not infective for humans until they pass outside the body and spend days to weeks undergoing transformation into infectious filariform larvae. In individuals who are chronically ill (protein-calorie malnutrition, burns, tuberculosis, syphilis) or immunosuppressed (lymphoma, renal transplant, AIDS, corticosteroid therapy, irradiation, or chemotherapy), however, this transformation may occur within the patient's own gastrointestinal tract, leading to overwhelming autoinfection with *Strongyloides*.[182,183] In many cases, the underlying parasitic infection may have been completely asymptomatic prior to the onset of disseminated strongyloidiasis.

Presenting symptoms of disseminated strongyloidiasis include severe generalized abdominal pain, distension, jaundice, and signs of sepsis.[181–183] Invasion of the lungs may produce asthma-like symptoms, with cough, wheezing, and eosinophilia. Parasites migrating from the gut often carry enteric bacteria into various tissues around the body, resulting in the appearance of polymicrobial bacteremia and septic shock.[181] CNS involvement often results in acute mental status deterioration associated with signs of pyogenic meningitis, with progression to coma[184] (Fig. 41-11). Alternatively, the process may be subacute, resulting in a picture of cerebritis or chronic meningoencephalitis, which may be mistaken for CNS vasculitis.[185] Diagnosis of CNS strongyloidiasis is usually clinical, based on the results of stool examinations for larvae and the presenting systemic symptoms. Therapy is primarily supportive, addressed to the symptoms induced by inflammation and bacterial superinfection. It is important to bear in mind, however, that corticosteroids may exacerbate the process of *Strongyloides* autoinfection.[182,183] Concomitant thiabendazole or mebendazole therapy should be ini-

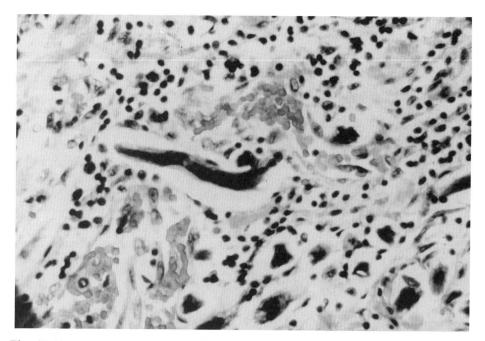

Fig. 41-11 *Strongyloides stercoralis* in the meninges, with acute hyperemia and inflammatory cell infiltration.

tiated to eliminate or suppress parasitic infection within the gut.[181,186,187] In immunosuppressed individuals, it may not be possible to eradicate infection; but if immunosuppression can be suspended or reduced during antiparasitic therapy, the effectiveness of antihelminthics may be improved.[181] Otherwise, suppressive doses of thiabendazole should be given on a monthly basis. Disseminated strongyloidiasis can be prevented in some cases by screening the stool of patients at risk prior to the initiation of immunosuppressive therapy. In AIDS-endemic areas, it would be prudent to screen and treat all HIV-infected individuals for *Strongyloides* infection prior to the onset of AIDS.

TRICHINOSIS

Trichinella spiralis infection is found worldwide and is acquired by ingestion of contaminated pork or other meat (e.g., bear meat). Infectious cysts within striated muscle tissue are digested, releasing maturing adult forms of *Trichinella* within the gastrointestinal tract.[188] Days to weeks later, these adult forms release living infective larvae in the gut. These immature forms penetrate the bowel wall, enter the circulation, and initiate the clinical syndrome of trichinosis by invading various body tissues.

Trichinosis is characterized by fevers, headache, myalgias, eosinophilia, and periorbital edema, and may be complicated by carditis or respiratory failure through direct involvement of cardiac and respiratory muscles.[188,189] Neurological disease occurs as a consequence of larval invasion of the CNS and can be associated with seizures, meningoencephalitis, focal infarction or hemorrhage, or cranial vessel thrombosis.[190–194] Progression of infarction may lead to severe cerebral edema, herniation, and death.[193]

Muscle biopsy for the demonstration of *Trichinella* larvae (Fig. 41-12) is the diagnostic procedure of choice, in that serological response may lag several weeks behind the onset of infection.[188] In some cases larvae may be demonstrated in sediments of centrifuged CSF. CT scanning and MRI may reveal multiple infarcts or hemorrhagic lesions, either in areas corresponding to focal motor deficits or throughout the brain.[189,191] In some cases, CT findings, angiography, and electroencephalography (EEG) may be entirely nondiagnostic.[190]

Optimal treatment of trichinosis has not been es-

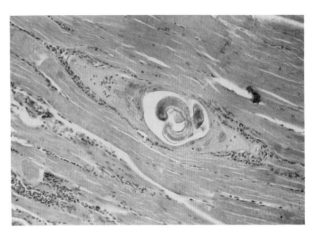

Fig. 41-12 *Trichinella spiralis:* larva encysted in human striated muscle.

tablished. The benefit of corticosteroid administration is unproved. Corticosteroid therapy is frequently used to control symptoms of trichinosis although, as with strongyloidiasis, it has the potential to enhance larval dissemination. Thiabendazole has been used to eliminate the source of invading larvae (i.e., adult worms within the gut). This therapy has limited value, however, in the patient already suffering from severe tissue involvement.[188]

EOSINOPHILIC MENINGITIS: ANGIOSTRONGYLIASIS, GNATHOSTOMIASIS AND VISCERAL LARVA MIGRANS

When humans are exposed to parasites of domestic or wild animals, an acute or subacute illness may result.[195] Because humans are not successful or "patent" hosts for these parasites, adult parasites do not develop within the body. Nevertheless, immature larvae may migrate for weeks within host tissues before dying. In the unnatural human host, the inflammatory response to tissue invasion by these parasites may be much more severe than the response noted in the normal, patent animal host.

Human CNS disease is common following infection by the rat lungworm *Angiostrongylus cantonensis,* which is transmitted by ingestion of snails, slugs, or undercooked prawns or crab.[196] Neurological disorders are also common with infection caused by *Gnathostoma* parasites of dogs and cats, which are transmitted by ingestion of undercooked freshwater fish or of frog, bird, or snake meat.[197] Angiostrongyliasis is found in Southeast Asia, Indonesia, Japan, the Philippines, Taiwan, southern areas of the Pacific, Egypt, Cuba, and Hawaii[196] and may potentially be transmitted by snails in North America.[198] Gnathostomiasis has been reported in Japan, China, Malaysia, Indonesia, India, Bangladesh, and Israel.[197]

With both parasites, symptoms occur 1 to 3 weeks after exposure and may be associated with creeping skin eruptions, abdominal and pleural symptoms, fever, and eosinophilia.[197,199] CNS invasion is marked by headache, meningismus, cranial nerve palsies, and paresthesias, which may be protracted and severe.[199–202] Spinal cord involvement may present as radiculomyeloencephalitis.[201,203]

The CSF examination is remarkable for intense eosinophilic pleocytosis (up to 90 percent), with mildly elevated CSF protein and normal or low-normal glucose concentrations. CSF cytology occasionally reveals parasite larvae,[204] but the specific diagnosis is more frequently based on clinical presentation, exposure history, and serological evidence. Optimal therapy for these parasites is not established.[196,197,199] Thiabendazole and corticosteroids have been used to alleviate symptoms of angiostrongyliasis; quinine and corticosteroids have been used to treat systemic gnathostomiasis. Both infections are self-limited in nature, although neurological deficits may persist for months to years.

Visceral larva migrans is a common US parasitic infection that must be included in the differential diagnosis of eosinophilic meningitis. It is caused by inadvertent ingestion of the eggs of animal roundworms, most frequently *Toxocara canis* and *Toxocara cati*.[205] Infection is frequently seen in children with pica who ingest contaminated soil. Developing larvae hatch within the gut and may migrate into the CNS or eyes.[205] Neurological symptoms are rare but may include absence attacks, generalized convulsions, focal sensorimotor deficits, and paraplegia, depending on the species of parasite.[206,207] Focal retinal inflammation may be mistaken for retinoblastoma, leading to unnecessary enucleation of the eye.[205] Systemically, infection may be characterized by fever, hepatomegaly, eosinophilia, and symptoms of pulmonary infection. Diagnosis is established by history of animal exposure and by serological studies, although by itself ocular disease may yield only low or

nonspecific anti-*Toxocara* titers in the serum.[205] A CSF eosinophilic pleocytosis may also be noted.[207] Treatment with corticosteroids is frequently used to alleviate inflammatory symptoms. Specific antiparasitic therapy with diethylcarbamazine or thiabendazole has been associated with improvement of symptoms in some cases.[205] Such therapy is not recommended in all cases because the outcome of most infections is generally benign.

ONCHOCERCIASIS AND LOIASIS

The filarial nematode parasites *Onchocerca volvulus* and *Loa loa* are transmitted from human to human by biting flies, with an obligate developmental stage in the intermediate vector fly.[208,209] Onchocerciasis is found in Central and West Africa, Central and South America, and in Yemen.[209] Loiasis is localized to the western portion of Central Africa.[208] In both diseases, developing filarial adults release their offspring as living microfilariae within the body, and it is the host reaction to these widely distributed larval forms that causes CNS disease.

Onchocerciasis is the fourth leading cause of blindness in the world. Microfilarial invasion of the eye tissues results in conjunctivitis, keratitis, anterior uveitis, significant chorioretinitis, and occasionally optic atrophy.[209,210] In some areas, retinal findings may be the predominant presenting sign (Fig. 41-13). Individuals from areas with endemic HIV infection should be evaluated by an experienced ophthalmologist to exclude opportunistic cytomegalovirus infection and toxoplasmosis.

Diagnosis of onchocerciasis is made by examination of skin snips for microfilariae.[209] Therapy is problematic in that the standard treatments, diethylcarbamazine and suramin, are associated with enhanced ocular inflammation.[211,212] Recent work with the drug ivermectin has shown promise in controlling microfilarial load without exacerbation of eye symptoms.[213]

Loa loa infection is usually associated with angioedematous skin reactions called calabar swellings.[208] Rare patients may develop nephropathy, cardiomyopathy, and encephalopathy associated with heavy infection and circulation of microfilariae in the bloodstream. In many cases, CNS symptoms are brought on by attempted antimicrofilarial therapy with diethylcarbamazine. The encephalopathic state is marked

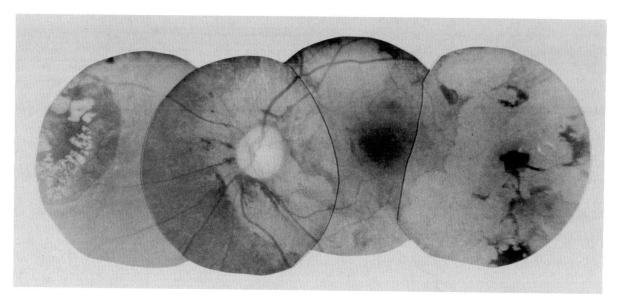

Fig. 41-13 Onchocercal chorioretinitis. Composite photograph of a patient from West Africa.

by insomnia, headache, and depression, and may be followed by coma and death in patients with severe microfilaremia.[214] Some patients manifest microfilaria in the CSF. Postmortem examination reveals both diffuse acute cerebral edema and a granulomatous reaction surrounding degenerating larvae. Effective therapy for this CNS syndrome has not been established. It is recommended, however, that patients with heavy microfilaremia be given prophylactic corticosteroids prior to and during the course of antiparasitic treatment in order to prevent severe ocular and CNS complications.[208]

Trematodes

SCHISTOSOMIASIS

Schistosoma species are trematode parasites transmitted to humans in contact with fresh water. The infectious larvae (cercariae) are released by parasitized snails, which serve as intermediate hosts.[215] There are three major species: *S. mansoni* is common to Africa and Brazil; *S. haematobium* is found in Egypt, in the Mideast, and throughout tropical Africa; and *S. japonicum* is found in Asia, Indonesia, and the Philippines.

After cercariae penetrate the skin, developing worms migrate to the mesenteric blood vessels (*S. mansoni* and *S. japonicum*) or to the venous system surrounding the ureters and bladder (*S. haematobium*). Host morbidity results from release of parasite eggs into surrounding host tissues, with resultant granulomatous inflammation and scar formation. CNS disease is relatively rare in schistosomiasis and appears to result from aberrant deposition of eggs within nervous tissues, either by migration of adults into the CNS or by transport of eggs into the CNS circulation via collateral veins.

The syndrome of cerebral schistosomiasis is most common in *S. japonicum* infection, affecting up to 2 to 4 percent of patients.[215] It is characterized by focal motor and sensory deficits, seizures (jacksonian or generalized) with EEG abnormalities, and hyperdense, multinodular enhancing lesions on CT scans, with surrounding edema.[216,217] In uncontrolled trials, treatment with praziquantel (60 mg/kg) has been associated with improvement or cure of seizures and resolution of CT abnormalities.[216]

By contrast, cerebral schistosomiasis is rarely seen with infections due to other schistosome species.[215] With *S. mansoni* infection, cerebral involvement often appears with acute infection, manifesting as a febrile meningoencephalitic reaction that may be associated with a cutaneous allergic reaction.[218] Chronic CNS disease may show evidence of vasculitis[219] or mass lesions.[220]

Spinal cord syndromes appear to be more common in patients with *S. mansoni* or *S. haematobium* infection.[221-225] Presentation may be acute or subacute and may be associated with cutaneous deposition of eggs at the level of spinal cord involvement.[226,227] Presenting syndromes include low back pain, paraparesis, sensory loss, and bladder dysfunction.[221-225] Acute vascular compromise may result in myelonecrosis,[224] or expanding granulomatous inflammation may lead to cord compression with evidence of CSF blockage on myelography or CT scanning.[221] The course may vary from one of rapid deterioration[224] to one of gradual improvement and resolution after antiparasitic therapy.[220,228]

Diagnosis should include parasitological or serological evidence of schistosome exposure,[215] and must exclude other causes of myelitis found in areas endemic for schistosomiasis.[229] Because developing areas also pose significant hazards in terms of chemical and venomous toxins as well as endemic polio and coxsackievirus infection, it may not be possible to determine with certainty the etiology of a patient's CNS disease without biopsy or autopsy diagnosis.[229]

Therapy with praziquantel will provide eradication of infection in more than 80 percent of patients.[215] Symptomatic treatment with corticosteroids, surgical decompression, or both may be necessary to control acute CNS symptoms and prevent tissue injury.

PARAGONIMIASIS AND FASCIOLIASIS

Tissue trematodes (flukes) infect humans who consume larval metacercaria in undercooked crustaceans or raw water plants.[230] *Paragonimus* species are endemic in areas of Asia and South and Central America,[230,231] but paragonimiasis has also been transmitted within the United States.[232] Fascioliasis is cosmopolitan in its distribution and is common to many sheep- and cattle-raising areas. Disease occurs as maturing larvae migrate through host tissues from the gastrointestinal tract to the lungs (paragonimiasis) or liver (fascioliasis). CNS disease is frequent in paragonimiasis but rare in fascioliasis, occurring when ectopic parasite localization takes place within the brain or spinal cord.[230,231] Presenting CNS syndromes may include acute and chronic meningitis, mass lesions, hemorrhage, infarction, or ocular abnormalities (papilledema, hemianopia, nystagmus, and optic atro-

phy). Frequent symptoms include seizures, headache, and visual disturbance.[230] Intellectual deterioration and vomiting may also be noted.

Diagnosis depends on a positive exposure history, along with parasitological, serological, or biopsy evidence of infection.[230] Sputum examination for ova is appropriate for the lung fluke *P. westermani,* the most common cause of paragonimiasis in Asia, whereas stool examination for ova is appropriate for the diagnosis of the liver fluke *Fasciola hepatica.* Radiographic examination of the lungs may show typical lesions of concurrent *Paragonimus* infection; retrograde cholangiography and bile duct aspiration may confirm exposure to or infection with liver flukes. Skull radiographs may show localized punctate or nodular calcification. CT examination may reveal ventricular dilatation and multiple lesions within brain tissues.[231,233] CSF examination often shows lymphocytic pleocytosis and elevated protein concentration, but eosinophils are found in fewer than 10 percent of CSF samples examined.[234]

Effective therapies for CNS paragonimiasis or CNS fascioliasis are not established. A combination of surgical removal of the parasite, along with praziquantel therapy, has been recommended.[231,234] Symptomatic therapy with corticosteroids, anticonvulsants, or ventricular shunting may be necessary.

REFERENCES

1. Wyler DJ: Malaria—resurgence, resistance, and research. N Engl J Med 308:875, 934 (two parts), 1983
2. Wyler DT: Plasmodium species (malaria). p. 2056. In Mandell GL, Douglas RG, Bennett JE (eds): Principles and Practice of Infectious Diseases. 3rd Ed. Churchill Livingstone, New York, 1990
3. Miller LH: Malaria. p. 245. In Warren KS, Mahmoud AAF (eds): Tropical and Geographic Medicine. 2nd Ed. McGraw-Hill, New York, 1990
4. Sein KK, Maeno Y, Thuc HV, et al: Differential sequestration of parasitized erythrocytes in the cerebrum and cerebellum in human cerebral malaria. Am J Trop Med Hyg 48:504, 1993
5. Oo MM, Aikawa M, Than T, et al: Human cerebral malaria: a pathologic study. J Neuropathol Exp Neurol 46:223, 1987
6. Walker O, Salako LA, Sowunmi A, et al: Prognostic risk factors and post mortem findings in cerebral malaria in children. Trans Roy Soc Trop Med Hyg 86: 491, 1992

7. Lobel HO, Campbell CC, Schwartz IK, Roberts JM: Recent trends in the importation of malaria caused by Plasmodium falciparum into the United States from Africa. J Infect Dis 152:613, 1985

8. Lobel HO, Campbell CC, Roberts JM: Fatal malaria in US citizens. Lancet 1:873, 1985

9. Bruce-Chwatt LJ: Imported malaria: an uninvited guest. Br Med Bull 38:179, 1982

10. Centers for Disease Control: Imported malaria among travelers—United States. MMWR 33:388, 1984

11. Guerrero IC, Weniger BC, Shultz MG: Transfusion malaria in the United States, 1972–1981. Ann Intern Med 99:221, 1983

12. Dover AS, Schultz ME: Transfusion-induced malaria. Transfusion 11:353, 1971

13. Miller LH, Howard RJ, Carter R, et al: Research toward malaria vaccines. Science 234:1349, 1986

14. Miller LH, Haynes JD, McAuliffe FM, et al: Evidence for differences in erythrocyte surface receptors for the malarial parasites, Plasmodium falciparum and Plasmodium Knowlesi. J Exp Med 146:277, 1977

15. Perkins M: Inhibitory effects of erythrocyte membrane proteins on the in vitro invasion of the human-malaria parasite (Plasmodium falciparum) into its host cell. J Cell Biol 90:563, 1981

16. White NH, Ho M: The pathophysiology of malaria. Adv Parasitol 31:83, 1992

17. Walzer PD, Gibson JJ, Schultz MG: Malaria fatalities in the United States. Am J Trop Med Hyg 23:328, 1974

18. Sheehy TW, Reba RC: Complications of falciparum malaria and their treatment. Ann Intern Med 66:807, 1967

19. Feldman RM, Singer C: Noncardiogenic pulmonary edema and pulmonary fibrosis in falciparum malaria. Rev Infect Dis 9:134, 1987

20. Warrell DA, Looareesuwan S, Warrell MJ, et al: Dexamethasone proves deleterious in cerebral malaria: a double-blind trial in 100 comatose patients. N Engl J Med 306:313, 1982

21. White NJ, Warrell DA, Looareesuwan S, et al: Pathophysiological and prognostic significance of cerebrospinal-fluid lactate in cerebral malaria. Lancet 1:776, 1985

22. Kilejian A: Characterization of a protein correlated with the production of knob-like protrusions on membranes of erythrocytes infected with Plasmodium falciparum. Proc Natl Acad Sci USA 76:4650, 1979

23. Igarashi I, Oo MM, Stanley H, et al: Knob antigen deposition in cerebral malaria. Am J Trop Med Hyg 37:511, 1987

24. Clark IA, Rockett RA, Cowden WB: TNF in cerebral malaria. Q J Med 86:217, 1993

25. Grau GE, Fajardo LF, Piguet P-F, et al: Tumor necrosis factor as an essential mediator in murine cerebral malaria. Science 237:1210, 1987

26. Looareesuwan S, Warrell DA, White NJ, et al: Do patients with cerebral malaria have cerebral oedema? A computed tomography study. Lancet 1:434, 1983

27. Chipman M, Cadigan FC, Benjapongse W: Involvement of the nervous system in malaria in Thailand. Trop Georg Med 19:8, 1967

28. Fitz-Hugh T, Pepper DS, Hopkins HU: The cerebral form of malaria. Bull US Army Med Dept 83:39, 1944

29. Warrell DA, Looareesuwan S, Phillips RE, et al: Function of the blood-cerebrospinal fluid barrier in human cerebral malaria: rejection of the permeability hypothesis. Am J Trop Med Hyg 35:882, 1986

30. Kean BH, Reilly PC: Malaria—the mime. Am J Med 61:159, 1976

31. White NJ, Warrell DA, Chanthavanich P, et al: Severe hypoglycemia and hyperinsulinemia in falciparum malaria. N Engl J Med 309:61, 1983

32. Krogstad DJ, Pfaler MA: Prophylaxis and treatment of malaria. Curr Clin Topics Infect Dis 4:56, 1984

33. Bruce-Chwatt LJ: Essential Malariology. Heinemann, New York, 1980

34. Centers for Disease Control: Revised recommendations for preventing malaria in travelers to areas with chloroquine-resistant Plasmodium falciparum. MMWR 34:185, 1985

35. Centers for Disease Control: Chloroquine-resistant Plasmodium falciparum malaria in West Africa. MMWR 36:13, 1987

36. Phillips RE: Management of Plasmodium falciparum malaria. Med J Aust 141:511, 1984

37. Bruce-Chwatt LJ: Quinine and quinidine in malaria. The old and the new! Trav Med Int 5:3, 1987

38. Colwell EJ, Hickman RL, Kosakal S: Tetracycline treatment of chloroquine-resistant falciparum malaria in Thailand. JAMA 220:684, 1972

39. Reacher M, Campbell CC, Freeman J, et al: Drug therapy for Plasmodium falciparum malaria resistant to pyrimethamine-sulfadoxine (Fansidar). Lancet 2:1066, 1981

40. Meek SR, Doberstyn EB, Gauzere BA, et al: Treatment of falciparum malaria with quinine and tetracycline or combined mefloquine/sulfadoxine/pyrimethamine on the Thai-Kampuchean border. Am J Trop Med Hyg 35:246, 1986

41. Miller KD, Greenberg AE, Campbell CC: Treatment of severe malaria in the United States with a continuous infusion of quinidine gluconate and exchange transfusion. N Engl J Med 321:65, 1989

42. Main EK, Main DM, Krogstad DJ: Treatment of chloroquine-resistant malaria during pregnancy. JAMA 249:3207, 1983

43. White NJ, Looareesuwan S, Warrell DA, et al: Quinine pharmacokinetics and toxicity in cerebral and uncomplicated falciparum malaria. Am J Med 73:564, 1982

44. White NJ, Loareesuwan S, Warrell DA, et al: Quinidine in falciparum malaria. Lancet 2:1069, 1981

45. Phillip RE, Warrell DA, White NJ, et al: Intravenous quindine for the treatment of severe falciparum malaria. N Engl J Med 312:1273, 1985

46. White NJ, Watt G, Bergqvist Y, Njelesani EK: Parenteral chloroquine for treating falciparum malaria. J Infect Dis 155:192, 1987

47. Rieckmann KH: Falciparum malaria: the urgent need for safe and effective drugs. Annu Rev Med 34:321, 1983

48. Dixon KE, Pitaktong U, Phintuyothin P: A clinical trial of mefloquine in the treatment of plasmodium vivax malaria. Am J Trop Med Hyg 34:435, 1985

49. Doberstyn EB, Phintuyothin P, Noeypatimanondh S, Teerakiartkamjorn C: Single-dose therapy of falciparum malaria with mefloquine or pyrimethamine-sulfadoxine. Bull WHO 57:275, 1979

50. Trenholme GM, Williams RL, Desjardin RE, et al: Mefloquine (WR 142,490) in the treatment of human malaria. Science 190:792, 1975

51. Roncoroni AJ, Martino OA: Therapeutic use of exchange transfusion in malaria. Am J Trop Med Hyg 28:440, 1979

52. Kramer SL, Campbell CC, Moncrieff RE: Fulminant Plasmodium falciparum infection treated with exchange blood transfusion. JAMA 249:244, 1983

53. Files JC, Case CJ, Morrison FS: Automated erythrocyte exchange in fulminant falciparum malaria. Ann Intern Med 100:396, 1984

54. Remington JS: Toxoplasmosis. p. 309. In Warren KS, Mahmoud AAF (eds): Tropical and Geographic Medicine. 2nd Ed. McGraw-Hill, New York, 1990

55. McCabe RE, Remington JS: Toxoplasma gondii. p. 2090. In Mandell GL, Douglas RE, Bennett JE (eds): Principles and Practice of Infectious Diseases. 3rd Ed. Churchill Livingstone, New York, 1990

56. Krick JA, Remington JS: Toxoplasmosis in the adult—an overview. N Engl J Med 298:550, 1978

57. Ruskin J, Remington JS: Toxoplasmosis in the compromised host. Ann Intern Med 84:193, 1976

58. Remington JS, Desmonts G: Toxoplasmosis. p. 143. In Remington JS, Klein JO (eds): Infectious Diseases of the Fetus and Newborn Infant. WB Saunders, Philadelphia, 1983

59. Wallace GD: The role of the cat in the natural history of Toxoplasma gondii. Am J Trop Med Hyg 22:313, 1973

60. Neu HC: Toxoplasmosis transmitted at autopsy. JAMA 202:844, 1967

61. Siegel SE, Lunde MN, Gelderman AH, et al: Transmission of toxoplasmosis by leukocyte transfusion. Blood 37:388, 1971

62. Britt RH, Enzmann DR, Remington JS: Intracranial infection in cardiac transplant recipients. Ann Neurol 9:107, 1981

63. Hofflin JM, Potasman R, Baldwin JC, et al: Infectious complications in heart transplant recipients receiving cyclosporine and corticosteroids. Ann Intern Med 106:209, 1987

64. Luft BJ, Noat Y, Aruajo FG, et al: Primary and reactivated Toxoplasma infection in patients with cardiac transplants. Ann Intern Med 99:27, 1983

65. Wong B: Parasitic diseases in immunocompromised hosts. Am J Med 76:479, 1984

66. Rubin RH, Wolfson JS, Cosimi AB, Tolkoff-Rubin NE: Infection in the renal transplant recipient. Am J Med 70:405, 1981

67. Frenkel JK: Pathology and pathogenesis of congenital toxoplasmosis. Bull NY Acad Med 50:182, 1974

68. O'Connor GR: The influence of hypersensitivity on the pathogenesis of ocular toxoplasmosis. Trans Am Ophthalmol Soc 68:501, 1970

69. O'Connor GR: Manifestations and management of ocular toxoplasmosis. Bull NY Acad Med 50:192, 1974

70. Lake KB, Van Dyke JJ, Abts RM, Moyes DR: Lympho-glandular toxoplasmosis: a diagnosis often missed. Postgrad Med 65:110, 1979

71. Kean BH: Clinical toxoplasmosis—50 years. Trans R Soc Trop Med Hyg 66:549, 1972

72. Sheagren JN, Lunde MN, Simon HB: Chronic lymphadenopathic toxoplasmosis: a case with hyperglobulinemia and impaired delayed hypersensitivity responses during active infection. Am J Med 60:300, 1976

73. Gump DW, Holden RA: Acquired chorioretinitis due to toxoplasmosis. Ann Intern Med 90:58, 1979

74. Perkins ES: Ocular toxoplasmosis. Br J Ophthalmol 57:1, 1973

75. Porter SB, Sande MA: Toxoplasmosis of the central nervous system in the acquired immunodeficiency syndrome. N Engl J Med 327:1643, 1992

76. Luft BJ, Remington JS: Toxoplasmic encephalitis in AIDS. Clin Infect Dis 15:211, 1992

77. Reynold C, Sugar A, Chave JP, et al: Toxoplasma encephalitis in patients with the acquired immunodeficiency syndrome. Medicine (Baltimore) 71:224, 1992

78. Wanke C, Tuazon CU, Kovacs A, et al: Toxoplasma encephalitis in patients with acquired immune deficiency syndrome: diagnosis and response to therapy. Am J Trop Med Hyg 36:509, 1987

79. Levy RM, Bredesen DE, Rosenblum ML: Neurological manifestations of the acquired immunodeficiency syndrome (AIDS): experience at UCSF and review of the literature. J Neurosurg 62:475, 1985

80. McArthur JC: Neurologic manifestations of AIDS. Medicine (Baltimore) 66:407, 1987

81. Luft BJ, Hafner R, Korzun AH, et al: Toxoplasmic encephalitis in patients with the acquired immunodeficiency syndrome. N Engl J Med 329:995, 1993

82. Conley FK, Jenkins HT, Remington JS: Toxoplasma gondii infection of the central nervous system. Hum Pathol 12:690, 1981

83. Sabin AB, Feldman HA: Dyes as microchemical indicators of a new immunity phenomenon affecting a protozoal parasite (Toxoplasma). Science 108:660, 1948

84. Welch PC, Masur H, Jones TC, Remington JS: Serologic diagnosis of acute lymphadenopathic toxoplasmosis. J Infect Dis 142:256, 1980

85. Siegel JP, Remington JS: Comparison of methods for quantitating antigen-specific immunoglobulin antibody M with a reverse enzyme-linked immunosorbent assay. J Clin Microbiol 18;63, 1983

86. Remington JS, Eimstad WM, Araujo FG: Detection of immunoglobulin M antibodies with antigen-tagged latex particles in an immunosorbent assay. J Clin Microbiol 17:939, 1983

87. Luft BJ, Brooks RG, Conley FK, et al: Toxoplasmic encephalitis in patients with acquired immunodeficiency syndrome. JAMA 252:913, 1984

88. Levy RM, Rosenbloom S, Perrett LV: Neuroradiologic findings in AIDS: a review of 200 cases. AJR 147:977, 1986

89. Orefice G, Carrieri PB, Chirianni A, et al: Cerebral toxoplasmosis and AIDS: clinical, neuroradiological and immunological findings in 15 patients. Acta Neurol (Napoli) 14:493, 1992

90. Haverkos HW: Assessment of therapy for toxoplasma encephalitis. Am J Med 82:907, 1987

91. Ghartey KN, Brockhurst RJ: Photocoagulation of active Toxoplasma retinochoroiditis. Am J Ophthalmol 89:858, 1980

92. Iannucci AA, Hart LL: Clindamycin in the treatment of toxoplasmosis in AIDS. Ann Pharmacol 26:645, 1992

93. Kovacs JA, Allegra CJ, Chabner BA, et al: Potent effect of trimetrexate, a lipid soluble antifolate, on Toxoplasma gondii. J Infect Dis 155:1027, 1987

94. Kirchhoff LV: Trypanosoma species (African sleeping sickness). p. 2085. In Mandell GL, Douglas RG, Bennett JE (eds): Principles and Practice of Infectious Diseases. 3rd Ed. Churchill Livingstone, New York, 1990

95. Englund PT, Smith DM: African trypanosomiasis. p. 268. In Warren KS, Mahmoud AAF (eds): Tropical and Geographic Medicine. 2nd Ed. McGraw-Hill, New York, 1990

96. Quinn TC, Hill CD: African trypanosomiasis in an American hunter in East Africa. Arch Intern Med 143:1021, 1983

97. Buyst H: The epidemiology of sleeping sickness in the historical Luangwa Valley. Ann Soc Belg Med Trop 57:349, 1977

98. Apten DIC: Clinical manifestations and diagnosis of sleeping sickness. p. 661. In Mulligan HW (ed): The African Trypanosomes. John Wiley & Sons, New York, 1970

99. Englund PT, Hadjuk SL, Marini JC: The molecular biology of trypanosomes. Annu Rev Biochem 51:695, 1982

100. Turner M: Antigenic variation in the trypanosome. Nature 298:606, 1982

101. Whittle HC, Greenwood BM, Bidwell DE, et al: IgM and antibody measurement in the diagnosis and management of Gambian trypanosomiasis. Am J Trop Med Hyg 26:1129, 1977

102. Lambert PH, Berney M, Kazyumba G: Immune complexes in serum and in cerebrospinal fluid in African trypanosomiasis. J Clin Invest 67:77, 1981

103. Greenwood BM, Whittle HC: Cerebrospinal-fluid IgM in patients with sleeping-sickness. Lancet 2:525, 1973

104. Duggan AJ, Hutchinson MP: Sleeping sickness in Europeans: a review of 109 cases. J Trop Med Hyg 69:124, 1966

105. Spencer HC, Gibson JJ, Brodsky RE, Schultz MG: Imported African trypanosomiasis in the United States. Ann Intern Med 82:633, 1975

106. Buyst H: The diagnosis of sleeping sickness. Trop Doct 3:110, 1973

107. Wery M, Wery-Paskoff S, Van Wettere N: The diagnosis of human African trypanosomiasis (T. gambiense) by the use of fluorescent antibody test. Ann Soc Belg Med Trop 50:613, 1970

108. Ruitenberg EJ, Buys J: Application of the enzyme-linked immunosorbent assay (ELISA) for the diagnosis of human African trypanosomiasis (sleeping sickness). Am J Trop Med Hyg 26:31, 1977

109. Williamson J: Chemotherapy of African trypanosomiasis. Trans R Soc Trop Med Hyg 70:117, 1976

110. Pearson RD, Hewlett EL: Pentamidine for the treatment of Pneumocystis carinii pneumonia and other protozoal diseases. Ann Intern Med 103:782, 1985

111. Evans DA: African trypanosomes. Antibiot Chemother 30:272, 1981

112. McCann PP, Bacchi CJ, Clarkson AB, et al: Further

studies on difluoromethylornithine in African trypa-nosomes. Med Biol 59:434, 1981

113. Clarkson AB, Bienen EJ, Bacchi CJ, et al: New drug combination for experimental late-stage African try-panosomiasis: DL-alpha-difluoromethylornithine (DFMO) with suramin. Am J Trop Med Hyg 33:1073, 1984

114. Taelman H, Schechter PJ, Marcelis L, et al: Difluoro-methylornithine, an effective new treatment of Gam-bian trypanosomiasis. Am J Med 82:607, 1987

115. Duma RJ: Primary amebic meningoencephalitis. p. 321. In Warren KS, Mahmoud AAF (eds): Tropical and Geographic Medicine. 2nd Ed. McGraw-Hill, New York, 1990

116. Ma P, Visvesvara GS, Martinez AJ, et al: Naegleria and Acanthamoeba infections: review. Rev Infect Dis 12:490, 1990

117. Fowler M, Carter RF: Acute pyogenic meningitis probably due to Acanthamoeba sp. Br Med J 2:740, 1965

118. Neva FA: Amebic meningoencephalitis—a new dis-ease? N Engl J Med 282:450, 1970

119. Martinez AJ: Infection of the central nervous system due to Acanthamoeba. Rev Infect Dis 13, suppl 5: S399, 1991

120. Di Gregorio C, Rivasi F, Mongiardo N, et al: Acanth-amoeba meningoencephalitis in a patient with ac-quired immunodeficiency syndrome. Arch Pathol Lab Med 116:1363, 1992

121. Wang SS, Feldman HA: Isolation of hartmannella spe-cies from human throats. N Engl J Med 277:1174, 1967

122. Martinez J, Duma RJ, Nelson EC, Moretto FL: Ex-perimental Naegleria meningoencephalitis in mice; penetration of the olfactory mucosal epithelium by Naegleria and pathologic changes produced: a light and electron microscopic study. Lab Invest 29:121, 1973

123. Gullett J, Mills J, Hodley K, et al: Disseminated gran-ulomatous acanthamoeba infection presenting as an unusual skin lesion. Am J Med 67:891, 1979

124. Duma RJ, Ferrell HW, Nelson CE, Jones MM: Pri-mary amebic meningoencephalitis. N Engl J Med 281:1315, 1969

125. Hysmith RM, Franson RC: Elevated levels of cellular and extracellular phospholipases from pathogenic Naegleria fowleri. Biochim Biophys Acta 711:26, 1982

126. Whiteman LY, Marciano-Cabral F: Susceptibility of pathogenic and nonpathogenic Naegleria spp. to com-plement-mediated lysis. Infect Immun 55:2442, 1987

127. Cleland PG, Lawande RV, Onyemelukwe G, Whittle HC: Chronic amebic meningoencephalitis. Arch Neurol 39:56, 1982

128. Stevens AR, Shulman ST, Lansen TA, et al: Primary amebic meningoencephalitis: a report of two cases and antibiotic and immunologic studies. J Infect Dis 143:193, 1981

129. Chang SL: Small, free-living amebas: cultivation, quantitation, identification, classification, pathogene-sis, and resistance. Curr Top Comp Pathobiol 1:201, 1974

130. Martinez AJ: Acanthamoebiasis and immunosuppres-sion. J Neuropathol Exp Neurol 41:548, 1982

131. Seidel JS, Harmatz P, Visvesvara GS, et al: Successful treatment of primary amebic meningoencephalitis. N Engl J Med 306:346, 1982

132. Centers for Disease Control: Primary amebic menin-goencephalitis: California, Florida, New York. MMWR 27:343, 1978

133. Duma RJ, Finley R: In vitro susceptibility of patho-genic Naegleria and Acanthamoeba species to a vari-ety of therapeutic agents. Antimicrob Agents Chemo-ther 10:370, 1976

134. Banerjee AK, Bhatnagar RK, Bhusnurmath SR: Sec-ondary cerebral amebiasis. Trop Geogr Med 35:333, 1983

135. Lombardo L, Alonso P, Arroyo LS, et al: Cerebral amebiasis. J Neurosurg 21:704, 1964

136. Orbison JA, Reeves N, Leedham CL, Blumberg JM: Amebic brain abscess. Medicine (Baltimore) 30:247, 1951

137. Hughes FB, Faehnle ST, Simon J: Multiple cerebral abscesses complicating hepatopulmonary amebiasis. J Pediatr 86:95, 1975

138. Reed SL: Amebiasis: an update. Clin Infect Dis 14:385, 1992

139. Juniper K Jr: Amebiasis in the United States. Bull NY Acad Med 47:448, 1971

140. Ravdin JI, Petri WA Jr: Amebiasis. In Mandell GL, Douglas RG, Bennett JE (eds): Principles and Practice of Infectious Diseases. 3rd Ed. Churchill Livingstone, New York, 1990

141. Ravdin JI, Guerrant RL: Current problems in diagno-sis and treatment of amebic infections. Curr Clin Top Infect Dis 7:82, 1986

142. Perez-Tamayo R, Brandt H: Amebiasis. p. 145. In Marcial-Rojas RA (ed): Pathology of Protozoal and Helminthic Diseases. Williams & Wilkins, Baltimore, 1971

143. Ellner JJ, Mahmoud AAF: Phagocytes and worms: David and Goliath revisited. Rev Infect Dis 4:698, 1982

144. Editorial: Parasites which migrate to the brain. Lancet 1:1116, 1976

145. Brown WJ, Voge M: Cysticercosis: a modern day plague. Pediatr Clin North Am 32:953, 1985

146. Pawlowski ZS: Cestodiases: taeniasis, diphyllobothriasis, hymenolepiasis and others. p. 490. In Warren KS, Mahmoud AAF (eds): Tropical and Geographical Medicine. 2nd Ed. McGraw-Hill, New York, 1990

147. Shanley JD, Jordan MC: Clinical aspects of CNS cysticercosis. Arch Intern Med 140:1309, 1980

148. Loo L, Braude A: Cerebral cysticercosis in San Diego: a report of 23 cases and a review of the literature. Medicine (Baltimore) 61:341, 1982

149. McCormick GF, Zee C-S, Heiden J: Cysticercosis cerebri: review of 127 cases. Arch Neurol 39:534, 1982

150. Schantz PM, Moore AC, Munoz JL, et al: Neurocysticercosis in an Orthodox Jewish community in New York City. N Engl J Med 327:692, 1992

151. Brown WJ, Voge M: Neuropathology of Parasitic Infections. Oxford University Press, Oxford, 1982

152. MacArthur WP: Cysticercosis as seen in the British army, with special reference to the production of epilepsy. Trans R Soc Med Hyg 27:343, 1934

153. Rabiela-Cervantes MT, Rivas-Hernandez A, Rodriguez-Ibarra J, et al: Anatomopathological aspects of human brain cysticercosis. p. 179. In Flisser A, Willms K, Laclette JP, Larralde C (eds): Cysticercosis: Present State of Knowledge and Perspectives. Academic Press, London, 1982

154. Keane JR: Death from cysticercosis: seven patients with unrecognized obstructive hydrocephalus. West J Med 140:787, 1984

155. Torrealba G, Del Villar S, Tagle P, et al: Cysticercosis of the central nervous system: clinical and therapeutic considerations. J Neurol Neurosurg Psychiatry 47:784, 1984

156. Rangel R, Torres B, Del Bruto O, Sotelo J: Cysticercotic encephalitis: a severe form in young females. Am J Trop Med Hyg 36:387, 1987

157. Sotelo J, Escobedo F, Rodriguez-Carbajal J, et al: Therapy of parenchymal brain cysticercosis with praziquantel. N Engl J Med 310:1001, 1984

158. Zee CS, Segall HD, Miller C, et al: Unusual neuroradiological features of intracranial cysticercosis. Radiology 137:397, 1980

159. Sharma K, Gupta RK: Scan-negative neurocysticercosis. Pediatr Neurosurg 19:206, 1993

160. Rhee RS, Kumasaki DY, Sarwar M, et al: MR imaging of intraventricular cysticercosis. J Comput Assist Tomogr 11:598, 1987

161. Ramos-Kuri M, Montoya RM, Padilla A, et al: Immunodiagnosis of neurocysticercosis: disappointing performance of serology (enzyme-linked immunosorbent assay) in an unbiased sample of neurological patients. Arch Neurol 49:633, 1992

162. deGhetaldi LD, Norman RM, Douville AW Jr: Cerebral cysticercosis treated biphasically with dexamethasone and praziquantel. Ann Intern Med 99:179, 1983

163. Sotelo J, Torres B, Rubio-Donnadieu F, et al: Praziquantel in the treatment of neurocysticercosis: long term follow-up. Neurology 35:752, 1985

164. Vasconcelos D, Cruz-Segura H, Mateos-Gomez H, Zenteno Alanis G: Selective indications for the use of praziquantel in the treatment of brain cysticercosis. J Neurol Neurosurg Psychiatry 50:383, 1987

165. Takayanagui OM, Jardim E: Therapy for neurocysticercosis: comparison between albendazole and praziquantel. Arch Neurol 49:290, 1992

166. Apuzzo ML, Dobkin WR, Zee C-S, et al: Surgical considerations in treatment of intraventricular cysticercosis: an analysis of 45 cases. J Neurosurg 60:400, 1984

167. Schantz PM, Okelo GBA: Echinococcosis (hydatidosis). p. 505. In Warren KS, Mahmoud AAF (eds): Tropical and Geographical Medicine. 2nd Ed. McGraw-Hill, New York, 1990

168. Williams JF, Lopez Adaros H, Trejos A: Current prevalence and distribution of hydatidosis with special reference to the Americas. Am J Trop Med Hyg 20:224, 1971

169. Pamir MN, Akalan N, Ozgen T, Erbengi A: Spinal hydatid cysts. Surg Neurol 21:53, 1984

170. Hira PR, Shweiki HM, Siboo R, Behbehani K: Counterimmunoelectrophoresis using an arc 5 antigen for the rapid diagnosis of hydatidosis and comparison with the indirect hemagglutination test. Am J Trop Med Hyg 36:592, 1987

171. Craig PS, Zeyhle E, Romig T: Hydatid disease: research and control in Turkana: II. The role of immunological techniques for the diagnosis of hydatid disease. Trans R Soc Trop Med Hyg 80:183, 1986

172. Bryceson ADM, Cowie AGA, Macleod C, et al: Experience with mebendazole in the treatment of inoperable hydatid disease in England. Trans R Soc Trop Med Hyg 76:510, 1982

173. Woodtli W, Bircher J, Witassek F, et al: Effect of plasma mebendazole concentrations in the treatment of human echinococcosis. Am J Trop Med Hyg 34:754, 1985

174. Saimot AG, Meulemans A, Cremieux AC, et al: Albendazole as a potential treatment for human hydatidosis. Lancet 2:652, 1983

175. Horton RJ: Chemotherapy of Echinococcus infection in man with albendazole. Trans R Soc Trop Med Hyg 83:97, 1989

176. Singounas EG, Leventis AS, Sakas DE, et al: Successful treatment of intracerebral hydatid cysts with albendazole: case report and review of the literature. Neurosurgery 31:571, 1992

177. Hunter GW, Swartzwelder JC, Clyde DF: Cestodes. p. 593. In Hunter GW, Swartzwelder JC, Clyde DF

(eds): Tropical Medicine. 5th Ed. WB Saunders, Philadelphia, 1976

178. Tsai MD, Chang CN, Ho YS, Wang AD: Cerebral sparganosis diagnosed and treated with stereotactic techniques: report of two cases. J Neurosurg 78:129, 1993

179. Holodniy M, Almenoff J, Loutit J, Steinberg GK: Cerebral sparganosis: case report and review. Rev Infect Dis 13:155, 1991

180. Torres JR, Noya OO, Noya BA, et al: Treatment of proliferative sparganosis with mebendazole and praziquantel. Trans R Soc Trop Med Hyg 75:846, 1981

181. Grove DI: Strongyloidiasis. p. 393. In Warren KS, Mahmoud AAF (eds): Tropical and Geographic Medicine. 2nd Ed. McGraw-Hill, New York, 1990

182. Scowden EB, Schaffner W, Stone WJ: Overwhelming strongyloidiasis: an unappreciated opportunistic infection. Medicine (Baltimore) 57:527, 1978

183. Igra-Siegman Y, Kapila R, Sen P, et al: Syndrome of hyperinfection with Strongyloides stercoralis. Rev Infect Dis 3:397, 1981

184. Meltzer RS, Singer C, Armstrong D, et al: Case report: antemortem diagnosis of central nervous system strongyloidiasis. Am J Med Sci 277:91, 1979

185. Wachter RM, Burke AM, MacGregor RR: Strongyloides stercoralis hyperinfection masquerading as cerebral vasculitis. Arch Neurol 41:1213, 1984

186. Vishwanath S, Baker RA, Mansheim BJ: Strongyloides infection and meningitis in an immunocompromised host. Am J Trop Med Hyg 31:857, 1982

187. Berger R, Kraman S, Paciotti M: Pulmonary strongyloidiasis complicating therapy with corticosteroids: report of a case with secondary bacterial infections. Am J Trop Med Hyg 29:31, 1980

188. Kazura JW: Trichinosis. p. 442. In Warren KS, Mahmoud AAF (eds): Tropical and Geographical Medicine. 2nd Ed. McGraw-Hill, New York, 1990

189. Brashear RE, Martin RR, Glover JL: Trichinosis and respiratory failure. Am Rev Respir Dis 104:245, 1971

190. Ryczak M, Sorber WA, Kandora TF, et al: Difficulties in diagnosing Trichinella encephalitis. Am J Trop Med Hyg 36:573, 1987

191. Ellrodt A, Halfon P, LeBras P, et al: Multifocal central nervous system lesions in three patients with trichinosis. Arch Neurol 44:432, 1987

192. Barr R: Human trichinosis: report of four cases, with emphasis on central nervous system involvement, and a survey of 500 consecutive autopsies at the Ottawa Civic Hospital. Can Med Assoc J 95:912, 1966

193. Gay T, Pankey GA, Beckman EN, et al: Fatal CNS trichinosis. JAMA 247:1024, 1982

194. Fourestie V, Douceron H, Brugieres P, et al: Neurotrichinosis: a cerebrovascular disease associated with myocardial injury and hypereosinophilia. Brain 116:603, 1993

195. Elliot DL, Tolle SW, Goldberg L, Miller JB: Pet-associated illness. N Engl J Med 313:985, 1985

196. Rosen L: Angiostrongyliasis. p. 438. In Warren KS, Mahmoud AAF (eds): Tropical and Geographical Medicine. McGraw-Hill, New York, 1984

197. Hunter GW, Swartzwelder JC, Clyde DF: Other tissue-inhabiting nematodes: gnathostomiasis p. 533. In Hunter GW, Swartzwelder JC, Clyde DF (eds): Tropical Medicine. 5th Ed. WB Saunders, Philadelphia, 1976

198. Kocan AA: Some common North American aquatic snails as experimental hosts of Angiostrongylus cantonensis—with special reference to Lymnaea palustris. J Parasitol 58:186, 1972

199. Punyagupta S, Juttijudata P, Bunnag T: Eosinophilic meningitis in Thailand: clinical studies of 484 typical cases probably caused by Angiostronglylus cantonensis. Am J Trop Med Hyg 24:921, 1975

200. Yii C-Y, Chen C-Y, Chen E-R, et al: Epidemiologic studies of eosinophilic meningitis in southern Taiwan. Am J Trop Med Hyg 24:447, 1975

201. Vejjajiva A: Parasitic diseases of the nervous system in Thailand. Clin Exp Neurol 15:92, 1978

202. Kuberski T, Wallace GD: Clinical manifestations of eosinophilic meningitis due to Angiostrongylus cantonensis. Neurology 29:1566, 1979

203. Kawamura J, Kohri Y, Oka N: Eosinophilic meningoradiculomyelitis caused by Gnathostoma spinigerum: a case report. Arch Neurol 40:583, 1983

204. Nitidandhaprabhas P, Harnsomburana K, Thepsitthar P: Angiostrongylus cantonensis in the cerebrospinal fluid of an adult male patient with eosinophilic meningitis in Thailand. Am J Trop Med Hyg 24:711, 1975

205. Glickman LT: Toxocariasis. p. 431. In Warren KS, Mahmoud AAF (eds): Tropical and Geographical Medicine. McGraw-Hill, New York, 1984

206. Glickman LT, Cypess RH, Crumrine PK, Gitline DA: Toxocara infection and epilepsy in children. J Pediatr 94:75, 1979

207. Fox AS, Kazacos KR, Gould NS, et al: Fatal eosinophilic meningoencephalitis and visceral larva migrans caused by the raccoon ascarid Bayliascaris procyonis. N Engl J Med 312:1619, 1985

208. Ottessen EA: Filariases and tropical eosinophilia. p. 407. In Warren KS, Mahmoud AAF (eds): Tropical and Geographical Medicine. 2nd Ed. McGraw-Hill, New York, 1990

209. Greene BM: Oncocerciasis. p. 429. In Warren KS, Mahmoud AAF (eds): Tropical and Geographical Medicine. 2nd Ed. McGraw-Hill, New York, 1990

210. Bird AC, Anderson J, Fuglsang H: Morphology of posterior segment lesions of the eye in patients with onchocerciasis. Br J Ophthalmol 60:2, 1976
211. Anderson J, Fuglsang H, De C Marshall TF: Effects of diethylcarbamazine on ocular onchocerciasis. Tropenmed Parasitol 27:263, 1976
212. Thylefors B, Rolland A: The risk of optic atrophy following suramin treatment of ocular onchocerciasis. Bull WHO 57:479, 1979
213. Taylor HR, Murphy RP, Newland HS, et al: Treatment of onchocerciasis: the ocular effects of ivermectin and diethylcarbamazine. Arch Ophthalmol 104:863, 1986
214. Carme B, Boulesteix J, Boutes H, Puruehnce MF: Five cases of encephalitis during treatment of loiasis with diethylcarbamazine. Am J Trop Med Hyg 44:684, 1991
215. Mahmoud AAF: Schistosomiasis p. 458. In Warren KS, Mahmoud AAF (eds): Tropical and Geographical Medicine. 2nd Ed. McGraw-Hill, New York, 1990
216. Watt G, Adapon B, Long GW, et al: Praziquantel in treatment of cerebral schistosomiasis. Lancet 2:529, 1986
217. Kirchhoff LV, Nash TE: A case of schistosomiasis japonica: resolution of CAT-scan detected cerebral abnormalities without specific therapy. Am J Trop Med Hyg 33:1155, 1984
218. Bissessur S, Minderhoud JM: Two cases of schistosomiasis. Clin Neurol Neurosurg 87:213, 1985
219. Pittella JEH: Vascular changes in cerebral schistosomiasis mansoni: a histopathological study of fifteen cases. Am J Trop Med Hyg 34:898, 1985
220. Bambirra EA, de Souza Andrade J, Cesarini I, et al: The tumoral form of schistosomiasis: report of a case with cerebellar involvement. Am J Trop Med Hyg 33:76, 1984
221. Centers for Disease Control: Acute schistosomiasis with transverse myelitis in American students returning from Kenya. MMWR 33:445, 1984
222. Lechtenberg R, Vaida GA: Schistosomiasis of the spinal cord. Neurology 27:55, 1977
223. Centers for Disease Control: Schistosomiasis in U.S. Peace Corps volunteers—Malawi, 1992. MMWR 42:565, 1993
224. Queiroz L de S, Nucci A, Facure NO, Facure JJ: Massive spinal cord necrosis in schistosomiasis. Arch Neurol 36:517, 1979
225. Cohen J, Capildeo R, Rose FC, Pallis C: Schistosomal myelopathy. Br Med J 1:1258, 1977
226. Wood MG, Srolovitz H, Schetman D: Schistosomiasis: paraplegia and ectopic skin lesions as admission symptoms. Arch Dermatol 112:690, 1975
227. Saxe N, Gordon W: Schistosomiasis of spinal cord and skin. S Afr Med J 49:57, 1975
228. Scrimgeour EM: Spinal cord disease due to Schistosoma mansoni successfully treated with oxamniquine. Br Med J 289:625, 1984
229. Gear JHS: Nonpolio causes of polio-like paralytic syndromes. Rev Infect Dis 6, suppl 2:S379, 1984
230. Harinasuta T, Bunnag D: Liver, lung and intestinal trematodiasis. p. 473. In Warren KS, Mahmoud AAF (eds): Tropical and Geographical Medicine. 2nd Ed. McGraw-Hill, New York, 1990
231. Kusner DJ, King CH: Cerebral paragonimiasis. Semin Neurol 13:201, 1993
232. Pachucki CT, Levandowski RA, Brown VA, et al: American paragonimiasis treated with praziquantel. N Engl J Med 311:582, 1984
233. Yoshida M, Moritaka K, Kuga S, Anegawa S: CT findings of cerebral paragonimiasis in the chronic state. J Comput Assist Tomogr 6:195, 1982
234. Patterson TF, Patterson JE, Barry M, Bia FJ: Parasitic infections of the central nervous system. p. 234. In Schlossberg D (ed): Infections of the Nervous System. Springer-Verlag, New York, 1990

42

Neurological Complications of Immunization

Gerald M. Fenichel

Assigning fault for vaccine injuries to specific antigens becomes more difficult as immunization schedules emphasize the use of multiple simultaneous vaccines (Table 42-1). Three methods are available for assigning fault for vaccine injuries: case reports, analytical population-based (epidemiological) studies, and randomized double-blind placebo-controlled studies. Randomized double-blind placebo-controlled studies provide the most conclusive information but are rarely done because it is unethical to withhold immunization from a population at risk.

Case reports are instructive when adverse reactions to immunization are different from disorders occurring naturally, for example, paralytic poliomyelitis following administration of oral poliomyelitis vaccine (OPV). Unfortunately, neurological complications attributed to immunization are often identical to naturally occurring disease, and it is not possible, in a specific case, to determine if the neurological disorder and the immunization are related or coincidental.

Epidemiological studies are useful to study the "relative risk" of vaccine injuries. However, they rarely detect a small increase in the frequency of a common, naturally occurring disorder and cannot exclude the possibility of a "one-in-a-million" reaction. Fortunately, one-in-a-million risks are generally accepted (and are exemplified by the risk of death when driving 400 miles on an interstate highway).

Government-sponsored surveillance programs of vaccine injury were initiated after the 1976 influenza vaccine program. The initial program administered by the Centers for Disease Control (CDC) was called the Monitoring System of Adverse Events Following Immunization (MSAEFI). This was replaced in 1988 by the Vaccine Adverse Event Reporting System (VAERS). Both are stimulated passive reporting systems. The information received is fragmentary, cannot be fully confirmed, and lacks follow-up. The assignment of cause is confounded by the simultaneous administration of several vaccines; adverse events must be assigned equally to all vaccines. Thus, the most frequently reported adverse reaction to oral polio vaccine is a sore arm, because DPT is given simultaneously.

VACCINES

Five types of vaccines are available (Table 42-2).

1. *Whole killed organisms:* These were the first vaccines. Injection of denatured bacterial or viral antigens does not cause the natural disease but provokes an antibody response that prevents disease but not infection. Immune-mediated reactions have been attributed to vaccines made from whole killed organism.

Table 42-1 Types of Vaccines

Killed organisms
  Influenza
  Japanese encephalitis
  Pertussis (P)
  Poliomyelitis (IPV)
  Rabies

Live attenuated viruses
  Measles
  Mumps
  Poliomyelitis (OPV)
  Rubella
  Varicella

Toxoids or components
  Diphtheria (D)
  Pertussis acellular (Pa)
  Tetanus (T)

Conjugated
  Hemophilus influenza type B (Hib)

Recombinant
  Hepatitis B (HBV)
  Smallpox

Table 42-2 Schedule of Routine Immunization of Healthy Infants and Children (Based on Recommendations of the American Academy of Pediatrics or The Advisory Committee on Immunization Practices)

Recommended Age	Immunizations
Birth	HBV[a]
2 months	DTP, HBV, HiB,[b] OPV
4 months	DTP, HiB, OPV
6 months	DTP, HiB
6–18 months	HBV
15 months	DTaP, OPV, HiB, MMR
4–6 years	DTaP, OPV, MMR
11–12 years	MMR

Abbreviations: DTaP, diphtheria and tetanus toxoids and acellular pertussis vaccine; DTP, diphtheria and tetanus toxoids and pertussis vaccine; HBV, hepatitis B vaccine; Hib, *Hemophilus influenzae* type B vaccine; MMR, measles, mumps, and rubella vaccines; OPV, oral polio vaccine.

[a] Two options are available for HBV immunization: (1) Birth, 2 months, and 6–18 months (shown above) or (2) 1–2 months, 4 months, and 6–18 months.

[b] Two options are available for HiB immunization: (1) 2 months, 4 months, 6 months, and 15 months (shown above) or (2) 1–2 months, 4 months, and 12 months.

2. *Live attenuated virus vaccines:* These newer vaccines are intended to cause an asymptomatic infection. The advantage of asymptomatic infection is that immunity may be lifelong (like having the natural disease). However, even properly constituted vaccines can sometimes cause symptomatic infection and the expected complications of the natural disease.

3. *Toxoid vaccines:* Toxoids are denatured bacterial toxins. They can be used when the toxin that causes disease is known. Toxoids prevent disease but not infection. These vaccines have the best safety record and are almost free of neurological complications. The new acellular pertussis vaccines contain denatured components and toxins of *Bordetella pertussis* and can be considered toxoids.

4. *Conjugated vaccines:* Hemophilus influenzae type b (Hib) vaccine is the only example of this group. The purified capsular polysaccharide, polyribosylribitolphosphate (PRP), is conjugated to other compounds to enhance immunogenicity.

5. *Recombinant vaccines:* Hepatitis B and smallpox vaccines are genetically engineered. This methodology represents the future of vaccine production and is unlikely to cause adverse reactions.

WHOLE KILLED ORGANISMS

Influenza, pertussis, and inactivated poliomyelitis vaccines are the only vaccines prepared from killed organisms that are used regularly in the United States.

Other important vaccines made from whole killed organisms are for Japanese B encephalitis and rabies. Japanese B encephalitis is epidemic in Asia. Two doses of the vaccine have been shown to produce appreciable protection among children without any adverse effects.[1]

The present Merieux HDCV rabies vaccine, used in this country since 1986, has an excellent safety record.[2] It is prepared by inactivating rabies virus grown on human diploid cells. Unfortunately, many underdeveloped countries continue to prepare rabies vaccine by inactivation of virus grown in the brains or spinal cords of mature animals (Semple vaccine). Myelin basic protein is present in Semple vaccine and is responsible for producing encephalomyelitis and polyneuritis.

Influenza

Annual vaccination against influenza is recommended for the elderly and the infirm. A new vaccine is constituted each year based on virus strains that are circulating in the world and expected to appear in the United States the following winter. Neurological complications of influenza immunization were rarely noted prior to 1976. In 1976, a national program to immunize the entire population against "swine flu" was initiated. A small increase in the incidence of Guillain-Barré syndrome was seen during the 6 weeks following immunization in the civilian population but not in the military.[3] The significance of this association was questioned but later confirmed.[4] Vaccine programs after 1976 were not associated with an increased incidence of Guillain-Barré syndrome or with any other neurological complication. However, the absolute risk of a flu-like illness without sequelae is 5.5 percent higher during the first week after immunization among elderly people.[5]

Pertussis

The present whole-cell vaccine was standardized in 1947 and is a suspension of inactivated *B. pertussis* bacteria. The whole cell was used and is still in use, because the components of the organism required for immunity have never been fully established. A new generation of pertussis vaccines that consist of one or more purified components of *B. pertussis,* referred to as acellular pertussis (aP) vaccines, have been licensed in the United States for the fourth and fifth immunizations (see Table 42-2). The acellular vaccines have lower rates of local reactions and fever than the whole-cell vaccine and are recommended for children at increased risk for febrile seizures.[6]

Pertussis vaccine is ordinarily combined with diphtheria and tetanus toxoids (DTP), and almost all studies of adverse reactions are based on DTP and not pertussis vaccine alone.

The Institute of Medicine has critically reviewed and analyzed the studies concerned with a possible association of whole-cell pertussis vaccine and neurological illness[7] and the Child Neurology Society has prepared a Consensus Statement[8] that contains many of the same conclusions. These are as follows:

1. Administration of pertussis vaccine is associated with a short-term increased risk of seizures, most of these being febrile seizures, and complete recovery is expected.

2. Case reports have raised the question as to whether there is an association between pertussis vaccine and progressive or chronic neurological disorders, but controlled studies have failed to prove such an association.

3. At the present time, there is no means by which a diagnosis of encephalopathy related to pertussis vaccine can be established in an individual case.

Inactivated Poliomyelitis Vaccine

An inactivated poliomyelitis virus vaccine (IPV) administered by injection was introduced in 1955 and resulted in an immediate decline in reported cases of poliomyelitis. In 1961, IPV was replaced in the United States by a live attenuated virus vaccine administered orally (OPV). OPV replaced IPV because it was more easily administered, conferred intestinal as well as serum immunity, and could be spread from immunized to nonimmunized persons. Both vaccines are trivalent and effective. An enhanced-potency IPV is the preferred vaccine in most European countries because it cannot cause paralytic disease. The relative virtues of IPV and OPV have been regularly debated by responsible advisory bodies in the United States.[9] Presently, IPV is only recommended in the United States for individuals who are immunosuppressed or who live in households with others who are immunosuppressed.

LIVE ATTENUATED VIRUSES

Measles

Measles is the most common vaccine-preventable cause of death among children in the world; 1.5 million children were estimated to die annually from measles in 1989.[10] The currently licensed vaccine in the United States is the Moraten strain, derived from the Edmonston B strain by prolonged passage in chicken embryo cell culture. It is ordinarily combined with mumps and rubella vaccines (MMR), and most studies of adverse events have looked at MMR rather than measles alone.

A double-blind placebo-controlled crossover study of MMR was performed in twins living in the same household in order to determine the true incidence of adverse reactions.[11] Significant differences between placebo and control occurred only in the second week and could be attributed to the development of measles: high fever, rash, conjunctivitis, and unusual behavior.

Seizures may occur 7 to 14 days following measles-mumps-rubella immunization. These are almost always simple febrile seizures and are not associated with permanent neurological sequelae.[12] However, individuals who develop systemic symptoms of measles and encephalopathy in the second week following immunization should be considered to have a vaccine-related illness.

Mumps

The present live attenuated vaccine used in the United States is derived by repeated passages of the Jeryl Lynn strain in chicken embryo cells. It is 90 percent effective and produces an immune response which closely parallels the natural infection.[13] The vaccine has almost completely eliminated natural mumps infection in the United States. Reports have suggested an association of mumps vaccines and aseptic meningitis and sensorineural deafness.[14,15] The aseptic meningitis, and probably the sensorineural hearing loss, is associated with the Urabe mumps strain (1 case of aseptic meningitis in 11,000 doses) and not with the Jeryl Lynn strain used in the United States. The onset of aseptic meningitis is 15 to 35 days after vaccine administration, and recovery is always complete. No other adverse neurological events have been established, but studies of adverse reactions to mumps vaccine alone are difficult because it is always combined with measles and rubella vaccines (MMR).

Rubella

The present vaccine (RA27/3), prepared in human diploid cell culture, replaced other rubella vaccines in 1979. The Institute of Medicine reviewed studies that associate rubella vaccine with neurological illness and concluded that there is insufficient evidence to indicate a causal relation between the present rubella vaccine and radiculoneuritis and other neuropathies.[7] Up to 40 percent of people receiving the present rubella vaccine may develop transitory arthralgias and paresthesias beginning 7 to 21 days after immunization and lasting from 1 to 3 days. These symptoms are mild and are more often seen in adults than children.

Rubella virus vaccine is safe and effective. It has almost eradicated rubella embryopathy. The CDC maintained a registry of women accidentally immunized from 3 months before to 3 months after conception until 1989; none resulted in congenital rubella syndrome.[16]

Oral Poliomyelitis Vaccine

In 1961, IPV was replaced in the United States by a live attenuated virus vaccine administered orally (OPV). The main disadvantage of OPV is that it may be associated with paralytic disease, whereas IPV produces only low-grade fever for the first 2 days in 5 percent of children.

Since 1980, all cases of paralytic polio in the United States have been vaccine-related.[17] The overall frequency of vaccine-related paralytic disease is 1 per 2.5 million doses of OPV distributed. The groups at risk are infants receiving their first immunization (90 percent of cases occur after the first dose), persons in contact with OPV-recipients, and immunologically compromised individuals who either receive OPV or are in contact with OPV recipients. The suggestion has been made that enhanced-potency IPV should be administered prior to OPV immunization in order to reduce the risk of vaccine-related disease.

The interval between vaccine administration and onset of illness ranges from 11 to 58 days. Healthy individuals tend to have a shorter latency than immunosuppressed individuals.

One epidemiological study suggested that OPV could trigger Guillain-Barré syndrome in adults.[18] Unfortunately, the study used 10 weeks as the risk interval. Only 6 of 10 patients developed the Guillain-Barré syndrome within 3 weeks of immunization; the interval in the remainder was 6 weeks or longer. The Institute of Medicine in their analysis of the data concluded that "the evidence favors acceptance of a causal relation between OPV and Guillain-Barré syndrome,"[19] but I do not accept the evidence as compelling.

Varicella

A live attenuated varicella vaccine was developed in 1974 and will eventually be licensed for routine immunization after 1 year of age. It is safe and immunogenic in normal and immunocompromised children and has been used to protect children with acute lymphocytic leukemia from natural infection.[20] Neurological complications have not been reported.

TOXOIDS

Diphtheria and tetanus toxoids are almost always given together, and it is difficult to distinguish which adverse events should be assigned to one or the other. The toxin elaborated by the two organisms is inactivated, and the antigens are absorbed on aluminum phosphate and preserved with thimerosal, a mercury derivative.

A man developed three episodes of Guillain-Barré syndrome, each following administration of tetanus toxoid, separated by 9 and 5 years; the intervals between immunization and onset of symptoms were 3 weeks, 2 weeks, and 9 days.[21] A child with two episodes of Guillain-Barré syndrome following two tetanus immunizations was reported to the national Vaccine Injury Compensation Program. These individuals clearly have a unique sensitivity to tetanus toxoid; however, the association between tetanus toxoid and Guillain-Barré syndrome in the general population has not been studied.

CONJUGATED VACCINES

The original *H. influenzae* type b vaccine (Hib) was a component vaccine consisting of the purified capsular polysaccharide, polyribosylribitolphosphate (PRP). Because PRP vaccine was not effective in children less than 18 months of age, the age when children are at greatest risk for *H. influenzae* meningitis, PRP was conjugated with other compounds to increase efficacy. PRP may be linked to the outer membrane protein complex of *Neisseria meningitidis* (PRP-OMPC) or to diphtheria toxoid (PRP-D). These vaccines have decreased the incidence of *H. influenza* type B disease in children by 90 percent.[22]

Adverse reactions to HiB vaccines are unusual; sore arms and fever occur in less than 2 percent of children when the vaccine is given alone.[23] Four children less than 5 years of age have developed Guillain-Barré syndrome within 10 days of PRP-D vaccine adminis-

tration.[24,25] One had simultaneously received DTP and OPV. The causal link between Hib immunization and Guillain-Barré syndrome is not established by this small number of reports.[19]

RECOMBINANT VACCINES

Recombinant technology is the future of vaccine development. A smallpox vaccine, used only by people working with the virus in laboratories, was the first recombinant vaccine. Hepatitis B vaccine is the only recombinant vaccine presently licensed in the United States. A portion of the hepatitis B virus gene coding for the surface antigen is cloned into yeast, and the vaccine is produced from cultures of the recombinant yeast strain.

A plasma-derived hepatitis B vaccine was used from 1982 to 1988; the recombinant product was initially used in late 1987. The incidence of pain at injection site, fatigue, fever, and headache among those receiving the vaccine was no greater than in those receiving placebo in controlled trials. There are reports of Guillain-Barré syndrome following vaccination, especially the plasma-derived vaccine, but a cause-and-effect association has not been established.[19]

REFERENCES

1. Hoke CH, Nisalak A, Sangawhipa N, et al: Protection against Japanese encephalitis by inactivated vaccines. N Engl J Med 319:608, 1988
2. Bernard KW, Smith PW, Kader FJ, et al: Neuroparalytic illness and human diploid cell rabies vaccine. JAMA 248:3136, 1982
3. Johnson DE: Guillain-Barré syndrome in the US Army. Arch Neurol 39:21, 1982
4. Safranek TJ, Lawrence DN, Kurland LT, et al: Reassessment of the association between Guillain-Barré syndrome and receipt of swine influenza vaccine in 1976–1977: results of a two-state study. Am J Epidemiol 133:940, 1991
5. Margolis KL, Poland GA, Nichol KL, et al: Frequency of adverse reactions after influenza vaccination. Am J Med 88:27, 1990
6. Centers for Disease Control: Pertussis vaccination: acellular pertussis vaccine for reinforcing and booster use—supplementary ACIP statement: recommenda-

tions of the Immunizations Practice Advisory Committee (ACIP). MMWR 41(RR-1):1, 1992

7. Institute of Medicine: Adverse Effects of Pertussis and Rubella Vaccines. National Academy Press, Washington, DC, 1991

8. Child Neurology Society Consensus Report: Pertussis immunization and the central nervous system. Ann Neurol 29:458, 1991

9. Kimpen JLL, Ogra PL: Poliovirus vaccines: a continuing challenge. Pediatr Clin North Am 37:627, 1990

10. Markowitz LE, Orenstein WA: Measles vaccines. Pediatr Clin North Am 37:603, 1990

11. Peltola H, Heinonen OP: Frequency of true adverse reactions to measles-mumps-rubella vaccine. Lancet 1: 939, 1986

12. Griffin MR, Ray WA, Mortimer EA, et al: Risk of seizures after measles-mumps-rubella immunization. Pediatrics 88:881, 1991

13. Bakshi SS, Cooper LZ: Rubella and mumps vaccines. Pediatr Clin North Am 37:651, 1990

14. Miller E, Goldacre M, Pugh S, et al: Risk of aseptic meningitis after measles, mumps, and rubella vaccine in UK children. Lancet 341:979, 1993

15. Stewart BJA, Prabhu PU: Reports of sensorineural deafness after measles, mumps, and rubella immunization. Arch Dis Child 69:153, 1993

16. Centers for Disease Control: Rubella vaccination during pregnancy 1971–1988. MMWR 39:287, 1989

17. Strebel PM, Sutter RW, Cochi SL, et al: Epidemiology of poliomyelitis in the United States one decade after the last reported case of indigenous wild virus-associated disease. Clin Infect Dis 14:568, 1992

18. Kinnunen E, Farkkila M, Hovi T, et al: Incidence of Guillain-Barré syndrome during a nationwide oral poliovirus vaccine campaign. Neurology 39:1034, 1989

19. Institute of Medicine: Adverse Events Associated with Childhood Vaccines. National Academy Press, Washington, DC, 1993

20. White CJ, Kuter BJ, Hildebrand CS, et al: Varicella vaccine (VARIVAX) in healthy children and adolescents: results from clinical trials, 1987 to 1989. Pediatrics 87:604, 1991

21. Pollard JD, Selby G: Relapsing neuropathy due to tetanus toxoid. J Neurol Sci 37:113, 1978

22. Murphy TV, White KE, Pastor P, et al: Declining incidence of Haemophilus influenzae type B disease since introduction of vaccination. JAMA 269:246, 1993

23. Vadheim CM, Greenberg DP, Marcy SM, et al: Safety evaluation of PRP-D Haemophilus influenzae type b conjugate vaccine in children immunized at 18 months of age and older: follow-up study of 30,000 children. Pediatr Infect Dis 9:555, 1990

24. D'Cruz OF, Shapiro ED, Spiegelman KN, et al: Acute inflammatory demyelinating polyradiculoneuropathy (Guillain-Barré syndrome) after immunization with Haemophilus influenzae type b conjugate vaccine. J Pediatr 115:743, 1989

25. Gervaix A, Caflisch M, Suter A, et al: Guillain-Barré syndrome following immunisation with Haemophilus influenzae type b conjugate vaccine. Eur J Pediatr 152: 613, 1993

43

Sarcoidosis of the Nervous System

Donald H. Silberberg

Sarcoidosis was first noticed as an unusual skin granuloma toward the end of the nineteenth century. At first a connection with tuberculosis was suspected because of the similarity of the skin lesions to those of cutaneous tuberculosis. It soon became evident, however, that the condition also affected bone, lymph nodes, spleen, lung, conjunctiva, iris, and other internal organs. The names of noted physicians are attached to various syndromes describing groups of cases with similar clinical pictures, understood by later workers to have resulted from sarcoidosis. An eponym worth noting for neurologists is Heerfordt's syndrome; in 1909 Heerfordt described patients with enlargement of the parotid and sometimes other salivary glands, chronic or subacute uveitis, and in many cases paresis from cranial nerve involvement, especially the facial nerve.[1] Heerfordt thought that it was chronic mumps, but later accounts of the histological picture made it clear that he was describing a somewhat unusual presentation of sarcoidosis. His was one of the first clinical descriptions of sarcoid involvement of the nervous system.

DEFINITION

Sarcoidosis is a systemic disease of unknown etiology with protean manifestations. It is necessary to define the limits of what can be considered sarcoido-

sis. Scadding has suggested that "sarcoidosis is a disease characterized by the presence in all or several affected organs or tissues of epithelioid cell tubercles, without caseation, though some fibrinoid necrosis may be present at the centers of a few tubercles, proceeding either to resolution or to conversion of the epithelioid cell tubercles into avascular acellular hyaline fibrous tissue."[2] He added as an explanatory note that "the organs most frequently involved are the lymph nodes, lungs, liver, spleen, skin, eyes, small bones of the hands and feet and salivary glands, though every organ and tissue, with the possible exception of the adrenal gland, has been reported to be involved." This description leads to the conclusion that the criterion that would be accepted by all or nearly all informed observers as definitive for the diagnosis of sarcoidosis is the demonstration in several affected organs of the typical granuloma.

Sarcoidosis must be distinguished from the nonspecific, localized sarcoid tissue reaction. Sarcoid tissue reaction may occur in response to a variety of stimuli and is distinguished by the fact that it usually involves only one system; moreover, affected patients have normal calcium metabolism and are not anergic to skin testing.

CLINICAL PRESENTATION

The patient with sarcoidosis most commonly consults a physician after being told that a routine chest

847

radiograph is abnormal. In several survey series the prevalence of chest roentgenogram findings highly suggestive of sarcoidosis outnumbered the prevalence of symptomatic cases by more than four to one. Approximately 25 percent of patients seek medical help because of respiratory symptoms, often dyspnea. Ocular symptoms bring more than 10 percent of sarcoid patients to the physician. Skin changes occur initially in approximately 5 percent of patients and enlargement of superficial lymph nodes, sufficient to be noticed initially by the patient, in slightly fewer patients. Less frequently, involvement of the nervous system, the hypothalamic-pituitary system, or muscle is the first sign of sarcoidosis.

EPIDEMIOLOGY

Prevalence

National prevalence rates of sarcoidosis vary widely from country to country and among different ethnic groups within countries. Some of these differences are due to varying degrees of awareness of sarcoidosis and some to differing diagnostic methods—from the incomplete method of miniature chest roentgenogram surveys to careful medical workup including biopsy for histological examination. A high prevalence rate was recorded for Sweden: a rate of 64/100,000 was based on radiographic study of approximately 2 million persons between 1953 and 1960. Prevalence rates vary widely from one area of Sweden to another, ranging from 4/100,000 to 137/100,000 population.[3] Other countries with high prevalence rates include Norway, Denmark, The Netherlands, Great Britain, and the United States. Low prevalence rates are recorded for Canada, Australia, Scotland, Finland, Japan, Czechoslovakia, Israel, Uruguay, Brazil, Argentina, and Portugal.[4] It has been difficult to determine the overall prevalence in the United States, although sarcoid seems to be 10 to 20 times more frequent in blacks than in whites.

Age and Sex Incidence

Sarcoidosis is slightly more frequent in women than in men. The peak incidence in both sexes is around the age of 25 to 30 years. Sarcoidosis is rare below the age of 15 and still more unusual below the age of 9, although the diagnosis has been made on histological evidence in infants.

HISTOPATHOLOGY OF SARCOIDOSIS

The pathological change that identifies sarcoidosis is the appearance of characteristic sarcoid tubercles in affected organs. The sarcoid tubercle is characterized by (1) a rounded collection of large epithelioid cells with pale-staining nuclei; (2) the sparsity of lymphocytes, which tend to be more numerous at the periphery of the tubercle; and (3) the absence of necrosis. Variable numbers of giant cells are present, but their frequency does not help to distinguish sarcoid from the other diseases in which tubercles are found.

The giant cells may be either the typical Langerhans' type, which contain nuclei in a circle or semicircle around a central granular zone, or the foreign-body type, in which the nuclei are found scattered throughout the cytoplasm. These giant cells may contain one of several varieties of inclusions; the origin of the inclusions is not clear, and their forms are not specific for sarcoidosis.

Epithelioid cells are mononuclear phagocytes modified by enlargement of both cytoplasm and nucleus. The nucleus appears pale because the chromatin does not increase proportionately. The origin of the mononuclear phagocyte is from either blood monocytes or tissue histiocytes. Giant cells are also formed from mononuclear phagocytes by fusion of individual cells or by nuclear division in the absence of cytoplasmic replication. The tubercle of tuberculosis is distinguished by necrosis in the center of the tubercle or in the center of a group of tubercles; autolysis is incomplete, and the result is a histological picture of caseation. Similar tubercles occur with less frequency in cryptococcosis, histoplasmosis, coccidioidomycosis, blastomycosis, syphilis, lymphogranuloma inguinale, leprosy, brucellosis, and tularemia.

Sarcoid tubercles may resolve completely. When they do not, they may cause production of a characteristic amorphous mass of avascular and acellular fibrous tissue, often with surviving sarcoid tubercles identifiable at various points in the mass.

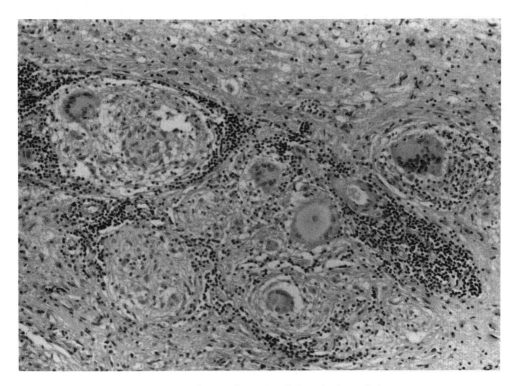

Fig. 43-1 Sarcoid granuloma involving the hypothalamus.

Virtually all organs of the body except the adrenal glands have been reported to be involved histologically. The omission is of interest but not yet explained. The appearance of the sarcoid tubercles does not vary from organ to organ, but each tissue responds with its own histological reaction to the intruding granuloma (Fig. 43-1).

IMMUNOLOGICAL AND OTHER LABORATORY FEATURES OF SARCOIDOSIS

Granuloma Formation

In lung tissue it appears that granuloma formation is preceded by an infiltration of mononuclear cells, many of which are T lymphocytes that show morphological features and surface markers of activation.[5] Macrophages coalesce into giant cells and epithelioid cell granulomas. T-helper lymphocytes mobilized by this activity interact with macrophages, leading to B lymphocyte overactivity. The activated B cells produce immunoglobulins. The granulomas secrete a variety of enzymes, including angiotensin-converting enzyme, and detection of this enzyme in blood and cerebrospinal fluid (CSF) helps in the diagnosis. Angiotensin-converting enzyme is elevated in about 60 percent of patients with active sarcoidosis.[6] Levels tend to return to normal with spontaneous or corticosteroid-induced remissions. However, the level may be falsely positive in up to 10 percent of individuals tested, so this is not a good diagnostic test. Its main value is for monitoring the progress of known sarcoidosis. Additionally, CSF angiotensin-converting enzyme may prove to be a valid marker of sarcoidosis within the central neuraxis.[7,8]

Immunological Alterations

The major immunological alterations of sarcoidosis include suppression of delayed-type hypersensitivity, elevated serum immunoglobulins, and a positive response to the Kveim-Siltzbach antigen. In 1916 Boeck noted that two of his original three patients showed no skin reaction to tuberculin testing.[2] Many workers have since found that the proportion of patients with sarcoidosis who have a positive tuberculin skin test is much lower than that of comparable population groups who do not have sarcoidosis. Patients with sarcoid are similarly nonreactive to other agents causing delayed hypersensitivity skin reactions. Antigens tested include mumps virus, pertussis, *Candida albicans, Trichophyton,* oidiomycin, pine pollen, dinitrochlorobenzene (DNCB), and keyhole limpet hemocyanin (KLH).[9] The reason for the impairment of delayed skin sensitivity is not clear. Anergy tends to correlate with lymphopenia and the extent of involvement outside the chest as well as with overall disease activity.

In contrast to the impairment in delayed-type hypersensitivity, patients with sarcoidosis have a normal capacity for producing circulating antibodies in response to appropriate antigenic stimulation and a normal incidence of allergic disorders. Formation of circulating antibodies has been tested with pertussis and typhoid-paratyphoid vaccines. The combination of normal circulating antibodies and poor skin responsivity has been used as the basis for a presumptive test for sarcoidosis: most normal adults show both a positive complement-fixation test and a positive skin test to mumps virus antigen. Virtually all patients with sarcoidosis have a positive complement-fixation test but less commonly have a positive skin test. Increased circulating antibody levels to Epstein-Barr virus, herpes simplex, rubella, and parainfluenza viruses and an increased antibody response to mismatched blood occur among patients with sarcoidosis, perhaps in correlation with increased immunoglobulin levels.

Immunoglobulin (Ig) levels are abnormally elevated in approximately 80 percent of patients with sarcoidosis. Serum IgG is most commonly raised; IgA, IgM, and IgE are raised in somewhat fewer patients.[9] The levels do not correlate with the organ systems involved, the clinical stage of the disease, or the response to Kviem-Siltzbach antigen. Patients do not have increased frequency of circulating autoantibodies to gastric, thyroid, antimitochondrial, or antinuclear factors compared with a normal population.[7] That a relative immune deficiency is part of sarcoidosis is suggested by the occurrence in patients with this disorder of opportunistic infections such as tuberculous meningitis,[10] cryptococcal meningitis,[11] progressive multifocal leukoencephalopathy,[12] and herpes simplex encephalitis.[13]

Kveim-Siltzbach Test

Kveim found that intradermal injection of a heated suspension of tissue homogenate prepared from a sarcoid lymph node resulted in the formation of a nodule within 4 weeks in 12 of 13 patients with sarcoidosis.[14] The nodules often increased in size for several weeks and persisted for several months. Biopsy showed histological changes resembling sarcoidosis. Kveim reported that this reaction did not occur in control subjects. Numerous investigators have reproduced the work with various refinements in the preparation of the antigen. Problems of routine clinical use of this test include the low but definite number of apparently normal people who have a positive tissue reaction and the fact that in 15 to 25 percent of patients with sarcoidosis the test is negative.

Attempts to isolate the active component have been unsuccessful. It is particulate and not water-soluble, and it does not pass a Berkefeld or Seitz filter. Particles sedimenting within 15 minutes after centrifugation at 5,500 × g have the highest activity. Lipid extraction does not reduce activity. Removal of nucleoprotein does not reduce potency, but exposure to alkaloid destroys potency. Spleen is the most convenient tissue for preparing antigen in large quantities.

It is of considerable epidemiological significance that sarcoid patients all over the world have been shown to react to a single Kveim antigen.[9] The lack of success in standardizing the antigen has led clinicians in the United States to use the Kveim test less often, although it is still in widespread use throughout Europe.

Hypercalcemia

Many patients with sarcoidosis develop an elevated serum calcium level at some time during their illness, and they may develop renal calculi. Corneal, conjunctival, and occasionally other soft tissue calcifications may develop as a result of the hypercalcemia.

The hypercalcemia occurs for reasons that are not clear. Patients with sarcoidosis convert 25-hydroxycholecalciferol to the highly active 1,25-dihydroxycholecalciferol (calcitriol). Calcitriol produces increased absorption of calcium from the gut, leading to hypercalcemia and hypercalciuria. In sarcoidosis, enhanced synthesis of calcitriol is induced by sunlight and is reversed by corticosteroid therapy.

ETIOLOGY

The cause of sarcoidosis is unknown, although many theories have been put forward. The concept that sarcoidosis is an unusual phase in the development of tuberculosis was popular until the 1940s. There are two major reasons for the modern belief that there is no obvious link between tuberculosis and sarcoid. First, the prevalence of tuberculosis in many areas throughout the world has dropped drastically in the past 20 years, whereas the prevalence of sarcoidosis has remained static. As tuberculosis becomes less common, the apparent evolution of sarcoidosis into pulmonary tuberculosis, said to occur in 10 to 25 percent of patients before World War II, has become an uncommon event. Second, the effective antituberculous drugs that are now available have no clinical effect on sarcoidosis.

It is possible that the development of sarcoidosis requires that abnormal immune regulation exist before the disease is contracted. Sarcoid arthritis, erythema nodosum, and anterior uveitis are more common in individuals who are HLA-A1-B8 positive. HLA-B13 is more likely to be associated with chronic disease.[15]

Overt immunocompromise as a predisposing factor seems to be excluded by the finding that, among a group of British schoolchildren receiving bacille Calmette-Guérin (BCG) vaccination, 52 patients who later developed sarcoidosis had developed positive tuberculin skin tests with the same frequency as vaccinated patients who did not develop sarcoidosis.[16]

Hormonal factors may play a part in predisposition, as erythema nodosum due to sarcoidosis commonly occurs in women during childbearing years and early pregnancy as well as in women using oral contraceptives. Although it is possible that *Mycobacterium tuberculosis* or "atypical" mycobacteria are somehow inciting etiological agents of sarcoidosis, no convincing evidence of an infectious etiology has been forthcoming.

INVOLVEMENT OF THE NERVOUS SYSTEM

Heerfordt's description of uveoparotid fever was one of the first studies of sarcoidosis of the nervous system.[1] He described three patients who complained of malaise, fever, parotid swelling, and uveitis. One man had polyuria and polydipsia with a mild CSF pleocytosis. Two patients had optic neuritis with transient dysphagia, and one also had paresthesias suggestive of mononeuritis multiplex. Two years after the report, one of the younger patients developed an acute retrobulbar neuritis. Since then, many patients have been described with various central nervous system (CNS), peripheral, and muscle manifestations of sarcoidosis,[17–36] as summarized in Table 43-1.

Estimates of the proportion of patients with neurological involvement vary greatly among the series reported. The highest incidence of neurological involvement in a series of patients with histologically proved sarcoidosis is 14 percent.[32] Other series average 4 to 8 percent of patients. These figures are derived from sarcoid clinics and of course do not allow for the occasional patient in whom there are insufficient systemic signs or laboratory findings to establish the diagnosis with certainty and in whom the neurological site of primary involvement is not suitable for biopsy. Most patients with neurosarcoidosis are those with previously diagnosed systemic sarcoidosis who develop signs of neurological involvement during the course of their illness. A smaller proportion initially exhibit neurological signs, and a still smaller proportion never develop clear signs of involvement of other organ systems.

The sites of clinical involvement, in decreasing order of frequency, are (1) meningeal (including most patients with cranial nerve palsies and involvement of the pituitary and hypothalamus); (2) peripheral nerve; (3) muscle; and (4) parenchymal regions (brain and spinal cord) (Table 43-1). If only histological features were used as criteria for involvement, muscle would rank first; muscle involvement is frequent in patients with no complaint of weakness.

Meningeal and Cranial Nerve Involvement

Facial nerve palsy is the most common neurological sign of sarcoidosis, occurring in about 50 percent of patients who develop neurological involvement. It is ordinarily transient and frequently bilateral. When the parotid gland is swollen (in which case there is often an accompanying iritis), the facial nerve is frequently involved. However, facial paresis also occurs without

Table 43-1 Reported Incidences of Neurological Manifestations of Sarcoidosis

Study	Location	Total	No. of Patients — Site of Involvement — Intracranial	Hypo-thalamic & Pituitary	Spinal cord	Peripheral Nerve	Cranial Nerve	Percent with Neurological Involvement
Longcope[17] (1941)	Baltimore	31	2	1	1	—	—	13
Gravesen[18] (1942)	Scandinavia	150	—	1	—	—	5	5
Reisner[19] (1944)	New York	35	—	—	1	—	1	6
Fisher[20] (1947)	Baltimore	94	—	1	2	—	6	10
Ricker & Clark[21] (1949)	Washington DC	195	3	—	—	—	—	1.5
Riley[22] (1950)	New York	52	1	—	—	1	1	6
Longcope[23] (1952)	Baltimore	90	—	1	—	1	3	6
Freiman[23] (1952)	Boston	70	1	—	—	—	—	1.4
Gendel et al[24] (1952)	Memphis	24	—	1	1	—	4	29
Nitter[25] (1953)	Oslo	90	—	—	—	—	3	3
Cowdell[26] (1954)	Oxford	90	1	3	—	1	—	6
Israel & Sones[27] (1958)	Philadelphia	160	2	2	—	—	3	4
Goodson[28] (1960)	Nashville	63	1	—	—	1	2	6
Douglas[29] (1961)	Scotland	100	—	2	—	—	6	8
Bacharach[30] (1961)	Denver	111	1	—	—	—	—	1
Rudberg-Roos[31] (1962)	Ostersund, Sweden	296	4	1	—	4	4	6
Mayock et al[32] (1963)	Philadelphia	145	10	—	2	10	3	16
Silverstein et al[33] (1965)	New York	450	5	—	1	4	8	4
James et al[34] (1976)	Worldwide	3,676	—	—	—	—	—	4
James & Williams[35] (1984)	London	818	—	—	—	—	—	9
Stern et al[36] (1985)	Baltimore	649	0	5	2	2	24	5

parotid swelling or may subside even as parotid swelling increases. Frequently the sense of taste is lost along with the power of the facial muscles, indicating that the lesion is not in the parotid gland but above the exit of the chorda tympani. Occasionally there is no parotid swelling or loss of taste sense and no other sign of involvement of the meninges of the base of the skull, so that the cause of the seventh nerve malfunction cannot be determined. It is important to re-

member that sarcoid-induced facial nerve palsy frequently subsided completely before corticosteroids were available. The occurrence of facial paresis in otherwise asymptomatic patients with sarcoidosis is sufficiently frequent to warrant the suggestion that all patients with facial palsy of unknown etiology should have a chest radiograph to exclude hilar adenopathy.[33]

When one includes the optic disc, the optic nerve

is the second most commonly involved cranial nerve. Approximately 30 percent of patients with sarcoidosis have ocular involvement.[37] Before corticosteroids were available for treating iritis, the media of the eye were frequently too hazy to allow a good ophthalmoscopic view of the posterior pole of the eye. Now that the anterior inflammation can be controlled fairly readily, many observers are reporting the appearance of papilledema, optic atrophy, or visual field defects.[37–41] Papilledema may result from posterior choroiditis involving the peripapillary area. It probably reflects invasion of the meningeal coverings of the optic nerves by sarcoid granulation tissue or, judging by occasional acute retrobulbar neuritis or other visual field defects, sometimes of the parenchyma of the nerve itself. In addition, papilledema may of course reflect increased intracranial pressure from either diffuse involvement of the meninges by sarcoid tissue or obstructive hydrocephalus due to interference with CSF flow at the base of the skull. Blain and associates estimated that 15 percent of patients with sarcoidosis have fundus involvement and that 5 percent have an abnormality of the optic disc.[37] Conversely, Gould and Kaufman estimated that 40 percent of patients with fundus lesions have neurological involvement.[38]

Dysphagia and paralysis of one or both vocal cords are also frequent cranial nerve manifestations of sarcoidosis. They commonly occur together with other cranial neuropathies.

The eighth cranial nerve is the next most frequently affected, and there are a number of reports of either unilateral or bilateral neural deafness or decreased vestibular response. Almost as frequent is involvement of either the sensory or motor divisions of the trigeminal nerve. Patients with sensory symptoms have been described more frequently than those with weakness of the muscles of mastication. This finding may reflect the considerable reserve in strength of the jaw muscles compared with the sensitivity of paresthesias in reflecting neurological dysfunction. Only scattered reports exist of involvement of the olfactory, oculomotor, trochlear, abducens, spinal accessory, or hypoglossal nerve.

Cranial nerve palsies frequently occur together, often with iritis and parotid swelling. Simultaneous involvement of several cranial nerves on one side strongly suggests granuloma infiltration of the meninges at the base of the brain. CSF protein concentra-

tion and cells are elevated in only some patients and hence are not helpful for the diagnosis. Ordinarily, the only histopathological findings are those obtained at autopsy, and the tissue most available for examination is that of the basal meninges. Everything from barely visible opacification and thickening of the meninges and origin of the cranial nerves to gross tumor formation with displacement of the optic chiasm or other structures has been reported. There has been little opportunity to examine the course of the cranial nerves once they leave the base of the skull, so the frequency of infiltration in the more peripheral part of the cranial nerves is not known. It is of interest that the Argyll-Robertson pupil (miosis, absent light reflex, intact accommodation reflex) has been reported in patients with neurosarcoidosis in a variety of clinical settings.[42,43]

Meningeal Sarcoidosis

Meningeal involvement may occur in virtually any region of the CNS. Involvement at the base of the brain was discussed above in terms of the production of cranial nerve dysfunction. Details concerning other areas related to the meninges follow.

PITUITARY-HYPOTHALAMIC SARCOIDOSIS

The pituitary-hypothalamic system is the most frequently involved of any endocrine tissue in sarcoidosis.[44]

Diabetes Insipidus

Polydipsia and polyuria have been reported frequently. Sarcoid granulomas have been found in the pituitary glands over a wide age range, from a 1-year-old infant[45] to a 77-year-old woman.[46] To date, diabetes insipidus has been reported in somewhat more than 10 percent of patients with neurosarcoidosis. The figures from cases without histological confirmation of the diagnosis are less valid, as polydipsia and polyuria may also be secondary to hypercalcemia, nephrocalcinosis, or nephrogenic diabetes insipidus of sarcoidosis.[47]

Most patients with sarcoidosis and diabetes insipidus have obvious involvement of other organ systems, but occasionally the hypothalamic-pituitary symptoms are the initial manifestations of the disease. They present obvious diagnostic difficulties. Most patients also have visual disturbances reflecting involvement of the optic chiasm, somnolence, hyperthermia, impotence, or amenorrhea as other manifestations of hypothalamic-pituitary disease. Frequently the entire optic chiasm, pituitary gland, and floor of the third ventricle including the hypothalamus are diffusely infiltrated by sarcoid granulomas. However, diabetes insipidus may result from involvement of the hypothalamus that has spared the pituitary gland and infundibulum. Conversely, involvement of the pituitary may occur without producing symptoms, which is consistent with the observation that diabetes insipidus does not ordinarily result from injury to the supraopticohypophyseal tract below the median eminence.[48]

Hypopituitarism

Winnacker and associates reviewed the reports of 19 randomly selected cases of sarcoidosis in which pituitary function was adequately evaluated; they found diabetes insipidus in 14 cases and deficiency of one or more anterior pituitary hormones in 17 cases.[44] Deficiencies of gonadotropin, thyroid-stimulating hormone, and ACTH were most common, in decreasing order of frequency. It therefore seems probable that the infrequency with which hypopituitarism was mentioned in earlier reports was due to inadequate laboratory evaluation of anterior pituitary function. Furthermore, the symptoms of hypopituitarism are subtle and slowly progressive compared to the rapid and dramatic polydipsia and polyuria, and they are often overshadowed by more serious involvement of other systems. Other reported manifestations of hypopituitarism in sarcoidosis have included fatal hypoglycemia, pituitary dwarfism, hypogonadism manifesting as infantilism or Frohlich's syndrome, and, in one patient at autopsy, an empty sella turcica.

Histologically, the granulomas are usually perivascular, suggesting that vascular channels are important in the pathogenesis of sarcoidosis in this region as well as elsewhere. However, cases have been reported with infiltration of the pituitary capsule but without involvement of the gland parenchyma, suggesting that transmission of the causative agent is through the CSF in some patients.

Hypothalamic Sarcoidosis

Involvement of the hypothalamus has been well documented at autopsy (Fig. 43-1). In addition to diabetes insipidus and hypopituitarism, the clinical results have included somnolence, insomnia, extreme variations in body temperature, progressive obesity, and marked personality changes.

As alluded to previously, definite diagnosis in isolated involvement of this region of the CNS presents a problem. As in other instances of meningeal involvement, the CSF protein concentration is frequently increased, with an associated lymphocytic pleocytosis and occasionally a low glucose content. Radiological evidence is often nonspecific. However, calcification in or above the pituitary gland is evidence against the diagnosis of intracranial sarcoidosis, as the sarcoid granulomas rarely develop gross calcification.

CEREBRAL SARCOIDOSIS

The site of meningeal invasion over the surface of the brain may act as a seizure focus. If involvement is generalized, mental changes, photophobia, and nuchal rigidity may mimic bacterial or fungal meningitis. Rarely a locus of granuloma enlarges sufficiently to act as a space-occupying lesion, producing the signs of a brain tumor referable to the area involved. "Tumors" occupying all regions of the brain have been reported.[49,50] Granulomas are readily detected and followed by computed tomography (CT) scanning or magnetic resonance imaging (MRI).

SPINAL CORD SARCOIDOSIS

Focal involvement of spinal arachnoid or dura usually produces the picture of a transverse myelopathy. Fortunately such involvement is unusual, because in this area the response to treatment is often incomplete at best. Some patients developing transverse myelopathy do not show abnormalities on myelography. MRI often shows meningeal thickening or, by gadolinium enhancement, inflammation. Unexpected parenchymal granulomas are also seen by MRI.[51]

Spinal fluid abnormalities are common in patients with meningeal involvement, as would be expected. Pleocytosis varies from a few to several hundred lymphocytes. Protein concentrations are almost always elevated and have been recorded as high as 560 mg/dl. CSF glucose concentration is often reduced in sarcoid of the meninges.

Peripheral Neuropathy

Peripheral nerves are involved in 25 percent[33] to 50 percent[32] of all patients with neurosarcoidosis. Motor and sensory symptoms occur with approximately equal frequency. The pattern of involvement varies from a symmetrical peripheral neuropathy to a mononeuropathy multiplex. In general, at least two mechanisms for involvement of peripheral nerves exist. Those patients with diffuse symmetrical involvement probably have an extension of meningeal sarcoidosis to involve the nerve roots, which would account for the instances in which no histological abnormality is found on peripheral nerve biopsy. Alternatively, occasional patients have gross thickening of the nerves. Inflammatory perineural changes and infiltration between nerve fibers of typical sarcoid granuloma have been described.[2]

As with other manifestations of sarcoidosis, the symptoms may be transient. CSF pleocytosis tends to be slight in these patients, whereas elevations of protein concentration are considerable, ranging up to 720 mg/dl. CSF glucose has been normal in patients with peripheral neuropathy (in contrast to the decreased glucose concentration often found with meningeal involvement). Some cases are clinically indistinguishable from acute Guillain-Barré syndrome.

Parenchymal Sarcoid

Reports of tumor formation within the brain or spinal cord, without obvious meningeal involvement, are rare. Ordinarily it is presumed that infiltration occurs via the Virchow-Robin spaces. However, it is possible that occasionally blood-borne foci of granuloma formation occur. As mentioned, neurosurgeons have reported finding sarcoid granuloma as an unexpected tumor at craniotomy in patients with signs of a brain tumor.[47,49,50] In addition to focal loss of function, focal or generalized seizures are frequently a severe problem with these lesions. With parenchymal involvement, the CSF is less likely to be abnormal because the lesion may not be near a CSF–brain interface.

Myopathy

An occasional patient shows muscle weakness that cannot be attributed to peripheral nerve or CNS involvement. Some have palpable nodules in the muscles, and stiffness and pain or soreness of the muscles may make it more obvious that the patient has a myopathy. Proximal muscle atrophy is frequent.

When a patient with known sarcoidosis develops symptoms referable to the muscles, the chances are excellent of finding the lesions histologically on muscle biopsy, allowing for the fact that a given biopsy sample is only a small portion of the total muscle mass. Of more interest is the fact that muscle biopsy yields typical sarcoid tubercles in up to 50 percent of patients with established sarcoidosis who do not have signs and symptoms of myopathy. Of 42 patients whose diagnosis was established by biopsy elsewhere but who did not have signs indicating muscle involvement, 23 showed sarcoid lesions on random biopsy from skeletal muscle.[52] Because muscle can be biopsied without risk, it has been proposed as a routine biopsy site. The wider the dissemination of the sarcoidosis, the more likely is the muscle biopsy to show sarcoid lesions.

NATURAL HISTORY OF NEUROSARCOIDOSIS

Cranial and peripheral nerve and meningeal involvement most commonly occur during the first 2 years of the disease.[33] Spontaneous remission occurs in about two-thirds of patients who develop neurological involvement; about one-third progress if untreated.[36,53,54] Resolution is likely in young patients with sarcoid of sudden onset and a short history. Once a remission has lasted for some time, it is unusual for new symptoms to occur in the same area; occasionally, however, a flareup occurs years after the initial symptoms. Parenchymal involvement frequently occurs in the patient who has had known sarcoid for several years. Sarcoid granulomas appearing as brain tumors are obvious exceptions when they occur in patients without apparent systemic involvement. Spontaneous remission of brain or spinal cord masses is much less likely than remission of peripheral lesions. Infarction and demyelination distal to arteries strangled by sarcoid tissues are well-known histological findings and probably account for much continuing or unremitting damage within the CNS. Other problems may arise without actual new granuloma formation. Meningeal involvement may lead to scarring and eventually to obstructive hydrocephalus, with consequent ataxia and dementia. Epilepsy may continue as a sign of previous granuloma involvement even though the process is no longer active.

DIAGNOSIS OF NEUROSARCOIDOSIS

Various areas of involvement frequently occur simultaneously, making neurosarcoidosis one of the more challenging diagnostic problems of modern neurology. The diagnosis is most secure when clinical and radiological evidence of multisystem involvement is supported by histological evidence of noncaseating epithelioid cell granulomas.

Neuroimaging studies, especially CT scanning and MRI, are helpful in detecting and localizing lesions.[55,56] On CT scans, lesions may have either increased or reduced densities; on MRI, they often appear with mixed signal intensities on T_1-weighted images and with increased signal intensity on T_2 scans. The two techniques may provide complementary information.[56] Gadolinium-enhanced MRI is important in detecting meningeal involvement. Diagnostic studies should almost always include an effort to secure histological confirmation. Biopsy of a clinically affected organ is most likely to be positive. Studies are also performed to determine that granulomas found in one system are part of a multisystemic disorder and not just a nonspecific local sarcoid tissue reaction. Other findings include elevated serum angiotensin-converting enzyme, elevated serum immunoglobulins, hypercalcemia, and elevated serum alkaline phosphatase (denoting hepatic involvement). The value of an elevated level of CSF angiotensin-converting enzyme is still being evaluated. With meningeal involvement, CSF findings often include increased content of mononuclear cells, elevated total protein concentration and sometimes oligoclonal bands on electrophoresis, and sometimes a reduced glucose concentration.

TREATMENT

No controlled trials have been reported for the treatment of sarcoidosis affecting the nervous system. However, because systemic sarcoidosis is usually responsive to treatment with corticosteroids, these preparations are often used successfully for treating neurosarcoidosis. Any assessment of efficacy must take into account the fact that about two-thirds of patients with neurosarcoidosis remit spontaneously, apparently suffering from a self-limited disorder. Because the overall prognosis of sarcoid is often excellent,[57] it seems reasonable to initiate treatment with corticosteroids at an early stage in order to try to prevent the development of the extensive fibrosis that may be the consequence of the inflammatory process.

We generally treat patients with systemic sarcoidosis with an initial dose of prednisone 0.5 mg/kg/d. The dose is adjusted upward or downward according to the clinical course, with a view to treatment for only a limited period of time. Patients who develop hydrocephalus as a result of meningeal thickening at the base of the skull may require neurosurgical shunting. Mass lesions in brain or spinal cord are occasionally operated on, usually because the nature of the lesion is not clear. It seems more reasonable otherwise to attempt to reduce the size of the lesion with corticosteroids rather than by surgical removal because sarcoid mass lesions are often responsive to corticosteroid therapy. Treatment of the infrequent corticosteroid-nonresponsive patient with a variety of immunosuppressant agents has had mixed results. Thus, cyclosporine has been well tolerated and helpful in the experience of some authors[57,58] but not others,[59] and methotrexate has similarly yielded conflicting results.[57,60,61] Treatment of resistant cases with radiation therapy is another option that may be helpful.[62–66]

REFERENCES

1. Heerfordt CF: Uber eine Febris uveo-parotidea subchronica. Graef Arch Klin Exp Ophthalmol 70:254, 1909
2. Scadding JG: Sarcoidosis. Eyre & Spottiswoode, London, 1967
3. Bauer HJ, Wyksstroem S: Sarcoidosis prevalence in Sweden. Acta Med Scand 176, suppl 425:112, 1964

4. Teirstein AS, Lesser M: Worldwide distribution and epidemiology of sarcoidosis. p. 103. In Fanburg BL (ed): Sarcoidosis and Other Granulomatous Diseases of the Lung. Marcel Dekker, New York, 1983

5. Daniele RP, Rossman MD, Kern JA, Elias JA: Pathogenesis of sarcoidosis: state of the art. Chest 89:174S, 1986

6. James DG: Sarcoidosis. p. 432. In Wyngaarden JB, Smith LH (eds): Cecil Textbook of Medicine. WB Saunders, Philadelphia, 1985

7. Chann Seem CP, Norfolk G, Spokes EG: CSF angiotensin-converting enzyme in neurosarcoidosis. Lancet 1:456, 1985

8. Oksanen V, Fyhrquist F, Gronhagen-Riska C, Somer H: CSF angiotensin-converting enzyme in neurosarcoidosis. Lancet 1:1050, 1985

9. James DG, Neville E, Walker A: Immunology of sarcoidosis. Am J Med 59:388, 1975

10. Hokins A: Tuberculous meningitis as a complication of sarcoidosis. J Neurol Neurosurg Psychiatry 37:644, 1974

11. Spickard A, Butler WA, Andriole V, Utz JP: The improved prognosis of cryptococcal meningitis with amphotericin B therapy. Ann Intern Med 58:66, 1963

12. Rosenbloom MA, Uphoff DF: The association of progressive multifocal leukoencephalopathy and sarcoidosis. Chest 83:572, 1983

13. Sweeney EC, McDonnell L: Herpes simplex encephalitis and sarcoidosis. Ir J Med Sci 148:54, 1979

14. Kveim A: En my og spesifikk kutan-reaksjon ved. Boecks Sarcoid. Nord Med 9:169, 1941

15. James DG, Williams WJ: Immunology of sarcoidosis. Am J Med 72:5, 1982

16. Sutherland I, Mitchell DN, D'Arcy Hart P: Incidence of intrathoracic sarcoidosis among young adults participating in a trial of tuberculosis vaccines. Br Med J 2:497, 1965

17. Longcope WT: Sarcoidosis or Besnier-Boeck-Schaumann disease. JAMA 117:1321, 1941

18. Gravesen PB, cited by Hook O: Sarcoidosis with involvement of nervous system. Arch Neurol Psychiatry 71:554, 1954

19. Reisner D: Boeck's sarcoid and systemic sarcoidosis (Besnier-Boeck-Schaumann disease). Am Rev Tuberc 49:289, 1944

20. Fisher AM: Some clinical and pathologic features observed in sarcoidosis. Trans Am Clin Climatol Assoc 59:58, 1947

21. Ricker W, Clark M: Sarcoidosis: clinicopathologic review of 300 cases including 22 autopsies. Am J Clin Pathol 19:725, 1949

22. Riley EA: Boeck's sarcoid: review based upon clinical study of 52 cases. Am Rev Tuberc 62:231, 1950

23. Longcope WT, Freiman D: Study of sarcoidosis, based on combined investigations of 160 cases including 30 autopsies. Medicine (Baltimore) 31:1, 1952

24. Gendel BR, Young JM, Greiner DJ: Sarcoidosis: review with 24 additional cases. Am J Med 12:205, 1952

25. Nitter L: Changes in chest roentgenograms in Boeck's sarcoid of the lungs. Acta Radiol Suppl (Stockh) 105:1, 1953

26. Cowdell RH: Sarcoidosis with special reference to diagnosis and prognosis. Q J Med 23:29, 1954

27. Israel HL, Sones M: Sarcoidosis. Arch Intern Med 102:766, 1958

28. Goodson WH JR: Neurologic manifestations of sarcoidosis. South Med J 53:1111, 1960

29. Douglas AC: Sarcoidosis in Scotland. Am Rev Respir Dis 84:143, 1961

30. Bacharach T: Sarcoidosis: clinical review of 111 cases. Am Rev Respir Dis 84:12, 1961

31. Rudberg-Roos I: Course and prognosis of sarcoidosis as observed in 296 cases. Acta Tuberc Scand 41, suppl 52:1, 1962

32. Mayock RL, Bertrand P, Morrison CE, Scott JH: Manifestations of sarcoidosis. Am J Med 35:67, 1963

33. Silverstein A, Feuer MM, Siltzbach LE: Neurologic sarcoidosis. Arch Neurol 12:1, 1965

34. James DG, Neville E, Siltzbach LE, et al: A worldwide review of sarcoidosis. Ann NY Acad Sci 278:321, 1976

35. James DG, Williams W: Sarcoidosis and Other Granulomatous Disorders. WB Saunders, Philadelphia, 1984

36. Stern BJ, Krumholz A, Johns C, et al: Sarcoidosis and its neurological manifestations. Arch Neurol 42:909, 1985

37. Blain JG, Riley W, Logothetis J: Optic nerve manifestations of sarcoidosis. Arch Neurol 13:307, 1965

38. Gould H, Kaufman H: Sarcoid of the fundus. Arch Ophthalmol 65:453, 1961

39. James DG, Zatouroff MA, Trowell J, Rose FC: Papilloedema in sarcoidosis. Br J Ophthalmol 51:526, 1967

40. Rush JA: Retrobulbar optic neuropathy in sarcoidosis. Ann Ophthalmol 12:390, 1980

41. Graham EM, Ellis CJ, Sanders MD, McDonald WI: Optic neuropathy in sarcoidosis. J Neurol Neurosurg Psychiatry 49:756, 1986

42. Matthews WB: Sarcoidosis of the nervous system. J Neurol Neurosurg Psychiatry 28:23, 1965

43. Poole CJM: Argyll-Robertson pupils due to neurosarcoidosis: evidence for site of lesion. Br Med J 289:356, 1984

44. Winnacker JL, Becker KL, Katz S: Endocrine aspects of sarcoidosis. N Engl J Med 278:483, 1968

45. Posner I: Sarcoidosis: case report. J Pediatr 20:486, 1942

46. Bleisch VR, Robbins SL: Sarcoid-like granulomata of pituitary gland. Arch Intern Med 89:877, 1952

47. Panitz F, Shinaberger JH: Nephrogenic diabetes insipidus due to sarcoidosis without hypercalcemia. Arch Intern Med 62:113, 1965

48. Coggins CH, Leaf A: Diabetes insipidus. Am J Med 42:807, 1967

49. Skillicorn SA, Garrity RW: Intracranial Boeck's sarcoid tumor resembling meningioma. J Neuosurg 12:407, 1955

50. Clark WC, Acker JD, Dohan FC, Robertson JH: Presentation of central nervous system sarcoidosis as intracranial tumors. J Neurosurg 63:851, 1985

51. Sauter MK, Panitch HS, Kristt DA: Myelopathic neurosarcoidosis: diagnostic value of enhanced MRI. Neurology 41:150, 1991

52. Wallace SL, Lattes R, Malia JP, Ragan C: Muscle involvement in Boeck's sarcoid. Ann Intern Med 48:497, 1958

53. Oksanen V: Neurosarcoidosis: clinical presentations and course in 50 patients. Acta Neurol Scand 73:283, 1986

54. Luke RA, Stern BJ, Krumholz A, Johns C: Neurosarcoidosis: the long-term clinical course. Neurology 37:461, 1987

55. Miller DH, Kendall BE, Barter S, et al: Magnetic resonance imaging in central nervous system sarcoidosis. Neurology 38:378, 1988

56. Hayes WS, Sherman JL, Stern BJ, et al: MR and CT evaluation of intracranial sarcoidosis. AJNR 8:841, 1987

57. Chapelon C, Ziza JM, Piette JC, et al: Neurosarcoidosis: signs, course and treatment in 35 confirmed cases. Medicine (Baltimore) 69:261, 1990

58. Kavanaugh AF, Andrew SL, Cooper B, et al: Cyclosporine therapy of central nervous system sarcoidosis. Am J Med 82:387, 1987

59. Cunnah D, Chew S, Wass J: Cyclosporin for central nervous system sarcoidosis. Am J Med 85:580, 1988

60. Soriano FG, Caramelli P, Nitrini R, Rocha AS: Neurosarcoidosis: therapeutic success with methotrexate. Postgrad Med J 66:142, 1990

61. Raoult D, Guibout M, Jaquet P, et al: Neuro-endocrine sarcoidosis: one case. Ann Med Interne (Paris) 135:149, 1981

62. Bejar JM, Kerby GR, Ziegler DK, Festoff BW: Treatment of central nervous system sarcoidosis with radiotherapy. Ann Neurol 18:258, 1985

63. Rubinstein I, Gray TA, Moldofsky H, Hoffstein V: Neurosarcoidosis associated with hypersomnolence treated with corticosteroids and brain irradiation. Chest 94:205, 1988

64. Garcia-Monco C, Berciano J: Sarcoid meningitis, high adenosine deaminase levels in CSF and results of cranial irradiation. J Neurol Neurosurg Psychiatry 51:1594, 1988

65. Feibelman RY, Harman EM: Sarcoid meningoencephalitis treated with high-dosage steroids and radiation. Ann Intern Med 102:136, 1985

66. Gelwan MJ, Kellen RI, Burde RM, Kupersmith MJ: Sarcoidosis of the anterior visual pathway: successes and failures. J Neurol Neurosurg Psychiatry 51:1473, 1988

44

Neurological Complications in Critically Ill Patients

Charles F. Bolton
G. Bryan Young

The term *critical illness* has been widely used for many years to describe the condition of any patient with illness severe enough to be considered at risk of death. However, it has now been given a more specific meaning and designated a syndrome comprising sepsis and multiple organ failure.[1] This syndrome has probably always been a component of preterminal illness, but before the advent of modern methods of treatment, the syndrome evolved so quickly that the nature of the preterminal events was not considered. However, with the use of intravenous transfusions, antibiotics, and particularly assisted ventilation, these patients are now kept alive for days, weeks, and even months in intensive or critical care units, and up to 40 percent recover.[2] The incidence of the syndrome in major medical or surgical intensive care units is 20 to 50 percent,[3] and it remains common on general hospital wards. It is now possible to study the syndrome in detail, but despite considerable attention to several major organ systems, there has been little attention to the nervous system.

Sepsis, an almost invariable component of the syndrome, may be defined as the systemic response to dividing and invading microorganisms of all types.[4] However, in many instances the offending organism cannot be cultured. For example, blood cultures are negative in one-half the patients suspected of being septic.[4] Moreover, the criteria for diagnosing sepsis

based on systemic responses are still unsettled. Bone has defined the septic syndrome as increased respiratory and heart rate, elevated or depressed body temperature, and inadequate organ perfusion[5] (Table 44-1). It may be more appropriate to call this the *systemic inflammatory response syndrome* when infection is an underlying cause and *septic syndrome* when trauma or burns are the underlying cause.[6]

The mechanisms by which the various organ systems are affected are still poorly understood but probably involve the release of cytokines and disturbances of the microcirculation of various organs.[7] There is no known specific treatment; however, it is known that if the underlying sepsis can be brought under control by either medical or surgical means, the various manifestations of the syndrome quickly disappear and full recovery is possible.[8]

Patients who are most susceptible are those suffering from multiple injuries or severe medical illness or who have just had major surgery, particularly if they are elderly or have serious underlying disease that may affect their resistance to infection. Early intubation and transfer to the critical care unit is usually necessary. In the course of time, various intravascular lines are inserted, either for treatment or to monitor vital function. There is little doubt that these invasive procedures induce the state of sepsis if it was not already present. Thus, it generally recognized that pa-

859

Table 44-1 Definition of the Septic Syndrome

1. Clinical evidence of infection
2. Respiratory rate >20/min. If mechanically ventilated, >10 L/min
3. Heart rate >90/min
4. Temperature >38.3°C or <35.1°C
5. Inadequate organ perfusion with one or more of the following:
   a. $PaO_2/FiO_2 \leq 280$ without pulmonary or cardiovascular disease
   b. Elevated plasma lactate
   c. Oliguria (urine output <0.5 ml/kg body weight for at least 1 hour)

(Modified from Bone RC, Fisher CJ, Clemmer TP, et al: Sepsis syndrome: a valid clinical entity. Crit Care Med 17:389, 1989, with permission.)

tients in the unit for more than 5 days almost invariably become septic and, if that is not controlled, soon develop the syndrome of multiple organ failure.

We have studied the nervous system manifestations of this syndrome in some detail, and a definite pattern has emerged,[9] as illustrated in Figure 44-1). Within hours of a patient becoming septic, a mild encepha-

lopathy develops. When deterioration to a state of multiple organ failure occurs, this encephalopathy becomes severe, but it soon subsides if the sepsis is successfully treated. However, it is then noted that it is difficult to wean the patient from the mechanical ventilator. If primary lung disease is excluded, we have shown that polyneuropathy is almost always the cause of this circumstance. However, as with the encephalopathy, the polyneuropathy eventually disappears if the sepsis does not recur and the patient survives. The recovery phase for the polyneuropathy is longer (a matter of months) than for the encephalopathy (a matter of weeks). A myopathy may also occur in patients with prolonged sepsis and presumably improves in the same way as the neuropathy, but its true nature is complex and is still being explored.

SEPTIC ENCEPHALOPATHY

We use the term *septic encephalopathy* to refer to altered brain function related to the presence of microorganisms or their toxins in the blood. This condi-

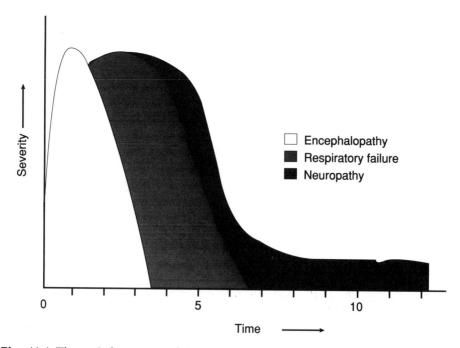

Fig. 44-1 The typical sequence of the nervous system complications of sepsis. The time course may be in weeks or months. (From Bolton CF, Young GB, Zochodne DW: The neurological complications of sepsis. Ann Neurol 33:94, 1993, with permission.)

tion has been recognized by surgeons and internists as a component of multiple organ failure, but it has received little systematic study.

Clinical Features

The clinical diagnosis of septic encephalopathy is one of exclusion. Altered brain function in the febrile patient can be due to a number of conditions other than the sepsis itself (Table 44-2). Space does not allow a complete discussion of the differential diagnosis, but other entities can usually be ruled out by history, physical examination, and laboratory tests. It is often necessary to perform a lumbar puncture to exclude bacterial meningitis.

We carried out a retrospective study on 12 autopsied patients[10] and a separate clinical, prospective study.[11,12] Patients with a fever and either a positive blood culture or a localized bacterial or fungal infection were included for both studies. We excluded patients less than 16 years old and those with central nervous system (CNS) disorders unrelated to the febrile illness, preexisting metabolic disorders, and conditions that affect the brain other than by a septic mechanism. In the prospective study we also excluded patients receiving heavy sedation or analgesics and those on skeletal muscle relaxants. For this study, using an arbitrary set of bedside criteria, patients were classified as nonencephalopathic, mildly encephalopathic, and severely encephalopathic. Basically, nonencephalopathic patients cooperated with testing and passed a series of tests of attention, concentration, orientation, and short-term memory. The mildly encephalopathic patients completed testing but failed to "pass," and the severely encephalopathic patients were too obtunded to test.

The clinical picture is similar to that of diffuse or multifocal encephalopathy in general.[13] The level of consciousness varied from clouding of consciousness to coma. Delirium occurred infrequently, preceding stupor or coma. Mildly encephalopathic patients often showed considerable fluctuation in their clinical state, and older individuals became especially confused at night. Attention, concentration, and memory were impaired. Writing disturbances occurred, as in other acute confusional states.[14] Paratonic rigidity, or gegenhalten, was almost universal in encephalopathic patients. This condition is a resistance to passive movement of a limb, part of a limb, or the neck. It

Table 44-2 Causes of Encephalopathy in Febrile Patients

Infections
Central nervous system
Bacterial: meningitis, cerebritis, brain abscess, subdural/epidural empyema
Viral: encephalitis
Other: spirochetal, rickettsial, protozoal, helminthic
Intracranial thrombophlebitis
Bacterial endocarditis: may produce embolism, meningitis, mycotic aneurysm
Systemic infection
Direct organ damage, e.g, hepatitis
Septic encephalopathy

Vascular Accidents
Pulmonary emboli
CNS: vertebrobasilar stroke, intracranial hemorrhage

Mechanical causes (trauma)
Cerebral injury
Fat embolism (fractures of long bones)

Immunological conditions
Drug fever
Acetylsalicylic acid toxicity
Connective tissue disease

Heat stroke

Metabolic conditions
Acute adrenal failure
Thyroid storm (hyperthyroidism)
Porphyria

Reye's syndrome (children)

Neoplasms
Systemic malignancy with organ failure
Brain tumors, primary or secondary: affecting thermoregulation

Hematological causes
Hemolytic episodes, e.g., sickle cell disease
Leukemia

Increased muscular activity
Convulsive seizures
Malignant neuroleptic syndrome

is felt throughout the range of movement, like parkinsonian rigidity, but differs from rigidity in that it disappears when the body part is moved very slowly.[13] We found tremor, asterixis, and multifocal myoclonus in 10 to 25 percent of noncomatose encephalopathic patients, but not in nonencephalopathic or comatose patients.

None of our patients showed any alteration of pupillary size or reaction or abnormalities of individual cranial nerves. None of the encephalopathic patients in our prospective study showed focal neurological signs or convulsive seizures. Hemiparesis or gaze palsy were found in 6, and focal or generalized convulsive seizures occurred in 5 of the 12 patients in our retrospective (autopsy) series. The difference may be accounted for in part by the duration of sepsis in the autopsy group and the pathological findings (discussed below).

As expected, the mortality rate was significantly greater among the severely encephalopathic patients than the other groups. Nearly half of the severely encephalopathic but none of the nonencephalopathic patients died. About 25 percent of the nonencephalopathic patients had clinical and electrophysiological evidence of mild peripheral neuropathy. Among the moderately and severely encephalopathic patients, 50 percent and 75 percent, respectively, had neuropathy; among the patients in the latter group, the neuropathy was usually severe. The time course of the encephalopathy and the neuropathy often differed. The encephalopathy peaked earlier and cleared long before the neuropathy in the course of the septic illness. Some severely encephalopathic patients were obtunded for a month or more, but CNS function improved soon after the infection and systemic metabolic problems were controlled or resolved.

There was a strong association of adult respiratory distress syndrome with severe encephalopathy. Transient hypotension was more common at the onset of sepsis in the severely encephalopathic patients, although there was no difference in blood pressure among the three groups at their initial neurological assessment. The degree of prior hypotension was not sufficient to account for the neurological findings. Interestingly, none of the following correlated with severity of encephalopathy: age (a trend for correlation of age and degree of encephalopathy did not achieve statistical significance), sex, temperature, or type of organism (no difference between gram-positive and gram-negative organisms, but patients with *Candida,* although few in number, were more severely affected).

Laboratory Features

The electroencephalogram (EEG) is a sensitive monitor of septic encephalopathy. We found it more sensitive than our arbitrary clinical assessment of mental status in that some nonencephalopathic patients had mild EEG abnormalities that resolved on subsequent recordings. The mildest EEG change consisted of mild, generalized slowing (rhythms more than 3 Hz but less than 8 Hz). More severe EEG abnormalities, which correlated with more profound depression of consciousness, consisted of greater slowing (less than 3 Hz), triphasic waves, or a burst-suppression pattern (Figs. 44-2 and 44-3).

Serum levels of creatinine and bilirubin showed a direct, linear correlation with the severity of the encephalopathy (Fig. 44-4). Although hyperventilation is a feature of sepsis, there were no significant differences in blood pH, bicarbonate, or PCO_2 among the three groups. In our retrospective study, a drop in platelet count was associated with the development of brain purpura and neurological signs.

We did not find any abnormalities in the cerebrospinal fluid (CSF) or on unenhanced computed tomographic (CT) brain scans in any of our patients, including those who showed microabscesses at autopsy (see below).

Autopsy Findings

In our autopsy series, 8 of the 12 patients had disseminated microabscesses in the brain, chiefly in the cerebral cortex and subcortical white matter. Because there was some reaction in the brain around the microabscesses, these lesions did not appear to be just agonal phenomena.

Four patients had increased protoplasmic astrocytes in the cerebral cortex. They were unrelated to the microabscesses and probably reflected a metabolic encephalopathy. Three patients had central pontine myelinolysis, a condition that has been related to overcorrection of hyponatremia,[15] as discussed in Chapter 17. Vascular lesions were found in six patients: five had multiple cerebral infarcts (one terminal), and one, who had thrombocytopenia before death, had brain purpura. We have had only two autopsies in our prospective series, and neither has shown abnormalities in the brain.

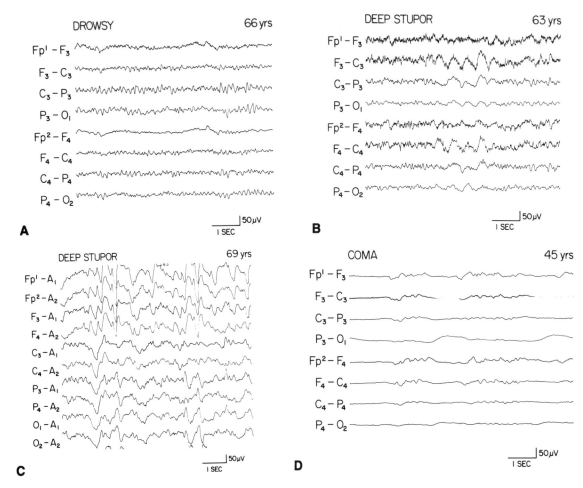

Fig. 44-2 EEGs from patients with septic encephalopathy. **(A)** Patient with mild encephalopathy. The EEG shows a mild excess of low-voltage 6- to 7-Hz theta rhythms in both left (odd-numbered electrode placements) and right (even-numbered placements) hemispheres. **(B–D)** Severely encephalopathic patients. **(B)** Bilateral intermittent rhythmic delta (<3 Hz) waves on a background of mild slowing. **(C)** Triphasic waves. **(D)** Burst-suppression pattern.

The significance of the above pathological findings is not clear, mainly because these patients had been septic for weeks. There is no way of knowing with certainty when the lesions found at autopsy actually developed. It is possible that focal signs and seizures could have been produced by the lesions, but the microabscesses and vascular lesions were small and multifocal. Furthermore, occasionally focal signs and focal seizures can occur in metabolic encephalopathies.[13]

In a literature search, we could not find a study of encephalopathy in septic humans comparable to ours. McGovern and Tiller in 1980 reported "watershed" cerebral infarctions in patients who died of septic shock,[16] but they provided no clinical correlations. Such watershed infarcts are ischemic lesions at or near the terminal portions of the anterior, middle, and posterior cerebral arteries, and they are typically associated clinically with bibrachial paralysis, which we have never encountered in our patients. Pendlebury and associates chose cases with microabscesses at postmortem examination rather than starting with clinically septic patients.[17] There is one report of a patient dying of sepsis due to a breast abscess who showed sagittal sinus thrombosis and thrombophlebitis of cerebral cortical veins.[18]

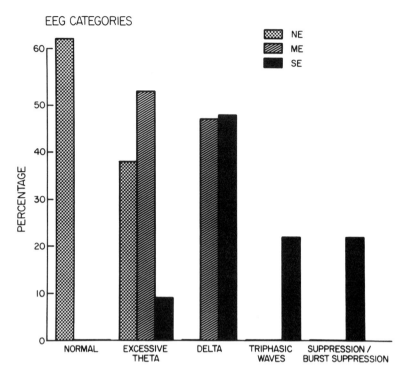

Fig. 44-3 Histogram of EEG findings in septic encephalopathy. NE, nonencephalopathic group; ME, mildly encephalopathic group; SE, severely encephalopathic group. Note that although most nonencephalopathic patients had normal EEGs, 38 percent were mildly abnormal. Severely encephalopathic patients showed the most marked abnormalities.

Pathogenesis of Septic Encephalopathy

Although the pathogenesis of septic encephalopathy remains to be conclusively established, it is unlikely that a single mechanism applies to all cases. The mechanisms shown in Figure 44-5 are not mutually exclusive.

The early, reversible encephalopathy is probably metabolic in nature (i.e., caused by a chemical imbalance that does not cause structural damage or neuronal death). With more advanced sepsis, structural changes including vascular lesions and microabscesses become more important.

The principal chemical mediators of the sepsis syndrome are cytokines, chemical messengers released from lymphocytes and macrophages.[5] These produce systemic capillary leakage and tissue edema, interfere with the microcirculation, and have direct effects on cellular metabolism. It seems reasonable to ask whether these substances may also affect the brain. They probably account for the patchy increase in brain capillary permeability that occurs within the first few hours of sepsis.[19] Transport of amino acids across the blood-brain barrier is altered in sepsis (i.e., there is an alteration in transcapillary transport systems).[20] These factors could alter the chemical milieu of the brain cells. Substances normally excluded from the brain may gain access to neuronal receptors; this includes drugs as well as the relative amounts of certain endogenous substances. The latter include relative ratios of aromatic to branched-chain amino acids (increased in the plasma and in the brain[21]) and increased exposure to other peptides and hormones. Such changes may play a role in the documented alteration of certain putative neurotransmitters in sepsis, such as serotonin, norepinephrine, and dopamine.[22]

Cytokines themselves may directly affect brain function. Again, their access to the brain may be facilitated by alterations in blood-brain barrier function. When directly injected into the brain or ventricles of experimental animals, interleukins-1 and -2 alter behavior and EEG frequencies.[23,24] Interleukin-1 facili-

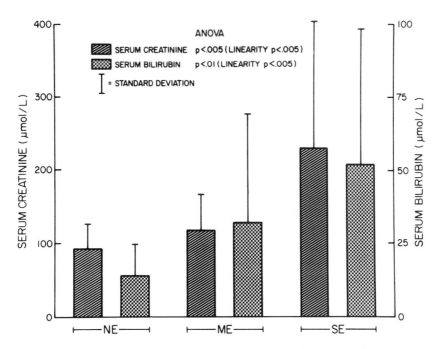

Fig. 44-4 Histogram showing the correlation of serum creatinine and bilirubin levels with the encephalopathic grade. NE, nonencephalopathic group; ME, mildly encephalopathic group; SE, severely encephalopathic group; ANOVA, analysis of variance.

tates sleep and induces fever by its effects on the hypothalamus.[25] Some of these effects relate to activation of opiate receptors in the brain; the possibility of effects on other peptide systems in the brain remains to be further explored.

Disturbances in the microcirculation of the brain may relate to endothelial injury.[26] The impairment in oxygen uptake by tissues can be at least partly corrected by prostacyclin infusion.[27] Such effects on the systemic microcirculation may affect the brain without the full picture of disseminated intravascular coagulation, an uncommon event in sepsis.[28] These findings may explain the small brain infarctions found in fatal cases.

Activation of "adhesion molecules," the selectin and integrin group, causes leukocyte adherence or "rolling leukocytes," which may be an early cause of endothelial cell damage.[7] This may then affect nitric oxide synthesis by the endothelium (not shown in Fig. 44-5). It has been shown that nitric oxide is the "vascular relaxing factor."[29] The synthesis of this mediator by nitric oxide synthetase is increased by endotoxin and cytokines in sepsis, leading to reduced peripheral vascular resistance and hypotension.[30]

Although this seems counterproductive, such multifocal vasodilatation helps to ensure adequate organ perfusion in sepsis; inhibition of nitric oxide production can lead to decreased organ perfusion and a fall in oxygen extraction by tissues.[31] Nitric oxide plays an important role in regulating brain circulation and the permeability of the blood-brain barrier.[32] Endothelial damage in sepsis may then compromise regional cerebral blood flow and account for the multifocal, dynamic increases in blood-brain (and possibly blood-nerve) permeability mentioned above.

Nitric oxide is also thought to act as a neurotransmitter and may mediate, at least in part, excitotoxic brain damage.[33] Whether nitric oxide synthesis and release are increased in the brain in sepsis remains to be explored.

The brain may also be affected indirectly, because of failure of or altered metabolism of other organ systems. Within 5 hours from the onset of sepsis, the liver shows impaired ability to clear indocyanine green.[34] We have also found an elevation of serum bilirubin in sepsis; there is a linear relationship of serum bilirubin concentration to the severity of the

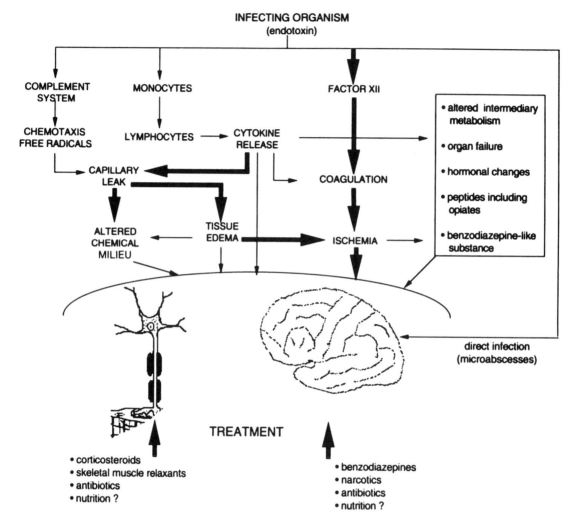

Fig. 44-5 Possible mechanisms for septic encephalopathy and critical illness polyneuropathy. Arrows pointing to the curved line indicate mechanisms that may apply to both the central and peripheral nervous systems independently. The heavy arrows highlight the most likely mechanisms. These hypotheses are complex but involve the infecting organism inducing chemical, microvascular, metabolic, or treatment effects that may act independently or in concert. The release of cytokines from macrophages and thence from T lymphocytes may directly affect the brain or act indirectly on the blood-brain barrier and microcirculation. Such vascular effects are abetted by activation of the complement system and factor XII. The encephalopathy may also be due to the failure of other organs or to direct infection of the brain, with the formation of microabscesses. Critical illness polyneuropathy may be due to disturbances of the microcirculation of peripheral nerve through vascular effects similar to those affecting the brain. Various treatments used in the critical care unit may play an additive role for both the encephalopathy and the polyneuropathy. (From Bolton CF, Young GB, Zochodne DW: The neurological complications of sepsis. Ann Neurol 33:94, 1993, with permission.)

encephalopathy.[11] The alteration in liver function, along with altered metabolism in muscle, probably produces the increase in aromatic branched-chain amino acids in sepsis.[35] The pattern is similar to that found in hepatic encephalopathy.[36] Endogenous benzodiazepine-like substance is also increased in hepatic failure.[37] Although this has not been explored in sepsis, we have found that some patients with septic encephalopathy may improve with flumazenil, the gamma amino butyric acid–A antagonist, even in the absence of exogenous benzodiazepines (unpublished observations).

In advanced sepsis, the failure of other organs (e.g., kidneys or heart) may, in turn, affect brain function and lead to an encephalopathy.

In intensive care units, iatrogenic factors should always be considered. Sedative drugs, particularly opiates and benzodiazepines, are commonly used to ease the use of assisted ventilation. If renal impairment occurs, opiate clearance is reduced, and this may lead to prolonged obtundation.[38] Brain function of critically ill patients, as reflected by the EEG, is very sensitive to midazolam[39]; this probably applies to other benzodiazepines. Total parenteral nutrition is sometimes associated with hypophosphatemia or hyperosmolality, both of which may cause coma.[40] High serum levels of penicillin, usually in association with renal impairment, may cause seizures,[41] as may the new antibiotic imipenem.[42] Central pontine myelinolysis may complicate the sudden increases of plasma osmolality in critically ill patients.[43]

DIFFERENTIAL DIAGNOSIS OF NEUROMUSCULAR PROBLEMS IN THE CRITICAL CARE UNIT

The list of conditions that can affect the neuromuscular system in patients in the critical care unit is remarkably long and potentially involves dysfunction of the entire nervous system (Table 44-3). To pinpoint the site of dysfunction may be remarkably difficult, especially in the setting of the critical care unit. History taking is often impossible, as an endotracheal tube prevents speech, and the often associated encephalopathy prevents reliable communication of any type. The limbs are not easily assessed due to the presence of intravenous lines, splints, bandages, and so forth. Thus, although a neurological examination

Table 44-3 Differential Diagnosis of Neuromuscular Signs in Critically Ill Patients

Encephalopathy
Septic
Anoxic-ischemic
Other

Myelopathy
Anoxic-ischemic
Traumatic
Other

Neuropathy
Critical illness polyneuropathy
Thiamine deficiency
Vitamin E deficiency
Nonspecific nutritional deficiency
Pyridoxine abuse
Hypophosphatemia
Aminoglycoside toxicity
Penicillin toxicity
Guillain-Barré syndrome
Motor neuron disease
Porphyria
Carcinomatous polyneuropathy
Compression neuropathy
Diphtheria

Neuromuscular Transmission Defects
Anesthetic drugs
Aminoglycoside toxicity
Myasthenia gravis
Lambert-Eaton myasthenic syndrome
Hypocalcemia
Hypomagnesemia
Organophosphate poisoning
Wound botulism
Tick-bite paralysis

Myopathy
"Septic myopathy"
Cachexia
Panfascicular fiber necrosis
Thick filament myopathy
Water and electrolyte disturbances: potassium, phosphate, calcium, magnesium
Corticosteroid myopathy
Muscular dystrophy
Polymyositis
Acid maltase deficiency

tailored to the comatose patient may provide some assessment of the nervous system, we have found that the presence and severity of either brain or peripheral nervous system dysfunction is often difficult to document by purely clinical methods. Electrophysiological tests have therefore been of particular value in this regard, and we now rely on them routinely to assess such patients.

Using electrophysiological tests, we have found that both septic encephalopathy and critical illness polyneuropathy are almost invariable manifestations of the sepsis and multiple organ failure syndrome, and the other conditions listed in the table are only rarely involved. In fact, these other conditions are usually evident before the patient has been admitted to the critical care unit and are the obvious reason for neuromuscular respiratory failure. Myasthenia gravis and Guillain–Barré syndrome are good examples, although in some instances it is necessary to rule these conditions out systematically. Studies involving repetitive nerve stimulation, for example, may be required to investigate for a defect in neuromuscular transmission, and muscle biopsy may be necessary to rule out primary myopathies such as polymyositis or a metabolic disturbance such as acid maltase deficiency. Except for critical illness polyneuropathy, the Guillain–Barré syndrome is, in our experience, the most common neuromuscular problem seen in the unit. It can almost invariably be recognized by the pattern of abnormalities on electromyograhy (EMG) and nerve conduction studies and by CSF examinations.[44]

In this section we will also discuss recent reports implicating neuromuscular blocking agents and corticosteroids as important causes of muscle weakness among patients in critical care units.

Critical Illness Polyneuropathy

Among patients who have the septic syndrome, 70 percent develop critical illness polyneuropathy,[45] the neuropathy being more severe the longer the patient has been in the unit (Fig. 44-6). It has been observed in other centers and at times attributed to other causes: gentamycin,[46] pancuronium bromide,[47] Guillain–Barré syndrome,[48] and pancreatic disease.[49] Others have linked the neuropathy to the septic syndrome.[50-55]

The first, and often the only, clinical sign is respira-

tory muscle weakness, manifest as a difficulty in weaning from the mechanical ventilator. Of 29 patients studied in our unit who had difficulty in weaning from the ventilator that on a clinical basis appeared neuromuscular, 28 were indeed found to have a neuromuscular problem. In addition to standard electrophysiological studies of peripheral nerve and muscle, we performed phrenic nerve conduction studies and needle electromyography of the diaphragm. The majority of these patients had critical illness polyneuropathy, others having trauma to the phrenic nerve, evidence of neuromuscular transmission defect, primary myopathy, or disorders of central drive due to an associated encephalopathy.[56] However, severe critical illness polyneuropathy is usually evident from the clinical examination alone. Such patients have weak or absent movements of the limbs, even when the limbs are stimulated distally by pressure over the nail beds. Tendon reflexes that were previously present cannot be elicited. By contrast, head, face, and jaw movements are relatively preserved. In two of our patients, this absence of movement in the extremities but preservation of movement of the head had erroneously been diagnosed as due to high cervical spinal cord disease. Lesser degrees of neuropathy show more equivocal signs, with variably weak muscles, particularly distally, and reduced or absent tendon reflexes, notably the ankle jerks. However, most patients have no clear-cut signs of neuromuscular disease.

Electrophysiological studies clearly establish the presence of a peripheral neuropathy and document its severity. Upper and lower limb motor and sensory conduction studies initially reveal only a reduction in the amplitude of compound muscle and sensory nerve action potentials, with no change in latency or conduction velocity (Fig. 44-7). Then within a matter of 2 weeks or so, fibrillation potentials and positive sharp waves appear in muscle, and sensory and compound muscle action potentials are further reduced. Even in the more advanced stages of critical illness polyneuropathy, conduction velocity and distal latencies remain relatively normal, emphasizing the purely axonal, degenerative nature of the neuropathy.

Comprehensive examination of the entire nervous system at autopsy, plus nerve and muscle biopsy, has revealed that there is a primary axonal degeneration of motor and sensory fibers, particularly involving

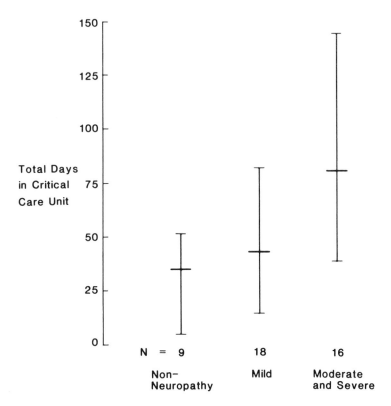

Fig. 44-6 Incidence, severity, and relation of neuropathy to time spent in the critical care unit for 43 patients who had sepsis and multiple organ failure, studied prospectively between 1983 and 1985. *Mild, moderate,* and *severe* refer to the neuropathy. The range of time spent in the critical care unit is shown by the bars.

distal nerve fibers (Figs. 44-8 and 44-9).[57] There is a resulting denervation atrophy of muscle; histopathological examination during the acute phase reveals scattered, angulated fibers and later shows grouped atrophy (Fig. 44-10). Neither the nerve nor the muscle shows any inflammatory change. Aside from chromatolysis of the anterior horn cells secondary to the peripheral axonal injury, the CNS is spared.

The mechanism of the polyneuropathy is not known. However, our investigations have excluded potential causes for polyneuropathy, including Guillain-Barré syndrome, various toxins, drugs (particularly antibiotics), and nutritional deficiency.[57] It is our belief that the neuropathy is probably caused by the same fundamental defect that affects all organ systems in the critical illness syndrome. We speculate that the primary axonal damage may be due to involvement of axonal transport systems, which are known to be

energy-dependent[58]; this fact may explain why predominantly distal nerve segments are involved.[59] Moreover, it is known that the blood-nerve barrier, in contrast to the blood-brain barrier, shows increased permeability to histamine and serotonin.[60] Several mediators of the septic syndrome are known to have histamine-like action.[61] Circulating "toxins" could potentially gain access to the endoneural space and directly damage the axon. It is also possible that disturbance of the microcirculation, as has been postulated to occur in sepsis and multiple organ failure, is the mechanism by which these events in peripheral nerve are initiated.

Our studies provide no evidence that the use of antibiotics causes the polyneuropathy. Indeed, because successful treatment of the sepsis results in improvement in the polyneuropathy, we advise that all medical and surgical means to improve the sepsis and

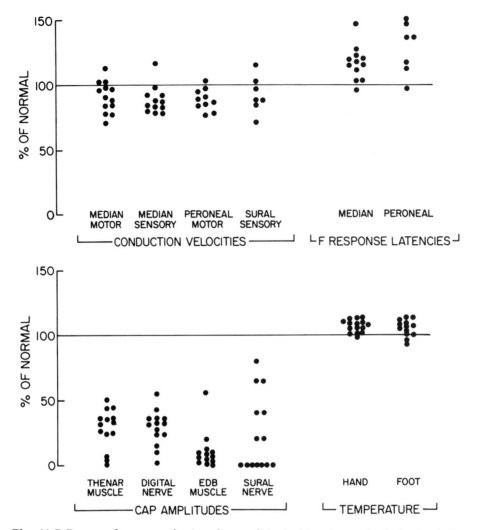

Fig. 44-7 Pattern of nerve conduction abnormalities in 14 patients who had critical illness polyneuropathy, studied between 1977 and 1981. All patients had evidence of denervation of muscle on needle EMG studies. Note the elevated distal skin temperature, consistent with sepsis. CAP, compound action potential.

multiple organ failure be instituted. Moreover, all critical care units should use whatever methods are necessary to avoid sepsis (e.g., use of sterile techniques and avoidance of invasive procedures unless absolutely necessary). Although we have no evidence that the neuropathy is due to nutritional deficiency, it seems prudent to administer total parenteral or enteral nutrition from the start of critical illness. Those responsible for physical therapy and rehabilitation should be aware of the nature and severity of the poly-neuropathy, so that they will take it into account as the patient gradually recovers.

Myopathy

For some years, it has been assumed that the muscle wasting that accompanies prolonged sepsis, which was observed by Osler in 1892,[62] is due to excessive breakdown of muscle proteins (i.e., represents a catabolic myopathy). It was believed that it accounted

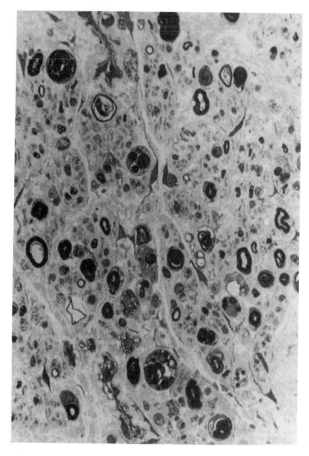

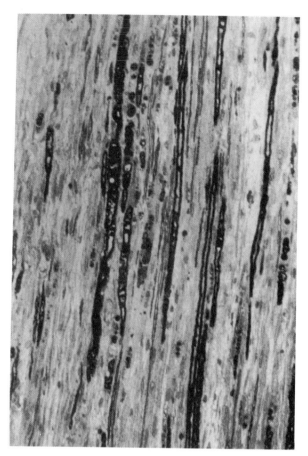

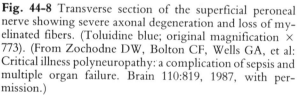

Fig. 44-8 Transverse section of the superficial peroneal nerve showing severe axonal degeneration and loss of myelinated fibers. (Toluidine blue; original magnification × 773). (From Zochodne DW, Bolton CF, Wells GA, et al: Critical illness polyneuropathy: a complication of sepsis and multiple organ failure. Brain 110:819, 1987, with permission.)

Fig. 44-9 Longitudinal section of the deep peroneal nerve demonstrating axonal degeneration and loss of myelinated fibers. (Toluidine blue; original magnification × 778). (From Zochodne DW, Bolton CF, Wells GA, et al: Critical illness polyneuropathy: a complication of sepsis and multiple organ failure. Brain 110:819, 1987, with permission.)

for early respiratory weakness, ultimately leading to intubation and assisted ventilation. It has also been thought to be the reason for any difficulty in weaning from the ventilator as the sepsis syndrome comes under control. There is evidence for a disturbance in intermediary metabolism affecting muscle, such that interleukin-1, stimulated by the macrophage system, causes an increase in prostaglandin-E$_2$ production, thereby activating lysosomal proteases in muscle.[63,64] Increased levels of catecholamine and cortisol may also increase muscle catabolism.

However, our studies strongly suggest that the muscle weakness and wasting is mainly due to dener-vation atrophy. As already noted, such changes have been seen regularly in muscles sampled at autopsy or by biopsy. The occasional section of muscle shows necrosis, suggesting an associated primary myopathy, but this finding is as yet equivocal. We investigated the disturbance of muscle by utilizing P31 nuclear magnetic resonance studies. In two patients these studies showed a marked reduction in the concentration of high-energy phosphate in muscle, an abnormality that improved with alleviation of the sepsis and the associated polyneuropathy.[65] However, in an earlier study, we noted that severe denervation of muscle alone may cause significant reductions in these high-energy phosphates.[66] Thus, in

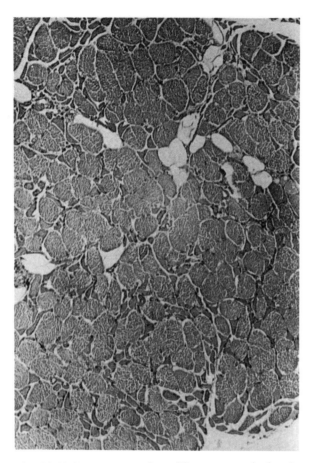

Fig. 44-10 Transverse section of iliopsoas muscle showing scattered and grouped atrophic fibers consistent with denervation atrophy. (Hematoxylin and eosin; original magnification ×195). (From Zochodne DW, Bolton CF, Wells GA, et al: Critical illness polyneuropathy: a complication of sepsis and multiple organ failure. Brain 110:819, 1987, with permission.)

practical terms, critical illness polyneuropathy should now be regarded as the main cause of muscle wasting and weakness in these patients.

However, other conditions occur. Due to prolonged recumbency in the critical care unit, myopathy in patients with sepsis and multiple organ failure may be due to cachexia or disuse atrophy of muscle. The EMG and serum creatine kinase levels are normal. Muscle biopsy shows atrophy of type II fibers. However, no systematic studies to determine this have yet been made.

A rare complication of infection is panfascicular

muscle fiber necrosis.[67,68] There is sudden, generalized weakness of muscles accompanied by marked elevation of serum creatine kinase concentration, and occasionally myoglobinuria. There may or may not be abnormal spontaneous activity on needle EMG of muscle, and muscle biopsy may be normal in the early stages. Later, however, findings of muscle fiber necrosis are evident and, in severe cases, there is panfascicular muscle fiber necrosis. An inflammatory reaction may be secondary to the necrotic muscle fibers. Recovery is usually quite prompt and occurs spontaneously. This condition represents an unusual reaction on the part of muscle to a variety of insulting agents in addition to sepsis, such as acute physical trauma and certain chemicals.[67] Due to the high incidence of infection and trauma in patients being managed in critical care units, this myopathy may be more common than is recognized.

Neuromuscular Transmission Defects

During retrospective and prospective studies to characterize critical illness polyneuropathy, we performed repetitive nerve stimulation studies and found no evidence for a defect in neuromuscular transmission associated with sepsis.[44,56] At those times, neuromuscular blocking agents to ease ventilation were used uncommonly and could not be implicated as causing polyneuropathy.[45] The experience of Coronel and colleagues in France has been similar.[69] In the last 5 years, these agents, particularly the shorter-acting ones such as vecuronium, have been used somewhat more frequently in our critical care unit, rarely for prolonged periods of time. We are now observing the occasional patient who has the septic syndrome and suddenly develops weakness in the limbs, lasting for more than several hours, after a single injection of a neuromuscular blocking agent. Repetitive nerve stimulation studies show a typical decremental response, indicating a neuromuscular transmission defect induced by the drug. At initial testing in such a patient, the compound muscle action potential is quite small, indicating that in addition to the neuromuscular block, a polyneuropathy is also probably present. Denervation potentials subsequently appear in muscle. Thus, the main problem is critical illness polyneuropathy, the neuromuscular blocking agent simply exacerbating the problem and bringing it to clinical attention.

We have also observed the occasional patient who has had severe, generalized muscular weakness induced by a combination of prolonged treatment with neuromuscular blocking agents and high-dose corticosteroids for acute, severe asthma. Such patients, clinically and electrophysiologically, have findings of a primary myopathy. Sepsis could well be an important underlying factor in these and other cases reported in the literature.

Thus, in our experience, and in regard to a number of reports in the literature, there have been two relatively distinct syndromes associated with the use of neuromuscular blocking agents in the critical care unit. Either vecuronium or pancuronium bromide have usually been implicated. In the first of these,[47,70–74] patients who have sepsis and multiple organ failure are given neuromuscular blocking agents for several days, and after this medication is discontinued the patient is noted to be quadriplegic. There are clinical and electrophysiological signs of a primary axonal degeneration of motor fibers, with denervation atrophy of muscle, and repetitive nerve stimulation studies may also show a defect in neuromuscular transmission which, if present, is transient. There is elevation of serum creatine kinase to moderate or high levels; muscle biopsy usually shows evidence of denervation and, at times, necrosis. Again, it is likely that the predominant factor was sepsis and critical illness polyneuropathy, but the neuromuscular blocking agent may have had an additive toxic effect.

The second syndrome is that in which a patient presents with acute, severe asthma that requires the use of high-dose corticosteroids and neuromuscular blocking agents for several days.[75–77] When the patient is taken off these medications, it is noted that there is quadriplegia and difficulty in weaning from the ventilator. Whereas some cases have suggested a motor neuropathy, others have been indicative of a primary myopathy. Repetitive nerve stimulation studies sometimes show a defect in neuromuscular transmission. Creatine kinase levels in the serum may be considerably elevated. Muscle biopsy shows with certain stains the distinctive features of a loss of structure centrally in muscle fibers, and within this area, under electron microscopy, there is a loss of the thick filaments (myosin) normally present in muscle.[75]

There may also be a variable degree of denervation atrophy and necrosis. These morphological changes are similar to those that can be induced in animals when muscle is experimentally denervated in conjunction with high-dose corticosteroid treatment.[78] These experimental results provide support for the clinical findings. Sepsis may induce first a critical illness polyneuropathy resulting in denervation of muscle and then, with the combination of high-dose corticosteroids and neuromuscular blocking agents, a primary myopathy with its distinctive features.

In both of these syndromes, if the patient survives the sepsis, recovery from the neuromuscular problem always occurs, although this may require a number of weeks in more severe cases.

Finally, prolonged weakness induced by neuromuscular blocking drugs may be due purely to the neuromuscular transmission defect, particularly in the presence of renal failure.[79] However, reversal then occurs in a matter of hours or days, with no evidence of either neuropathy or myopathy, although systematic studies to exclude neuropathy or myopathy have usually not been performed.

Theories to Explain Neuromuscular Syndromes

While the precise mechanisms of critical illness polyneuropathy and the additional effects of neuromuscular blocking agents and corticosteroids are not known, some speculation is possible. As discussed in the section on critical illness polyneuropathy, the septic syndrome may be due to a disturbance in the microcirculation of various organs. If this were to affect peripheral nerve, energy depletion would produce the distal axonal degeneration typical of critical illness polyneuropathy. Increased capillary permeability may be a prominent feature of the microcirculatory disturbance. Potentially toxic substances such as neuromuscular blocking agents or their metabolites could thereby gain entry to the endoneurial space and cause further direct damage to nerve axons.

These mechanisms may also apply to muscle. Animal experiments show that the effects of corticosteroids on denervated muscle are to cause a loss of thick (myosin) filaments,[78] typical of that seen in human cases.[75] One could speculate that, in human cases, the

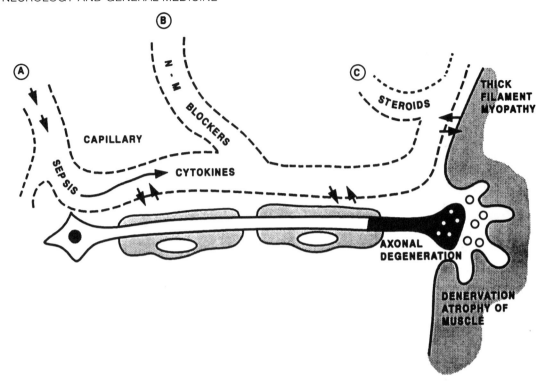

Fig. 44-11 Theoretical mechanisms of medication-induced neuropathy and myopathy in septic patients. Through the release of cytokines from macrophages, sepsis induces capillary permeability. This and other vascular disturbances may induce endoneurial edema, hypoxia, and, hence, a distal axonal degeneration typical of critical illness polyneuropathy **(A)**. However, the increased capillary permeability may also allow the entry of known toxins, such as neuromuscular blocking agents or their metabolites, which may further induce neuropathy **(B)**. The entry of steroids into muscle may have the additional effect of inducing a myosin filament myopathy **(C)**. (From Bolton CF: The polyneuropathy of critical illness. J Intens Care Med, in press, with permission.)

muscle is first denervated by critical illness polyneuropathy and then by neuromuscular blocking agents; the entry of corticosteroids completes the toxic effect (Fig. 44-11).

These mechanisms theoretically explain the three main types of neuromuscular conditions that have been seen in humans: (1) polyneuropathy due to sepsis alone (critical illness polyneuropathy); (2) polyneuropathy due to sepsis plus neuromuscular blocking agents; and (3) polymyopathy due to sepsis, neuromuscular blocking agents, and corticosteroids. Combinations of all three may occur in the same patient. Only prospective studies in humans and animals will unravel these complex neuromuscular events.

A SUMMARY OF THE APPROACH TO THE INVESTIGATION OF MUSCLE WEAKNESS IN CRITICALLY ILL PATIENTS

A review of the history is important, particularly in relationship to possible underlying sepsis and the use of medications, such as neuromuscular blocking agents and corticosteroids. The physical examination is difficult due to mechanical ventilation, sedation, vascular lines, etc., and electrophysiological studies are always indicated. Serum levels of creatine kinase give some indication of the degree of muscle fiber breakdown. Muscle biopsy may be necessary. The

Table 44-4 The Differentiating Features of Neuromuscular Disorders in Critically Ill Patients

Condition	Antecedent Illness	Clinical features	Electrophysiology	Morphology	Treatment	Prognosis
Critical illness polyneuropathy	Sepsis	Absent, or signs of mainly motor neuropathy	Consistent with a primary axonal degeneration of mainly motor fibers	Primary axonal degeneration of nerve, denervation atrophy of muscle	Treat septic syndrome	Good in 40 percent who survive sepsis and organ failure
Neuromuscular blocking agents and neuropathy	Sepsis	Acute quadriplegia	Neuromuscular transmission defect and/or axonal motor neuropathy	Normal or denervation atrophy on muscle biopsy	None	Good
Neuromuscular blocking agents, corticosteroids and myopathy	Sepsis ?	Acute quadriplegia	Neuromuscular transmission defect and/or myopathy	Thick myosin filament loss	None	Good
Panfascicular muscle fiber necrosis	Transient infection, trauma, etc.	Severe muscle weakness, increased serum creatine kinase, often myoglobinuria	Positive sharp waves and fibrillation potentials on needle EMG	Panfascicular muscle fiber necrosis	None, or hemo-dialysis for myoglobinuria	Good
Cachectic myopathy	Severe systemic illness, prolonged recumbency	Diffuse muscle wasting	Normal	Type II fiber atrophy on muscle biopsy	Physiotherapy, improved nutrition	Good

same patient may have combinations of the conditions described above. A summary of how these different neuromuscular syndromes associated with sepsis can be differentiated is provided in Table 44-4.

REFERENCES

1. Shoemaker WC, Thompson WL, Holbrook PR (eds): Textbook of Critical Care. WB Saunders, Philadelphia, 1984
2. Pine RW, Wertz MJ, Lennard ES, et al: Determinants of organ malfunction or death in patients with intra-abdominal sepsis: a discriminant analysis. Arch Surg 118:242, 1983
3. Tran DD, Groeneveld AAJB, van der Meulen J, et al: Age, chronic disease, sepsis, organ system failure, and mortality in a medical intensive care unit. Crit Care Med 18:474, 1990
4. Ayres SM: Sepsis and septic shock—a synthesis of ideas and proposals for the direction of future research. p. 375. In Sibbald WJ, Sprung CL (eds): New Horizons: Perspectives on Sepsis and Septic Shock. Society of Critical Care Medicine, Fullerton, CA, 1986
5. Bone RC, Fisher CJ, Clemmer TP, et al: Sepsis syndrome: a valid clinical entity. Crit Care Med 17:389, 1989
6. Bone RC, Sprung CL, Sibbald WJ: Definitions for sepsis and organ failure. Crit Care Med 20:724, 1992
7. Glauser MP, Zanetti G, Baumgartner JD, Cohen J: Septic shock: pathogenesis. Lancet 338:732, 1991
8. Meakins JL: Host-defense response to sepsis and septic shock. p. 113. In Sibbald WJ, Sprung CL (eds): New

Horizons: Perspectives on Sepsis and Septic Shock. Society of Critical Care Medicine, Fullerton, CA, 1986

9. Bolton CF, Young GB, Zochodne DW: The neurological complications of sepsis. Ann Neurol 33:94, 1993

10. Jackson AC, Gilbert JJ, Young GB, Bolton CF: The encephalopathy of sepsis. Can J Neurol Sci 12:303, 1985

11. Young GB, Bolton CF, Austin TW, et al: The electroencephalogram (EEG) in sepsis. Can J Neurol Sci 13:164, 1986

12. Young GB, Bolton CF, Austin TW, et al: The encephalopathy associated with septic illness. Clin Invest Med 13:297, 1990

13. Plum F, Posner JB: The Diagnosis of Stupor and Coma. 3rd Ed. FA Davis, Philadelphia, 1980

14. Chedru F, Geschwind N: Writing disturbances in acute confusional states. Neuropsychologia 10:343, 1972

15. Ayus JC, Krothapalli RK, Arieff AI: Changing concepts in treatment of severe symptomatic hyponatremia. Am J Med 78:897, 1985

16. McGovern VJ, Tiller DJ: Shock: A Clinico-Pathological Correlation. Masson, New York, 1980

17. Pendlebury WW, Perl DP, Karibo RM, McQuillen JB: Disseminated microabscesses of the central nervous system. Neurology 33,suppl 2:223, 1983

18. Blackwood W, McMenemy WF, Meyer A, et al: Greenfield's Neuropathology. 2nd Ed. Edward Arnold, London, 1963

19. du Moulin GC, Paterson D, Hedley-Whyte J, Broitman SA: E. coli peritonitis and bacteremia cause increased blood-brain barrier permeability. Brain Res 340:261, 1985

20. Jeppsson B, Freund HR, Gimmon Z, et al: Blood-brain barrier dysfunction in sepsis: cause of septic encephalopathy? Am J Surg 141:136, 1981

21. Fernstrom JD, Wurtman RJ: Brain serotonin content: physiological regulation by plasma neutral amino acids. Science 178:414, 1972

22. Freund HR, Muggia-Sullam M, Peiser J, Melamed E: Brain neurotransmitter profile is deranged during sepsis and septic encephalopathy in the rat. J Surg Res 38:267, 1985

23. Krueger JM, Walter J, Dinarello CA, et al: Sleep-promoting effects of endogenous pyrogen (interleukin-1). Am J Physiol 246:R994, 1984

24. De Sarro GB, Masuda Y, Ascioti C, et al: Behavioural and ECoG spectrum changes induced by intracerebral infusion of interferons and interleukin 2 in rats are antagonized by naloxone. Neuropharmacology 29:167, 1990

25. Dinarello CA: Interleukin-1. Rev Infect Dis 6:51, 1984

26. Meyrick B, Brigham KL: Acute effects of Escherichia coli endotoxin on the pulmonary microcirculation of anesthetized sheep—structure-function relationships. Lab Invest 48:458, 1983

27. Bihari D, Smithies M, Gimson A, Tinker J: The effects of vasodilation with prostacyclin on oxygen delivery and uptake in critically ill patients. N Engl J Med 317:397, 1987

28. Riedler GF, Straub PW, Frick PG: Thrombocytopenia in septicemia. Helv Med Acta 36:23, 1971

29. Palmer RMJ, Ferrige AG, Moncada S: Nitric oxide release accounts for the biological activity of endothelium-derived relaxing factor. Nature 327:524, 1987

30. Nava E, Palmer RMF, Moncada S: Inhibition of nitric oxide synthesis in septic shock: how much is beneficial? Lancet 338:1557, 1991

31. Lorente JE, Landin L, Renes E, Esteban A: Regulation of vascular tone in sepsis. Intens Care World 10:58, 1993

32. Tanaka K, Gotoh F, Gomi S, et al: Inhibition of nitric oxide synthesis induces a significant reduction in local cerebral blood flow in the rat. Neurosci Lett 127:129, 1991

33. Vincent SR, Hope BT: Neurons that say NO. Trends Neurosci 15:108, 1992

34. Chaudry IH, Schleck S, Clemens MG, et al: Altered hepatocellular active transport: an early change in peritonitis. Arch Surg 117:151, 1982

35. Duff JH, Viidik T, Marchuk JB, et al: Femoral arteriovenous amino acid differences in septic patients. Surgery 85:344, 1979

36. Fraser CL, Arieff AI: Hepatic encephalopathy. N Engl J Med 313:865, 1985

37. Olasmaa M, Rothstein JD, Guidotti A, et al: Endogenous benzodiazepine receptor ligands in human and animal hepatic encephalopathy. J Neurochem 55:2015, 1990

38. Ball M, McQuay HJ, Moore RA, et al: Renal failure and the use of morphine in the intensive care unit. Lancet 1:784, 1985

39. Herkes GK, Wszolek ZK, Westmoreland BF, Klass DW: Effects of midazolam on electroencephalograms of seriously ill patients. Mayo Clin Proc 67:334, 1992

40. Chudley AE, Ninan A, Young GB: Neurologic signs and hypophosphatemia with total parenteral nutrition. Can Med Assoc J 125:604, 1981

41. Weinstein L: Antimicrobial agents: penicillins and cephalosporins. p. 1130. In Goodman KS, Gilman A (eds): The Pharmacological Basis of Therapeutics. 5th Ed. Macmillan, New York, 1975

42. Leo RJ, Ballow CH: Seizure activity associated with imipenem use: clinical case reports and review of the literature. DICP 25:351, 1991

43. McKee AC, Winkelman MD, Banker BQ: Central

pontine myelinolysis in severely burned patients: relationship to serum hyperosmolality. Neurology 38: 1211, 1988

44. Bolton CF, Laverty DA, Brown JD, et al: Critically ill polyneuropathy: electrophysiological studies and differentiation from Guillain-Barré syndrome. J Neurol Neurosurg Psychiatry 49:563, 1986

45. Witt N, Zochodne DW, Bolton CF, et al: Peripheral nerve function in sepsis and multiple organ failure. Chest 99:176, 1991

46. Bischoff A, Meier C, Roth F: Gentamicin-neurotoxizitat (polyneuropathie-enzephalopathie). Schweiz Med Wochenschr 107:3, 1977

47. Op de Coul AAW, Lambregts PCLA, Koeman J, et al: Neuromuscular complications in patients given Pavulon (pancuronium bromide) during artificial respiration. Clin Neurol Neurosurg 87:17, 1985

48. Covert CR, Brodie SB, Zimmerman JE: Weaning failure due to acute neuromuscular disease. Crit Care Med 14:307, 1986

49. Gross ML, Fowler CJ, Ho R, et al: Peripheral neuropathy complicatng pancreatitis and major pancreatic surgery. J Neurol Neurosurg Psychiatry 51:1341, 1988

50. Roelofs RI, Cerra F, Bielka N, et al: Prolonged respiratory insufficiency due to acute motor neuropathy: a new syndrome? Neurology 33, suppl 2:240, 1983

51. Couturier JC, Robert D, Monier P: Polynevrites compliquant des sejours prolonges en reanimation: a propos de 11 cas d'etiologie encore inconnue. Lyon Med 252: 247, 1984

52. Williams AC, Sturman S, Kelsey S, et al: The neuropathy of the critically ill. Br Med J 293:790, 1986

53. Barat M, Brochet B, Vital C, et al: Polyneuropathies au cours de sejours prolonges en reanimation. Rev Neurol (Paris) 143:823, 1987

54. Lycklama J, Nijeholt A, Troost J: Critical illness polyneuropathy. p. 575. In Matthews WB (ed): Handbook of Clinical Neurology. Vol 51. Elsevier, Amsterdam, 1987

55. Bolton CF: Electrophysiologic studies of critically ill patients. Muscle Nerve 10:129, 1987

56. Maher J, Rutledge F, Remtulla H, et al: Neurophysiological assessment of failure to wean from a ventilator. Can J Neurol Sci 20,suppl 2:S28, 1993

57. Zochodne DW, Bolton CF, Wells GA, et al: Critical illness polyneuropathy: a complication of sepsis and multiple organ failure. Brain 110:819, 1987

58. Ochs S: Basic properties of axoplasmic transport. p. 453. In Dyck PJ, Thomas PK, Lambert EH, Bunge R (eds): Peripheral Neuropathy. 2nd Ed. WB Saunders, Philadelphia, 1984

59. Spencer PS, Schaumburg HH: Experimental models of primary axonal disease induced by toxic chemicals. p. 636. In Dyck PJ, Thomas PK, Lambert EH, Bunge R (eds): Peripheral Neuropathy. 2nd Ed. WB Saunders, Philadelphia, 1984

60. Olsson Y: Studies on vascular permeability in peripheral nerves: I. Distribution of circulating fluorescent serum albumin in normal, crushed and sectioned rat sciatic nerve. Acta Neuropathol (Berl) 7:1, 1966

61. Lefer AM: Eicosanoids as mediators of ischemia and shock. Fed Proc 44:275, 1985

62. Osler W: The Principles and Practice of Medicine. Appleton, New York, 1892

63. Baracos V, Rodemann HP, Dinarello CA, Goldberg AL: Stimulation of muscle protein degradation and prostaglandin E_2 release by leukocytic pyrogen (interleukin-1). N Engl J Med 308:553, 1983

64. Clowes GHA, George BC, Villee CA, Saravis CA: Muscle proteolysis induced by a circulating peptide in patients with sepsis of trauma. N Engl J Med 308:545, 1983

65. Zochodne DW, Bolton CF, Thompson RT, et al: Myopathy in critical illness. Muscle Nerve 9:652, 1986

66. Zochodne DW, Thompson RT, Driedger AA, et al: Topical P31 NMR spectroscopy in human forearm denervation. Neurology 36,suppl 1:138, 1986

67. Penn AS: Myoglobinuria. p. 1792. In Engel AG, Banker BQ (eds): Myology. McGraw-Hill, New York, 1986

68. Lannigan R, Austin TW, Vestrup J: Myositis and rhabdomyolysis due to Staphylococcus aureus septicemia. J Infect Dis 150:784, 1984

69. Coronel B, Mercatello A, Couturier J-C, et al: Polyneuropathy: potential cause of difficult weaning. Crit Care Med 18:486, 1990

70. Op de Coul AAW, Verheul GAM, Leyten ACM, et al: Critical illness polyneuromyopathy after artificial respiration. Clin Neurol Neurosurg 93:27, 1991

71. Subramony SH, Carpenter DE, Raju S, et al: Myopathy and prolonged neuromuscular blockade after lung transplant. Crit Care Med 19:1580, 1991

72. Rossiter A, Souney PF, McGowan S, Carvajal P: Pancuronium-induced prolonged neuromuscular blockade. Crit Care Med 19:1583, 1991

73. Gooch JL, Suchyta MR, Balbierz JM, et al: Prolonged paralysis after treatment with neuromuscular junction blocking agents. Crit Care Med 19:1125, 1991

74. Kupfer Y, Namba T, Kaldawi E, Tessler S: Prolonged weakness after long-term infusion of vecuronium bromide. Ann Intern Med 117:484, 1992

75. Danon MJ, Carpenter S: Myopathy with thick filament (myosin) loss following prolonged paralysis with vecuronium during steroid treatment. Muscle Nerve 14: 1131, 1991

76. Douglass JA, Tuxen DV, Horne M, et al: Myopathy in severe asthma. Am Rev Respir Dis 146:517, 1992

77. Hirano M, Ott BR, Raps EC, et al: Acute quadriplegic myopathy: a complication of treatment with steroids, nondepolarizing blocking agents, or both. Neurology 42:2082, 1992

78. Karpati G, Carpenter S, Eisen AA: Experimental core-like lesions and nemaline rods: a correlative morphological and physiological study. Arch Neurol 27:237, 1972

79. Segredo V, Caldwell JE, Matthay MA, et al: Persistent paralysis in critically ill patients after long-term administration of vecuronium. N Engl J Med 327:524, 1992

45

Neurological Complications of Imaging Procedures

Howard A. Rowley
Christopher F. Dowd
William P. Dillon

Neurological complications of imaging procedures are varied and largely related to either local complications of an invasive procedure or complications arising from the systemic use of intravenous contrast agents. In this chapter a summary is provided of neurological complications related to those imaging procedures that are commonly performed in modern radiological practices. Some historical perspective has been presented as well, and the reader must be aware that changes in the practice of radiological procedures will affect the kinds of complications and their incidence over time.

COMPLICATIONS OF INTRAVENOUS INJECTION OF CONTRAST MATERIAL

Radiographic contrast agents have been in use for over 60 years and are employed in approximately 10 million radiographic procedures annually in the United States. They find wide use in the evaluation of disease processes both within the central nervous system (CNS) and throughout the body. Contrast material helps to define normal vascular anatomy as well as to pinpoint patterns of abnormal contrast enhancement indicative of pathological processes. Most patients tolerate radiographic contrast with little or no side effects.

Iodinated Contrast Media

The toxicity of ionic radiocontrast media is well documented.[1] Two general categories of reactions have been described. The idiosyncratic reactions may occur on first or subsequent contrast administration and consist of hives, edema, bronchospasm, hypotension, and other anaphylactic reactions. A second category of complications is mainly dose-related and includes cardiovascular depression and renal failure. Secondary neurological symptoms and signs may result when significant cardiorenal dysfunction occurs. Life-threatening reactions occur on the order of 0.05 to 0.10 percent of injections, with deaths occurring approximately once in every 75,000 injections.[2]

Major direct neurological complications ascribed to contrast media relate to seizures, usually in patients with known primary or metastatic tumors.[3,4] Seizures and parkinsonian symptoms have also been identified following overdose of contrast medium during cardiac catheterization performed with diatrizoate meglumine 66 percent and diatrizoate sodium 10 percent.[5] It has been postulated that a time- and dose-related breakdown of blood-brain barrier leads to subsequent direct neuronal toxicity.

Cortical blindness has also been reported following use of contrast medium, usually related to cardiac catheterization or other angiographic procedures. This is most commonly seen with vertebral angiography (0.3 to 1 percent incidence)[6] or rarely after other angiographic procedures.[7] This syndrome is usually transient and has been associated with abnormal retention of contrast medium within the occipital cortex.[6]

Hematological effects of injection of contrast medium have been reported, including increased sickling of red blood cells in patients with sickle cell anemia and clumping of red blood cells in patients with apparently normal hemoglobin. These laboratory observations have had no clear clinical implications, however.

Aggravation of myasthenia gravis is a potential risk of ionic contrast administration[8] but appears to be somewhat less frequent with the nonionic formulations.

Extravasation of x-ray contrast medium can occur, leading to local tissue injury, including peripheral nerve damage. Swelling, which attends severe extravasation injuries, can also lead to compartment syndromes and therefore to injury of the peripheral nervous system. The risk of severe soft tissue extravasation injury appears to be greatest with ionic contrast agents which have been injected via power injectors.[9]

Contrast Media for Magnetic Resonance Imaging

Contrast media for magnetic resonance imaging (MRI) generally have lower toxicity profiles and much higher patient tolerance than their x-ray contrast counterparts. The most widely employed by far are chelates of gadolinium, a lanthanide metal. This metal in its free form is toxic, but through chelation is safely distributed and then eliminated from the body via renal clearance. Both ionic and nonionic formulations of gadolinium are available, with the incidence of complications being approximately 1 percent or less.[2,10] Minor side effects are sometimes noted during injection, including headache, nausea, and vomiting, but the risk of anaphylaxis appears to be extremely low,[11,12] on the order of 1 per several 100,000 injections. Death has been reported due to anaphylaxis. Gadolinium agents do cross the placenta, with undetermined effects on developing fetuses; therefore they are not approved for use during pregnancy. To our knowledge, there have been no reports of gadolinium-based contrast agents causing seizures.

Other contrast agents for MRI are entering clinical application. These include chelates of dysprosium, a related lanthanide metal. Chelates of manganese (manganese dpdp) are beginning to find use in liver imaging. Free manganese has a theoretical risk of parkinsonian complications, but the chelated compound was found to cause no serious side effects during phase 2 clinical trials.[13]

Miscellaneous Complications of Contrast Media

Reflux of ionic x-ray contrast medium has been reported into the abdominal port of a ventriculoperitoneal shunt after bladder rupture sustained during voiding cisternourethrography. This extravasated contrast medium then tracked up the ventriculoperitoneal shunt, causing seizures and ventriculitis.[14]

Venous air embolism has occasionally been documented in relation to infusion of contrast medium, either due to scalp vein malposition or inadvertent trapping of air within power injectors or tubing. Two separate reports of malpositioning of scalp vein catheters point to the risk of sagittal sinus and cavernous sinus venous air emboli.[15,16] These can be a cause of stroke, especially in infants with patent cardiac foramen ovale or other right-to-left shunts. The presence of iatrogenic air within the venous sinuses is important to recognize and distinguish from infectious causes.

NONINVASIVE IMAGING PROCEDURES

Computed Tomography

Direct and acute neurological effects from computed tomography (CT) itself have not been described. Neurological complications related to x-ray

CT are usually incidental to the procedure itself and related instead to complications of sedation, mechanical falls, or other mishaps that incidentally attended the procedure. There is a theoretical risk of causing cataracts or radiation-induced tumors with multiple CT studies carried out over time. For this reason, MRI may be a better method of following patients who require repeated imaging procedures if they are able to tolerate this examination.

Xenon CT

Inhalation of inert xenon[133] gas mixed with oxygen has been used for determination of cerebral blood flow and perfusion. Stable xenon is a highly lipid-soluble, freely diffusible tracer which is distributed according to local cerebral blood flow and can be imaged using the standard clinical CT scanner. In a retrospective review of 1,830 xenon-enhanced CT examinations, headaches (0.4 percent), seizures (0.2 percent), nausea and vomiting (0.2 percent), and change in sensorium (0.1 percent) were noted.[17] No serious respiratory depression, transient ischemic attacks, or permanent neurological deficits were observed in this study group.

Magnetic Resonance Imaging

MRI has rapidly gained wide acceptance in the imaging of the CNS as well as for musculoskeletal and many cardiac and general body applications. Images are produced by placing a patient in an extremely strong applied static magnetic field (on the order of 30,000 times the earth's gravitational field) and then changing the magnetic relaxation properties of water protons within the body using radiofrequency pulses; computer mathematical manipulation allows the production of images.

Because of the need for a very strong continuous magnetic field, the presence of metal in or around the imaging environment can be quite hazardous. Patients, staff, and others coming into proximity of the magnet are therefore routinely screened for potential ferromagnetic objects. The major contraindications to MRI include prior placement of a ferromagnetic aneurysm clip and the presence of cardiac pacemakers, intraocular metallic foreign bodies and some types of prosthetic cardiac valves, electronic or magnetically activated medical devices, and any other

large, potentially ferromagnetic foreign body.[18,19] The hazard of aneurysm clips deserves special attention. The vast majority of currently used aneurysm clips are felt to have little if any ferromagnetic properties, as judged by lack of deflection within a magnetic field when tested in vitro. At least one instance of fatal clip movement in a patient has, however, been reported, in this case due to inaccurate information supplied during the screening process.[20,21] The performance of MRI in patients with aneurysm clips is therefore currently a matter of controversy. The potential information to be gained from the procedure must be carefully balanced against the potential danger of clip movement. Although the metal from the clip may cause significant artifact on the examination, useful information can often still be gleaned by appropriately tailoring the examination.

Screening of patients and others referred for MRI is primarily via a questionnaire regarding any of the potential contraindications mentioned above. When in doubt, the specific medical device must be documented precisely and in writing prior to entry of the patient into the magnet. This information can be checked against the known magnetic deflection properties of the device, as appropriate. In patients with a history of possible metallic ocular foreign body, plain x-ray of the orbit or orbital CT can be used to exclude the presence of significant metal fragments.[22,23]

Some monitoring devices are also potentially dangerous because looped metallic wires may develop induced currents, resulting in burns to the skin attachment sites. For this reason, all physiological monitoring equipment and other devices must be carefully screened and approved specifically for use during MRI.

Another potential hazard related to the static magnetic field required for MRI is that of missile injury. The missile effect is perhaps the most serious potential hazard, as many clinicians entering the MR environment are not aware that the magnet is always "on." Paper clips, scissors, vacuum cleaners, oxygen tanks, and other ferromagnetic metallic items have been rapidly pulled into the bore of a magnet when inappropriately brought in close proximity to it, sometimes with fatal results. Proper introduction to safety precautions for visitors is important.

The rapid switching of the gradient coils used in MRI causes a loud vibration or banging noise. This has been estimated at between 65 and 95 dB. Hyperacusis is reported very commonly following MRI. Both temporary and permanent instances of hearing loss have also been reported; for these reasons, patients are routinely offered the use of earplugs before their examination commences. These are especially to be recommended in cases requiring very rapid switching of gradients coils, as with most magnetic resonance angiography sequences and ultrafast techniques such as fast spin echo and echo planar techniques.

Tissue heating is also a potential but to date not real complication of MRI. Radiofrequency energy deposition is limited by the FDA to 0.4 W/kg. In animal studies, levels at 10 times this rate over a 75-minute period raise the skin and eye temperature of a sheep by only 1.5°C, with no observed side effects.

MYELOGRAPHY AND INTRATHECAL INJECTIONS OF CONTRAST MEDIA

The number of myelographic procedures has dramatically diminished since the introduction of MRI and CT. In our own institution, the rapid acceptance of MRI resulted in a 48 percent decrease in the number of myelograms between 1981 and 1986 and a further 75 percent reduction from 1986 through 1988.[24] This trend, while substantial for all regions of the spine, has been most pronounced for thoracic and lumbar myelography. CT and more recently MRI have largely replaced myelography in the evaluation of the spinal cord and lumbar spine. MRI has clearly been established as superior to myelography in the evaluation of lumbar disc disease,[25,26] discitis and vertebral osteomyelitis,[27] and extra- and intradural spinal lesions.[28,29] Myelography is limited compared with CT and MRI as a single investigation of lumbar disc disease because of its insensitivity to extraforaminal, paraspinous, and lateral disc disease. In such a setting, if CT is used as the modality of first choice, the number of myelograms is decreased by over 60 percent.[25,26,30]

Low-dose CT myelography is preferred to plain-film myelography for evaluating the thecal sac in those patients who cannot tolerate MRI due to severe claustrophobia or the presence of a pacemaker or implanted metallic devices such as aneurysm clips.[25,26] In addition, some patients with severe spondylitic disease of the spine or postoperative changes with prominent osteophytes are best studied by low-dose CT myelography. In such instances, a lumbar puncture is performed and a low-dose injection (5 to 8 ml) of contrast is instilled prior to CT scanning.

There are very few indications left for traditional plain-film (high-dose) myelography. Suspected cerebrospinal fluid (CSF) loculations, arachnoid cysts, or arachnoiditis may still be studied by myelography, as the septations separating these CSF-filled structures can be difficult to detect on MRI. In addition, myelography is occasionally required to locate precisely the site of a CSF leak, and is better than MRI or CT in verifying the presence of dural arteriovenous fistula.[31]

The reduction in numbers of myelograms performed at major institutions has reduced the exposure of this procedure to trainees in radiology. As with any procedure, the incidence of complications associated with a procedure relates to the experience of the practitioner. In the case of myelography, it is our impression that the rate of complications is on the rise due to the decrease in experience of recent trainees. It is therefore appropriate to review the neurological complications of myelography and intrathecal injections of contrast material despite their decline in use in recent years.

Terminology

Myelography consists of plain films following intrathecal instillation of contrast media via either a lumbar puncture or a cervical puncture at the C1-C2 level, posterior to the spinal cord. Water-soluble nonionic contrast agents are currently used. Using a tilt-table and fluoroscopy, the contrast is positioned via gravity into the area of interest. Cervical, thoracic, and lumbar myelography as well as "total" intrathecal opacification can be accomplished through a single needle puncture. Prior to MRI, the choice of a lumbar or C1-C2 puncture was largely determined on the basis of clinical symptomatology. In recent years, low-dose (lower than routinely administered for plain-film myelography) injections prior to CT scanning, so called *CT myelography,* has gained in popularity and in many institutions has replaced formal plain-film myelography. This is helped by current helical high-speed CT scanners that are capable of high-resolution 1-mm contiguous scans through the entire cervical region in less than 5 minutes. Occasionally contrast must be positioned intracranially to opacify the CSF cisterns. *CT cisternography* has now largely been replaced by MRI, but it is still used occasionally to evaluate for CSF leak and intracranial arachnoid cyst.

Technique

There are several approaches for performing intrathecal injections. Generally a 22-gauge or smaller spinal needle is positioned via fluoroscopy in the lumbar or cervical subarachnoid space. This requires topical and subcutaneous anesthesia and is contraindicated in those with bleeding disorders. If required, a C1-C2 puncture is most safely performed using lateral fluoroscopy so that the needle can be placed without patient movement. The needle enters the lateral neck just below the mastoid tip and is fluoroscopically positioned in the posterior aspect of the cervical subarachnoid space, which is *usually* rather capacious, behind the cervical spinal cord. As will be discussed, C1-C2 puncture carries a risk of cervical cord puncture, and efforts must be taken to avoid this by proper positioning of the patient and careful technique. If CT is required, a low-dose injection of contrast medium may be performed from either C1-C2 or the lumbar route, but this is done more safely and with fewer potential complications from a lumbar puncture. CT is performed immediately following instillation of contrast medium. Delayed CT has been used in the past to evaluate syringomyelia, but this condition is now best evaluated by MRI.

Cisternal puncture in the suboccipital region is rarely if ever performed. The authors have never performed this procedure themselves and see little indication for its use in the current era of MRI.

Complications

The neurological complications of myelography and intrathecal injections can be divided into those related to intrathecal needle puncture itself and those related to instillation of intrathecal contrast material.

COMPLICATIONS OF INTRATHECAL PUNCTURE

Vasovagal Response
Vasovagal syncope occurs infrequently during lumbar puncture. Its occurrence can be anticipated by communication with the patient and by noting the initial appearance of diaphoresis. This generally occurs during head elevation and can be countered by promptly lowering the patient's head.

Headache
Headache and associated nausea and vomiting are the most frequent complications of lumbar puncture and myelography.[32–38] The etiology of headache is often obscure and may be related to a variety of complications. These include neurotoxic effects of the contrast agent, persistent CSF leak at the puncture site with postural low-pressure headache syndrome, intracranial hematomas, and psychological factors. Postural headache is usually due to persistent CSF leakage from the puncture site and is related to the size of the needle.[32,34,39] The incidence of headache following myelography has decreased with the development of nonionic water-soluble contrast agents compared to the ionic version (metrizamide).

In a study by Skalpe and Nakstad, 1,000 myelograms performed with nonionic water-soluble agent (iohexol) were reviewed for adverse effects.[33] Headache occurred in 38 percent of patients and was most frequent following cervical myelography with a lumbar puncture technique and with the patient placed horizontally after the examination. The lowest frequency of headache occurred following cervical myelography with the C1-C2 puncture technique, with the patient placed in bed and the head elevated 20°. The frequency of headache during lumbar myelography performed on an outpatient basis was 49 percent; however, no serious complications were encountered in this group. Many authors feel that the occurrence of headache, nausea, and vomiting are probably more related to spinal puncture and persistent leakage of CSF than to the toxicity of myelographic contrast media.[34,36,37,40]

Following myelography, it is current practice to keep patients in a supine position, with the head elevated approximately 25 to 45°, for a period of 4 to 6 hours.[41,42] Adequate oral hydration is important to reduce the incidence of headache. Autologous epidural blood patch and intravenous hydration is indicated in those patients with severe headache persisting for longer than 48 hours after myelography.[38,43]

Psychological factors may also play a role in the etiology of headache. Lee and Lui studied the psychological aspects of headache after lumbar puncture in

100 consecutive patients undergoing myelography.[44] Headache was found to be strongly associated with a normal examination and showed an association with hospital anxiety depression score. Sex and age have also been studied with regard to the incidence of adverse reactions to myelography. Maly studied a prospective group of over 1,700 patients undergoing myelography.[45] Regardless of the type of contrast medium or type of myelography, adverse reactions were 1.4 to 3.0 times as frequent in women as in men. Headache was more frequent in both women and men aged 26 to 50 years compared with older patients. The reason for this difference is unclear.

Hearing Loss

Hearing loss has been described as an adverse reaction following lumbar puncture as well as myelography.[46–49] Nine cases of hearing loss following myelography, lumbar puncture, and spinal anesthesia were reported by Michel and Brusis.[46–48] In six of the nine patients, bilateral impairment was present; recovery of normal hearing occurred in six patients. They speculate that this complication relates to patency of the cochlear aqueduct; altered pressure equilibrium between CSF and perilymph results in a release of perilymphatic fluid into the subarachnoid space. Alternatively, a direct toxic effect of contrast material on the inner ear may be a factor in hearing loss. They recommend the use of fine-gauge needles to reduce the leakage of CSF through the dural puncture. Mizuno and colleagues reported two cases of vestibular disturbances caused by residual oily contrast media in the internal auditory canal after myelography.[50] They speculate that the contrast medium, in this case, iophendylate (Pantopaque), acted as an irritant to the vestibular nerve. Steiner and co-workers, in a review of the neurological complications in diabetics after metrizamide lumbar myelography, found that auditory and visual hallucinations were increased in incidence in diabetics compared with a nondiabetic control group.[51] The use of nonionic myelographic agents may prove "safer in this population."

Epidermoid Tumors

Iatrogenic intraspinal epidermoid tumors have been reported as a sequela of lumbar puncture.[52,53] It is believed that implantation of epithelial cells from the skin into the thecal sac or epidermal space during lumbar puncture may allow this benign tumor to grow gradually. The incidence of iatrogenic epidermoid tumors has become exceedingly rare, probably related to improved needle design for lumbar punctures.[54] Epidermoid tumors appear on MRI as masses with signal characteristics similar to CSF. Lumbar puncture with myelography or CT would demonstrate them as a CSF-density mass filling the thecal sac. The presence of this rare tumor should arouse suspicions to possible iatrogenic causes, and a history of prior lumbar puncture should be sought.

Hemorrhage

Hemorrhagic sequela of myelography have been well documented.[55–61] In all likelihood, most of the hemorrhagic complications of myelography relate to persistent CSF leakage and low intracranial CSF pressure, which then result in the production of subdural hematomas. Subdural hematomas occur in response to low CSF pressure as a result of tearing of bridging veins or possibly as a response to accommodate the loss of intracranial volume. Subdural hematomas have also been recognized as a complication of spontaneous CSF leakage.[62,63] The possibility of subdural hematoma should be considered in patients who complain of prolonged headache or who develop neurological signs after lumbar puncture or myelography, especially if large quantities of CSF have been removed. Acute epidural hematoma complicating myelography in a normotensive patient with normal blood coagulability has been reported by Stevens and colleagues,[55] and bilateral intraparenchymal hemorrhages in a 38-year-old woman 7 days after lumbar myelography has been reported by Van de Kelft and associates.[56] The etiology of these hematomas remains obscure.

When spinal punctures are followed by anticoagulation, there is an increased risk of paraparesis or severe pain unless anticoagulation is delayed for at least 1 hour following the puncture.[64] These complications are usually related to epidural hematomas.

Puncture of the Conus Medullaris

While uncommon, puncture of the conus medullaris has been described.[65] This complication can be avoided by restricting lumbar punctures to below the L3 level. Low-lying conus and tethered cord may increase the risk of conus puncture, but these anatomical abnormalities can be detected by MRI.

COMPLICATIONS RELATED TO C1-C2 PUNCTURE

The frequency and approach to cervical myelography has been revolutionized with the wide acceptance of MRI. Cervical myelography via the C1-C2 level approach was routine for many years and was felt in experienced hands to be a safe alternative to the lumbar approach for cervical myelography. However, complications related to the C1-C2 approach have been well documented in the literature and include those associated with direct puncture of the spinal cord, laceration of epidural and vertebral venous and arterial structures, and complications related to neck hyperextension during the procedure. The indications for C1-C2 puncture are now quite infrequent. In those patients who cannot undergo MRI but who require cervical myelography, low-dose CT myelography via a lumbar puncture often suffices. This route of administration has been associated with a slightly higher incidence of headache, nausea, and vomiting than with C1-C2 puncture; however, with the use of low-dose nonionic water-soluble agents, these complications have been reduced to an acceptable level. Therefore, in our view, there are few if any indications for the C1-C2 approach in current neuroradiological practice.

The complications of C1-C2 puncture are nevertheless worthy of discussion. Katoh and co-workers documented the complications of lateral C1-C2 puncture myelography in 112 patients.[66] Spinal cord and blood vessel punctures were the most serious encountered. The authors point out that these complications principally depended on incorrect positioning of the patient's neck and misdirection of the x-ray beam. Spinal cord puncture is the most serious complication.[66-70] The injection of contrast material into the spinal cord may be associated with hemorrhagic necrosis of the gray matter and acute neurological decline. We have personally experienced one case of spinal cord injection and seen two cases from other institutions, resulting in acute and permanent trigeminal dysesthesia and quadriparesis. The important factor in avoiding this complication is proper patient positioning during myelography. A free flow of CSF should be documented prior to contrast injection.

The patient should experience no pain during the instillation of contrast media. If there *is* pain, the procedure should be terminated immediately and the cause of the pain assessed. Katoh and associates also documented three cases of epidural injection during a C1-C2 puncture,[66] a complication we have also seen in our own practice. Injection into the epidural venous plexus, and intra-arterial injection into an aberrant vertebral artery have been documented.[71,72] In approximately 2 percent of patients, the vertebral artery swings inferiorly into the posterior C1-C2 interspace[71]; an approach by lateral C1-C2 puncture may then inadvertently lacerate or puncture it. Rogers reported the death of a patient following C1-C2 myelography due to acute subdural hemorrhage as a consequence of laceration of an anomalous intraspinal vertebral artery.[73]

Robertson and Smith documented 68 major complications of cervical myelography.[69] Two-thirds of the complications were attributed to cervical spine hyperextension during the procedure and one-third to lateral C1-C2 puncture. The narrow sagittal diameter of the spinal canal and severe cervical spondylosis were frequent contributing factors to hyperextension injury of the cervical spinal cord. These authors recommend that MRI be performed first in patients with suspected spinal canal stenosis, severe spondylosis, or myelopathy of any cause. Should cervical CT myelography then be required, it is our view that a low-dose lumbar injection followed by thin-section CT is a safer alternative than C1-C2 puncture.

COMPLICATIONS OF MYELOGRAPHY RELATED TO CONTRAST AGENT

Neurological complications related to the intrathecal administration of contrast agents range from aseptic meningitis to encephalopathy and seizures. Other reported complications include hyperthermia, hallucinations, depression and anxiety states, and headache. The development of nonionic water-soluble contrast agents has reduced these neurotoxic side effects significantly.[74-76]

Aseptic Meningitis

One of the neurotoxic side effects that is clearly unrelated to dose is aseptic meningitis. Bacterial meningitis must be excluded in such cases, which are characterized by the abrupt onset of fever, usually within 24 hours after the intrathecal instillation of contrast. Transient CSF pleocytosis (neutrophils and lymphocytes) and elevated protein concentrations accompany symptoms that appear very similar to those of bacterial meningitis.[77–80] Once a bacterial infection has been excluded, the use of corticosteroids may be useful.

Seizures

Intrathecal contrast material may cause other less frequent but potentially serious complications. Encephalopathy, seizures, and focal neurological deficits have all been reported following myelography, presumably due to reflux of contrast material into the brain.[74,81] The risk of seizures is on the order of 0.1 to 0.3 percent with the nonionic water-soluble contrast agent iopamidol.[82] Increased risk of seizures is present when the total dose of iodine is greater than 4,500 mg, there is a preexisting seizure disorder, a cervical route of injection is chosen, or the patient is concurrently on drugs known to lower the seizure threshold.

Inadvertent administration of the ionic contrast media used for urography or angiography during myelography causes convulsions that probably arise within the spinal cord itself as well as the brain.[83,84] These water-soluble ionic contrast agents are visually indistinguishable from the nonionic contrasts used for myelography; therefore great care must be taken in identifying the specific brand and subtype chosen for myelography. Due to these serious complications, the FDA has introduced new guidelines that will require specific warning labels to be attached to water-soluble ionic contrasts.[83]

Arachnoiditis

Arachnoiditis or inflammation of the leptomeninges has also been ascribed to the use of contrast agents for myelography. Iophendylate, an oil-soluble contrast agent, was first noted to cause arachnoiditis, especially when associated with subarachnoid blood (i.e., following a traumatic tap). In many cases it is difficult to ascribe this syndrome with any confidence to the contrast agent, because confounding variables such as trauma, surgery, infection, or bleeding may have occurred within the spinal subarachnoid space and have also been associated with arachnoiditis.[85] The issue is further complicated by the observation that

arachnoiditis can be induced by intrathecal corticosteroid injections.[86] Contrast-related arachnoiditis may appear months or years following the instillation of the compound. Clinically, patients generally present with symptoms of constant low back pain aggravated by movement. Evidence of multifocal radiculopathy is found on examination. On repeat myelography or MRI, the nerve roots of the cauda equina appear thickened, clumped, and adherent to the periphery of the thecal sac, giving rise to locutions of contrast centrally. The incidence of arachnoiditis with the new water-soluble nonionic contrast agents appears to be much lower than with iophendylate or with ionic water-soluble agents (metrizamide).

The pathogenesis of postmyelographic arachnoiditis is unclear. One group found that after 8 days, animals undergoing metrizamide myelography developed progressively more severe arachnoid fibrosis.[87] However, no iodine was found in the arachnoid after 24 hours following myelography. Therefore the chronic effects of water-soluble media on the arachnoid are apparently not mediated by contrast media persisting in the arachnoid or by immune complexes. Clinical reports have suggested that myelography and laminectomy may produce more arachnoiditis than myelography alone; however, others have disputed this point.[88] We have witnessed at least two cases of acute, severe arachnoiditis following myelography and laminectomy. In these instances, MRI demonstrated prominent enhancement of intrathecal nerve roots. Clinically, patients responded to corticosteroids and conservative therapy.

DISCOGRAPHY

Discography is a procedure that involves the placement of a needle within the nucleus pulposus of a lumbar or cervical disc and the injection therein of water-soluble contrast agents. CT can be performed following discography for added spatial resolution. However, the value of discography is primarily as a provocative test—an attempt is made to recreate the patient's pain syndrome and to isolate a symptomatic disc that may not be abnormal on MRI or CT. Its usefulness is controversial, but discography is performed quite frequently throughout the United States. Horton and Daftari found that while MRI and discography correlated in many instances, MRI could not reliably predict which disc was the cause of a patient's pain.[89] Complications with discography are rare and are mainly related to the introduction of infection into the disc space through nonsterile technique. Disc space infections following discography have been clearly documented, although their incidence is low.[90] Both septic and aseptic discitis are potential side effects. In our experience, the incidence of discitis may be related to the length of the procedure, the use of the same needle for multiple discs, and breaks in sterile technique. Johnson found no evidence that diagnostic discography injured normal discs.[91]

ANGIOGRAPHY

Angiography is essential in the diagnostic evaluation of many patients with vascular pathology, but it carries the greatest risk of morbidity among diagnostic imaging procedures. This risk is generated by the necessity of inserting a catheter into a blood vessel, directing the catheter to the required location, injecting contrast material to visualize the vessel, and removing the catheter while maintaining hemostasis. Skill, experience, and judgment are elements that help to reduce the risk of this invasive procedure, but risk cannot be eliminated. Moreover, therapeutic transcatheter procedures (embolizations) have become important definitive and adjunctive therapies in patients with cerebrovascular, visceral, and peripheral vascular disease. The decision to undertake a diagnostic or therapeutic angiographic procedure requires sober assessment of the goals of the investigation and its risks.

Neurological complications of angiography or embolization are the most feared because of the relative permanence of the deficit, which can profoundly impair the patient. Neurological sequelae are encountered most often in angiographic procedures undertaken to evaluate or treat the vessels of the brain and spinal cord, but they can result from procedures undertaken to evaluate vascular disease elsewhere.

Cerebral and Aortic Angiography

Most aortic arch, carotid, and vertebral arteriograms are carried out via transfemoral arterial access. A common femoral arterial puncture provides retrograde access via the aorta to the aortic arch and great vessels. Arch aortography can be performed using a pigtail catheter, and selective catheterization of the carotid or vertebral arteries can be accomplished with a wide variety of catheter–guide wire combinations.

The most feared complication of cerebral angiography is stroke. Thrombus can form on or inside the tip of the catheter, especially if the catheter is not flushed properly with heparinized saline at regular intervals. Atherosclerotic intimal plaque may be present along the arterial wall, especially at the common carotid bifurcation. This thrombus or plaque can embolize distally into the cerebral circulation by force of injection or from dislodgment of plaque by the catheter or guide wire. The duration and extent of the resulting ischemic neurological deficit depends on the size and length of the embolus, its composition (fresh thrombus is thought to fragment more readily), its location, and the available collateral circulation. Identified risk factors for ischemic complications include lack of experience on the part of the angiographer,[92] atherosclerosis, vasospasm, low cardiac output, decreased oxygen-carrying capacity, advanced age, and possibly migraine.[93] The risk of a neurological complication has been estimated by many authors and is variable.[93–97] Hankey and colleagues reviewed eight prospective and seven retrospective studies involving over 8,000 patients with known cerebrovascular ischemic disease and estimated the risk of cerebral angiography at 4 percent for transient ischemic attack (TIA) and stroke, 1 percent for permanent deficit, and very low (<0.1 percent) for death.[97]

Ischemic complications can also result from intimal dissection of the carotid or vertebral artery by direct trauma from the tip of the catheter or guide wire. If the thin intimal lining is torn, it can allow a pocket of blood to form beneath it, resulting in extension of the intima dissection, narrowing or occlusion of the arterial lumen, and production of thromboemboli within the stagnant trapped pool of blood between the intima and media. Catheter-induced spasm of an artery also raises the potential for neurological complication. Although usually temporary, this phenomenon can result in a transient deficit if the spasm prevents adequate blood flow distally. One must identify the presence of spasm before injection of contrast agent, because such an injection into the stenotic spastic segment can result in dissection and possibly in permanent deficit.

Intravascular contrast material injected into the cerebral vasculature may have a toxic effect on the brain. In particular, patients with dolichoectasia of the basilar artery may suffer reversible brainstem dysfunction and acute short-term memory loss after multiple contrast injections into the vertebrobasilar system. It is postulated that the contrast bathes the perforating arteries of the brainstem on the dependent dorsal aspect of the basilar artery, because of its irregular dolichoectatic configuration. Limiting contrast injections into the vertebrobasilar system will limit the occurrence of this phenomenon.

Rarely, an intracranial aneurysm will rupture during an angiographic contrast injection,[98] causing subarachnoid hemorrhage. This is reported to result from the force of the injection, although this theory is not accepted universally.

Prior to catheter insertion into the common femoral artery, the local soft tissues must be infiltrated with an anesthetic agent, usually lidocaine. If the anesthetic agent is inadvertently injected into the femoral nerve, this may cause transient dysesthesias along the course of the nerve, which lies medial to the common femoral artery in the inguinal space. This rare phenomenon is usually self-limited.

In decades past, common practice dictated the use of a direct carotid artery puncture for the performance of cerebral angiography. Although this technique is now outmoded, there are rare circumstances that might require its use. Administration of local anesthesia for such a procedure may result in direct intracarotid injection of lidocaine, which can cause generalized seizures. Moreover, intimal damage may occur at the puncture site from the puncture needle or from subintimal contrast or saline injection, the most common cause of a neurological deficit occurring during direct carotid angiography.[93] Poor hemostatic control of the carotid puncture site may cause an expanding hematoma, which can deviate the trachea.

Axillary or brachial artery approaches are also used for cerebral angiography when the transfemoral route is not possible. These access routes will be discussed below.

Spinal Angiography

Spinal angiography may be indicated to evaluate vascular malformations and tumors and to identify the artery of Adamkiewicz prior to aortic aneurysm repair. Although the procedure requires the use of relatively large volumes of contrast and is tedious and lengthy in comparison to most other angiographic procedures, the incidence of complications is low. Forbes and colleagues evaluated 134 consecutive spinal angiograms prospectively and found only 3 neurological complications (2.2 percent), 2 recovering fully within 24 hours and 1 recovering fully within 1 week.[99] These adverse events included paraparesis, subjective visual blurring, and speech changes. Formerly, contrast material was implicated in the production of spasms during injection, but this phenomenon seems to occur rarely with newer contrast agents.

Peripheral Angiography

Peripheral (noncerebral–noncardiac) angiography also utilizes a transfemoral approach where possible. Although the cerebral vasculature is not examined per se, there is a risk of producing a cerebral embolic event if the subclavian or axillary arteries require examination, because of the adjacent origins of the vertebral and carotid arteries. Catheter manipulations are sometimes performed in the descending aortic arch in order to form special loops in the catheter's distal segment, and this may produce a neurological deficit by dislodging plaque from great vessels or by thrombus forming on the catheter tip.

Many patients undergo peripheral angiography to evaluate atherosclerotic disease of the abdominal aorta and iliofemoral system, which itself may preclude the use of a femoral artery puncture. If transfemoral access is not possible due to severe atherosclerosis, the axillary or brachial routes may be used. Each has its own set of risks.[100–103] An axillary puncture is performed with the arm abducted. The axillary artery is palpated and the puncture is made as deep into the axilla as possible. The left axilla is chosen for most examinations of the descending aorta and its branches; the right axilla is preferred when studying the carotid and vertebral arteries. For peripheral angiography, an axillary approach carries a two-[104] to fourfold[105] greater risk of neurological complications than a transfemoral approach. Stroke can result from dislodgment of an atherosclerotic plaque at the origin of the vertebral artery during catheter passage to the aorta. Hemostasis at the puncture site is a much more crucial issue than with a femoral puncture: the axillary artery is more difficult to compress after removal of the catheter, and an expanding hematoma may injure the brachial plexus.

Brachial artery access requires the use of a smaller-diameter catheter because of the smaller size of the artery. Puncture is made in the antecubital fossa and the catheter is navigated retrogradely through the brachial, axillary, and subclavian arteries to the aorta. Risks of cerebral thromboemboli exist as with the transaxillary route. The median nerve can be damaged by needle puncture[93] or by compression from a developing hematoma.

EMBOLIZATION PROCEDURES

The development of new materials and techniques has advanced the relatively young and small field of interventional neuroradiology, providing new therapeutic options for patients with difficult neurovascular problems. A variety of procedures is available, including detachable coil or balloon therapy for aneurysms, particulate or liquid adhesive embolization of arteriovenous malformations (AVMs), balloon angioplasty of stenosis or vasospasm, transarterial or transvenous embolization of dural arteriovenous fistulas, balloon occlusion of carotid-cavernous and vertebral fistulas, endovascular treatment of vein of Galen malformations, preoperative embolization of tumors, and thrombolysis of acute arterial or venous thrombosis. Many of these diseases place the patient at high risk of cerebral hemorrhage, stroke, or death. These endovascular treatments have their own risks, and therapy should be tailored to the disease risk of individual patients. The therapeutic risks are closer to the neurosurgical risks than the radiological risks.

The highest complication rates are found predictably with therapies geared to treating the highest-risk diseases. Among potential complications of endovascular aneurysm therapy are aneurysmal rupture, stroke from thromboemboli or from migration of the balloon or coil, and death. In a large series of surgically difficult intracranial aneurysms treated with detachable balloons, Higashida and colleagues reported a 7.4 percent incidence of stroke and a 9.8 percent death rate.[106,107] These figures must be considered in light of the high morbidity and mortality among patients with untreated and surgically unapproachable aneurysms, a patient population posing very high

risks. The advent of the electrolytically detachable coil[108,109] may reduce these rates, but endovascular therapy remains largely reserved for the more difficult aneurysms not amenable to standard craniotomy and surgical clipping.

Endovascular treatment of AVMs is frequently used as a preoperative adjunct to surgical resection or stereotactic radiosurgery. Embolic materials include liquid adhesives, polyvinyl alcohol (PVA) particles, and fibered coils. Therapeutic risks include AVM rupture with intracerebral hemorrhage; inadvertent embolization of normal arteries, causing stroke; and gluing the catheter into the embolized artery.[110] In separate studies using different embolic agents (liquid adhesives and PVA particles) for AVM embolization, the permanent neurological complication rate was 8 percent in each.[111,112]

Endovascular therapy is also applicable to vascular problems involving the spinal cord. In the treatment of intramedullary AVMs, which often present with hemorrhage, embolization may provide definitive, palliative, or adjunctive therapy. The major risk is occlusion of a normal portion of the anterior or posterolateral spinal arteries with the embolic material. Casasco and colleagues have estimated the risk of a permanent therapy-related neurological deficit at 5.7 percent.[113] This risk is similar in the treatment of perimedullary spinal arteriovenous fistulas. The spinal dural arteriovenous fistula represents a shunt between a dural artery on the nerve root sleeve and an adjacent radicular vein that drains toward the spinal cord, resulting in a venous engorgement syndrome. The risk involved in endovascular treatment of this dural process is lower, because spinal arteries are not involved directly.

Although advances in imaging capabilities, catheters, and embolic materials will advance endovascular capabilities, the knowledge, judgment, and experience of the angiographer will have the greatest effect in diminishing the risks of endovascular therapy.

REFERENCES

1. Junck L, Marshall WH: Neurotoxicity of radiological contrast agents. Ann Neurol 13:469, 1983
2. Bush WH, Swanson DP: Acute reactions to intravascular contrast media: types, risk factors, recognition, and specific treatment. AJR 157:1153, 1991

3. LoZito JC: Convulsions: a complication of contrast enhancement in computerized tomography. Arch Neurol 34:649, 1977

4. Haslam RH, Cochrane DD, Amundson GM, Johns RD: Neurotoxic complications of contrast computed tomography in children. J Pediatr 111:837, 1987

5. May EF, Ling GS, Geyer CA, Jabbari B: Contrast agent overdose causing brain retention of contrast, seizures and parkinsonism. Neurology 43:836, 1993

6. Lantos G: Cortical blindness due to osmotic disruption of the blood-brain barrier by angiographic contrast material: CT and MRI studies. Neurology 39:567, 1989

7. Kinn RM, Breisblatt WM: Cortical blindness after coronary angiography: a rare but reversible complication. Cathet Cardiovasc Diagn 22:177, 1991

8. Schwaninger M, Patt S, Henningsen P, Schmidt D: Spinal canal metastases: a late complication of glioblastoma. J Neurooncol 12:93, 1992

9. Memolo M, Dyer R, Zagoria RJ: Extravasation injury with nonionic contrast material. AJR 160:203, 1993

10. Chuang S: Contrast agents in pediatric neuroimaging. AJNR 13:785, 1992

11. Takebayashi S, Sugiyama M, Nagase M, Matsubara S: Severe adverse reaction to IV gadopentetate dimeglumine. AJR 160:659, 1993

12. Shellock FG, Hahn HP, Mink JH, Itskovich E: Adverse reaction to intravenous gadoteridol. Radiology 189:151, 1993

13. Øksendal AN, Hals PA: Biodistribution and toxicity of MR imaging contrast media. J Magn Reson Imaging 3:157, 1993

14. Dalkin B, Franco I, Reda EF, et al: Contrast-induced central nervous system toxicity after radiographic evaluation of the lower urinary tract in myelodysplastic patients with ventriculoperitoneal shunts. J Urol 148:120, 1992

15. Peled N, Blaser SI, Moore A, Harwood-Nash D: Computerized tomography appearance of accidental infusion of air into the venous sinuses. Pediatr Neurosurg 17:251, 1991

16. Adams M, Quint DJ, Eldevik OP: Iatrogenic air in the cavernous sinus. AJR 159:189, 1992

17. Latchaw RE, Yonas H, Pentheny SL, Gur D: Adverse reactions to xenon-enhanced CT cerebral blood flow determination. Radiology 163:251, 1987

18. Teitelbaum GP, Lin MC, Watanabe AT, et al: Ferromagnetism and MR imaging: safety of carotid vascular clamps. AJNR 11:267, 1990

19. Shellock FG, Curtis JS: MR imaging and biomedical implants, materials, and devices: an updated review. Radiology 180:541, 1991

20. Klucznik RP, Carrier DA, Pyka R, Haid RW: Placement of a ferromagnetic intracerebral aneurysm clip in a magnetic field with a fatal outcome. Radiology 187:855, 1993

21. Kanal E, Shellock FG: MR imaging of patients with intracranial aneurysm clips. Radiology 187:612, 1993

22. Otto PM, Otto RA, Virapongse C, et al: Screening test for detection of metallic foreign objects in the orbit before magnetic resonance imaging. Invest Radiol 27:308, 1992

23. Williams S, Char DH, Dillon WP, et al: Ferrous intraocular foreign bodies and magnetic resonance imaging. Am J Ophthalmol 105:398, 1988

24. Dillon WP: Myelography: in memoriam. Perspect Radiol 1:131, 1988

25. Modic MT, Masaryk TJ, Ross JS, Carter JR: Imaging of degenerative disk disease. Radiology 168:177, 1988

26. Modic MT, Masaryk T, Boumphrey F, et al: Lumbar herniated disk disease and canal stenosis: prospective evaluation by surface coil MR, CT, and myelography. AJR 147:757, 1986

27. Modic MT, Feiglin DH, Piraino DW, et al: Vertebral osteomyelitis: assessment using MR. Radiology 157:175, 1985

28. Sze G, Krol G, Zimmerman RD, Deck MD: Malignant extradural spinal tumors: MR imaging with Gd-DTPA. Radiology 167:217, 1988

29. Dillon WP, Norman D, Newton TH, et al: Intradural spinal cord lesions: Gd-DTPA-enhanced MR imaging. Radiology 170:229, 1989

30. Schipper J, Kardaun JW, Braakman R, et al: Lumbar disk herniation: diagnosis with CT or myelography. Radiology 165:227, 1987

31. Gaensler EH, Dillon WP: Vascular malformation of the spinal cord: MR spectrum and pitfalls. Presented at American Society of Neuroradiology, Orlando, Florida, 1989

32. Urso S, Giannini S, Migliorini A, Donnetti L: The incidence of postural headache in in- and outpatients following lumbar myelography (needles of different gauges and headache). Radiol Med (Torino) 77:165, 1989

33. Skalpe IO, Nakstad P: Myelography with iohexol (Omnipaque); a clinical report with special reference to the adverse effects. Neuroradiology 30:169, 1988

34. Tourtellotte WW, Henderson WG, Tucker RP, et al: A randomized, double-blind clinical trial comparing the 22 versus 26 gauge needle in the production of the post-lumbar puncture syndrome in normal individuals. Headache 12:73, 1972

35. Sand T: Which factors affect reported headache incidences after lumbar myelography? A statistical analysis of publications in the literature. Neuroradiology 31:55, 1989

36. Sand T, Myhr G, Stovner LJ, et al: Side effects after ambulatory lumbar iohexol myelography. Neuroradiology 31:49, 1989
37. Nestvold K, Sortland O: Lumbar myelography with iohexol: adverse effects compared with spinal puncture. Acta Radiol 29:637, 1988
38. Quinn CM, O'Sullivan PS, Patterson ET: Effects of route of fluid administration on severity of side effects with post-metrizamide myelogram. J Neurosci Nurs 19:261, 1987
39. Wilkinson AG, Sellar RJ: The influence of needle size and other factors on the incidence of adverse effects caused by myelography. Clin Radiol 44:338, 1991
40. Sand T, Stovner LJ, Dale L, Salvesen R: Side effects after diagnostic lumbar puncture and lumbar iohexol myelography. Neuroradiology 29:385, 1987
41. Kuuliala IK, Goransson HJ: Adverse reactions after iohexol lumbar myelography: influence of postprocedural positioning. AJR 149:389, 1987
42. Jones AG, Meinecke E, Becker J, Spoo K: Side effects following metrizamide myelography and lumbar laminectomy. J Neurosci Nurs 19:90, 1987
43. Wilton NC, Globerson JH, des Rosayro AM: Epidural blood patch for postdural puncture headache: it's never too late. Anesth Analg 65:895, 1986
44. Lee ST, Lui TN: Acute paraplegia resulting from haemorrhage into a spinal neurofibroma. Paraplegia 30:445, 1992
45. Maly P: Sex and age related differences in postmyelographic adverse reactions: a prospective study of 1765 myelographies. Neuroradiology 31:331, 1989
46. Michel O, Brusis T, Loennecken I, Matthias R: Inner ear hearing loss following cerebrospinal fluid puncture: a too little appreciated complication? HNO 38:71, 1990
47. Michel O, Brusis T: Hearing disorders following spinal anesthesia. Reg Anaesth 14:92, 1991
48. Michel O, Brusis T: Hearing loss as a sequel of lumbar puncture. Ann Otol Rhinol Laryngol 101:390, 1992
49. Nelson M, Lamb JT: Vestibulo-cochlear symptoms after myelography. Br J Radiol 58:388, 1985
50. Mizuno M, Yamasoba T, Nomura Y: Vestibular disturbance after myelography: contrast media in the internal auditory canal. ORL J Otorhinolaryngol Relat Spec 54:113, 1992
51. Steiner E, Simon JH, Ekholm SE, et al: Neurologic complications in diabetics after metrizamide lumbar myelography. AJR 146:1057, 1986
52. Batnitzky S, Keucher TR, Mealey J Jr, Campbell RL: Iatrogenic intraspinal epidermoid tumors. JAMA 237:148, 1977
53. McDonald JV, Klump TE: Intraspinal epidermoid tumors caused by lumbar puncture. Arch Neurol 43:936, 1986
54. Visciani A, Savoiardo M, Balestrini MR, Solero CL: Iatrogenic intraspinal epidermoid tumor: myelo-CT and MRI diagnosis. Neuroradiology 31:273, 1989
55. Stevens JM, Kendall BE, Gedroyc W: Acute epidural haematoma complicating myelography in a normotensive patient with normal blood coagulability. Br J Radiol 64:860, 1991
56. Van de Kelft E, Bosmans J, Parizel PM, et al: Intracerebral hemorrhage after lumbar myelography with iohexol: report of a case and review of the literature. Neurosurgery 28:570, 1991
57. Manji H, Birley H: Subdural haematoma—a complication of myelography in a patient with AIDS. AIDS 4:698, 1990
58. Overbeek HC, Keyser A: Multiple subcortical haemorrhages following lumbar metrizamide myelography. J Neurol 234:177, 1987
59. Gupta SR, Naheedy MH, Rubino FA: Cranial subdural hematoma following lumbar myelography. Comput Radiol 9:129, 1985
60. Dan NG: Intracranial subdural haematoma after metrizamide myelography. Med J Aust 140:289, 1984
61. Dohrmann PJ, Elrick WL, Siu KH: Intracranial subdural hematoma after lumbar myelography. Neurosurgery 12:694, 1983
62. Rando TA, Fishman RA: Spontaneous intracranial hypotension: report of two cases and review of the literature. Neurology 42:481, 1992
63. Fishman RA, Dillon WP: Dural enhancement and cerebral displacement secondary to intracranial hypotension. Neurology 43:609, 1993
64. Ruff RL, Dougherty JH Jr: Complications of lumbar puncture followed by anticoagulation. Stroke 12:879, 1981
65. Nelson DA: Dangers of lumbar spinal needle placement. Ann Neurol 25:310, 1989
66. Katoh Y, Itoh T, Tsuji H, et al: Complications of lateral C1–2 puncture myelography. Spine 15:1085, 1990
67. Farese MG, Martinez CR, Fisher CH: Inadvertent cervical cord puncture during myelography via C1–C2 approach. J Fla Med Assoc 77:91, 1990
68. Muller Vahl H, Vogelsang H: Spinal cord injury caused by a lateral C1–2 puncture for cervical myelography. Eur J Radiol 6:160, 1986
69. Robertson HJ, Smith RD: Cervical myelography: survey of modes of practice and major complications. Radiology 174:79, 1990
70. Nakstad PH, Kjartansson O: Accidental spinal cord injection of contrast material during cervical myelography with lateral C1–C2 puncture. AJNR 9:410, 1988
71. Kowada M, Yamaguchi K, Takahashi H: Fenestration

of the vertebral artery with a review of 23 cases in Japan. Radiology 103:343, 1972

72. Kowada M, Takahashi M, Gito Y, Kishikawa T: Fenestration of the vertebral artery: report of 2 cases demonstrated by angiography. Neuroradiology 6:110, 1973

73. Rogers LA: Acute subdural hematoma and death following lateral cervical spinal puncture: case report. J Neurosurg 58:284, 1983

74. Donaghy M, Fletcher NA, Schott GD: Encephalopathy after iohexol myelography. Lancet 2:887, 1985

75. Wang YS, Jiang YH, Hou ZY: Intrathecal injection of iohexol for routine myelography and CT myelography in 1,000 cases. [Published erratum appears in Chin Med J (Engl) 103:898, 1990.] Chin Med J (Engl) 103:497, 1990

76. Dobrzynska L, Mierzejewska E, Sokol A: Clinical and electroencephalographic signs of side effects in patients after myelography using "Amipaque." Neurol Neurochir Pol 19:221, 1985

77. Nakakoshi T, Moriwaka F, Tashiro K, et al: Aseptic meningitis complicating iotrolan myelography. AJNR 12:173, 1991

78. Alexiou J, Deloffre D, Vandresse JH, et al: Post-myelographic meningeal irritation with iohexol. Neuroradiology 33:85, 1991

79. Damani NN, Chin AT: Streptococcus pyogenes meningitis after myelography. J Pak Med Assoc 38:197, 1988

80. Schelkun SR, Wagner KF, Blanks JA, Reinert CM: Bacterial meningitis following Pantopaque myelography: a case report and literature review. Orthopedics 8:73, 1985

81. Reynolds DJN: Meningoencephalopathy following iopamidol myelography. J Neurol Neurosurg Psychiatry 52:410, 1989

82. Levey AI, Weiss H, Yu R, et al: Seizures following myelography with iopamidol. Ann Neurol 23:397, 1988

83. McClennan BL: Contrast media alert. Radiology 189: 35, 1993

84. Bøhn HP, Reich L, Suljaga Petchel K: Inadvertent intrathecal use of ionic contrast media for myelography. AJNR 13:1515, 1992

85. Esses SI, Morley TP: Spinal arachnoiditis. Can J Neurol Sci 10:2, 1983

86. Roche J: Steroid-induced arachnoiditis. Med J Aust 140:281, 1984

87. Garancis JC, Haughton VM: Pathogenesis of postmyelographic arachnoiditis. Invest Radiol 20:85, 1985

88. Johansen JG, Barthelemy CR, Haughton VM, et al: Arachnoiditis from myelography and laminectomy in experimental animals. AJNR 5:97, 1984

89. Horton WC, Daftari TK: Which disc as visualized by magnetic resonance imaging is actually a source of pain? A correlation between magnetic resonance imaging and discography. Spine 17, suppl: S164, 1992

90. Wiley JJ, Macnab I, Wortzman G: Lumbar discography and its clinical applications. Can J Surg 11:280, 1968

91. Johnson RG: Does discography injure normal discs? An analysis of repeat discograms. Spine 14:424, 1989

92. McIvor J, Steiner TJ, Perkin GD, et al: Neurological morbidity of arch and carotid arteriography in cerebrovascular disease: the influence of contrast medium and radiologist. Br J Radiol 60:117, 1987

93. Howieson J: Complications of cerebral angiography. p. 1034. In Newton TH, Potts DG (eds): Radiology of the Skull and Brain. Vol 2, Book 1. Angiography: Technical Aspects. CV Mosby, St Louis, 1974

94. Mani RL, Eisenberg RL: Complications of catheter cerebral arteriography: analysis of 5,000 procedures: II. Relations of complication rates to clinical and arteriographic diagnoses. AJR 131:867, 1978

95. Kerber CW, Cromwell LD, Drayer BP, Bank WO: Cerebral ischemia: I. Current angiographic techniques, complications, and safety. AJR 130:1097, 1978

96. Earnest F 4th, Forbes G, Sandok BA, et al: Complications of cerebral angiography: prospective assessment of risk. AJR 142:247, 1984

97. Hankey GJ, Warlow CP, Sellar RJ: Cerebral angiographic risk in mild cerebrovascular disease. Stroke 21:209, 1990

98. Allcock JM: Aneurysms. p. 2435. In Newton TH, Potts DG (eds): Radiology of the Skull and Brain. Vol 2. Book 4. Angiography: Specific Disease Processes. CV Mosby, St Louis, 1974

99. Forbes G, Nichols DA, Jack CR Jr, et al: Complications of spinal cord arteriography: prospective assessment of risk for diagnostic procedures. Radiology 169:479, 1988

100. Gordon RL, Haskell L: Iatrogenic disease: interventional radiology. p. 165. In Prager L (ed): Iatrogenic Disease. Vol 2. CRC Press, Boca Raton, FL, 1986

101. Hessel SJ, Adams DF, Abrams HL: Complications of angiography. Radiology 138:273, 1981

102. Molnar W, Paul DJ: Complications of axillary arteriotomies: an analysis of 1,762 consecutive studies. Radiology 104:269, 1972

103. Hessel SJ: Complications of angiography and other catheter procedures. p. 1041. In Abrams HL (ed): Abrams Angiography: Vascular and Interventional Radiology. 3rd Ed. Vol 2. Little, Brown, Boston, 1983

104. Kadir S: Complications of angiography. p. 679. In Diagnostic Angiography. WB Saunders, Philadelphia, 1986

105. Head RM, Robboy SJ: Embolic stroke from mural thrombi, a fatal complication of axillary artery catheterization. Radiology 102:307, 1972

106. Higashida RT, Halbach VV, Dowd CF, et al: Intracranial aneurysms: interventional neurovascular treatment with detachable balloons—results in 215 cases. Radiology 178:663, 1991

107. Higashida RT, Halbach VV, Hieshima GB: Endovascular therapy of intracranial aneurysms. p. 51. In Viñuela F, Halbach VV, Dion JE (eds): Interventional Neuroradiology: Endovascular Therapy of the Central Nervous System. Raven Press, New York, 1992

108. Guglielmi G, Viñuela F, Dion J, Duckwiler G: Electrothrombosis of saccular aneurysms via endovascular approach: Part 2. Preliminary clinical experience. J Neurosurg 75:8, 1991

109. Guglielmi G: Embolization of intracranial aneurysms with detachable coils and electrothrombosis. p. 63. In Viñuela F, Halbach VV, Dion JE (eds): Interventional Neuroradiology: Endovascular Therapy of the Central Nervous System. Raven Press, New York, 1992

110. Viñuela F: Functional evaluation and embolization of intracranial arteriovenous malformations. p. 77. In Viñuela F, Halbach VV, Dion JE (eds): Interventional Neuroradiology: Endovascular Therapy of the Central Nervous System. Raven Press, New York, 1992

111. Fournier D, Ter Brugge KG, Willinsky R, et al: Endovascular treatment of intracerebral arteriovenous malformations: experience in 49 cases. J Neurosurg 75: 228, 1991

112. Purdy PD, Samson D, Batjer HH, Risser RC: Preoperative embolization of cerebral arteriovenous malformations with polyvinyl alcohol particles: experience in 51 adults. AJNR 11:501, 1990

113. Casasco AE, Houdart E, Gobin YP, et al: Embolization of spinal vascular malformations. Neuroimaging Clin North Am 2:337, 1992

46

Neurological Complications of Anesthesia

David L. Brown

Neurological complications related to anesthesia often evoke powerful images, such as the vegetative patient who has sustained intraoperative cerebral hypoxia or the paraplegic patient whose neurological deficit is thought to be a result of spinal or epidural anesthesia. Most neurological complications of anesthesia are neither so sensational nor as clear in causation. The remarkable safety of modern anesthetic practice, due both to more sophisticated monitoring of hypoxemia and improvements in drugs and techniques, necessarily requires us to focus on many less severe complications, perhaps better termed side effects, rather than simply focusing on the dramatic central nervous system (CNS) injuries that may occur. In an effort to simplify the coverage of neurological complications of anesthesia, this chapter is arranged by symptom complexes that physicians are asked to deliberate upon, rather than simply providing a list of different complications. The conditions that will be covered include (1) mental status changes associated with anesthesia; (2) perioperative sensorimotor neurological deficits; (3) perioperative neurological excitation, including seizures and myoclonus; (4) perioperative headache; (5) perioperative visual changes; and (6) perioperative auditory changes.

PERIOPERATIVE MENTAL STATUS CHANGES

The administration of anesthesia is designed to produce an altered mental status for a circumscribed length of time. When mental status changes persist beyond the immediate perioperative period, it is necessary to verify that there are no reversible causes for it. In order to better understand the most typical alterations of mental status that may be identified perioperatively, three such changes will be discussed: (1) intraoperative awareness, (2) postoperative confusion, and (3) delayed or absent awakening (postoperative coma).

Intraoperative Awareness

One of patients' primary clinical fears as they approach surgery is that they may "be awake" during the surgical procedure. Prior to the introduction of clinically useful muscle relaxants (curare) in 1942, patient movement with surgical stimulation often alerted the anesthesiologist to an inadequate depth of anesthesia. The introduction of muscle relaxants has allowed many high-risk patients to undergo a surgical procedure safely and successfully. However, as patient movement does not occur, the anesthesiologist may be unaware of an inadequate depth of anesthesia.[1]

The incidence of recall depends upon which group of patients is being discussed. It seems evident that severely traumatized patients, whose anesthetic may be minimized due to hemodynamic instability, have a higher incidence of recall than healthy patients undergoing elective surgery.[2] Another group of patients that report awareness more frequently than others are obstetrical patients, whose anesthetic may be required urgently to facilitate surgical care for either the mother or the infant.[3] Four features have been identified by Blacher that may alert physicians to the postoperative syndrome of intraoperative awareness: (1) anxiety and irritability, (2) repetitive nightmares, (3) a preoccupation with death, and (4) a reluctance by patients to discuss their symptoms less they be thought insane.[4,5] Blacher believes that the best treatment for intraoperative awareness is simply telling the patient that it probably did occur. He states that a simple discussion of the matter with the patient invariably serves as a cure. The frequency of intraoperative awareness appears to be decreasing, but the methodology between studies makes this statement necessarily speculative. Table 46-1 highlights a number of studies over the last 30 years suggesting that the current incidence is approximately 2 per 1,000. This seems higher than in my clinical experience. The two patients included in the study by Liu and colleagues were said to remember events shortly after the induction of anesthesia rather than during the operative procedure itself.[10]

Postoperative Confusion

Many investigations of postoperative confusion have concentrated on elderly patients, in whom prolonged mental status changes are thought to be frequent following anesthesia. Nevertheless, the frequency of postoperative confusion remains ill defined. As Table 46-2 highlights, there are physiological, environmental, and psychosocial factors that need to be considered when a patient develops confusion perioperatively.[11] The immediate concern is to identify those reversible causes that may be related to cerebral hypoxia. Although this etiology must be evaluated, it is an infrequent cause of postoperative confusion, especially since the advent of intraopera-

Table 46-1 Incidence of Awareness with Recall and Dreaming in Studies using a Structured Postoperative Interview

Study	Awareness (%)	Dreaming (%)	Sample Size
Hutchinson,[6] 1961	1.2	3.0	656
Harris et al,[7] 1971	1.6	26.0	120
McKenna and Wilton,[8] 1973	1.5	—	200
Wilson et al,[9] 1975	0.8	7.7	490
Liu et al,[10] 1991	0.2	0.9	1000

tive and immediate postoperative pulse oximetry. Many studies have been performed comparing general and regional anesthetic techniques for the elderly, in an effort to clarify the relationship between anesthetic choice and postoperative confusion.[12–15] It seems clear that anesthetic prescription probably affects perioperative mental status in only a small proportion of cases. There are many who believe that regional anesthetic techniques decrease the risk of deterioration in mental status, but there are no definitive randomized studies to support the conclusion.[16] What does seem clear is that patient variables are the most important determinants of postoperative mental status deterioration. Specifically, a history of mental depression and the preoperative use of drugs with an anticholinergic effect (antidepressants) are found to correlate most closely with the development of postoperative confusion.[12] Postoperative hypoxemia also correlates with confusion.[12] Some of the difficulty in analyzing postoperative confusion relates to the postoperative analgesia techniques that are prescribed following the anesthetic. It is likely that development of perioperative confusion will be further clarified once the interaction between intraoperative anesthetic and postoperative analgesia techniques is better understood.

Delayed or Absent Awakening

Failure to awaken promptly after general anesthesia has been attributed by Denlinger to three principal causes: (1) prolonged drug action, (2) metabolic encephalopathy, and (3) cerebral injury (Table 46-3).[17] Once again, the most important approach to managing a patient failing to awaken from anesthesia is to

Table 46-2 Factors in Postoperative Delirium

Physiological factors	Environmental and psychosocial factors
Factors that principally decrease cerebral oxygen delivery Decreased cardiac output (hypotension, arrhythmias, hypovolemia) Cerebrovascular insufficiency (occlusive or embolic) Hypoxemia or anemia Hyperviscosity or coagulopathy Increased intracranial pressure **Factors that principally increase cerebral oxygen demand** Stress Hyperpyrexia Infection Hyperthyroidism Hypercarbia or acidosis Seizures **Factors that alter cerebral metabolism or function** Malignant hypertension Metabolic factors Hepatic or renal dysfunction Ionic imbalances (e.g., of glucose, sodium, calcium, potassium) Endocrine imbalances (hypothyroidism, adrenal insufficiency) Drug toxicity Heavy metals, thiamine, or carbon monoxide Ketamine, neuroleptics, opiates, sedatives, anticholinergics, hallucinogens Withdrawal from alcohol, barbiturates, hallucinogens, opiates, benzodiazepines Neuroleptic malignant syndrome Allergic or idiopathic reaction to administered drugs CNS disease processes Dementia or chronic organic brain syndrome, Parkinson's disease, multiple sclerosis Meningoencephalitis (bacterial, viral, fungal) Cerebral contusion or injury	**Factors that principally affect normal sensory integration** Sleep deprivation Impaired ability to communicate Sensory deprivation, monotony, or physical isolation Impaired mobility **Factors that can increase fear and anxiety** Pain and discomfort Incisional pain Gastric or bladder distention Enviromental factors including noise, frightening activities, etc. Bad previous experience in a similar setting Surgical procedure Position Extremes of age Preoperative vocational or retirement-related problems Feelings of dependence, hopelessness, and loss of dignity **Psychiatric factors** Underlying psychotic or neurotic (especially paranoid) disorder Endogenous depression Postpartum psychosis Conversion reaction Inadequate preoperative defenses and coping mechanisms Morbid or pessimistic expectations Body image distortion

(From Weinger MB, Swerdlow NR, Millar WL: Acute postoperative delirium and extrapyramidal signs in a previously healthy parturient. Anesth Analg 67:291, 1988 with permission.)

exclude reversible and important causes, such as hypoxemia, hypercapnia, hypoglycemia, and electrolyte abnormalities. It seems clear that the most common cause of delayed awakening is prolonged anesthetic effect. Nevertheless, passage of time is the only practical method of evaluating this etiology, although pharmacological antagonists such as naloxone, flumazenil, and physostigmine are often administered in an effort to hasten awakening. For a nonanesthesiologist, the most important issue to understand is what type of anesthetic was administered to the patient who is failing to regain consciousness.

Table 46-3 Differential Diagnosis of Prolonged Recovery and Failure to Regain Consciousness

Prolonged drug action
 Overdose
 Increased central sensitivity
  Age
  Biological variation
  Metabolic effects
 Decreased protein binding
 Delayed anesthetic excretion
 Anesthetic redistribution
 Decreased hepatic metabolism, drug interaction, and
  biotransformation

Metabolic encephalopathy
 Hepatic, renal, endocrine, and neurological disorders
 Hypoxia and hypercapnia
 Acidosis
 Hypoglycemia
 Hyperosmolar syndrome
 Electrolyte imbalance (Na^+, Ca^{++}, Mg^{++}), water in-
  toxication
 Hypothermia and hyperthermia
 Neurotoxic drugs

Neurological injury
 Cerebral ischemia
 Intracranial hemorrhage
 Cerebral embolus (air, calcium, fibrin, fat)
 Hypoxia and cerebral edema

(From Denlinger JK: Prolonged emergence and failure to regain consciousness. p. 369. In Orkin FK, Cooperman LH (eds): Complications in Anesthesiology. JB Lippincott, Philadelphia, 1983 with permission.)

Many of the more recently introduced anesthetics—such as intravenous propofol and the inhalational agent desflurane—are much shorter-acting drugs than previous anesthetics, the barbiturates and older inhalational agents, respectively.

POSTOPERATIVE NEUROLOGICAL DEFICITS

There are few physicians other than anesthesiologists who fully understand modern anesthetic techniques. When sensorimotor neurological deficits appear perioperatively, it is intuitively appealing for many to relate the deficit to some aspect of anesthetic or surgical care. A recent case report highlighting a healthy 47-year-old woman who developed complete transverse myelitis after an uncomplicated general an-

esthetic for a total abdominal hysterectomy and bilateral salpingo-oophorectomy is an excellent example to consider in contemplating the linkage between a perioperative neurological deficit and the anesthetic or surgical procedure.[18] As the authors of this report highlight, had this neurological injury developed after regional anesthesia (i.e., the administration of a local anesthetic to produce nerve block centrally or in the peripheral nervous system), the causal relationship would seem to have been established simply because a needle has been inserted near the neuraxis. In considering the CNS injuries that may result from anesthetic and surgical procedures, one practical way of categorizing the injuries is related to anesthetic type (i.e., whether general or regional anesthesia was used).

Central Nervous System Injury Related to General Anesthesia

The administration of general anesthesia is rarely accompanied by development of an unexpected CNS deficit postoperatively.[19,20] There are specific higher-risk surgical procedures, such as aortic,[21,22] spinal cord,[23,24] or cardiovascular procedures requiring cardiopulmonary bypass,[25] that are the most frequent causes of the injuries associated with general anesthesia.

Those patients who undergo surgical procedures with a significant incidence of spinal cord injury often have somatosensory evoked potentials (SEPs) utilized for intraoperative monitoring of spinal cord function. Function of the anterior spinal cord is difficult to evaluate intraoperatively, however, because SEPs primarily focus on posterior column function.

In addition to specific procedure-associated CNS injuries, both intracerebral and cervical spinal cord injuries have been produced during attempts at tracheal intubation. These injuries occur most often in severely injured patients requiring urgent tracheal intubation, but patients undergoing elective surgery (such as patients with rheumatoid arthritis or Down's syndrome) may also develop cord injury following tracheal intubation.[26] It seems clear from work by Magnaes that pressure on the spinal cord may increase by approximately 15-fold during routine tracheal intubation in patients with cervical spondylosis.[27] Intracranial injuries related to nasal intubation have occurred in patients with basilar skull fractures who

Table 46-4 The Frequency of Cerebrovascular Accidents After General Surgery in Representative Studies

Study	Material	Number of Patients	Incidence of CVA
Knapp et al,[30] 1962	Men over 50 years; R	8,949	34 (0.4%)
Cooperman et al,[31] 1978	Vascular surgery; R	566	4 (0.7%)
Goldman et al,[32] 1979	Elective—patients over 40 years; P	617	1 (0.2%)
Ropper et al,[33] 1982	Elective—patients over 55 years; P	568	0 (0.0%)
Larsen et al,[29] 1988	Elective + acute patients over 40 years; P	2,463	6 (0.2%)

Abbreviations: CVA, cerebrovascular accident; R, retrospective study; P, prospective study.
(From Larsen SF, Zaric D, Boysen G: Postoperative cerebrovascular accidents in general surgery. Acta Anaesthesiol Scand 32:698, 1988 with permission.)

were undergoing nasogastric, and presumably nasotracheal, intubation, in a "blind" fashion.[28] In such patients the tracheal tube may be unintentionally passed into the cranium via the basilar skull fracture. Due to the rarity of this injury, prospective data are not available; but with the introduction of easy-to-use fiberoptic laryngoscopes, it is likely that the incidence of this rare complication is decreasing.

The occurrence of a perioperative stroke may be detected by failure of the patient to awaken promptly following a general anesthetic or by the development of typical unilateral sensorimotor deficits. In general surgical patients (i.e., adults undergoing surgery not involving the heart or carotid arteries), the incidence of strokes in the perioperative period[29] is approximately 2 per 1,000 (Table 46-4). In the most recent study by Larsen and co-workers, 6 strokes developed in 2,463 patients, and they all appeared late in the postoperative period (i.e., 5 to 26 days postoperatively).[29] Thus, none of these strokes seemed directly related to the anesthetic or surgical procedure. Strokes were more frequent after emergency surgery compared with elective operation. Patients developing strokes were older and had a higher incidence of cerebrovascular, cardiac, and peripheral vascular diseases as well as hypertension than did those not developing stroke. Another group that is at higher risk of stroke than other adults are pregnant patients, who appear to be approximately 13 times more likely than nonpregnant women of the same age to develop a perioperative stroke.[34]

Regional Anesthesia and Injury to the Neuraxis

A central deficit following spinal or epidural anesthesia does occur, but less frequently than many physicians believe, and much less frequently than most patients' level of anxiety justifies. Nevertheless, the development of sensorimotor deficits following an epidural or a spinal anesthetic requires prompt evaluation and treatment in the hope of preventing permanent deficits.

It seems probable to many that if a needle catheter is inserted near the neuraxis and weakness or sensory change is found postoperatively, the most likely cause of the neurological deficit is the anesthetic.[35] Marinacci reviewed 542 patients who were believed to have neurological deficits related to spinal anesthesia during the 1950s and found that in only 4 could deficits be attributed to the spinal anesthetic.[36] When the incidence of permanent and profound neurological deficit following spinal and epidural anesthesia is surveyed, it appears that in large series (Table 46-5) the figure ranges from 1 in 5,000 to 1 in 65,000 patients. If milder neurological deficits are the focus, such as symptoms of cauda equine dysfunction, a Swedish survey from 1980 to 1984 suggests that the incidence is approximately 1 in 12,820 patients undergoing spinal epidural or caudal anesthesia.[41] Table 46-6 highlights the different complications in this Swedish series.

Schreiner and colleagues reported on three cases of major paralysis following general anesthesia in an effort to highlight the lack of connection between neurological deficit and anesthetic technique.[42] The differential diagnosis of perioperative paralysis is outlined in Table 46-7; although regional anesthesia is not listed as a specific cause, the table shows the circumstances in which it may be of etiological importance. Patients must be evaluated with urgency. Those CNS deficits that are related to space-occupying lesions, such as epidural hematoma, demand immediate decompression if permanent neurological injury is to be minimized. In a recent literature review

Table 46-5 Incidence of Permanent Neurological Deficit Following Spinal or Epidural Block

Year	Permanent CNS Sequelae	Incidence	Cases	Type of Anesthesia	Reference No.
1969	0	0	10,440	Spinal	37
1971	0	0	78,746	Spinal	38
1973	7	1:4,571	32,000	Epidural	39
1981	3	1:16,666	>50,000	Epidural	40
1981	1	1:65,000	65,000	Spinal	40
1988	39[a]	1:12,820	500,000	Spinal and epidural	41

[a] Milder neurological deficits were included in this series.

of epidural abscesses,[43] the time of recognition of the lesion ranged from 72 hours to 5 months after presentation. In this group of 16 patients, approximately half had complete neurological recovery. Most patients with epidural hematomas will have complete return of neurological function if decompression is carried out within 4 to 8 hours; evaluation must therefore be rapid and imaging studies performed promptly.

Too often, nonanesthesiologists seem to believe that spinal and epidural anesthesia are quite similar and that it matters little what drug or technique is used. If involved in consultation in an urgent situation, it is incumbent upon the physician evaluating the patient to contact the anesthesiologist to find out what type of drug or vasoconstrictor was used and what the anesthesiologist's expectation is for length of motor and sensory block. In those patients at high-

est risk for developing epidural hematomas, it may be prudent to use the shortest-acting agent possible in order to avoid confounding the postoperative diagnosis of lower extremity weakness. Most anecdotal reports of epidural hematomas suggest that back pain is prominent during their development. If a local anesthetic is utilized and the sensory level is more cephalad than the level of the hematoma, however, any back pain produced by the hematoma may be masked.

Delayed Neurological Symptoms Following Spinal and Epidural Anesthesia

In considering the etiology of neurological changes that occur at some time (i.e., days to weeks) after spinal and epidural anesthesia, the clinical conditions

Table 46-6 Complications Attributed to Spinal or Epidural Block by Patients and Legal Advisers and Reported to Swedish Patient Insurance Database during 1980–1984

Complication	Type of Anesthesia			
	Epidural Block	Intrathecal Block	Caudal Block	Block and General Anesthesia in Combination
Deaths	1	—	—	—
Brain damage	1	—	—	1
Symptoms of cauda equina lesions	12	20	2	5
Spinal/epidural hematoma	2	—	—	—
Subdural hematoma	—	2	—	—
Subarachnoid hemorrhage	1	—	—	—
Significant paresis	10	7	—	—
Purulent meningitis	—	2	—	—
Deep local infection	—	1	—	—
Somatosensory disturbances	18	21	—	4
Chronic back pain	7	8	1	2

(From Puke M, Arnér S, Norlander O: Complications of regional anaesthesia, with special reference to epidural, spinal and caudal anaesthesia. p. 1106. In Nunn JF, Utting JE, Brown BR Jr (eds): General Anaesthesia. 5th Ed. Butterworths, London, 1989 with permission.)

Table 46-7 Differential Diagnosis of Perioperative Central Paralysis after Regional Anesthesia

Congenital	Spinal cysts, syringomyelia, arteriovenous abnormalities of cord
New growth	Secondary neoplastic deposits in spinal canal Primary spinal cord tumors Implanted dermoids (long induction period)
Infection	Epidural abscess, intrinsic-metastatic or extrinsic infection[a] Tuberculosis of spine Meningitis[a] Viral encephalomyelitis
Degeneration	Prolapsed intervertebral disc Paget's disease Spinal stenosis
Vascular	Anterior spinal artery syndrome[a] Epidural haematoma[a] Venous infarction from inferior vena caval obstruction Air embolism Post–cardiac arrest or anoxic hypoxia
Trauma	Direct injury to cord, section or cauterization of cord vasculature[a]
Chemical	Unintentional injection of irritant solutions[a] Radiological—angiography of cord with hyperosmolar contrast media

[a] Regional anesthetic may be etiological.
(Modified from Schreiner EJ, Lipson SF, Bromage PR, Camporesi EM: Neurological complications following general anaesthesia. Anaesthesia 38:226 1983 with permission.)

that must be considered include cauda equina syndrome, aseptic meningitis, adhesive arachnoiditis, and epidural abscess (Table 46-8).

Cauda equina syndrome has recently received considerable notoriety with a report by Riegler and colleagues, who described its development following continuous spinal anesthesia techniques in four patients.[44] There was a 1- to 2-week delay in diagnosis in all these patients. The authors speculated that a maldistribution of local anesthetic was responsible for the development of a neurotoxic reaction to the subarachnoid injection of drug. The cauda equina syndrome may develop after either spinal or epidural anesthesia (see Table 46-6). When members of the

Table 46-8 Patterns of Onset and Resolution of Four Neurological Syndromes Found in Rare Patients Following Spinal or Epidural Block

Neurological Syndrome	Onset of Symptoms	Resolution of Symptoms
Aseptic meningitis	<24 hours	<7–10 days
Cauda equina syndrome	Immediate or several days delay	Permanent or temporary
Adhesive arachnoiditis	Weeks after block	Permanent
Epidural abscess	Days to months after block	Permanent or temporary

American Society of Anesthesiologists were surveyed in 1992, it was clear that this syndrome has been noted following both single-shot and continuous spinal anesthesia techniques as well as epidural techniques (Table 46-9). Regarding spinal techniques in which hyperbaric anesthetic drugs are utilized, it has been postulated that the transient neurological change that some patients report as S1 root pain may be due to the anatomical location of the S1 roots.[45] These roots are located most posteriorly when the patient assumes the supine position, and the hyperbaric drug may concentrate in their vicinity, causing mild, transient S1 irritation. There is evidence, both clinical and from bench work,[46] that a number of the commonly used local anesthetics, if given in high enough concentra-

Table 46-9 Partial Listing of Anesthetic Technique and Development of Cauda Equina Syndrome Reported During Retrospective Survey Carried out by American Society of Regional Anesthesia in 1992

Technique	Number
Single-shot spinal	
Lidocaine	3
Tetracaine	5
Continuous spinal	
Lidocaine/small catheter	6[a]
Tetracaine/small catheter	1
Tetracine/large catheter	2
Lidocaine + tetracaine/large catheter	2

[a] One patient also had an opioid added to local anesthetic mixture.
(Personal communication: Gale E. Thompson, 1992.)

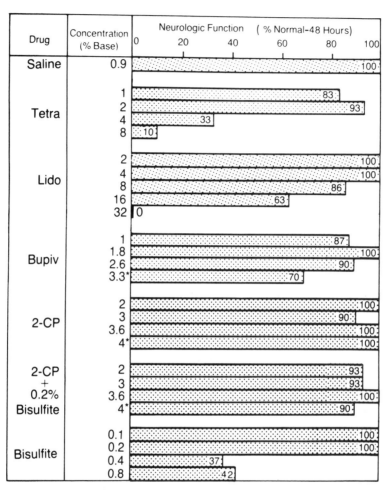

Fig. 46-1. Neurological function in rabbits as a percent of normal, 48 hours after intrathecal injection of varied concentrations of local anesthetics, using a three-component neurological examination (ability to hop, "toe spread," and cutaneous sensation). Each bar represents the cumulative scores of five rabbits. ★ Approximate solubility limit. Tetra, tetracaine; Lido, lidocaine; Bupiv, bupivacaine; 2-CP, 2-chloroprocaine. (From Ready LB, Plumer MH, Haschke RH, et al: Neurotoxicity of intrathecal local anesthetics in rabbits. Anesthesiology 63:364, 1985, with permission.)

tion (i.e., 4 to 8 times usual concentration) may be neurotoxic (Fig. 46-1). If some situation develops preventing free flow of the local anesthetic in the cerebropsinal fluid, a higher-than-usual concentration may be present near neural structures.

Epidural Abscess

Epidural abscesses may develop following instrumentation of the epidural space. In surgical epidural anesthesia, this is exceedingly unusual. For example,

in a review of 43 cases of bacterial spinal epidural abscesses noted from 1981 to 1991 in four Houston teaching hospitals, there were no cases directly related to spinal or epidural anesthesia for surgical care.[47] About one-third of these cases did develop after instrumentation related to the neuraxis (i.e., after laminectomy, discography, or epidural steroid injection for chronic pain therapy). Table 46-10 highlights patient and other predisposing factors that were found in these 43 patients.

With regard to anesthetic-related epidural ab-

Table 46-10 Predisposing Factors Associated With Epidural Abscess in 43 Patients

	Number of Patients
Underlying disease	
Diabetes mellitus	8
Alcoholism	7
Cirrhosis	2
Para/quadriplegia	4
Miscellaneous	4[a]
Total	21[b]
Potential source of infection	
Skin and soft-tissue infection	8
Urinary tract infection	5
Documented sepsis	3
Intravenous drug abuse	4
Vascular catheter	1
Total	17[c]
Abnormality of vertebral spine	
Underlying local	
Degenerative joint disease, spondylosis, remote surgery	10
Precipitating local	
Post-procedure	6[d]
Nonpenetrating trauma	6
Total	22
No predisposing factor	8

[a] One patient each had HIV infection, renal insufficiency, thrombotic thrombocytopenic purpura, and Crohn's disease (+ steroids + total parenteral nutrition).
[b] Four patients each had two diseases.
[c] Includes four para/quadriplegic patients who had both decubitus ulcers and urinary tract infection.
[d] Laminectomy in four, injection of dye into disc space in one, and epidural steroid injection in one. (These patients all had underlying local abnormality as well but are not also included in that category.)
(Modified from Darouiche RO, Hamill RJ, Greenberg SB, et al: Bacterial spinal epidural abscess. Review of 43 cases and literature survey. Medicine (Baltimore) 71:369, 1992 with permission.)

scesses, Ngan Kee and colleagues in New Zealand reported on an epidural abscess developing in an obstetrical patient 5 days after the anesthetic and reviewed 15 other published cases.[43] They noted that most of these epidural abscesses involved catheters that were in place for less than 5 days, and they believed that thoracic catheters may have been associated with higher rates of abscess development than those found in lumbar sites. Symptoms progressed

from (1) spinal ache, to (2) nerve root pain, to (3) weakness, and finally to (4) paralysis. Positive blood cultures correlate with the organisms found in the epidural abscess in 25 percent of patients.[48] The imaging study most useful for the diagnosis of epidural abscess is magnetic resonance imaging.[47,49,50]

Injury of the Peripheral Nervous System

It has long been emphasized that peripheral nerve injuries are related primarily to "malpositioning" of patients intraoperatively.[51] A retrospective study by Parks involving general surgical patients at Colorado General Hospital promoted this concept after a review of approximately 50,000 patients who developed 72 perioperative neuropathies.[52] As noted in Table 46-11, 70 percent of the neuropathies involved the upper extremity, and the majority of the lower extremity lesions involved the peroneal nerve. Parks suggested that the use of muscle relaxants allowed "un-natural" positions to be adopted more easily intraoperatively, thus increasing the incidence of neuropathy. Somewhat similar data were reported by Duhnèr at the Karolinska Institute covering the years 1940 to 1945.[53] When the American Society of Anesthesiologists reviewed closed malpractice claims, approximately 15 percent of anesthesia-related malpractice claims involved neural injury.[54] As shown in

Table 46-11 Incidence of Postoperative Neuropathy in Approximately 50,000 General Surgical Patients From 1957–1969

Nerve	Number of Patients
Upper extremity: 70% of total	
Brachial plexus	28
Radial	11
Ulnar	9
Median	2
Lower extremity: 30% of total	
Peroneal	15
Sciatic	4
Femoral cutaneous	3

(Modified from Parks BJ: Postoperative peripheral neuropathies. Surgery 74:348, 1973, with permission.)

Table 46-12 Claims for Noncerebral Neurological Injury in American Society of Anesthesiologists Closed Claims Database, Circa 1989

Nerve	Number of Claims	Percent of 227
Ulnar	77	34
Brachial plexus	53	23
Lumbosacral nerve root	36	16
Spinal cord	13	6
Sciatic	11	5
Median	9	4
Radial	6	3
Femoral	6	3
Multiple nerves[a]	5	2
Other nerves[a]	11	5
Total	227	100

[a] Includes phrenic, pudendal, perineal, facial, long thoracic and optic nerves, and unspecified other nerves, each with a frequency of less than 1 percent.
(Modified from Kroll DA, Caplan RA, Posner K, et al: Nerve injury associated with anesthesia. Anesthesiology 73:202, 1990 with permission.)

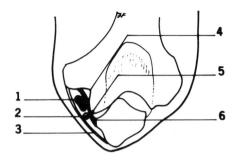

Fig. 46-2. Anatomical disposition of cubital tunnel and its content (right elbow flexed): *(1)* ulnar nerve, *(2)* ulnar collateral artery, *(3)* triangular arcuate ligament, *(4)* medical epicondylar groove, *(5)* medial lip of trochlea, *(6)* medial ligament of elbow. (From Perreault L, Drolet P, Farny J: Ulnar nerve palsy at the elbow after general anaesthesia. Can J Anaesth 39:499, 1992, with permission.)

Table 46-12, most peripheral nerve injuries involved upper extremity nerves, especially the ulnar nerve. In many cases the exact mechanism of specific nerve injuries could not be identified, and very often the standard of care for protection of upper extremity sites had been met in patients developing perioperative neuropathy.[54]

In a community hospital practice, more than 6,500 patients undergoing operation were followed prospectively, and 17 patients developed ulnar nerve palsy (0.26 percent incidence). Of these patients, 50 percent were undergoing orthopedic surgery, and 33 percent were undergoing coronary bypass grafting.[55] The cubital tunnel (Figs. 46-2 and 46-3), through which the ulnar nerve passes on its way from the arm to the forearm, is the region at which most perioperative ulnar neuropathies develop, and either accentuated extension or flexion may be involved in compression injury at this site.[56] A predominance of ulnar nerve injury in males suggests that there is an anatomical predisposition associated with the male body habitus.[56,57]

When patients undergoing coronary artery bypass graft (CABG) procedures are monitored with SEPs perioperatively, up to 6 percent of the patients may

have evidence of nerve deficits at 1 week postoperatively.[58] Almost 70 percent of patients undergoing CABG may show SEP changes during the procedure when surgical retractors are in use. Other data suggest that circulatory compromise of nerve blood flow occurs with approximately 8 percent stretch of a nerve; complete nerve ischemia occurs with approximately

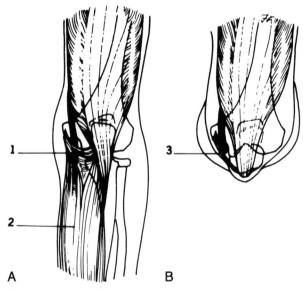

Fig. 46-3. Cubital tunnel in **(A)** extension and **(B)** 90° flexion: *(1)* slack arcuate ligament; *(2)* flexor carpi ulnaris; *(3)* taut arcuate ligament. (From Perreault L, Drolet P, Farny J: Ulnar nerve palsy at the elbow after general anaesthesia. Can J Anaesth 39:499, 1992, with permission.)

15 percent stretch in length of the nerve.[59,60] Small nerve fibers are less vulnerable to compression injuries than large fibers.[61] There is evidence that A fibers rely on aerobic metabolism to a greater extent than C fibers, and this is consistent with the clinical observation that motor function and tactile sensations are lost long before pain sensation is lost in perioperative neuropathies related to nerve ischemia from stretch or positioning.[62]

When a tourniquet is used during surgical procedures, arbitrary decisions are often made about the length of time it can be in place as well as the level of pressure chosen to occlude blood flow to the limb. Many suggest that after 2 hours of tourniquet inflation the blood flow be reestablished for 10 to 15 minutes in order to minimize perioperative neuropathy, although there is little evidence that the 2 hour limit has any physiological basis. There are data to suggest that 3 hours is a "reasonable" upper limit for safe application of automatic tourniquet.[63] In any event, tourniquet time should be individualized and decisions based on patient as well as surgical factors.

When peripheral nerve blocks are utilized during surgical procedures and a neural deficit develops, the regional anesthetic is often suspected to be the cause. Selander and associates have concluded that "when performing a nerve block, paresthesia should be elicited with care, or if possible avoided, in order to reduce the risk of post-block nerve lesions."[64] The data on which these authors based their conclusions involved a study performed in parallel in two different institutions, with one group of anesthesiologists exclusively performing paresthesia-seeking regional block while the other group performed nonparesthesia-seeking blocks. No randomization of patients was possible, and there was no statistically significant different in outcome in the patients in the two groups. In these patients, the incidence of neuropathy following upper extremity operation was 1 in 30 when the patients were prospectively evaluated. This is in contrast to other data from private practitioners utilizing brachial blocks for upper extremity surgery, who identified only 3 neuropathies in 854 surgical patients, giving an incidence of 0.36 percent. This 10-fold difference in incidence in prospective evaluation remains unexplained.[65]

Selander and colleagues have also recommended that epinephrine not be utilized in peripheral nerve blocks. They base this on an in vitro rabbit nerve investigation during experiments in which they determined that epinephrine would "increase the risk of neurologic sequela once the nerve was injured."[66] Again, this recommendation needs perspective because other investigators have reported on large series of patients in whom epinephrine-containing local anesthetics have been used without apparent problem.[67]

Cardiovascular Monitoring

Anesthesiologists are often involved in insertion of central venous catheters for cardiovascular monitoring perioperatively. There are numerous reports of neural injury related to central venous cannulation.[68–72] As shown in Figure 46-4, there are numerous neural structures that can be injured during cardiovascular cannulation. It may be that significant injury is more likely with cannulation in patients already anesthetized, because they are unable to describe pain or paresthesias during the insertion.

PERIOPERATIVE SEIZURES

There are numerous reasons for patients to exhibit changes in mental status as well as abnormal motor activity in the perioperative period. These include simple "faints" during intravenous cannulation and seizures induced by inhalational agents or related to systemic toxicity of local anesthetics. Simple faints or symptoms compatible with vagal reactions during intravenous cannulation may occur in up to 17 percent of ambulatory patients below the age of 40 years.[73] It can sometimes be difficult to determine if an idiopathic seizure has occurred preoperatively or whether the patient has experienced a simple faint. It does seem clear that younger patients are more likely to experience these perioperative events and that the greater the number of attempts to place the intravenous cannula, the higher the incidence of such events.[73] Perioperative seizure may also be psychogenic in origin.[74] Although psychogenic seizures are exceedingly rare in this setting, there are patients in whom this diagnosis needs to be considered.

As shown in Table 46-13, a number of anesthetic drugs are proconvulsants, with a significant number of these also being identified as anticonvulsants depending upon dose and rate and route of administration.[75] In considering inhalational anesthetic agents, the drug that has been linked to seizure activity most

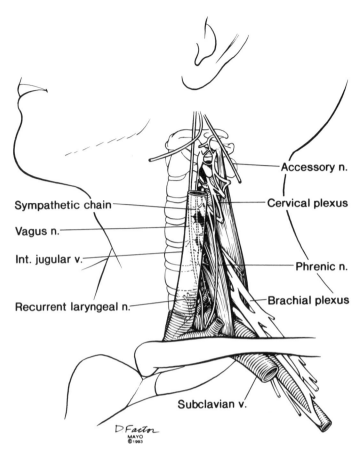

Fig. 46-4. Left oblique view of nerves in the neck and supraclavicular fossa that may be injected during both internal jugular and subclavian central venous techniques. (With permission of Mayo Foundation.)

often is enflurane. The tendency of enflurane to produce seizure or electroencephalographic (EEG) spike activity is influenced by both its concentration and $PaCO_2$.[76,77] During normocarbic states, EEG spiking is maximal at inspired enflurane concentrations of 2 to 3 percent. Although infrequent, patients have evidenced abnormal twitching of individual muscle groups, and even tonic-clonic activity, during enflurane anesthesia.[78,79] When patients are hyperventilated, the frequency, magnitude, and synchrony of the EEG abnormalities increase for a given level of inspired enflurane concentration.[80]

Intravenous anesthetic agents have also been implicated in perioperative seizures. Meperidine neurotoxicity, manifesting itself clinically as shakiness, tremors, myoclonus, and seizures, is the most frequent cause of opioid-induced seizure activity.[81] The accentuation of abnormal motor movements is attributed to its N-demethylated metabolite, normeperidine.[82] Myoclonus generally precedes seizures in this setting, and both will resolve with discontinuation of the meperidine administration.[83,84] Other opioids have also been implicated, but it is clear that meperidine is the one most frequently involved.

An anesthetic drug, ketamine, that is frequently used in trauma patients undergoing surgery has been linked to the activation of epileptogenic foci in patients with known seizure disorders.[85,86] It appears that doses larger than 2 mg/kg of intravenous ketamine are needed to influence the incidence of seizures in these patients.

In addition to frank seizure activity, some general anesthetics may produce abnormal neurological findings persisting for 40 to 60 minutes after cessation of

Table 46-13 Anesthetics and Analgesics Reported to Cause or Suppress Seizure Activity in Humans

Proconvulsants	Anticonvulsants
Nitrous oxide	Halothane
Halothane	Enflurane
Enflurane	Isoflurane
Isoflurane	Thiopental
Morphine	Etomidate
Meperidine	Diazepam
Fentanyl	Lorazepam
Sufentanil	Midazolam
Methohexital	Ketamine
Etomidate	Propofol
Diazepam	Local anesthetics
Ketamine	
Propofol	
Local anesthetics	

(Modified from Modica PA, Tempelhoff R, White PF: Pro- and anticonvulsant effects of anesthetics (Part I). Anesth Analg 70:303, 1990 with permission.)

the anesthetic. In a prospective study, it was found that transient hyperreflexia and transient Babinski responses can be found for up to nearly 1 hour in patients undergoing enflurane–nitrous oxide anesthetics as well at a lesser frequency with halothane–nitrous oxide anesthetics, and even less frequently with nitrous oxide–narcotic anesthetics. These neurological findings were most marked when patients remained unresponsive[87] and persisted for longer periods in selected patients. In one healthy, 38-year-old woman undergoing arthroscopy of the knee, myoclonic jerks involving multiple muscle groups (except those innervated by cranial nerves) occurred over the first 48 hours postoperatively; neurological findings after this period were normal.[88]

Seizures Induced by Regional Anesthetics

A variety of CNS effects may occur when local anesthetics are used for regional block. These effects, which include restlessness, dizziness, nervousness, apprehension, perioral numbness, nausea, tinnitus, a metallic taste, and visual and auditory hallucinations, may precede the development of seizures.[89,90] Objective signs that may precede the occurrence of such seizures include euphoria, dysarthria, nystagmus,

sweating, vomiting, pugnaciousness, loquaciousness, and an inability to respond to reason.[91] Stimulation of the CNS by local anesthetics may occur from intravascular injection or rapid systemic uptake from the regional block site. The initial excitatory phase is due to selective inhibition of inhibitory neurons in the cerebral cortex, thus allowing facilitatory neurons to discharge in an unopposed fashion.[92] Once blood levels of local anesthetic increase to a certain point, both inhibitory and facilitatory pathways are inhibited, leading to CNS depression. Many of the toxic, systemic premonitory signs and symptoms mimic the presentation of temporal lobe epilepsy.[93] A number of investigators have published on the incidence of seizures secondary to the clinical use of local anesthetics, and those centers most experienced in the use of regional block report a figure of approximately 0.1 to 0.33 percent.[91] As seen in Figure 46-4, there is a predictable pattern of peak serum levels depending on the site of regional block, but most systemic toxic reactions are from direct intravascular injection of local anesthetic rather than rapid systemic uptake.[94]

If signs of CNS toxicity or frank convulsions occur, a number of steps must be followed if adverse outcomes are to be prevented. With seizures induced by local anesthetics, hypoxemia, hypercarbia, and acidosis rapidly develop, and symptomatic treatment of the toxicity must involve treatment of these factors. Oxygen should be given via a bag and mask; tracheal intubation is not mandated unless ventilation is ineffective.[95] The next step in therapy remains controversial, involving administration of either succinylcholine or anticonvulsant drugs. Succinylcholine is often recommended because seizures are usually short-lived, and pharmacologically induced muscle relaxation facilitates ventilation and decreases the magnitude of metabolic acidosis. Nevertheless, it does not prevent seizures or decrease cerebral metabolism. In addition to the toxic CNS effects, cardiovascular collapse and arrhythmias may also result from a systemic reaction to local anesthetics. It was originally postulated that toxicity (both CNS and cardiovascular) of local anesthetics parallels anesthetic potency; current information suggests that the potent and long-acting agents bupivacaine and etidocaine are proportionately more cardiotoxic than their anesthetic potency predicts.[96–99] This relative increase in cardiotoxicity appears to result from more potent effects on the sodium channels by long-acting drugs. Thus, if a seizure and cardiovascular collapse occur due to a local anesthetic, resuscitation from the cardiovascular collapse may require 1 to 2 hours of resuscitation because it may take an extended period of time to "wash out" the long-acting local anesthetic from the myocardium during the low-flow states that are produced with cardiopulmonary resuscitation.

PERIOPERATIVE HEADACHE

Chronic headaches occur in 10 percent of the general population. Since approximately 25 million people undergo surgery in the United States each year, a considerable number of these patients will have chronic headaches. When headaches occur perioperatively, it is important to determine whether they correspond to prior headache patterns or represent an entirely new symptom complex.

Table 46-14 lists some causes of perioperative headache. The perioperative period is stressful, and tension and stress-related headaches may be exacerbated during this time. A significant percentage of the population consume caffeine-containing drinks on a regular basis, and the perioperative period often limits their caffeine intake. One review of 287 patients undergoing minor elective procedures during general anesthesia suggests that headaches related to caffeine withdrawal may begin 24 hours after cessation of caffeine intake and last for up to 5 or 6 days.[100,101] The use of nitrous oxide in patients with inflamed sinuses or air-containing middle-ear spaces may result in sinus or ear block—and thus headache—related to increases in pressure from nitrous oxide equilibrating with the air contained in these structures; the diagnosis is often made by exclusion. General anesthesia may be accomplished by the use of masks that produce pressure upon terminal trigeminal nerve branches, such as the supraorbital or infraorbital nerve; long-standing headaches may then result from compression neuropathy.[102] Other causes of headache are intracranial mass lesions that may occur in patients at any time; these need to be distinguished from benign causes of new-onset headache in the perioperative period. The complicating feature is that spinal anesthesia (with dural puncture) may be associated with headaches in from 1 to 5 percent of patients, depending upon gender, age, and type of needle utilized for the anesthetic. Headaches are more common in women than men and in the young than the elderly; they are also more common when a large needle is used for dural puncture, especially when the bevel of the needle results in dural fibers being cut transversely.[103,104] It should be emphasized that an arbitrary period of recumbency after spinal anesthesia has not been found to decrease the incidence of such headache,[105] and some data indicate that early ambulation may actually decrease the incidence of postdural puncture headache.[106,107] It is estimated that approximately 50 percent of these headaches do not interfere with daily activities, whereas 35 percent are severe enough that daily activities are affected and the patient must rest intermittently[108] and 15 percent are severe enough that patients cannot attend to normal daily functions.[105] The headache related to dural puncture (decreased intracranial pressure) is probably related to traction on trigeminal, glossopharyngeal, or vagal fibers.[109,110]

It is important that patients with headaches related to dural puncture are referred when appropriate for definitive treatment by epidural blood patch. The safety and efficacy of this approach (greater than 90 percent efficacy in relieving headache per epidural patch) have been well documented.[111–113] If an epidural blood patch is not successful in relieving headaches ascribed to dural puncture, further questioning should ascertain whether the headaches have the "postural hallmarks" of being dramatically relieved in the supine position. In selected patients, it may be clinically appropriate to administer a second epidural blood patch without further diagnostic evaluation, but if a headache does not respond to this second patch, further consultation should be undertaken to exclude underlying structural lesions.

Table 46-14 Potential Causes of Headaches in Perioperative Period

Preexisting chronic headache
Myofascial headache
Caffeine-withdrawal headache
Closed air-space headache (e.g., N₂O effects on inflamed sinus or middle ear)
Compression neuropathy of terminal trigeminal nerve branch (e.g., supraorbital)
Structural intracranial cause
Postdural puncture headaches
Infectious cause

PERIOPERATIVE VISUAL CHANGES

Visual changes can occur after both general and regional anesthesia. Following general anesthesia, visual changes can occur from pressure being transmitted to the globe of the eye to a level that occludes retinal artery flow while the patient is anesthetized. This can evidence itself as postoperative blindness. Dural puncture may be followed by cranial nerve palsies, the most frequent involving the abducens nerve (bilaterally on rare occasion).[114,115] The most commonly proposed explanation for the predominance of sixth cranial nerve changes following development of low CSF pressure is that the nerve's relatively long intracranial course renders it susceptible to both pressure and stretch. Others promote the concept that the abducens palsy is due to increased venous pressure in the cavernous sinus, as the nerve courses through this site. It is true that venous dilatation occurs in the cranium in compensation for a decrease in CSF pressure, which may occur following spinal anesthesia. When larger spinal needles were used and the incidence of headache after dural puncture was 11 percent, the incidence of ocular difficulties was 0.4 percent.[116] Thus, with the incidence of such headache now being between 1 and 4 percent with the use of small-gauge conical-tipped spinal needles, the incidence of abducens palsy following spinal anesthesia is probably between 0.1 and 0.2 percent.

Pupillary changes may follow epidural and spinal anesthesia. There are numerous case reports of Horner's syndrome developing following epidural block.[117–120] These are related to local anesthetic effects upon sympathetic nerves, but the level of the central block surprisingly does not correlate with the development of Horner's syndrome, at least in the parturient.[119] Among 150 parturients undergoing epidural anesthesia for cesarean section or labor, the frequency of Horner's syndrome was 1.3 percent for labor analgesia and 4 percent when the epidural block was used for cesarean section.[119] The Horner's syndrome occurs only for the duration of local anesthetic block, and accordingly should not confound postoperative pupillary assessment except in rare circumstances. Horner's syndrome has also been noted with other regional techniques, and continuous brachial catheter local anesthetic infusions have also been associated with its development.[121] Thus, if postoperative pupillary changes complicate neurological diagnosis,

attempts should be made to determine whether a regional block technique may have produced a Horner's syndrome. Trigeminal nerve changes have also been found following epidural anesthesia and analgesia.[118] Once again, this is an unpredictable accompaniment of the epidural local anesthetic, and time will clarify its relationship to the regional block.

One final ocular alteration that may confuse neurological diagnosis in the immediate perioperative period is the pupillary dilatation that follows "total" spinal anesthesia. This most frequently occurs when an intended epidural anesthetic injection is unintentionally administered into the subarachnoid space. This produces unconsciousness as well as markedly dilated pupils. Symptomatic support of the circulation and ventilation is necessary, and time ($1\frac{1}{2}$ to 4 hours) will help clarify the patient's clinical course. It is important to understand that these pupillary changes are a predictable accompaniment of unintentional "total spinal" anesthesia and diagnosticians should not be misled by the unusual appearance of the widely dilated pupils.

PERIOPERATIVE AUDITORY CHANGES

Similar to visual changes following anesthesia, auditory changes can accompany either general or regional anesthetic techniques. Auditory changes following general anesthesia are most commonly related to "ear block" that develops following the use of nitrous oxide in patients susceptible to eustachian tube obstruction.[122] The ear block that develops is similar to that found after ear blocks associated with air travel. Symptoms resolve with time, although nasopharyngeal decongestants may also help reduce mucosal edema to the point that the ear block can be cleared.

Patients who have undergone spinal anesthesia and who are not experiencing headaches from dural puncture may show a decrease in ability to hear if sensitive testing is used. Fog and colleagues studied 28 patients receiving spinal anesthesia for transurethral resection of the prostate and found that as larger needles were utilized, more marked (perhaps subclinical) changes in auditory function were found.[123] None of their patients had headaches; thus, decreased hearing may occur in isolation. The decrease in hearing may relate to a decrease in cerebrospinal fluid volume that reduces the perilymphatic pressure; as the endolymphatic pressure equilibrates slowly compared to the perilymphatic pressure, an endolymphatic hydrops results. Thus, a decrease in intralabyrinthine pressure probably causes the transient hearing loss. Hyperacusis may also develop following spinal anesthesia.[124]

EVALUATION OF PERIOPERATIVE NEUROLOGICAL COMPLICATIONS

When neurological changes occur postoperatively, many physicians and nurses assume that "something" must have gone wrong intraoperatively. As the American Society of Anesthesiologists closed-claims analysis of perioperative injury indicates, many perioperative neuropathies have no ready explanation, and our inability to define the etiology of such nerve injuries probably reflects an incomplete understanding of perioperative nerve function. The first step in managing a perioperative neurological change is to obtain a comprehensive evaluation by a skilled neurologist. It is also important to minimize speculation in the medical record and simply document facts. Time is often helpful in identifying the etiology of neurological changes and early electrodiagnostic studies should also be considered, when appropriate, since preexisting nerve damage may evidence itself in the perioperative period.[125] This is important because abnormal spontaneous activity is unlikely to appear in affected muscles until $2\frac{1}{2}$ to 3 weeks following nerve injury; the presence of such activity in the immediate postoperative period suggests that the nerve lesion existed before operation.

Time is of the essence if a major injury of the neuraxis is being evaluated. If concern is present about an epidural hematoma following either epidural or spinal anesthesia, imaging studies should be obtained immediately, since recovery of neural function is related to length of time of neural compression by the hematoma.

Finally, if perioperative neural changes are present, both the surgeons and anesthesiologists involved in the patient's care should be included in consultation. Contemporary surgical and anesthetic care has become complex, and these individuals may have unique insights into predictable perioperative changes that nonsurgical physicians or anesthesiologists would find difficult to uncover.

REFERENCES

1. Blacher RS: Editorial views: awareness during surgery. Anesthesiology 61:1, 1984
2. Bogetz MS, Katz JA: Recall of surgery for major trauma. Anesthesiology 61:6, 1984
3. Bogod DG, Orton JK, Yau HM, Oh TE: Detecting awareness during general anaesthetic caesarean section: an evaluation of two methods. Anaesthesia 45:279, 1990
4. Blacher RS: On awakening paralyzed during surgery: a syndrome of traumatic neurosis. JAMA 234:67, 1975
5. Howard JF: Incidents of auditory perception during anaesthesia with traumatic sequelae. Med J Aust 146:44, 1987
6. Hutchinson R: Awareness during surgery: a study of its incidence. Br J Anaesth 33:463, 1961
7. Harris TJB, Brice DD, Hetherington RR, Utting JE: Dreaming associated with anaesthesia: the influence of morphine premedication and two volatile adjuvants. Br J Anaesth 43:172, 1971
8. McKenna T, Wilton TNP: Awareness during endotracheal intubation. Anaesthesia 28:599, 1973
9. Wilson SL, Vaughan RW, Stephen CR: Awareness, dreams and hallucinations associated with general anesthesia. Anesth Analg 54:609, 1975
10. Liu WHD, Thorp TAS, Graham SG, Aitkenhead AR: Incidence of awareness with recall during general anaesthesia. Anaesthesia 46:435, 1991
11. Weinger MB, Swerdlow NR, Millar WL: Acute postoperative delirium and extrapyramidal signs in a previously healthy parturient. Anesth Analg 67:291, 1988
12. Berggren D, Gustafson Y, Eriksson B, et al: Postoperative confusion after anesthesia in elderly patients with femoral neck fractures. Anesth Analg 66:497, 1987
13. Nielson WR, Gelb AW, Casey JE, et al: Long-term cognitive and social sequelae of general versus regional anesthesia during arthroplasty in the elderly. Anesthesiology 73:1103, 1990
14. Chung FF, Chung A, Meier RH, et al: Comparison of perioperative mental function after general anaesthesia and spinal anaesthesia with intravenous sedation. Can J Anaesth 36:382, 1989
15. Asbjorn J, Jakobsen BW, Pilegaard HK, et al: Mental function in elderly men after surgery during epidural analgesia. Acta Anaesthesiol Scand 33:369, 1989
16. Brown DL: Anesthetic choice. p. 202. In Brown DL

(ed): Risk and Outcome in Anesthesia. 2nd Ed. JB Lippincott, Philadelphia, 1992

17. Denlinger JK: Prolonged emergence and failure to regain consciousness. p. 369. In Orkin FK, Cooperman LH (eds): Complications in Anesthesiology. JB Lippincott, Philadelphia, 1983

18. Gutowski NJ, Davies AO: Transverse myelitis following general anaesthesia. Anaesthesia 48:44, 1993

19. Newberry JM: Paraplegia following general anaesthesia. Anaesthesia 32:78, 1977

20. Kitching A, Taylor S: A postoperative neurological problem. Anaesthesia 44:695, 1989

21. Grace RR, Mattox KL: Anterior spinal artery syndrome following abdominal aortic aneurysmectomy. Arch Surg 112:813, 1977

22. Gloviczki P, Cross SA, Stanson AW, et al: Ischemic injury to the spinal cord or lumbosacral plexus after aorto-iliac reconstruction. Am J Surg 162:131, 1991

23. Kalkman CJ, Been HD, Ongerboer de Visser BW: Intraoperative monitoring of spinal cord function. Acta Orthop Scand 64:114, 1993

24. Purnell RJ: Scoliosis correction and epidural analgesia. Anaesthesia 37:1115, 1982

25. Wong DHW: Perioperative stroke: Part II. Cardiac surgery and cardiogenic embolic stroke. Can J Anaesth 38:471, 1991

26. Hastings RH, Marks JD: Airway management for trauma patients with potential cervical spine injuries. Anesth Analg 73:471, 1991

27. Magnaes B: Clinical recording of pressure on the spinal cord and cauda equina. J Neurosurg 57:64, 1982

28. Seebacher J, Rozik D, Mathieu A: Inadvertent intracranial introduction of a nasogastric tube, a complication of severe maxillofacial trauma. Anesthesiology 42:100, 1975

29. Larsen SF, Zaric D, Boysen G: Postoperative cerebrovascular accidents in general surgery. Acta Anaesthesiol Scand 32:698, 1988

30. Knapp RB, Topkins MJ, Artusio JF: The cerebrovascular accident and coronary occlusion in anesthesia. AMA 182:332, 1962

31. Cooperman M, Pflug B, Martin EW, Evans WE: Cardiovascular risk factors in patients with peripheral vascular disease. Surgery 84:505, 1978

32. Goldman I, Caldera DI, Southwick FS, et al: Cardiac risk factors and complications in noncardiac surgery. Medicine (Baltimore) 57:357, 1978

33. Ropper AH, Wechsler IR, Wilson IS: Carotid bruit and the risk of stroke in elective surgery. N Engl J Med 307:1388, 1982

34. Fox MW, Harms RW, Davis DH: Selected neurologic complications of pregnancy. Mayo Clin Proc 65:1595, 1990

35. Wildsmith JAW, Lee JA: Neurological sequelae of spinal anaesthesia. Br J Anaesth 63:505, 1989

36. Marinacci AA: Neurological aspects of complications of spinal anesthesia. Bull Los Angeles Neurol Soc 25: 170, 1960

37. Phillips OC, Ebner H, Nelson AT, Black MH: Neurologic complications following spinal anesthesia with lidocaine: a prospective review of 10,440 cases. Anesthesiology 30:284, 1969

38. Noble AB, Murray JG: A review of the complications of spinal anaesthesia with experiences in Canadian teaching hospitals from 1959 to 1969. Can Anaesth Soc J 18:5, 1971

39. Editorial: Neurological complications following epidural blockade. Anaesthesia 29:527, 1974

40. Kane RE: Neurologic deficits following epidural or spinal anesthesia. Anesth Analg 60:150, 1981

41. Puke M, Arnér S, Norlander O: Complications of regional anaesthesia, with special reference to epidural, spinal and caudal anaesthesia. p. 1106. In Nunn JF, Utting JE, Brown BR Jr (eds): General Anaesthesia. 5th Ed. Butterworths, London, 1989

42. Schreiner EJ, Lipson SF, Bromage PR, Camporesi EM: Neurological complications following general anaesthesia. Anaesthesia 38:226, 1983

43. Ngan Kee WD, Jones MR, Thomas P, Worth RJ: Extradural abscess complicating extradural anaesthesia for caesarean section. Br J Anaesth 69:647, 1992

44. Rigler ML, Drasner K, Krejcie TC, et al: Cauda equina syndrome after continuous spinal anesthesia. Anesth Analg 72:275, 1991

45. Schneider M, Ettlin T, Kaufmann M, et al: Transient neurologic toxicity after hyperbaric subarachnoid anesthesia with 5% lidocaine. Anesth Analg 76:1154, 1993

46. Ready LB, Plumer MH, Haschke RH, et al: Neurotoxicity of intrathecal local anesthetics in rabbits. Anesthesiology 63:364, 1985

47. Darouiche RO, Hamill RJ, Greenberg SB, et al: Bacterial spinal epidural abscess: review of 43 cases and literature survey. Medicine (Baltimore) 71:369, 1992

48. Verner EF, Musher DM: Spinal epidural abscess. Med Clin North Am 69:375, 1985

49. Nordström O, Sandin R: Delayed presentation of an extradural abscess in a patient with alcohol abuse. Br J Anaesth 70:368, 1993

50. Mamourian AC, Dickman CA, Drayer BP, Sonntag KH: Spinal epidural abscess: three cases following spinal epidural injection demonstrated with magnetic resonance imaging. Anesthesiology 78:204, 1993

51. Navalgund AA, Jahr JS, Gieraerts R, et al: Multiple nerve palsies after anesthesia and surgery. Anesth Analg 67:1002, 1988

52. Parks BJ: Postoperative peripheral neuropathies. Surgery 74:348, 1973
53. Dhunèr KG: Nerve injuries following operations: a survey of cases occurring during a six-year period. Anesthesiology 11:289, 1950
54. Kroll DA, Caplan RA, Posner K, et al: Nerve injury associated with anesthesia. Anesthesiology 73:202, 1990
55. Alvine FG, Schurrer ME: Postoperative ulnar-nerve palsy: are there predisposing factors? J Bone Joint Surg [Am] 69:255, 1987
56. Perreault L, Drolet P, Farny J: Ulnar nerve palsy at the elbow after general anaesthesia. Can J Anaesth 39:499, 1992
57. Cameron MGP, Stewart OJ: Ulnar nerve injury associated with anaesthesia. Can Anaesth Soc J 22:253, 1975
58. Hickey C, Gugino LD, Aglio LS, et al: Intraoperative somatosensory evoked potential monitoring predicts peripheral nerve injury during cardiac surgery. Anesthesiology 78:29, 1993
59. Lundborg G, Rydevik B: Effects of stretching the tibial nerve of the rabbit. J Bone Joine Surg [Br] 55:390, 1973
60. Lundborg G: Structure and function of the intraneural microvessels as related to trauma, edema formation, and nerve function. J Bone Joint Surg [Am] 57:938, 1975
61. Sunderland S: Nerves and Nerve Injuries. 2nd Ed. Churchill Livingstone, Edinburgh, 1978
62. Fink BR, Cairns AM: A bioenergetic basis for peripheral nerve fiber dissociation. Pain 12:307, 1982
63. Klenerman L, Biswas M, Hulands GH, Rhodes AM: Systemic and local effects of the application of a tourniquet. J Bone Joint Surg [Br] 62:385, 1980
64. Selander D, Edshage S, Wolff T: Paresthesiae or no paresthesiae? Nerve lesions after axillary blocks. Acta Anaesthesiol Scand 23:27, 1979
65. Winchell SW, Wolfe R: The incidence of neuropathy following upper extremity nerve blocks. Reg Anaesth 10:12, 1985
66. Selander D, Brattsand R, Lundborg G, et al: Local anesthetics: importance of mode of application, concentration and adrenaline for the appearance of nerve lesions. Acta Anaesthiol Scand 23:127, 1979
67. Moore DC, Bridenbaugh LD, Thompson GE, et al: Bupivacaine: a review of 11,080 cases. Anesth Analg 57:42, 1978
68. Paschall RM, Mandel S: Brachial plexus injury from percutaneous cannulation of the internal jugular vein. Ann Emerg Med 12:58, 1983
69. Hoffman JC: Permanent paralysis of the accessory nerve after cannulation of the internal jugular vein. Anesthesiology 58:583, 1983
70. Frasquet FJ, Belda FJ: Permanent paralysis of C-5 after cannulation of the internal jugular vein. Anesthesiology 54:528, 1981
71. Drachler DH, Koepke GH, Weg JG: Phrenic nerve injury from subclavian vein catheterization. JAMA 236:2880, 1976
72. Vaswani S, Garvin L, Matuschak GM: Postganglionic Horner's syndrome after insertion of a pulmonary artery catheter through the internal jugular vein. Crit Care Med 19:1215, 1991
73. Pavlin DJ, Links S, Rapp SE, et al: Vaso-vagal reactions in an ambulatory surgery center. Anesth Analg 76:931, 1993
74. Parry T, Nirsch N: Psychogenic seizures after general anaesthesia. Anaesthesia 47:534, 1992
75. Modica PA, Tempelhoff R, White PF: Pro- and anti-convulsant effects of anesthetics (Part I). Anesth Analg 70:303, 1990
76. Lebowitz MH, Blitt CD, Dillon JB: Enflurane-induced central nervous system excitation and its relation to carbon dioxide tension. Anesth Analg 51:355, 1972
77. Neigh JL, Garman JK, Harp JR: The electroencephalographic pattern during anesthesia with ethrane: effects of depth anesthesia, $PaCO_2$, and nitrous oxide. Anesthesiology 35:482, 1971
78. Virtue RW, Lund LO, Phelps M Jr, et al: Difluoromethyl 1,1,2-trifluoro-2 chlorethyl ether as an anesthetic agent: results with dogs, and a preliminary note on observations in man. Can Anaesth Soc J 13:233, 1966
79. Botty C, Brown B, Stanley V, Stephan CR: Clinical experiences with compound 347, a halogenated anesthetic agent. Anesth Analg 47:477, 1968
80. Lebowitz MH, Blitt CD, Dillon JB: Enflurane-induced central nervous system excitation and its relation to carbon dioxide tension. Anesth Analg 51:355, 1972
81. Goetting MG, Thirman MJ: Neurotoxicity of meperidine. Ann Emerg Med 14:1007, 1985
82. Szeto HH, Inturrisi CE, Houde R, et al: Accumulation of normeperidine, an active metabolite of meperidine in patients with renal failure and cancer. Ann Intern Med 86:738, 1977
83. Kaiko RF, Foley KM, Grabinski PY: Central nervous system excitatory effects of meperidine in cancer patients. Ann Neurol 13:180, 1983
84. Hochman MS: Meperidine-associated myoclonus and seizures in long-term hemodialysis patients. Ann Neurol 14:593, 1983
85. Ferrer-Allado T, Brechner VL, Dymond A, et al: Ketamine-induced electroconvulsive phenomena in the human limbic and thalamic regions. Anesthesiology 38:333, 1973

86. Bennett DR, Madsen JA, Jordan WS, Wiser WC: Ketamine anesthesia in brain-damaged epileptics: electroencephalographic and clinical observations. Neurology 23:449, 1973
87. Rosenberg H, Clofine R, Bialik O: Neurologic changes during awakening from anesthesia. Anesthesiology 54:125, 1981
88. Ng ATH: Prolonged myoclonic contractions after enflurane anaesthesia—a case report. Can Anaesth Soc J 27:502, 1980
89. DeJong RH: Local anesthetic seizures. Anesthesiology 30:5, 1969
90. Moore DC: Local anesthetic drugs: tissue and systemic toxicity. Acta Anaesthesiol Scand 4:283, 1981
91. Garfield JM, Gugino L: Effects of local anesthetics on electrical activity of the brain. p. 254. In Strichartz GR (ed): Local Anesthetics. Handbook of Experimental Pharmacology. Vol 81. Springer-Verlag, Berlin, 1987
92. Tanaka K, Yamasaki M: Blocking of cortical inhibitory synapses by intravenous lidocaine. Nature 209:207, 1966
93. DeJong RH: Central nervous system effects. p. 84. In: Local Anesthetics. 2nd Ed. Charles C Thomas, Springfield, IL, 1977
94. Covino BG, Vassallo HG: Local Anesthetics. Grune & Stratton, Orlando, FL, 1976
95. Moore DC, Bridenbaugh LD: Oxygen: the antidote for systemic toxic reactions from local anesthetic drugs. JAMA 174:842, 1960
96. Munson ES, Tucker WK, Ausinsch B, Malagodi MH: Etidocaine, bupivacaine, and lidocaine seizure thresholds in monkeys. Anesthesiology 42:471, 1975
97. Block A, Covino B: Effect of local anesthetic agents on cardiac conduction and contractility. Reg Anaesth 6:55, 1981
98. deJong RH, Ronfeld RA, DeRosa RA: Cardiovascular effects of convulsant and supraconvulsant doses of amide local anesthetics. Anesth Analg 61:3, 1982
99. Kotelko DM, Shnider SM, Daily PA, et al: Bupivacaine-induced cardiac arrhythmias in sheep. Anesthesiology 60:10, 1984
100. Griffiths RR, Bigelow GE, Liebson IA: Human coffee drinking: reinforcing and physical dependence producing effects of caffeine. J Pharmacol Exp Ther 230:416, 1986
101. Fennelly M, Galletly DC, Purdie GI: Is caffeine withdrawal the mechanism of postoperative headache? Anesth Analg 72:449, 1991
102. Klein DS, Schmidt RE Jr: Chronic headache resulting from postoperative supraorbital neuralgia. Anesth Analg 73:490, 1991
103. Brown DL: Spinal, epidural, and caudal anesthesia. p. 1505. In Miller RD (ed): Anesthesia. 4th Ed. Churchill Livingstone, New York, 1994
104. Denny N, Masters R, Pearson D, et al: Postdural puncture headache after continuous spinal anesthesia. Anesth Analg 66:791, 1987
105. Jones RJ: The role of recumbency in the prevention and treatment of postspinal headache. Anesth Analg 53:788, 1974
106. Thornberry EA, Thomas TA: Posture and post-spinal headache: a controlled trial in 80 obstetric patients. Br J Anaesth 60:195, 1988
107. Baumgarten RK: Should caffeine become the firstline treatment for postdural puncture headache? Anesth Analg 66:913, 1987
108. Murphy TM, O'Keeffe D: Complications of spinal, epidural, and caudal anesthesia. p. 38. In Benumof JL, Saidman LJ (eds): Anesthesia and Perioperative Complications. Mosby-Year Book, St Louis, 1992
109. Atkinson RS, Lee JA: Spinal anaesthesia and day care surgery. Anaesthesia 40:1059, 1985
110. Bonica JJ: The Management of Pain. Lea & Febiger, Philadelphia, 1953
111. DiGiovanni AJ, Dunbar BS: Epidural injections of autologous blood for post-lumbar puncture headache. Anesth Analg 49:268, 1970
112. DiGiovanni AJ, Galbert MW, Wahle WM: Epidural injection of autologous blood for post-lumbar puncture headache: II. Additional clinical experiences and laboratory investigation. Anesth Analg 51:226, 1972
113. Ostheimer GW, Palahniuk RJ, Shnider SM: Epidural blood patch for post-lumbar-puncture headache. Anesthesiology 41:307, 1974
114. Vandam LD: Symptoms following lumbar puncture may be related to decreased cerebrospinal fluid pressure and/or venous dilation. Anesthesiology 76:321, 1992
115. Dripps RD, Vandam LD: Hazards of lumbar puncture. JAMA 147:1118, 1951
116. Vandam LD, Dripps RD: Long-term follow-up of patients who received 10,098 spinal anesthetics: syndrome of decreased intracranial pressure (headache and ocular and auditory difficulties). JAMA 161:586, 1956
117. Evans JM, Gauci CA, Watkins G: Horner's syndrome as a complication of lumbar epidural block. Anaesthesia 30:774, 1975
118. Sprung J, Haddox JD, Maitra-D'Cruze AM: Horner's syndrome and trigeminal nerve palsy following epidural anaesthesia for obstetrics. Can J Anaesth 38:767, 1991
119. Clayton KC: The incidence of Horner's syndrome during lumbar extradural for elective Caesarean section and provision of analgesia during labour. Anaesthesia 38:583, 1983
120. Tabatabia M, Mazloomdoost M, Kirimli B: Bilateral

Horner's syndrome and hoarseness complicating lumbar epidural anesthesia. Reg Anaesth 14:10, 1989

121. Lennon RL, Gammel S: Horner's syndrome associated with brachial plexus anesthesia using an axillary catheter. Anesth Analg 74:311, 1992

122. Hochermann M, Reimer A: Hearing loss after general anaesthesia: a case report and review of literature. J Laryngol Otol 101:1079, 1987

123. Wang LP, Fog J, Bove M: Transient hearing loss following spinal anaesthesia. Anaesthesia 42:1258, 1987

124. Gordon AG: Hyperacusis after spinal anesthesia. Anesth Analg 73:502, 1991

125. Bralliear F: Electromyography: its use and misuse in peripheral nerve injuries. Orthop Clin North Am 12: 229, 1981

47

Neurological Complications of Thermal and Electrical Burns

Marc D. Winkelman

The United States has the highest incidence of burn injuries in the world.[1] Each year 2.5 million people seek medical attention for a burn: 100,000 are hospitalized and 12,000 die. Among Americans, 1 in 70 is hospitalized for a burn at some time. Only automobile accidents cause more accidental deaths. That serious neurological complications can follow a burn has been known since the nineteenth century.[2] The complications of thermal burns differ considerably from those of electrical burns, and they will therefore be treated separately. Electricity is encountered in two forms—lightning and man-made current. The neurological effects of these two forms are much the same and they will be considered together.

THERMAL BURNS

In this chapter the term *thermal burn* refers to a burn caused by contact with flames, hot metal, or hot water or by the flash of radiant heat from an explosion. The extent of a burn is expressed as the percentage of the total body surface area involved. The depth is gauged as *full thickness* when the dermal appendages are destroyed and *partial thickness* when they are spared. Patients with extensive, full-thickness burns are more likely to die and to suffer neurological complications than those with less severe burns. These are the ones who require the intensive care of a burns unit and with whom this chapter is concerned.

Neurological diagnosis is difficult, because extensively burned patients are hard to examine. Their burned eyelids are swollen shut; their faces are swollen and move poorly. It is hard for the patient to move swollen and bandaged limbs and for the doctor to assess their tone and reflexes. Under these circumstances a detailed neurological examination cannot be performed; hence, focal signs may escape detection. Peripheral neuropathies may go unnoticed, and symptoms of focal, structural cerebral lesions may be attributed to metabolic or toxic encephalopathies. The limitations of the neurological examination must be appreciated; cerebral imaging, examination of the cerebrospinal fluid (CSF), and nerve conduction studies may be required more often than with other types of patient.

Central Nervous System Complications

Because the brain and spinal cord lie deep in the body, they are not injured by the heat of flash or flame. Most victims are neurologically normal immediately after their burn. Those who are not have usually suffered head trauma or anoxic encephalopathy caused by carbon monoxide poisoning or cardiopulmonary arrest due to smoke inhalation.[3,4] Most disorders of the central nervous system (CNS) arise later, during hospitalization, not as a direct consequence of the burn but as a result of some other complication: a systemic infection, disseminated intravascular coagulation (DIC), hypotension, or metabolic abnormalities.[4] Most of these bear a characteristic temporal relationship to the burn, and this may provide a valuable clue to diagnosis.

The overall frequency of CNS complications was 5, 6.6, and 14 percent in reports of three large clinical series of patients with burns.[2,5,6] Metabolic encephalopathies, cerebrovascular lesions, and CNS infections are the major types of complication and occur in that order of frequency.[2,4,6] Adults and children are equally affected.[4] Many patients have more than one CNS complication.[4] There are several reasons for this. First, a systemic infection can affect the brain by direct invasion, by an intermediary mechanism of disease (such as DIC or septic shock), and by leading to systemic metabolic abnormalities. A patient may thus be affected in more than one way. Second, patients may have several independent CNS complications, infectious and noninfectious, metabolic and structural. And third, elderly patients may have coexisting cerebral diseases in addition to complications of their burn. Often a single diagnosis is an adequate but incomplete explanation for a cerebral symptom. For example, a patient with an atherosclerotic cerebral infarct or a metabolic encephalopathy may also have a CNS infection. For that reason, diagnostic evaluations have to be extensive, and the response to treatment may be hard to interpret.

METABOLIC ENCEPHALOPATHIES

Burned patients are liable to a variety of metabolic derangements, many of which cause encephalopathy. Anoxemia, hyponatremia, serum hyperosmolality, and uremia, treated in detail below, are the major ones, but there are others. Hypernatremia, due to insensible water loss through the burn wound, is the most common electrolyte abnormality.[7] A burn causes a marked increase in metabolic rate.[8] There is increased production of glucose, and this may lead to hyperglycemia. Insulin resistance and intravenous hyperalimentation are other causes of hyperglycemia in this setting. Hypoglycemia is usually associated with overwhelming systemic infection.[8] Sequestration of calcium in burned skin may cause hypocalcemia,[8] which in turn can lead to seizures and confusion.[2] Hypomagnesemia, with muscle cramps or hallucinations, occurs occasionally.[9]

Anoxic Encephalopathy

A severe burn is attended by the rapid and massive accumulation of edema in the burned and unburned skin ("burn edema").[7] Intravascular volume depletion and hypotension follow, leading to ischemic tissue damage. This state is called "burn shock." Anoxic encephalopathy is the most common neurological complication of a burn, and burn shock is its most common cause in the first few days after a burn.[4,6] After the first week, septic shock becomes the major cause.[4]

Hyponatremic Encephalopathy

Fluid resuscitation for burn shock can result in dilutional hyponatremia, the commonest cause of early confusion and seizures in burned patients, especially children.[5,6,10] Later in the hospital course, hyponatremia is most often associated with systemic infection.[7]

Uremic and Hepatic Encephalopathy

Uremic encephalopathy is most often due to acute renal failure, which in turn is caused by acute tubular necrosis or DIC.[4] The causes of acute tubular necrosis are much the same as those of anoxic encephalopathy. Patients with chronic liver disease can develop hepatic encephalopathy during convalescence from a burn.[4] Precipitating causes include a systemic infection, narcotic analgesics, hypovolemia, and bleeding from a Curling ulcer of the stomach.[8]

Central Pontine Myelinolysis

Burned patients, like alcoholics, are especially susceptible to central pontine myelinolysis. In a retrospective autopsy study, this disorder was found 25 times more often in burned patients than in the general population.[11] It was associated with a prolonged period (at least 3 days) of extreme serum hyperosmolality (at least 360 mOsm/kg), but not with hyponatremia or the correction of hyponatremia. An infection was a major factor in the genesis of the hypernatremia, azotemia, and hyperglycemia that contributed to hyperosmolality. Central pontine myelinolysis was a late complication; it began after the second hospital week in most cases, and never in the first week. The lesions were often small and asymptomatic. Even when the lesion is large, diagnosis is difficult. Metabolic coma may hide the motor signs of central pontine myelinolysis, or they may be missed as a result of the difficulties of neurological examination described earlier. Late development of quadriplegia, pseudobulbar palsy, the locked-in syndrome,[12] or coma unresponsive to correction of serum hyperosmolality suggests the diagnosis. Magnetic resonance imaging (MRI) can confirm it.

CENTRAL NERVOUS SYSTEM INFECTIONS

Infection is the most common cause of morbidity and mortality in burned patients because they are immunocompromised.[8] The burn destroys the skin barrier to microorganisms, and the devitalized eschar of the burn wound makes an ideal culture medium. Inhalation of smoke injures the local defense mechanisms of the tracheobronchial tree. Intravenous and urethral catheters and endotracheal tubes promote intraluminal ingress of organisms. In addition, both the cellular and humoral immune systems suffer complex impairments.[8]

CNS infection is the result of hematogenous spread of microorganisms from a source outside the nervous system.[4] Burn-wound infection, pneumonia, suppurative thrombophlebitis, and infective endocarditis are the most common sources; *Candida* species, *Pseudomonas aeruginosa,* and *Staphylococcus aureus* the commonest pathogens.[4] Most CNS infections arise in the second and third weeks after the burn; they occur only rarely in the first week and never in the first few days.[4,6] This delay occurs because the CNS is a secondary rather than a primary target of invading microorganisms. Serious infections, including those of the CNS, are a complication of extensive, deep burns—full-thickness burns that involve at least 30 percent of total body surface area.[13]

The foregoing facts may help in neurological diagnosis. A week or more after extensive burns, a patient with a systemic infection is at high risk for developing a CNS infection. In contrast, patients without a known site of infection, positive blood cultures, or systemic signs of infection, and those in the first week after their burn are unlikely to have an infection of the CNS.[4] Similarly, a patient with a burn involving less than 30 percent of total body surface is unlikely to have a CNS infection, even if there is a systemic source.[4] Such patients have less suppression of systemic immune function than those with a major burn and are better able to contain a local infection.[14,15]

Pseudomonas Aeruginosa

Bacterial meningitis develops in 1 to 4 percent of extensively burned patients.[4,6] *P. aeruginosa* is the most common etiology.[4,6] Moreover, in a recent autopsy series, meningitis developed in 15 percent of burned patients who had a systemic *Pseudomonas* infection.[4] A burn-wound infection was the most common source. Blood cultures were positive. This is the only CNS infection that has been reported to begin in the first week after a burn.[4,6] Other gram-negative enteric organisms, such as *Escherichia coli,* but no gram-positive bacteria or fungi have been reported to cause meningitis during the first week in burned patients.[4] Gram-negative rods have not caused other patterns of intracranial infection, such as brain abscess.[4,6]

The diagnosis of meningitis may be difficult, because the burn surgeon will probably have initiated treatment of the primary infection by the time of neurological consultation. This may eliminate the headache and stiff neck of meningitis without eradicating the infection. In some patients only confusion, stupor, or coma is found. Hence, a metabolic or septic[16] encephalopathy may be diagnosed. However, a gram-negative infection outside the CNS, especially one due to *P. aeruginosa,* occurring in the context of an extensive burn that is more than 1 week old, should prompt lumbar puncture. Evidence of meningitis, perhaps partially treated, may be found. If cultures and smears of CSF are negative, antibiotics effective against *P. aeruginosa* meningitis should be prescribed, because that is the likeliest pathogen. Many burned patients have more than one systemic infection.[4] Adequate coverage should also be provided for meningitis due to all other microorganisms grown in systemic culture, even *S. aureus* and *Candida* species, because they too can cause meningitis, although rarely.[17–19]

If the skin of the back is burned, it may be impossible to do a lumbar or cervical puncture. It is in the most extensively burned patients that this will be the case. Unfortunately, these are the patients who are most likely to develop meningitis. If such a patient has a systemic infection due to a gram-negative rod, particularly *P. aeruginosa,* an antibiotic with good CSF penetration should be prescribed so that meningitis, although impossible to document, does not go untreated.

Candida Species

The frequency of *Candida* infections is increasing among burned patients—a result of the use of broad-spectrum antibiotics for bacterial infections, longer survival of older and more extensively burned patients, and the use of central intravenous catheters and intravenous hyperalimentation.[4,8,20,21] Half the patients with invasive candidiasis have cerebral involvement at autopsy.[4,22] This most often takes the form of disseminated microabscesses; large abscesses, meningitis, and mycotic aneurysms are much less common.[4,18,19,22,23] Patients infected with *Candida* have almost always had at least one previous treated bacterial infection.[4,20] This is reflected in the relatively late onset of cerebral candidiasis–usually late in the second hospital week and never in the first week.[4]

The premortem diagnosis of disseminated cerebral microabscesses is notoriously difficult.[19,24] They typically produce drowsiness, confusion, stupor, or coma. Fixed, focal cerebral signs and focal seizures are unusual. The CSF remains normal. Often less than 3 mm in diameter, the abscesses are too small to be detected by computed tomographic (CT) scanning but do appear as small, bright foci on T_2-weighted MRI[25] and probably enhance with contrast. Thus, it may require MRI to distinguish multiple cerebral microabscesses from a metabolic or septic[16] encephalopathy.

The diagnosis of cerebral candidiasis may be difficult because the CSF is usually normal, and the diagnosis therefore requires the demonstration of infection outside the CNS.[26,27] The primary site of infection may not be apparent, and metastatic foci of infection may be hidden in the myocardium or kidney.[22] Pneumonia, which can be seen on a chest radiograph, is not common.[19] Positive urine, sputum, fecal, and wound cultures can mean colonization rather than infection. Blood cultures are often nega-

tive. Without candidemia, the diagnosis is usually made only after death.[4,27] There is currently no single test that identifies every case of invasive candidiasis. The diagnosis begins with a high index of suspicion in patients with unexplained systemic signs of infection; deep, extensive burns; and a prior bacterial infection. Blood cultures, biopsy of the burn wound (the most frequent site of infection), serological tests, and repeated clinical evaluation for involvement of the skin and eye may help with diagnosis.[8,26] In a recent autopsy study, almost half the burned patients with candidemia had cerebral involvement.[4] Therefore, a positive blood culture should prompt systemic antifungal therapy.

Staphylococcus aureus

This organism spreads to the brain by way of endocarditis in burned patients. Intracranial spread from other sites has not been reported in this group of patients and seldom occurs in other groups.[28] The sequence of events is burn-wound infection, bacteremia, infection of a heart valve, and thence embolism of infected material to the brain, with infarction or microabscess formation.[4] Other cerebral complications of endocarditis, such as meningitis and mycotic aneurysm, may presumably occur in burned patients but have not been reported. Intracranial staphylococcal infections begin relatively late—in most cases more than 10 days after the burn—presumably because the brain is infected after the burn wound and endocardium.[4] The frequency of CNS infection with this organism has declined in the past 25 years, because better antibiotic treatment of burn-wound infections prevents the development of endocarditis.[4] The diagnosis of staphylococcal cerebral microabscesses is as hard as that of abscesses due to *Candida,* but the identification of *S. aureus* as the cause is easier, because blood cultures are positive.[4] This diagnosis should prompt a search for endocarditis. Cerebral infarction and *S. aureus* infections are discussed below. A full discussion of the neurological complications of infective endocarditis can be found in Chapter 6.

CEREBROVASCULAR DISEASE

Cerebrovascular lesions typically present as a stroke (i.e., with the sudden onset of a focal neurological deficit), but in burned patients this is often not the case, for three reasons. First, there is the difficulty of neurological examination, described earlier. Second, multiple cerebral complications, the general debility of patients, and the use of narcotic analgesics may obscure the acute onset of cerebrovascular accidents. And third, cerebral infarcts and hemorrhages are often multiple and bilateral in patients with burns.[4] This can turn an asymmetrical neurological picture into one of relative symmetry. Thus, an infarct or hemorrhage may not present as a stroke but in the guise of a metabolic encephalopathy. Therefore, any unexplained cerebral symptom or sign should lead to MRI or CT scan of the brain.

Septic Infarction

Cerebral infarction is more often due to complications of the burn than to atherosclerosis, atrial fibrillation, and other premorbid conditions unrelated to the burn.[4] Each major infection discussed earlier can cause septic occlusion of cerebral blood vessels, with infarction of brain. Meningeal infection can extend into the walls of arteries and veins that run through the subarachnoid space, leading to inflammation and occlusion of affected vessels. This is a common complication of *P. aeruginosa* meningitis and can occur in the first week of disease.[4] Embolism of infected material with occlusion of cerebral arteries is a classic complication of infective endocarditis.[29] Only one burned patient with cerebral aspergillosis has been reported, but this fungus is a common cause of systemic infection in patients with burns.[4,8] *Aspergillus* and *Candida* species invade and occlude blood vessels at their portal of entry.[18,22] Thence the fungi spread through the bloodstream, causing inflammation and thrombosis of blood vessels in distant organs.[18] In the brain, infarction is the major pathological effect of *Aspergillus*.[30,31] *Candida* causes mainly microabscesses; infarcts are fewer.[4,23]

Radiological features do not serve to distinguish septic infarcts from those caused by premorbid vascular disease, but certain clinical points are helpful.[4] Septic infarction may affect patients of any age and does not occur during the first week after a burn. Patients have extensive burns and systemic signs of sepsis. Focal neurological deficits do not improve. Infarction caused by premorbid conditions, however, may occur at any point during the hospital course, regardless of the severity of the burn or the presence of systemic infection; patients are usually elderly,

have conventional risk factors for cerebral infarction, and may have had previous cerebral infarcts or coronary or peripheral vascular disease.

When a burned patient has a cerebral infarct and a septic cause seems likely, it is important to determine the mechanism involved—meningitis, endocarditis, or fungal invasion of a vessel—and the responsible microorganism. If the patient was neurologically normal before cerebral infarction, meningitis is unlikely. Physical signs of meningitis, infective endocarditis, or disseminated candidiasis may be found. The mechanism and etiology of septic infarcts correlate with one another. Cerebral infarction in a patient with *S. aureus* bacteremia suggests the presence of endocarditis. A systemic *P. aeruginosa* infection suggests that meningitis due to that organism underlies the infarct. If meningitis is found, it is the likely mechanism of infarction, and *P. aeruginosa* is the probable cause. Thus, examination of the CSF should always be considered. If evidence for neither meningitis nor endocarditis is found, fungal invasion of cerebral blood vessels should be suspected. Cerebral infarction in a patient with invasive candidiasis or aspergillosis suggests that spread to the brain has occurred. Infarction in a patient with systemic signs of sepsis but negative cultures suggests the possibility of infection with *Candida* or *Aspergillus*.

Disseminated Intravascular Coagulation

DIC is a well-known complication of burns.[32] Bacteremia or fungemia with or without hypotension is the cause.[4,32–34] Fibrin thrombi occlude capillaries and small arteries and veins throughout the body.[35] In the brain, disseminated hemorrhagic infarcts and microinfarcts are the result.[4,36] These may or may not produce focal cerebral signs.[36,37] DIC, like disseminated microabscesses, may simulate a metabolic or toxic encephalopathy. CT scanning will detect the larger infarcts. The microinfarcts may appear as small, bright foci on T_2-weighted MRI, and their hemorrhagic character helps to distinguish them from microabscesses. DIC is unlikely to be the cause of early neurological symptoms. It usually begins later than the first week after a burn and never before the fourth day.[4,32,33]

The diagnosis of DIC can be difficult in a patient with burns. A bleeding diathesis may be absent.[4,38]

None of the elements of the typical coagulation profile is specific for DIC. Consumption of platelets and clotting factors in the burn wound itself may result in thrombocytopenia and prolonged clotting times.[39] Bacteremia per se and certain drugs may cause a thrombocytopenia. Nutritional deficiency and antibiotic-induced alteration of the flora of the gut may deplete the body of vitamin K and consequently of vitamin K–dependent clotting factors. Moreover, titers of fibrin degradation products are elevated early in all patients with burns.[32] Helpful findings in the diagnosis of DIC are a sudden decline in the plasma concentration of fibrinogen (sometimes from an elevated level into the normal range) and a positive biopsy of unburned skin.[32,36] Heparin has not proved helpful in treating DIC in patients with burns.[33,39–41] Treatment of the infection and hypotension underlying the DIC is therefore the recommended approach.

Border-Zone Infarction
Cerebral infarction in the arterial border zone occurs early as a complication of burn shock, and later in the hospital course with septic shock.[4] The location of the infarcts on CT scan and the clinical setting point to the diagnosis.[42]

Venous Infarction
Cerebral infarction caused by occlusion of dural sinuses and large and small cerebral veins has been reported.[43] Meningitis was not associated, but DIC or intravascular volume depletion may have been responsible. Magnetic resonance venography or simple MRI can document occlusion of large venous channels.

Nonbacterial thrombotic endocarditis and deep vein thrombosis with paradoxical embolism are possible but unreported causes of cerebral infarction in burned patients.

Intracranial Hemorrhage
Intracranial hemorrhage occurs much less often than cerebral infarction.[4] Lobar hemorrhage, subarachnoid hemorrhage, and widespread parenchymal petechiae ("brain purpura") have been reported.[4,44] A bleeding diathesis related to DIC or thrombocytopenia, resulting, in turn, from bacteremia, is the cause.[4] Cerebral hematomas and hemorrhagic infarcts may be adjacent to each other in patients with DIC.[4]

Peripheral Nervous System Complications

MONONEUROPATHIES

In a prospective study, 26 percent of hospitalized patients with burns developed a mononeuropathy.[45] The figure would be more meaningful and useful if electrical burns had been distinguished from thermal burns. Heat may cause coagulation necrosis of nerve trunks involved in a thermal burn.[46] Superficial nerves, such as the ulnar nerve at the elbow and the sensory branch of the radial nerve in the hand, are more liable than deep nerves to thermal damage. Such injuries cannot be treated surgically. Many limbs burned deeply enough to involve nerves ultimately require amputation. Blunt trauma from a fall is another cause of nerve injury during a burn and may affect nerves in unburned or burned limbs.

Reference was made earlier to burn edema, the massive swelling that follows a serious burn. When the indistensible eschar of a burn surrounds a limb, the hydrostatic pressure within may be sufficient to shut off the flow of blood. Thus, in a circumferential burn, a tourniquet effect may lead to ischemic necrosis of distal muscle and nerve.[46] This is the major nerve injury that presents in the first day or so after a burn. Loss of peripheral pulses or Doppler-audible flow in the distal vascular arches and digital arteries of a limb is an indication for immediate escharotomy.[46] In very deep burns, edema develops below the skin and subcutaneous fat, inside the osteofascial compartments that envelop muscle and nerve.[47] Blood flow may be obstructed to such an extent that ischemic necrosis of tissue results, but the deep fascia, not the burn eschar, is responsible, and fasciotomy, not escharotomy, is the appropriate treatment. These compartment syndromes are rare in thermal burns but common in electrical burns; they are discussed further on p. 923.

Most nerve injuries occur as complications of treatment.[46,48] Nerves can be lacerated during escharotomy if the procedure is not done carefully. The ulnar nerve at the elbow, the peroneal nerve as it winds around the head of the fibula, and the sensory branch of the radial nerve are especially vulnerable because they are superficial. The same nerves are liable to compression by tight dressings or malpositioning. Improper positioning of the patient can lead to a variety of other traction or compression neuropathies, which are described in standard textbooks, as are also the neurological consequences of misplaced intramuscular injections.

Heterotopic bone formation can cause a mononeuropathy late in the hospital course.[46] The ossification is usually periarticular. The elbow is the joint affected most often: the ulnar nerve may be compressed. Treatment consists of decompression and transposition of the nerve. The cause of heterotopic bone formation is unknown. Recurrence is common.

Marquez and associates recently reported several patients with multiple mononeuropathies in burned and unburned limbs which could not be attributed to the mechanisms of injury discussed above.[49] They speculated that a circulating neurotoxin derived from burned tissue, or thrombosis of the vasa nervorum, was responsible, but they had no supportive evidence.

POLYNEUROPATHY

Two prospective studies of polyneuropathy in severely burned patients have been published.[45,50] Generalized polyneuropathy was said to develop in 15 and 29 percent of patients, but the available data do not allow distinction between the syndromes of polyneuropathy and multiple mononeuropathy.[49]

Helm and co-workers studied 74 patients with burns who developed neuromuscular symptoms during hospitalization.[48] Among these patients, 52 percent were found to have a polyneuropathy. Weakness in the distal muscles of the extremities was the major neurological sign; sensation was normal in most patients. Polyneuropathy was more prevalent among patients with extensive rather than minor burns. Most patients recovered after their burns had healed, and the cause of the neuropathy was not determined.

In recent years a polyneuropathy associated with sepsis and multiple organ failure has been described and designated *critical illness polyneuropathy*.[51] The polyneuropathy, as well as the acute pulmonary, cardiac, hepatic, and renal failure that attend it, has been attributed to sepsis[52]; the clinical features of the disorder are discussed in Chapter 44. Two burned patients with this polyneuropathy have been reported.[49,53] A

third patient, with pneumonia, gram-negative bacteremia, adult respiratory distress syndrome, and acute renal failure is probably another example.[54] Sepsis and multiple organ failure are prevalent among seriously burned patients. It is likely that critical illness polyneuropathy is also prevalent among them and accounts for many of the cases of polyneuropathy in the study of Helm and associates.[48]

ELECTRICITY AND LIGHTNING

Serious electrical injuries are much less common than serious thermal burns. They make up only 3 to 7 percent of admissions to burn units.[55–57] Electricity causes three types of burn. High-voltage current often jumps a gap between its source and a victim. This "arc" can attain a temperature of 4,000°C and cause a severe burn, identical to a flash burn. Ignition of the victim's clothing may cause a flame burn. These thermal burns make the victim of electrical trauma liable to the neurological complications discussed earlier. The third type of burn is produced only when the victim becomes part of an electrical circuit, and current flows through the body on its way to ground. Burns mark the points of entry and exit. These "contact burns" are much deeper than flash and flame burns and often involve nerves. Organs between the entry and exit wounds, including nerves, spinal cord, and brain, conduct the current and suffer its direct effects, as is discussed below. Of importance also are two indirect mechanisms of neurological damage—cardiac arrest and trauma. Passage of an electrical current through the heart causes asystole or ventricular fibrillation, with syncope or anoxic encephalopathy occurring as a result. An electrical shock often causes the victim to fall, and this may result in head injury. Moreover, emanating from the axis of a lightning channel is a cylindrical shock wave of expanded, displaced, and returning air.[58,59] This, like the force of an explosion, may cause trauma directly or by throwing the victim to the ground.

The Effect of Electricity on the Nervous System

Man-made electricity or lightning can injure any structure in the peripheral or central nervous system through which it passes. The degree of damage is directly related to the amount of current.[56,60,61] A small current produces only a derangement of function; clinical manifestations are transient. Larger currents cause structural damage that may be reversible or irreversible; neurological deficits may be permanent or may resolve with time.

The quantity of current varies directly with its voltage and the duration of its passage and inversely with the resistance of the skin, which it must breach before it reaches neural structures.[62] An arbitrary division is made at 1,000 V between high-tension and low-tension electrical current. Household current is 110 or 220 V; high-tension wires carry current of several thousand volts. Alternating current causes muscle tetany, and this may prolong an electrical shock by, for example, causing the victim's hand to grip the contact. Thus, alternating current is more dangerous than direct current. A high-tension circuit will often be completed by arcing before contact is made. A massive contraction of axial and limb musculature ensues, and this can throw the victim to safety. Thus, low-tension alternating current may cause more damage to the nervous system than high-tension current.

Electricity takes the shortest pathway through the body to ground.[63] Identifying the entry and exit wounds is important, because the current injures only structures between them. When current travels from hand to hand, the nerves and muscles in the arms, the brachial plexus, and the cervical spinal cord lie in its pathway; the brain does not. A current pathway from head to feet includes the brain, the entire spinal cord, and the nerves and muscles in the legs.[63]

A bolt of lightning can exceed 200 million V, which is far larger than the highest-tension wire of man-made electricity. A direct stroke need not, however, be fatal, for two reasons. First, the duration of the electrical discharge is short, approximately one-thousandth of a second.[64] And second, most of the current flows over the surface of the body, not through it.[62] Lightning, considerably attenuated after striking a tree, can "splash or spray" onto a nearby person. Moreover, once lightning has struck the ground, the weakened current can run up one leg and down the other leg of a bystander (stride potential). Such phenomena probably explain how one bolt of lightning can injure many people gathered together.[65,66] In addition to entrance and exit burns, lightning figures may be present on the skin. These are arborescent red lines that indicate the path of lightning over the surface of the body.[67] As they fade, they may leave pigmentary changes in their place. Their presence on a victim's back may help account for a myelopathy after a stroke of lightning.

As current flows through the resistance of tissue, electrical energy is turned into heat (Joule effect). This is the cause of many electrical lesions of the nervous system, but some may be due to nonthermal effects. Three arguments support this idea. First, the peripheral nerve and brain of animals can be damaged experimentally by electrical current without an appreciable rise in temperature.[56,61,68] Second, some victims of electrical trauma are left with a neuropathy or myelopathy but no electrical burn.[56,67] And third, neurological symptoms may begin a considerable time after an electrical shock. Lee and co-workers have suggested electrical breakdown of cell membranes—electroporation—as a nonthermal mechanism of tissue injury.[69] Perforations in the plasma membrane large enough to alter the electrochemical balance between the intracellular and extracellular compartments would result in a cellular metabolic disorder that might cause the eventual rather than the immediate death of a cell.

Clinical Syndromes

TRANSIENT LOSS OF CONSCIOUSNESS

Lightning or man-made electrical current passing through the head causes immediate loss of consciousness. Patients awaken in minutes to hours. Agitation, confusion, retrograde amnesia, headache, and even a convulsive seizure often follow, but complete recovery is to be expected.[56,65,67,70] Some of these patients may have suffered cerebral concussion caused by a fall or the cylindrical pressure wave of the lightning bolt, but electrically induced seizure activity or inhibition of cerebral function is the likely pathophysiological mechanism in most cases. Brief loss of consciousness often follows passage of lightning or high-tension current outside the head. Transient cardiac asystole, ventilatory failure caused by tetanic contraction or paralysis of the thoracic musculature, acute intracranial hypertension, and loops of current that find their way into the head are possible mechanisms.[56,67,68,71] Loss of consciousness is sometimes delayed rather than immediate, or it may occur immediately and then again somewhat later.[67,71,72] A similar phenomenon can follow mild head trauma and probably represents vasodepressor syncope.[12] Patients who lose consciousness for more than a few hours or develop focal cerebral signs do not fall into this category; anoxic encephalopathy or a serious head injury should be suspected.

TRANSIENT PARALYSIS

Immediate and transitory sensorimotor paralysis is the neurological syndrome that typically results from the passage of lightning. Charcot coined the term *keraunoparalysis* (lightning paralysis). Symptoms and signs correspond to the sites in the peripheral nervous system, spinal cord, and occasionally the brain through which the lightning has passed. Paraplegia is most common, but quadriplegia, monoplegia, bibrachial paralysis, hemiplegia, ventilatory paralysis, cranial neuropathies, and aphasia have been reported.[67,73,74] Signs of involvement of the autonomic nervous system are common and include pupillary abnormalities and loss of peripheral pulses, as well as coldness and pallor or cyanosis of the weak limbs. Prolonged ventilatory paralysis and binocular mydriasis can simulate death. This accounts for the clinical dictum that some patients who "die" after lightning stroke can "live again" if given cardiopulmonary resuscitation for long enough.[75] Lightning paralysis lasts for minutes to hours and seldom for more than a day, although minor paresthesias may linger for weeks.[65,72,76] High-tension man-made electrical current can produce the same syndrome.[56,57,71,77]

INJURY TO PERIPHERAL AND CRANIAL NERVES

High-Tension Current

A focal peripheral neuropathy is the most common serious neurological complication of a high-tension electrical burn.[57] In three large series of patients, the frequency was 13, 22, and 34 percent.[55,57,78] The lesion is usually located in the midst of a contact burn but may be elsewhere in the pathway of the current.[56] It consists of *coagulation necrosis* and is caused by heat.[79] Its severity parallels that of thermal damage to surrounding muscle, blood vessels, and tendons.[56] Symptoms begin immediately. If the nerve sheath and vasculature are intact, some function may re-

turn.[57] Permanent damage to peripheral nerves does not extend beyond the area of local tissue damage.[56] Care must be taken to distinguish this disorder from neuropathy resulting from a fall, compartment syndrome, or acute entrapment. A delay between the electrical shock and onset of the neuropathy, worsening of a neuropathy after the shock, or the presence of severe pain suggests a compartment syndrome or entrapment neuropathy.

High-tension electrical current, including lightning,[80] causes coagulation necrosis of muscle in its pathway. Swelling begins within hours. Massively swollen muscles, encased in compartments of fascia and bone, may compress adjacent blood vessels. The result is ischemic necrosis of tissue, including muscle and nerve. The diagnosis of this *compartment syndrome* can be difficult. Unburned skin may cover a vast extent of burned muscle ("hidden muscle damage"). The swollen muscle is confined by fascia, over which the skin may be loose, not taut. Distal pulses may be present. Myoglobinuria and acute renal failure are clues to the diagnosis. More than one peripheral nerve may be affected—the median, musculocutaneous, and radial nerves in the anterior arm and the median and ulnar nerves in the anterior forearm.[81] Wick catheters (to measure the pressure inside a muscle compartment) and nerve conduction studies may help in diagnosis,[81,82] but most surgeons perform emergency fasciotomy upon clinical indication.

Swelling of burned tissue can cause *acute entrapment* of nerves that pass through tight anatomical canals. The median nerve may be affected in the carpal tunnel or between the heads of the pronator teres muscle (pronator syndrome), the ulnar nerve in Guyon's canal or the cubital tunnel, and the posterior interosseous nerve in the arcade of Frohse. Most often the clinical problem is that of a deep burn of the anterior wrist associated with a median or ulnar neuropathy. Many surgeons routinely open the carpal tunnel and Guyon's canal in such circumstances.[46,83] Patients who respond presumably have a compressive neuropathy; those who do not may have a primary electrical neuropathy.

Scar tissue in healing electrical burns may grow around or within a peripheral nerve, thereby impeding regeneration or causing a new mononeuropathy late in the hospital course. This happens most often with deep burns of the wrist.[56] The responsible scar is usually apparent on the surface of the body.

Low-Tension Current

Peripheral nerve injury by low-tension current is uncommon but can occur when the resistance of the skin is lowered by water or when contact is prolonged.[77,84,85] Electrical burns, if present, are minor, and the neural lesion lies far from where current entered the body. For example, current flow from hand to hand may cause a brachial plexopathy.[85] Usually only one nerve is involved. Pain in the limb begins with the shock. Muscle weakness appears instantly or after an hour or so. In one case there was a delay of 2 weeks.[77] Symptoms may worsen over several hours. Full or almost full spontaneous recovery is the rule. Whether a nonthermal mechanism is responsible or nerve is more vulnerable than surrounding tissue to heat is unknown.

Experimental studies illustrate the probable physiological and anatomical changes that occur. When low-tension electrical current was applied to the sciatic nerve of the cat, limb paralysis and electrophysiological abnormalities increased in duration from minutes to weeks and then became permanent as the quantity of current increased.[56,61] No morphological change was found after very brief periods of paralysis. Demyelination of axons was associated with paralysis that lasted for 2 to 3 weeks; recovery of strength was probably due to remyelination. In animals with permanent paralysis, there was destruction of axons as well as myelin.

Lightning

Limb neuropathies have been reported more often than cranial neuropathies with man-made electricity, but with lightning the reverse is true. This is probably because lightning often involves the head. These cranial neuropathies resemble low-tension rather than high-tension electrical neuropathies in two important respects. First, they are usually reversible, probably because most of the current flows *over* the victim, and burns tend to be superficial.[62] And second, their onset may be delayed for a few days.[86] Ocular palsies, Horner's syndrome, internal ophthalmoplegia, and lesions of the facial, vagus, and glossopharyngeal nerves have been recorded.[64,86,87] Deafness is especially common.[65] In one patient, autopsy showed loss of hair cells from the organ of Corti,[88] but most victims have conductive deafness caused by thermal injury of the tympanic membrane or middle ear.[58,89]

SPINAL CORD INJURY

Delayed Electrical Myelopathy

This is the most characteristic neurological effect of electricity. Estimates of its frequency range from less than 1 to 6 percent of victims.[57,90-92] The following analysis is based on a review of 20 patients.[88,90-100] High-tension current (usually more than 5,000 V) or lightning, a current pathway crossing or running the length of the spinal cord, and at least some deep electrical burns are typical. If the victim's skin is wet, enough household current can flow to damage the spinal cord.[97] Neurological symptoms may appear immediately, but a delay of between 1 day and 6 weeks—1 week on the average—is typical. Neurological signs worsen for between 2 and 14 days, usually for about 5 days. In one patient they progressed for 2 years.[95] One-third of patients recover fully, one-third make a partial recovery, and one-third do not recover at all. Those with signs of a complete spinal cord lesion or with prolonged progression of signs do not recover completely. Almost all patients have pyramidal signs (i.e., paraparesis or quadriparesis with spasticity, hyperreflexia, and Babinski signs). A few develop atrophy of muscle innervated by segments of the spinal cord through which the current flowed. Sensory are less prominent than motor abnormalities and may be transitory. Joint position sense and vibratory sense are affected more than pain and temperature. Sphincter paralysis is uncommon. One patient developed only a Lhermitte sign.[77]

Five patients have had postmortem examinations.[88,92-95] The abnormal portion of the spinal cord corresponded to the pathway of the current. The white matter was more affected than the gray matter, and the lateral and posterior columns were most affected of all. These showed demyelination with relative preservation of axons. Central chromatolysis, necrosis, and mild loss of anterior horn cells were also found. In three patients, some segments of the cord were necrotic. There were no vascular changes. The preponderance of long tract signs over muscle atrophy correlates with that of damage to white matter over gray matter. Regeneration of the myelin of demyelinated tracts may underlie the functional recovery in some patients.[88]

The delay in onset of symptoms has prompted a comparison to delayed radiation myelopathy,[12,101] but the differences are greater than any similarities.

The latent period of radiation myelopathy is measured in months rather than days, and the subsequent course is usually progressive rather than self-limited. Furthermore, the normality of the blood vessels distinguishes electrical from radiation myelopathy, in which parenchymal necrosis may relate, at least in part, to vascular changes.[12,102] Although the reason for the delayed onset of symptoms is unknown, it is unlikely to represent a fundamental pathogenetic difference among electrical injuries: with or without a delay, the location, clinical course, and pathological features of accidental or experimental[103] electrical myelopathies are the same.

Spinal cord compression due to fracture of the spine—usually the thoracic spine—is the major differential diagnosis.[104,105] This can result from a fall or from tetanic contraction of the paraspinal muscles during electrical shock. The absence of pain in electrical myelopathy is a useful diagnostic point.

Spinal Atrophic Paralysis

Panse coined the term *spinal atrophic paralysis* for a syndrome of focal muscular atrophy occurring after a shock from man-made electricity.[67] No figures of its frequency are available, but it must be quite rare in that no new case has been published since Panse's review in 1955.[67] Low-tension current, a pathway from hand to hand (across the cervical spinal cord), and either minor or no burns typify the context in which the syndrome occurs, but it may also follow lightning stroke. Pain or paresthesias in the arm through which current entered begins at once but disappears within days or weeks. Weakness begins immediately or after a few days' or weeks' delay. Muscle wasting becomes evident weeks to months later. The muscles of the shoulder girdle or the hand are affected (i.e., those supplied by the middle or lower cervical segments). Involvement is usually unilateral. Some but not all patients have weakness and spasticity in the legs. Sensory signs may be present in the arms or legs. Horner's syndrome and cyanosis, coolness, and trophic changes in the fingernails are occasionally present, as is sphincter incontinence. The weakness and muscle atrophy worsen for a few months but then stabilize or improve. If the current flows from hand to foot or from foot to foot, the muscles of the leg may atrophy.

Panse contrasted the syndrome to that of delayed electrical myelopathy.[67] In the latter disorder, high-tension current injures mainly the white matter of the spinal cord by means of heat; the gray matter is relatively spared. In spinal atrophic paralysis, low-tension current injures mainly the gray matter of the cord—specifically, the anterior horn cells—by a nonthermal mechanism, and the white matter is relatively spared. There are no postmortem studies of the disorder, but Langworthy found experimentally that the anterior horn cells of the spinal cord are especially vulnerable to electrical current.[60]

Amyotrophic Lateral Sclerosis

Delayed electrical myelopathy and spinal atrophic paralysis resemble amyotrophic lateral sclerosis (ALS) in some respects—there are upper and lower motor neuron signs, whereas sensory and sphincter functions are often spared. Reports of patients with progressive rather than self-limited disease have advanced the idea of an association between electrical shock and ALS.[67,106–108] These patients developed signs pointing to parts of the brain and spinal cord outside the pathway of electrical current. Hence, a direct effect of current could not have caused them. Patten wondered about an autoimmune mechanism.[108] Epidemiological studies have found electrical shock and lightning stroke, like other types of trauma, to be more frequent in ALS than in control patients.[109] The meaning of this finding is unclear, because all these retrospective analyses depend on adequate memory of events by subjects and on valid selection of the control population.[109]

BRAIN INJURY

Electrical Burns of the Skull

The skull's resistance to electrical current protects the brain from electrical injury. Only high-voltage current passes through the skull. The heat generated by this passage causes coagulation of the blood in the underlying dural sinuses and coagulation necrosis of the underlying brain.[56,67,104,110] Distant cerebral structures in the pathway of the current may also be affected. For example, a man with an electrical burn of the occipital bone is reported to have developed thrombosis of the torcula and necrosis of the cerebellum as well as necrosis of the optic nerves.[111]

Skull burns with open dura are conducive to the

development of meningitis[55,78] and necrotic skull bones (not yet sequestered) to epidural abscess formation.[56,67]

Lightning Stroke to the Head

This is fatal in most victims.[67] Most survivors suffer no cerebral damage, but several cases of cerebellar ataxia have been reported.[67,112,113] In experimental animals, cerebellar Purkinje cells seem to be particularly vulnerable to electrical current.[60,68] This may be the pathological basis of the clinical syndrome in humans. Parkinsonian signs and hemiplegia have also been reported, but no pathological or neuroimaging data are available.[67,70,74] Some of these patients may have had the syndrome of delayed parkinsonism after cardiac arrest.[114]

Cerebrovascular Complications

A small number of reported patients have suffered cerebral infarction, subarachnoid hemorrhage, or intracerebral hemorrhage after electrical shock or lightning stroke.[67,77,115-120] The precise cause of these complications is unclear. It is noteworthy, however, that intense constriction of the lumen for 1 to 10 minutes follows the experimental passage of current through an artery.[68,103,121] Structural changes also occur. Heat causes coagulation necrosis of the endothelium and muscular coat, but the adventitia is little changed.[121,122] Deprived of the support of the intima and media, the artery becomes dilated, and a fusiform aneurysm may develop. Complications include thrombosis, the formation and embolism of mural thrombi, and rupture with hemorrhage.[123] These could lead to intracranial hemorrhage or cerebral infarction soon or long after an electrical current had passed through the head.[67,77] Dural sinus thrombosis may also cause venous infarction of the brain.[124] Other mechanisms may also lead to cerebrovascular complications. For example, an electrical shock can induce acute hypertension, up to 400 mmHg in animals,[67,125] and such effects on the blood pressure may lead to cerebral hemorrhage.[115] Trauma, caused by a fall or the cylindrical shock wave of a lightning bolt, may also lead to intracerebral or subarachnoid bleeding or to arterial dissection with cerebral infarction.[59,116-119] Cardiac arrest may cause cerebral infarction in the arterial border zone.[119] Finally, a patient may have a stroke soon after—but unrelated to—an electrical shock.[120]

ACKNOWLEDGMENT

I am grateful to Monroe Cole, MD, for translating references 94 and 95.

REFERENCES

1. Deitch EA: The management of burns. N Engl J Med 323:1249, 1990
2. Mohnot D, Snead OC III, Benton JW Jr: Burn encephalopathy in children. Ann Neurol 12:42, 1982
3. Hawtof DB: Intracranial hemorrhage in burned patients: report of four cases. J Trauma 6:503, 1966
4. Winkelman MD, Galloway PG: Central nervous system complications of thermal burns: a postmortem study of 139 patients. Medicine (Baltimore) 71:271, 1992
5. McManus WF, Hunt JL, Pruitt BA: Postburn convulsive disorders in children. J Trauma 14:396, 1974
6. Antoon AY, Volpe JJ, Crawford JD: Burn encephalopathy in children. Pediatrics 50:609, 1972
7. Pruitt BA Jr: The burn patient: I. Initial care. Curr Probl Surg 16(4):1, 1979
8. Pruitt BA Jr: The burn patient: II. Later care and complications of thermal injury. Curr Probl Surg 16(5): 1, 1979
9. Broughton A, Anderson IRM, Bowden CH: Magnesium-deficiency syndrome in burns. Lancet 2:1156, 1968
10. Hughes JR, Cayaffa JJ, Pruitt BA, et al: Seizures following burns of the skin. Dis Nerv Syst 34:347, 1973
11. McKee AC, Winkelman MD, Banker BQ: Central pontine myelinolysis in severely burned patients: relationship to serum hyperosmolality. Neurology 38: 1211, 1988
12. Adams RD, Victor M: Principles of Neurology. 5th Ed. McGraw-Hill, New York, 1993
13. Pruitt BA Jr: The diagnosis and treatment of infection in the burn patient. Burns Incl Therm Inj 11:79, 1984
14. Deitch EA, Gelder F, McDonald JC: Sequential prospective analysis of the nonspecific host defense system after thermal injury. Arch Surg 119:83, 1984
15. Munster A, Eurenius K, Katz RM, et al: Cell-mediated immunity after thermal injury. Ann Surg 177: 139, 1973
16. Jackson AC, Gilbert JJ, Young GB, Bolton CF: The

encephalopathy of sepsis. Can J Neurol Sci 12:303, 1985

17. Schlesinger LS, Ross SC, Schaberg DR: Staphylococcus aureus meningitis: a broad-based epidemiologic study. Medicine (Baltimore) 66:148, 1987
18. Fetter BF, Klintworth GK, Hendry WS: Mycoses of the Central Nervous System. Williams & Wilkins, Baltimore, 1967
19. Walsh TJ, Hier DB, Caplan LR: Fungal infections of the central nervous system: comparative analysis of risk factors and clinical signs in 57 patients. Neurology 35:1654, 1985
20. Pensler JM, Herndon DN, Ptak H, et al: Fungal sepsis: an increasing problem in major thermal injuries. J Burn Care Rehabil 7:488, 1986
21. Prasad JK, Feller I, Thomson PD: A ten-year review of Candida sepsis and mortality in burn patients. Surgery 101:213, 1987
22. Parker JC, McCloskey JJ, Knauer KA: Pathobiologic features of human candidiasis: a common deep mycosis of the brain, heart, and kidney in the altered host. Am J Clin Pathol 65:991, 1976
23. Parker JC, McCloskey JJ, Lee RS: Human cerebral candidosis—a postmortem evaluation of 19 patients. Hum Pathol 12:23, 1981
24. Pendlebury WW, Perl DP, Munoz DG: Multiple microabscesses in the central nervous system: a clinicopathologic study. J Neuropathol Exp Neurol 48:290, 1989
25. Kuhn JM, Taveras JM: Small bright foci on T2-weighted magnetic resonance images and associated disorders. Chap 40, p. 1. In Taveras JM, Ferrucci JT (eds): Radiology: Diagnosis, Imaging, Intervention. Vol 3. JB Lippincott, Philadelphia, 1989
26. Edwards JE: Invasive candida infections: evolution of a fungal pathogen. N Engl J Med 324:1060, 1991
27. Edwards JE: Candida species. p. 1943. In Mandell GL, Douglas RG, Bennett JE (eds): Principles and Practice of Infectious Diseases. 3rd Ed. Churchill Livingstone, New York, 1990
28. Wilson R, Hamburger M: Fifteen years' experience with staphylococcal septicemia in a large city hospital. Am J Med 22:437, 1957
29. Pruitt AA, Rubin RH, Karchmer AW, Duncan GW: Neurologic complications of bacterial endocarditis. Medicine (Baltimore) 57:329, 1978
30. Walsh TJ, Hier DB, Caplan LR: Aspergillosis of the central nervous system: clinicopathological analysis of 17 patients. Ann Neurol 18:574, 1985
31. Beal MF, O'Carroll CP, Kleinman GM, Grossman RI: Aspergillosis of the nervous system. Neurology 32:473, 1982
32. McManus WF, Eurenius K, Pruitt BA: Disseminated intravascular coagulation in burned patients. J Trauma 13:416, 1973
33. Caprini JA, Lipp V, Zuckerman L, et al: Hematologic changes following burns. J Surg Res 22:626, 1977
34. Hergt K: Blood levels of thrombocytes in burned patients: observations on their behavior in relation to the clinical condition of the patient. J Trauma 12:599, 1972
35. Robboy SJ, Major MC, Colman RW, Minna JD: Pathology of disseminated intravascular coagulation (DIC): analysis of 26 cases. Hum Pathol 3:327, 1972
36. Collins RC, Al-Mondhiry H, Chernik NL, Posner JB: Neurologic manifestations of intravascular coagulation in patients with cancer. Neurology 25:795, 1975
37. Schwartzman RJ, Hill JB: Neurologic complications of disseminated intravascular coagulation. Neurology 32:791, 1982
38. Graus F, Rogers LR, Posner JB: Cerebrovascular complications in patients with cancer. Medicine (Baltimore) 64:16, 1985
39. Simon TL, Curreri PW, Harker LA: Kinetic characterization of hemostasis in thermal injury. J Lab Clin Med 89:702, 1977
40. Curreri PW, Wilterdink ME, Baxter CR: Coagulation dynamics following thermal injury: effect of heparin and protamine sulfate. Ann Surg 181:161, 1975
41. Curreri PW, Wilterdink ME, Baxter CR: Characterization of elevated fibrin split products following thermal injury. Ann Surg 181:157, 1975
42. Toole J: Cerebrovascular Disorders. 3rd Ed. Raven Press, New York, 1984
43. Sevitt S: The nervous system. p. 276. In: Burns: Pathology and Therapeutic Applications. Butterworths, London, 1957
44. Gregorios JB: Leukoencephalopathy associated with extensive burns. J Neurol Neurosurg Psychiatry 45: 898, 1982
45. Helm PA, Johnson ER, Carlton AM: Peripheral neurological problems in the acute burn patient. Burns 3: 123, 1977
46. Salisbury RE, Dingeldein GP: Peripheral nerve complications following burn injury. Clin Orthop 163:92, 1982
47. Asch MJ, Flemma RJ, Pruitt BA: Ischemic necrosis of tibialis anterior muscle in burn patients: report of three cases. Surgery 66:846, 1969
48. Helm PA, Pandian G, Heck E: Neuromuscular problems in the burn patient: cause and prevention. Arch Phys Med Rehabil 66:451, 1985
49. Marquez S, Turley JJE, Peters WJ: Neuropathy in burn patients. Brain 116:471, 1993
50. Henderson B, Koepke GH, Feller I: Peripheral polyneuropathy among patients with burns. Arch Phys Med Rehabil 52:149, 1971

51. Zochodne DW, Bolton CF, Wells GA, et al: Critical illness polyneuropathy: a complication of sepsis and multiple organ failure. Brain 110:819, 1987

52. Witt NJ, Zochodne DW, Bolton CF, et al: Peripheral nerve function in sepsis and multiple organ failure. Chest 99:176, 1991

53. Carver N, Logan A: Critically ill polyneuropathy associated with burns: a case report. Burns 15:179, 1989

54. Anastakis DJ, Peters WJ, Lee KC: Severe peripheral burn polyneuropathy: a case report. Burns 13:232, 1987

55. DiVincenti FC, Moncrief JA, Pruitt BA: Electrical injuries: a review of 65 cases. J Trauma 9:497, 1969

56. Ugland OM: Electrical burns: a clinical and experimental study with special reference to peripheral nerve injury. Scand J Plast Reconstr Surg Suppl 2:1, 1967

57. Grube BJ, Heimbach DM, Engrav LH, Copass MK: Neurologic consequences of electrical burns. J Trauma 30:254, 1990

58. Wright JW, Silk KL: Acoustic and vestibular defects in lightning survivors. Laryngoscope 84:1378, 1974

59. Hanson GC, McIlwraith: Lightning injury: two case histories and a review of management. Br Med J 4:271, 1973

60. Langworthy OR: Abnormalities produced in the central nervous system by electrical injuries. J Exp Med 51:943, 1930

61. Alexander L: Electrical injuries of the nervous system. J Nerv Ment Dis 94:622, 1941

62. Cooper MA: Electrical and lightning injuries. Emerg Med Clin North Am 2:489, 1984

63. Weeks AW, Alexander L: The distribution of electric current in the animal body: an experimental investigation of 60 cycle alternating current. J Indust Hyg Toxicol 21:517, 1939

64. Critchley M: The effects of lightning: with special reference to the nervous system. Bristol Med Chir J 49:285, 1932

65. Arden GP, Harrison SH, Lister J, Mandsley RH: Lightning accident at Ascot. Br Med J 1:1450, 1956

66. Cwinn AA, Cantrill SV: Lightning injuries. J Emerg Med 2:379, 1985

67. Panse F: Electrical lesions of the nervous system. p. 344. In Vinken PJ, Bruyn GW (eds): Handbook of Clinical Neurology. Vol 7. North-Holland, Amsterdam, 1970

68. Morrison LR, Weeks A, Cobb S: Histopathology of different types of electric shock on mammalian brains. J Indust Hyg 12:324, 1930

69. Lee RC, Kolodney MS: Electrical injury mechanisms: electrical breakdown of cell membranes. Plast Reconstr Surg 80:672, 1987

70. Langworthy OR: Neurological abnormalities produced by electricity. J Nerv Ment Dis 84:13, 1936

71. Silversides J: The neurological sequelae of electrical injury. Can Med Assoc J 91:195, 1964

72. Critchley M: Neurological effects of lightning and electricity. Lancet 1:68, 1934

73. Currens JH: Arterial spasm and transient paralysis resulting from lightning striking an airplane. J Aviat Med 16:275, 1945

74. Paterson JH, Turner JWA: Lightning and the central nervous system. J R Army Med Corps 82:73, 1944

75. Taussig HB: "Death" from lightning—and the possibility of living again. Ann Intern Med 68:1345, 1968

76. ten Duis HJ, Klasen HJ: Keraunoparalysis, a "specific" lightning injury. Burns 12:54, 1985

77. Critchley M: Industrial electrical accidents in their neurological aspect. J State Med 40:459, 1932

78. Solem L, Fischer RP, Strate RG: The natural history of electrical injury. J Trauma 17:487, 1977

79. Koshima I, Moriguchi T, Soeda S, Murashita T: High-voltage electrical injury: electron microscopic findings of injured vessel, nerve, and muscle. Ann Plast Surg 26:587, 1991

80. Yost JW, Holmes FF: Myoglobinuria following lightning stroke. JAMA 228:1147, 1974

81. Matsen FA: Compartmental Syndromes. Grune & Stratton, Orlando, FL, 1980

82. Shields RW Jr, Root KE, Wilbourn AJ: Compartment syndromes and compression neuropathies in coma. Neurology 36:1370, 1986

83. Engrav LH, Gottlieb JR, Walkinshaw MD, et al: Outcome and treatment of electrical injury with immediate median and ulnar palsy at the wrist: a retrospective review and a survey of members of the American Burn Association. Ann Plast Surg 25:166, 1990

84. Savitsky N, Gerson MJ: Peripheral nerve injury following electrical trauma: axillary and radial nerve involvement. J Nerv Ment Dis 96:635, 1942

85. Suematsu N, Matsuura J, Atsuta Y: Brachial plexus injury caused by electric current through the ulnar nerve: case report and review of the literature. Arch Orthop Trauma Surg 108:400, 1989

86. Richards A: Traumatic facial palsy. Proc R Soc Med 66:556, 1973

87. Saddler MC, Thomas JE: Temporary bulbar palsy following lightning strike. Cent Afr J Med 36:161, 1990

88. Davidson GS, Deck JH: Delayed myelopathy following lightning strike: a demyelinating process. Acta Neuropathol (Berl) 77:104, 1988

89. Jones DT, Ogren FP, Roh LH, Moore GF: Lightning and its effects on the auditory system. Laryngoscope 101:830, 1991

90. Koller J, Orsagh J: Delayed neurological sequelae of high-tension electrical burns. Burns 15:175, 1989

91. Varghese G, Mani MM, Redford JB: Spinal cord inju-

ries following electrical accidents. Paraplegia 24:159, 1986

92. Levine NS, Atkins A, McKeel DW, et al: Spinal cord injury following electrical accidents: case reports. J Trauma 15:459, 1975

93. Jackson FE, Martin R, Davis R: Delayed quadriplegia following electrical burn. Milit Med 130:60, 1965

94. Komar J, Komar G: Paralysie spinale atrophiante due au traumatisme electrique du chat. Schweiz Arch Tierheilk 108:325, 1966

95. Gerhard L, Spancken E: Chronische Ruckenmarksschadigung nach Starkstrom-unfall. Acta Neuropathol (Berl) 20:357, 1972

96. Christensen JA, Sherman RT, Balis GA, Wuamett JD: Delayed neurologic injury secondary to high-voltage current, with recovery. J Trauma 20:166, 1980

97. So SC, Lee MLK: Spastic quadriplegia due to electric shock. Br Med J 2:590, 1973

98. Holbrook LA, Beach FXM, Silver JR: Delayed myelopathy: a rare complication of severe electrical burns. Br Med J 4:659, 1970

99. Sharma M, Smith A: Paraplegia as a result of lightning injury. Br Med J 2:1464, 1978

100. Alexander L: Clinical and neuropathological aspects of electrical injuries. J Indust Hyg Toxicol 20:191, 1938

101. Farrell DF, Starr A: Delayed neurological sequelae of electrical injuries. Neurology 18:601, 1968

102. Delattre JY, Rosenblum MK, Thaler HT, et al: A model of radiation myelopathy in the rat: pathology, regional capillary permeability changes and treatment with dexamethasone. Brain 111:1319, 1988

103. MacMahon HE: Electric shock. Am J Pathol 5:33, 1929

104. Skoog T: Electrical injuries. J Trauma 10:816, 1970

105. Steffen DJ, Schoneweis DA, Nelssen JL: Hind limb paralysis from electrical shock in three gilts. J Am Vet Med Assoc 200:812, 1992

106. Sirdofsky MD, Hawley RJ, Manz H: Progressive motor neuron disease associated with electrical injury. Muscle Nerve 14:977, 1991

107. Karnosh LJ: The neurological aspects of industrial electrocution. Ohio State Med J 28:786, 1932

108. Patten BM: Lightning and electrical injuries. Neurol Clin 10:1047, 1992

109. Tandan R, Bradley WG: Amyotrophic lateral sclerosis: Part 2. Etiopathogenesis. Ann Neurol 18:419, 1985

110. Gardner WJ: Electrical burns of the brain. J Neurosurg 5:90, 1948

111. North JP: Electric burns of the head and arm with residual damage to eyes and brain. Am J Surg 76:631, 1948

112. Cherington M, Yarnell P, Hallmark D: MRI in lightning encephalopathy. Neurology 43:1437, 1993

113. Suri ML, Vijayan GP: Neurological sequelae of lightning. J Assoc Physicians India 26:209, 1978

114. Boylan KB, Chin JH, DeArmond SJ: Progressive dystonia following resuscitation from cardiac arrest. Neurology 40:1458, 1990

115. Stanley LD, Suss RA: Intracerebral hematoma secondary to lightning stroke: case report and review of the literature. Neurosurgery 16:686, 1985

116. Mann H, Kozic Z, Boulos M: CT of lightning injury. AJNR 4:976, 1983

117. Morgan ZV, Headley RN, Alexander E, Sawyer CG: Atrial fibrillation and epidural hematoma associated with lightning stroke. N Engl J Med 259:956, 1958

118. Strasser EJ, Davis RM, Menchey MJ: Lightning injuries. J Trauma 17:315, 1977

119. Cherington M, Yarnell P, Lammmereste D: Lightning strikes: nature of neurological damage in patients evaluated in hospital emergency departments. Ann Emerg Med 21:575, 1992

120. Haase E, Luhan JA: Protracted coma from delayed thrombosis of basilar artery following electrical injury. Arch Neurol 1:195, 1959

121. Jaffe RH, Willis D, Bachem A: The effect of electric current on the arteries. Arch Pathol 7:244, 1929

122. Ponten B, Erikson U, Johansson SH, Olding L: New observations on tissue changes along the pathway of the current in an electrical injury: case report. Scand J Plast Reconstr Surg 4:75, 1970

123. Muir IFK: The treatment of electrical burns. Br J Plast Surg 10:292, 1958

124. Patel A, Lo R: Electric injury with cerebral venous thrombosis: case report and review of the literature. Stroke 24:903, 1993

125. Urquhart RWI: Experimental electric shock. J Indust Hyg 9:140, 1927

48

Abnormalities of Thermal Regulation and the Nervous System

Douglas Gelb

The human thermoregulatory system serves to maintain the body temperature near 37°C (98.6°F). Both the central nervous system (CNS) and the peripheral nervous system are important for thermoregulation, so a variety of neurological disorders may produce thermoregulatory abnormalities. At the same time, the nervous system is very sensitive to the effects of body temperature, so thermoregulatory disorders may produce a variety of neurological problems. This chapter covers both the neurological conditions that produce thermoregulatory disorders and the neurological conditions that may result from abnormal temperature regulation.

THE THERMOREGULATORY SYSTEM

A thermoregulatory "center" in the preoptic and anterior hypothalamus is believed to integrate thermal inputs and to produce an output that adjusts body temperature to match a set point.[1–3] Thermoregulatory disorders may be produced either by malfunction of this thermoregulatory system or by conditions that overwhelm the capacity of the system. Thermo-

regulatory disorders should be distinguished from other causes of abnormal body temperature, in which the thermoregulatory system functions properly but the set point is shifted. The most common condition of this type is fever, which is thought to be produced by an abnormal upward shift of the set point.[4–10] Shifts in the set point may also be responsible for variations of body temperature with the menstrual cycle and for diurnal temperature fluctuations.[3,11]

The afferent limb of the thermoregulatory system is primarily concerned with the core body temperature. In particular, there are neurons in the preoptic and anterior hypothalamic areas that are sensitive to the temperature conditions existing in the thermoregulatory center itself.[1,2,12] There are also thermosensitive neurons in the brainstem and spinal cord and possibly in the abdominal viscera.[1,7,13,14] The specific cold and warm thermoreceptors in the skin contribute relatively little to thermal equilibrium (though rapid, transient thermoregulatory responses may follow rapid changes in skin temperature before any significant change in brain temperature occurs).[1,3]

The efferent limb of the system serves to generate or dissipate heat, as necessary. Heat generation is achieved primarily by shivering.[3,15] Heat is also produced as a function of basal metabolic activity, but this is not significantly modulated with thermoregulation. Brown adipose tissue contributes to heat production in neonates exposed to cold, but not in older individuals.[16,17] Heat dissipation is achieved by evaporation (sweating) and by nonevaporative heat loss (conduction, convection, and radiation). Evaporative heat loss is the most important of these mechanisms in most clinical situations.[3,18] Nonevaporative heat loss can occur only when the ambient temperature is lower than the skin temperature. When that is the case, the amount of heat dissipated is a function of vasomotor activity: increased skin blood flow promotes heat dissipation, whereas reduced skin blood flow minimizes heat dissipation. These thermoregulatory vasomotor effects are controlled by both the hypothalamus and local reflexes. The local vasomotor reflexes can override the hypothalamic regulation when there are sufficiently extreme local temperature conditions.[7,14,19–21]

NEUROLOGICAL CAUSES OF ABNORMAL THERMOREGULATION

In principle, thermoregulatory disorders could be produced by abnormal function of the thermoregulatory center or by interruption of its afferent or efferent connections. In practice, because the major afferent input comes from neurons that are themselves located in the hypothalamus, afferent disruption is not a significant concern. Consequently, the main neurological causes of abnormal thermoregulation are diseases of the hypothalamus and its autonomic outflow. In addition, a few neurological disorders result in excessive heat production that overwhelms the thermoregulatory system. Tables 48-1 and 48-2 summarize the main causes of hyperthermia and hypothermia, respectively.

Hypothalamic Lesions

Hypothalamic lesions may produce either hyperthermia or hypothermia, though hypothermia is more common.[22,23] Hyperthermia has been described with hypothalamic tumors,[24–27] stroke,[28] and encephalitis.[26,28] Head trauma and brain surgery involving the hypothalamus may also produce hyperther-

Table 48-1 Causes of Hyperthermia

Malfunction of the thermoregulatory system
  Hypothalamic disorders
    Tumor
    Stroke
    Encephalitis
    Head trauma
    Surgery
  Other lesions
    Hydrocephalus
    Posterior fossa surgery

Interruption of effector pathways
  Spinal cord lesions
  Autonomic neuropathies

Overwhelming heat production or exposure
  Neurological conditions
    Status epilepticus
    Delirium tremens
    Tetanus
    Malignant hyperthermia
    Neuroleptic malignant syndrome
  Nonneurological conditions
    Heat stress disorders
      Heat shock
      Heat exhaustion
    Endocrine disorders
      Thyrotoxicosis
      Pheochromocytoma
    Drugs

Inadequate heat dissipation
  Dehydration
  Skin disorders
  Occlusive dressings
  Drugs

mia.[25] Hypothermia has been reported with hypothalamic tumors,[24,26,28] strokes,[29] subarachnoid hemorrhage,[30] sarcoidosis,[29,31] and idiopathic gliosis.[32] It is common in Wernicke's encephalopathy and may be the presenting feature.[33–36] Its occurrence in Wernicke's encephalopathy has been attributed to lesions in the posterolateral hypothalamus and in the floor of the fourth ventricle.[36] In contrast, while fever is also common in Wernicke's encephalopathy (occurring in about 12 percent of patients), an infection is almost always found to account for it.[36] Accidental hypothermia has been seen in two patients with Parkinson's disease[37]; again, this has been attributed to hypothalamic abnormalities.[37,38] Prominent abnor-

Table 48-2 Causes of Hypothermia

Malfunction of the thermoregulatory system
  Hypothalamic disorders
    Tumors
    Strokes
    Subarachnoid hemorrhage
    Sarcoidosis
    Wernicke's encephalopathy
    Parkinson's disease
    Primary autonomic failure
    Multisystem atrophy
    Multiple sclerosis
  Agenesis of the corpus callosum (Shapiro's syndrome)
  Disease at the mesencephalic-diencephalic junction

Interruption of effector pathways
  Spinal cord lesions
  Autonomic neuropathies
  Neuromuscular causes of weakness

Inadequate heat production
  Accidental hypothermia (exposure)
  Endocrine disorders
    Hypothyroidism
    Hypoadrenalism
    Hypopituitarism
  Derangements of glucose regulation
    Hypoglycemia
    Diabetic ketoacidosis
    Hyperosmolar coma
  Malnutrition
  Drugs

Excessive heat dissipation
  Severe burns
  Exfoliative dermatitis

malities of sweating (anhidrosis or hypohidrosis) have been described both in primary autonomic failure and in multisystem atrophy,[39-41] and hyperthermia may be of major concern when patients with these disorders live in hot climates without air conditioning.

Lesions of Effector Pathways

Interruption of the autonomic outflow from the hypothalamus may produce either hyperthermia or hypothermia by impairing the effector mechanisms necessary for heat dissipation or production, respectively.[42] Lesions of the spinal cord above the high thoracic level may interrupt descending pathways

that influence the intermediolateral cell column, producing both vasomotor abnormalities and disorders of sweating.[43,44] Spinal cord lesions also interrupt descending input to anterior horn cells, impairing or eliminating shivering below the level of the lesion.[43-46] Any neuromuscular disease that is severe enough to cause profound weakness may produce the same result.[47] Finally, both acquired and hereditary polyneuropathies may involve autonomic fibers and produce abnormalities of vasomotor activity and sweating.[48-50] Either hypothermia or hyperthermia may result. Hypothermia is more common in diabetic patients than in normal subjects,[51] for example, probably because of impaired vasomotor reflexes.[49] In contrast, some diabetics manifest a syndrome of heat intolerance that is attributed to anhidrosis. Since the autonomic nerve involvement in diabetes is usually predominantly distal, these patients sometimes exhibit profuse sweating over the head and upper trunk ("compensatory hyperhidrosis").[48,52,53]

Miscellaneous Lesions

Abnormal thermoregulation resulting from pathology elsewhere in the nervous system is less well established. Hypothermia has been seen in patients with multiple sclerosis,[54,55] and in one instance, careful pathological examination of the hypothalamus failed to reveal any abnormality.[55] One patient has been reported in whom a syndrome like Wernicke's encephalopathy (with hypothermia and eye movement abnormalities) was attributed to a hematoma at the mesencephalic-diencephalic junction.[56]

Agenesis of the corpus callosum may be associated with episodic hyperhidrosis and hypothermia (Shapiro's syndrome).[57,58] There may also be associated abnormalities in the septal region, cingulate gyrus, and posterior hypothalamus. A similar syndrome has occasionally been seen without any associated abnormality of the corpus callosum.[58-61] The periods of sweating may last from minutes to hours, and the hypothermia may last from 30 minutes up to several weeks. Episodes may be separated by intervals of months to years. There is often ataxia and impaired cognition during the hypothermic episodes. Some of these patients have been found to have abnormalities in the anterior hypothalamus or infundibular nuclei. Recurrent hypothermia has also been attributed to "diencephalic epilepsy," but electrographic seizures have not been demonstrated.[58]

Hyperthermia has been reported after operations in the posterior fossa[25] and in patients with acute hydrocephalus.[62,63] It is difficult to make inferences about localization from such patients, however, because of the presence of mass effect. Hyperthermia associated with ischemic lesions in the posterior fossa has also been reported, but the details provided were insufficient to judge the extent of pathological involvement.[64] As a general rule, even when a patient has CNS disease, hyperthermia should not be attributed to "neurogenic factors" unless there is clear involvement of the hypothalamus or effector pathways.

Neurological Causes of Thermoregulatory System Overload

Several neurological diseases produce thermoregulatory disorders by creating conditions that overwhelm the capacity of the thermoregulatory system. Just as paralysis may eliminate effective shivering and result in hypothermia, muscle hyperactivity may result in hyperthermia. Elevated body temperatures are common after generalized seizures,[65] for example, and are of prognostic relevance in patients in generalized status epilepticus.[66] Generalized tetanus, delirium tremens, and catatonia are also associated with hyperthermia.[9] Two noteworthy examples of hyperthermia associated with increased muscle activity are malignant hyperthermia and neuroleptic malignant syndrome.

MALIGNANT HYPERTHERMIA

Malignant hyperthermia is an inherited condition characterized by vigorous muscle contractions and abrupt increase in temperature on exposure to certain drugs, notably inhalation anesthetics and succinylcholine.[67,68] The hyperthermia is probably a direct result of the heat produced by sustained muscle activity, which, in turn, is thought to be due to a defect in the sarcoplasmic reticulum resulting in defective regulation of intracellular free calcium. Patients with primary muscle disorders, notably central core disease and Duchenne muscular dystrophy, have an increased incidence of malignant hyperthermia.[69–72] While patients with myotonic dystrophy may also

have adverse effects from anesthesia (contractures after administration of succinylcholine, and increased susceptibility to respiratory depression after receiving barbiturates or opiates), they do not appear to have an increased risk of malignant hyperthermia.[68]

NEUROLEPTIC MALIGNANT SYNDROME

Neuroleptic malignant syndrome is also characterized by hyperthermia and muscle rigidity, though altered consciousness and cardiovascular liability are cardinal features as well.[73] While the elevated body temperatures are at least partly due to the muscle activity, there may also be an elevation of the hypothalamic temperature set point. This condition is typically triggered by exposure to neuroleptic agents, but it has also been described in patients being treated for presumed Parkinson's disease after sudden withdrawal of dopamine.[74,75] When associated with neuroleptics, the condition typically arises within 2 weeks of starting therapy or increasing the dose, but at times it may begin within hours or after a delay of months.

NEUROLOGICAL CONSEQUENCES OF ABNORMAL THERMOREGULATION

Most cases of abnormal thermoregulation occur in individuals without a primary neurological disease. These individuals are exposed to external temperature conditions (or, less commonly, to internal metabolic derangements) that overwhelm the thermoregulatory system. Regardless of the underlying cause of the hyperthermia or hypothermia, neurological manifestations are prominent.

Neuronal function is significantly affected by even moderate changes in temperature. Basic electrical parameters such as membrane capacitance, axoplasmic resistance, maximum sodium and potassium conductances, and ion channel rate constants vary systematically with temperature. Consequently, the amplitude, duration, maximum rate of rise, net ionic movements, and conduction velocity of the action potential are all affected by temperature.[76] These parameters, in turn, determine the likelihood of propagation or conduction block.[77] Such considerations apply to both central and peripheral neurons. With respect to the peripheral nervous system, these effects have long been recognized because of their impact on clinical electrophysiological tests.[78–82] For example, the maximum motor conduction velocity of human ulnar nerve falls by 2.4 m/s for every 1°C fall in temperature.[79] Compound action potential amplitudes increase with falling temperatures.[78,81] The duration of motor unit action potentials increases and mean amplitude declines as temperature drops, and polyphasic potentials become more frequent.[82]

While these alterations in function can have significant clinical consequences, they do not represent actual injury to the nervous system. At extreme temperatures, however, such injury does occur. Direct thermal injury to the brain and spinal cord produces cell death, edema, and hemorrhage.[83] Cerebellar Purkinje cells are particularly vulnerable. There is an increase in the cerebral metabolic rate at temperatures between 38°C and 42°C, but at 43°C cerebral metabolic rate is decreased.[84] Cerebral oxygen metabolism also increases with rising temperature up to 42°C but declines as temperatures rise further.[85,86]

With extreme reduction in temperature, there is a roughly exponential decline in metabolic rate, with a reduction of approximately 50 percent in the rate of chemical reactions for every 10°C.[87–89] There is a corresponding reduction in cerebral oxygen consumption by about 50 percent for every 10°C decline in temperature. This reduction in metabolic rate is protective, but neural damage still occurs. In experimental studies using hippocampal slices, the critical survival time for complete recovery of neural activity after oxygen and glucose deprivation was 10 minutes at 37°C, 15 minutes at 28°C, and 45 minutes at 21°C.[89] In patients who die from hypothermia, autopsy reveals perivascular hemorrhages in the region of the third ventricle, with chromatolysis of ganglion cells.[90]

It is difficult to know to what extent these metabolic and pathological abnormalities result from direct damage to neural elements and to what extent they reflect systemic effects (including cardiovascular collapse) that secondarily injure the nervous system. It is clear, however, that they are associated with symptomatic manifestations that often dominate the clinical course of both hyperthermia and hypothermia.

HYPERTHERMIA

The neurological causes of hyperthermia are considered above.

Nonneurological Causes of Hyperthermia

Conditions in which the thermoregulatory system is overwhelmed by extremely high external temperatures are called *heat stress disorders*.[9,22,91,92] The most severe form of heat stress disorder is heat stroke, which is defined by three criteria: severe hyperthermia (core body temperature greater than 41°C), disturbances of the CNS, and hot, dry skin.[93,94] Heat exhaustion is a milder form of heat stress disorder, characterized by progressive lethargy, headache, vomiting, tachycardia, and hypotension; the main distinguishing feature is that the level of consciousness is depressed in heat stroke but not in heat exhaustion.[22,91,93–95] These two conditions form a continuum: if untreated, heat exhaustion may progress to heat stroke.

The term *classic heat stroke* refers to the disorder that results from prolonged exposure to high environmental temperatures while undertaking normal activities; the term *exertional heat stroke* applies in situations of physical exertion.[9,22,92,96,97] Exertional heat stroke typically occurs in healthy young individuals, often athletes and military personnel. Inadequate cardiovascular conditioning, poor acclimatization, dehydration, heavy clothing, low work efficiency, and reduced ratio of skin area to body mass all are risk factors. Congenital or acquired abnormalities of sweat gland function may contribute.[98,99] Classic heat stroke, in contrast, is typically seen in the elderly, especially those with chronic diseases such as alcoholism, malnutrition, diabetes, cardiovascular dysfunction, and obesity. Anticholinergic and diuretic medications are predisposing factors. Lower socioeconomic groups are at particular risk, especially those living in urban areas, because they are exposed to a greater thermal load and often live in apartments with inadequate ventilation.[9,22,92]

The most common cause of hyperthermia is simple dehydration, because it results in vasoconstriction and decreased sweating, thereby interfering with heat dissipation.[9,96] Heat dissipation may also be impaired in advanced scleroderma,[100] miliaria,[101] or by extensive

Table 48-3 Pharmacological Agents That Promote Hyperthermia

	Excess Heat Production		Impaired Heat Dissipation		
Agent(s)	Occurrence	Cause or Comment	Occurrence	Cause	Other Mechanisms
Anticholinergic agents			+		
Vasoconstricting agents			+		
β-blockers			+		
Diuretics			+		
Antihistamines			+		
Alcohol			+		
Tricyclic antidepressants	+	Increased motor activity	+	Anticholinergic effects	
Cocaine	+				
Amphetamines	+				
Opiates	+				
Lysergic acid diethylamide (LSD)	+				
Cannabinoids	+				
Phenothiazines	+	Neuroleptic malignant syndrome	+	Anticholinergic effects	Possible effect on hypothalamus
Butyrophenones	+	Neuroleptic malignant syndrome			Failure to recognize thirst, possible effect on hypothalamus
Salicylate overdose	+				
Methyldopa					Idiosyncratic
Propylthiouracil					Idiosyncratic
Inhalational anesthetics	+	Malignant hyperthermia			
Monoamine oxidase inhibitors (overdose in conjunction with meperidine or in conjunction with biogenic amine precursors)	+				

use of occlusive dressings.[9] Thyrotoxicosis (mainly during thyroid storm)[102] and pheochromocytoma[103] can both cause hyperthermia on the basis of hypermetabolism. Drug exposure can produce hyperthermia in several ways, including increased metabolic rate, hyperactivity, and impaired heat dissipation (Table 48-3).[9,22,92,104–106]

Neurological Manifestations of Hyperthermia

The earliest neurological manifestations of hyperthermia include thirst, weakness, and fatigue.[22,92–94] Skeletal muscle cramps may occur in the exertional heat stress disorders and are probably due to hyponatremia.[22,91,92] Patients with heat exhaustion are frequently agitated and may develop delirium and incoordination.[92] Paresthesias or tetany sometimes occur from hyperventilation.[22,92,94]

In general, hyperthermia that is severe enough to cause stupor or coma occurs only with heat stroke.[107] Heat stroke may present with the sudden onset of stupor or coma, or patients may pass through a prodromal period that can include headache, drowsiness, confusion, agitation, and delirium.[92,97,104,108] Seizures occur in 60 to 70 percent of patients.[94,109] Examination reveals pupils that are usually small and often pinpoint.[97,108,109] Caloric responses are intact except terminally.[107] There is commonly diffuse hypertonia, but flaccidity has also been described.[94,108]

Hemiplegia, cerebellar deficits, and papilledema may also be found.[93,94,104] Cerebrospinal fluid (CSF) from patients with heat stroke is usually normal but may show an increased protein concentration, xanthochromia, and a mild lymphocytic pleocytosis.[93,94,104,108] Slowing of the electroencephalogram (EEG) occurs at temperatures above 42°C.[85]

Most patients who recover from heat stroke have no permanent neurological sequelae, but some develop a syndrome of ataxia and dysarthria,[110–114] and a few cases of persistent hemiparesis, myelopathy, or quadriparesis have been reported.[94,110,114] Persistent polyneuropathy was reported in 4 of 14 patients who were treated with whole-body hyperthermia for cancer.[115] Survivors of severe heat stroke may also develop premature cataracts, attributed to dehydration.[116]

Systemic Manifestations of Hyperthermia

The mildest manifestations of heat stress disorders are mild dependent edema and syncope.[92] Possible explanations for the edema include salt supplementation, heat-induced vasodilatation with consequent oliguria, and increased aldosterone production. Syncope has been attributed to vasodilatation, postural pooling of blood, diminished venous return to the heart, reduced cardiac output, and a global reduction in cerebral perfusion. Skeletal muscle cramps also occur in mild heat stress disorder, as noted above.

Heat stroke is associated with diffuse systemic derangements.[92–94,96,104,109] Respiratory alkalosis is almost always present, and tetany may occur. Hypoxia, metabolic acidosis, hypokalemia, hyperkalemia, hypernatremia, hypophosphatemia, hypomagnesemia, and hypoglycemia may each be seen. A peripheral leukocytosis in the range of 20,000 to 30,000 cells/mm^3 is common.

Cardiovascular manifestations include low cardiac output and low diastolic pressure. Subendocardial hemorrhages may occur. Minor electrocardiographic changes (transient conduction abnormalities and inverted or flattened T waves) are sometimes found. Apart from the respiratory alkalosis, pulmonary manifestations may include pulmonary edema and adult respiratory distress syndrome in the presence of disseminated intravascular coagulation (DIC).

Rhabdomyolysis is almost universal in exertional heat stroke but uncommon in classic heat stroke. Elevated serum creatine kinase levels occur in both conditions. Acute renal failure occurs in about 25 percent of patients with exertional heat stroke but is uncommon in classic heat stroke. Elevated serum amylase levels are common. Serum concentrations of liver enzymes are often elevated also, and cholestasis and patchy hepatic necrosis have been described. Diarrhea and vomiting are common; hematemesis and melena may occur in severe cases.

Clinically significant coagulopathies are common. Contributing factors include abnormal hepatic function with resultant impairment in clotting factor synthesis, thermal activation of either clotting factors or platelets, thrombocytopenia, and fibrinolysis. In severe heat shock, DIC is almost always present.

Patient Management

There are three components to the management of the hyperthermic patient: treatment of the underlying cause (when possible), cooling, and treatment or prevention of common complications.[92,93,96,104,109]

Most of the hypothalamic causes of hyperthermia are not amenable to acute treatment, though dexamethasone administration is appropriate when there is vasogenic edema. Certain spinal cord lesions associated with hyperthermia (e.g., epidural hematoma or abscess) may require immediate treatment, but no acute treatment is possible for other lesions. Hyperthermia causes by excessive muscle activity is treated by reducing or eliminating the muscle activity. Patients in status epilepticus may require neuromuscular blockade (in addition to continuing measures to control their seizures) if temperatures exceed 40°C for a prolonged period.[117] Patients with malignant hyperthermia are treated by stopping the responsible anesthesia, hyperoxygenation, and intravenous administration of dantrolene.[67,96,118] Dantrolene is a skeletal muscle relaxant that uncouples excitation and contraction by preventing the release of calcium from the sarcoplasmic reticulum.[67] It has also been used successfully to treat neuroleptic malignant syndrome.[119–122] Because of the apparent role of dopaminergic systems in neuroleptic malignant syndrome, bromocriptine and amantadine have also been tried therapeutically, and favorable results have been reported.[73,122–126]

Nonneurological causes of hyperthermia may also

be amenable to specific treatment. Thyrotoxic crisis is treated with β-adrenergic antagonists, glucocorticoids (because of increased requirement and reduced adrenal reserve), and large doses of an antithyroid agent such as propylthiouracil.[102] Patients with pheochromocytoma are treated with α-adrenergic antagonists. Dehydrated patients are rehydrated as necessary. For hyperthermic patients in whom a precipitating drug can be identified, treatment is directed at minimizing the drug's toxicity. Patients in delirium tremens require large doses of benzodiazepines. For the hyperthermia of heat stress disorders, treatment of the underlying cause simply consists of removing the patient from the hot environment.

Cooling may be achieved by either evaporative or direct external methods.[22,92,96,106,109,127] *Evaporative methods* involve wetting the skin with tepid water and directing bedside fans at the patient. *Direct external cooling* involves immersion of the patient in ice water, use of a hypothermic mattress, or packing the patient in ice. Vigorous skin massage should accompany these direct external cooling techniques, because low skin temperatures produce vasoconstriction and thus impede removal of heat from the core. Cooling is more rapid and more effective with direct external methods than with evaporative methods, but evaporative techniques are often adequate and permit more convenient patient management and monitoring. In rare instances, neither method is sufficient; treatment may then necessitate peritoneal lavage with iced saline, gastric lavage or enemas with ice water, or hemodialysis or cardiopulmonary bypass with external cooling of blood.[9,96]

Regardless of the cooling method used, shivering often occurs as the body temperature falls. It can be treated with phenothiazines, benzodiazepines, or nondepolarizing muscle relaxants. As the patient's core temperature reaches 38°C or 39°C, cooling is stopped to avoid overshoot hypothermia.

Centrally acting antipyretic medications act by lowering the temperature set point. They are therefore appropriate for use in fever, where the set point is abnormally high. In thermoregulatory disorders, however, the problem lies not in the set point itself but in the system's inability to attain it. It follows that manipulation of the set point has no effect on body temperature, so central antipyretic medications are of no help in this situation.

The most important complication of hyperthermia

is hypotension, which should be treated with fluid administration.[92,96] Isoproterenol may be used if necessary.[96] Dopaminergic and α-adrenergic agonists should be avoided because of their tendency to produce vasoconstriction. Patients should receive 100 percent oxygen until adequate oxygenation is documented. Serum electrolyte and glucose concentrations should be assessed frequently and treated as necessary. To promote urine output, patients are given an initial dose of mannitol and subsequent doses of diuretics as necessary.[92,96,109] If DIC occurs, it should be treated in the same way as in any other setting. When seizures occur, they are usually treated with benzodiazepines.[109]

The prognosis for patients with hyperthermia depends on the peak temperature reached and the duration of symptoms before initiation of treatment.[94,104,109] Mortality rates as high as 70 percent have been reported in the past,[93,106] but most recent series suggest a mortality rate of 5 to 10 percent with appropriate management.[9,92,108,109]

HYPOTHERMIA

Neurological causes of hypothermia are discussed earlier (p. 932).

Nonneurological Causes of Hypothermia

As with hyperthermia, hypothermia (defined as a core temperature below 35°C) is usually due to conditions that overwhelm the thermoregulatory system rather than to a primary malfunction in the system. Accidental hypothermia is defined as "a spontaneous decrease in core temperature, usually in a cold environment and associated with an acute problem without primary pathology of the temperature regulatory center."[128] It is most commonly seen in neonates, the elderly, and those who are unconscious or immobile, especially because of drug exposure. In the United States, hypothermia is seen most frequently in alcoholics.[128–131] Alcohol is a vasodilator, a central nervous system depressant, an anesthetic, and a risk factor for trauma and environmental exposure, all of which increase the risk of hypothermia. Other drugs predispose to hypothermia in various ways, including depression of the hypothalamic center, inhibition of

Table 48-4 Pharmacological Agents That Promote Hypothermia

Agent(s)	Impaired Heat Production	Excessive Heat Loss	Other Mechanisms
Alcohol	+	+	Possible effect on hypothalamus
Barbiturates	+		
General anesthetics	+		
Phenothiazines	+		
Benzodiazepines	+		
Tricyclic antidepressants		$+^a$	
Vasodilating agents		+	
Bromocriptine			Possible effect on hypothalamus
Reserpine			Possible effect on hypothalamus
Acetaminophen			Possible effect on hypothalamus

^{a} Hyperhydrosis in some subjects.

shivering by neuromuscular blockade, and vasodilatation (Table 48-4).[22,128–132]

Patients with severe burns, exfoliative dermatitis, or other dermatological conditions may develop hypothermia because of increases in both evaporative and nonevaporative heat loss and the inability to regulate these processes through vasoconstriction.[133–137] Hypothermia may also occur in the setting of several endocrine disorders that impair metabolism, including hypothyroidism,[90,102,129,131,138,139] hypoadrenalism,[132] and hypopituitarism.[128,132,140] Hypoglycemia, diabetic ketoacidosis, and hyperosmolar coma are also associated with hypothermia,[129,131,140,141] but it is not clear whether this is because of a hypometabolic state or a direct effect on the hypothalamic thermoregulatory center. Malnutrition may be complicated by fatal hypothermia, presumably on the basis of hypometabolism, hypoglycemia, and loss of subcutaneous tissue.[128,132]

Neurological Manifestations of Hypothermia

The neurological manifestations of hypothermia progress in a fairly predictable manner.[131,142,143] Thought processes may be normal with rectal temperatures as low as 34°C, but below this temperature most patients exhibit psychomotor retardation, speech perseveration, lethargy, or confusion. A few patients have been described as alert with rectal temperatures as low as 31°C, but this is uncommon. Dysarthria develops below 33.5°C, and below 28°C most patients only grunt in response to questions, though some patients remain verbally responsive at temperatures as low as 23.5°C. Most patients still make purposeful responses to noxious stimuli even with temperatures approaching 20°C.

Pupillary size is not affected by hypothermia in a consistent way, but pupillary reaction to light becomes progressively more sluggish as temperatures fall below about 32°C. Eye movement abnormalities were frequent in one series[131] but did not correlate with temperature; they may have reflected the presence of Wernicke's encephalopathy, since they occurred mainly in alcoholic patients.

Deep tendon reflexes are typically normal or even increased at temperatures as low as 29.5°C, but they become progressively diminished at lower temperatures. Extensor plantar responses are rare at any temperature. Increased muscle tone is frequent even in mild hypothermia, and it is universal at temperatures below 29.5°C. Myotonia is common. Focal dystonias and dyskinesias are rare, but patients may exhibit a characteristic posture consisting of flexion in all four limbs, with the limbs held close to the torso.

Even in hypothermic patients who have a stiff neck, examination of the CSF fails to reveal a pleocytosis.[131] Hypothermia produces a fall in CSF pressure because of reduced cerebral blood flow[88,144]; it has also been shown experimentally to reduce CSF secretion in animals.[145] The EEG frequency spectrum changes with hypothermia, with increased beta and theta activity and reduced alpha activity.[146,147] Triphasic waves have been reported in a patient whose rectal temperature was 34°C.[148] At temperatures below 28°C, there is progressive slowing in the record. As the temperature falls further, a burst-suppression pattern appears, and the EEG becomes isoelectric below 10°C to 20°C.[87,88,149] Brainstem auditory evoked potentials (BAEPs) show increasing latencies of waves I, III, and V as temperature decreases.[150] Visual evoked potential (VEP) latencies also increase progressively as temperature declines.[146,151] The changes that occur in electromyographic (EMG) and nerve conduction studies have already been discussed.

Patients who recover from hypothermia usually have no long-term neurological problems.

Systemic Manifestations of Hypothermia

During the shivering phase (typically between 35°C and 30°C) there is an initial rise in metabolic rate and oxygen consumption, but at temperatures below about 30°C shivering ceases and there is a rapid decline in metabolic rate and oxygen consumption.[128,130,132,152,153] As shivering abates, respiration slows and becomes shallow. This is primarily a reflection of reduced respiratory requirements rather than pathologically depressed respiratory drive.[88,128,130,152] Similarly, cardiac output falls with decreasing temperatures, but it is sufficient to meet systemic metabolic requirements. Clinically significant hypotension does not occur until temperatures of 25°C and below are reached.[88,128,130,152] The principal cardiac concern is the risk of arrhythmia. Arrhythmia is preceded by characteristic J-point elevation that appears at about 33°C.[128,130,132,152] The J wave (or "Osborne wave") becomes increasingly prominent as the temperature falls and is consistently present below 25°C. Atrial fibrillation is common below 33°C.[88,130,152] Prolongation of PR and QT intervals occurs, with progressively more advanced degrees of heart block or bradycardia as the temperature continues to fall. Below 28°C the myocardium becomes extremely irritable, and ventricular fibrillation may occur.[88,128,130,132,152]

Hypothermia results in an increase in peripheral vascular resistance and central redistribution of intravascular blood volume. There is consequently a reduction in renal blood flow and glomerular filtration rate.[88,130,152,154] Even so, urine output increases in response to the increased core intravascular volume and also because of blunted response to antidiuretic hormone.[88,130,152,154] The hematocrit may be increased because of hemoconcentration.[130,132,152] Platelet count is reduced and function is impaired, producing a coagulopathy.[130,152,155] Granulocytopenia may occur with temperatures below 28°C.[130,152,155]

Moderate elevations in serum glucose concentration are sometimes seen.[130,152] Endocrine functions generally remain normal. Ileus frequently occurs in hypothermia,[130,152] and asymptomatic pancreatitis is common (based on elevated serum amylase levels and on autopsy findings).[90,156] Hepatic detoxification and conjugation functions are impaired, resulting in prolonged drug half-lives.[88] Because the depressed level of consciousness blunts protective airway reflexes, there is a high incidence of pneumonia.

Patient Management

The management of hypothermia is analogous to the management of hyperthermia. It involves treatment of the underlying cause (when possible), rewarming, and treatment or prevention of common complications.

The comments made previously regarding treatment of hypothalamic and spinal cord pathology causing hyperthermia also apply to hypothermia from these causes. In addition, thiamine should be given routinely to hypothermic patients unless Wernicke's encephalopathy can be excluded with confidence. The spells of some patients with episodic hyperhidrosis and hypothermia have reportedly responded to cyproheptadine, clonidine, anticonvulsants, or peripheral muscarinic blockade with oxybutinin.[58,61,157,158]

With regard to nonneurological causes of hypothermia, naloxone should be routinely administered to hypothermic patients in coma because of the high incidence of drug exposure in this setting and the lack of evidence for any harmful effect of naloxone in hypothermia. Any metabolic derangement predisposing to hypothermia should be corrected. In particular, exogenous thyroxine is usually required in treating myxedema coma[102,138,139]; when it is not given, the mortality rate is high. For patients with dermatological conditions and those without any predisposition to hypothermia other than environmental exposure, treatment of the underlying cause consists of simply drying them and removing them from the cold environment.

There are three rewarming methods: passive external rewarming, active external rewarming, and active central rewarming.[90,128–130,132,152,159–162] *Passive external rewarming* is the slowest and least invasive of these techniques. Patients are placed in a warm environment and covered with blankets, and intravenous fluids are warmed to a temperature of 36°C to 39°C.[152] This technique is usually adequate for patients with a core temperature of 32°C or above as long as the external hypothermic stresses are removed. Caution is necessary in patients who must avoid the cardiovascular stress of shivering, however. Active rewarming may be indicated in such patients; alternatively, shivering can be suppressed by giving meperidine or eliminated by inducing neuromuscular blockade (in patients who are already sedated and receiving mechanical ventilation).

Active external rewarming consists of heating the skin with heating pads, heated blankets, or hot water bottles or by immersion in warm water. Concern has been raised about these methods, however, because warming the skin before the core may result in peripheral vasodilatation and consequent hypotension. It may also cause an abrupt return of blood to the core from relatively hypoperfused regions, resulting in acidosis.

Active central rewarming techniques include the administration of heated oxygen by face mask or endotracheal tube, warm gastric or bladder irrigation, peritoneal lavage, pleural lavage, and hemodialysis or cardiopulmonary bypass with extracorporeal blood rewarming. The most effective of these methods are peritoneal lavage, pleural lavage, and extracorporeal blood rewarming, but these are also the most invasive procedures. In general, they should be reserved for patients with temperatures below 30°C, though decisions in individual cases will be influenced by cardiopulmonary status and underlying disease.

Because aspiration and pneumonia are common complications of hypothermia, all patients with depressed level of consciousness should be intubated. Patients should receive 100 percent oxygen until adequate oxygenation has been documented. Blood gas interpretation is complicated in these patients, be-

cause blood pH increases by 0.015 for each 1°C drop in temperature, while PCO_2 drops by 4.4 percent and PO_2 by 7.2 percent. Thus, if blood is warmed to 37°C before analysis, the measured PCO_2 and PO_2 values will be higher than actually exist in the patient. Even so, the pH and PCO_2 do not need to be corrected for the patient's body temperature.[130,152] Human acid-base regulation changes with falling body temperature to produce an alkaline shift by relative hyperventilation. This adaptation helps to preserve protein and enzyme function as temperatures drop. In effect, the "normal" values of pH and PCO_2 change with falling body temperature in just such a way as to cancel out the changes that occur in anaerobically warmed blood. However, PO_2 must be corrected for body temperature or the value will be overestimated.

Hypotension in hypothermic patients is generally due to dehydration, which, in turn, results from increased urine output. Fluid resuscitation is usually adequate. When it is not, more aggressive rewarming may be necessary, since dobutamine and dopamine have reduced efficacy in this situation and they are arrhythmogenic. Similarly, cardiac arrhythmias in hypothermic patients are resistant to many pharmacological agents, pacing efforts, and defibrillation. Aggressive rewarming techniques may provide the only hope for effective treatment. In particular, electrical defibrillation is usually ineffective at temperatures below 30°C. Lidocaine and procainamide have been of little benefit in this situation, though bretylium may be effective.[130]

Electrolyte concentrations in the blood must be monitored closely and abnormalities managed as necessary. Potassium levels vary greatly during treatment. Treatment may also produce hypophosphatemia. Patients should be assessed for coagulopathy, including DIC, and treated as necessary. A nasogastric tube should be inserted and serum amylase level checked because of the risk of pancreatitis and ileus.

The prognosis in hypothermia is influenced more by the patient's age and underlying disease than by the magnitude of the temperature drop.[129,130,132] Patients have been successfully resuscitated after 2 hours of apparent arrest, and others have survived temperatures below 20°C. This has prompted some to advocate warming all patients to normal temperatures before concluding that resuscitation is futile ("nobody is dead unless they are warm and dead"). While this recommendation puts appropriate emphasis on the marked protective effects of hypothermia, it is probably best to judge each case based on the specific clinical situation.

REFERENCES

1. Cabanac M: Temperature regulation. Annu Rev Physiol 37:415, 1975
2. Boulant JA: Hypothalamic mechanisms in thermoregulation. Fed Proc 40:2843, 1981
3. Ogawa T, Low PA: Autonomic regulation of temperature and sweating. p. 79. In Low PA (ed): Clinical Autonomic Disorders, Evaluation and Management. Little, Brown, Boston, 1993
4. Stitt JT: Neurophysiology of fever. Fed Proc 40:2835, 1981
5. Dinarello CA, Wolff SM: Pathogenesis of fever in man. N Engl J Med 298:607, 1978
6. Hellon R, Townsend Y, Laburn HP, Mitchell D: Mechanisms of fever. p. 19. In Schönbaum E, Lomax P (eds): Thermoregulation: Pathology, Pharmacology and Therapy. Pergamon Press, New York, 1991
7. Hensel H: Thermoreception and Temperature Regulation. (Physiological Society Monographs: No. 38). Academic Press, London, 1981
8. Veale WL, Ruwe WD, Cooper KE: Mechanism of fever and antipyresis. p. 79. In Khogali M, Hales JRS (eds): Heat Stroke and Temperature Regulation. Academic Press Australia, Sydney, 1983
9. Simon HB: Hyperthermia. N Engl J Med 329:483, 1993
10. Dinarello CA, Cannon JG, Wolff SM: New concepts on the pathogenesis of fever. Rev Infect Dis 10:168, 1988
11. Attia M, Khogali M: Set-point shift in thermoregulatory adaptation and heat stroke. p. 65. In Khogali M, Hales JRS (eds): Heat Stroke and Temperature Regulation. Academic Press Australia, Sydney, 1983
12. Hellon RF: Hypothalamic neurons responding to changes in hypothalamic and ambient temperatures. p. 463. In Hardy JD, Gagge AP, Stolwijk JAJ (eds): Physiological and Behavioral Temperature Regulation. Charles C Thomas, Springfield, IL, 1970
13. Thauer R: Thermosensitivity of the spinal cord. p. 472. In Hardy JD, Gagge AP, Stolwijk JAJ (eds): Physiological and Behavioral Temperature Regulation. Charles C Thomas, Springfield, IL, 1970
14. Jessen C: Thermal afferents in the control of body temperature. p. 153. In Schönbaum E, Lomax P (eds): Thermoregulation: Physiology and Biochemistry. Pergamon Press, New York, 1990
15. Kleinebeckel D, Klussmann FW: Shivering. p. 235. In Schönbaum E, Lomax P (eds): Thermoregulation: Physiology and Biochemistry. Pergamon Press, New York, 1990
16. Brück K, Wünnenberg W: "Meshed" control of two effector systems: nonshivering and shivering thermogenesis. p. 562. In Hardy JD, Gagge AP, Stolwijk JAJ (eds): Physiological and Behavioral Temperature Regulation. Charles C Thomas, Springfield, IL, 1970
17. Himms-Hagen J: Brown adipose tissue thermogenesis: role in thermoregulation, energy regulation and obesity. p. 327. In Schönbaum E, Lomax P (eds): Thermoregulation: Physiology and Biochemistry. Pergamon Press, New York, 1990
18. Houdas Y, Ring EFJ: Human Body Temperature: Its Measurement and Regulation. Plenum Press, New York, 1982
19. Grayson J: Responses of the microcirculation to hot and cold environments. p. 221. In Schönbaum E, Lomax P (eds): Thermoregulation: Physiology and Biochemistry. Pergamon Press, New York, 1990
20. Kerslake DM, Cooper KE: Vasodilatation in the hand in response to heating the skin elsewhere. Clin Sci 9: 31, 1950
21. Bryce-Smith R, Coles DR, Cooper KE, et al: The effects of intravenous pyrogen upon the radiant heat induced vasodilatation in man. J Physiol (Lond) 145: 77, 1959
22. Ingall TJ: Hyperthermia and hypothermia. p. 713. In Low PA (ed): Clinical Autonomic Disorders, Evaluation and Management. Little, Brown, Boston, 1993
23. Carmel PW: Vegetative dysfunctions of the hypothalamus. Acta Neurochir (Wien) 75:113, 1985
24. Davison C, Demuth EL: Disturbances in sleep mechanism: a clinicopathologic study: III. Lesions at the diencephalic level (hypothalamus). Arch Neurol Psychiatry 55:111, 1946
25. Erickson TC: Neurogenic hyperthermia (a clinical syndrome and its treatment). Brain 62:172, 1939
26. Bauer HG: Endocrine and other clinical manifestations of hypothalamic disease: a survey of 60 cases, with autopsies. J Clin Endocrinol Metab 14:13, 1954
27. Alpers BJ: Hyperthermia due to lesions in the hypothalamus. Arch Neurol Psychiatry 35:30, 1936
28. Wechsler IS: Hypothalamic syndromes. Br Med J 2: 375, 1956
29. Branch EF, Burger PC, Brewer DL: Hypothermia in a case of hypothalamic infarction and sarcoidosis. Arch Neurol 25:245, 1971
30. Spiro SG, Jenkins JS: Adipsia and hypothermia after subarachnoid haemorrhage. Br Med J 3:411, 1971
31. Johnson RH, Delahunt JW, Robinson BJ: Do thermoregulatory reflexes pass through the hypothalamus?

Studies of chronic hypothermia due to hypothalamic lesion. Aust NZ J Med 20:154, 1990

32. Fox RH, Davies TW, Marsh FP, Urich H: Hypothermia in a young man with an anterior hypothalamic lesion. Lancet 2:185, 1970

33. Harper C: Wernicke's encephalopathy: a more common disease than realised. A neuropathological study of 51 cases. J Neurol Neurosurg Psychiatry 42:226, 1979

34. Haak HR, vanHilten JJ, Roos RAC, Meinders AE: Functional hypothalamic derangement in a case of Wernicke's encephalopathy. Neth J Med 36:291, 1990

35. Philip G, Smith JF: Hypothermia and Wernicke's encephalopathy. Lancet 2:122, 1973

36. Victor M, Adams RD, Collins GH: The Wernicke-Korsakoff Syndrome and Related Neurologic Disorders Due to Alcoholism and Malnutrition. FA Davis, Philadelphia, 1989

37. Gubbay SS, Barwick DD: Two cases of accidental hypothermia in Parkinson's disease with unusual E.E.G. findings. J Neurol Neurosurg Psychiatry 29:459, 1966

38. Appenzeller O, Goss JE: Autonomic deficits in Parkinson's syndrome. Arch Neurol 24:50, 1971

39. Cohen J, Low P, Fealey R, et al: Somatic and autonomic function in progressive autonomic failure and multiple system atrophy. Ann Neurol 22:692, 1987

40. Quinn N: Multiple system atrophy—the nature of the beast. J Neurol Neurosurg Psychiatry special suppl: 78, 1989

41. Baser SM, Meer J, Polinsky RJ, Hallett M: Sudomotor function in autonomic failure. Neurology 41:1564, 1991

42. Lipton JM, Dwyer PE, Fossler DE: Effects of brainstem lesions on temperature regulation in hot and cold environments. Am J Physiol 226:1356, 1974

43. Pledger HG: Disorders of temperature regulation in acute traumatic tetraplegia. J Bone Joint Surg [Br] 44:110, 1962

44. Schmidt KD, Chan CW: Thermoregulation and fever in normal persons and in those with spinal cord injuries. Mayo Clin Proc 67:469, 1992

45. Birzis L, Hemingway A: Descending brain stem connections controlling shivering in cat. J Neurophysiol 19:37, 1956

46. Altus P, Hickman JW, Nord HJ: Accidental hypothermia in a healthy quadriplegic patient. Neurology 35:427, 1985

47. Exton-Smith AN: Accidental hypothermia. Br Med J 4:727, 1973

48. Fealey RD, Low PA, Thomas JE: Thermoregulatory sweating abnormalities in diabetes mellitus. Mayo Clin Proc 64:617, 1989

49. Scott AR, MacDonald IA, Bennett T, Tattersall RB: Abnormal thermoregulation in diabetic autonomic neuropathy. Diabetes 37:961, 1988

50. Dyck PJ: Neuronal atrophy and degeneration predominantly affecting peripheral sensory and autonomic neurons. p. 1065. In Dyck PJ, Thomas PK, Griffin JW, et al (eds): Peripheral Neuropathy. Vol 2. WB Saunders, Philadelphia, 1993

51. Neil HAW, Dawson JA, Baker JE: Risk of hypothermia in elderly patients with diabetes. Br Med J 293:416, 1986

52. Rundles RW: Diabetic neuropathy: general review with report of 125 cases. Medicine (Baltimore) 24:111, 1945

53. Goodman JI: Diabetic anhidrosis. Am J Med 41:831, 1966

54. Sullivan F, Hutchinson M, Bahandeka S, Moore RE: Chronic hypothermia in multiple sclerosis. J Neurol Neurosurg Psychiatry 50:813, 1987

55. Lammens M, Lissoir F, Carton H: Hypothermia in three patients with multiple sclerosis. Clin Neurol Neurosurg 91:117, 1989

56. Gaymard G, Cambon H, Dormont D, et al: Hypothermia in a mesodiencephalic haematoma. J Neurol Neurosurg Psychiatry 53:1014, 1990

57. Shapiro WR, Williams GH, Plum F: Spontaneous recurrent hypothermia accompanying agenesis of the corpus callosum. Brain 92:423, 1969

58. LeWitt PA, Newman RP, Greenberg HS, et al: Episodic hyperhidrosis, hypothermia, and agenesis of corpus callosum. Neurology 33:1122, 1983

59. Thomas DJ, Green ID: Periodic hypothermia. Br Med J 2:696, 1973

60. Fox RH, Wilkins DC, Bell JA, et al: Spontaneous periodic hypothermia: diencephalic epilepsy. Br Med J 2:693, 1973

61. Arroyo HA, DiBlasi AM, Grinszpan GJ: A syndrome of hyperhidrosis, hypothermia, and bradycardia possibly due to central monoaminergic dysfunction. Neurology 40:556, 1990

62. Davison C, Demut EL: Disturbances in sleep mechanism: a clinicopathologic study: IV. Lesions at the mesencephalometencephalic level. Arch Neurol Psychiatry 55:126, 1946

63. Talman WT, Florek G, Bullard DE: A hyperthermic syndrome in two subjects with acute hydrocephalus. Arch Neurol 45:1037, 1988

64. Khurana RK: Autonomic dysfunction in pontomedullary stroke. Ann Neurol 12:86, 1982

65. Wachtel TJ, Steele GH, Day JA: Natural history of fever following seizure. Arch Intern Med 147:1153, 1987

66. Aminoff MJ, Simon RP: Status epilepticus: causes,

clinical features and consequences in 98 patients. Am J Med 69:657, 1980

67. Britt BA: Malignant hyperthermia—a review. p. 179. In Schönbaum E, Lomax P (eds): Thermoregulation: Pathology, Pharmacology and Therapy. Pergamon Press, New York, 1991

68. Gronert GA: Malignant hyperthermia. p. 1763. In Engel AG, Banker BQ (eds): Myology: Basic and Clinical. McGraw-Hill, New York, 1986

69. Schiller HH: Chronic viral myopathy and malignant hyperthermia. N Engl J Med 292:1409, 1975

70. Frank JP, Harati Y, Butler IJ, et al: Central core disease and malignant hyperthermia syndrome. Ann Neurol 7:11, 1980

71. Oka S, Igarashi Y, Takagi A, et al: Malignant hyperpyrexia and Duchenne muscular dystrophy: a case report. Can Anaesth Soc J 29:627, 1982

72. Wedel DJ: Malignant hyperthermia and neuromuscular disease. Neuromus Disord 2:157, 1992

73. Caroff SN, Mann SC: Neuroleptic malignant syndrome. Med Clin North Am 77:185, 1993

74. Figà-Talamanca L, Gualandi C, DiMeo L, et al: Hyperthermia after discontinuance of levodopa and bromocriptine therapy: impaired dopamine receptors a possible cause. Neurology 35:258, 1985

75. Toru M, Matsuda O, Makiguchi K, Sugano K: Neuroleptic malignant syndrome-like state following a withdrawal of antiparkinsonian drugs. J Nerv Ment Dis 169:324, 1981

76. Joyner RW: Temperature effects on neuronal elements. Fed Proc 40:2814, 1981

77. Bénita M, Condé H: Effects of local cooling upon conduction and synaptic transmission. Brain Res 36:133, 1972

78. Buchthal F, Rosenfalck A: Evoked action potentials and conduction velocity in human sensory nerves. Brain Res 3:1, 1966

79. Kaeser HE: Nerve conduction velocity measurements. p. 116. In Vinken PJ, Bruyn GW (eds): Handbook of Clinical Neurology. Vol 7. North Holland, Amsterdam, 1970

80. Halar EM, DeLisa JA, Soine TL: Nerve conduction studies in upper extremities: skin temperature corrections. Arch Phys Med Rehabil 64:412, 1983

81. Bolton CF, Sawa GM, Carter K: The effects of temperature on human compound action potentials. J Neurol Neurosurg Psychiatry 44:407, 1981

82. Buchthal F, Pinelli P, Rosenfalck P: Action potential parameters in normal human muscle and their physiological determinants. Acta Physiol Scand 32:219, 1954

83. Dobin NB, Neymann CA, Osborne SL: Pathologic changes in the central nervous system resulting from experimentally produced hyperpyrexia. J Neuropathol Exp Neurol 8:295, 1949

84. Nemoto EM, Frankel HM: Cerebral oxygenation and metabolism during progressive hyperthermia. Am J Physiol 219:1784, 1970

85. Meyer JS, Handa J: Cerebral blood flow and metabolism during experimental hyperthermia (fever). Minn Med 50:37, 1967

86. Carlsson C, Hägerdal M, Siesjö BK: The effect of hyperthermia upon oxygen consumption and upon organic phosphates, glycolytic metabolites, citric acid cycle intermediates and associated amino acids in rat cerebral cortex. J Neurochem 26:1001, 1976

87. Michenfelder JD: Anesthesia and the Brain: Clinical, Functional, Metabolic, and Vascular Correlates. Churchill Livingstone, New York, 1988

88. Blair E: Clinical Hypothermia. McGraw-Hill, New York, 1964

89. Tanimoto M, Okada Y: The protective effect of hypothermia on hippocampal slices from guinea pig during deprivation of oxygen and glucose. Brain Res 417:239, 1987

90. Duguid H, Simpson RG, Stowers JM: Accidental hypothermia. Lancet 2:1213, 1961

91. Sutton JR: Hyperthermia and temperature regulation. p. 237. In Arieff AI, Griggs RC (eds): Metabolic Brain Dysfunction in Systemic Disorders. Little, Brown, Boston, 1992

92. Knochel JP: Heat stroke and related heat stress disorders. DM 35:301, 1989

93. Clowes GHA, O'Donnell TF: Heat stroke. N Engl J Med 291:564, 1974

94. Malamud N, Haymaker W, Custer RP: Heat stroke: a clinico-pathologic study of 125 fatal cases. Milit Surg 99:397, 1946

95. Lind AR: Pathophysiology of heat exhaustion and heat stroke. p. 179. In Khogali M, Hales JRS (eds): Heat Stroke and Temperature Regulation. Academic Press Australia, Sydney, 1983

96. Curley FJ, Irwin RS: Disorders of temperature control: Part 2. Hyperthermia. p. 674. In Rippe JM, Irwin RS, Alpert JS, Fink MP (eds): Intensive Care Medicine. 2nd Ed. Little, Brown, Boston, 1991

97. Khogali M: Heat stroke: an overview. p. 1. In Khogali M, Hales JRS (eds): Heat Stroke and Temperature Regulation. Academic Press Australia, Sydney, 1983

98. Low PA, Fealey RD, Sheps SG, et al: Chronic idiopathic anhidrosis. Ann Neurol 18:344, 1985

99. Murakami K, Sobue G, Terao S, Mitsuma T: Acquired idiopathic generalized anhidrosis: a distinctive clinical syndrome. J Neurol 235:428, 1988

100. Buchwald I, Davis PJ: Scleroderma with fatal heat stroke. JAMA 201:270, 1967

101. Pandolf KB, Griffin TB, Munro EH, Goldman RF: Persistence of impaired heat tolerance from artificially induced miliaria rubra. Am J Physiol 239:R226, 1980

102. Gavin LA: Thyroid crises. Med Clin North Am 75: 179, 1991
103. Simon HB, Daniels GH: Hormonal hyperthermia: endocrinologic causes of fever. Am J Med 66:257, 1979
104. Shibolet S, Lancaster MC, Danon Y: Heat stroke: a review. Aviat Space Environ Med 47:280, 1976
105. Clark WG, Lipton JM: Drug-related heatstroke. p. 125. In Schönbaum E, Lomax P (eds): Thermoregulation: Pathology, Pharmacology and Therapy. Pergamon Press, New York, 1991
106. Tek D, Olshaker JS: Heat illness. Emerg Med Clin North Am 10:299, 1992
107. Plum F, Posner JB: The Diagnosis of Stupor and Coma. 3rd Ed. FA Davis, Philadelphia, 1980
108. Al-Khawashki MI, Mustafa MKY, Khogali M, El-Sayed H: Clinical presentation of 172 heat stroke cases seen at Mina and Arafat—September, 1982. p. 99. In Khogali M, Hales JRS (eds): Heat Stroke and Temperature Regulation. Academic Press Australia, Sydney, 1983
109. Shapiro Y, Seidman DS: Field and clinical observations of exertional heat stroke patients. Med Sci Sports Exerc 22:6, 1990
110. Salem SN: Neurological complications of heat-stroke in Kuwait. Ann Trop Med Parasitol 60:393, 1966
111. Freeman W, Dumoff E: Cerebellar syndrome following heat stroke. Arch Neurol Psychiatry 51:67, 1944
112. Freedman DA, Schenthal JE: A parenchymatous cerebellar syndrome following protracted high body temperature. Neurology 3:513, 1953
113. Mehta AC, Baker RN: Persistent neurological deficits in heat stroke. Neurology 20:336, 1970
114. Lin J, Chang M, Sheu Y, et al: Permanent neurologic deficits in heat stroke. Chin Med J (Taipei) 47:133, 1991
115. Bull JM, Lees D, Schuette W, et al: Whole body hyperthermia: a phase-I trial of a potential adjuvant to chemotherapy. Ann Intern Med 90:317, 1979
116. Minassian DC, Mehra V, Jones BR: Dehydrational crises from severe diarrhoea or heatstroke and risk of cataract. Lancet 1:751, 1984
117. Simon RP: Management of status epilepticus. p. 137. In Pedley TA, Meldrum BS (eds): Recent Advances in Epilepsy. Churchill Livingstone, Edinburgh, 1985
118. Bristow G, Patel L: Hyperthermia. p. 858. In Hall JB, Schmidt GA, Wood LDH (eds): Principles of Critical Care. McGraw-Hill, New York, 1992
119. Coons DJ, Hillman FJ, Marshall RW: Treatment of neuroleptic malignant syndrome with dantrolene sodium: a case report. Am J Psychiatry 139:944, 1982
120. Goekoop JG, Carbaat PAT: Treatment of neuroleptic malignant syndrome with dantrolene. Lancet 2:49, 1982
121. Daoudal P, Delacour JL: Treatment of neuroleptic malignant syndrome with dantrolene. Lancet 2:217, 1982
122. Granato JE, Stern BJ, Ringel A, et al: Neuroleptic malignant syndrome: successful treatment with dantrolene and bromocriptine. Ann Neurol 14:89, 1983
123. Mueller PS, Vester JW, Fermaglich J: Neuroleptic malignant syndrome: successful treatment with bromocriptine. JAMA 249:386, 1983
124. Dhib-Jalbut S, Hesselbrock R, Brott T, Silbergeld D: Treatment of the neuroleptic malignant syndrome with bromocriptine. JAMA 250:484, 1983
125. Zubenko G, Pope HG: Management of a case of neuroleptic malignant syndrome with bromocriptine. Am J Psychiatry 140:1619, 1983
126. McCarron MM, Boettger ML, Peck JJ: A case of neuroleptic malignant syndrome successfully treated with amantadine. J Clin Psychiatry 43:381, 1982
127. Costrini A: Emergency treatment of exertional heatstroke and comparison of whole body cooling techniques. Med Sci Sports Exerc 22:15, 1990
128. Reuler JB: Hypothermia: pathophysiology, clinical settings, and management. Ann Intern Med 89:519, 1978
129. Fitzgerald FT, Jessop C: Accidental hypothermia: a report of 22 cases and review of the literature. Adv Intern Med 27:127, 1982
130. Curley FJ, Irwin RS: Disorders of temperature control: Part 1. Hypothermia. p. 658. In Rippe JM, Irwin RS, Alpert JS, Fink MP (eds): Intensive Care Medicine. 2nd Ed. Little, Brown, Boston, 1991
131. Fischbeck KH, Simon RP: Neurological manifestations of accidental hypothermia. Ann Neurol 10:384, 1981
132. Paton BC: Accidental hypothermia. p. 397. In Schönbaum E, Lomax P (eds): Thermoregulation: Pathology, Pharmacology and Therapy. Pergamon Press, New York, 1991
133. Stoner HB: Mechanism of body temperature changes after burns and other injuries. Ann NY Acad Sci 150: 722, 1968
134. Moncrief JA: Burns. N Engl J Med 288:444, 1973
135. Krook G: Hypothermia in patients with exfoliative dermatitis. Acta Derm Venereol (Stockh) 40:142, 1960
136. Grice KA, Bettley FR: Skin water loss and accidental hypothermia in psoriasis, ichthyosis, and erythroderma. Br Med J 4:195, 1967
137. Magnusson B: Exfoliative dermatitis with hypothermia. Acta Derm Venereol (Stockh) 40:161, 1960
138. Forester CF: Coma in myxedema. Arch Intern Med 111:734, 1963
139. Angel JH, Sash L: Hypothermic coma in myxoedema. Br Med J 1:1855, 1960

140. Davidson M, Grant E: Accidental hypothermia: a community hospital perspective. Postgrad Med 70: 42, 1981

141. Strauch BS, Felig P, Baxter JD, Schimpff SC: Hypothermia in hypoglycemia. JAMA 210:345, 1969

142. Fay T, Smith GW: Observations on reflex responses during prolonged periods of human refrigeration. Arch Neurol Psychiatry 45:215, 1941

143. Holtzman DM, Simon RP: Neurologic manifestatiosn of hypothermia. p. 217. In Arieff AI, Griggs RC (eds): Metabolic Brain Dysfunction in Systemic Disorders. Little, Brown, Boston, 1992

144. Rosomoff HL: Hypothermia and the central nervous system. p. 253. In Dripps RD (ed): The Physiology of Induced Hypothermia. National Academy of Sciences—National Research Council, Washington, DC, 1956

145. Fenstermacher JD, Li C, Levin VA: Extracellular space of the cerebral cortex of normothermic and hypothermic cats. Exp Neurol 27:101, 1970

146. FitzGibbon T, Hayward JS, Walker D: EEG and visual evoked potentials of conscious man during moderate hypothermia. Electroencephalogr Clin Neurophysiol 58:48, 1984

147. McQueen JD: Effects of cold on the nervous system. p. 243. In Dripps RD (ed): The Physiology of Induced Hypothermia. National Academy of Sciences—National Research Council, Washington, DC, 1956

148. Reutens DC, Dunne JW, Gubbay SS: Triphasic waves in accidental hypothermia. Electroencephalogr Clin Neurophysiol 76:370, 1990

149. Pagni CA, Courjon J: Electroencephalographic modifications induced by moderate and deep hypothermia in man. Acta Neurochir Suppl (Wien) 13:35, 1964

150. Markand ON, Lee BI, Warren C, et al: Effects of hypothermia on brainstem auditory evoked potentials in humans. Ann Neurol 22:507, 1987

151. Russ W, Kling D, Loesevitz A, Hempelmann G: Effect of hypothermia on visual evoked potentials (VEP) in humans. Anesthesiology 61:207, 1984

152. Keamy MF, Hall J: Hypothermia. p. 848. In Hall JB, Schmidt GA, Wood LDH (eds): Principles of Critical Care. McGraw-Hill, New York, 1992

153. Horvath SM, Spurr GB: Effects of hypothermia on general metabolism. p. 8. In Dripps RD (ed): The Physiology of Induced Hypothermia. National Academy of Sciences—National Research Council, Washington, DC, 1956

154. Moyer JH, Morris GC, DeBakey ME: Renal functional response to hypothermia and ischemia in man and dog. p. 199. In Dripps RD (ed): The Physiology of Induced Hypothermia. National Academy of Sciences—National Research Council, Washington, DC, 1956

155. Villalobos TJ, Adelson E, Riley P: The effect of hypothermia on platelets and white cells in dogs. p. 186. In Dripps RD (ed): The Physiology of Induced Hypothermia. National Academy of Sciences—National Research Council, Washington, DC, 1956

156. Maclean D, Murison J, Griffiths PD: Acute pancreatitis and diabetic ketoacidosis in accidental hypothermia and hypothermic myxoedema. Br Med J 4:757, 1973

157. LeWitt P: Hyperhidrosis and hypothermia responsive to oxybutynin. Neurology 38:506, 1988

158. Sanfield JA, Linares OA, Cahalan DD, et al: Altered norepinephrine metabolism in Shapiro's syndrome. Arch Neurol 46:53, 1989

159. Bohn DJ: Treatment of hypothermia: in the hospital. p. 286. In Sutton JR, Houston CS, Coates G (eds): Hypoxia and Cold. Praeger, New York, 1987

160. Paton BC: Accidental hypothermia—update 1988. p. 444. In Schönbaum E, Lomax P (eds): Thermoregulation: Pathology, Pharmacology and Therapy. Pergamon Press, New York, 1991

161. Weinberg AD: Hypothermia. Ann Emerg Med 22: 370, 1993

162. Jolly BT, Ghezzi KT: Accidental hypothermia. Emerg Med Clin North Am 10:311, 1992

49

The Neurology of Aging

Richard K. Olney

The diagnosis of neurological disease requires the recognition of symptoms and signs that are not present in normal individuals of comparable age. The clinician's diagnostic acumen is especially challenged when he or she is confronted with a patient over 65 years of age, because the phenomenology of numerous normal age-related changes that occur in the nervous system differs more quantitatively than qualitatively from certain common neurological diseases of older individuals. This chapter reviews the normal age-related changes that occur in the findings on neurological examination and certain common neurological diseases that are associated with aging, emphasizing their distinguishing features.

AGE-RELATED CHANGES IN THE FINDINGS ON NEUROLOGICAL EXAMINATION

Normal age-related changes are defined as progressive and irreversible changes in the neurological examination that develop with advancing age in most individuals without overt disease. These changes are observed with variable frequency and severity depending on the study design and the rigor with which associated diseases are excluded. With regard to study design, cross-sectional studies tend to magnify the frequency and severity of age-related changes, in part because it is difficult to exclude the increasingly common effects of associated diseases and differences in

social, educational, and environmental factors. Longitudinal studies minimize age-related effects, in part because long-term follow-up is more readily attained in those individuals who maintain normal function and because subjects who develop overt disease are later excluded. Thus, although they are described with variable magnitude and frequency, there are a number of important changes in the normal neurological examination with advancing age.[1,2]

Decline in Cognitive Function

The normal age-related decline in cognitive function has been characterized with increasing accuracy and precision over the past three decades. Since the late nineteenth century, measures of intelligence have been identified that reach a peak in young adulthood and then decline throughout the remainder of life.[3] In the 1950s, intelligence quotients (IQs) derived from the Wechsler Adult Intelligence Scale (WAIS) were interpreted to support this belief, because performance IQs declined more than 40 percent and verbal IQs decreased half as much with increasing age from the late twenties to the early seventies. Subsequently, the effect of slower motor responses on timed performance tasks and the confounding influence of cohort differences were recognized as factors that cause an overestimation of the measured age-related decline in intelligence in cross-sectional studies.[3] Longitudinal studies have generally demonstrated stability rather than decline in verbal intelligence prior to the age of 60 years.[4] Verbal intelligence often declines thereafter by an average of less than 5 percent through the seventh decade and by less than 10 percent through the eighth decade.[4] Cognitive function is even relatively stable in most individuals during the ninth decade.[5]

With regard to specific aspects of cognitive function that decline with aging, the influence of speed on successful completion of the task is an important consideration. Apart from slowness of movements (discussed below), the speed of central processing is reduced with advancing age. This can be demonstrated neuropsychologically as slowness of perceptual processing and neurophysiologically as a delay in event-related evoked potentials. Slowness of perceptual processing, dissociated from motor response time, has been most convincingly shown with backward masking experiments. If paired stimuli are presented sufficiently close together that the second stimulus blocks perception of the first, backward masking is said to have occurred. In this type of experiment, the speed of central perceptual processing can also be separated from peripheral processing by delivering target and masking visual stimuli to opposite eyes.[6] When comparing subjects in their sixties with those in their late teens, the interstimulus interval necessary to prevent such backward masking is increased by 20 to 30 percent.[6] Recent experiments with visual word identification have shown that this slowness of processing does not develop abruptly in old age but occurs continuously with aging from the third through the eighth decades of life.[7] Other experimental studies demonstrate similar degrees of slowing for processing of language and information and longer retrieval time for information from short- and long-term memory.[8-11]

Reduction in the speed of central processing with advancing age can also be demonstrated neurophysiologically. An event-related evoked potential is the electrocerebral activity that occurs in response to the information content of a specified signal or event. These potentials are often recorded as the response evoked by an infrequent auditory signal that is inserted at random into a sequence of more frequent auditory signals of a different pitch. The event-related evoked response occurs between 200 and 500 ms after the infrequent auditory signal, and attention is usually directed at the peak of the positive waveform at around 300 ms (the P300). The mean latency for this component is around 300 ms in the third decade of

life. Thereafter, as reflected in several recent studies, the latency increases by 9 to 17 ms per decade with aging, so that the mean latency is 350 to 380 ms by the age of 70 years.[12] Thus, both neurophysiological and neuropsychological investigations support the general concept that the speed of central processing is reduced with advancing age.

Mild memory impairment is another specific aspect of cognitive function that declines with advancing age. Although slowness of central processing underlies many aspects of the measured age-related decline in cognitive function, the deficit in recent memory and learning can be demonstrated apart from processing speed with untimed supraspan learning tasks. A supraspan is an amount of information just beyond that which can be recalled immediately from the working memory. An example of a supraspan memory test is serial digit learning, in which a subject is given 12 trials to learn and recall eight or nine digits in a standardized but untimed protocol. Published normative data for this test reflects mild impairment in recent memory and learning in older individuals, with subjects aged 65 to 74 years generally scoring 10 percent lower than younger subjects with similar educational backgrounds.[13] As recently reviewed, memory impairment with aging can be demonstrated for speed of search in short-term memory, memory span, list recall, paired associated recall, and prose recall.[11]

The terms *benign senescent forgetfulness* and *age-associated memory impairment* were coined in recognition that the mild impairment in memory with normal aging is distinct from early dementia. This is manifest clinically as difficulty in retrieving the name of a vague acquaintance, remembering to buy every needed item at the grocery store without a list, or recalling where an object was placed—rather than as difficulty in remembering significant personal events. Such common complaints of the elderly are due more to decreased learning than to increased forgetfulness. In evaluating the memory function of 161 community-dwelling, cognitively normal individuals ranging in age from 62 to 100 years, learning or acquisition of memory for pictures and words declined uniformly with advancing age; however, delayed recall or forgetfulness was similar at all ages if adjusted for number of initially learned objects.[14] This reinforces the observation that preservation of delayed recall discriminates normal older individuals from those with mild dementia better than other cognitive attributes among a large battery of neuropsychological tests.[15,16]

Thus it is generally agreed that there is an age-related decline in the speed of central processing, performance on timed tasks, and recent memory and learning, whereas verbal intelligence is well preserved at least through the seventies. Several short, standardized tests are available which are clinically useful for distinguishing these normal age-related changes in cognitive function from mild dementia. Two of the more commonly used tests are the Mini-Mental State and the six-item Orientation-Memory-Concentration Test.[17-19] The Mini-Mental State tests language and praxis in addition to memory, and thus contains items that have low sensitivity in distinguishing normal aging from early dementia.[20-22] The six-item Orientation-Memory-Concentration Test was derived from questions on the 26-item Blessed Dementia Scale and has been shown to correlate with the density of neuritic plaques at autopsy.[17] It is especially useful in differentiating normality from mild dementia.[17,19] On this test, normal subjects ranging in age from 67 to 93 years score 6 or fewer out of 24 possible errors, with their errors usually involving the memory phase that contains a name and address; however, normal subjects remain oriented to time of day, month, and year, and retain normal concentration for the ability to count backward from 20 and name the months backward.[17]

Changes in Cranial Nerve Function

Changes in the cranial nerve examination relate primarily to an age-related decline in sensory functions, especially for vision and hearing.[23-30] With regard to vision, contrast sensitivity and visual acuity decline with advancing age.[23,24] The pupils become progressively smaller with age and are less reactive to light and accommodation, reducing the amount of light that reaches the retina.[24,25] Increasing opacity of the lens and vitreous further decreases the visual input, and increasing rigidity of the lens reduces its accommodative ability.[24-26] These preretinal and retinal factors are the major causes of presbyopia.

A restriction in the range of eye movements, especially vertically, develops with advancing age.[25,27] Whereas young adults normally have 35° to 45° of upgaze, 15° to 20° of upgaze is normal in those in their eighth decade.[25] When limited upgaze and diminished visual acuity are combined with decreased mobility of the neck, vision above the horizontal may be functionally impaired (e.g., with loss of ability to read signs mounted high on the walls or hung from the ceiling).[28]

Presbycusis is produced by a progressive elevation of the auditory threshold, especially for higher frequencies. This produces a decline in speech discrimination, because high-frequency perception is important for the recognition of many consonants.[29] Loss of hair cells in the organ of Corti, thickening of the basilar membrane, atrophy of the stria vascularis, degeneration of cells in the spiral ganglion, and degeneration of neurons in the cochlear nuclei have all been implicated in presbycusis.[29,30] However, the primary lesion seems to be the degeneration of hair cells, as this is the most severe and consistent abnormality.[30]

Changes in the Findings on Examination of the Motor System

A progressive decline in the bulk and strength of muscles and in the speed and coordination of movement has long been recognized as an accompaniment of aging. The muscular wasting occurs diffusely but is most notable in intrinsic hand and foot muscles.[25] In cross-sectional studies, strength consistently and progressively declines with increasing age.[31-33] In one comprehensive cross-sectional study of 61 normal men ranging in age from 20 to 80 years, the maximal force that could be exerted by various arm and leg muscles decreased across the age range by 21 to 45 percent, with hip extension showing the greatest decline.[31] As expected from previously discussed design considerations, diminished strength with advancing age is less prominent in longitudinal studies but still quite apparent.[32] Grip strength did not decline in only 15 percent of subjects over the age of 60 years during this recently published 9-year longitudinal study.[32] Declining strength and progressive loss of muscle mass accompany each other with advancing age, but the loss of muscle bulk is insufficient to explain the degree of decreased strength.[32,33]

The pathophysiology of this mild generalized weakness is multifactorial, but a neurogenic basis is of prime importance. Electromyographic studies have consistently shown features of chronic partial denervation with reinnervation as the usual accompaniment of advancing age.[34] Neuropathological studies on muscle biopsies of normal elderly subjects are consistently but mildly abnormal. Features of neurogenic change (fiber type grouping and grouped atrophy) are far more prominent in most studies than other features, such as those of disuse, fibrosis, and myopathic change (type II atrophy, increased numbers of central nuclei, and other nonspecific features of myopathy).[35] The mild but widespread neurogenic component of these generalized changes in muscle is largely due to a mild amount of anterior horn cell degeneration.[35]

In addition to strength, the speed and coordination of movements decline with advancing age.[25] Thus it has been shown that the speed of simple tasks (e.g., hand and foot tapping) slows by 20 to 24 percent from ages 20 to 80, and coordination for the manipulation of small objects and for tracking decreases by 14 to 27 percent.[31] Activities of daily living (e.g., putting on a shirt, zipping a garment, and rising from a chair) required 31 to 40 percent more time in older individuals.[31] On the routine neurological examination, these changes are manifest as mild bradykinesia with all motor tasks and as mild incoordination without dysmetria on the finger-to-nose and heel-to-shin tests.

Changes in Station and Gait

The station and gait show conspicuous changes with advancing age.[25,36] Both are dependent on adequate sensory input, efficient integration of this input with motor control programming, and an adequate motor response.[25,36] In a comprehensive cross-sectional study of the normal changes that occur in neurological function with aging, the single greatest change among the 128 tests occurred in the ability to maintain balance on one leg with the eyes closed. Whereas most young adults could maintain station under these conditions for the full test time of 30 seconds, few older subjects could perform the task for more than a few seconds.[31] Although increased postural sway with various tests of station is virtually universal with advanced age,[31,37–40] postural righting reflexes are preserved in most older subjects.[38,39] Increased postural sway correlates well with diminished sensation in the legs but not with visual or vestibular changes with age.[37] In addition to increased postural sway, dynamic posturography demonstrates a diminished capacity to process conflicting sensory input with aging.[40]

Although changes in gait among the elderly are well recognized,[25,36] quantitation of these changes has been difficult. Timing tandem-walking without support for a specified distance[31]; quantifying the variability in step length, stride width, and stride time[41]; and other techniques have not been successful in objectively quantitating the normal age-related change in walking. Qualitatively, the normal gait of an octogenarian is usually described with the same adjectives as are used to describe a parkinsonian gait.[25] Thus the gait is slightly broadened and the steps mildly shortened, with a modest diminution in the arm swing and a slightly stooped posture. However, this type of gait was found in fewer than half of 181 subjects with a mean age of 80 years in one study.[42] Applying a multivariate analysis of stride length, walking speed, vibratory sensitivity at the ankle, and the degree of spine anteroflexion, three groups were found. Half of the elderly subjects fell into one group with normal results on all measurements. The other half had reduced stride length and walking speed but were equally divided between two patterns. One of these groups had vibratory impairment with erect posture, while the other had the parkinsonian pattern of a flexed posture without impairment of vibratory sensitivity.[42]

Changes in Tendon Reflexes and the Sensory System

The most prominent age-related change in the findings on sensory examination is a decrease in the sensitivity of vibratory perception, especially distally in the legs.[25,31,43] Although vibratory threshold is elevated by 52 to 58 percent at 80 years compared with 20 years at the clavicle, shoulder, and elbow, the change is 64 to 67 percent at the tibia and wrist, 86 percent at the ankle, and 97 percent at the toe.[31] A less prominent distal diminution in the perception of painful and tactile stimuli is described in some but not other cross-sectional studies.[25,31,43]

Changes in the deep tendon reflexes are similar to those described for vibration, with a mild generalized reflex depression and a more marked depression or absence of the Achilles tendon reflex. The reported prevalence of absent ankle reflexes in individuals over the age of 65 years is usually less than 20 percent when

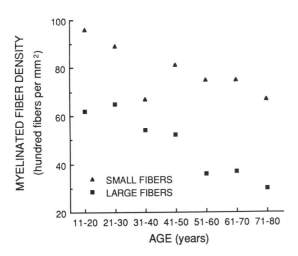

Fig. 49-1 Fiber density of large and small myelinated axons in human sural nerve at different ages. (Data derived from Tohgi and colleagues.[47]).

observations are made on active, healthy individuals living in the community.[27,44,45] Although absent Achilles tendon reflexes are observed in a few individuals over 70 years, depression of the ankle relative to the knee reflex is more common and was observed in nearly all subjects in one study.[44]

This distal depression of deep tendon reflexes and sensory function is primarily due to distal degeneration of sensory axons. The most striking electrophysiological change with advancing age is a reduction in the amplitude of sensory nerve action potentials, which correlates with a loss of sensory axons.[46] Neuropathologically, degeneration of both myelinated and unmyelinated sensory fibers has been identified with advancing age in sural nerve biopsies (Fig. 49-1).[47–49] The average 80-year-old has about one-half the number of large myelinated axons in the sural nerve as a 20-year-old.[47] Similar axonal degeneration has been described in mixed sensorimotor nerves.

Reappearance of Release Signs

Although the reappearance of release signs may support the concept that a loss of cortical suppression has occurred, the prevalence of these signs in normal individuals is important to recognize. Although considered a release sign, the palmomental reflex is present in 20 to 27 percent of adults between the ages of 20 and 50 years,[50] and its prevalence is 20 to 60 percent in patients aged from 60 to 93 years.[50–53] The snout reflex may similarly be present in 13 percent of adults aged from 40 to 57 years and in up to 54 percent of subjects over the age of 60 years.[50–53] The suck reflex may be elicited in 5 percent of normal subjects aged over 65 years,[27] but the grasp reflex was rarely observed in normal subjects.[27,51,53] Thus a positive palmomental, snout, or even suck reflex should be interpreted with caution, because these reflexes may be observed in normal individuals. Only the reappearance of the grasp reflex is a reliable sign that more cortical suppression has been lost than is normal for age.

Pathological Reflexes

An extensor plantar response is not a normal age-related change in the neurological examination but reflects some underlying pathology. There are occasional reports of this sign in small numbers (less than 5 percent) of "normal" subjects. However, such patients generally have other neurological abnormalities (e.g., incontinence or cognitive impairment), suggesting that the extensor plantar responses are of pathological significance and that the subjects have underlying neurological disease.

Senile Tremor

A patient with an essential tremor typically presents to medical attention during middle life, although a similar tremor may also develop with advanced age and is frequently labeled a senile tremor. This tremor often causes a fine titubation of the head as well as an action tremor in the arms. Although essential tremor during middle life usually has a frequency of about 10 Hz, senile tremor and the lower-amplitude physiological tremor often have a frequency of about 6 Hz in subjects over the age of 60 years.

NEUROLOGICAL DISEASES THAT ARE COMMON WITH AGING

Alzheimer's Disease and Vascular Dementia

Alzheimer's disease is a dementia with insidious onset and progression that usually occurs in middle or late life. The diagnosis can be definitively confirmed only by histopathological examination of the brain. The disease was initially described in a 51-year-old woman by Alzheimer in 1907 and was considered a presenile dementia for the first half of this century. However, a broader definition that is independent of age has become accepted.[54] Based upon clinical or pathological criteria or both, the incidence of Alzheimer's disease is 123 per 100,000 per year in adults over the age of 29 years, with the incidence of dementia of all types being 187 per 100,000 per year.[55] However, the incidence of Alzheimer's disease increases exponentially with advancing age at least through the ninth decade, so that the incidence at 80 years is 100 times greater than at 50 years.[55] The prevalence of Alzheimer's disease increases from 1 to 15 percent from 65 to 85 years of age, and more than half of the residents of nursing homes have this disease.[56]

Clinical criteria for the diagnosis of *probable* Alzheimer's disease have been proposed by the Work Group on the Diagnosis of Alzheimer's Disease, established by the National Institute of Neurological and Communicative Disorders and Stroke (NINCDS) and the Alzheimer's Disease and Related Disorders Association (ADRDA).[57] Dementia of any type is diagnosed clinically by behavioral changes that include a decline in memory and other cognitive functions. The clinical diagnosis of dementia cannot be made while an alteration in the level of consciousness is present because drowsiness and agitation interfere with the assessment of cognitive function. If the patient is alert, possible decline in cognitive function is determined by comparing the present and previous levels of performance as well as by neurological and neuropsychological examinations. Specifically, deficits in two or more areas of cognition must be established, and progressive worsening of memory and other cognitive functions must be documented. Impaired recall of recently learned material is usually the first sign of an early dementia.[14–16] Neuropsychological examinations are important to document objectively that two or more areas of function are impaired quantitatively to a greater extent than normal for age and that these cognitive deficits are progressive over time. The Mini-Mental State and the Blessed Dementia Scale are two specifically recommended tests that may be used clinically to aid in this determination.[17–19] The Blessed Dementia Scale or a shorter derived form of it, the six-item Orientation-Memory-Concentration Test, are particularly useful in identifying a mildly demented patient.[17,19] The estimate of severity of dementia based on either of the Blessed tests also correlates with the number of neuritic plaques documented neuropathologically, so either of these tests has utility in staging the severity of dementia.[17] The Mini-Mental State examination is particularly useful in staging the severity of dementia, because it assesses language and praxis in addition to memory, and its scores correlate well with the neuropathological estimates of synaptic density in the frontal lobes.[20,58–60]

More extensive neuropsychological testing is important for documentation of the range and severity of cognitive impairment in the clinical setting of an early or uncertain diagnosis and in research studies. The Consortium to Establish a Registry for Alzheimer's Disease (CERAD) was developed to identify and standardize the most efficient battery of neuropsychological tests.[20] As they had previously shown, impairment of delayed recall was verified as the most sensitive measure to distinguish early dementia from normal aging, but measures of learning and memory were not useful in staging the severity of dementia.[61] Combined measurements of fluency, praxis, and recognition memory best differentiated mild from moderate or severe dementia.[61]

Once the presence of dementia is documented, other criteria for the clinical diagnosis of probable Alzheimer's disease include an insidious onset between the ages of 40 and 90 years and the absence of systemic disorders or other brain diseases than in and of themselves may account for the progressive deficits in memory and cognition.[54,57] The diagnosis is further supported by documentation of impairment in activities of daily living and alteration in behavioral patterns. A positive family history is obtained in about 5 percent of cases. Laboratory tests are important to confirm other specific causes for dementia. Normal cerebrospinal fluid (CSF), an electroencephalogram (EEG) that is either normal or shows nonspecific abnormalities, and evidence for cerebral atrophy with computed tomographic (CT) scanning or magnetic resonance imaging (MRI) are supportive of probable Alzheimer's disease.

Neuropathologically, neuronal cell loss is present in the brains of patients with Alzheimer's disease relative to age-matched controls,[62] and this loss is primarily seen in the large neurons that have cross-sectional areas of more than 90 μm^2.[56,60] Furthermore, this neuronal cell loss is particularly seen in the cholinergic cells of the nucleus basalis and the serotonergic cells of the raphe.[60] However, the degree of cognitive impairment correlates better with the reduction of synaptic density in the frontal lobes than with the decrease in neuronal count or the accumulation of amyloid plaques.[58–60] Despite recognition of these observations, measurement of neuritic plaques and neurofibrillary tangles remains the routine basis for pathological confirmation of Alzheimer's disease.

The diagnosis of *definite* Alzheimer's disease requires confirmation of the characteristic neuropathological features, which primarily consist of an abnormal number of neuritic plaques (Fig. 49-2) and neurofibrillary tangles (Fig. 49-3). Although often present in small numbers in normal elderly subjects, numerous neuritic plaques and neurofibrillary tangles are present in Alzheimer's disease (Fig. 49-4),[63,64] The necessary brain sites in which the pathognomonic neuritic plaques and neurofibrillary tangles must exist to confirm the diagnosis are less uniformly accepted.[63,64] Whereas some neuropathologists require only lesions in the hippocampus, others demand involvement of the neocortex with or without hippo-

campal lesions. The frequency of pathological confirmation of the clinical diagnosis of probable Alzheimer's disease, based upon the NINCDS-ADRDA criteria, has been studied. In 57 cases, an increased concentration of plaques and tangles was found more often in the hippocampus than in the neocortex of cases with probable Alzheimer's disease; an increased number of lesions was never found in the neocortex without a concomitant increase in the hippocampus.[64] The clinical diagnostic criteria proposed by the NINCDS-ADRDA Work Group resulted in pathological confirmation in 84 to 100 percent of cases with examination of the hippocampus.[63,64]

Whereas pure Alzheimer's disease accounts for 50 to 60 percent of cases, multi-infarct dementia is the second most frequent cause of dementia and is the primary pathology in 10 to 20 percent of cases.[54,56] The two disorders coexist in another 10 to 20 percent of cases.[54,56] Recently the concept of multi-infarct dementia has been expanded to include a broader array of vascular disease that is capable of producing dementia.[65,66] When such a broader definition of vascular dementia is utilized, Alzheimer's disease and vas-

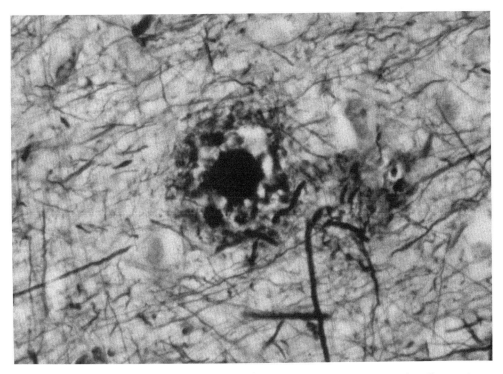

Fig. 49-2 Neuritic plaque with central core of amyloid protein. (Bielschowsky silver stain, original ×250, photographically enlarged ×2.) (Courtesy of Dr. M. F. Gonzales.)

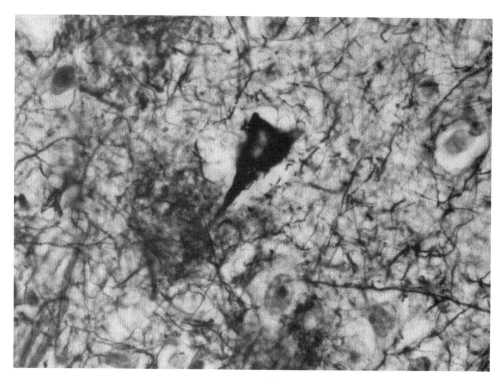

Fig. 49-3 Neurofibrillary tangle. (Bielschowsky silver stain, original ×250, photographically enlarged ×2.) (Courtesy of Dr. M. F. Gonzales.)

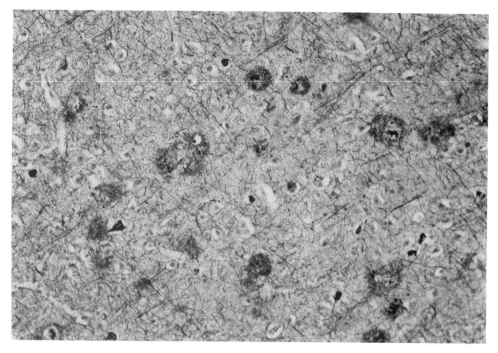

Fig. 49-4 Numerous neuritic plaques and neurofibrillary tangles in advanced Alzheimer's disease. (Bielschowsky silver stain, original ×100.) (Courtesy of Dr. M. F. Gonzales.)

cular dementia have similar age-specific prevalences under the age of 80 years, but Alzheimer's disease has a higher prevalence in older ages.[67] The criteria for vascular dementia that were proposed at an International Workshop sponsored by National Institute of Neurological Disorders and Stroke (NINDS) and the Association Internationale pour la Recherche et l'Enseignement en Neurosciences (AIREN) are listed in Table 49-1.[66] Clinical criteria for probable vascular dementia are the presence of dementia, the presence of cerebrovascular disease, and a temporal relationship between the two. Dementia is diagnosed in a manner similar to that for Alzheimer's disease. The diagnosis of cerebrovascular disease requires the presence of focal neurological signs and abnormal brain imaging that supports vascular disease. The findings on brain imaging may consist of multiple large-vessel infarcts, a single strategically placed infarct (e.g., involving the angular gyrus, thalamus, or basal forebrain), multiple lacunae, extensive periventricular white matter lesions, or combinations of these. The temporal relationship may consist of onset of dementia within 3 months following a recognized stroke or of a course that is not insidiously progressive. The criteria for definite vascular dementia include the preceding probable clinical criteria and pathological confirmation of vascular and no other disease.

In recent years, the relationship between dementia and white matter lesions that are seen on CT scans or MRI has been clarified. Such white matter lesions do correlate with cognitive impairment if they are large or confluent, but are not relevant to dementia if they are less extensive.[66,68–70] Furthermore, the prevalence of small white matter lesions in patients with Alzheimer's disease is not significantly different from that in age-matched healthy control subjects if both groups are screened equally to exclude cerebrovascular disease risk factors.[71] Not surprisingly, then, in a neuropathological study, the exclusion of only those cases with vascular lesions larger than 50 ml from pure Alzheimer's disease produced the highest agreement with the clinical diagnosis of probable Alzheimer's disease by the NINCDS-ADRDA criteria (88 percent accuracy).[64]

The pathophysiology of dementia of the Alzheimer's type remains uncertain, but Alzheimer's disease may represent a syndrome in which the cumulative effects of one or more different pathophysiologies converge to produce a consistent clinical picture.[60] In some individuals, the predominant pathophysiology may involve a molecular genetic abnormality, such as a point mutation in the amyloid precursor protein. In others, abnormalities of tau protein or mitochondrial function may be more relevant to loss of synaptic density on cholinergic cells of the nucleus basalis or serotonergic cells of the raphe. Treatment strategies may have to be multifactorial and individualized for each patient. Recently, the US Food and Drug Administration has approved the release of the first drug shown to be beneficial for symptomatic treatment of some patients with Alzheimer's disease. Tacrine, a reversible inhibitor of butylcholinesterase and acetylcholinesterase, may modestly improve cognitive function and functional activities in some patients.[72] Treatments that alter the course of the disease have not yet been developed, but future efforts may involve use of nerve growth factor or drugs that inhibit

Table 49-1 Criteria Proposed for the Diagnosis of Vascular Dementia

I. Criteria for *probable* vascular dementia—all of the following:
  1. Dementia
  2. Cerebrovascular disease
    a. Focal neurological signs
    b. Abnormal brain imaging—one or more of the following:
      i. Multiple large-vessel infarcts
      ii. Single strategically placed infarct
      iii. Multiple lacunae
      iv. Extensive periventricular white matter lesions
  3. A relationship between the dementia and the cerebrovascular disease
    a. Onset of dementia within 3 months following a recognized stroke
    b. Abrupt deterioration in cognitive function or fluctuating, stepwise progression of cognitive deficits

II. Criteria for *definite* vascular dementia—all of the following:
  1. Clinical criteria for probable vascular dementia
  2. Histopathological evidence of cerebrovascular disease (biopsy or autopsy)
  3. Absence of neurofibrillary tangles and neuritic plaques exceeding those expected for age
  4. Absence of other clinical or pathological disorder capable of producing dementia

(Based on recomendations of Roman and colleagues.[66])

excitatory amino acids or the production of amyloid.[73]

Metabolic Encephalopathy

Metabolic encephalopathy is a diffuse but potentially reversible disorder of cerebral function that often impairs the state of arousal and cognitive function and is due to a metabolic or toxic cause. When such a metabolic disturbance develops acutely, an alteration in arousal with either drowsiness or agitation is common. This state alerts the clinician that evaluation of metabolic factors may be etiologically important and at the same time precludes the diagnosis of dementia. However, when the metabolic disturbance develops insidiously over weeks or months, arousal is often not affected. Metabolic encephalopathy may then be difficult to distinguish from dementia. Furthermore, the two disorders commonly coexist in the elderly. When they are coexistent, chronic metabolic encephalopathy is the remediable aspect of cognitive impairment in an insidiously developing dementia.

The incidence of metabolic encephalopathy in 200 elderly outpatients with suspected dementia has been studied prospectively with follow-up of outcome.[74] The patients had a mean age of 76 years, with a range from 60 to 94 years; more than 89 percent lived in the community, either alone or with a relative. Whereas Alzheimer's disease was diagnosed clinically in 75 percent, a total of 248 medical diagnoses were made in 124 of the 200 patients, and more than 30 percent had more than one condition contributing to their dementia-like presentation. Metabolic encephalopathy was the primary reason for cognitive impairment in 18 patients. It resulted from adverse drug reactions (10 patients), hypothyroidism (3), hyperparathyroidism (2), hyponatremia (2), and hypoglycemia (1). Even after excluding depression, 45 of the 200 patients experienced cognitive improvement for 1 month or longer due to treatment of the identified medical condition.[74]

Adverse drug reactions as the cause of cognitive impairment were the focus of a subsequent report by the same group.[75] Of 308 elderly patients, 35 were identified who had cognitive impairment for over 3 months without alteration in the level of arousal and who improved with discontinuation of the causal drug. The most common offending drugs were benzodiazepines (13 patients), other sedative or tranquilizing drugs (9), antihypertensives (5), and cimetidine (3). The patients with these adverse drug reactions took an average of twice the number of prescription drugs as the others (an average of four versus two).

Parkinson's Disease

This section reviews those aspects of Parkinson's disease that deserve special consideration in the elderly; it is not intended to be a comprehensive review.

The average annual incidence of Parkinson's disease is about 20 per 100,000, or about one-sixth of that for Alzheimer's disease.[76,77] In contrast to the incidence of Alzheimer's disease, which increases throughout life,[55] the incidence of Parkinson's disease increases with advancing age until it reaches a peak at around the age of 75 years.[76,77] Although the incidence of Parkinson's disease is lower during the ninth than during the eighth decade,[76,77] the prevalence continues to increase through the ninth decade, since long-term survival is common.[76,77] The mortality rate of patients with Parkinson's disease who are treated with levodopa is only slightly greater than that of age- and sex-matched controls,[76] with early levodopa treatment having a significant effect in lowering the mortality rate.[78]

Although a considerable number of elderly subjects have a slow, shuffling gait with a stooped posture,[42,79] these parkinsonian features are not considered adequate by many clinicians to establish the diagnosis of Parkinson's disease in the elderly.[80,81] A resting tremor, rigidity, and an exaggerated glabellar reflex or a definite beneficial response to levodopa, or both, are usually necessary to diagnose Parkinson's disease with confidence.[80,81] The tremor due to Parkinson's disease may also be different in the elderly than in younger adults. There is often a 4- to 6-Hz postural tremor that has an amplitude greater than any resting tremor in the untreated elderly patient with Parkinson's disease,[82] in contrast to a 4- to 6-Hz postural tremor without a resting component in the elderly with a normal physiological tremor. Otherwise, the features of Parkinson's disease are similar in the elderly and in the middle-aged adult.

The treatment of Parkinson's disease requires special consideration in the elderly, primarily due to the greater sensitivity of elderly patients to adverse drug reactions. Confusion is a major side effect of anticholinergic medications, especially in the elderly with preexisting minor cognitive impairment. Constipation in both sexes and urinary retention in men are two other frequent side effects of anticholinergic medications. Hallucinations, delusions, and chorea are often dose-limiting side effects of dopaminergic medications, especially in the elderly, whether levodopa or dopamine agonists are prescribed. In contrast to the anticholinergic medications, the dosage of dopaminergic treatment can usually be adjusted to provide functional improvement with fewer adverse effects. Thus, treatment of Parkinson's disease in the elderly often requires the slow introduction and careful adjustment of levodopa/carbidopa therapy and avoidance of anticholinergic drugs.[83]

Nonparkinsonian Gait Disorders

Various gait disorders are seen in elderly patients.[36,42] One general pattern is associated with decreased arm swing and other signs of bradykinesia. Some patients with this general pattern of gait disorder also have the specific, previously discussed, diagnostic features of Parkinson's disease or Alzheimer's disease. However, a large number of elderly patients with this gait disturbance lack these specific diagnostic features, leaving a nonspecific bradykinetic senile gait as the presumptive diagnosis by exclusion.[42,79] The distinction between this nonspecific bradykinetic senile gait and a mildly parkinsonian-appearing "normal" gait is largely based upon clinical experience and judgment.

A second type of disorder is the cautious gait.[36] In some series, this is the most common pattern.[36] Patients with a cautious gait do not hesitate to initiate walking, but do so slowly, with a short stride and a normal or slightly broadened base. Although turns are en bloc, the normal cadence and quick initiation of walking distinguish this from the previous pattern.

A third pattern is a gait with ataxia or disequilibrium.[36,42] This gait may be associated with other signs of cerebellar, posterior column, or peripheral nerve disease. However, elderly patients often have falls and an ataxic gait that is associated with decreased proprioception and vibratory perception but not with other signs of a specific neurological disease.[42] Thus

classification of an abnormal senile gait may be difficult even in a patient with frequent falls.[72]

Peripheral Neuropathy

The distinction of polyneuropathy, especially distal axonal polyneuropathy, from normal age-related changes that occur in the peripheral nervous system is often a quantitative one.[84] Normal changes with aging do not produce positive symptoms (e.g., paresthesias or dysesthesias) or significant negative symptoms (e.g., weakness that interferes with activities of daily living). Although distal sensory impairment for vibration and depressed or absent Achilles tendon reflexes are often found in normal elderly subjects, the development of a painless pressure sore on a foot or bilateral partial footdrop indicates a severity of distal axonal degeneration that is far greater than normal for age. Diabetes mellitus is the most common cause of distal axonal polyneuropathy in the elderly, as it is in middle-aged and younger adults.[85–87] Alcoholic and nutritional deficiency polyneuropathies are also common causes, as observed in two series that were restricted to polyneuropathy in elderly patients.[86,87]

Orthostatic Hypotension

Orthostatic hypotension is present in 10 to 30 percent of subjects over the age of 65 years if defined as a decline of more than 20 mmHg in systolic pressure and 10 mmHg in diastolic pressure for more than 1 minute.[88] A significant factor underlying this increasing frequency of orthostatic hypotension may be diminution in baroreceptor sensitivity with advancing age.[89] The elderly not only have less reduction in heart rate in response to pressor drugs[89] but also a blunted increase in heart rate with standing even in the absence of hypotension.[90] In addition to blunting of the autonomic response as a predisposing factor to orthostatic hypotension, compensatory mechanisms that restrict volume depletion are also impaired in the elderly.[91]

Syncope becomes more common with advancing age, and orthostatic hypotension is a common cause. However, this diagnosis is accepted only when postural changes in blood pressure can be demonstrated by examination. Further discussion of autonomic function in the elderly is provided in Chapter 8.

Falls

Injuries are the sixth most common reason for death in subjects over the age of 75 years, with falls accounting for most of these injuries.[92] Falls are responsible for nearly 10,000 deaths and approximately 200,000 hip fractures annually in the United States among patients over the age of 65 years.[92] When a fall at home causes a hip fracture, placement in a nursing home at discharge from the hospital is commonly a permanent move.[93] Thus falls in the elderly have a special significant as a cause of morbidity and mortality and as a sign of impending loss of independence.

The potential etiologies for falls include a large number of differential diagnostic possibilities. Syncope due to orthostatic hypotension is one identifiable cause. Although one series estimates an incidence of nearly 20 percent, most large series document postural hypotension in only 3 to 4 percent of patients with a history of recent falls.[94] Although other causes account for some of the other 5 to 15 percent of patients with syncope, impairment of station and gait for any reason is implicated as the most common cause of falls.[95] Additional risk factors for falls include cognitive impairment, loss of vision, and peripheral neuropathy.[96-98]

Hypothermia and Hyperthermia

The ability to maintain thermal homeostasis diminishes as age increases, with hypothermia recognized as a cause of death nearly twice as often as hyperthermia.[99] Hypothermia is defined as a core body temperature below 35°C. Annual mortality from hypothermia increases from 1.3 per million between the ages of 15 and 24 years to 23.1 per million over the age of 74 years.[99] In the elderly, both heat production and heat conservation are impaired.[99,100] The basal metabolic rate and the ability to produce heat through shivering and other muscular activity become lower with advancing age.[99] Likewise, the ability to conserve heat is diminished through a decreased ability to vasoconstrict peripherally.[100]

Hyperthermia is defined as a core temperature above 41.1°C—or above 40.7°C with anhidrosis or altered mental status. Impairment of heat loss in a warm environment is the cause of hyperthermia.[99] Inadequate sweating was often implicated in earlier studies, but more recent studies provide evidence that reduced peripheral vasodilatation is more important than diminished sweating.[101,102] Further discussion of this topic is provided in Chapter 48.

Sleep Disorders

The pattern of daily sleep normally changes with advancing age.[103] Typically, elderly subjects report a shorter nocturnal sleep duration with more frequent arousals during the night and earlier awakening in the morning, but they also nap more frequently in the daytime. Polysomnography indicates that normal elderly subjects have a marked decrease in stage IV sleep time, a moderate reduction in total sleep and rapid eye movement (REM) sleep times, and more frequent nocturnal awakenings. Non-REM and REM sleep cycles are similar to those of young adults except for a shorter first cycle due to the reduction in stage IV sleep. Thus normal sleep in the elderly may be described as having a weaker monophasic circadian rhythm.

Disorders of sleep are common in the elderly.[103] Because these disorders do not differ in elderly and younger subjects, the reader is referred to Chapter 25 for a review of sleep disorders in general. Two aspects, however, warrant particular consideration in the elderly. First, the possible effect of an enforced cycle must be considered in evaluating a complaint of insomnia or excessive daytime drowsiness in the institutionalized elderly patient. Nursing home environments typically require all patients to retire and awaken on a predetermined schedule. Although this strong environmental pattern successfully induces synchronized circadian rhythms in most of the population, such synchronization may be difficult for some individuals, resulting in complaints of disordered sleep. Second, although the sleep apnea syndrome is among the most common causes for excessive daytime somnolence, sleep-disordered breathing is common in normal elderly subjects, and different criteria need to be defined for the diagnosis of sleep apnea in older patients. The sleep apnea syndrome may be diagnosed in young adults when five or more apneic or hypopneic episodes occur during one night. However, 27 percent of healthy, asymptomatic subjects over 60 years of age have five or more such episodes of sleep-disordered breathing per night.[104] Furthermore, elderly subjects with and without sleep-disordered breathing are similar in terms of daytime alertness and cognitive function.[104]

OTHER NEUROLOGICAL DISEASES

The epidemiology of many neurological diseases changes with advancing age. Cerebrovascular disease becomes particularly common with advancing age. Because discussion of these disorders is provided in standard neurological textbooks, they are not considered here.

REFERENCES

1. Katzman R, Terry R (eds): The Neurology of Aging. FA Davis, Philadelphia, 1983
2. Tallis R (ed): The Clinical Neurology of Old Age. John Wiley & Sons, Chichester, England, 1989
3. Parker KCH: Changes with age, year-of-birth cohort, age by year-of-birth cohort interaction, and standardization of the Wechsler Adult Intelligence Tests. Hum Dev 29:209, 1986
4. Schaie KW, Hertzog C: Fourteen-year cohort-sequential analyses of adult intellectual development. Dev Psychol 19:531, 1983
5. Johansson B, Zarit SH, Berg S: Changes in cognitive functioning of the oldest old. J Gerontol 47:P75, 1992
6. Walsh DA: Age differences in central perceptual processing: a dichoptic backward masking investigation. J Gerontol 31:178, 1976
7. Madden DJ: Four to ten milliseconds per year: age-related slowing of visual word identification. J Gerontol 47:P59, 1992
8. Bowles NL, Poon LW: Aging and retrieval of words in semantic memory. J Gerontol 40:71, 1985
9. Madden DJ: Age-related slowing in the retrieval of information from long-term memory. J Gerontol 40:208, 1985
10. Wingfield A, Poon LW, Lombardi L, Lowe D: Speed of processing in normal aging: effects of speech rate, linguistic structure, and processing time. J Gerontol 40:579, 1985
11. Verhaeghen P, Marcoen A, Goossens L: Facts and fiction about memory aging: a quantitative integration of research findings. J Gerontol 48:P157, 1993
12. Goodin DS: Event-related (endogenous) potentials. p. 627. In Aminoff MJ (ed): Electrodiagnosis in Clinical Neurology. 3rd Ed. Churchill Livingstone, New York, 1992
13. Benton AL, Hamsher K deS, Varney NR, Spreen O: Contributions to Neuropsychological Assessment: A Clinical Manual. Oxford University Press, New York, 1983
14. Petersen RC, Smith G, Kokmen E, et al: Memory function in normal aging. Neurology 42:396, 1992
15. Grober E, Buschke H, Crystal H, et al: Screening for dementia by memory testing. Neurology 38:900, 1988
16. Welsh K, Butters N, Hughes J, et al: Detection of abnormal memory decline in mild cases of Alzheimer's disease using CERAD neuropsychological measures. Arch Neurol 48:278, 1991
17. Katzman R, Brown T, Fuld P, et al: Validation of a short orientation-memory concentration test of cognitive impairment. Am J Psychiatry 140:734, 1983
18. Giordani B, Boivin MJ, Hall AL, et al: The utility and generality of Mini-Mental State Examination scores in Alzheimer's disease. Neurology 40:1894, 1990
19. Pittman J, Andrews H, Tatemichi T, et al: Diagnosis of dementia in a heterogeneous population. Arch Neurol 49:461, 1992
20. Morris JC, Heyman A, Mohs RC, et al: The Consortium to Establish a Registry for Alzheimer's Disease (CERAD): Part I. Clinical and neuropsychological assessment of Alzheimer's disease. Neurology 39:1159, 1989
21. Feher EP, Mahurin RK, Doody RS, et al: Establishing the limits of the Mini-Mental State: examination of 'subtests.' Arch Neurol 49:87, 1992
22. Braekhus A, Laake K, Engedal K: The Mini-Mental State Examination: identifying the most efficient variables for detecting cognitive impairment in the elderly. J Am Geriatr Soc 40:1139, 1992
23. Scialfa CT, Garvey PM, Tyrrell RA, Leibowitz HW: Age differences in dynamic contrast thresholds. J Gerontol 47:P172, 1992
24. Chisholm I: Visual failure. In Tallis R (ed): The Clinical Neurology of Old Age. John Wiley & Sons, Chicheter, England, 1989
25. Wolfson LI, Katzman R: The neurologic consultation at age 80. p. 221. In Katzman R, Terry R (eds): The Neurology of Aging. FA Davis, Philadelphia, 1983
26. Wright BE, Henkind P: Aging changes and the eye. p. 149. In Katzman R, Terry R (eds): The Neurology of Aging. FA Davis, Philadelphia, 1983
27. Benassi G, D'Alessandro R, Gallassi R, et al: Neurological examination in subjects over 65 years: an epidemiological survey. Neuroepidemiology 9:27, 1990
28. Hutton JT, Shapiro I, Christians B: Functional significance of restricted upgaze. Arch Phys Med Rehabil 63:617, 1982

29. Mader S: Hearing impairment in elderly persons. J Am Geriatr Soc 32:548, 1984

30. Souceck S, Michaels L, Frohlich A: Evidence for hair cell degeneration as the primary lesion in hearing loss of the elderly. J Otolaryngol 15:175, 1986

31. Potvin AR, Syndulko K, Tourtellotte WW, et al: Human neurologic function and the aging process. J Am Geriatr Soc 28:1, 1980

32. Kallman DA, Plato CC, Tobin JD: The role of muscle loss in the age-related decline of grip strength: cross-sectional and longitudinal perspectives. J Gerontol 45:M82, 1990

33. Overend TJ, Cunningham DA, Kramer JF, et al: Knee extensor and knee flexor strength: cross-sectional area ratios in young and elderly men. J Gerontol 47:M204, 1992

34. Howard JE, McGill KC, Dorfman LJ: Age effects on properties of motor unit action potentials: ADEMG analysis. Ann Neurol 24:207, 1988

35. Hubbard BM, Squier M: The physical ageing of the neuromuscular system. p. 3. In Tallis R (ed): The Clinical Neurology of Old Age. John Wiley & Sons, Chichester, England, 1989

36. Nutt JG, Marsden CD, Thompson PD: Human walking and higher-level gait disorders, particularly in the elderly. Neurology 43:268, 1993

37. Brockelhurst JC, Robertson D, James-Groom P: Clinical correlates of sway in old age—sensory modalities. Age Ageing 11:1, 1982

38. Weiner WJ, Nora LM, Glantz RH: Elderly inpatients: postural reflex impairment. Neurology 34:945, 1984

39. Era P, Hiekkinen E: Postural sway during standing and unexpected disturbance of balance in random samples of men of different ages. J Gerontol 40:287, 1985

40. Wolfson L, Whipple R, Derby CA, et al: A dynamic posturography study of balance in healthy elderly. Neurology 42:2069, 1992

41. Gabell A, Nayak USL: The effect of age on variability in gait. J Gerontol 39:662, 1984

42. Delwaide PJ, Delmotte P: Distinct patterns of senile gait revealed by multiparametric analysis. Neurology 38, suppl 1:289, 1988

43. Kenshalo DR: Somesthetic sensitivity in young and elderly humans. J Gerontol 41:732, 1986

44. Olney RK, Bromberg S, Baumbach NJ: Age-related changes in monosynaptic reflex function. Muscle Nerve 6:529, 1983

45. Impallomeni M, Kenny RA, Flynn MD, et al: The elderly and their ankle jerks. Lancet 1:670, 1984

46. Taylor PK: Non-linear effects of age on nerve conduction in adults. J Neurol Sci 66:223, 1984

47. Tohgi H, Tsukagoshi H, Toyokura Y: Quantitative changes with age in normal sural nerves. Acta Neuropathol (Berl) 38:213, 1977

48. Jacobs JM, Love S: Qualitative and quantitative morphology of human sural nerve at different ages. Brain 108:897, 1985

49. Vital A, Vital C, Rigal B, et al: Morphological study of the aging human peripheral nerve. Clin Neuropathol 9:10, 1990

50. Jacobs L, Gossman MD: Three primitive reflexes in normal adults. Neurology 30:184, 1980

51. Koller WC, Glatt S, Wilson RS, Fox JH: Primitive reflexes and cognitive function in the elderly. Ann Neurol 12:302, 1982

52. Jenkyn LR, Reeves AG, Warren T, et al: Neurologic signs in senescence. Arch Neurol 42:1154, 1985

53. Galasko D, Kwo-on-Yuen PF, Klauber MR, Thal LJ: Neurological findings in Alzheimer's disease and normal aging. Arch Neurol 47:625, 1990

54. Friedland RP: Alzheimer's disease: clinical features and differential diagnosis. Neurol 43, suppl 4:S45, 1993

55. Schoenberg BS, Kokmen E, Okazaki H: Alzheimer's disease and other dementing illnesses in a defined United States population: incidence rates and clinical features. Ann Neurol 22:724, 1987

56. Katzman R: Alzheimer's disease. N Engl J Med 314:964, 1986

57. McKhann G, Drachman D, Folstein M, et al: Clinical diagnosis of Alzheimer's disease: report of the NINCDS-ADRDA Work Group under the auspices of Department of Health and Human Services Task Force on Alzheimer's Disease. Neurology 34:949, 1984

58. Terry RD, Masliah E, Salmon DP, et al: Physical basis of cognitive alterations in Alzheimer's disease: synapse loss is the major correlate of cognitive impairment. Ann Neurol 30:572, 1991

59. DeKofsky ST, Scheff SW: Synapse loss in frontal cortex biopsies in Alzheimer's disease: correlation with cognitive severity. Ann Neurol 27:457, 1990

60. Blass JP: Pathophysiology of Alzheimer's syndrome. Neurology 43, suppl 4:S25, 1993

61. Welsh KA, Butters N, Hughes JP, et al: Detection and staging of dementia in Alzheimer's disease. Arch Neurol 49:448, 1992

62. Terry RD, DeTeresa R, Hansen LA: Neocortical cell counts in normal human adult aging. Ann Neurol 21:530, 1987

63. Morris JC, McKeel DW, Fulling K, et al: Validation of clinical diagnostic criteria for Alzheimer's disease. Ann Neurol 24:17, 1988

64. Tierney MC, Fisher RH, Lewis AJ, et al: The NINCDS-ADRDA Work Group criteria for the clini-

cal diagnosis of probable Alzheimer's disease: a clinicopathologic study of 57 cases. Neurology 38:359, 1988

65. Chui HC, Victoroff JI, Margolin D, et al: Criteria for the diagnosis of ischemic vascular dementia proposed by the State of California Alzheimer's disease diagnostic and treatment centers. Neurology 42:473, 1992

66. Roman GC, Tatemichi TK, Erkinjuntti T, et al: Vascular dementia: diagnostic criteria for research studies. Neurology 43:250, 1993

67. Rocca WA, Hofman A, Brayne C, et al: The prevalence of vascular dementia in Europe: facts and fragments from 1980–1990 studies. Ann Neurol 30:817, 1991

68. van Swieten JC, Geyskes GG, Derix MMA, et al: Hypertension in the elderly is associated with white matter lesions and cognitive decline. Ann Neurol 30: 825, 1991

69. Boone KB, Miller BL, Lesser IM, et al: Neuropsychological correlates of white-matter lesions in healthy elderly subjects. Arch Neurol 49:549, 1992

70. Ylikoski R, Ylikoski A, Erkinjuntti T, et al: White matter changes in healthy elderly persons correlates with attention and speed of mental processing. Arch Neurol 50:818, 1993

71. Kozachuk WE, DeCarli C, Schapiro MB, et al: White matter hyperintensities in dementia of Alzheimer's type and in healthy subjects without cerebrovascular risk factors. Arch Neurol 47:1306, 1990

72. Schneider LS: Clinical pharmacology of aminoacridines in Alzheimer's disease. Neurology 43, suppl 4: S64, 1993

73. Davis KL, Haroutunian V: Strategies for the treatment of Alzheimer's disease. Neurology 43, suppl 4: S52, 1993

74. Larson EB, Reifler BV, Sumi SM, et al: Diagnostic evaluation of 200 elderly outpatients with suspected dementia. J Gerontol 40:536, 1985

75. Larson EB, Kukull WA, Buchner D, Reifler BV: Adverse drug reactions associated with global cognitive impairment in elderly persons. Ann Intern Med 107: 169, 1987

76. Rajput AH, Offord KP, Beard M, Kurland LT: Epidemiology of parkinsonism: incidence, classification, and mortality. Ann Neurol 16:278, 1984

77. Schoenberg B: Descriptive epidemiology of Parkinson's disease: disease distribution and hypothesis formulation. Adv Neurol 45:277, 1986

78. Diamond SG, Markham CH, Hoehn MM, et al: Multi-center study of Parkinson mortality with early versus later dopa treatment. Ann Neurol 22:8, 1987

79. Koller WC, Glatt SL, Fox JH: Senile gait: a distinct neurologic entity. Clin Geriatr Med 1:661, 1985

80. Newman RP, LeWitt PA, Jaffe M, et al: Motor function in the normal aging population: treatment with levodopa. Neurology 35:571, 1985

81. Koller W, O'Hara R, Weiner W, et al: Relationship of aging to Parkinson's disease. Adv Neurol 45:317, 1986

82. Griffiths RA, Dalziel JA, Sinclair KGA, et al: Tremor and senile parkinsonism. J Gerontol 36:170, 1981

83. Aminoff MJ: Parkinson's disease in the elderly: current management strategies. Geriatrics 42:31, 1987

84. Olney RK: Age-related changes in peripheral nerve function. Geriatr Med Today 4:76, 1985

85. Olney RK: Diseases of peripheral nerve. p. 171. In Tallis R (ed): The Clinical Neurology of Old Age. John Wiley & Sons. Chichester, England, 1989

86. Huang CY: Peripheral neuropathy in the elderly: a clinical and electrophysiologic study. J Am Geriatr Soc 29:49, 1981

87. George J, Twomey JA: Causes of polyneuropathy in the elderly. Age Ageing 15:247, 1986

88. Robbins AS, Rubenstein LZ: Postural hypotension in the elderly. J Am Geriatr Soc 32:769, 1984

89. Low PA, Opfer-Gehrking TL, Proper CJ, Zimmerman I: The effect of aging on cardiac autonomic and postganglionic sudomotor function. Muscle Nerve 13:152, 1990

90. White NJ: Heart-rate changes on standing in elderly patients with orthostatic hypotension. Clin Sci 58: 411, 1980

91. Lye M: Autonomic dysfunction and abnormal vascular reflexes. p. 191. In Tallis R (ed): The Clinical Neurology of Old Age. John Wiley & Sons, Chichester, England, 1989

92. Baker SP, Harvey AH: Fall injuries in the elderly. Clin Geriatr Med 1:501, 1985

93. Keene JS, Anderson CA: Hip fractures in the elderly: discharge predictions with a functional rating scale. JAMA 248:564, 1982

94. Lipsitz LA: Abnormalities in blood pressure homeostasis that contribute to falls in the elderly. Clin Geriatr Med 1:637, 1985

95. Issacs B: Clinical and laboratory studies of falls in old people. Clin Geriatr Med 1:513, 1985

96. Nevitt MC, Cummings SR, Hudes ES: Risk factors for injurious falls: a prospective study. J Gerontol 46: M164, 1991

97. Lord SR, Clark RD, Webster IW: Physiological factors associated with falls in an elderly population. J Am Geriatr Soc 39:1194, 1991

98. Richardson JK, Ching C, Hurvitz EA: The relation-

ship between electromyographically documented peripheral neuropathy and falls. J Am Geriatr Soc 40: 1008, 1992

99. Lybarger JA, Kilbourne EM: Hyperthermia and hypothermia in the elderly: an epidemiologic review. p. 149. In Davis BB, Wood WG (eds): Homeostatic Function and Aging. Raven Press, New York, 1985

100. Jennings JR, Reynolds CF, Houck PR, et al: Age and sleep modify finger temperature responses to facial cooling. J Gerontol 48:M108, 1993

101. Sagawa S, Shiraki K, Yousef MK, Miki K: Sweating and cardiovascular responses of aged men to heat exposure. J Gerontol 43:M1, 1988

102. Evans E, Rendell M, Bartek J, et al: Thermally-induced cutaneous vasodilatation in aging. J Gerontol 48:M53, 1993

103. Prinz PN, Vitiello MV, Raskind MA, Thorpy MJ: Geriatrics: sleep disorders and aging. N Engl J Med 323:520, 1990

104. Berry DTR, Phillips BA, Cook YR, et al: Sleep-disordered breathing in healthy aged persons: possible daytime sequelae. J Gerontol 42:620, 1987

Index

Page numbers followed by f indicate figures; those followed by t indicate tables

Lyme disease. *See* Lyme neuroborreliosis
Lyme neuroborreliosis, 695–700
    causative organism of, 696–697
    clinical features of, 695–696, 697–698
    diagnosis of, 698–699
      serological tests for, 698–699
    treatment of, 699–700
Lymphoma. *See also* Hodgkin's disease
    Burkitt's, neurological manifestations of,
      232–233
    neurological manifestations of, 231–232
    primary intracerebral, neurological mani-
      festations of, 233f, 233–234,
      313–314, 768
Lymphomatous meningitis, in AIDS, 762,
    762t

M

McLeod's syndrome, 223
Macroglobulinemia, neurological manifesta-
    tions of, 230–231
Magnesium, disturbances of, 327–328
Magnetic resonance imaging (MRI). *See also*
    individual disorders
    in AIDS dementia, 764
    of brain abscess, 678f, 679
    of cardiogenic embolism, 78
    in cerebral infarction, 124, 125, 128f
    of cerebral mycotic aneurysm, 104–105
    in chemotherapy-induced encephalopa-
      thy, 428, 431f
    contrast media for, neurological complica-
      tions of, 880
    in cysticercosis, 626
    in diabetes insipidus, 386
    in intracranial hemorrhage, 130
    myelographic procedures of, neurological
      complications of, 882
    neurological complications of, 881–882
    for outcome prediction in cardiac arrest,
      170
    of progressive multifocal leukoen-
      cephalopathy, 742f, 742–743
    radiation damage and, 435, 436f, 437
    of spinal epidural abscess, 683, 684f
    in subdural empyema????, 681
    in toxoplasmosis, 765, 766f, 819
    in trichinosis, 829
    in tuberculous meningitis, 708
    of tuberous sclerosis, 207, 208f
Malabsorption
    congenital folate, 221
    hypomagnesemia and, 328
    of vitamin B$_{12}$, 294
    vitamin D deficiency and, 295
    vitamin E deficiency and, 295

in Whipple's disease, 263
Malaria, cerebral, 811, 813f, 813–816,
    814f
Malignant hyperpyrexia, iatrogenic,
    608–609
Malignant hyperthermia, neurological causes
    of, 934
Manganese intoxication, 645, 656
Manic psychoses, 479
Man-in-the-barrel syndrome, 165
Manometry, anal, 526
Marantic endocarditis. *See* Nonbacterial
    thrombotic endocarditis
Marchiafava-Bignami disease, 259, 296–297,
    618
Marcus-Gunn phenomenon, 747
Marfan's syndrome, 44
Marijuana, abuse, neurological complications
    of, 634
Masturbation, 546, 547, 550
Mayo Clinic muscle strength grading system,
    357t
MDEA (3,4-methylenedioxyethylam-
    phetamine), 637
MDMA (3,4-methylenedioxymetham-
    phetamine), 637
Measles, neurological complications of, 732,
    733t, 741, 744t, 745
Measles mumps and rubella vaccine (MMR),
    843–844
Measles vaccine, 843–844
Medical Research Council (MRC), muscle
    strength grading system, 356–357,
    357t
Medium-chain acyl-CoA dehydrogenase
    deficiency, 256, 260
Medullary center, ventilation and, 9, 10f,
    11–12
Mees' lines, 655
Megacolon, 539
Memory
    age-associated impairment of, 948
    in frontal lobe syndromes, 475–476
Meningeal leukemia, 224
Meningeal lymphoma, 231–232, 762
Meningiomas
    depressive illness and, 487
    frontal lobe damage and, 476
    in neurofibromatosis, 203
    pregnancy and, 570–571
    sex hormones and, 393
Meningitis
    in AIDS, 758–759
    aseptic. *See* Aseptic meningitis
    bacterial. *See* Bacterial meningitis
    chronic, 797–798, 798t
    eosinophilic, 827, 829–830
    fungal. *See* Fungal meningitis

in infective endocarditis, 97, 98, 102, 105,
    107
    Lyme disease and, 697–698, 699
    lymphomatous, 232, 762, 762t
    syphilitic, 692
    transplantation, 62
    tuberculous. *See* Tuberculous meningitis
    viral. *See* Viral meningitis
Meningoencephalitis. *See also* Encephalitis;
    individual diseases and causal agents;
    Meningitis
    in endocarditis, 105, 107
    maternal infections and, 575–576
    primary amebic, 822–824
Menstruation, migraine and, 390
Mental changes. *See individual disorders*
Mental neuropathy, 224
Meralgia paresthetica, in pregnancy, 579
Mercaptans, hepatic encephalopathy and, 255
Mercury exposure, 645, 655
Merieux HDCV rabies vaccine, 842
MERRF (myoclonic epilepsy and ragged red
    fibers), 17
Mesial temporal sclerosis, 481
Metabolic encephalopathy. *See* Encephalo-
    pathy
Metamphetamine, neurological complications
    of, 632–634
Methcathinone, 637
Methotrexate, adverse neurological effects of,
    227, 423t, 426–428, 427t, 589t, 591,
    600
N-Methyl-D-aspartate (NMDA), 11, 12
3,4-Methylenedioxyethylamphetamine
    (MDEA), 637
3,4-Methylenedioxymethamphetamine
    (MDMA), 637
Methylphenidate
    for narcolepsy, 512
    neurotoxicity of, 501t, 589t, 595, 596
1-Methyl-4-phenyl-4-propionoxypiperidine
    (MPPP), 637
1-Methyl-4-phenyl-1,2,3,6-tetrahydropyri-
    dine (MPTP), 637
Metoclopramide
    for gastrointestinal mobility disorders,
    281
    neurotoxicity of, 593, 594, 594t, 595
    for postural hypotension, 152t, 154
Metronidazole
    for bacterial meningitis, 674
    for cerebral amebiasis, 824
    neurotoxicity of, 600, 601, 602t
Miconazole
    for coccidioidal meningitis, 805
    for fungal infections, 801
    for primary amebic meningoencephalitis,
    824